Medical Radiology

Diagnostic Imaging

For further volumes:
http://www.springer.com/series/4354

Jan Bogaert • Steven Dymarkowski
Andrew M. Taylor • Vivek Muthurangu
Editors

Clinical Cardiac MRI

Foreword by
Maximilian Reiser

Springer

Prof. Dr. Jan Bogaert
Department of Radiology
Katholieke Universiteit Leuven
University Hospital Leuven
Herestraat 49
3000 Leuven
Belgium

Prof. Dr. Steven Dymarkowski
Department of Radiology
Katholieke Universiteit Leuven
University Hospital Leuven
Herestraat 49
3000 Leuven
Belgium

Prof. Andrew M. Taylor
Cardio-respiratory Unit
Hospital for Children
Great Ormond Street
London WC1N 3JH
UK

Dr. Vivek Muthurangu
Cardio-respiratory Unit
Hospital for Children
Great Ormond Street
London WC1N 3JH
UK

Additional material to this book can be downloaded from http://extras.springer.com/

ISBN 978-3-662-49978-8
ISBN 978-3-642-23035-6 (eBook)
DOI 10.1007/978-3-642-23035-6
Springer Heidelberg New York Dordrecht London

Printed on acid-free paper

Springer is part of Springer Science+Business Media (www.springer.com)

Foreword

For this second edition of the highly successful reference book on *Clinical Cardiac* MRI the editorial team has been enlarged and several chapters have been added or rewritten in order to take the developments of the last 7 years into account. MRI has only recently been established as diagnostic as well as prognostic method in cardiovascular imaging and is now also used for cardiovascular intervention.

Cardiovascular diseases are the leading cause of death, counting for about 30% percent of global deaths. The value of an up to date, thoroughly researched and comprehensive textbook on cardiac imaging written by leading international experts in the field can therefore not be overestimated.

Clinical Cardiac MRI includes chapters on physics, anatomy, cardiac functions as well as MRI imaging techniques, contrast agents, guidelines for imaging interpretation and—where applicable-interventions for all common cardiac pathologies. Additionally 100 life cases can be found in the online material for the book. These also include less frequent cardiac diseases.

I would like to sincerely thank the editors as well as the authors of this textbook for their time and expertise and am very confident that this edition will, as its predecessor, be a very useful tool for everyone involved in cardiac MRI imaging.

Maximilian Reiser

Preface

By the time a book preface is written, usually most of the work has been accomplished, chapter proofs have been forwarded for correction to the authors, while the book index is still waiting to be finished. It is also the moment the editors get a first glimpse whether the book will match their expectations. About 7 years after the first edition, and almost two years after we agreed with Springer to edit a second edition of our textbook on 'Clinical Cardiac MRI', we are pleased to present you with a new, completely updated textbook. The decision to write a second version was largely driven by the huge success of the first edition, with almost exclusively positive comments not only by reviewers but by the many readers of our book throughout the world, readers that appreciated our book for being a highly useful guide for daily use, for the high-quality of the images and the addition of a CD ROM with 50 real-life cases. Their enthusiasm has been the strongest drive to edit a new version, while their comments have been most helpful to prepare an improved second edition.

For the new edition, we welcome Dr. Vivek Muthurangu, from Great Ormond Street Hospital for Children, London as the fourth member of the editorial board. Dr. Muthurangu has great expertise in the field of cardiac MR physics, pulmonary hypertension and cardiac modeling.

At the end of 2004, when the first edition of 'Clinical Cardiac MRI' was released, cardiac MRI had been through five truly exciting years that had caused a paradigm shift in cardiovascular imaging. Balanced steady-state free precession bright imaging had rapidly become the reference technique to assess cardiac function, and moreover yielded promise for other applications such as coronary artery imaging. Non-invasive comprehensive cardiac tissue characterization was no longer a far off dream. For instance, T2-weighted imaging offered the possibility of in-vivo imaging of reversible myocardial injury, while the nature of the underlying disease could often be deduced by the pattern of myocardial enhancement using (inversion-recovery) contrast-enhanced imaging, thus obviating the need for other, more invasive procedures. Besides its diagnostic role, cardiac MRI was beginning to show promise as a prognostic tool that could provide predictive information about future cardiac events.

Ever since MRI was proposed to have a role in the assessment of cardiovascular disease, cardiac MRI has experienced some resistance from the broader cardiology community with regard to its clinical value and the daily use of this 'exotic' technique. Fortunately, things have moved in the right direction. Cardiac MRI has now become the technique of choice when it comes to the depiction of therapeutic effects (e.g. regenerative cell therapy), and for an increasing number of clinical indications a cardiac MRI study is becoming a crucial investigation that guides patients care. This is due in great extent to an increased visibility and awareness of cardiac MRI at congress meetings and in scientific journals, and the integration of this technique into appropriateness criteria and guidelines. Also the availability of dedicated textbooks has helped toward a broader recognition of cardiac MRI.

For this edition, a new chapter on cardiac modeling has been added; the chapter on heart failure, pulmonary hypertension and heart transplantation has been split in two separate chapters, yielding a total of twenty chapters. Some of the chapters have been extensively rewritten and also extended, aiming to appropriately highlight the rapidly evolving role of cardiac MRI. In particular, this was the case for ischemic heart disease and heart muscle diseases. For other chapters, such as the chapter on congenital heart disease, the emphasis is now on daily clinical applications to investigate simple and more complex cardiac malformations. Throughout the textbook, practical schemes are provided indicating how to apply cardiac MRI for a wide variety of cardiac diseases. And last, but by no mean least, a series on 100 new clinical cases is available as online material. These cases cover a wide spectrum of cardiac diseases, including some less frequent cardiac abnormalities, which have been selected to underscore the added value of cardiac MRI. The online material has the advantage of bringing the dynamic features of cardiac MRI (e.g., functional or stress imaging).

We sincerely hope that readers will receive this edition with the same enthusiasm as our first effort.

Jan Bogaert
Steven Dymarkowski
Andrew M. Taylor
Vivek Muthurangu

Contents

Cardiac MRI Physics 1
Vivek Muthurangu and Steven Dymarkowski

MR Contrast Agents for Cardiac Imaging 31
Yicheng Ni

Practical Set-Up 53
S. Dymarkowski

Cardiac Anatomy 69
J. Bogaert and A. M. Taylor

Cardiovascular MR Imaging Planes and Segmentation 93
A. M. Taylor and J. Bogaert

Cardiac Function 109
J. Bogaert

Myocardial Perfusion 167
J. Bogaert and K. Goetschalckx

Ischemic Heart Disease 203
J. Bogaert and S. Dymarkowski

Heart Muscle Diseases 275
J. Bogaert and A. M. Taylor

Pulmonary Hypertension 355
Shahin Moledina and Vivek Muthurangu

Heart Failure and Heart Transplantation 367
S. Dymarkowski and J. Bogaert

Pericardial Disease 383
J. Bogaert and A. M. Taylor

Cardiac Masses 411
J. Bogaert and S. Dymarkowski

Valvular Heart Disease 465
Andrew M. Taylor, Steven Dymarkowski, and Jan Bogaert

Coronary Artery Diseases 511
S. Dymarkowski, J. Bogaert, and A. M. Taylor

Congenital Heart Disease 553
Marina L. Hughes, Vivek Muthurangu, and Andrew M. Taylor

Imaging of Great Vessels 611
Oliver R. Tann, Jan Bogaert, Andrew M. Taylor, and Vivek Muthurangu

MR Guided Cardiac Catheterization 657
Vivek Muthurangu and Andrew M. Taylor

Cardiovascular Modeling 669
Giovanni Biglino, Silvia Schievano, Vivek Muthurangu,
and Andrew Taylor

General Conclusions 695
J. Bogaert, S. Dymarkowski, A. M. Taylor, and V. Muthurangu

Index 701

Contributors

G. Biglino Centre for Cardiovascular Imaging, UCL Institute of Cardiovascular Science and Great Ormond Street Hospital for Children, Great Ormond Street, WC1N 3JH, London, UK

J. Bogaert Department of Radiology and Medical Imaging Research Center (MIRC), University Hospitals Leuven, Catholic University Leuven, Herestraat 49, 3000, Leuven, Belgium, e-mail: jan.bogaert@uzleuven.be

Steven Dymarkowski Department of Radiology and Medical Imaging Research Center (MIRC), University Hospitals Leuven, Catholic University Leuven, Herestraat 49, 3000, Leuven, Belgium, e-mail: steven.dymarkowski@uzleuven.be

K. Goetschalckx Department of Cardiovascular Diseases, University Hospitals Leuven, Catholic University Leuven, Herestraat 49, 3000, Leuven, Belgium, e-mail: kaatje.goetschalckx@uzleuven.be

Marina L. Hughes Centre for Cardiovascular Imaging, UCL Institute of Cardiovascular Science and Great Ormond Street Hospital for Children, Great Ormond Street, WC1N 3JH, London, UK

Shahin Moledina, UCL Centre for Cardiovascular Imaging and Great Ormond Street Hospital for Children, London, WC1N 3JH, UK

Vivek Muthurangu Cardio-respiratory Unit, Hospital for Children, Great Ormond Street, London, WC1N 3JH, UK; Centre for Cardiovascular Imaging, UCL Institute of Cardiovascular Science and Great Ormond Street Hospital for Children, Great Ormond Street, WC1N 3JH, London, UK

Yicheng Ni Department of Radiology, University Hospitals Leuven, Catholic University Leuven, Herestraat 49, 3000, Leuven, Belgium, e-mail: yicheng.ni@med.kuleuven.be

Silvia Schievano Centre for Cardiovascular Imaging, UCL Institute of Cardiovascular Science and Great Ormond Street Hospital for Children, Great Ormond Street, WC1N 3JH, London, UK

Oliver R. Tann Consultant in Cardiovascular Imaging, Cardio-Respiratory Unit, Great Ormond Street Hospital for Children, London, WC1N 3JH, UK

Andrew M. Taylor Centre for Cardiovascular Imaging, UCL Institute of Cardiovascular Science and Great Ormond Street Hospital for Children, London, UK, e-mail: a.taylor76@ucl.ac.uk

Cardiac MRI Physics

Vivek Muthurangu and Steven Dymarkowski

Contents

1	**Basic Physics**	1
1.1	Spin	1
1.2	Resonance	2
1.3	The MR Signal	2
1.4	Relaxation	3
2	**Magnetization Preparation Pulses**	4
2.1	Inversion Recovery	4
2.2	Saturation Recovery	7
2.3	T2 Preparation	8
3	**Spatial Encoding and Image Construction**	8
3.1	*k*-Space	9
3.2	*k*-Space Filling Strategies	12
3.3	Parallel Imaging	15
4	**Motion Compensation**	16
4.1	Cardiac Gating	16
4.2	Multi-Phase Acquisitions	17
4.3	Respiratory Gating	18
4.4	Single Shot and Real-Time Acquisitions	20
5	**Cardiac MRI Sequences**	20
5.1	Spin Echo Sequences	20
5.2	Spoiled Gradient Echo Sequences	22
5.3	Balanced Steady-State Free Precession	25
6	**Conclusion**	28
7	**Key Points**	29
References		29

V. Muthurangu (✉)
Cardio-Respiratory Unit, Great Ormond Street, Hospital for Children, Great Ormond Street, London, WC1N 3JH, UK
e-mail: v.muthurangu@ucl.ac.uk

S. Dymarkowski
Department of Radiology, University Hospital Leuven, Katholieke Universiteit Leuven, Herestraat 49, 3000 Leuven, Belgium

Abstract

This chapter addresses the use of MRI and to a lesser extent CT in the diagnosis and management of pulmonary hypertension. The basics of pulmonary hypertension will be addressed, including epidemiology and treatment strategies. Then different MRI techniques will be discussed in the context of their relevance to pulmonary hypertension. Finally the role of CT in pulmonary hypertension will be discussed. By the end of the chapter the reader should have a better understanding of how to use cross-sectional imaging in pulmonary hypertension.

1 Basic Physics

The basic principles of magnetic resonance imaging (MRI) are the same irrespective of the part of the body that is being imaged. However, there are specific areas of MRI physics that are particularly important for cardiac MRI specialists to understand. Thus, in this chapter we will review both basic MRI physics (i.e. generation of the MR signal and spatial encoding), as well as more cardiac-specific topics (i.e. motion compensation and cardiac relevant MRI sequences). The purpose of this chapter is to enable the reader to better understand and optimize their MR imaging.

1.1 Spin

Nuclei with unpaired protons or neutrons (i.e. an odd proton or neutron numbers) possess a property called quantum spin, which makes them 'MR active'. The most common of these 'MR active' nuclei is ^{1}H, but

J. Bogaert et al. (eds.), *Clinical Cardiac MRI*, Medical Radiology. Diagnostic Imaging,
DOI: 10.1007/174_2011_412,

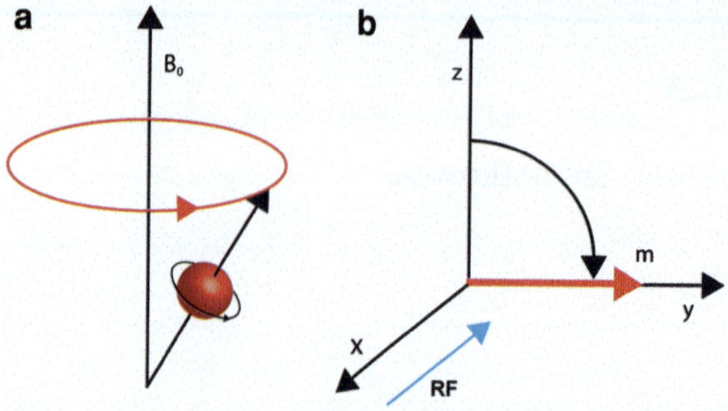

Fig. 1 **a** Proton spinning around its own axis while precessing around the *z*-axis (i.e. the direction of the static field). **b** RF excitation causing flipping of *z* magnetization into the *x*–*y* plane

other nuclei are used in MRI (e.g. ^{19}F, ^{13}C and ^{23}Na). In the rest of this chapter only the ^1H nucleus (essentially a single proton) will be considered. In Newtonian terms, nuclei with spin can be thought of as spheres spinning on their own axis (much like the earth spinning around the polar axis). As these nuclei have a net positive charge (due to their proton component) they generate a magnetic field as they spin, giving rise to their popular analogy as bar magnets. At rest, the protons are randomly arranged in the body. However, in the presence of an external magnetic field (B_0) protons will become aligned. In quantum terms, nuclei align either parallel or antiparallel to the B_0 field due to the fact that protons can occupy multiple energy states. Low-energy protons line up parallel to B_0 while high-energy protons line up antiparallel. At room temperature there is always a small excess of parallel protons and thus the net magnetic vector (NMV) is in the direction of the B_0 field. The exact excess of parallel protons, and thus the magnitude of the NMV, is governed by the Boltzmann distribution. This states that as field strength increases, and temperature decreases, the magnitude of NMV increases. This explains the greater signal at higher field strengths. Although MR is a quantum phenomenon from this point forward it is easier to think of the magnetic moments in purely Newtonian terms. This is because it simplifies the explanation of precession, resonance and spatial encoding.

In the presence of a B_0 field the protons do not simply line up, they actually precess or 'wobble' around the B_0 axis (Fig. 1a). This is analogous to the motion of a spinning top, which spins around its own axis, while also precessing around its surface point of contact. The precessional frequency (ω) of a MR active nucleus is given by the Larmor equation: $\omega = \gamma B_0$, where γ is the gyromagentic constant, a nuclei specific constant. Hydrogen exposed to a 1.5T field precess around the B_0 axis at approximately 64 MHz. However, as they are out of phase with each other, the NMV does not precess and only has a component in the direction of the B_0 field. It is in this state that radiofrequency (RF) energy can be inputted into the system causing the NMV to move toward a plane perpendicular to the B_0 field.

1.2 Resonance

RF energy is transmitted as an electromagnetic wave and its magnetic component (the B_1 field) can interact with the magnetic moments of spinning protons. If the B_0 field is assumed to be in the *z* direction (along the bore of the MR scanner), then a perpendicular RF pulse is in the *x*–*y* plane. Unlike the B_0 field, the B_1 field oscillates and it is this fact that forms the basis of resonance. Resonance only occurs if the frequency of the RF pulse equals the precessional frequency of the hydrogen nucleus at the given field strength. On transmission of a resonant RF pulse, protons, which were previously precessing around the *z*-axis will line up and start precessing around the axis of the B_1 field. This leads to two important changes in the NMV (M_0). Firstly, because the protons have aligned with the B_1 field they precess around the z-axis in phase. This is important, as now M_0 possesses coherent *x*−*y* magnetization. Secondly, the precession of protons around both the *z* and B_1 axis causes the M_0 to nutate or spiral into the *x*–*y* plane. The spiral motion during nutation is difficult to visualize and therefore resonance is usually described in the rotating frame of reference (i.e. the observer is rotating around the *z*-axis at the same frequency as the protons). In the rotating frame of reference, nutation becomes a simple flip into the *x*–*y* plane (Fig. 1b). The flip angle is dependent on the strength and duration of RF pulse, with a 90° flip placing all the longitudinal magnetization into the transverse plane. The flipped magnetization vector now has a transverse component, which forms the basis of the MR signal.

1.3 The MR Signal

Faraday's law of electromagnetic induction states voltage will be induced in a conductor exposed to a changing magnetic field. Longitudinal magnetization

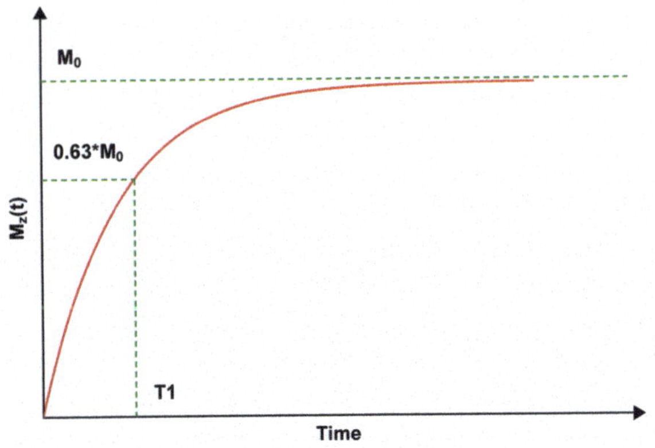

Fig. 2 T1 relaxation curve—note that at time = T1 the z magnetization has relaxed back to 0.63 times its original value

does not change and therefore it cannot induce a voltage. Transverse magnetization on the other hand rotates in the x–y plane and therefore it will induce a voltage in a conductor. This is an important point to note: only the transverse component of M_0 induces voltage. As the transverse magnetization rotates at the Larmor frequency, the induced voltage will also oscillate at the same frequency. However it is not in this form that the data is ultimately used. The sinusoidally varying voltage undergoes a process called complex demodulation, which essentially converts the data into the rotating frame of reference. Thus, the resultant MR signal has a magnitude (the amplitude of the varying voltage) and a phase, which after RF excitation is zero. It can easily be represented as a hand on a clock face, whose size is equal to the magnitude and whose position is equal to the phase. It is within this signal that spatial information must be encoded. However this signal does not stay the same indefinitely, but rather relaxes back to its resting state. It is this relaxation that forms the basis of MRI contrast.

1.4 Relaxation

Relaxation is the process by which magnetization returns to its resting state after RF excitation. There are two processes involved, both of which are dependent on the atomic arrangement within tissues. Thus, the rate of relaxation is tissue specific and can be used to develop tissue contrast. Longitudinal relaxation (or recovery) is due to transfer of energy from high-energy protons to the surrounding lattice (spin-lattice relaxation). This causes the NMV to flip back into the z direction; during this process longitudinal magnetization recovers exponentially (Fig. 2). The rate of longitudinal recovery is dependant on the rate constant T1. As T1 depends on the atomic structure of the tissue, it is a tissue-specific constant. In tissues with a short T1 (such as fat) longitudinal magnetization will be recovered more quickly than in tissue with a longer T1 (such as muscle). This is important in the generation of T1-weighted contrast, which will be discussed later in this chapter. The nature of the exponential recovery curve means that when time equals T1, 63% of z magnetization will have recovered. Recently T1 mapping has become a great interest in cardiac MRI. In T1 mapping, multiple images are acquired at different times after an excitation pulse (or more usually after an inversion pulse which will be discussed in more detail later in this chapter). This allows reconstruction of the T1 recovery curve and calculation of the tissue T1. The reason that T1 mapping has become of great interest is that there is evidence to suggest that after contrast administration the tissue T1 correlates with the amount of myocardial fibrosis. This will be addressed in more detail in "Heart Muscle Diseases".

The other relaxation process is transverse relaxation and is due to dephasing of the individual spins leading to a reduction in coherent transverse magnetization. This is due to the interaction between the magnetic fields of adjacent protons (spin–spin interactions) and results in different protons precessing at different rates. In the rotating frame of reference, this variation in frequency is seen as dephasing. Thus, the coherent magnetization vector in the x–y plane starts to fan out resulting in a reduction in the net transverse magnetization. Transverse relaxation results in exponential decay of coherent transverse magnetization at a rate governed by T2 (Fig. 3). Thus, when time equals T2, transverse magnetization will have decayed to 37% of its original value. Much like T1, T2 also depends on the atomic structure of the tissue, and is therefore an independent tissue-specific constant. In tissues with a long T2 (such as tissue with a high water content) transverse magnetization will persist longer than tissue in tissue with a shorter T2 (such as fat). This is important in the generation of T2-weighted contrast, which will be discussed later in this chapter. However, there is a second process that results in loss of transverse magnetization. This is B_0

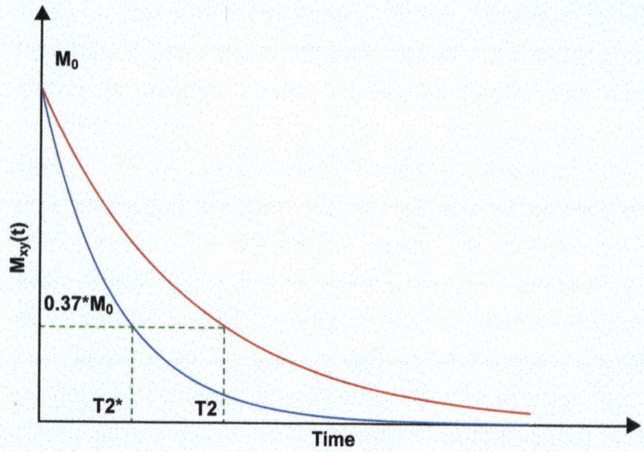

Fig. 3 T2 and T2* relaxation curves—note that the transverse magnetization has fallen to 0.37 times its original value at time = T2/T2*

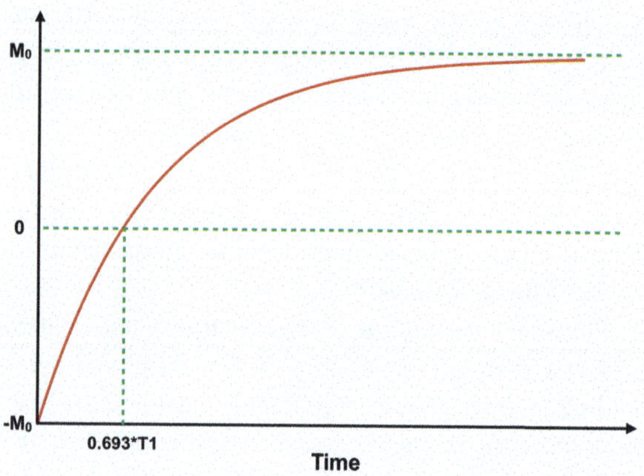

Fig. 4 Inversion recovery curve—note that *z*-axis magnetization passes through 0 at time = 0.693 times the T1 of the tissue

field inhomogeneity, which also results in dephasing. This accelerated dephasing is encapsulated in the time constant $T2^*$. The $T2^*$ value is dependant on the underlying T2 and any field inhomogeneity and is therefore not purely a tissue constant. One way to improve field homogeneity is to shim. Shimming is a process by which either metal is used to distort the magnetic field (passive shimming) or shim coils are used to generate a corrective magnetic field (active shimming). These techniques can be used together and active shimming is vital for some newer cardiac MR sequence. In the same way that one can measure the T1 of myocardium, one can also measure myocardial T2 or T2*. Quantification of T2 is useful when trying to quantify myocardial edema, while T2* is useful when assessing iron overload (iron causes local field inhomogeneity). Mapping T2 or T2* is done by acquiring multiple images at different times after the excitation pulse. This allows reconstruction of the T2/T2* decay curve.

With prior knowledge of tissue T1 and T2, timing parameters (i.e. TR and TE) can be altered to provide specific tissue contrasts. Other ways to change contrast are to add exogenous contrast agents or to prepare magnetization prior to imaging. The next section will discuss in detail the use of magnetization preparation to change MR contrast.

2 Magnetization Preparation Pulses

Magnetization preparation is the process by which the magnetic vector is manipulated prior to imaging in order to produce specific tissue contrast. This technique is used heavily in cardiac MRI and the most common techniques are described below.

2.1 Inversion Recovery

The most commonly used form of magnetization preparation is inversion recovery (IR). IR depends on the fact that different tissues have different T1 characteristics. In IR sequences, an 180° RF pulse (or inversion pulse) is used to flip the magnetization into the opposite direction along the *z*-axis. From this position the magnetization relaxes back to its original state following the T1 curve of the tissue (Fig. 4). At a time of approximately T1 * Ln2 (0.693) the longitudinal magnetization will pass through zero (i.e. the magnetization will be completely in the *x*–*y* plane). As different tissues have different T1 characteristics, each tissue will pass through zero (or the null point) at different times. During RF excitation (which is applied some time after the IR pulse) only tissues with non-zero longitudinal magnetization will produce an MR signal. Therefore if the time between inversion and imaging (TI) is chosen carefully, signal from a given tissue can be completely abolished. All IR sequences work on this principle, and that different tissues can be nulled by choosing specific TI's.

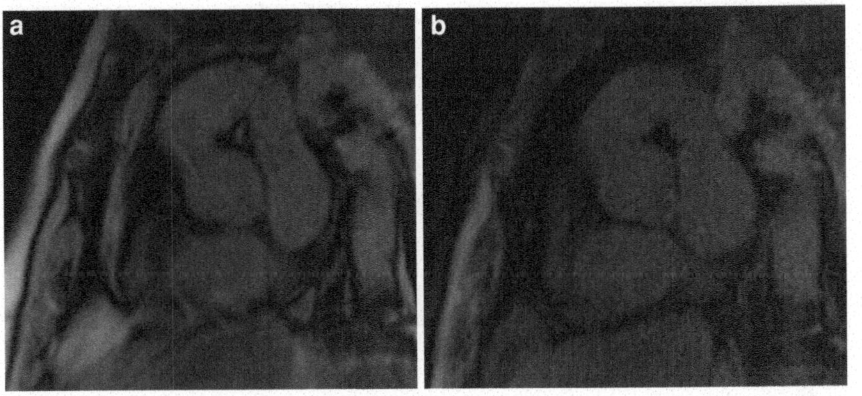

Fig. 5 **a** Short axis view through the atria with no fat saturation. **b** STIR sequence in the same image plane—note that the anterior and pericardial fat are nulled because of the inversion pulse (TI = 160 ms)

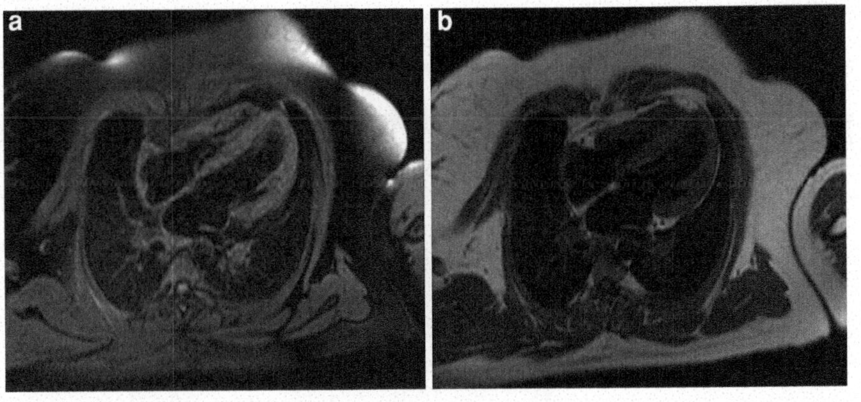

Fig. 6 **a** SPIR dark blood sequence—note the inhomogeneous nulling of the fat when using spectrally selective inversion pulses. **b** Non-fat saturated dark blood image in the same image plane

2.1.1 Short Tau Inversion Recovery

Fat suppression can be an important requirement in cardiac MRI. A robust method of fat suppression is STIR (Simonetti et al. 1996), which relies on the short T1 of fat compared to other tissues. Therefore, the fat magnetization will pass through null point of an IR sequence before the tissue of interest. If imaging is performed at the null point of fat, the signal from the fat will be suppressed. As the T1 of fat is around 230 ms, a TI of between 150 and 170 ms can be used to robustly suppress fat. Of course the magnetization from other tissue (such as muscle) will also be recovering and thus the signal produced will be lower than if no inversion had been performed. This is particularly true for tissue with short T1's. Nevertheless STIR is frequently used in cardiac MRI due to its robustness and the fact that it can be combined with most imaging sequences (Fig. 5).

2.1.2 Spectral Inversion Recovery

The problem with STIR is the loss of signal to noise ratio (SNR); this can be overcome by the use of SPIR sequences (Kaldoudi et al. 1993). Spectral selective pulses rely on the fact that water and fat precess at slightly different frequencies (approximately 220 Hz difference at 1.5T). Therefore a special RF pulse can be used that only excites fat. In SPIR a spectrally selective 180° pulse is used to invert only the fat magnetization. The water magnetization is unchanged by the spectrally selective 180° pulse. The fat magnetization is then allowed to recover and a TI is chosen that coincides with the null point of fat. Unlike STIR, at the onset of imaging all of the water magnetization is in the longitudinal axis and therefore there is no loss in SNR (Fig. 6). However, SPIR techniques are very susceptible to magnetic field inhomogeneity and shimming is important. In real-world applications of SPIR an inversion pulse of between 90 ° and 180° is used.

2.1.3 Contrast-Enhanced Inversion Recovery

Contrast-enhanced inversion recovery is an extremely important technique in cardiac MRI (Kim et al. 2000). It relies on the fact that tissue containing gadolinium

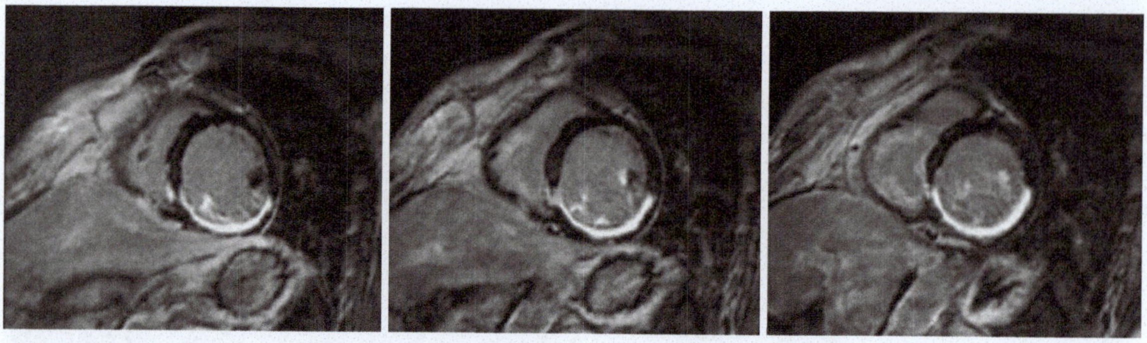

Fig. 7 Late Gd image of an inferior myocardial infarct. Note that the inversion pulse has nulled the myocardium. However, the presence of Gadolinium in the scar tissue leads to a shorter T1 and therefore *z*-axis magnetization is present and produces a bright signal in the infarct

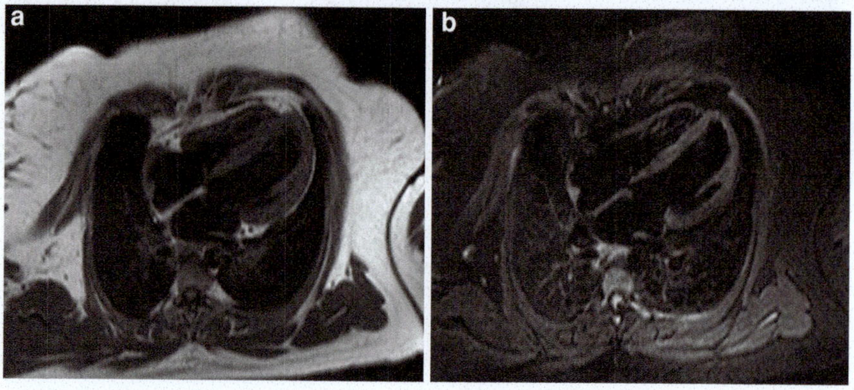

Fig. 8 **a** Double inversion turbo spin echo sequence creating a black blood image of the heart. **b** Triple inversion recovery turbo spin echo sequence creating a black blood image with fat suppression

will have a shorter T1 than tissue not containing gadolinium. It is known that gadolinium (Gd) concentration in infarcted myocardium is higher than in normal myocardium. Therefore by the time the magnetization from the normal myocardium passes through the null point of an IR sequence, the infarcted myocardium will already have regained positive longitudinal magnetization. Consequently, if the TI is chosen to coincide with myocardial nulling, infarcted tissue will appear bright (Fig. 7). Unlike STIR imaging the TI in contrast- enhanced IR cannot be predefined, as it is dependent on parameters such as patient weight, contrast dose, renal function and time contrast of administration. Contrast-enhanced IR forms the basis of early and late Gd imaging, which will be discussed in more detail in later chapters of this book.

2.1.4 Double Inversion Recovery

Double inversion recovery (DIR) techniques are used to produce 'black blood' contrast (Stehling et al. 1996). As the name implies DIR sequences include two inversion pulses. The first pulse is nonspatially selective and therefore inverts all magnetization in the body. The second pulse is slice selective and re-inverts magnetization only in the slice to be imaged. At the end of the DIR module all magnetization outside the imaging slice is inverted, while magnetization in the slice is all in the normal *z*-axis. Any blood that flows into the slice will therefore carry with it this inverted magnetization. If a TI is chosen to coincide with the null point of blood, any blood that has flowed into the imaging slice will produce no signal (Fig. 8a). Thus flowing blood appears black, while surrounding tissues produce normal signal as their magnetization is in the *z*-axis prior to excitation. The optimal TI between the DIR module and image acquisition is patient and blood flow dependent. However, a TI of about 600 ms is a good compromise. DIR sequences are used heavily in assessing cardiovascular morphology, particularly when slow flowing blood is present (Stehling et al. 1996).

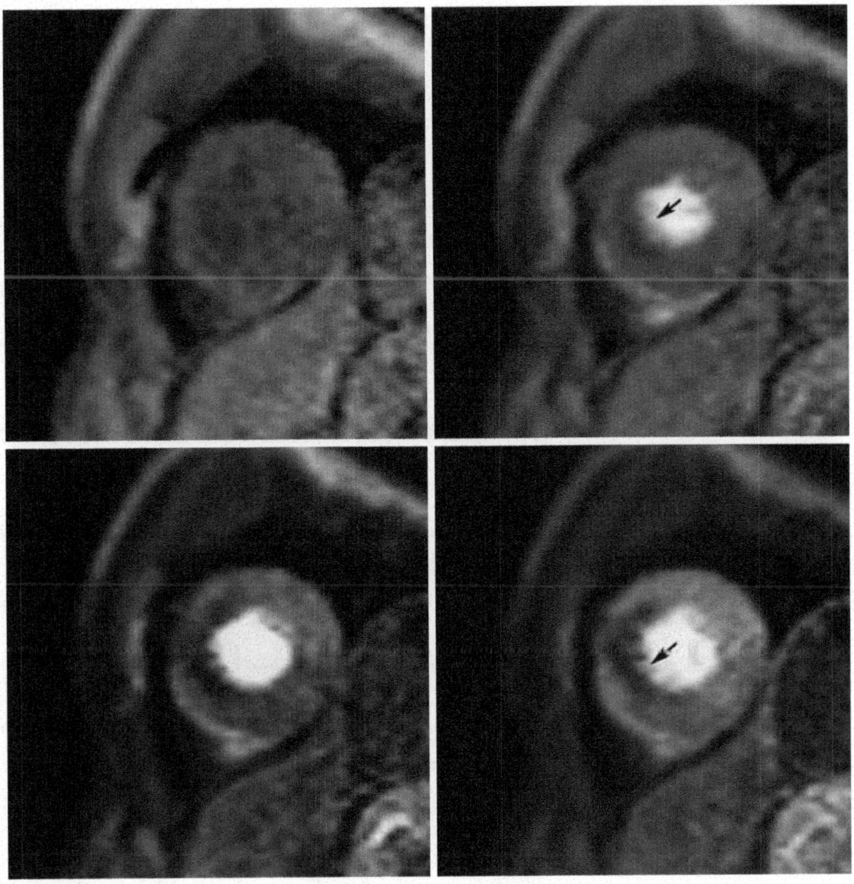

Fig. 9 Set of saturation recovery spoiled gradient echo images. The arrows point to an area in anteroseptal segment with reduced signal. This is a perfusion defect and is due to reduced gadolinium in the area of the myocardium

2.1.5 Triple Inversion Recovery

Triple inversion recovery (TIR) sequences are a combination of DIR and STIR (Simonetti et al. 1996). Essentially, after the DIR module a further slice selective 180° pulse is used to re-invert the magnetization in the slice. This magnetization then relaxes along a T1 recovery curve and imaging is performed when the fat magnetization crosses the null point. However because of the preceding DIR module inflowing blood is also nulled. Therefore, TIR sequences provide fat suppressed black blood contrast (Fig. 8b). The timing of the 180° pulses is important to ensure nulling of both fat and blood. Usually the first TI is set at approximately 600 ms and the second at between 150 and 170 ms.

2.2 Saturation Recovery

As with IR techniques, saturation recovery (SR) techniques depend on the T1 characteristics of tissue. In SR imaging, a 90° pulse is used to flip magnetization into the *x*–*y* plane. This magnetization is then dephased by a large magnetic gradient so that it produces no signal (a process known as spoiling). The dephased magnetization then recovers according to the tissue T1 characteristics and the shorter the T1 the more magnetization can be flipped into *x*–*y* during imaging. Thus, SR provides improved T1 contrast. However, IR sequences are better at producing T1 contrast and therefore slice selective SR sequences are only used in situations where time is important. The most obvious of these is myocardial perfusion imaging (Ding et al. 1998). Areas of poor perfusion contain less Gd and thus have longer T1 values. After the SR module, poorly perfused tissue will not recover as much longitudinal magnetization and will appear dark compared to normal myocardium (Fig. 9). Even though slice selective SR is not used extensively outside perfusion imaging, spatially selective saturation pulses (saturation bands) are still important in cardiac MRI. Saturation bands are volumes of tissue within the imaging slice that have

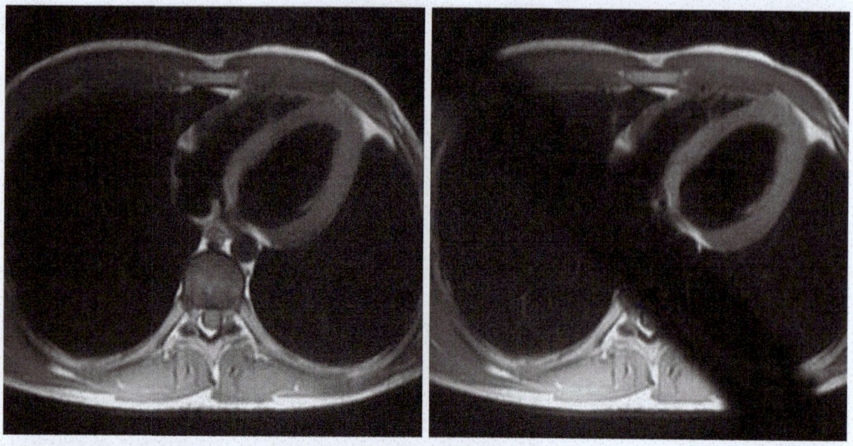

Fig. 10 Dark blood sequence with a saturation band added in the second image. Note the almost complete signal loss in the vicinity of the band

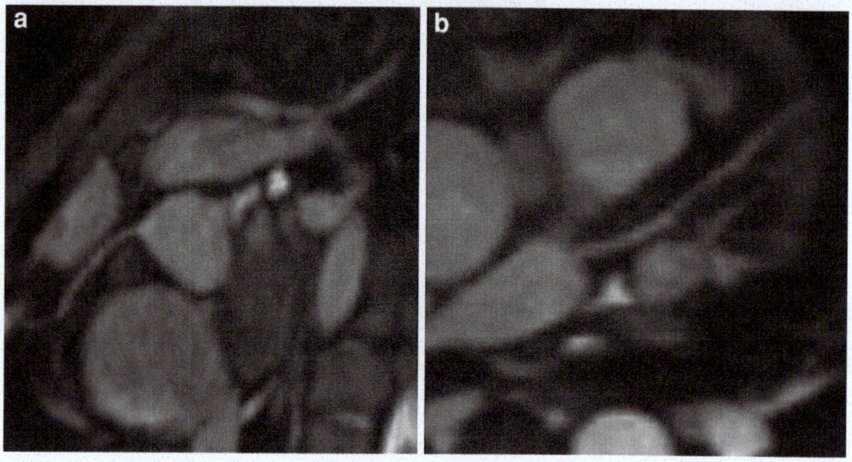

Fig. 11 3D cardiac gated SSFP sequence with T2 prep. Note the excellent delineation of the (**a**) *right* coronary artery (**b**) *left* coronary artery

been exposed to a saturation pulse. If imaging occurs immediately after the saturation band is applied, tissue in this area will be effectively suppressed (Fig. 10). This technique is often used to suppress motion-related or ghosting artefacts arising from tissue not related to the object of interest. One good example is placing a saturation band over the spine during late Gd imaging, as it prevents ghosting artifact that may confuse the late Gd signal.

2.3 T2 Preparation

So far we have discussed magnetization preparation that is dependant on T1 properties. However, magnetization preparation can also improve T2 contrast (Botnar et al. 1999). T2 preparation (T2 prep) consists of a 90° pulse that flips all magnetization into the *x–y* plane, an 180° pulse that inverts the magnetization in the *x–y* plane and a final −90° pulse that flips all magnetization back into the *z*-axis. During these multiple flips, T2 relaxation will have occurred and the resulting magnetization in the *z*-axis is dependant on the tissue T2 and the time between the pulses. This technique is particularly useful in suppressing myocardial signal in coronary imaging as the myocardial T2 is around 50 ms compared to a blood T2 of 250 ms. When a T2 preparation time of 40 ms is chosen optimum contrast between coronary blood and the myocardium is produced (Fig. 11).

3 Spatial Encoding and Image Construction

The basic purpose of imaging is to understand how an object occupies space. In all cases this requires interaction with the object and subsequent collection of

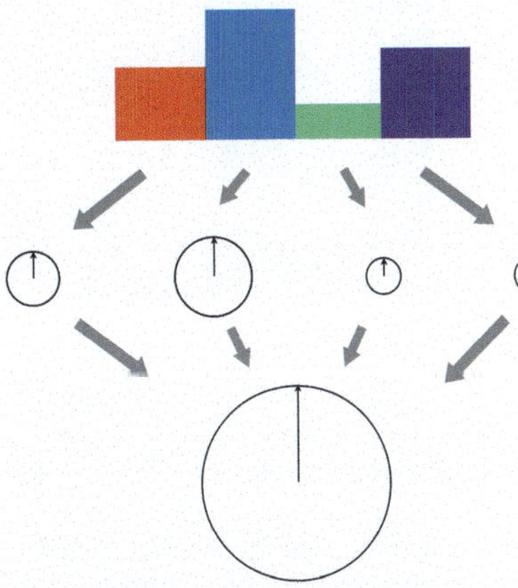

Fig. 12 Diagram of RF excitation of a one-dimensional object and summation of the to produce the total MR signal

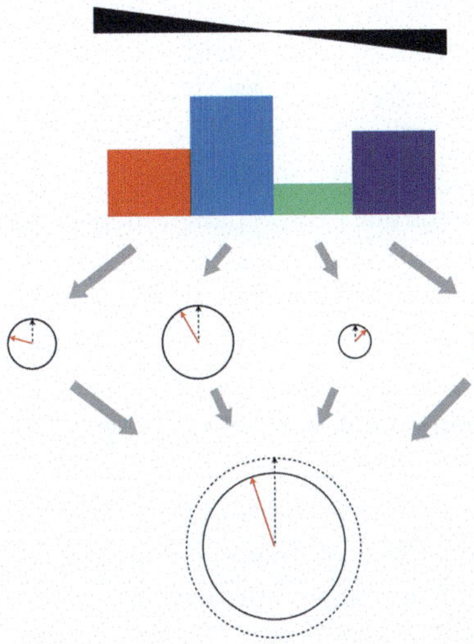

Fig. 13 Diagram of RF excitation of a one-dimensional object with an additional gradient. Note the individual MR signals are now dephased in relation to one another and the vectoral summation produce a different total MR signal than in Fig. 12

spatially encoded measurements. In MRI, the induced signal is spatially encoded by magnetic gradient fields. To better understand this process let us consider a one-dimensional (1D) object with four distinct areas with different proton densities (Fig. 12). After RF excitation each area produces an MR signal whose magnitude is proportional to the proton density (in realistic models also relaxation parameters and flip angle) and whose frequency is the resonant frequency of hydrogen (64 MHz at 1.5T). In the rotating frame of reference, the signal from each area has the same magnitude (as described above) and zero phase. The total MR signal from the object (which is what we record) is the vectoral sum of each individual signal (Fig. 12). However, because the phase is zero, the total signal is simply the sum of the magnitudes. In this example, the total MR signal provides us with information about how many protons are in the object, but not how they are distributed within the object.

Now consider what would happen if a magnetic gradient (a magnetic field whose strength varies with space) is applied to the object. As we know the precessional frequency is directly proportional to the magnetic field. Thus, a magnetic gradient results in a spatially varying precessional frequency. However, as already pointed out, the MR signal is actually in the rotating frame of reference. This means that frequency shifts will actually be exhibited as phase shifts. In the rotating frame of reference, a magnetic gradient results in a spatial variation in the phase of the MR signal from different areas (Fig. 13). The total MR signal is the vectoral sum of the signals from each area and will now be dependant on the spatial distribution of protons (Fig. 13). Is this enough to provide information about how protons are distributed in our example? No because it is conceivable that there is more than one distribution of protons that will give the same total MR signal. Intuitively, by performing more 'experiments' with different gradients we would ultimately reach a point where there was only one possible distribution that fits all the collected MR signals. In fact, to create an image with x number of pixels we have to perform x number of experiments or independent measurements. Each independent measurement requires an MR signal to be acquired under a different magnetic gradient (producing different amounts of spatially dependant dephasing). However, it should be noted that the actual dephasing caused by the gradient is dependent on both its strength and the amount of time the gradient is applied. For this reason the 'dephasing capability' of a gradient is described by its zeroth moment (the time integral of the gradient) not just its strength. In the next section the practical aspects of spatial encoding with gradient fields will be discussed.

3.1 *k*-Space

In the last section, we stated that the number of pixels in an image is determined by the number of

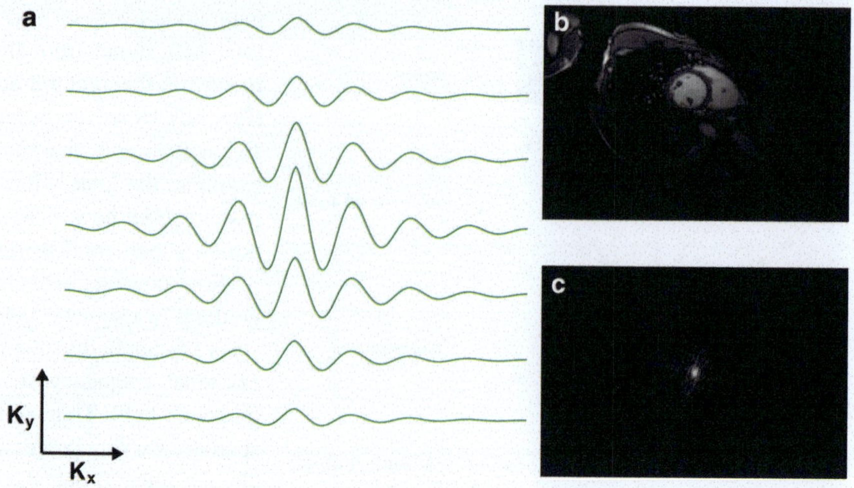

Fig. 14 **a** Diagram of *k*-space—note the increased amplitude in the middle of *k*-space. **b** A short axis view of the ventricles. **c** The corresponding *k*-space

independent MR measurements acquired. An extension of this idea is that each 'measurement' produces an equation with results (the MR signal), several unknowns (the proton density in each pixel) and a weight (the gradient). If the number of equations (or measurements) equals the number of unknowns (the number of pixels), we can reconstruct the image by solving the equations simultaneously. Simple sets of simultaneous linear equations (i.e. two equations and two unknowns) can be solved by hand. However, MR images often require more than 20,000 independent MRI measurements and obviously cannot be solved by hand or using simple computational methods. Thankfully, if the MR signals and the gradient moments are arranged in a specific way, solving the equations can be accomplished by a relatively simple inverse Fourier transformation. For this reason MRI signals are stored in a structure called *k*-space (Fig. 14). A position in *k*-space is proportional to the gradient moment, with the center of *k*-space coinciding with a zero zeroth moment (i.e. no gradient applied) and the edge with the highest moment. Thus for a given measurement, the MR signal produced is 'recorded' at the *k*-space position that corresponds to the gradient moment used for that measurement. Due to this very specific arrangement the application of an inverse Fourier transformation will produce data in which each point is the proton density in a given area of the object. This data set is better known as the MR image.

The properties of *k*-space can be difficult to understand and it is important to appreciate that *k*-space is a spatial frequency domain. Thus, a point in *k*-space represents a given spatial frequency, and not a point in the image. Furthermore, it is has both positive and negative parts in both axis. The central portions of *k*-space encode the low spatial frequencies and have the highest signal amplitude due to less gradient-dependant dephasing. These low spatial frequencies equate to the broad contrast in the image, essentially blobs of signal rather than defined objects (Fig. 15a). The outer portions of *k*-space encode the higher spatial frequencies and have the lowest amplitude (due to greater gradient dependent dephasing). High spatial frequencies define the edge of an image—the higher the frequency the sharper the edge (Fig. 15b). An important question is: how do *k*-space characteristics relate to measures such as resolution and field of view?

3.1.1 Field of View and Resolution

Field of view (FOV) and resolution determine both the gradient moments used during acquisition and the number of measurements recorded. To understand this let us consider our original 1D object. We use gradients to induce phase shifts in the different areas. However, if the gradient moment is too high, spins at the edge of the object may dephase so much that they start back at zero. This is called aliasing and will result in image foldover or wrap after inverse Fourier transformation (Fig. 16). To prevent this, a gradient moment must be chosen that produces a 360° phase shift over a distance greater than the object occupies. This means that spins at the edge of the object will be less than 360° apart and will not alias. The *k*-space

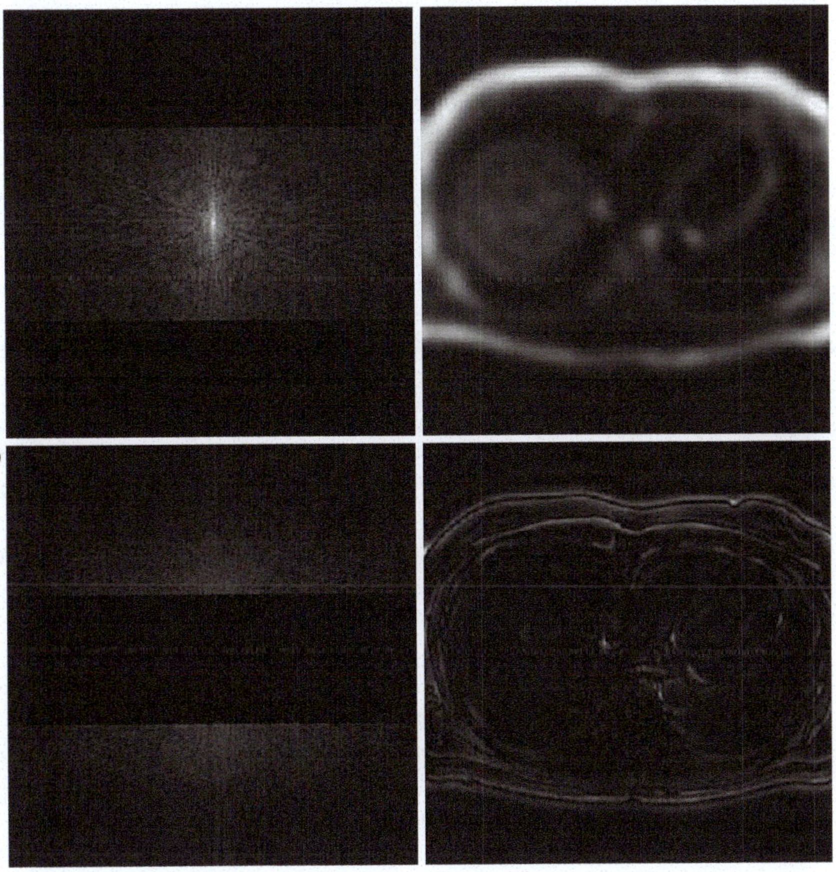

Fig. 15 **a** The center of k-space and its resultant image—note that its essentially a low resolution image. **b** The edge of k-space and its resultant image—note that this image is essentially the edges of the image

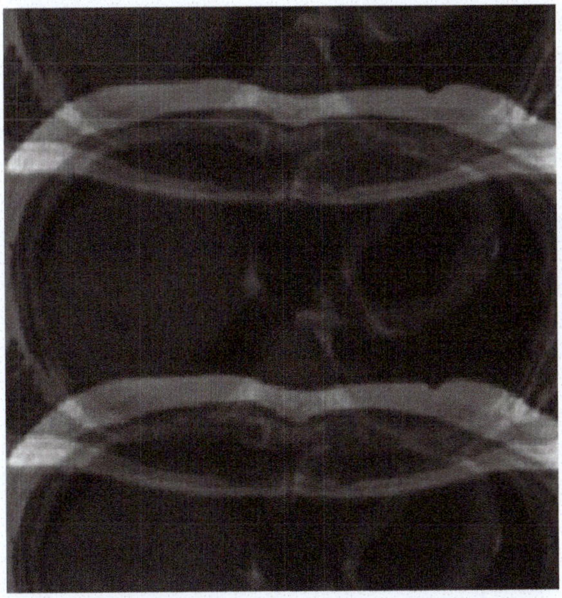

Fig. 16 Image foldover due to inadequate field of view

position that corresponds to this gradient moment is the first point from the center. However, as we have already stated x MR measurements must be acquired to reconstruct an image with x pixels. Each of these MR measurements will be made with higher gradient moments and will therefore be further out in k-space. The distance between subsequent k-space points (Δk) is usually the same as the distance between the center and the first point. Thus, the FOV equals $1/\Delta k$ and equates to the distance over which a 360° phase shift will be induced by the lowest gradient moment. If the object is larger than the FOV, the signal in k-space will contain aliased information and the image will wrap after inverse Fourier transformation. The other aspect that must be understood is the relationship between k-space and resolution. We have already stated that larger gradient moments encode high spatial frequencies and relate to positions further out in k-space. Therefore, the resolution of an image must be proportional to the extent of k-space (position of

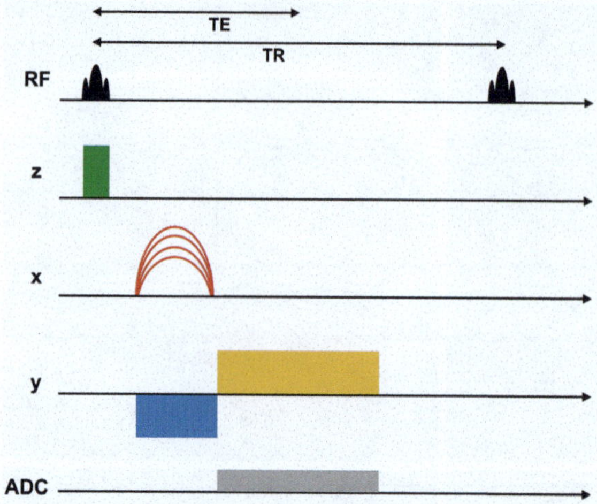

Fig. 17 Generic pulse sequence diagram. RF is the radiofrequency pulse, z is the slice selection axis, x is the phase encoding axis, y is the readout encoding axis and the ADC is the analog digital converter. The blocks represent the gradient (the height is the gradient strength and the length the time they are applied for)

the furthest point from the center). The position of this point will depend on the number of different measurements made and the distance between them i.e. Δk (or 1/FOV) multiplied by the number of measurements. One important point is that as resolution increases SNR decreases. Thus one of the main drawbacks of high spatial resolution imaging is low SNR. In the next section k-space filling will be addressed.

3.2 *k*-Space Filling Strategies

In this section the actual methods by which k-space is filled will be reviewed. The purpose is to allow the reader to better understand the physics of MR spatial encoding and thus allow better optimization.

3.2.1 Slice Selection

In two dimensional (2D) imaging we only want to obtain information from a single slice of tissue. Therefore some sort of selection must be performed that limits signal production to the required slice. In 2D MRI, this slice selection allows discrimination of spatial information in the slice direction (conventionally the z-axis) and is the first component of spatial encoding. As previously noted the resonant frequency is directly proportional to the magnetic field. Thus, a magnetic gradient field applied in the z-axis during RF excitation causes a linear variation of resonant frequencies. In this situation, a RF pulse of a given frequency only causes resonance at a certain position along the z-axis, thus selecting a slice within the volume. The RF pulse itself has a bandwidth that contains a small range of frequencies and slice thickness depends on both the RF bandwidth and the slope of the slice select gradient.

3.2.2 Cartesian Filling of *k*-Space

To perform 2D spatial encoding, multiple MR measurements must be acquired with different gradients moments in both the x and y directions. These MR measurements fill k-space and after inverse Fourier transformation produce an image. There are many ways in which k-space can be filled, but the most common is Cartesian or rectilinear filling. In Cartesian filling, gradient moments are changed in one direction by changing the time they are applied for and in the other by changing the gradient strength.

In the frequency (or readout) encoding direction a gradient of constant strength is applied for a certain length of time. During this period MR signals are continuously recorded and this data is referred to as the readout. Each MR signal in the readout is acquired with a different gradient moment because the time the gradient is applied for is always increasing. As previously pointed out the position in k-space is proportional to the gradient moment. Consequently, a single readout fills a single line in k-space. However to fill all of k-space, multiple readouts (or lines) are required with different position in the other axis. Different lines in k-space are acquired in the phase encoding direction by changing the gradient strength and keeping the application time constant. Thus in Cartesian filling, each line in k-space is filled using the same frequency encode gradient moments but different phase encode gradient moments. This is better understood by viewing the pulse sequence diagram.

3.2.3 Pulse Sequences Diagrams

Pulse sequence diagrams (PSD) include all processes performed in a given sequence and provide a complete understanding of the sequence. Figure 17 shows a generic pulse sequence diagram for a 2D Cartesian MRI sequence. The first process is RF excitation, which is classically shown on the first line. As previously mentioned in 2D imaging, a slice selection gradient is applied during RF excitation and this is shown on the second line. Although by convention this is the z-axis line, slices do not have to be acquired in the true z-axis of the scanner. The next stage is phase encoding which is shown as nested gradients implying the different gradient strengths used for different k-space lines. At the same time as the phase encoding gradient is applied, the negative lobe of the frequency encode gradient is applied (which is shown on the bottom line). This is necessary to make sure that the readout fills k-space from the edge. The next stage is the positive lobe of the frequency encode gradient and it is during this time that MR signals are acquired. This is usually shown by activation of the analog digital converter (ADC), which converts the voltage into a digital signal. Halfway through the readout the total moment in the readout direction is zero and therefore signal is highest at the halfway point of the line. This is because when the moment is zero there is no dephasing of the MR signal and therefore the transverse magnetization is at its most coherent. The time between the RF excitation and this point is called the echo time (TE). The time between successive excitatory RF pulses (or repetitions of the PSD) is called repetition time (TR). In Cartesian filling the time taken to fill k-space equals the TR multiplied by the number of k-space lines.

3.2.4 Rectangular Field of View and Partial Fourier

There are many benefits to Cartesian filling in k-space such as simple gradient design and minimal artefacts. Furthermore, Cartesian filling lends itself to mechanisms by which imaging can be easily accelerated. Previously we have stated that acquisition time is dependent on the TR and number of k-space lines. In cardiac imaging, the TR is often minimized and therefore the only way of shortening scan time is to reduce the number of k-space lines. Usually this would result in a reduction in resolution in the phase encode direction. However, as the thorax is an oblong structure, the FOV in the anterior–posterior direction can be decreased creating a rectangular FOV (RFOV). The creation of a RFOV does not in itself produce any reduction in scan time. Actually, all it does is result in a widening of the gap between k-space lines and increase the furthest extent of k-space. However as previously pointed out, this increases the spatial resolution in the phase encode direction. This is unnecessary and one can consequently acquire less k-space lines while still maintaining resolution. In fact if RFOV is reduced by x%, the same proportion of k-space lines can be discarded from the edge of k-space without a reduction in resolution. Thus the RFOV method can significantly reduce scan times depending on the dimensions of the patient. Unfortunately, this reduction in scan time does not come for free and it is always associated with a reduction in SNR. However for many cardiac MR sequences this reduction in SNR does not lead to a significant reduction in image quality.

Further reduction in the number of phase encode steps required to produce an image can be achieved by using partial Fourier techniques (also known as half scan or partial k-space). Partial Fourier techniques rely on k-space symmetry around the zero phase encode line axis. In a perfect world in which k-space is totally symmetrical, only half of k-space would be required to reconstruct an accurate image. In reality k-space is not completely symmetrical and reconstructing of one half of k-space would produce significant artefacts. Nevertheless, accurate images can be reconstructed with less than 100% of k-space. Usually when performing partial Fourier acquisitions, between 62.5 and 87.5% of k-space is sampled. The missing data occupies a proportion of one half of k-space in the phase encode direction and the middle of k-space is fully sampled. Reconstruction is then performed using either zero-filling of the missing part of k-space or the more accurate homodyne method. Partial Fourier techniques significantly reduce scan times, although as with RFOV they do cause a fall in SNR and occasionally additional artefacts. In cardiac MRI, RFOV and partial Fourier techniques are widely used as they lower scan times. This is important as many sequences are performed within a breath hold as will be discussed later in the chapter.

3.2.5 Echo-planar and Non-Cartesian Imaging

So far we have discussed classical Cartesian filling of k-space with each line in k-space being acquired with the same readout gradient and a different phase encode gradient. Although this is the simplest type of sequence to implement on a scanner, it is not the most time efficient way of filling k-space. In order to speed up acquisition, several more complex k-space filling strategies have been developed. Echo planar imaging (EPI) was the first methodology used to speed up

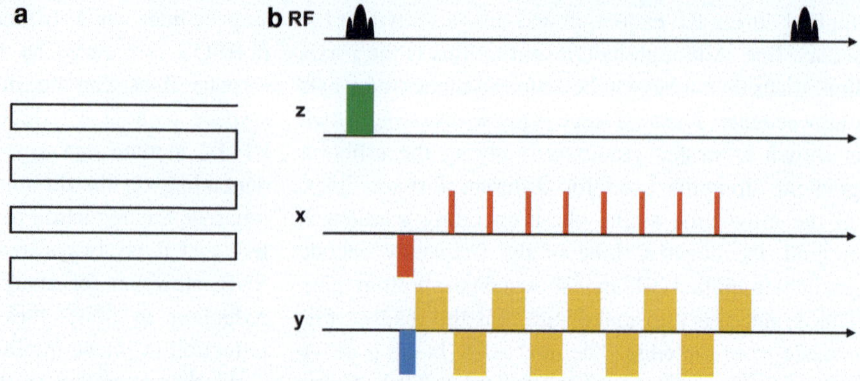

Fig. 18 **a** EPI trajectory, **b** pulse sequence diagram for an EPI sequence

acquisition (Chrispin et al. 1986). EPI is still essentially a Cartesian sequence. However in EPI, each readout fills several *k*-space lines as shown in Fig. 18a. The PSD for an EPI sequence demonstrates that this is done by reversing the readout gradient for each line while providing a phase encode 'blip' that move the trajectory from one line to another (Fig. 18b). Thus EPI is more time efficient, requiring less excitations to fill *k*-space. Theoretically, a whole *k*-space could be filled by one EPI readout. However, several factors prevent this happening in real-world situations. Firstly the readout still experiences T2/T2* effects and therefore readout length is limited by the amount of signal required. Furthermore, gradient waveforms are never accurately played out and this leads to trajectory errors that accumulate with time. These trajectory errors result in MR signals being placed in slightly incorrect positions in *k*-space, creating artefacts when long EPI readouts are used. Therefore, most EPI sequences rely on the use of interleaves: readouts that together fill *k*-space. EPI sequences are heavily used in perfusion (Wang et al. 2005) and real-time applications (Korperich et al. 2004) and have benefited from significant improvements in scanner hardware. Importantly as EPI is essentially a Cartesian technique, RFOV and partial Fourier can still be used to further reduce scan time.

A variation on EPI is spiral filling in *k*-space. In spiral imaging *k*-space is filled by spiral readouts that are produced by sinusoidally varying gradients in both the *x*- and *y*-axis. As spiral trajectories are circularly symmetric the terms phase encoding and frequency encoding become redundant and we simply refer to *x* and *y* directions. Spiral trajectories are the most time efficient way filling of *k*-space and are heavily used in high-end real-time applications (Steeden et al. 2010a, b). However, they suffer from all the problems of EPI sequences except to a much greater extent. This has limited their applications in routine clinical imaging. Another non-Cartesian trajectory is radial imaging in which *k*-space is filled by radial spokes. Radial filling is produced by simultaneously applying readout gradients in both the *x* and *y*-axis. By varying the relative strength of the gradients, different angles for the radial spokes can be produced. This form of *k*-space filling has the advantage of using separate lines in *k*-space and is therefore less sensitive to trajectory errors. The main benefit of radial acquisitions is that they have been shown to be less sensitive to motion artefacts and are thus very useful in morphological cardiac imaging (Kolbitsch et al. 2011). Furthermore, the center of *k*-space is relatively oversampled and as will be discussed later this has some important properties when performing *k*-space under sampling (Hansen et al. 2006).

3.2.6 3D Imaging

Previously it has been stated that *k*-space has the same dimensions as the resultant image. Thus in three dimensional (3D) imaging, *k*-space is also 3D and we have to perform spatial encoding in all 3 directions. To understand this, we need to extend the idea that multiple lines fill *k*-space, each acquired with a different phase encode gradient. In 2D imaging only one phase encode gradient is required; however, in 3D imaging, two phase encode gradients are required. This second phase encode gradient is usually referred to as the slice encode gradient and encodes spatial information in the slice direction. The resultant signal can then be inverse Fourier transformed to produce a 3D volume representing the object in question.

It should be understood that this is not the same as multi-slice 2D imaging, which consists of multiple 2D *k*-spaces. The major benefit of 3D encoding is that SNR is significantly greater than multi-slice approaches because of the greater volume of excitation. Although Cartesian 3D imaging is most common, non-Cartesian techniques have also been developed. These include stack of spirals/stars acquisitions and 3D radial acquisitions. However, few have entered routine clinical practice.

3.3 Parallel Imaging

Parallel imaging relies on the fact that most MRI is now performed with phased array coils that consist of multiple coil elements. Thus, each element receives signal in parallel. However because each element has a different spatial sensitivity the signal received in each coil is different. Thus, information about the spatial distribution of signal can be elucidated from the different coil images. This extra information can be used to speed up acquisition as it can essentially replace some of the MRI spatial encoding steps. Several different parallel imaging approaches have been suggested and in this section the most common will be reviewed.

3.3.1 Sensitivity Encoding

Sensitivity encoding (SENSE) is one of the most commonly used forms of parallel imaging and has proven to be a robust method of reducing scan time (Pruessmann et al. 1999, 2001). Acquisition time is directly proportional to the number of lines in *k*-space (or phase encode lines). Therefore, skipping alternate phase encode lines would halve scan time. However, skipping lines causes an increase in Δk and is the same as halving the FOV (Fig. 19). This results in foldover of signal from tissue outside the FOV, making the final image unusable. However, the foldover is different in each coil image and this can be use to unwrap the final image (Fig. 19). To understand this let us consider a single wrapped pixel. The pixel contains signal from both tissue at that point and from a known position outside the FOV. Unfortunately, we have no knowledge of the proportion of each and therefore the pixel cannot be unwrapped. Mathematically this can be described by an equation where we have two unknowns (the individual pixel intensities) each multiplied by the coil sensitivity at that position and one known quantity (the wrapped pixel intensity). This sort of problem cannot be solved with a single equation. However, it can be solved if there are two equations and the local coil sensitivities are known. In SENSE, each wrapped pixel is unwrapped using information from both the coil images and the local coil sensitivities. The coil sensitivities are usually derived from a low resolution filtered scan of the imaging volume. It should be obvious that if the number of unknowns is greater than the number of coil images, the final image cannot be fully unwrapped. Therefore, in SENSE the acceleration factor (i.e. the number of lines skipped = R) cannot be greater than the number of independent coil elements. However, in the current era of large element arrays (32 coil elements are now standard) high acceleration factors are used. It should be noted that acceleration factors cannot be increased indefinitely because in SENSE, the SNR is inversely proportional to $\sqrt{R}$. Therefore, as R increases SNR decreases and in reality, an acceleration factor greater than four is not useful in 2D imaging. SENSE can also be performed in 3D imaging, with under sampling in both the phase encode and slice encode direction.

3.3.2 Generalized Autocalibration Partially Parallel Acquisition

Generalized autocalibration partially parallel acquisition (GRAPPA) is another commonly used parallel imaging technique (Griswold et al. 2002). Unlike SENSE, which works in the image domain, GRAPPA works in *k*-space. The fundamental idea in GRAPPA is to synthesize the skipped *k*-space lines using the surrounding sampled parts of *k*-space. Importantly, this surrounding data is derived from all the coil elements, making this a parallel imaging technique. In order to synthesize missing *k*-space data some knowledge of the relationship between points in *k*-space is required. This is done by fitting the sampled *k*-space points in all the coils to the *k*-space equivalent of the low resolution coil sensitivity image. In GRAPPA, this is derived from the fully sampled center of *k*-space. Once these *k*-space relationships have been delineated, the missing lines in *k*-space can be synthesized and inverse Fourier transformation will produce an unwrapped image. Like SENSE, GRAPPA acceleration is restricted to the number of independent coil elements and as the center must be fully sampled the acceleration factors are

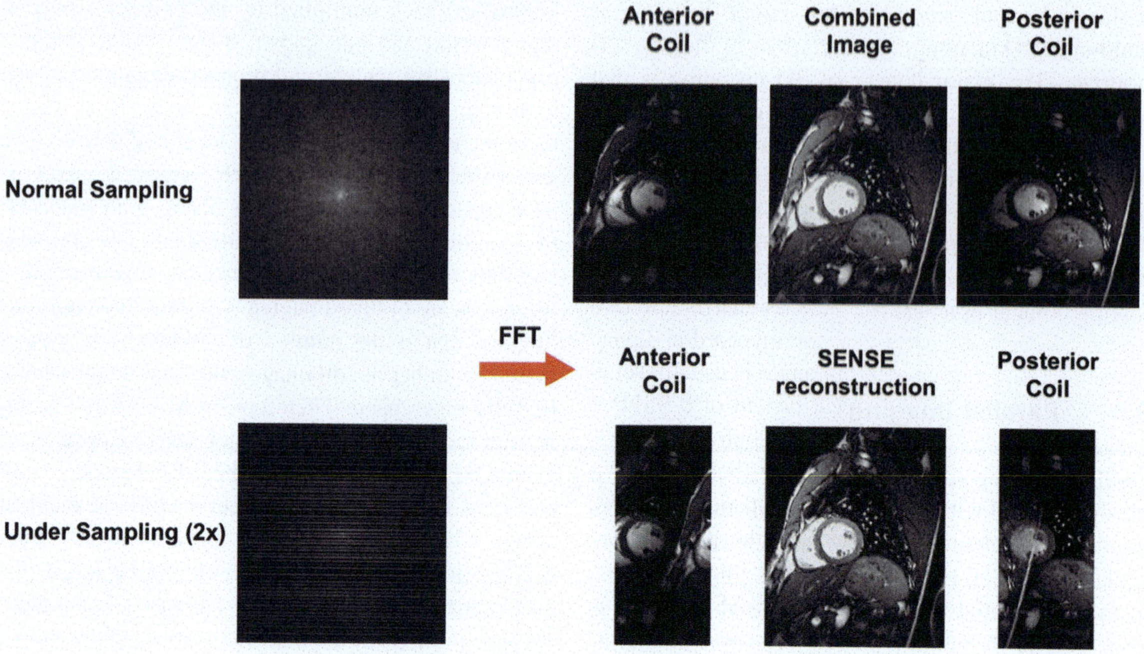

Fig. 19 SENSE reconstruction. When *k*-space is fully sampled there is no aliasing in the images from the anterior or posterior coils. When the coil images are combined there is therefore no aliasing. When *k*-space is under sampled the coil images are aliased. If they were combined normally the resultant image would also be aliased. However by using the SENSE reconstruction the aliasing is unwrapped

slightly lower than in SENSE. However, GRAPPA does have the benefit of not requiring a separate coil sensitivity scan.

3.3.3 *k-t* Methods

As the name suggests *k-t* methods involve dynamic imaging and they are not strictly a form of parallel imaging. However, they are a method of producing unwrapped images from under sampled data. In the original technique (*k-t* BLAST), spatio-temporal correlations in the data are determined using a low spatial resolution high temporal resolution 'training' data set (Tsao et al. 2005). These correlations are then used to unwrap a specifically under sampled high spatial resolution data set. The benefit of this technique is that it does not require multiple coils and does not have the same noise amplification problems as parallel imaging. Thus, the possible acceleration achievable with techniques such as *k-t* BLAST is greater than in traditional parallel imaging. However, as with parallel imaging there is a cost, which in *k-t* methods is blurring, particularly during periods of fast motion. One way to partly remedy this is to combine *k-t* and parallel methods in techniques such as *k-t* SENSE (Tsao et al. 2005; Muthurangu et al. 2008). These methods represent the best of both worlds with less blurring and noise than their single counterparts.

4 Motion Compensation

More than any other type of MRI, cardiac MRI has to compensate for motion in order to achieve acceptable image quality. Therefore, MRI sequences must be adjusted to account for cardio-respiratory motion. In this section the various strategies used to perform motion compensation will be reviewed.

4.1 Cardiac Gating

If conventional MRI protocols were used to image the heart during contraction, the images would be unusable due to overwhelming motion artefacts (Lanzer et al. 1984). In fact, in order to image the heart successfully cardiac motion must be 'frozen'. This can be achieved by synchronizing MRI acquisition to specific points in the cardiac cycle through ECG gating.

However, ECG acquisition within the MRI environment is difficult due to MRI-induced artefacts in the ECG signal. The major sources of ECG artefacts are RF pulses and gradient field switching as they induce voltages in the ECG leads. Improvements have been gained by using fiber optic connections to the scanner, which have resolved some of the problems of induced voltages in wires. However, these measures have not removed another significant source of artifact, namely the magnetohydrodynamic effect. The magnetohydrodynamic effect describes the induction of voltages caused by ions (flowing in the blood) moving through the magnetic field. This voltage artifact is mainly superimposed on the ST segment of the ECG coinciding with ejection of blood in systole. The increase in amplitude of the ST segment can cause a false QRS detection. To overcome this problem, modern scanners use the spatial information in a vector cardiogram (VCG) to improve *R*-wave detection. VCG triggering is now routinely used on most scanners and has significantly improved gating.

4.1.1 Segmented *k*-Space

The purpose of gating is to 'freeze' cardiac motion. The importance of this can be seen if we consider a simple *k*-space filling example. Consider a *k*-space with 128 phase encode lines and a TR of 2.5 ms. It would take 320 ms to fill one *k*-space and this represents more than 30% of an average *R–R* interval. Thus, it is impossible to freeze motion when performing traditional *k*-space filling. One way around this is to divide *k*-space into segments and fill each segment in successive *R–R* intervals. This is called a segmented *k*-space acquisition (Finn and Edelman 1993). Obviously any motion that occurs during the acquisition of a segment will lead to motion artifact. However, if the time taken to fill a segment is short or the myocardium is relatively still, motion is essentially frozen. The success of these techniques is highly dependent on the parameters chosen, particularly the time taken to fill a segment. This time equals the number of lines per segment multiplied by the TR. Thus, reducing the number of lines per segment should improve image sharpness. However, reducing the number of lines per segment increases the number of *k*-space segments. As each segment is acquired in a single *R–R* interval, increasing the number of segments increases total acquisition time. Consequently, choosing these parameters is a balancing act between image quality, motion and total scan time. The segmented *k*-space approach is the basis of cardiac gating for both single-phase and multi-phase acquisitions.

4.1.2 Single-Phase Acquisitions

In many types of cardiac MRI, such as morphological imaging (e.g. coronary MR angiography) or tissue characterization (e.g. late Gd) a static image of the heart is required. MRI data must therefore be acquired at a certain point of the cardiac cycle. The traditional approach is to image during diastasis, as this is the period in the cardiac cycle when the myocardium is most at rest. Diastasis occurs during mid to-late diastole and its length is inversely related to heart rate. Thus, to produce an image without motion artifact two decisions must be made: 1) How long after the R-wave should imaging start and 2) Over what time period should MR data be acquired. Firstly, the time between the r-wave and the start of image acquisition (i.e. trigger) should be decided. There are several different ways to calculate the precise timing of diastasis. One strategy is to calculate the time delay using the empirical method such as the Weissler formula. A much easier approach is to perform a cine MRI scan with very high temporal resolution and find the start of diastasis. Importantly, this approach reveals situations when diastasis is not the most quiescent period in the cardiac cycle. For instance, in children end systole is often a better period to perform imaging, as diastole is short and filling is continuous. The second decision that must be made is the length of time MR data should be acquired (data acquisition window). This is done by changing the number of lines per segment, such that the time taken to fill a segment equals the period of myocardial stillness. This can be done empirically by decreasing the lines per segment as heart rate increases. However, the cine MRI scan acquired to decide the trigger delay can also be used to decide the length of the quiescent period.

4.2 Multi-Phase Acquisitions

In multi-phase acquisitions, multiple *k*-spaces are acquired throughout the *R–R* interval. After inverse Fourier transformation this produces a multi-frame

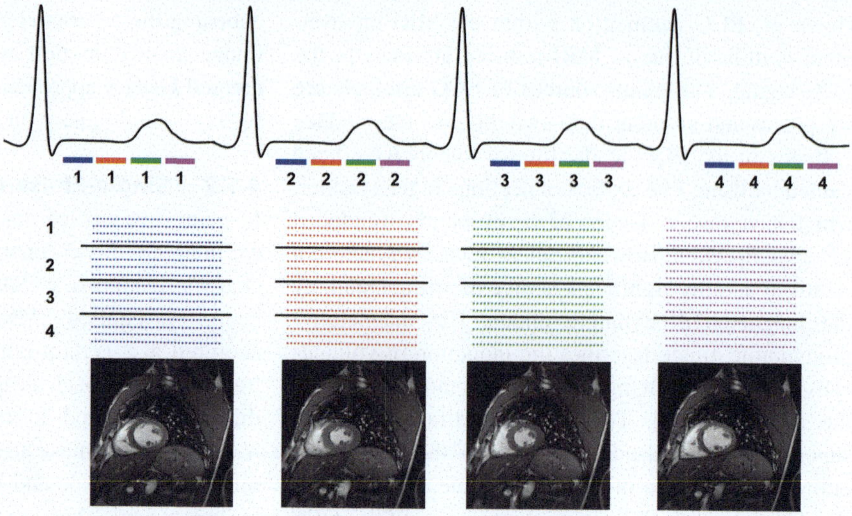

Fig. 20 Prospective multi-phase acquisition. In this example, *k*-space is divided into four segments—each of which is collected at the same point in the cardiac cycle in four *R–R* intervals. Each *k*-space is collected at a different point in the cardiac cycle. Together this data can be reconstructed into a cine image

cine of cardiac motion. In their simplest form, multi-phase acquisitions are extension of the single-phase segmented *k*-space technique. The easiest way to perform cine MRI is prospective gating. This can be understood by considering single-phase techniques in which data is acquired in a certain part of the cardiac cycle. If the trigger delay was set at 0 ms the single-phase technique would only acquire the first part of the cardiac cycle (Fig. 20). However, if data acquisition was continued another segment would be acquired and a second *k*-space would be filled in the same number of *R–R* intervals. Obviously this would represent the second frame in the cardiac cycle (Fig. 20). Consequently, if data was acquired during the whole *R–R* interval, one could produce a multi-phase cine loop of cardiac motion. In multi-phase sequences, the number of frames acquired depends on the time it takes to fill a segment (i.e. the line per segment). As the lines per segment go up, the number of frames is reduced and thus the temporal resolution falls. However if the lines per segment go down (improving the temporal resolution) the acquisition times goes up. Thus, in multi-phase imaging there must be a compromise between temporal resolution and acquisition time. Of course these decisions depend on individual patients and the clinical question being asked. Another important point with prospective gating is that to compensate for *R–R* interval variability there is a period of 'dead time' at the end of each cardiac cycle. This is referred to as the arrhythmia rejection window and prevents sampling during end diastole.

End diastole can be imaged if retrospective gating is used (Lenz et al. 1989). In retrospective gating, lines in *k*-space are continuously collected during the scan. Each line in *k*-space is then time stamped in relation to the *R–R* interval it is acquired in. At the end of the scan the average *R–R* interval is calculated and each individual *R–R* interval is stretched or compressed to this mean value. This deformation can either be done in a linear manner or in more complex ways in which diastole is stretched more than systole. The end result of this temporal deformation is that all lines in *k*-space are time stamped relative to the mean *R–R* interval. They can then be re-binned (in simplistic terms) to produce separate frames. Unfortunately complete filling of *k*-space requires a certain amount of redundancy, and therefore in retrospective gating more lines are sampled. Thus, retrospective gating has the advantage of imaging throughout the cardiac cycle, although at the cost of slightly longer scan durations.

4.3 Respiratory Gating

So far freezing cardiac motion has been discussed. However, the total acquisition times of gated scans can be several seconds long. Over this period respiratory motion would cause significant artefacts if not taken into consideration. In Cartesian imaging these artefacts are most obvious as ghosts in the phase encode direction. In this section the two main approaches to dealing with respiratory motion will be reviewed.

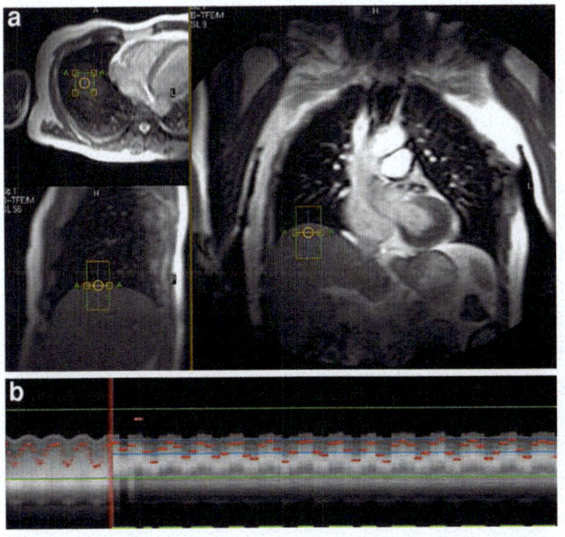

Fig. 21 **a** Pencil beam navigator placed on the dome of the right hemi-diaphragm. **b** Resultant navigator data that is used for respiratory gating

4.3.1 Breath Hold Imaging

The simplest method of dealing with breathing is to perform imaging during breath holds. With the development of newer faster MRI techniques (particularly ones that incorporate parallel imaging) breath holds have become the mainstay of cardiac MRI. Generally speaking, most patients can hold their breath for about 10–15 s. Of course in patients with more significant disease, maximum breath hold may only be a few seconds. Therefore, one of the main issues with breath hold scanning is patient specific optimization. Increasing either spatial or temporal resolution will lead to prolonged breath hold times. Thus, resolution may need to be sacrificed in order to achieve breath hold times that are achievable in sick patients. However, there are several methods that can be used to speed up scan time without losing spatial or temporal resolution. Often simple measures such as enabling RFOV or partial Fourier may be sufficient. In addition, under-sampling techniques such as SENSE or *k-t*-SENSE provide can also significantly reduce scan times. As discussed previously all these techniques result in loss of SNR and some artefacts. This must be taken into consideration prior to their application.

In some instances breath holding is simply not possible and an alternative approach is to use multiple signal averages during free breathing. This technique relies on the acquisition of the same data at different points of the respiratory cycle. The resulting image has less obvious respiratory artefacts and much-improved SNR. However edge sharpness will be reduced and therefore it is of less use when accurate delineation of anatomy is required. Nevertheless, it is heavily used in flow imaging as it does not seem to affect the accuracy of blood flow measurements.

4.3.2 Navigator Gating

In longer imaging sequences such as gated whole heart MR angiography, the above-mentioned strategies have little chance of success. These longer acquisitions need a different approach to respiratory motion compensation such as respiratory navigators (Keegan et al. 1999). Fundamentally these are simple MR measurements of diaphragmatic position that enable data acquisition to be restricted to certain points in the respiratory cycle. This technique will be briefly described here, since it is elaborated in "Coronary Artery Disease". A navigator usually consists of a 2D RF pulse that excites a cylinder of tissue (a so-called pencil beam excitation) and a single readout along the length of the cylinder. The navigator is usually placed on the dome of the right hemi-diaphragm with the position of the diaphragm being the same as liver-lung interface (Fig. 21a). Thus, when the navigator readout is inverse Fourier transformed, the position of the diaphragm can be determined. Consequently, if the navigator is interleaved with the imaging it can provide real-time measurement of the diaphragmatic excursion (Fig. 21b). Usually the navigator echo is acquired every *R–R* interval, immediately prior to data acquisition.

When using this navigator information, a range must be defined over which the MR data is accepted (the acceptance window). This range is set so that MR data is only accepted over a certain part of the respiratory cycle, for instance at end-expiration. The total length of acquisition depends on the acceptance window chosen and the respiratory pattern and is encapsulated into the concept of navigator efficiency. A narrow acceptance window will provide sharper imaging, but at the expense of longer scan times. Conversely a wide acceptance window will keep scan times short, although residual respiratory artifact maybe present. As with cardiac gating optimization of navigator efficiency depends on the patient and the

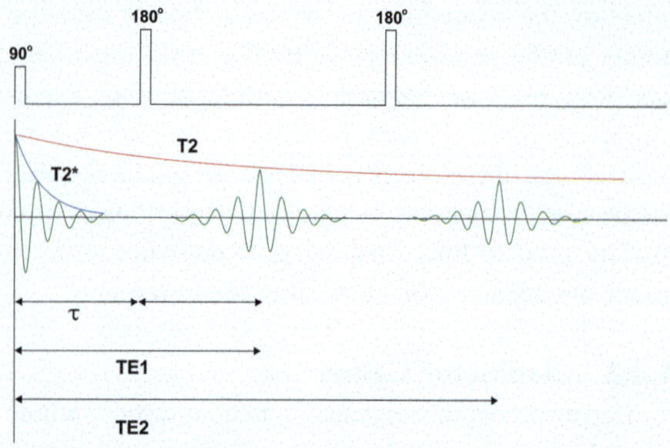

Fig. 22 Spin echo sequence—note the initial signal decay along a T2* curve; however the 180 pulse creates a spin echo at the TE. The spin echoes decay along a T2 curve

question being asked. Another issue with navigator gating is respiratory drift, which is a bulk change in diaphragmatic position (often due to the patient falling asleep). This can cause complete loss of data MR acceptance but is usually rectified by some sort of respiratory drift correction built into navigator algorithms.

4.4 Single Shot and Real-Time Acquisitions

A completely different approach to cardio-respiratory motion is to significantly speed up *k*-space filling and thus dispense with gating. As *k*-space is filled in a single *R–R* interval (i.e. it is not segmented) this technique is known as a single shot acquisition. In order to prevent motion artefacts, single shot *k*-space filling must be performed in less than 100 ms. In order to do this the number phase encode lines collected must be significantly reduced. This can be accomplished by lowering the spatial resolution and most single shot imaging is performed at much lower spatial resolution than gated MRI. Other techniques such as RFOV and partial Fourier can also be used to reduce acquisition times. Higher resolution single shot imaging requires more sophisticated methods to be used. For instance non-Cartesian trajectories can be used as they increase the temporal efficiency of *k*-space filling. Other techniques heavily used in single shot imaging are parallel imaging (i.e. SENSE) and if the data is dynamic *k-t* methods. Using these techniques, *k*-space filling can be reduced to as little as 30 ms. Unfortunately reconstruction of this data is computationally more intensive and real-time image display is difficult. Thankfully, the advent of parallel computing, particularly on graphical processing units, does open up the possibility of real-time reconstruction of heavily under sampled data (Hansen et al. 2008). As with cardiac gated sequences, single shot imaging can be performed as a single- or multi-phase technique. Single-phase single shot techniques are used for morphological imaging when breath holding is not possible. They are usually still triggered to a certain part of the cardiac cycle, although this is not a necessity. Examples are scout imaging, single shot late Gd imaging and HASTE imaging.

If a single shot technique is continuously run, it becomes real-time imaging. Real-time MRI is still relatively underutilized in cardiac MRI. However it does have the benefit of not requiring cardiac or respiratory gating. Its main uses have been in assessing cardiac function and flow in patients in whom breath holding is difficult. The temporal resolution of real-time techniques is entirely dependant on the time taken to fill *k*-space. Therefore most clinically useful real-time sequences employ non-Cartesian or EPI trajectories as well as parallel imaging and *k-t* methods. In the future better reconstruction algorithms may make the real-time imaging the standard for cardiac MRI. However, this future is still some years off.

5 Cardiac MRI Sequences

5.1 Spin Echo Sequences

The majority of MR imaging relies on echo formation at some point after the RF excitation. The earliest MR sequences (even prior to imaging) were spin echo (SE) sequences. As previously noted, magnetic field inhomogeneity leads to additional dephasing and loss of transverse magnetization. The spin echo sequence allows recovery of transverse magnetization that is lost due to field inhomogeneity. In fact in the early days of MR when fields were less powerful and less homogeneous, SE sequences were the only acquisitions that provided reasonable signal. Let us look at how a spin echo is formed (Fig. 22). At time τ after a 90° RF pulse a given amount of spin dephasing occurs due to B_0 inhomogeneity. If a 180° pulse is then

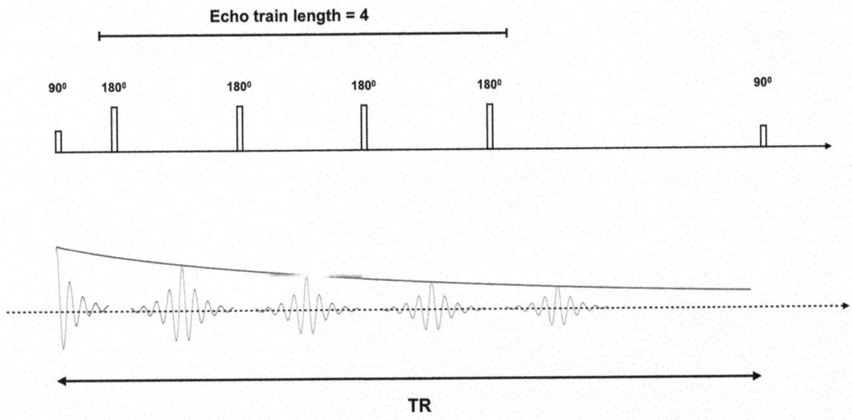

Fig. 23 Turbo spin echo sequence—each subsequent echo decays along a T2 curve. The number of echoes in each TR is the echo train length

applied, the spins precess in the opposite direction. The B_0 field inhomogeneity is still present; however, due to the reversal of precessional direction, it rephases rather than dephases spins. Thus, transverse magnetization refocuses, with full recovery occurring at time 2τ. Of course, the spin echo sequence does not compensate for T2 effects (spin–spin interactions) and the amplitude of the echo still exponentially decays with a T2 time constant. In SE sequences, the time taken for full refocusing (2τ) is the echo time (TE) and the time between 90° pulses is the repetition time (TR). If more than one 180° pulse is used, then more than one echo can be read out (Fig. 22).

5.1.1 Fast or Turbo Spin Echo

The traditional spin echo sequence takes a long time to acquire and is not classically used in cardiac MRI. More commonly a fast or turbo spin echo (FSE/TSE) sequence is used. In these sequences, more than one echo is created by multiple 180° pulses (Fig. 23), each of which fills a separate line in *k*-space (i.e. acquired with a different phase encoding gradient). The number of echoes acquired during a single TR is called the echo train length (ETL). This type of sequence allows *k*-space to be filled very rapidly, with acceleration dependant on the echo train length. However, it should be noted that T2 decay still occurs and this limits the maximum practical echo train length. In gated FSE, echo train lengths of between 9 and 15 are commonly used and this allows FSE sequences to be performed in a breath hold. FSE sequences can also be acquired as single shot images and in these sequences the echo train length equals the number of lines in *k*-space. To make the ETL shorter, single shot FSE is often combined with partial Fourier techniques to produce a half acquisition single shot turbo spin echo (HASTE) sequence. These sequences are heavily used for morphological imaging in patients who cannot hold their breath. Specific SE sequences are usually determined by their tissue contrast.

5.1.2 Specific Spin Echo Sequences

T1w MRI. For T1-weighting, SE sequences must have a short TE and importantly a short TR (<700 ms). This results in T1-weighting as only tissue with a short T1 will have recovered significant longitudinal magnetization to be flipped into *x*–*y* during the next excitation. In order to acquire data quickly, most T1-weighted SE sequences use FSE readouts. From now on T1-weighted FSE sequences will be refereed to as T1w MRI. T1w MRI is often used to assess cardiovascular morphology (Bogaert et al. 2000). However, in order to do this accurately, flowing blood must be nulled. All spin echo sequences intrinsically suppress flowing blood. This is because blood that flows out of the imaging plane after the 90° excitation pulse will not experience the 180° refocusing pulse and will not produce any signal. Obviously the amount of suppression will be dependant on how quickly blood flows out of the imaging slices. This form of 'black blood' imaging is particularly robust in areas of high flow such as the great vessels during systole. Unfortunately, intrinsic black blood contrast is not robust in areas of slow flowing blood (e.g. the atrial and ventricular cavities). For 'black blood' imaging in areas of slow flowing blood, a DIR preparation module is required (Fig. 24). This has been shown to provide more robust suppression of slow flowing blood than SE alone (Greenman et al. 2003). To ensure that the

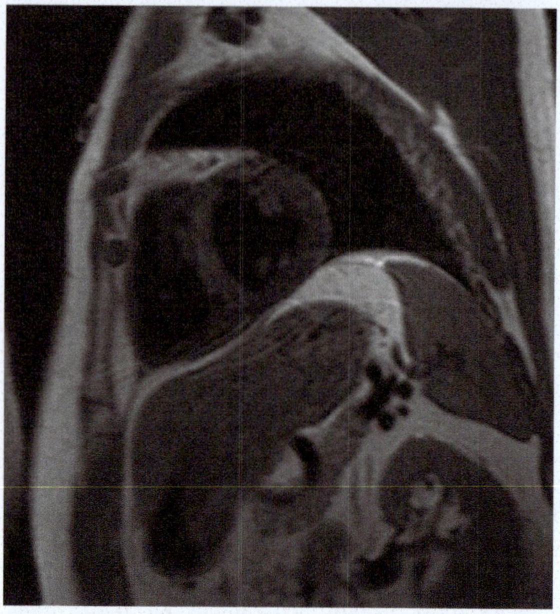

Fig. 24 T1-weighted double inversion recovery spin echo image (T1w MRI)

blood in the imaging slices is nulled, a TI of around 600 ms is required. Thus, DIR sequences can be difficult to gate and in adults are usually limited to diastole. In children or adults with a high heart rate more than one *R–R* interval maybe required in order to accommodate both DIR and image acquisition.

T2w MRI. Spin echo sequences are particularly well suited to T2-weighted imaging as the refocusing 180° pulse means that the signal envelope is controlled by T2 rather than T2*. For T2- weighting, SE sequences must have a long TE (>80 ms) and a long TR (>2,000 ms). The long TE ensures that only tissue with a long T2 has significant coherent transverse magnetization at the time of imaging. In cardiac MRI the main use of T2-weighted imaging is to perform myocardial edema imaging. This is because water has a long T2 and will therefore show up more brightly. Usually T2-weighted sequences are performed using an FSE readout. However, simply performing a FSE sequence with a long TE will not provide good T2-weighted imaging. This is for two reasons. Firstly, intra-cavity blood will still produce signal that can be confused with edema in the endocardial regions. Secondly, the pericardial fat signal can also be confused with edema in the epicardial regions. Thus, most T2w SE echo sequences include a TIR for 'black blood' and fat suppression (Simonetti et al. 1996). An example image is shown in Fig. 25. In the rest of this textbook this TIR T2 weight spin echo sequence will be referred to as T2w MRI. As with DIR T1w MRI, T2w MRI is often acquired over two *R–R* intervals, prolonging breath hold time.

5.2 Spoiled Gradient Echo Sequences

Gradient echo (GRE) sequences are commonly used to dynamically image the heart. The fundamental difference between GRE and SE sequences is the absence of a refocusing pulse, and the use of a partial flip angle (less than 90°). A consequence of partial flip angle is that there is significant longitudinal magnetization present even after a short TR. Shorter TR's translate into shorter scan duration, and it is for this reason that GRE is heavily used in cardiac MRI. However in GRE sequences, dephasing due to external field inhomogeneities is not recovered and the amplitude envelope is controlled by T2* rather than T2.

Tissue contrast is heavily influenced by TR and flip angle. Short TR's and high flip angles increase T1-weighting because they allow less magnetization to recover. In cardiac MR, TR is often kept short and therefore most GRE sequences are heavily T1-weighted. There is also a further contrast mechanism specific to GRE imaging known as flow-related enhancement. In GRE imaging with a short TR, longitudinal magnetization may not fully recover before the next RF pulse. Thus, the amount of magnetization able to be flipped back into the transverse plane is reduced. However, if the spins are moving (i.e. blood moving in the through plane direction) new unsaturated spins will be present in the slice during the next excitation. This increases the total magnetization available to be flipped into the transverse plane, increasing the signal. Thus, structures containing blood moving in the through plane direction will appear brighter than surrounding stationary tissue. An important aspect of GRE imaging is dealing with coherent transverse magnetization prior to the next RF excitation. If left, the coherent transverse magnetization would combine with the *x–y* magnetization from the next pulse in an unpredictable way and lead to image artefacts. Therefore at the end of each TR, transverse magnetization is spoiled using either RF or gradient spoiling. The result is that at the start of

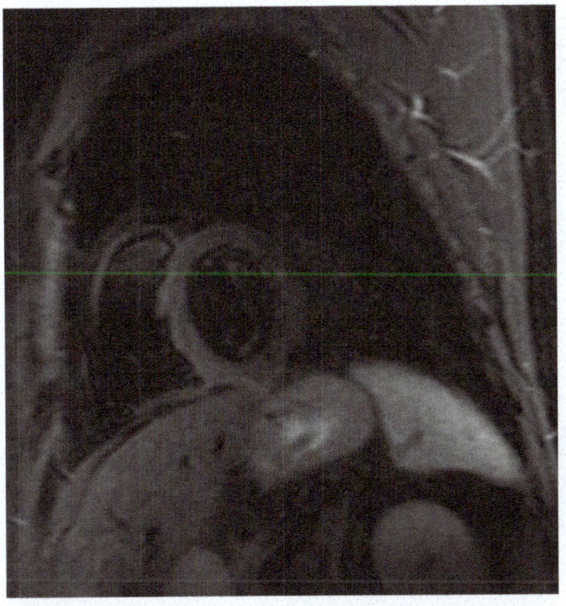

Fig. 25 T2-weighted triple inversion recovery spin echo image (T2w MRI)

the next TR there is no coherent magnetization left in *x–y*. This type of sequence is called a spoiled GRE (Sp-GRE) sequence. Spoiled GRE sequences were initially the mainstay of dynamic cardiac MRI. However due to poor myocardial blood pool contrast, they have been replaced by balanced steady state free precession (b-SSFP) imaging. Nevertheless, Sp-GRE sequences are still used in specific situations. In dynamic imaging Sp-GRE sequences are used in situations where b-SSFP imaging contains significant artefacts. Examples include: imaging inside and around stents (Nordmeyer et al. 2010), imaging around heart valves and imaging when there is retained metal within the thoracic cavity.

5.2.1 Specific Gradient Echo Sequences

ceMRA. Contrast-enhanced MR angiography (ceMRA) relies on the T1 shortening properties of Gadolinium. Gadolinium contrast will be discussed in more detail in the next chapter. However, in this chapter we will review the basic MR physics of the ceMRA sequence. In order to image blood vessels containing Gd, a heavily T1-weighted sequence is required. Furthermore to properly assess the vasculature, 3D imaging is required. Therefore, ceMRA is usually performed using a 3D Sp-GRE sequence with a TR of between 2 and 3 ms. The resolution used in these sequences depends on the structures being imaged. For great vessel imaging, a resolution of between 1.2 and 1.7 mm is usually sufficient. Often ceMRA is acquired with non-isotropic voxels. However, there are good reasons to keep pixels isotropic when assessing complex three-dimensional lesions in the thorax.

As Gd is an extracellular contrast agent, it will not stay in the blood pool indefinitely. In fact within 2–3 min it will have distributed throughout the extracellular space. Therefore, ceMRA must be performed as the Gd bolus travels through the vessel of interest. This means that total imaging time must be kept short and therefore ceMRA cannot be cardiac gated. In essence ceMRA is a 3D single shot technique triggered as the Gd bolus travels through a specific vessel. There are two main methods of determining the exact time to start the ceMRA acquisition after Gd injection. The first is to use a low dose test bolus and to perform a series of low resolution scouts at regular intervals. These can then be retrospectively viewed and the time to greatest vessel signal can be determined. The second method is to use some sort of real-time bolus tracking technology. Bolus tracking consists of continuous low resolution imaging that allows real-time visualization of the contrast bolus. When the operator visualizes high levels of contrast in the vessel of interest, the ceMRA is triggered (Fig. 26).

The most common *k*-space filling strategy for ceMRA is Cartesian. Thus, *k*-space is filled in 3D by multiple lines each with different phase and slice-encoding gradients. Usually *k*-space is filled from the center outward, which is known as centric ordering or filling. This is very important in bolus tracking as it ensures that the low frequencies are collected at the point of maximum contrast in the vessel of interest. In general, each ceMRA volume takes approximately 10–15 s to acquire (in a breath hold). It must remembered that this relatively short scan time is only achievable by utilizing techniques such as parallel imaging, partial Fourier and RFOV. In clinical practice, it is common to acquire two volumes to provide early and late vascular images. For instance, imaging could be triggered with Gd in the pulmonary artery. This would result in visualization of the pulmonary vasculature in the early images and imaging of the systemic arterial system in the late images (Fig. 27). Other *k*-space filling strategies are also used in

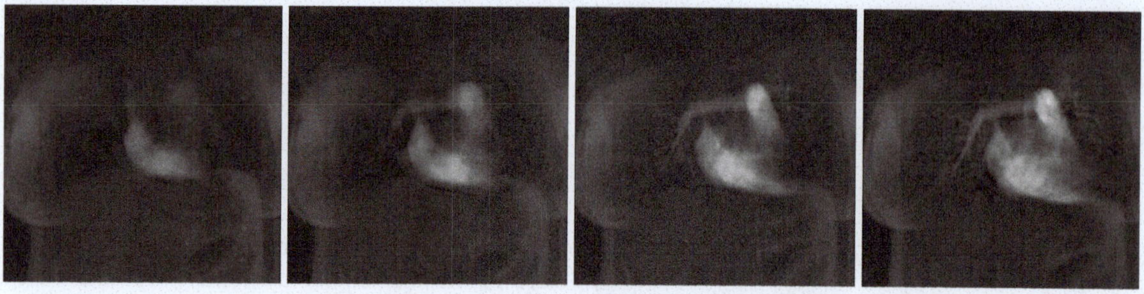

Fig. 26 Low-resolution thick slice single shot spoiled gradient echo sequence tracking contrast into the pulmonary arteries

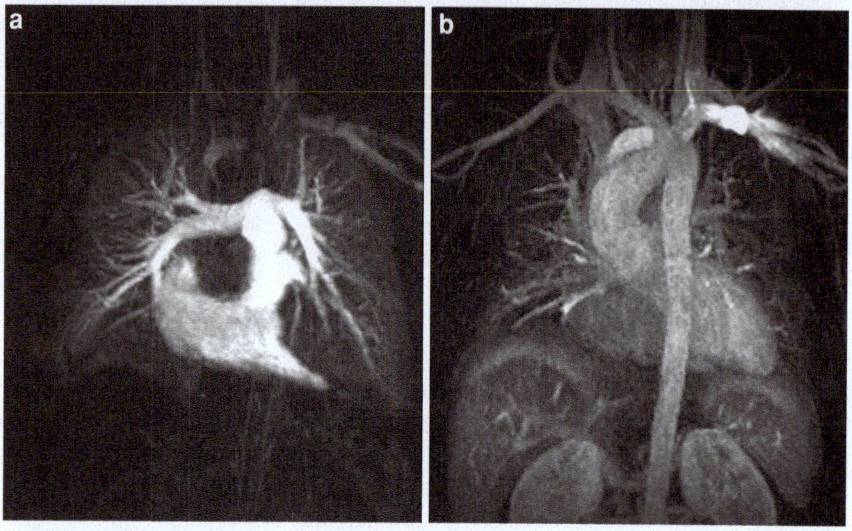

Fig. 27 Contrast-enhanced MRA. (**a**) Early with contrast in pulmonary arteries, (**b**) late with contrast in aorta

ceMRA. However, non-Cartesian trajectories tend to suffer from trajectories errors, which can cause image artefacts. Thus, their use is mainly confined to time resolved ceMRA. Time resolved MRA allows 3D visualization of the Gd bolus through the vasculature (Fenchel et al. 2007). To accomplish this each volume should be acquired in 1–3 s. In this situation, the improved temporal efficiency of non-Cartesian trajectories is of great benefit. Nevertheless, spatial resolution is usually sacrificed in order to image at a fast enough rate.

PC-MRI. velocity encoded phase contrast techniques enable non-invasive quantification of blood flow in major vessels. When magnetization is exposed to an additional magnetic gradient moment it accrues phase. Previously we have discussed this in relation to spatial encoding. However, gradients can also be used to encode any derivative of space (e.g. velocity or acceleration). Measuring blood flow depends on velocity-encoding and this section will concentrate on velocity encoded phase contrast MRI (PC-MRI). PC-MRI utilizes simple spoiled GRE sequences combined with an additional velocity-encoding gradient. This additional gradient creates a phase image in which pixel intensity is directly proportional to velocity. To understand this let us consider a vessel surrounded by static tissue (Fig. 28). After RF excitation all magnetization is coherent and in phase. If a gradient is then applied in the z direction, spins in the static tissue will dephase depending on their spatial position. This is akin to spatial encoding and the amount of phase accrued is proportional to the zeroth moment. Spins in the moving blood will also accrue phase, but because they are moving through the gradient field they will accrue more (or less depending on the direction of flow). So at this point static spins will have phase due to their spatial position, while moving spins will develop phase because of their position and velocity (Fig. 28a). If we now reverse the gradient the phase in the static tissue will return to zero. However,

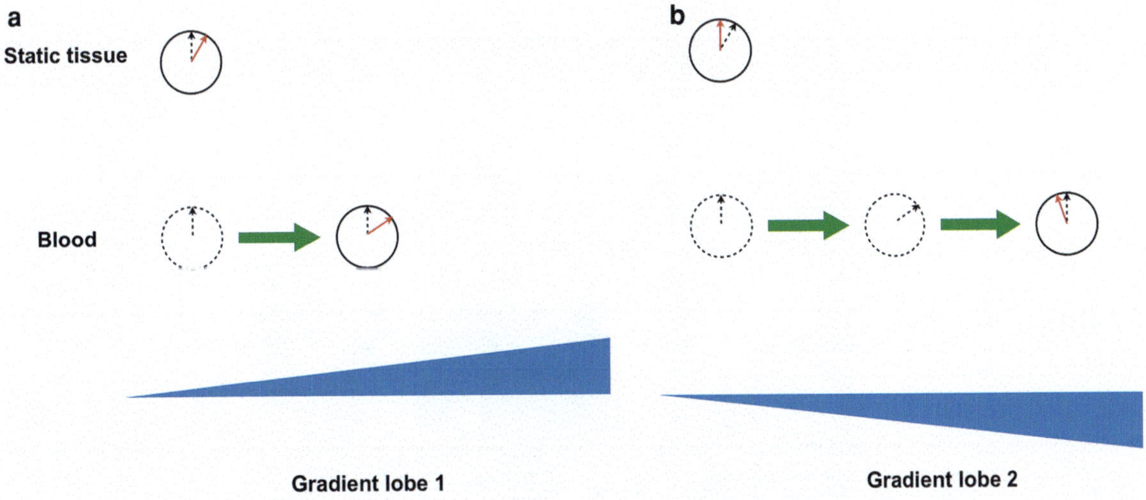

Fig. 28 The phase contrast experiment. **a** When a gradient is applied in the direction of flow the static tissue dephases; however in this case the moving spins diphase more because they are moving into a stronger magnetic field. **b** When the negative gradient is applied the static spins rephrase, however as the moving spins are moving into an even higher magnetic field they are left with residual phase at the end of the experiment

the phase in the moving blood will not go back to zero, rather it will be more or less than zero depending on direction of flow (Fig. 28b). This is because the spins in the moving blood are continuously traveling through a varying magnetic field. The end result of these two gradient lobes is that the phase of a spin population is directly proportional to their velocity. This gradient is known as a bipolar gradient it has a zero zeroth order moment and a non-zero first order moment. It is the first order moment that encodes velocity. One might think that this is all that is required in velocity-encoding. However, to negate phase shifts caused by other factors, a repeat measurement must be acquired without the velocity-encoding gradient (or by using two opposite gradients). The two measurements are subtracted eliminating phase secondary to other factors. This results in a phase difference solely dependent on the first order moment and the velocity of the moving spin (Fig. 29). It should be remembered that the phase difference is always within ±180° and therefore if the gradient moment is too high aliasing occurs. Thus, the strength of the velocity-encoding gradient moment must be set prior to acquisition. In clinical practice, it is usual to have some prior knowledge of the maximum velocity in a given situation. The first order gradient moment can then be set such that a velocity (v_{enc}), which is just greater than the maximum expected, will produce a phase shift of 180°. This will ensure no aliasing occurs. Lower strength gradients (higher v_{enc}) could also be used without the risk of aliasing. However, the use of higher v_{enc} leads to a reduced velocity to noise ratio.

Quantification of volume flow requires acquisition of a short axis view of a vessel with blood flow in the through plane direction. The phase map of such a slice can be used to calculate the average spin velocity in each pixel (v_{pix}) at time t. The pixel area multiplied by v_{pix} is the volume flow in each pixel (Q_{pix}) at time t. The sum of Q_{pix} within a region of interest (ROI) drawn around the vessel equals the volume flow at time t. As phase measurements are made at multiple time points within the cardiac cycle forward flow, regurgitant flow and cardiac output can then be calculated. Definition of the ROI is performed on the magnitude image as it allows better visualization of the vessel wall. PC-MRI will be dealt with in more detail in the flow and function chapter in this textbook.

5.3 Balanced Steady-State Free Precession

Balanced steady-state free precession (b-SSFP) is a GRE sequence that primarily relies on steady-state magnetization for signal production. If the TR is short, residual transverse magnetization will be present during subsequent excitations, eventually leading

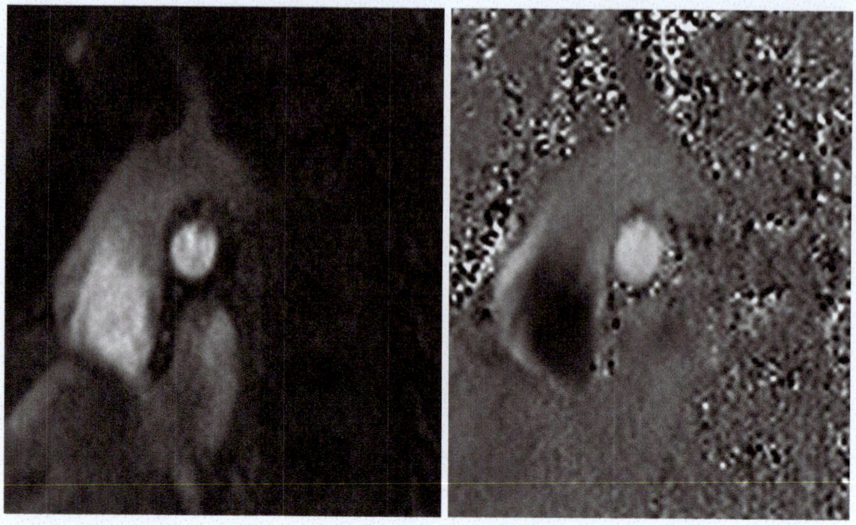

Fig. 29 Magnitude and phase images of the left pulmonary artery

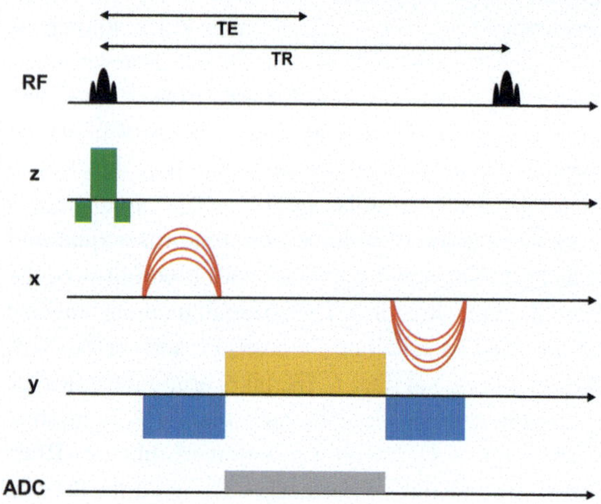

Fig. 30 Pulse sequence diagram of a b-SSFP sequence. Note that the net area of all the gradients is zero

to the evolution of steady state magnetization. In b-SSFP sequences, the steady state signal is optimized by both alternating excitation and balancing all the gradients (Fig. 30) (Scheffler and Lehnhardt 2003).

Sequence	Siemens	Philips	GE
Spin Echo	SE	SE	SE
Turbo spin Echo	TSE	TSE	FSE
Spoiled Gradient Echo	FLASH	T1-FFE	SPGR
Balanced steady state free precession	True FISP	bFFE	FIESTA

Balancing of the gradients is achieved as follows. The addition of a second negative lobe in the readout direction enables recovery of the echo that has been dephased during the second half of the readout gradient (Fig. 30). Dephasing due to phase encoding is compensated for by applying a second phase encode gradient in the opposite direction. This is sometimes referred to as the 'rewinder' gradient and is applied at the same time as the second negative lobe in the readout direction. In addition, the slice select gradient, which usually possesses a negative lobe to refocus spins in the slice select direction, is also fully balanced. The consequence of balancing the gradients is increased coherency of the magnetic vector prior to excitation. This makes the evolution of the signal produced by the RF excitation train more predictable. As the balancing gradient takes approximately the same time to apply as the encoding gradient, TR equals 2xTE in b-SSFP sequences.

In b-SSFP sequences, this coherent magnetization is flipped alternatively $+\alpha°$ and $-\alpha°$. Ultimately, this leads to the magnetization reaching a steady state at which point acquisition can commence. Prior to reaching the steady state, the complex trajectory of the NMV precludes inclusion in *k*-space.

Unlike Sp-GRE sequences, the signal in b-SSFP sequences is dependent on the square root of the T2/T1 ratio and the proton density. Thus, blood provides a much higher signal than myocardium (blood: T1 = 1,200 ms, T2 = 200 ms, myocardium: T1 = 867 ms, T2 = 57 ms) (Schar et al. 2004). The

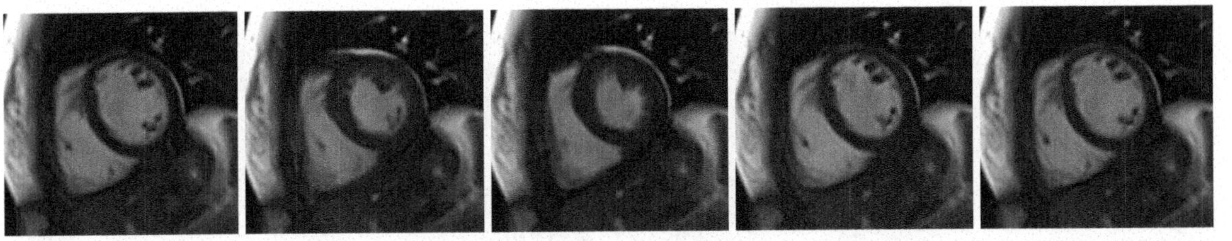

Fig. 31 Images from a cine sequence

signal is also dependent on the optimum flip angle, which is different for different tissues. The optimum flip angle for blood is 45° while for myocardium it is around 30°. Thus, when performing b-SSFP imaging with a flip angle of 45° the blood signal is approximately two times greater than the myocardial signal. In clinical applications, the flip angle is usually set to between 50° and 80°. The great benefit of b-SSFP is the excellent blood pool myocardial contrast, which is present throughout the cardiac cycle (because signal is not as dependant on flow related enhancement). For these reasons b-SSFP has become the predominant sequence used in cardiovascular MR imaging. However, there are some drawbacks with b-SSFP imaging. The main drawback is their well-described sensitivity to magnetic field inhomogeneity, which results in b-SSFP dark band artifact. Dark band artifact is caused by dephasing secondary to variations in the magnetic field. As dephasing approaches 180° there is almost 100% signal collapse. Of course local shimming reduces these artefacts as it reduces B_0 field inhomogeneity. Another important method of reducing the amount of dephasing is to keep TR short, as this reduces the amount of time for phase accrual. In clinical practice TR's of about 2–3 ms optimal for b-SSFP imaging. Unfortunately, there are also other sources of magnetic field inhomogeneity. The most obvious is metal inside the thoracic cavity in the form of stents, sternal wires or clips. These create localized signal drop that are often much larger than the structure themselves. The exact size of the signal dropout will depend on the type of metal and often orientation in the magnetic field. If the signal dropout encompasses an area of interest, other sequences may be required such as Sp-GRE or SE. Dephasing can also occurs in the presence of high flow, which can cause significant signal dropout with stenotic jets or valvar regurgitation. The last drawback of b-SFFP sequences is the high-energy deposition due to the large flip angle and short TR's. At 1.5T this is not a significant problem, however at higher field strengths excess energy deposition often precludes b-SSFP imaging.

5.3.1 Specific b-SSFP Sequences

Cine MRI. One of the most important uses of b-SSFP imaging is dynamic imaging of the heart (Fig. 31). As previously noted b-SSFP provides excellent contrast throughout the cardiac cycle. For this reason b-SSFP has replaced Sp-GRE sequences as the sequence of choice for dynamic imaging. In most units cine MRI will be performed with retrospective gating as this allows assessment of the heart throughout the entire cardiac cycle. In order to perform imaging in an acceptable breath hold, cine MRI is often combined with parallel imaging or *k-t* methods. Using these methods, a cine with 1.5 mm spatial resolution and approximately 40 ms temporal resolution can be acquired in less than 10 s. If cine imaging includes high velocity flow during systole, all measures must be taken to reduce dephasing. These include ensuring that the TR is between 2 and 3 ms and optimizing local shim.

3D MRA. The majority of MR angiography is performed using ce-MRA sequences. However, increasingly non-contrast angiography is being used in cardiac MRI. This is for several reasons. Firstly, if the structure of interest experiences significant motion during the cardiac cycle, gated imaging must be used. This precludes the use of ce-MRA as it is essentially a 3D single shot technique. Obvious examples of structures that move significantly during the cardiac cycle are the coronary arteries. In fact, gated non-contrast angiography was developed in order to visualize coronary arteries (MRCA). A more timely reason to reduce the use of ce-MRA sequences is the increasing concern regarding the safety profile of Gd contrast agents.

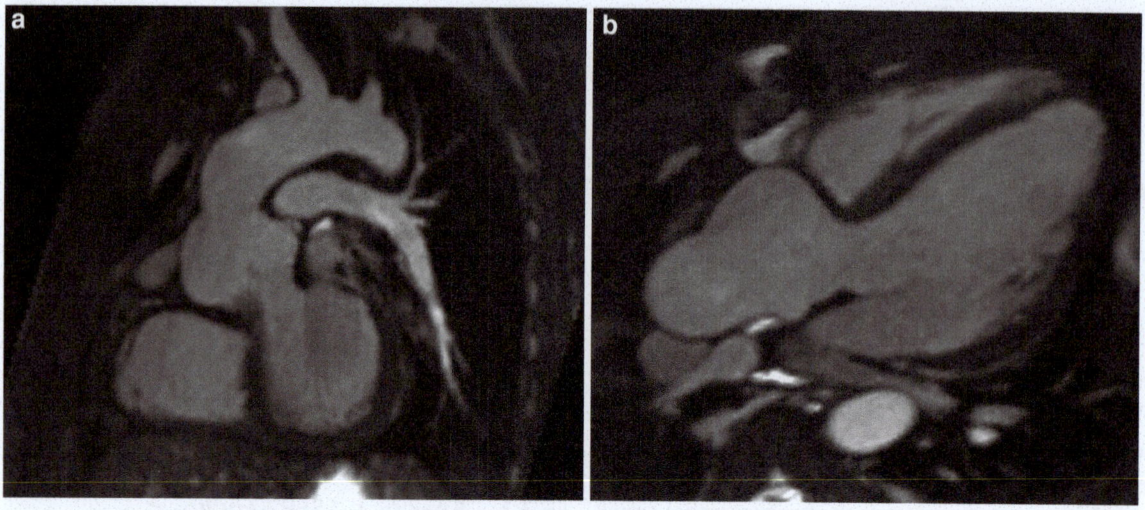

Fig. 32 3D Whole heart T2 prepared b-SSFP sequence in a patient who has had the Ross operation. **a** Coronal oblique view of the left ventricular outflow tract—note the excellent blood pool to myocardial contrast. **b** Axial oblique view of the left ventricular outflow tract

As previously pointed out, b-SSFP sequences provide excellent blood pool to myocardial contrast and are therefore well suited to angiography (Fig. 32a). As with ce-MRA, angiographic b-SSFP imaging employs 3D *k*-space filling. However, because 3D MRA must be cardiac gated, acquisition time is long. Even with the use of parallel imaging 3D MRA sequences cannot be performed in a breath hold. Therefore, navigators are often used to compensate for respiratory motion, further increasing scan time. Due to the long scan times, thin 3D slabs were traditionally placed over the coronary arteries in MRCA. The problem with this approach is that planning can often be difficult, and SNR is limited because of the small volume of excitation. An alternative approach is whole-heart imaging, which was facilitated by the advent of faster hardware and parallel imaging. In whole-heart imaging, no planning is required as the imaging volume is simply placed over the heart. The major drawback of this technique is that scan times are long often between 10 and 15 min. Nevertheless, this technique is heavily used particularly in congenital heart disease where it provides excellent delineation of intra-cardiac and great vessel anatomy (Sorensen et al. 2004) (Fig. 32b).

In order to improve contrast, several magnetization preparation schemes are utilized. The first is T2 preparation, which significantly improves myocardial blood pool contrast. This is important in 3D techniques, as SSFP contrast is lower than in 2D techniques. The second is fat saturation usually using SPIR. This reduces pericardial fat signal and is particularly important when imaging the coronary arteries. These magnetization preparation pulses are interleaved with the navigator pulse prior to image acquisition. In adults, acquisition is triggered in diastalic diastasis to reduce motion artifact. However, in children end systole may be a better point in the cardiac cycle to trigger. In both adults and children timing can be elucidated using a high temporal resolution cine MRI in the four-chamber plane. Although, Cartesian filling is overwhelmingly used in 3D MRA, other techniques have also been tried. The most promising are 3D radial acquisition. This is because radial *k*-space filling benefits from less motion insensitivity, which reduces artifact when trying to assess small fast moving structures.

6 Conclusion

To conclude the purpose of this chapter is to provide a better understanding of MRI physics. However, it is only a foundation and in order to be proficient at sequence optimization, one must gain experience through trail and error. Therefore the author suggests that constant questioning of scan parameters and attempts at optimization are prerequisites to good cardiac MRI.

7 Key Points

- A wide variety of prepulses, segmentation algorithms and triggering techniques are used to adapt MRI sequences to the specific requirements for cardiac studies.
- Parallel imaging and real-time MRI are recent evolutions that contribute significantly to the interactive nature of a cardiac MRI examination.
- Careful choice of sequences and the knowledge of the tissue properties they reveal allow comprehensive studies of cardiac pathology.

References

Bogaert J, Kuzo R, Dymarkowski S, Janssen L, Celis I, Budts W, Gewillig M (2000) Follow-up of patients with previous treatment for coarctation of the thoracic aorta: comparison between contrast-enhanced MR angiography and fast spin-echo MR imaging. Eur Radiol 10:1847–1854

Botnar RM, Stuber M, Danias PG, Kissinger KV, Manning WJ (1999) Improved coronary artery definition with T2-weighted, free-breathing, three-dimensional coronary MRA. Circulation 99:3139–3148

Chrispin A, Small P, Rutter N, Coupland RE, Doyle M, Chapman B, Coxon R, Guilfoyle D, Cawley M, Mansfield P (1986) Echo planar imaging of normal and abnormal connections of the heart and great arteries. Pediatr Radiol 16:289–292

Ding S, Wolff SD, Epstein FH (1998) Improved coverage in dynamic contrast-enhanced cardiac MRI using interleaved gradient-echo EPI. Magn Reson Med Off J Soc Magn Reson Med/Soc Magn Reson Med 39:514–519

Fenchel M, Saleh R, Dinh H, Lee MH, Nael K, Krishnam M, Ruehm SG, Miller S, Child J, Finn JP (2007) Juvenile and adult congenital heart disease: time-resolved 3D contrast-enhanced MR angiography. Radiology 244:399–410

Finn JP, Edelman RR (1993) Black-blood and segmented k-space magnetic resonance angiography. Magn Reson Imaging Clin North Am 1:349–357

Greenman RL, Shirosky JE, Mulkern RV, Rofsky NM (2003) Double inversion black-blood fast spin-echo imaging of the human heart: a comparison between 1.5T and 3.0T. J Magn Reson Imaging JMRI 17:648–655

Griswold MA, Jakob PM, Heidemann RM, Nittka M, Jellus V, Wang J, Kiefer B, Haase A (2002) Generalized autocalibrating partially parallel acquisitions (GRAPPA). Magn Reson Med Off J Soc Magn Reson Med/Soc Magn Reson Med 47:1202–1210

Hansen MS, Atkinson D, Sorensen TS (2008) Cartesian SENSE and k-t SENSE reconstruction using commodity graphics hardware. Magn Reson Med Off J Soc Magn Reson Med/Soc Magn Reson Med 59:463–468

Hansen MS, Baltes C, Tsao J, Kozerke S, Pruessmann KP, Eggers H (2006) k-t BLAST reconstruction from non-Cartesian k-t space sampling. Magn Reson Med Off J Soc Magn Reson Med/Soc Magn Reson Med 55:85–91

Kaldoudi E, Williams SC, Barker GJ, Tofts PS (1993) A chemical shift selective inversion recovery sequence for fat-suppressed MRI: theory and experimental validation. Magn Reson Imaging 11:341–355

Keegan J, Gatehouse PD, Taylor AM, Yang GZ, Jhooti P, Firmin DN (1999) Coronary artery imaging in a 0.5-Tesla scanner: implementation of real-time, navigator echo-controlled segmented k-space FLASH and interleaved-spiral sequences. Magn Reson Med Off J Soc Magn Reson Med/Soc Magn Reson Med 41:392–399

Kim RJ, Wu E, Rafael A, Chen EL, Parker MA, Simonetti O, Klocke FJ, Bonow RO, Judd RM (2000) The use of contrast-enhanced magnetic resonance imaging to identify reversible myocardial dysfunction. N Engl J Med 343:1445–1453

Kolbitsch C, Prieto C, Smink J, Schaeffter T (2011) Highly efficient whole-heart imaging using radial phase encoding-phase ordering with automatic window selection. Magn Reson Med 66(4):1008–1018

Korperich H, Gieseke J, Barth P, Hoogeveen R, Esdorn H, Peterschroder A, Meyer H, Beerbaum P (2004) Flow volume and shunt quantification in pediatric congenital heart disease by real-time magnetic resonance velocity mapping: a validation study. Circulation 109:1987–1993

Lanzer P, Botvinick EH, Schiller NB, Crooks LE, Arakawa M, Kaufman L, Davis PL, Herfkens R, Lipton MJ, Higgins CB (1984) Cardiac imaging using gated magnetic resonance. Radiology 150:121–127

Lenz GW, Haacke EM, White RD (1989) Retrospective cardiac gating: a review of technical aspects and future directions. Magn Reson Imaging 7:445–455

Muthurangu V, Lurz P, Critchely JD, Deanfield JE, Taylor AM, Hansen MS (2008) Real-time assessment of right and left ventricular volumes and function in patients with congenital heart disease by using high spatiotemporal resolution radial k-t SENSE. Radiology 248:782–791

Nordmeyer J, Gaudin R, Tann OR, Lurz PC, Bonhoeffer P, Taylor AM, Muthurangu V (2010) MRI may be sufficient for noninvasive assessment of great vessel stents: an in vitro comparison of MRI, CT, and conventional angiography. Am J Roentgenol 195:865–871

Pruessmann KP, Weiger M, Boesiger P (2001) Sensitivity encoded cardiac MRI. J Cardiovasc Magn Reson Off J Soc Cardiovasc Magn Reson 3:1–9

Pruessmann KP, Weiger M, Scheidegger MB, Boesiger P (1999) SENSE: sensitivity encoding for fast MRI. Magn Reson Med Off J Soc Magn Reson Med/Soc Magn Reson Med 42:952–962

Schar M, Kozerke S, Fischer SE, Boesiger P (2004) Cardiac SSFP imaging at 3 Tesla. Magn Reson Med 51:799–806

Scheffler K, Lehnhardt S (2003) Principles and applications of balanced SSFP techniques. Eur Radiol 13:2409–2418

Simonetti OP, Finn JP, White RD, Laub G, Henry DA (1996) "Black blood" T2-weighted inversion-recovery MR imaging of the heart. Radiology 199:49–57

Sorensen TS, Korperich H, Greil GF, Eichhorn J, Barth P, Meyer H, Pedersen EM, Beerbaum P (2004) Operator-independent isotropic three-dimensional magnetic resonance imaging for morphology in congenital heart disease: a validation study. Circulation 110:163–169

Steeden JA, Atkinson D, Taylor AM, Muthurangu V (2010a) Assessing vascular response to exercise using a combination of real-time spiral phase contrast MR and noninvasive blood pressure measurements. J Magn Reson Imaging 31:997–1003

Steeden JA, Atkinson D, Taylor AM, Muthurangu V (2010b) Split-acquisition real-time CINE phase-contrast MR flow measurements. Magn Reson Med Off J Soc Magn Reson Med/Soc Magn Reson Med 64:1664–1670

Stehling MK, Holzknecht NG, Laub G, Bohm D, Von Smekal A, Reiser M (1996) Single-shot T1- and T2-weighted magnetic resonance imaging of the heart with black blood: preliminary experience. Magma 4:231–240

Tsao J, Kozerke S, Boesiger P, Pruessmann KP (2005) Optimizing spatiotemporal sampling for k-t BLAST and k-t SENSE: application to high-resolution real-time cardiac steady-state free precession. Magn Reson Med Off J Soc Magn Reson Med/Soc Magn Reson Med 53:1372–1382

Wang Y, Moin K, Akinboboye O, Reichek N (2005) Myocardial first pass perfusion: steady-state free precession versus spoiled gradient echo and segmented echo planar imaging. Magn Reson Med Off J Soc Magn Reson Med/Soc Magn Reson Med 54:1123–1129

MR Contrast Agents for Cardiac Imaging

Yicheng Ni

Contents

1 Introduction 31

2 Basic Principle of MR Contrast Agents 32
2.1 Origins of Imaging Signals for Current Clinical MR 32
2.2 Unique Mechanisms of MRI Contrast Agents 33
2.3 Dosage in Relation to Contrast Enhancing Efficacy 35

3 Classifications of Contrast Agents for Cardiac MRI 35
3.1 Extracellular Fluid Space Contrast Agents 35
3.2 Blood-Pool Contrast Agents 37
3.3 Intracellular Contrast Agents 39
3.4 Necrosis-Avid or Multipurpose Contrast Agents? ... 39
3.5 Potential Plaque- and Thrombus-Specific Contrast Agents 44
3.6 Emerging Molecular Imaging Contrast Agents 45

4 Application Scopes of MR Contrast Agents for Cardiac Imaging 45

5 Conclusion 46

References 46

Abstract

Thanks to the ever-advancing technologies, cardiac magnetic resonance imaging (MRI) has become a major diagnostic tool in clinical cardiology for acquisition of morphological, functional and metabolic information. However, it is of no doubt that only when complemented with the use of contrast agents, can cardiac MRI fully play its pivotal roles in clinical diagnosis and therapeutic decision-making. In particular, MR coronary angiography, perfusion mapping, and cellular membrane integrity or myocardial viability assessment rely more on the use of appropriate contrast agents. The current chapter aims to provide an overview on the main topics related to MRI contrast agents including the mechanisms of MRI contrast and contrast agents, classification of both commercially available and preclinically investigational contrast agents useful for cardiac MRI, as well as the general scope of contrast agent applications in relevant clinical practice and experimental research.

1 Introduction

Magnetic resonance imaging (MRI) has rapidly evolved into a major player in the armamentarium of clinical diagnostic imaging. This development is a great symbol of contemporary medicine. Acknowledging its significance, the 2003 Nobel Prize in Physiology or Medicine was awarded jointly to Lauterbur and Mansfield for their pivotal contributions in the discovery and utility of MRI (Gore 2003).

Y. Ni (✉)
Department of Radiology,
Gasthuisberg University Hospital,
Herestraat 49, 3000 Leuven, Belgium
e-mail: yicheng.ni@med.kuleuven.be

J. Bogaert et al. (eds.), *Clinical Cardiac MRI*, Medical Radiology. Diagnostic Imaging,
DOI: 10.1007/174_2011_360, © Springer-Verlag Berlin Heidelberg 2012

Comparing with any other body structures, the ever-pumping heart in the respiration-tided thorax represents the most difficult organ to image. Nonetheless cardiac MRI is now entirely feasible thanks to the implemented techniques such as ECG triggering, respiration gating, ultrafast or even real-time imaging methods that have efficiently minimized or overcome cardiac and breathing motion artifacts (Kuhl et al. 2004). Over the last decade, there has been tremendous progress in MRI of both cardiac morphology and function. Further advances toward faster acquisition with real-time imaging, higher resolution for plaque imaging and quantitative analysis are taking place at a rapid pace.

Thus, for cardiac imaging, MRI has become advantageous over other modalities due to its versatile strengths, including noninvasiveness; nonionizing safety; superb spatial and temporal resolution; inherent 3D data acquisition with unlimited orientation; intrinsic contrast exploitable for tissue characterization; sensitivity to blood flow and cardiac wall motion; and potential for in vivo measurement of myocardial metabolism by using MR spectroscopy or MRS, as well as any further technical breakthroughs (Van der wall et al. 1996).

Despite all these strengths, it is of no doubt that only when complemented with the use of contrast agents, cardiac MRI can fully play its pivotal roles in clinical diagnosis and therapeutic decision-making. In fact, the potential and necessity of using contrast materials to promote MRI capacity was recognized soon after the invention of this imaging technology (Lauterbur et al. 1978). In particular, MR coronary angiography (MRCA), perfusion mapping and cellular membrane integrity or myocardial viability assessment rely more on the use of appropriate contrast agents for eased imaging acquisition, enhanced image quality and/or improved diagnostic sensitivity and specificity. In addition, contrast agents may be useful for MRI-guided interventional procedures such as angioplasty and localized delivery in gene or other advanced therapies in the future. Further research and development of more targeted MRI contrast agents at the cellular and molecular levels will help to more specifically identify different cardiovascular pathologies including ischemia, atherosclerosis, inflammation, necrosis and angiogenesis. Only by joining together all these indispensable elements, can the comprehensive "one-stop shop" cardiac MRI examination become the reality of clinical cardiology (Ni 1998).

The current chapter aims to provide an overview on the main topics related to MRI contrast agents including the mechanisms of MRI contrast and contrast agents, classification of both commercially available and preclinically investigational contrast agents useful for cardiac MRI, as well as the general scope of contrast agent applications in relevant clinical and experimental research. For the 2nd edition, more information has been updated and incorporated into this chapter since the 1st edition of this book was published 6 years ago.

2 Basic Principle of MR Contrast Agents

2.1 Origins of Imaging Signals for Current Clinical MR

About two-thirds of the human body consists of water that exists either freely or confined within the life molecules. Water is formed by one atom of oxygen bound with two atoms of hydrogen (^{1}H). Another more "MRI-discernible" body constituent is the fat, which is chemically composed of fatty acids such as stearic, palmitic, oleic, etc., covalently bound in various proportions with glyceryl, all are enriched with ^{1}H.

The imaging signals in the clinically applied MRI at present stem from the abundant ^{1}H in the human body, which is inherent in magnetic property due to its single positively charged proton. The similar property is also found in other less abundantly occurring isotopic nuclei such as ^{13}C, ^{19}F, ^{23}Na and ^{31}P with only odd numbers of protons, but not in ^{12}C, ^{14}N and ^{16}O, with even numbers of protons and neutrons.

When the body is exposed to a strong magnetic field, the ^{1}H nuclei in the tissue orient themselves within this magnetic field. While sending in a pulse of radio waves at a certain frequency, the energy content as well as the orientation of the nuclei changes, and, as they relax to their previous states, a resonance radio wave or an MRI signal is emitted. In 1971, Lauterbur pioneered spatial information encoding principles that made image formation possible by utilizing such emitted MRI signals. The further studies of Mansfield on the concept of echo-planar imaging dramatically decreased acquisition time and allowed functional and dynamic imaging (Gore 2003).

The frequencies of electromagnetic waves or radiations used for MRI are from 10^{6} to 10^{9} Hz approximately, i.e. within radiofrequency range, which are much lower than that of ionizing X-rays (10^{16}–10^{20} Hz) and γ-rays (10^{21}–10^{24} Hz) used for radiography and nuclear medicine, respectively and are therefore considered biologically safe.

Besides ^{1}H, other magnetic nuclei such as ^{23}Na, ^{13}C, ^{19}F and ^{31}P in the human body can also generate MRI signals, though normally with much less intensity but under much more technically demanding conditions and/or at much higher costs (Cannon et al. 1986; Fishman et al. 1987; Friedrich et al. 1995; Kim et al. 1997, 1999; Ardenkjaer-Larsen et al. 2003; Golman et al. 2003; Svensson et al. 2003). Some of these techniques are of particular cardiovascular relevance. The feasibility of obtaining cardiac ^{23}Na MRI at both 4.7 T animal and 1.5 T human scanners has been demonstrated using double-resonant ^{23}Na-^{1}H surface radiofrequency coils for myocardial viability determination (Cannon et al. 1986; Kim et al. 1997; Ouwerkerk et al. 2008). In this context, the dramatic alterations of extra-versus intracellular ^{23}Na concentration during myocardial ischemia or infarction were exploited as intrinsic source of contrast to identify irreversibly damaged myocytes due to disruption of sodium concentration gradient across cellular membranes. However, as the authors admitted, clinical feasibility does not imply clinical utility. Further efforts have to be made before cardiac ^{23}Na MRI can be incorporated as part of the clinical routine (Kim et al. 1999). On the other hand, ^{31}P chemical shift imaging may provide a profile of regional adenosine triphosphate (ATP) and phosphocreatine (PCr) contents, hence an estimation of energy status and viability of the myocardium (Friedrich et al. 1995). Recently a new revolutionary technology that utilizes biomolecules bearing certain prepared hyperpolarized (HP) nucleus such as HP ^{13}C-urea has shown the promise in ultrafast high-resolution MR angiography with unprecedented signal-to-noise (SNR) and contrast-to-noise (CNR) ratios even at very low magnetic field (e.g. 0.01 T). This may also open new horizon for molecular imaging with MRI (Ardenkjaer-Larsen et al. 2003; Golman et al. 2003; Svensson et al. 2003). Despite the high performance of such novel approaches (Bhattacharya et al. 2009), it is likely that conventional ^{1}H MRI will still serve as the mainstream method for providing the basic morphological and functional information of normal and diseased cardiovascular tissues.

2.2 Unique Mechanisms of MRI Contrast Agents

Image contrast is the basis for human visual perception to differentiate between regions on the object. Contrast media or agents denote extrinsic or intrinsic substances that are intended to improve the image contrast of the target tissues by means of increasing or decreasing the attenuation of X-rays in radiography, the signal intensity (SI) in MRI and the echo amplitude in ultrasonography. The radiopharmaceuticals can also be considered as contrast media to a certain extent. Since there is virtually no native radioactivity in the human body, introduction of a radiopharmaceutical into the body always increases positively the contrast of the target tissue over the background. Acceptable biotolerance remains one of the basic requirements for any potential contrast agents.

The main contrast determinants in MRI are ^{1}H proton density, longitudinal (T1) or transverse (T2) relaxation times of ^{1}H protons, and magnetic susceptibility. Since water content or ^{1}H proton density in the tissue is virtually unchangeable, magnetic properties of T1, T2 and susceptibility have therefore been the major parameters dominating the development of MRI contrast agents. Although T1 and T2 are generally prolonged in injured myocardium, there is considerable overlap of relaxation times between normal, reversibly injured and irreversibly damaged myocardium on native MRI, a fact stressing the need of contrast agents for cardiac MRI.

Some paramagnetic transition metal elements such as gadolinium (Gd^{3+}), manganese (Mn^{2+}), dysprosium (Dy^{3+}) and iron (Fe^{3+}) contain in their outer shells of the electron orbit a number of unpaired electron spins, which have relatively long electron spin relaxation time. The magnetic field produced by an electron is much stronger than that by a ^{1}H proton, and therefore these paramagnetic elements are ideal candidates for producing MRI contrast agents that affect T1 and T2 of tissue ^{1}H protons, hence the tissue SI and/or contrast. Contrast enhancement is achieved by either increasing or decreasing the SI of a tissue; thus its signal over background noise ratio (SNR), its contrast relative to another tissue (contrast ratio or CR) and/or to the background noise (contrast-to-noise ratio or CNR) can be enhanced.

Differing from the direct and linear principles of contrast formation with the high-density contrast

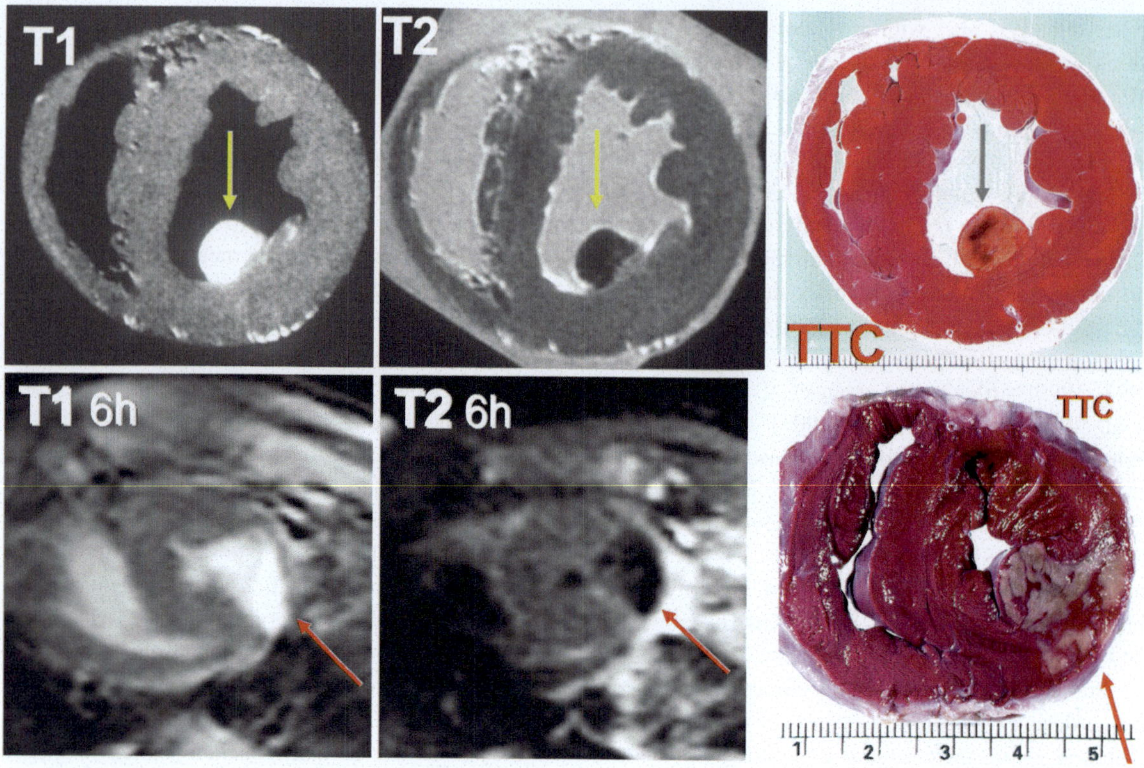

Fig. 1 Nonporphyrin necrosis-avid contrast agents (NACAs) at the same intravenous dose of 0.05 mmol/kg induced both T1 and T2 contrast enhancement (CE) with relevant MRI sequences in reperfused MI (*arrow*) on postmortem images of a dog overnight after injection of *bis*-Gd-DTPA-pamoic acid derivative (ECIII-60; *upper row*) and on in vivo images of a pig 6 h after injection of *bis*-Gd-DTPA-*bis*-indole derivative (ECIV-7; *lower row*), suggesting the chemotactic accumulation of NACAs in the necrotic myocardium as proven by the corresponding TTC stained specimen

media for radiography or the gamma ray emitting isotopes for nuclear scintigraphy, the mechanisms of the current MRI contrast agents are basically indirect and nonlinear, and much more complicated. They rest on the distinct magnetic properties and interactions of native ^{1}H protons toward introduced MRI contrast agents. Depending on influential factors, including the dose of the contrast agent and MRI sequence applied, either T1 shortening (positive) or T2 shortening (negative) contrast effect can be predominant.

The positive contrast agents are typically Gd- or Mn-containing paramagnetic chelates. They shorten both T1 and T2 of the tissue, but since T1 is much longer than T2, their predominant effect at low doses is T1 shortening. Therefore the tissue taking up such contrast agents becomes bright or hyperintense on T1 weighted MRI. However, when the local concentration of a T1 or positive contrast agent becomes very high, its T2 shortening effect appears or becomes even predominant as often seen in the renal pelvis shortly after an intravenous dosage, or as exemplified in the case of experimental acute myocardial infarction (AMI) enhanced with a necrosis-avid contrast agent (NACA; Fig. 1).

The negative contrast agents are often termed superparamagnetic or susceptibility contrast agents that can be created as small Fe_3O_4 particulate aggregates consisting of ferromagnetic or superparamagnetic crystals or particles smaller than 300 nm. They generate local magnetic field gradients that disrupt the homogeneity of the primary magnetic field over the tissue. Besides T2 shortening effect due to the diffusion of water through these field gradients, their more prominent effect is T2* shortening or susceptibility effect, both effects darken the region of interest or produce hypointense signals on T2, T2* and even T1 weighted MR images. However, depending on their particle size and coating, they can also produce substantial T1 shortening effect and function as positive contrast agents used, for example, for MR angiography (MRA).

There are also intrinsic MRI contrast substances such as hemoglobin. The paramagnetic property of deoxyhemoglobin to cause local magnetic field distortion and susceptibility has been exploited as the source of blood oxygen level dependent (BOLD) contrast for functional MRI of the brain (Turner 1997), heart (Manka et al. 2010) and tumor (Padhani 2010).

In principle, it is their magnetic impact on the ^{1}H proton relaxation rather than the MRI contrast agents themselves that create enhanced contrast on MR images. In other words, MRI contrast agents do not generate signals but only modify the amplitude of the signals generated by ^{1}H protons in the presence of magnetic field.

'Because of such an indirect mechanism of action, a lack of linear relation between the SI and the local concentration represents a drawback for accurate quantification of studied MRI contrast agents. Nevertheless, similar to radiopharmaceuticals or radiographic contrast media, in unconventional MRI when the scanner is tuned to the resonant frequencies for nuclei of ^{23}Na, ^{13}C, ^{19}F and ^{31}P, the generated images will only show regions where these nuclei are present, hence feasible for quantitative data analysis with a direct SI and nucleus concentration relationship.

2.3 Dosage in Relation to Contrast Enhancing Efficacy

Normally MRI contrast agents are chemically formulated in a manner similar to that for producing radiopharmaceuticals. Due to the fact that the sensitivity of ^{1}H MRI to detect CA induced effects visible on the image is higher than that of radiography but much lower than that of nuclear scintigraphy, the MRI contrast agents can be given with doses of micromoles per kilogram (about 5–300 μmol/kg), i.e. about 10^{2}–10^{3} times lower than that for radiographic contrast media at a millimoles-per-kilogram level, but 10^{4}–10^{6} times higher than that for radiopharmaceuticals at a nanomole- or even picomole-per-kilogram level. Usually, the physicians' knowledge and experience with CT contrast media can be extended to the use of clinically available MRI extracellular fluid (ECF) space contrast agents. However, as illustrated in Fig. 1, MRI contrast agents possess both T1- and T2-shortening effects and their positive or negative effects of contrast enhancement (CE) depend not only on the total dosage administered but also the local concentration of the accumulated agent in a given target tissue, as well as interaction between the contrast agent and the tissue components. Such a unique phenomenon differing from that with CT and nuclear imaging should be taken into account when contrast enhanced MRI is interpreted.

Based on the diagnostic purpose as well as safety considerations, the exact doses and manners of contrast agent administration vary among different cardiac MRI protocols. For a first-pass myocardial perfusion MRI, a bolus of a contrast agent at a relatively low dose of 0.005–0.05 mmol/kg is intravenously injected at a high speed (e.g. 3–5 ml/s) and flushed with certain volume of 0.9% saline by using a power injector. This is usually followed by another normal dose of contrast agent for delayed CE for estimation of MI or viability (Chiu et al. 2003). To compensate the unstable CE in the AMI due to the use of ECF contrast agents, a constant infusion of Gd-DTPA was recommended for more accurate determination of myocardial necrosis in a clinical setting (Pereira et al. 2000). Diversely, slow intravenous infusion is also a common practice for administration of Mn-based intracellular contrast agents but to avoid acute side-effect caused by calcium disturbance in myocardium (Bremerich et al. 2000; Flacke et al. 2003).

3 Classifications of Contrast Agents for Cardiac MRI

3.1 Extracellular Fluid Space Contrast Agents

The first generation MRI contrast agents including Gd-DTPA and Gd-DOTA (Table 1, Fig. 2) are created by chelating the lanthanide metal element gadolinium with linear or cyclic multidentate ligands (DTPA or DOTA) to form thermodynamically stable and biologically inert complex or coordination compounds so that the paramagnetic properties of gadolinium can be utilized for enhancing MRI contrast, whereas the toxicity of both gadolinium and the

Table 1 Contrast agents that could be used for Cardiac MRI

Category	Short name	Generic name	Trade name	Feature
Extracellular fluid space contrast agents[b]	Gd-DTPA	Gadopentetate dimeglumine	Magnevist	Positive[c]
	Gd-DOTA	Gadoterate meglumine	Dotarem	Positive
	Gd-DTPA-BMA	Gadodiamide injection	Omniscan	Positive
	Gd-HP-DO3A	Gadoteridol injection	ProHance	Positive
	Gd-DTPA-BMEA	Gadoversetamide	Optimark	Positive
	Gd-DO3A-butriol	Gadobutrol	Gadovist	Positive
	Gd-BOPTA	Gadobenate dimeglumine	Multi-Hance	Positive
	Porphyrin and Nonporphyrin NACAs			Positive
Blood pool contrast agents	NC-100150	PEG-feron (USPIO)	Clariscan	Positive
	SH U 555 C	Ferucarbotran (USPIO)	Supravist	Positive
	MS-325		Angiomark	Positive
	B-22956	Gadocoletic Acid		Positive
	Gadomer-17			Positive
	P792	Macromolecular Gd-DOTA derivate	Vistarem	Positive
	AMI-227	Ferumoxtran (USPIO)	Sinerem/combidex	Positive or negative
	Gd-BOPTA	Gadobenate dimeglumine	Multi-Hance	Positive
	Porphyrin and Nonporphyrin NACAs			Positive
Intracellular contrast agents	Mn-DPDP	Mangafodipir Trisodium	Teslascan	Intramyocytic uptake, positive
	$MnCl_2$, MP-680, CVP 1001-1			Experimental, positive
Necrosis-avid contrast agents (NACAs)	Bis-Gd-DTPA-mesoporphyrin		Gadophrin-2 Gadophrin-3[a]	Experimental, positive; Central chelation of Cu[a]
	ECIII-60	Gd-DTPA-pamoic acid derivative	Nonporphyrin NACA	Experimental, positive
	ECIV-7	Gd-DTPA-bisindole derivative	Nonporphyrin NACA	Experimental, positive
	Gadofluorine-M			Experimental, positive
Plaque-specific contrast agents	Gadofluorine-M			Experimental, positive
	Porphyrin and Nonporphyrin NACAs			Experimental, positive

Note
[a] Approved or in development
[b] All ECF space contrast agents are excreted via urine
[c] With high local concentration, negative contrast can be observed, e.g. first-pass perfusion

ligands, if each applied alone, can thus be avoided. After intravenous injection, these contrast agents randomly distribute in intravascular and interstitial ECF spaces, and are eliminated rapidly in their unchanged forms through glomerular filtration in the kidney (Fig. 2), which makes the "renal-specific" property exploitable for evaluation of renal function. These contrast agents also allow possible diagnosis of certain pathological conditions with altered distribution space at vascular level, such as hemangioma and blood–brain-barrier (BBB) breakdown, at interstitial level, such as inflammatory edema and regenerative fibrosis, and at cellular membrane integral level such as tissue necrosis or infarction, e.g. AMI. However, normally they do not allow definite histological diagnoses owing to the intrinsic feature of nonselective distribution over all the above-mentioned pathologies. Alternatively, analyses of enhancement kinetics have been elaborated for differential diagnosis between malignant and benign lesions (Heywang et al. 1989; Kaiser and Zeitler 1989), for quantitative assessment of tumor angiogenesis and microvascular density (Hawighorst et al. 1999), and for determination of cerebral blood flow and volume (Villringer et al. 1988). Lack of real tissue and/or disease specificity of these contrast agents have prompted further research and development of more specific MRI contrast agents. One noteworthy issue is that other, more advanced specific or targeting contrast agents always share more or less the nonspecific properties of the ECF contrast agents especially in their early systemic distribution phase, which has been explored for multipurpose applications of certain organ- or tissue-specific contrast agents such as the hepatobiliary Gd-BOPTA (Cavagna et al. 1997) and necrosis-avid contrast agents (NACAs) (Ni et al. 2002a, b, c, 2005a; Ni 2008) (Table 1).

3.2 Blood-Pool Contrast Agents

This unique type refers to a variety of contrast agents that are confined by purpose to the intravascular space and dedicated exclusively to cardiovascular applications. Such blood-pool (BP) property can be realized by controlling the distribution and elimination of the contrast agents, which in turn is determined by their size relative to the permeability of the capillary endothelium in different organs. Although BP contrast agents are partially or completely limited in passing through the endothelial membrane elsewhere, they can still be excreted by the kidneys (Fig. 2). Usually, the higher the molecular weight of macromolecular compounds, the slower the blood elimination half-life and total blood clearance. In tissues such as myocardium, the lumen of the continuous capillaries is lined with an uninterrupted endothelial layer, which only allow diffusion of drugs with small molecular weight such as Gd-DTPA (590 Da); whereas in the kidneys, glomerular capillaries are fenestrated with pores of 60–70 nm in diameter, which facilitate passage of any drug molecules weighted approximately below 20,000 Da. Above this molecular weight, renal excretion then depends on the lipophilicity and polarity of the agent as well as the pH of the environment. Molecules larger than 70,000 Da cannot pass the glomerular filter, but are metabolized before excretion (Brasch 1991).

Relative to the ECF contrast agents with a short period of peak vascular enhancement, BP contrast agents possess longer plasma half-life and render a higher intravascular signal, and therefore facilitate MR angiography (MRA) with improved flexibility, accuracy and versatility. With the use of BP contrast agents, the time interval between contrast injection and imaging acquisition becomes less crucial due to the resultant optimal imaging window in tens of minutes instead of seconds with the use of ECF contrast agents.

An adequate and uniform particulate size, a high ratio of T1 over T2 relaxivity, an initial intravascular space distribution, a sufficient eventual body clearance and a lack of toxicity and/or immunogenecity are the basic requirements for an ideal BP contrast agent. Several concepts dominate the development of BP contrast agents (Fig. 2). One approach is to synthesize large and median molecules of Gd-containing polymer for prolonged intravascular retention and slower extravasation during renal elimination, as represented by Gd-polylysine (Bogdanov et al. 1993), Gadomer-17 (Misselwitz et al. 2001) and P792 (Port et al. 2001; Taupitz et al. 2001), which may feature rapid urinary clearance kinetics. Another approach utilizes the reversible protein-binding property of certain small molecular Gd chelates to form a type of "semi-endogenous" BP markers, as represented by gadofosveset trisodium (formerly identified asMS-325 or Angiomark) (Lauffer et al.

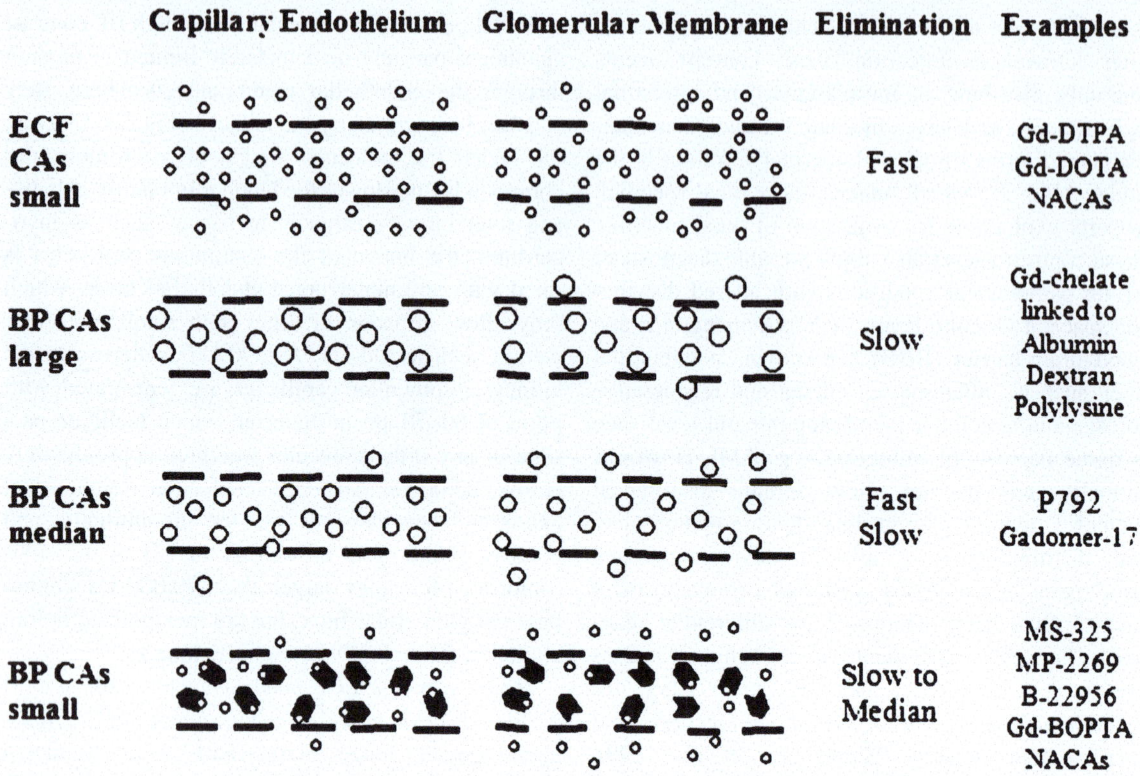

Fig. 2 Extracellular fluid space versus blood-pool contrast agents Note *BP* blood-pool; *CAs* contrast agents; *DTPA* diethylenetriaminepentaacetic acid; *ECF* extracellular fluid space; *Gd* gadolinium; *NACAs* necrosis-avid contrast agents; *DOTA* tetraazacyclododecanetetraacetic acid; *Gd-BOPTA* Gadobenate dimeglumine

1998), MP-2269 (Wallace et al. 1998) and B-22956 (La Noce et al. 2002), as well as other protein-binding (though perhaps somewhat weaker) agents such as Gd-BOPTA (Cavagna et al. 1997) and NACAs (Ni 1998; Ni et al. 2002a, b, c; Ni et al. 2005a; Ni 2008). MS-325 has been the most clinically advanced agent of this class (Lauffer et al. 1998). While all above BP contrast agents are based on paramagnetic gadolinium, the third class is based on small or ultrasmall superparamagnetic iron oxides (USPIO) optimized for blood retention and minimized for susceptibility effects (Chambon et al. 1993; Mayo-Smith et al. 1996; Stillman et al. 1996). Furthermore, clinical trials with starch-coated and stabilized iron oxide particles code-named NC 100150 (Clariscan) have been performed (Ahlstrom et al. 1999). These particulate contrast agents are slowly cleared up from the circulation and recycled through the mononuclear phagacytotic or reticuloendothelial system (MPS or RES), a metabolic route completely different from that used by gadolinium-based contrast agents. The potential cardiovascular applications of BP contrast agents include MRCA, assessment of myocardial perfusion, pulmonary and peripheral MRA, as well as evaluation of microvascular permeability in different pathological conditions. While a slower bolus of BP contrast agents is administered for dynamic arterial phase MRA, higher injection speed as a very fast bolus often necessary for myocardial first-pass perfusion MRI remains one of the safety concerns that have to be taken into account before BP contrast agents can be applied in clinical routine. The speed of injection appears to be crucial in acute toxicity effects of any contrast agents. However, the injection rate at about 1 ml/min used in laboratories to determine LD50 values in experimental animals is probably too slow to detect early deaths (within few minutes after administration), which are mainly caused by osmotic expansion of the plasma volume and failure of the cardiovascular circulation (de Haen et al. 1994). Other factors that are responsible for adverse reactions to contrast agents are chemotoxicity, osmotoxicity, ion toxicity, allergy and dose (Almen 1994).

3.3 Intracellular Contrast Agents

In nuclear scintigraphic tomography, active uptake of radioactive thallium-201 (^{201}Tl) as a potassium analog (Schoeder et al. 1993), and manganese 52 m (^{52m}Mn) and manganese 54 (^{54}Mn) as calcium antagonists (Chauncey et al. 1977; Atkins et al. 1979) by viable myocytes has been applied for assessment of myocardial viability (MV). Similar approach has been adopted in cardiac MRI using cold cation Mn^{2+} preparations as intracellular contrast agents for infarct imaging, since Mn^{2+} is potent for T1 shortening and is taken up only in cells capable of active calcium (Ca^{2+}) transport, and thereby provides an analog to ^{201}Tl imaging in cardiac scintigraphy (Bremerich et al. 2000; Karlsson et al. 2001; Flacke et al. 2003; Storey et al. 2003; Krombach et al. 2004). Mn^{2+} has an ionic radius similar to that of Ca^{2+} and is known to enter myocytes via voltage-facilitated calcium channels. These agents feature bifacial functions, i.e. for myocardial perfusion imaging with the initial blood-pool effect and as viability markers for functional myocytes at the equilibrium phase. Among these preparations, manganese chloride salt ($MnCl_2$) has shown the highest contrast enhancing efficacy with the ability even to identify stunned myocardium (Flacke et al. 2003; Krombach et al. 2004). However, because Mn^{2+} functions as a potent antagonist at the voltage-dependent Ca^{2+} channel across cellular membrane and competes with Ca^{2+} uptake of myocardium, concerns about the potential cardiac toxicity for negative inotropic effects or reduction of myocardial contractility have led to various formulations, all intended to lower cardiac toxicity, such as injection solution of $MnCl_2$ dissolved in calcium gluconate (Flacke et al. 2003) and chelated preparations as slower Mn^{2+} releasers including MP-680 or Mn[EDTA-bis(amino-propanediol)] (Flacke et al. 2003), EVP 1001-1 (Storey et al. 2003), and mangafodipir trisodium (manganese dipyridoxyl diphosphate or Mn-DPDP or Teslascan) (Bremerich et al. 2000; Flacke et al. 2003). The latter is already marketed for liver imaging with a plasma half-life <25 min (Hustvedt et al. 1997) and LD50 about 5.4 mmol/kg in mice (Elizondo et al. 1991).

Interestingly, recent experimental studies in pigs revealed that the metabolite from Mn-DPDP namely manganese dipyridoxyl ethyldiamine (MnPLED) could reduce postischemic reperfusion-induced cardiac dysfunction and infarct size (Karlsson et al. 2001). Therefore, the use of a Mn^{2+}-releasing contrast agents such as Mn-DPDP may be a promising multipurpose approach. In addition to the suggested therapeutic effects of antioxydative myocardial protection (Brurok et al. 1999; Karlsson et al. 2001), with noninvasive MRI, more functional information about myocardial metabolism and MV might be acquired by depicting differential patterns of T1 relaxation changes in relation to regional coronary flow, cellular cation uptake and retention, ion channel function and metabolism in patients with coronary heart disease. However, all these encouraging outcomes are still experimental. Before clinical cardiac MRI might enjoy the CE with an intracellular CA, its formulation, dosage, imaging protocol and especially biotolerance have to be optimized through further strenuous preclinical and clinical research.

3.4 Necrosis-Avid or Multipurpose Contrast Agents?

The ECF contrast agents such as Gd-DTPA have been widely applied to enhance cardiac MRI in both clinical practice and experimental research due to their immediate availability and general safety. Despite the considerable consensus to regard them as viability markers with "necrosis-specific" property to discriminate between viable and nonviable myocardium at delayed phase contrast enhanced MRI (Ramani et al. 1998; Kim et al. 2000; Pereira et al. 2001; Weinmann et al. 2003), inaccuracy, uncertainty, and dependency of using them on multiple influential factors, for imaging interpretation have also been evidenced (Ni et al. 2001b; Oshinski et al. 2001; Saeed et al. 2001; Choi et al. 2002; Judd and Kim 2002; Jin et al. 2007). Particularly, they are still incapable of making explicit distinctions between reversible and irreversible injured myocardium, between acute and chronic infarction, and between ischemic and inflammatory lesions, for which other nonspecific alternatives such as geographic patterns of CE had to be adopted (Hunold et al. 2005). A lack of accuracy in determination of therapeutic tumor necrosis with an ECF contrast agent was also evident in a more recent experimental study (Wang et al. 2011a, b). Therefore, there has been a continuing strategy for searching more specific contrast agents that can offer unambiguous and indisputable imaging diagnosis.

Phosphonate modified Gd-DTPA complexes could produce a persistent and strong CE in diffuse and occlusive MI due to their affinity for calcium-rich tissues and subsequent formation of insoluble calcium phosphate precipitates in the damaged myocardium. However, they may cause disordered calcium-homeostasis and consequently impaired ventricular contractility (Adzamli et al. 1993). Besides, studies with technetium-99 m pyrophosphate, a scintigraphic analogue of this type, showed a lack of specificity between ischemic and necrotic myocardium (Bianco et al. 1983) leading to a significant overestimation of the infarct (Khaw et al. 1987).

Anti-myosin antibody-labeled magnetopharmaceuticals denote an appealing approach. However, possible immunogenic side effects, insufficient expression of antigens or MRI sensitivity to the currently available relaxation enhancers, and complexity in preparation and handling of the agents challenge their clinical applicability (Weissleder et al. 1992).

What do X-rays, nylon, vaccination and penicillin have in common? They were discovered by accident or serendipitously. The word "serendipity" was first introduced in the middle of eighteenth century to express the phenomenon of discovery "by accident and sagacity" (Roberts 1989). What likely also belongs to this type is the discovery of another category of necrosis-targeting contrast agents, which represents an ongoing multiepisode story. To distinguish them from other antibody or receptor-mediated specific contrast agents with better-defined molecular targets, we proposed to nominate these newly discovered porphyrin and nonporphyrin species "necrosis-avid contrast agents" (NACAs) because of their remarkable affinity for necrotic and/or infarcted tissues (Ni et al. 1997a, 1999, 2001a, 2005a; Ni 1998, 2008; Pislaru et al. 1999; Cresens et al. 2001).

Porphyrin derivatives have been investigated for decades in diagnosis and treatment of malignant tumors (Kessel 1984; Gomer 1989; Nelson et al. 1990; Pass 1993). The rationales governing porphyrin-mediated cancer photodynamic therapy are based on "tumor-localizing" and photosensitizing properties of the agents. By analogy, the tumor "preferential uptake" of porphyrins has also been exploited for developing paramagnetic metalloporphyrins as "tumor-seeking" MRI contrast agents (Chen et al. 1984; Ogan et al. 1987; Furmanski and Longley 1988; Bockhorst et al. 1990; Fiel et al. 1990; Van Zijl et al. 1990; Nelson and Schmiedl 1991; Ebert et al. 1992; Place et al. 1992; Hindre et al. 1993; Young et al. 1994; Saini et al. 1995).

However, the research activities in this laboratory have dramatically converted metalloporphyrins from being used as tumor-seeking contrast agents into magnetic markers of MI (Ni et al. 1996; Ni 2008). During the early 1990s, in helping the former Institut für Diagnostikforschung, Berlin, Germany, to screen and confirm a few potentially tumor-specific porphyrin contrast agents, including bis-Gd-DTPA-mesoporphyrin (later named Gadophrin-2) and Mn-tetraphenylporphyrin (Mn-TPP), we conducted experiments on our well-established animal models of primary and secondary liver tumors (Ni et al. 1992). By using the methodologies dissimilar to those in the previous studies, we found that the notified "specific" CE could be attributed only to nonviable (typically necrotic) instead of viable tumor components (Ni et al. 1995), an observation contrary to the assumption raised by an earlier study (Ebert et al. 1992). To support our findings and to convince the believers in tumor-specificity of porphyrins that they are wrong, more metalloporphyrins were assessed in rats with various induced "benign" necroses and the so-called "tumor localizing" phenomenon could be reproduced without exceptions (Ni et al. 1997a). Furthermore, such a specific CE appeared more striking in pure necrosis than in tumors because the latter consist of necrosis only in proportion. Although, unfortunately, these contrast agents can no longer be considered tumor-specific, their superb necrosis targetability has elicited even more exciting, novel applications for MRI visualization of acute MI (Ni et al. 1994, 1998, 2001b Marchal et al. 1996; Herijgers et al. 1997; Pislaru et al. 1999; Marchal and Ni 2000) and brain infarction (Schneider et al. 1995). The local concentration of Gd is frequently over tens of times higher in infarcted compared with normal myocardium. Finally, the potent effects of Gadophrin-2 for labeling spontaneous and therapeutic necroses, including MI and lesions of radiofrequency ablation (RFA) on MRI, have been widely recognized a few years later, after multi-institutional reproducibility studies (Lim and Choi 1999; Saeed et al. 1999; Stillman et al. 1999; Wendland et al. 1999; Choi et al. 2000; Jeong et al. 2001; Saeed et al. 2001; Barkhausen et al. 2002; Ni et al. 2005c; Ni et al. 2006a).

Besides a normal intravenous dose at 0.05–0.1 mmol/kg for cardiac MRI to visualize MI with an extended imaging window of 3–48 h (Ni et al. 1994; Marchal et al. 1996, 2000; Herijgers et al. 1997; Ni 1998; Pislaru et al. 1999; Lim et al. 1999; Saeed et al. 1999; Stillman et al. 1999; Wendland et al. 1999; Choi et al. 2000; Jeong et al. 2001; Barkhausen et al. 2002), intracoronary delivery of a tiny dose at 0.005 mmol/kg in combination with the percutaneous transcatheter coronary angioplasty (PTCA) procedure served as a diagnostic adjuvant for MV determination and therapeutic assessment (Ni et al. 1998, 2001b; Jin et al. 2007).

So far, triphenyltetrazolium chloride (TTC) staining has been used as the only gold standard for macroscopic identification or quantification of acute MI. However, it is a post-mortem technique and not clinically applicable. Studies with both intravenous and intracoronary NACA injections have revealed that what is specifically enhanced on cardiac MRI corresponds exactly to what TTC dye does not stain on the excised heart, resulting in the same accuracy for MI delineation (Ni et al. 1994, 1998, 2001b; Marchal et al. 1996; Herijgers et al. 1997; Ni 1998; Lim et al. 1999; Pislaru et al. 1999; Saeed et al. 1999; Stillman et al. 1999; Wendland et al. 1999; Choi et al. 2000; Marchal and Ni 2000; Jeong et al. 2001; Jin et al. 2007) (Fig. 1). Experimentally, NACA enhanced MRI has been used as a surrogate of TTC histochemical staining or an in vivo viability gold standard for evaluation of medicinal myocardial protection (Lund et al. 2001), interventional RFA (Ni et al. 1997a, 2005c, 2006a) and drug-effects on inducing tumor necrosis (Wang et al. 2011a). By chelating a copper ion in the center of the cyclic tetrapyrrole ring, Gadophrin-3 has been introduced to improve its structural stability and safety yet still retain its targeting efficacy (Barkhausen et al. 2002; Schalla et al. 2004). Except for slight discoloration that faded considerably over 24 h, during animal experiments no detectable side effects have been reported with porphyrin agents at a 0.05–0.1 mmol/kg dose range (Ni et al. 1994, 1997a, 1998, 2001a Schneider et al. 1995; Marchal et al. 1996; Herijgers et al. 1997; Ni 1998; Lim et al. 1999; Pislaru et al. 1999; Saeed et al. 1999; Stillman et al. 1999; Wendland et al. 1999; Choi et al. 2000; Marchal et al. 2000; Jeong et al. 2001; Saeed et al. 2001). Nevertheless, despite optimistic expectations (Krombach et al. 2002), further commercial development of these colored porphyrin complexes has unfortunately been abandoned by the industry (Weinmann, Schering AG, personal communication) most likely due to the predicted unsatisfactory clinical tolerance resulting from unchangeable nature of dark-colored pigments of this type of chemicals (Fig. 3).

In order to overcome the discoloration, phototoxicity and other side effects related to the use of porphyrin derivatives, we have made continuing efforts to search for more effective, less toxic and less colored compounds. First, to verify whether the cyclic tetrapyrrole structure characteristic of all porphyrins is essential or not for the observed necrosis targeting, we checked more metalloporphyrins and found that four out of nine metalloporphyrins did not prove necrosis avid (Ni et al. 1999). Such unequal performances among different porphyrins, also occurring in cancer photodynamic therapy (Kessel 1984; Pass 1993) and tumor imaging (Ebert et al. 1992), suggest that the tetrapyrrole ring does not appear to be a common structural requirement for the specific targetability. Furthermore, other Gd chelates conjugated to either open-chain tetrapyrroles such as bilirubin and biliverdin or smaller constituents such as mono-, bis- and tri-pyrrole derivatives also failed to reveal a necrosis-specificity (Ni et al. 2002a). These findings not only disprove an inevitable link between porphyrin-related structures and the affinity for necrosis but also imply the possibility to generate totally different nonporphyrin molecules that could be more effective and less colored or even colorless and, therefore, deprived of any unwanted effects associated with porphyrins. Along this line, we have been able to successfully synthesize a few promising leading compounds such as the light yellowish ECIII-60 (bis-Gd-DTPA-pamoic acid) and the colorless ECIV-7 (bis-Gd-DTPA-bisindole) (Marchal et al. 1999; Cresens et al. 2001; Ni et al. 2002a, b; Ni 2008; Wang et al. 2011a), with both featuring extraordinary necrosis-avidity (Figs. 1 and 3). All studied NACAs, whether porphyrin or nonporphyrin species, allow differential diagnoses between reversible ischemic injury and irreversible infarct, acute and healing MI, and occlusive and reperfused MI (Saeed et al. 1999; Choi et al. 2000; Jeong et al. 2001; Ni et al. 2002c; Saeed et al. 2002; Jin et al. 2007). Even negative findings after CE with NACAs help to reliably exclude the presence of necrosis, which would also be of high significance for differential diagnosis (Marchal et al. 1996; Ni 1998, Ni 2008; Ni et al. 2005a).

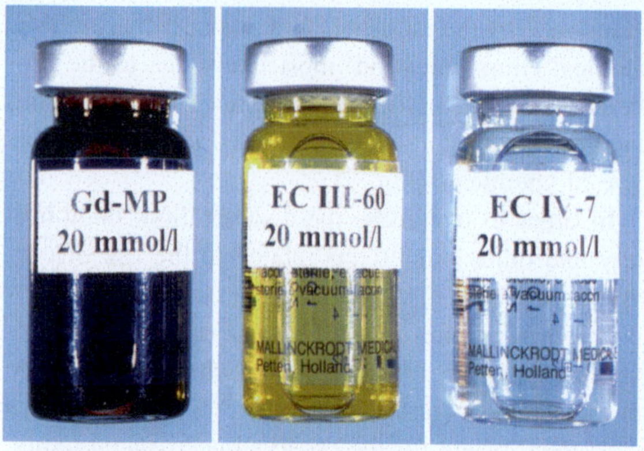

Fig. 3 Vials contain the porphyrin derived NACA Gadophrin-2 on the *left*, the nonporphyrin NACA *bis*-Gd-DTPA-pamoic acid derivative (ECIII-60) in the *middle* and the nonporphyrin NACA *bis*-Gd-DTPA-*bis*-indole derivative (ECIV-7) on the *right* at the same concentration of 20 mmol/L. In contrast to the nontransparent dark-colored pigment-like Gadophrin-2, nonporphyrin NACAs appear as either a transparent light yellowish (ECIII-60) or completely colorless (ECIV-7) water solutions

In a proposed "one-stop-shop" comprehensive package of cardiac MR for MV assessment, the NACA serves as the only key factor that can provide a clear-cut distinction between viable and necrotic myocardium (Ni 1998). In addition to the necrosis-targeting property, NACAs also share some exploitable features commonly seen with other existing contrast agents, for instance their relatively long plasma half-life due to protein binding facilitates their utility as BP contrast agents for MR angiography (Fig. 4) especially of coronary arteries; their amphiphilicity, as well as hepatobiliary and renal pathways, may render applications for liver and kidney specific CE. Therefore, with combined specific and nonspecific capacities, NACAs may serve well as versatile or multipurpose contrast enhancing agents (Ni et al. 2002b, 2005a; Ni 2008). A similar example can be found with Gd-BOPTA or trade-named MultiHance® (Cavagna et al. 1997), which is albeit void of necrosis acidity. (Table 1). Indeed, it appears that both porphyrin and nonporphyrin NACAs exert their necrosis-targeting function only when there exists denatured nonviable tissue debris in a living being, otherwise they just behaved like other less specific contrast agents such as ECF contrast agents used, e.g., for the first-pass myocardial perfusion, BP contrast agents used for MRCA, and hepatobiliary and urinary contrast agents for liver and kidney CE (Ni et al. 2005a; Ni 2008).

Nobel Prize laureate Arthur Kornberg (1918–2007) once thus described that you cannot prove a mechanism but you can only disprove a mechanism, which is exactly reflected by the current status of the mechanism research on NACAs. Hofmann et al. attributed the accumulation mechanism of Gadophrin-2 to its binding to albumin in the plasma and interstitium and subsequent trapping in intratumoral necrotic regions (Hofmann et al. 1999). However, this conclusion was disproved in another study in which only Gadophrin-2 but not the strong albumin-binding BP contrast agent MP2269 revealed in vivo necrosis-avidity (Ni et al. 2001). This finding suggests that only few albumin-binding contrast agents possess the NACA property, although to some extent most of the NACAs tend to bind plasma proteins (typically albumin); in other words, the necrosis-avidity is an outstanding feature beyond the general pharmacological process of albumin-binding-mediated drug transportation (Ni et al. 2005a; Ni 2008).

Hypothetically, NACA-induced necrosis targeting may arise in a seemingly chemotactic fashion as follows. While circulating in the blood pool after administration, the agents approach the necrotic region by a time-consuming process of perfusion through residual vessels, extravasation and interstitial diffusion, wherein reperfused infarction is more favorable than an occlusive one for NACA accumulation due to the ampler access. The disintegrated cell-membrane after autolysis facilitates contact and communication of NACAs with the tissue debris, which in turn may further augment the relaxivity due to macromolecular interactions leading always to a striking CE of the infarct (Lauffer 1991). Our recent studies suggest that such local interaction and retention seems strictly chemo-structure dependent rather than a simple trapping or sluggish wash-in and washout because either a slight modification or even an isomer transformation may drastically switch off the necrosis-targeting effect of certain NACA molecules (Ni et al. 2005a; Ni 2008). With respect to target tissues, the size and site of infarcted areas as well as the presence or absence of postischemic reperfusion determine what the NACA-induced necrosis-specific CE looks like (i.e. patchy or bulky, subendocardial or transmural and complete or rim-like) and how long it may persist. Unlike the "detrapping" process of nonspecific contrast agents in a few hours, the eventual clearance of NACAs from necrotic foci typically takes a few days after administration and parallels the

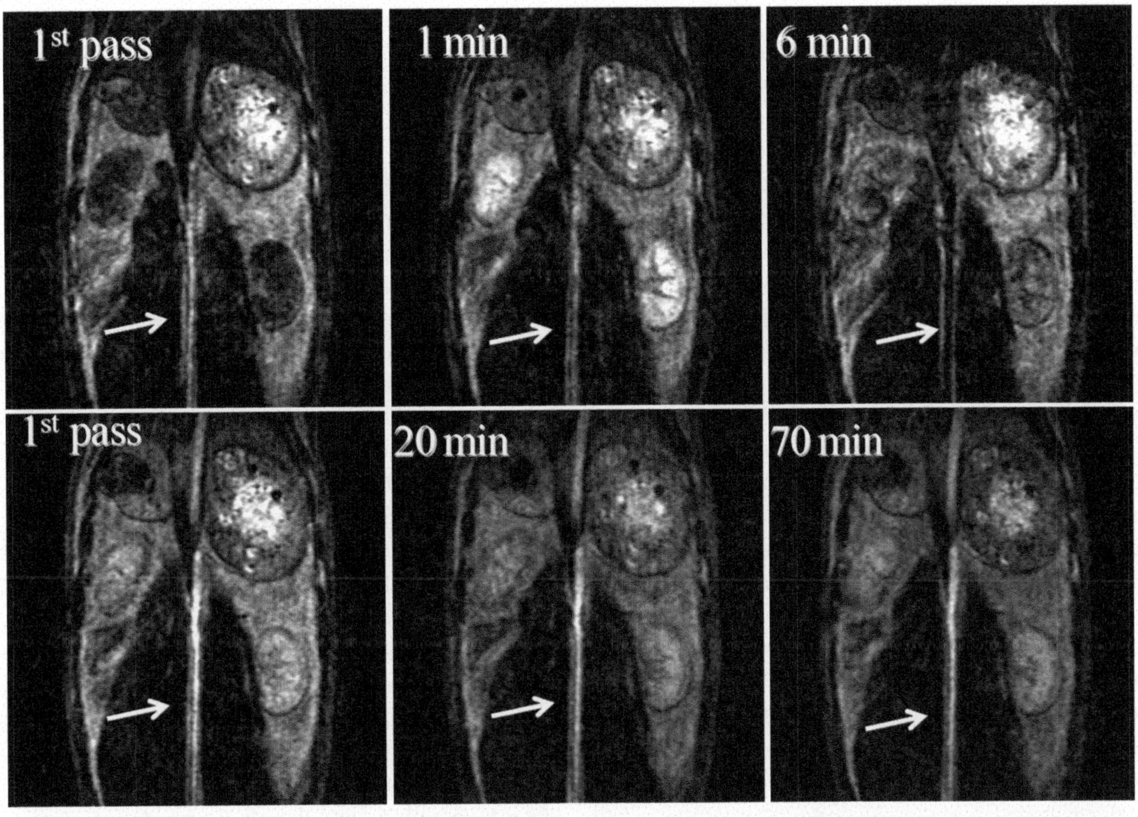

Fig. 4 MR angiography of rabbit aorta (*arrow*) comparing Gd-DTPA at 0.1 mmol/kg (*upper row*) and the nonporphyrin NACA ECIV-7 at 0.05 mmol/kg (*lower row*) display rapid clearance of Gd-DTPA from the circulation and blood-pool (BP) effect of ECIV-7 over 70 min

natural healing process, during which the necrotic tissues are progressively infiltrated and phagocytozed by inflammatory cells (mainly neutrophils, monocytes and/or macrophages) and replaced by the granulation tissue. Therefore the retained NACAs in necrosis are most likely removed together with necrotic materials by phagocytosis, which is supported by more recent results (Ni 2008). Questions remain as to whether the Gd-complex of NACAs is still stable after being taken up by macrophages and what the fate and consequence are of this small necrosis-binding fraction of NACAs in the human body (Ni 1998; Ni et al. 2001a, 2002a, b, 2005a). These have to be further elucidated (Ni 2008). Alternatively, to substitute the bio-incompatible lanthanide element Gd^{3+} with the physiological trace metal element Mn^{2+} in the complex of NACAs may eliminate the concerns about any potential side effects due to gadolinium body retention, which though has proven to be technically challenging until now.

In addition to the above identified porphyrin and nonporphyrin NACAs, there appears to be a large variety of synthetic or natural, endogenous or exogenous substances such as the organic dye Evans blue used for intravital staining (Hamer et al. 2002), the botanical extract hypericin derived from St. Johns Wort (Ni et al. 2005a, 2006b, 2007a, b; Ni 2008; Van de Putte et al. 2008a, b), the heme-related cofactor hematoporphyrin for oxygen transportation (Kessel 1984; Gomer 1989; Nelson et al. 1990; Nelson et al. 1991; Pass 1993), and the urinary-excretable glucarate catabolized from UDP (uridine diphosphate)-glucose (Orlandi et al. 1991), which all seem to share a common necrosis-avidity (Ni 2008). They may firmly bind to the denatured nonviable tissue components or subcellular organelle proteins found in necrotic debris (Ni et al. 2005a). However, unless being inherently colored or fluorescent, their existence can hardly be discerned prior to their labeling with detectable markers as to form radiopharmaceuticals (Ni et al. 2006b; Ni 2008), magnetopharmaceuticals (Ni et al. 1994, 1998, 2001a, b; Schneider et al. 1995; Marchal et al. 1996, 2000; Herijgers et al. 1997; Ni 1998; Lim et al. 1999; Pislaru et al. 1999; Saeed et al. 1999; Stillman et al. 1999; Wendland et al. 1999; Choi et al. 2000; Jeong et al. 2001; Saeed et al. 2001) and optical contrast media (Ni 2008; Van de Putte et al. 2008a, b).

Furthermore, such generally perceived structural diversity versus functional similarity supports our hypothesis that the avidity of certain chemicals to necrotic debris in the living body is an ever existing phenomenon as part of the natural wound healing process, which has never been well recognized yet deserves to be wisely exploited for medical purposes (Ni et al. 2002a, b, c; Ni et al. 2005a, b; Ni 2008). The key steps to realize this more close-to-nature strategy include understanding the underlying mechanisms of necrosis-avidity and identifying the exact local structural configuration responsible for such a strong physicochemical reaction through careful analyses on the structure–function relationship among all available NACA-like substances. Then, it might be possible to create dedicated, all-in-one, multifunctional contrast agents by purposely tailoring the chemical structures. In contrary to more aggressive and sophisticated approaches such as transgenic or cloning techniques that are prone to potential ecological hazards, such more biocompatible molecular engineering may render additional NACA targetability onto any known nontoxic substances that could be the more physiological life molecules such as vitamins, simple carbohydrates and amino acids, and/or even existing medications already in use such as anti-ischemic and thrombolytic drugs (Ni 2008).

Although side effects and adverse reactions from MRI CAs are much less common than their CT counterparts, one extremely rare adverse reaction from gadolinium-based contrast agents called nephrogenic systemic fibrosis (NSF), a disease of the skin and internal organs that could be debilitating and even fatal (Perazella 2007; Wang et al. 2011b), has drawn public attention and may hinder further development of Gd-based MRI contrast agents including NACAs. Alternatively, taking the advantage of high sensitivity and low toxicity of nuclear medicine, a necrosis-avid tracer agent based on the natural compound hypericin has been developed and validated for MV determination by combined use of single photon emission computed tomography (SPECT) and positron emission tomography (PET) (Ni et al. 2006b; Fonge et al. 2008). The strong affinity of hypericin to necrosis appears to be a few orders of magnitude higher than that of monoclonal antibodies and therefore has been further exploited for developing a novel targeted radiotherapy for the treatment of solid malignancies (Ni et al. 2007a; Li et al. 2011).

Development in this promising direction may open a new horizon certainly for the diagnosis and treatment of diseases including those in clinical cardiology, wherein interdisciplinary collaborations from both academics and industries are warranted. The ultimate beneficiaries would be the entire human society (Ni 2008).

3.5 Potential Plaque- and Thrombus-Specific Contrast Agents

Atherosclerosis and thrombosis are two sequential, interdependent processes causative for acute coronary syndrome (ACS) in patients with chronic cardiovascular disease. Noninvasive, high-resolution MRI may depict 3D microanatomy of the lumen and the vascular wall, characterize the composition of the atherosclerotic plaque, identify lesions vulnerable to erosion or rupture, and therefore provide information about not only the individual high-risk plaques but also overall plaque burden in each patient. These diagnostic messages are critical for making decisions in emergent therapeutic interventions and monitoring progression and regression of atherosclerosis during preventive treatment with, e.g., lipid-lowering drug regiments. It is believed that the high resolution of MRI in combination with sophisticated contrast agents under development may offer the promise of in vivo molecular imaging of the plaque (Fayad 2003).

There have been some developments in favor of plague and thrombus-specific contrast agents that can target either matrices or cellular compositions of the lesion (Table 1).

Fibrin-specific paramagnetic nanoparticles formulated with Gd-DTPA-bis-oleate (BOA) or Gd-DTPA-phosphatidylethanolamine (PE) are reported to have high affinity for fibrin-rich thrombus and the potential to sensitively detect active vulnerable plaques on T1 weighted MRI (Flacke et al. 2001).

Macrocyclic gadolinium-based Gadofluorines prone to form nanomicelles were originally intended for intravenous MR lymphography but have been found also to be able to accumulate in the deeper-layer intima (rich in foam cells and cellular debris) of the atherosclerotic aorta, leading to a strong positive CE in a genetically hyperlipidemic rabbit model one day after intravenous injection (Barkhausen et al. 2003). Gadofluorine B can also be regarded as another nonporphyrin NACA because of characteristic pharmacodynamic behaviors similar to those commonly seen with other NACAs (Misselwitz, Schering AG, personal communication).

Interestingly, porphyrins and an expanded porphyrin target atherosclerotic plaques too (Spokojny et al. 1986; Vever-Bizet et al. 1989; Young et al. 1994; Woodburn et al. 1996; Barkhausen et al. 2003). Given the clues collected in the studies on porphyrin and nonporphyrin species of NACAs as described in detail above, their multiple pyrrole ring structures are unlikely essential for their preferential accumulation in the nonviable matrices of the plaques. A secondary macrophage uptake following NACA-necrosis binding may also count for their local enrichment. Further studies may reveal that plaque-targeting could well be one of the NACAs' versatile functions.

Besides functioning as positive BP contrast agents for MR angiography and negative contrast agents for lesion delineation in the lymph node, liver and spleen, long-circulating USPIOs also accumulate in atherosclerotic plaques due to active uptake by localized monocytes and macrophages. At a relatively high intravenous dose (e.g., 1 mmol/kg), persistent hypointense signals could be detected over a few days in the wall of atherosclerotic arteries from the same rabbit atherosclerotic models (Schmitz et al. 2000; Ruehm et al. 2001; Kooi et al. 2003). Nonetheless, from the viewpoints of dose efficacy and safety, so far none of these agents have convincingly shown even their remote clinical feasibility.

3.6 Emerging Molecular Imaging Contrast Agents

Molecular imaging can be typically defined as the technology that is established for developing targeted and activatable imaging agents to exploit specific molecular markers, pathways or cellular processes to generate image contrast with appropriate imaging modalities (Jaffer and Weissleder 2004). Strictly speaking, what also fall well into this plausible definition would be many already existing MRI contrast agents, including albumin targeting BP contrast agents, Mn-based intracellular contrast agents and even NACAs that are involved in several pathophysiological processes such as protein binding, chemotactic interaction with necrotic tissues as well as hepatobiliary and renal pathways.

The underpinning hypothesis of this newer approach to imaging is that most disease processes have a molecular basis that can be exploited to (1) detect disease earlier, (2) stratify disease subsets (e.g., active versus inactive), (3) objectively monitor novel therapies by imaging molecular biomarkers and (4) prognosticate disease (Jaffer et al. 2004).

Although still far from the clinical reality in cardiac MRI, the research in this discipline is rapidly advancing with a few leading molecular probes already emerging from laboratory experiments for MRI monitoring cardiovascular pathologic processes or consequences such as atherosclerosis (Winter et al. 2003), thrombosis (Johansson et al. 2001) and heart failure (Schellenberger et al. 2002) as well as therapeutic intervention (Kraitchman et al. 2003; Yang 2010). It has been predicted that in the ensuing years fundamental aspects of cardiovascular biology will be detectable in vivo and that promising molecular imaging agents will be translated into the clinical arena to guide diagnosis and therapy of human cardiovascular illness (Jaffer et al. 2004). For an overview of the fundamentals of cardiovascular molecular imaging approaches, the latest advances in the areas of atherosclerosis, heart failure, and stem cell therapy, the future prospects of translational molecular imaging in the clinical cardiology, as well as future directions that will shape molecular imaging in the postgenomics era, the readers are directed to the details in a recent review article (Chen and Wu 2011). This would again offer opportunities for us to witness whether such anticipations could bring about the breakthroughs that are really beneficial to patients suffering from, and to clinicians fighting against, cardiovascular diseases.

4 Application Scopes of MR Contrast Agents for Cardiac Imaging

As demonstrated in many chapters throughout the contents in this book, the use of contrast agents has undoubtedly become an integral part of the daily practice

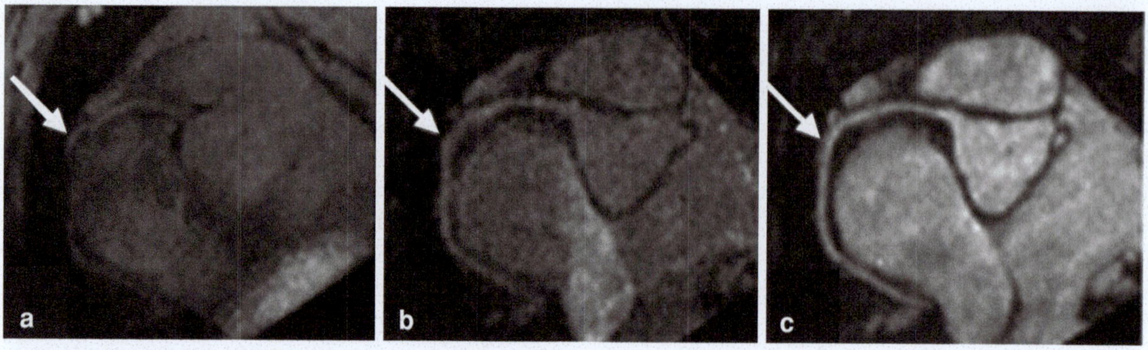

Fig. 5 Comparison of MR angiography of the right coronary artery (*arrow*) in the same pig without contrast agent injection (**a**), with an ECF agent Gd-DTPA at 0.2 mmol/kg (**b**) and with a blood-pool contrast agent Gadomer-17 at 0.1 mmol/kg (**c**) demonstrate the indispensable role of contrast agents especially the blood-pool contrast agent in MR coronary angiography. The images are displayed after multiplanar reconstruction. (by courtesy of Debiao Li, Biomedical Engineering Department, Northwestern University, Evanston, IL, USA; now Biomedical Imaging Research Institute, Cedars-Sinai Medical Center, University of California, Los Angeles, CA, USA)

of cardiac MRI because of their efficacy and their excellent tolerance profile. Their application scopes cover almost all aspects of cardiac MRI, including noninvasive depiction of cardiac anatomy ("Cardiac Anatomy") and real-time monitor of cardiac function ("Cardiac Function"), in particular myocardial perfusion ("Myocardial Perfusion") and cardiac output quantification. The indispensable role of contrast agents is exemplified in comprehensive diagnoses of ischemic ("Ischemic Heart Disease") and nonischemic ("Heart Muscle Diseases") heart diseases as well as heart failure ("Heart Failure and Heart Transplantation") and neoplasms ("Cardiac Masses"). More delicate evaluations with CE MRI on pericardial diseases and valvular heart diseases are addressed in "Pericardial Disease" and Chapter entitled "Valvular Heart Disease", respectively. The state-of-the-art techniques for MR coronary artery imaging is introduced in "Coronary Artery Disease". The images by courtesy of Dr. Debiao Li illustrate well the crucial added value of contrast agents by comparing MRCA in a swine without contrast agent, with an ECF contrast agent and with a BP contrast agent injection (Fig. 5). In addition, the usefulness of contrast agents has also been proven for clinical diagnoses of congenital heart diseases ("Congenital Heart Disease") and abnormalities in great vessels ("Great Vessels"). Similarly, it proves crucial to apply a contrast agent for MR guided catheterized cardiac interventions ("MR-Guided Cardiac Catheterization") and for studying cardiac modeling ("Cardiac Modelling–Future Perspectives").

5 Conclusion

Despite the appreciable maturity with continuing excellence over 30 years of age, it is encouragingly evident that MRI would still have its best years to come toward a "one-stop shop" final solution of noninvasive, 3D, high-resolution real-time imaging of the cardiovascular system particularly boosted by the new inventions and applications of MRI contrast agents.

References

Adzamli IK, Blau M, Pfeffer MA, Davis MA (1993) Phosphonate-modified Gd-DTPA complexes. III: The detection of myocardial infarction by MRI. Magn Reson Med 29:505–511

Ahlstrom KH, Johansson LO, Rodenburg JB, Ragnarsson AS, Akeson P, Borseth A (1999) Pulmonary MR angiography with ultrasmall superparamagnetic iron oxide particles as a blood pool agent and a navigator echo for respiratory gating: pilot study. Radiology 211:865–869

Almen T (1994) The etiology of contrast medium reactions. Invest Radiol 29(suppl 1):S37–S45

Ardenkjaer-Larsen JH, Fridlund B, Gram A et al (2003) Increase in signal-to-noise ratio of >10, 000 times in liquid-state NMR Molecular imaging with endogenous substances. Proc Natl Acad Sci U S A 100:10158–10163

Atkins H, Som LP, Fairchild RG et al (1979) Myocardial positron tomography with manganese-52 m. Radiology 133(3 Pt 1):769–774

Barkhausen J, Ebert W, Debatin JF, Weinmann HJ (2002) Imaging of myocardial infarction: comparison of magnevist and gadophrin-3 in rabbits. J Am Coll Cardiol 39(8):1392–1398

Barkhausen J, Ebert W, Heyer C, Debatin JF, Weinmann HJ (2003) Detection of atherosclerotic plaque with Gadofluorine-enhanced magnetic resonance imaging. Circulation 108(5):605–609

Bhattacharya P, Ross BD, Bunger R (2009) Cardiovascular applications of hyperpolarized contrast media and metabolic tracers. Exp Biol Med (Maywood) 234:1395–1416

Bianco JA, Kemper AJ, Taylor A, Lazewatsky J, Tow DE, Khuri SF (1983) Technetium-99m(Sn2+)pyrophosphate in ischemic and infarcted dog myocardium in early stages of acute coronary occlusion: histochemical and tissue-counting comparisons. J Nucl Med 24:485–491

Bockhorst K, Hohn-Berlage M et al (1990) Proton relaxation enhancement in experimental brain tumors–in vivo NMR study of manganese(III)TPPS in rat brain gliomas. Magn Reson Imaging 8(4):499–504

Bogdanov AA Jr, Weissleder R, Frank HW et al (1993) A new macromolecule as a contrast agent for MR angiography: preparation, properties, and animal studies. Radiology 187: 701–706

Brasch RC (1991) Rationale and applications for macromolecular Gd-based contrast agents. Magn Reson Med 22: 282–287 discussion 300–303

Bremerich J, Saeed M, Arheden H, Higgins CB, Wendland MF (2000) Normal and infarcted myocardium: differentiation with cellular uptake of manganese at MR imaging in a rat model. Radiology 216:524–530

Brurok H, Ardenkjaer-Larsen JH, Hansson G et al (1999) Manganese dipyridoxyl diphosphate: MRI contrast agent with antioxidative and cardioprotective properties? Biochem Biophys Res Commun 254:768–772

Cannon PJ, Maudsley AA, Hilal SK, Simon HE, Cassidy F (1986) Sodium nuclear magnetic resonance imaging of myocardial tissue of dogs after coronary artery occlusion and reperfusion. J Am Coll Cardiol 7:573–579

Cavagna FM, Maggioni F, Castelli PM et al (1997) Gadolinium chelates with weak binding to serum proteins. A new class of high-efficiency, general purpose contrast agents for magnetic resonance imaging. Invest Radiol 32:780–796

Chambon C, Clement O, Le Blanche A, Schouman-Claeys E, Frija G (1993) Superparamagnetic iron oxides as positive MR contrast agents: in vitro and in vivo evidence. Magn Reson Imaging 11:509–519

Chauncey DM Jr, Schelbert HR, Halpern SE et al (1977) Tissue distribution studies with radioactive manganese: a potential agent for myocardial imaging. J Nucl Med 18:933–936

Chen IY, Wu JC (2011) Cardiovascular molecular imaging: focus on clinical translation. Circulation 123:425–443

Chen CW, Cohen JS, Myers CE, Sohn M (1984) Paramagnetic metalloporphyrins as potential contrast agents in NMR imaging. FEBS Lett 168:70–74

Chiu CW, So NM, Lam WW, Chan KY, Sanderson JE (2003) Combined first-pass perfusion and viability study at MR imaging in patients with non-ST segment-elevation acute coronary syndromes: feasibility study. Radiology 226:717–722

Choi C (2002) Contrast washout by MRI identifies stunned myocardium in patients after reperfused myocardial infarction. J Cardiovasc Mag Res 4:19 (Abstract)

Choi SI, Choi SH, Kim ST et al (2000) Irreversibly damaged myocardium at MR imaging with a necrotic tissue-specific contrast agent in a cat model. Radiology 215:863–868

Cresens E, Ni Y et al (2001). Substituted bis-indole derivatives useful as contrast agents, pharmaceutical compositions containing them and intermediates for producing them. Patent Application number PCT/BE01/00192, USA patent 7081472

de Haen C, Morisetti A, Bertani F, Tirone P (1994) The factor time in acute intravenous toxicity studies of contrast media. Invest Radiol 29(suppl 2):S108–S110

Ebert E, Hofmann S (1992) Metallopophyrins: tumor-specific contrast agents? European Magnetic Resonance Forum Foundation. Hamburg, Germany

Elizondo G, Fretz CJ, Stark DD et al (1991) Preclinical evaluation of MnDPDP: new paramagnetic hepatobiliary contrast agent for MR imaging. Radiology 178:73–78

Fayad ZA (2003) MR imaging for the noninvasive assessment of atherothrombotic plaques. Magn Reson Imaging Clin N Am 11:101–113

Fiel RJ, Musser DA, Mark EH, Mazurchuk R, Alletto JJ (1990) A comparative study of manganese meso-sulfonatophenyl porphyrins: contrast-enhancing agents for tumors. Magn Reson Imaging 8:255–259

Fishman JE, Joseph PM, Floyd TF, Mukherji B, Sloviter HA (1987) Oxygen-sensitive 19F NMR imaging of the vascular system in vivo. Magn Reson Imaging 5:279–285

Flacke S, Fischer S, Scott MJ et al (2001) Novel MRI contrast agent for molecular imaging of fibrin: implications for detecting vulnerable plaques. Circulation 104:1280–1285

Flacke S, Allen JS, Chia JM et al (2003) Characterization of viable and nonviable myocardium at MR imaging: comparison of gadolinium-based extracellular and blood pool contrast materials versus manganese-based contrast materials in a rat myocardial infarction model. Radiology 226:731–738

Fonge H, Vunckx K, Wang H et al (2008) Non-invasive detection and quantification of acute myocardial infarction in rabbits using mono-[123I]iodohypericin microSPECT. Eur Heart J 29:260–269

Friedrich J, Apstein CS, Ingwall JS (1995) 31P nuclear magnetic resonance spectroscopic imaging of regions of remodeled myocardium in the infarcted rat heart. Circulation 92:3527–3538

Furmanski P, Longley C (1988) Metalloporphyrin enhancement of magnetic resonance imaging of human tumor xenografts in nude mice. Cancer Res 48:4604–4610

Golman K, Ardenkjaer-Larsen JH, Petersson J, Mansson S, Leunbach SI (2003) Molecular imaging with endogenous substances. Proc Natl Acad Sci U S A 100:10435–10439

Gomer CJ (1989) Photodynamic therapy in the treatment of malignancies. Semin Hematol 26:27–34

Gore J (2003) Out of the shadows—MRI and the Nobel Prize. N Engl J Med 349:2290–2292

Hamer PW, McGeachie JM, Davies MJ, Grounds MD (2002) Evans blue dye as an in vivo marker of myofibre damage: optimising parameters for detecting initial myofibre membrane permeability. J Anat 200(Pt 1):69–79

Hawighorst H, Knapstein PG, Knopp MV, Vaupel P, van Kaick G (1999) Cervical carcinoma: standard and pharmacokinetic analysis of time-intensity curves for assessment of tumor angiogenesis and patient survival. Magma 8:55–62

Herijgers P, Laycock SK, Ni Y et al (1997) Localization and determination of infarct size by Gd-Mesoporphyrin enhanced MRI in dogs. Int J Card Imaging 13:499–507

Heywang SH, Wolf A, Pruss E, Hilbertz T, Eiermann W, Permanetter W (1989) MR imaging of the breast with Gd-DTPA: use and limitations. Radiology 171:95–103

Hindre F, Le Plouzennec M, de Certaines JD, Foultier M, Patrice TT, Simonneaux G (1993) Tetra-p-aminophenylporphyrin conjugated with Gd-DTPA: tumor-specific contrast agent for MR imaging. J Magn Reson Imaging 3:59–65

Hofmann B, Bogdanov A Jr, Marecos E, Ebert W, Semmler W, Weissleder R (1999) Mechanism of gadophrin-2 accumulation in tumor necrosis. J Magn Reson Imaging 9:336–341

Hunold P, Schlosser T, Vogt FM et al (2005) Myocardial late enhancement in contrast-enhanced cardiac MRI: distinction between infarction scar and non-infarction-related disease. AJR Am J Roentgenol 184:1420–1426

Hustvedt SO, Grant D, Southon TE, Zech K (1997) Plasma pharmacokinetics, tissue distribution and excretion of MnDPDP in the rat and dog after intravenous administration. Acta Radiol 38(4 Pt 2):690–699

Jaffer FA, Weissleder R (2004) Seeing within: molecular imaging of the cardiovascular system. Circ Res 94: 433–435

Jeong AK, Choi SI, Kim DH et al (2001) Evaluation by contrast-enhanced MR imaging of the lateral border zone in reperfused myocardial infarction in a cat model. Korean J Radiol 2:21–27

Jin J, Teng G, Feng Y et al (2007) Magnetic resonance imaging of acute reperfused myocardial infarction: intraindividual comparison of ECIII-60 and Gd-DTPA in a swine model. Cardiovasc Intervent Radiol 30:248–256

Johansson LO, Bjornerud A, Ahlstrom HK, Ladd DL, Fujii DK (2001) A targeted contrast agent for magnetic resonance imaging of thrombus: implications of spatial resolution. J Magn Reson Imaging 13:615–618

Judd RM, Kim RJ (2002) Imaging time after Gd-DTPA injection is critical in using delayed enhancement to determine infarct size accurately with magnetic resonance imaging. Circulation 106 (e6) author reply e6

Kaiser WA, Zeitler E (1989) MR imaging of the breast: fast imaging sequences with and without Gd-DTPA. Preliminary observations. Radiology 170(3 Pt 1):681–686

Karlsson JO, Brurok H, Eriksen M et al (2001) Cardioprotective effects of the MR contrast agent MnDPDP and its metabolite MnPLED upon reperfusion of the ischemic porcine myocardium. Acta Radiol 42:540–547

Kessel D (1984) Porphyrin localization: a new modality for detection and therapy of tumors. Biochem Pharmacol 33:1389–1393

Khaw BA, Strauss HW, Moore R et al (1987) Myocardial damage delineated by indium-111 antimyosin Fab and technetium-99m pyrophosphate. J Nucl Med 28:76–82

Kim RJ, Lima JA, Chen EL et al (1997) Fast ^{23}Na magnetic resonance imaging of acute reperfused myocardial infarction. Potential to assess myocardial viability. Circulation 95:1877–1885

Kim RJ, Judd RM, Chen EL, Fieno DS, Parrish TB, Lima JA (1999) Relationship of elevated 23Na magnetic resonance image intensity to infarct size after acute reperfused myocardial infarction. Circulation 100:185–192

Kim RJ, Wu E, Rafael A et al (2000) The use of contrast-enhanced magnetic resonance imaging to identify reversible myocardial dysfunction. N Engl J Med 343:1445–1453

Kooi ME, Cappendijk VC, Cleutjens KB et al (2003) Accumulation of ultrasmall superparamagnetic particles of iron oxide in human atherosclerotic plaques can be detected by in vivo magnetic resonance imaging. Circulation 107:2453–2458

Kraitchman DL, Heldman AW, Atalar E et al (2003) In vivo magnetic resonance imaging of mesenchymal stem cells in myocardial infarction. Circulation 107:2290–2293

Krombach GA, Higgins CB, Gunther RW, Kuhne T, Saeed M (2002) MR contrast media for cardiovascular imaging. Rofo 174:819–829

Krombach GA, Saeed M, Higgins CB, Novikov V, Wendland MF (2004) Contrast-enhanced MR delineation of stunned myocardium with administration of MnCl(2) in rats. Radiology 230:183–190

Kuhl HP, Spuentrup E, Wall A et al (2004) Assessment of myocardial function with interactive non-breath-hold real-time MR imaging: comparison with echocardiography and breath-hold Cine MR imaging. Radiology 231:198–207

La Noce A, Stoelben S, Scheffler K et al (2002) B22956/1, a new intravascular contrast agent for MRI: first administration to humans—preliminary results. Acad Radiol 9(suppl 2):S404–S406

Lauffer RB (1991) Targeted relaxation enhancement agents for MRI. Magn Reson Med 22:339–342 (discussion 343–346)

Lauffer RB, Parmelee DJ, Dunham SU et al (1998) MS-325: albumin-targeted contrast agent for MR angiography. Radiology 207:529–538

Lauterbur P, Mendonca Dias H, Rudin A (1978) Augmentation of tissue proton spin-lattice relaxation rates by in vivo addition of paramagnetic ions. In: LJ Dutton PO, Scarpa A (eds) Frontiers of biological energetics. Academic Press, New York, pp 752–759

Li J, Sun Z, Zhang J, et al (2011) A dual targeting anticancer approach: soil and seed principle. Radiology, published online before print on June 28, doi:10.1148

Lim TH, Choi SI (1999) MRI of myocardial infarction. J Magn Reson Imaging 10:686–693

Lund GK, Higgins CB, Wendland MF, Watzinger N, Weinmann HJ, Saeed M (2001) Assessment of nicorandil therapy in ischemic myocardial injury by using contrast-enhanced and functional MR imaging. Radiology 221: 676–682

Manka R, Paetsch I, Schnackenburg B, Gebker R, Fleck E, Jahnke C (2010) BOLD cardiovascular magnetic resonance at 3.0 tesla in myocardial ischemia. J Cardiovasc Magn Reson 12:54

Marchal G and Ni Y (2000) Use of porphyrin-complex or expanded porphyrin-complex as an infarction localization diagnosticum. US patent No. 6,013,241

Marchal G, Ni Y, Herijgers P et al (1996) Paramagnetic metalloporphyrins: infarct avid contrast agents for diagnosis of acute myocardial infarction by MRI. Eur Radiol 6:2–8

Marchal G, Verbruggen A, Ni Y, Adriaens P, Cresens E (1999) Non-porphyrin compounds for use as a diagnosticum and/or pharmaceutical, Belgium, International application No. PCT/BE99/00104

Mayo-Smith WW, Saini S, Slater G, Kaufman JA, Sharma P, Hahn PF (1996) MR contrast material for vascular enhancement: value of superparamagnetic iron oxide. Am J Roentgenol 166:73–77

Misselwitz B, Schmitt-Willich H, Ebert W, Frenzel T, Weinmann HJ (2001) Pharmacokinetics of Gadomer-17, a new dendritic magnetic resonance contrast agent. Magma 12:128–134

Nelson JA, Schmiedl U (1991) Porphyrins as contrast media. Magn Reson Med 22:366–371 (discussion 378)

Nelson JA, Schmiedl U, Shankland EG (1990) Metalloporphyrins as tumor-seeking MRI contrast media and as potential selective treatment sensitizers. Invest Radiol 25(suppl 1):S71–S73

Ni Y (1998) Myocardial viability. In: Bogaert JDA, Rademakers FE (eds) Magnetic resonance of the heart and great vessels: clinical applications. Medical Radiology—diagnostic imaging and radiation oncology. Springer, Berlin, pp 113–132

Ni Y (2008) Metalloporphyrins and functional analogues as MRI contrast agents. Curr Med Imaging Rev 4:96–112

Ni Y, Marchal G, van Damme B et al (1992) Magnetic resonance imaging, microangiography, and histology in a rat model of primary liver cancer. Invest Radiol 27:689–697

Ni Y, Marchal G, Petré C et al (1994) Metalloporphyrin enhanced magnetic resonance imaging of acute myocardial infarction (abstract). Circulation 90:I–468

Ni Y, Marchal G, Yu J et al (1995) Localization of metalloporphyrin-induced "specific" enhancement in experimental liver tumors: comparison of magnetic resonance imaging, microangiographic, and histologic findings. Acad Radiol 2:687–699

Ni Y, Marchal G, Herijgers P et al (1996) Paramagnetic metalloporphyrins: from enhancers of malignant tumors to markers of myocardial infarcts. Acad Radiol 3(suppl 2): S395–S397

Ni Y, Miao Y, Bosmans H et al (1997a) Evaluation of interventional liver tumor ablation with Gd-mesoporphyrin enhanced magnetic resonance imaging (abstract). Radiology 205(P):319

Ni Y, Petre C, Miao Y et al (1997b) Magnetic resonance imaging-histomorphologic correlation studies on paramagnetic metalloporphyrins in rat models of necrosis. Invest Radiol 32:770–779

Ni Y, Pislaru C, Bosmans H et al (1998) Validation of intracoronary delivery of metalloporphyrin as an in vivo "histochemical staining" for myocardial infarction with MR imaging. Acad Radiol suppl 5(1):S37–S41 (discussion S45–S46)

Ni Y, Miao Y, Cresens E et al (1999) Paramagnetic metalloporphyrins: there exist necrosis-avid and non-avid species. 7th Annual Scientific Meeting for ISMRM, Philadelphia, Pennsylvania, USA

Ni Y, Adzamli K, Miao Y et al (2001a) MRI contrast enhancement of necrosis by MP-2269 and gadophrin-2 in a rat model of liver infarction. Invest Radiol 36:97–103

Ni Y, Pislaru C, Bosmans H et al (2001b) Intracoronary delivery of Gd-DTPA and Gadophrin-2 for determination of myocardial viability with MR imaging. Eur Radiol 11:876–883

Ni Y, Cresens E, Adriaens P et al (2002a) Necrosis-avid contrast agents: introducing nonporphyrin species. Acad Radiol 9(suppl 1):S98–S101

Ni Y, Cresens E, Adriaens P et al (2002b) Exploring multifunctional features of necrosis avid contrast agents. Acad Radiol 9(suppl 2):S488–S490

Ni Y, Dymarkowski S, Chen F, Bogaert J, Marchal G (2002c) Occlusive myocardial infarction enhanced or not enhanced with necrosis-avid contrast agents at MR imaging. Radiology 225:603–605

Ni Y, Bormans G, Chen F et al (2005a) Necrosis avid contrast agents: functional similarity versus structural diversity. Invest Radiol 40:526–535

Ni Y, Huyghe D, Chen F, Bormans G, Verbruggen G, Marchal G (2005b) Research on necrosis avid contrast agents: further expansion of scope. Acad Radiol 12(suppl 5):55–56

Ni Y, Mulier S, Miao Y, Michel L, Marchal G (2005c) A review of the general aspects of radiofrequency ablation. Abdom Imaging 30:381–400

Ni Y, Chen F, Mulier S et al (2006a) Magnetic resonance imaging after radiofrequency ablation in a rodent model of liver tumor: tissue characterization using a novel necrosis-avid contrast agent. Eur Radiol 16:1031–1040

Ni Y, Huyghe D, Verbeke K et al (2006b) First preclinical evaluation of mono-[^{123}I]iodohypericin as a necrosis-avid tracer agent. Eur J Nucl Med Mol Imaging 33:595–601

Ni Y, Van de Putte M, de Witte P, Verbruggen A, Marchal G, Sun Z (2007a) Targeted radiotherapy. Patent application PCT/BE2008/000099

Ni Y, Van de Putte M, Fonge H, Verbruggen A, de Witte P, Marchal G (2007b) Necrosis avid contrast agents (NACAs): evidence in favour of hypothetical mechanisms and new potential applications. Contrast Media Mol Imaging 2:276

Ogan MD, Revel D, Brasch RC (1987) Metalloporphyrin contrast enhancement of tumors in magnetic resonance imaging. A study of human carcinoma, lymphoma, and fibrosarcoma in mice. Invest Radiol 22:822–828

Orlandi C, Crane PD, Edwards DS et al (1991) Early scintigraphic detection of experimental myocardial infarction in dogs with technetium-99 m-glucaric acid. J Nucl Med 32:263–268

Oshinski JN, Yang Z, Jones JR, Mata JF, French BA (2001) Imaging time after Gd-DTPA injection is critical in using delayed enhancement to determine infarct size accurately with magnetic resonance imaging. Circulation 104:2838–2842

Ouwerkerk R, Bottomley PA, Solaiyappan M et al (2008) Tissue sodium concentration in myocardial infarction in humans: a quantitative ^{23}Na MR imaging study. Radiology 248:88–96

Padhani A (2010) Science to practice: what does MR oxygenation imaging tell us about human breast cancer hypoxia? Radiology 254:1–3

Pass HI (1993) Photodynamic therapy in oncology: mechanisms and clinical use. J Natl Cancer Inst 85:443–456

Perazella MA (2007) Nephrogenic systemic fibrosis, kidney disease, and gadolinium: is there a link? Clin J Am Soc Nephrol 2:200–202

Pereira RS, Wisenberg G, Prato FS, Yvorchuk K (2000) Clinical assessment of myocardial viability using MRI during a constant infusion of Gd-DTPA. MAGMA 11:104–113

Pereira RS, Prato FS, Wisenberg G, Sykes J, Yvorchuk KJ (2001) The use of Gd-DTPA as a marker of myocardial viability in reperfused acute myocardial infarction. Int J Cardiovasc Imaging 17:395–404

Pislaru SV, Ni Y, Pislaru C et al (1999) Noninvasive measurements of infarct size after thrombolysis with a necrosis-avid MRI contrast agent. Circulation 99:690–696

Place DA, Faustino PJ, Berghmans KK, van Zijl PC, Chesnick AS, Cohen JS (1992) MRI contrast-dose relationship of manganese(III)tetra(4-sulfonatophenyl) porphyrin with human xenograft tumors in nude mice at 2.0 T. Magn Reson Imaging 10:919–928

Port M, Corot C, Rousseaux O et al (2001) P792: a rapid clearance blood pool agent for magnetic resonance imaging: preliminary results. MAGMA 12:121–127

Ramani K, Judd RM, Holly TA et al (1998) Contrast magnetic resonance imaging in the assessment of myocardial viability in patients with stable coronary artery disease and left ventricular dysfunction. Circulation 98:2687–2694

Roberts R (1989) Serendipity: accidental discoveries in science. Wiley, New York

Ruehm SG, Corot C, Vogt P, Kolb S, Debatin JF (2001) Magnetic resonance imaging of atherosclerotic plaque with ultrasmall superparamagnetic particles of iron oxide in hyperlipidemic rabbits. Circulation 103:415–422

Saeed M, Bremerich J, Wendland MF, Wyttenbach R, Weinmann HJ, Higgins CB (1999) Reperfused myocardial infarction as seen with use of necrosis-specific versus standard extracellular MR contrast media in rats. Radiology 213:247–257

Saeed M, Lund G, Wendland MF, Bremerich J, Weinmann H, Higgins CB (2001) Magnetic resonance characterization of the peri-infarction zone of reperfused myocardial infarction with necrosis-specific and extracellular nonspecific contrast media. Circulation 103:871–876

Saeed M, Wendland MF, Bremerich GL, Weinmann HJ, Higgins CB (2002) Assessment of myocardial viability using standard extracellular and necrosis specific MR contrast media. Acad Radiol 9(suppl 1):S84–S87

Saini SK, Jena A, Dey J, Sharma AK, Singh R (1995) MnPcS4: a new MRI contrast enhancing agent for tumor localisation in mice. Magn Reson Imaging 13:985–990

Schalla S, Wendland MF, Higgins CB, Ebert W, Saeed M (2004) Accentuation of high susceptibility of hypertrophied myocardium to ischemia: complementary assessment of Gadophrin-enhancement and left ventricular function with MRI. Magn Reson Med 51:552–558

Schellenberger EA, Bogdanov A Jr, Hogemann D, Tait J, Weissleder R, Josephson L (2002) Annexin V-CLIO: a nanoparticle for detecting apoptosis by MRI. Mol Imaging 1:102–107

Schmitz SA, Coupland SE, Gust R et al (2000) Superparamagnetic iron oxide-enhanced MRI of atherosclerotic plaques in Watanabe hereditable hyperlipidemic rabbits. Invest Radiol 35:460–471

Schneider G, Hayd C, Mühler A et al (1995) Contrast enhanced MRI of experimentally induced brain infarctions in rabbits using Bis-Gd-MP as MR contrast agent. 3rd Annual Scientific Meeting. Society of Magnetic Resonance, Nice, France. Society of Magnetic Resonance, p 1144

Schoeder H, Friedrich M, Topp H et al (1993) Myocardial viability: what do we need? Eur J Nucl Med 20:792–803

Spokojny AM, Serur JR, Skillman J, Spears JR (1986) Uptake of hematoporphyrin derivative by atheromatous plaques: studies in human in vitro and rabbit in vivo. J Am Coll Cardiol 8:1387–1392

Stillman AE, Wilke N, Li D, Haacke M, McLachlan S (1996) Ultrasmall superparamagnetic iron oxide to enhance MRA of the renal and coronary arteries: studies in human patients. J Comput Assist Tomogr 20:51–55

Stillman AE, Wilke N, Jerosch-Herold M (1999) Myocardial viability. Radiol Clin North Am 37:361–378 vi

Storey P, Danias PG, Post M et al (2003) Preliminary evaluation of EVP 1001–1: a new cardiac-specific magnetic resonance contrast agent with kinetics suitable for steady-state imaging of the ischemic heart. Invest Radiol 38:642–652

Svensson J, Mansson S, Johansson E, Petersson JS, Olsson LE (2003) Hyperpolarized ^{13}C MR angiography using true-FISP. Magn Reson Med 50:256–262

Taupitz M, Schnorr J, Wagner S et al (2001) Coronary magnetic resonance angiography: experimental evaluation of the new rapid clearance blood pool contrast medium P792. Magn Reson Med 46:932–938

Turner R (1997) Signal sources in bold contrast fMRI. Adv Exp Med Biol 413:19–25

Van de Putte M, Wang H, Chen F, de Witte PA, Ni Y (2008a) Hypericin as a marker for determination of tissue viability after intratumoral ethanol injection in a murine liver tumor model. Acad Radiol 15:107–113

Van de Putte M, Wang H, Chen F, de Witte PA, Ni Y (2008b) Hypericin as a marker for determination of tissue viability after radiofrequency ablation in a murine liver tumor model. Oncol Rep 19:927–932

van der Wall EE, Vliegen HW, de Roos A, Bruschke AV (1996) Magnetic resonance techniques for assessment of myocardial viability. J Cardiovasc Pharmacol 28(suppl 1): S37–S44

van Zijl PC, Place DA, Cohen JS, Faustino PJ, Lyon RC, Patronas NJ (1990) Metalloporphyrin magnetic resonance contrast agents. Feasibility of tumor-specific magnetic resonance imaging. Acta Radiol (suppl) 374:75–79

Vever-Bizet C, L'Epine Y, Delettre E et al (1989) Photofrin II uptake by atheroma in atherosclerotic rabbits. Fluorescence and high performance liquid chromatographic analysis on post-mortem aorta. Photochem Photobiol 49:731–737

Villringer A, Rosen BR, Belliveau JW et al (1988) Dynamic imaging with lanthanide chelates in normal brain: contrast due to magnetic susceptibility effects. Magn Reson Med 6:164–174

Wallace RA, Haar JP Jr, Miller DB et al (1998) Synthesis and preliminary evaluation of MP-2269: a novel, nonaromatic small-molecule blood-pool MR contrast agent. Magn Reson Med 40:733–739

Wang H, Miranda Cona M, Chen F et al (2011a) Comparison between nonspecific and necrosis-avid gadolinium contrast agents in vascular disrupting agent-induced necrosis of rodent tumors at 3.0T. Invest Radiol May 13. (Epub ahead of print). PMID: 21577133

Wang Y, Alkasab TK, Narin O et al (2011b) Incidence of nephrogenic systemic fibrosis after adoption of restrictive gadolinium-based contrast agent guidelines. Radiology 260:105–111

Weinmann HJ, Ebert W, Misselwitz B, Schmitt-Willich H (2003) Tissue-specific MR contrast agents. Eur J Radiol 46:33–44

Weissleder R, Lee AS, Khaw BA, Shen T, Brady TJ (1992) Antimyosin-labeled monocrystalline iron oxide allows detection of myocardial infarct: MR antibody imaging. Radiology 182:381–385

Wendland MF, Saeed M, Lund G, Higgins CB (1999) Contrast-enhanced MRI for quantification of myocardial viability. J Magn Reson Imaging 10:694–702

Winter PM, Morawski AM, Caruthers SD et al (2003) Molecular imaging of angiogenesis in early-stage atherosclerosis with alpha(v)beta3-integrin-targeted nanoparticles. Circulation 108:2270–2274

Woodburn KW, Fan Q, Kessel D et al (1996) Phototherapy of cancer and atheromatous plaque with texaphyrins. J Clin Laser Med Surg 14:343–348

Yang X (2010) Interventional molecular imaging. Radiology 254:651–654

Young SW, Sidhu MK, Qing F et al (1994) Preclinical evaluation of gadolinium (III) texaphyrin complex. A new paramagnetic contrast agent for magnetic resonance imaging. Invest Radiol 29:330–338

Practical Set-Up

S. Dymarkowski

Contents

1 **Introduction** ... 53

2 **The Physical MRI Environment and Safety Issues** ... 54
2.1 Static Magnetic Field ... 54
2.2 Alternating Magnetic Field Gradients ... 55
2.3 Bioeffects of Radiofrequency Energy ... 55
2.4 Interaction with Medical Devices ... 58

3 **General Patient Preparation** ... 60
3.1 Patient Positioning and Coil Placement ... 60
3.2 ECG Monitoring ... 61
3.3 Breath-Holding and Free Breathing Scans ... 61

4 **Specific Patient Preparation** ... 61
4.1 Stress Testing ... 61
4.2 Pediatric and Neonatal Cardiac MRI ... 62

5 **Contrast Media-Related Precautions** ... 62

6 **MRI and Pregnancy** ... 63

7 **Claustrophobia** ... 66

8 **Contraindications to MRI** ... 66

References ... 66

Abstract

In performing a cardiovascular MRI examination, preparation is considered to be paramount to a successful subsequent image acquisition. Although seemingly trivial, this image acquisition and interpretation requires a working knowledge of adequate patient preparation, ECG lead placement, breath-hold instructions and contrast injection. This expertise should be accompanied by knowledge of safety issues and precautions in the MRI environment. The purpose of this chapter is to provide MRI users, in particular those who aim to perform cardiovascular MRI studies in daily clinical practice, a practical introduction to setting up and performing an MR scan.The safety issues in the MR suite will be discussed and ample attention is given to the specific patient preparation for patients undergoing cardiac MR. Several contra-indications and risks relating to pregnancy and contrast media will be discussed.

1 Introduction

In performing a cardiovascular MRI examination, preparation is considered to be paramount to a successful subsequent image acquisition. Although seemingly trivial, this image acquisition and interpretation requires a working knowledge of adequate patient preparation, ECG lead placement, breath-hold instructions and contrast injection. This expertise should be accompanied by knowledge of safety issues and precautions in the MRI environment, relating to the use of strong magnetic fields, radio frequency

S. Dymarkowski (✉)
Department of Radiology,
University Hospitals Gasthuisberg,
Catholic University of Leuven,
Herestraat 49, 3000 Leuven, Belgium
e-mail: steven.dymarkowski@uz.kuleuven.ac.be

J. Bogaert et al. (eds.), *Clinical Cardiac MRI*, Medical Radiology. Diagnostic Imaging,
DOI: 10.1007/174_2011_355, © Springer-Verlag Berlin Heidelberg 2012

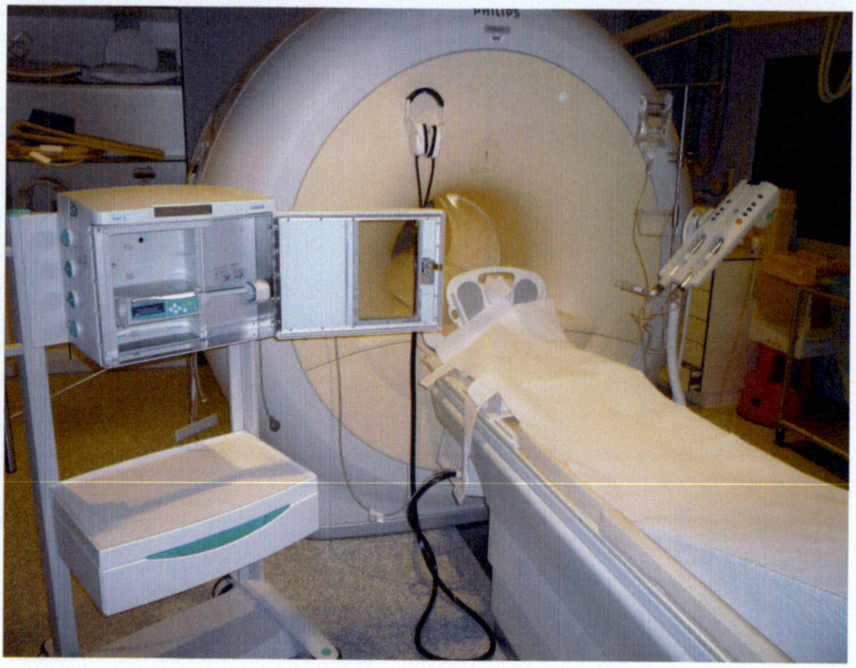

Fig. 1 Typical example of MRI unit equipped with power injector with dual injection system (contrast agent and saline) and MR compatible infusion system

(RF) energy, magnetic field gradients and cryogenic liquids.

The purpose of this chapter is to provide MRI users, in particular those who aim to perform cardiovascular MRI studies in daily clinical practise, a practical introduction to setting up and performing an MR scan.

2 The Physical MRI Environment and Safety Issues

As with other imaging techniques, MRI has its risks, and precautions need to be taken to ensure that potentially hazardous situations do not occur. Attraction of ferromagnetic objects due to the static magnetic field is the most important consideration, but the potential unwanted effects of RF induced heating and peripheral nerve stimulation in the MR environment should also be considered, in particular in patients with permanent pacemakers, automatic implantable cardiac defibrillators (AICDs), long lengths of temporary cardiac pacing wires, metallic stents and prosthetic valves.

Monitoring physiological parameters within the MR scanners can also be problematic. For example, use of MRI incompatible ECG electrodes may be associated with third degree burns, and distortion of the ECG by the magnetic field may interfere with monitoring of ischemic changes during MR examinations. Specifically designed hardware exists to provide monitoring under safe conditions (Fig. 1).

Thus, appropriate knowledge of the MR environment is essential to eliminate the risks that can be associated with the specific physical properties of MRI.

2.1 Static Magnetic Field

MRI personnel are expected to be familiar with the dangers associated with the presence of ferromagnetic objects in the vicinity of the strong static magnetic field of MR scanners. However, other medical professionals, insufficiently experienced with MRI, and patients themselves, may not be aware, and the trained MR staff should remain vigilant about MR safety.

The powerful magnetic field of an MR system will attract ferromagnetic objects and may cause them to move suddenly and with great force. This poses a considerable risk to the patient or anyone in an object's path. Precaution is necessary to prevent that any ferromagnetic objects, such as infusion stands and oxygen tanks, are brought into the MR suite. It is vital that patients themselves remove all metallic belongings in advance of any MRI examination, including jewelry, watches and any item of clothing that have metallic zippers, buttons or fasteners. Providing a patient with a disposable or washable gown may further prevent accidental introduction of hazardous material into the MR room.

Despite numerous safety warnings issued by the manufacturers and the medical profession, sad but true stories of objects being pulled into MR scanners circulate, with, in the extreme cases, fatal outcomes. Special consideration should be given to objects that are associated with patient management, for example oxygen cylinders, monitors, injection systems and drip stands (Fig. 2).

The physical boundary up to which ferromagnetic objects can be safely manipulated is indicated as the 5 Gauss line. In some MR suites, this is visually indicated on the floor to prevent accidental movement of these objects (Fig. 3).

Similar forces are at work on ferromagnetic metal implants or foreign matter inside those being imaged. These forces can pull on these objects cutting and compressing healthy tissue. For these reasons individuals with foreign metal objects such as shrapnel or older ferromagnetic implants are not imaged. Most centers will provide their patients with information brochures about the examination and will ask them to fill out a safety questionnaire prior to the examination to gain supplemental insight into potentially hazardous situations (Fig. 4). Furthermore, the internet contains a plethora of vulgarized information concerning MR examinations that can be consulted free of charge.

2.2 Alternating Magnetic Field Gradients

Part of the MR imaging process involves alternations of the magnetic field state of the gradient magnets necessary for spatial encoding. The rate with which the change of magnetic field occurs is dependent on the gradient power of the systems and is expressed as dB/dt. Gradient requirements are usually higher in high-application systems (e.g. for functional brain MRI and cardiovascular MRI), to enable sequence repetition time (TR) to be as short as possible. The United States Food and Drug Administration (FDA) has issued recommendations for dB/dt for each system to be at a level less than that required to produce peripheral nerve stimulation (Fig. 5).

The switching of these magnetic gradients also produces high acoustic noise levels, which has been limited by the FDA to 140 dB. It is also recommended that all patients should be provided with hearing protection in the form of earplugs or headphones.

2.3 Bioeffects of Radiofrequency Energy

The RF energy from an imaging sequence is nonionizing electromagnetic radiation in a high frequency range. Research has shown that the majority of the RF energy transmitted for MR imaging is dissipated as heat in the patient's tissues due to resistive losses. Such temperature changes are not felt by the patient. Nevertheless, MR imaging can potentially cause significant heating of body tissues, and the FDA recommends that the exposure to RF energy be limited. The limiting measure is the specific absorption rate (SAR) and is expressed as Joules of RF energy deposited per second per kilogram of body weight (i.e.Watts/kilogram). The recommended SAR limit depends on the anatomy being imaged. The SAR for the whole body must be less than 4 W/kg, and must be less than 3.2 W/kg averaged over the head. Any pulse sequence must not rise the temperature by more than 1°C and no greater than 38°C in the head, 39°C in the trunk and 40°C in the extremities.

The precise mechanism of tissue heating with MRI in not completely understood. It seems to be multifactorial in origin. Some organs are more sensitive than others to heating, and underlying medical conditions or drugs can influence the degree of heat accumulation within the human body. Normally, when heat accumulates in the body, it is dissipated by conduction, convection, evaporation and radiation. Disease states (hypertension, diabetes, …) or medication (sedatives, vasodilators, …) can impair the normal thermoregulatory responses to a heat challenge.

The heat interaction of pure biological phenomena is negligible. However, this is not true in the case of heating in association with devices inside the MR system. Thermal injuries, up to third degree burns, have been reported with the use of ECG leads, pulse oximeters and monitoring devices with wires

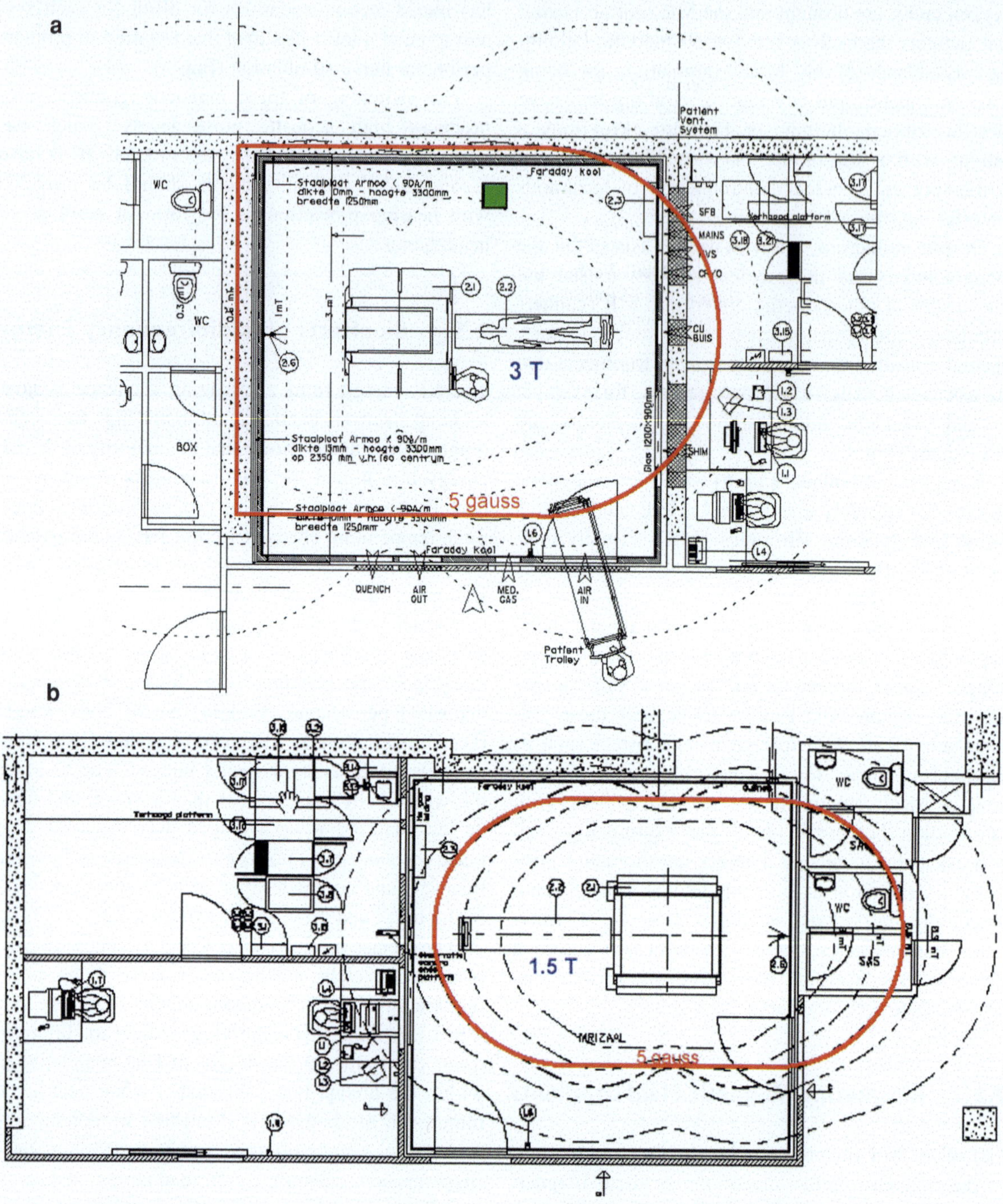

Fig. 2 **a** Siting diagram for a 3 T Unit. The 5 Gauss line is marked in *red*. Note that the public restrooms in the waiting hall (*arrows*) are separated from the magnetic field by a thick reinforced wall. **b** Similar, but less optimal siting diagram of a 1.5 T unit. The 5 Gauss line extends beyond the Faraday cage into the restrooms. People with pacemakers are potentially in danger when using this facility

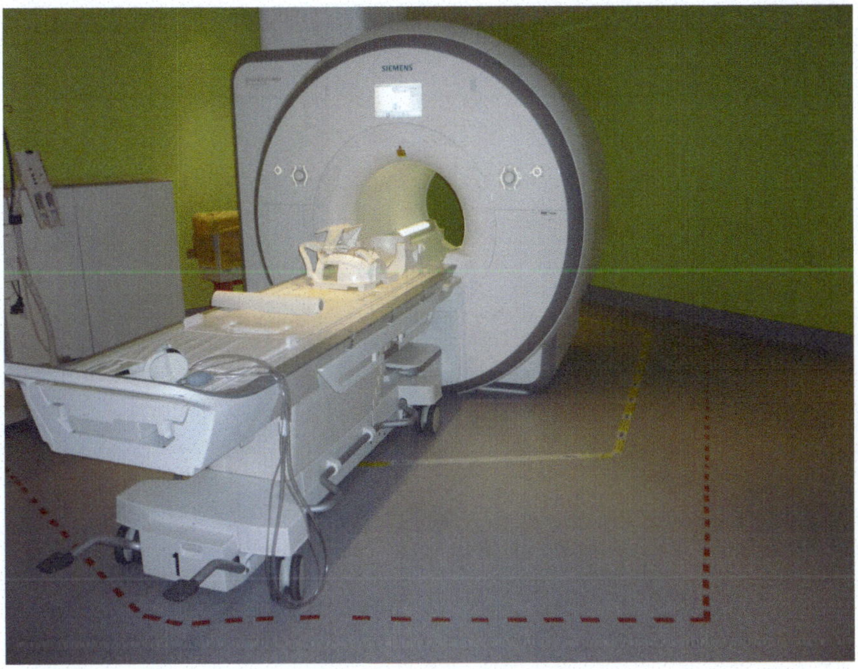

Fig. 3 Floor markings inside a 1.5 T suite mark the invisible boundary of the 5 and 10 Gauss lines (*yellow* and *red*, respectively). No additional monitoring unit or power injection, even MRI compatible ones may be positioned within this line for safety purposes

14 december 2010

UZ LEUVEN | RADIOLOGIE

Questionnaire for Magnetic Resonance/ MR patients :

With a view to establishing a medical diagnosis your GP has asked for a MR scan.

Due to the powerful magnetic field that you will be submitted to it is important for your own safety to accurately complete below questionnaire so that we can trace any possible contraindications for performing the scan.

Please bring this form with you and give it to the MRI technician.
If the document is not properly filled out the scan may be cancelled for your own safety.
If you have any further questions about the list below, please don't hesitate to address the MRI technician or call 016.347770 or 016.47771

- Do you have a pacemaker ? Yes ☐ No ☐
- Do you have a defibrillator? Yes ☐ No ☐
- Do you have an artificial heart valve ? Yes ☐ No ☐
- Do you have a dental or joint prosthesis ? Yes ☐ No ☐
- Do you have an hearing aid, ear implant, cohleair implant ? Yes ☐ No ☐
- Do you have an implanted pump or neurostimulator ? Yes ☐ No ☐
- Do you have a catheter port ? Yes ☐ No ☐
- Have you had brain surgery ? Yes ☐ No ☐
- Have you had blood vessel surgery ? Yes ☐ No ☐
- Do you have any medication patches or other on your body ? Yes ☐ No ☐
- Do you have a tattoo or a piercing ? Yes ☐ No ☐
- Do you have any metal objects :
  - in the eye (metal fragments) ? Yes ☐ No ☐
  - elsewhere in your body (shotgun pellets, bullet) ? Yes ☐ No ☐
- Are you a metal worker or a welder ? Yes ☐ No ☐

Please turn this page over, complete and sign. Thank you.

14 december 2010

- Are you suffering from any allergies ? Yes ☐ No ☐
- Are you pregnant or breastfeeding ? Yes ☐ No ☐
- Are you suffering from renal insufficiency ? Yes ☐ No ☐
- Are you claustrophobic ? Yes ☐ No ☐

Please indicate below where you have had surgery, if applicable :

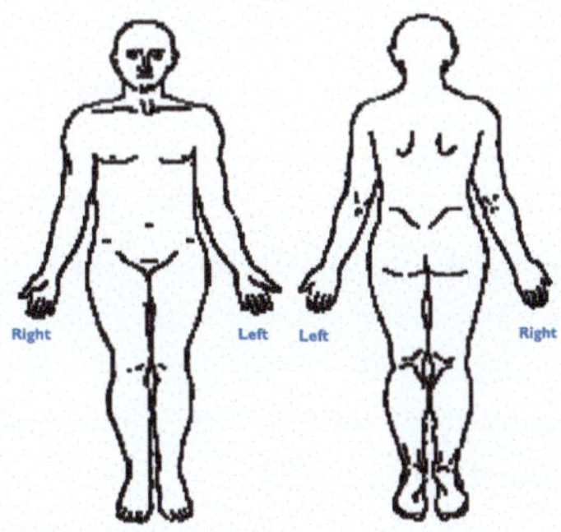

Please remove all metal objects (piercing and jewellery) from your body and leave these items in the changing room together with your ID card, bank cards, coins, belts, and keys.

Please don't hesitate to contact us, if you have any questions: 016.347770 or 016.47771

I HEREBY ACKNOWLEGDE THAT THE INFORMATION GIVEN IS ACCURATE AND TRUE ON THE DATE OF THE MR EXAM.

Name patient:.................................... Length:....m.....cm Weight:.........kg

Name (patient or parent/guardian) : Date : Signature :

..../...../........ ....

Fig. 4 MRI questionnaire filled out by patients prior to their scan

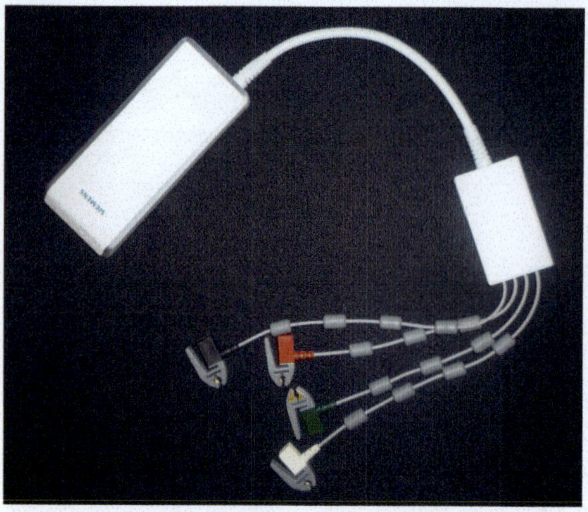

Fig. 5 Example of wireless ECG unit. Communication with the scanner is made using Bluetooth technology

made of conductive materials. Therefore, manufacturer's guidelines should be strictly enforced and if any doubt exists about safety of a certain device, this should not be used.

If leads are used they should not be looped and should not be placed immediately on the individual's bare skin. If available, leads with fiber-optic signal transmission and special outer shielding should be used.

2.4 Interaction with Medical Devices

2.4.1 Cardiac Pacemakers and AICD's

A cardiac pacemaker is the most common electrical implant that can be found across the patient population. A commonly asked question is therefore whether or not an MR procedure can be safely performed in patients with implanted cardiac pacemakers. It is generally assumed that presence of a pacemaker is a strict contraindication for MRI.

The effects of the MR environment on pacemakers are diverse and dependent on many factors such as the strength of the external magnetic field, the kind of sequences used and the body area that is to be imaged.

Practical experience has taught us that though many patients with pacemakers have been inadvertently placed into MR systems in the past, hazardous or fatal outcomes have only occurred in a small number of patients. The following facts, however, summarize the many dangers of performing MRI with pacemaker patients and provide evidence that such practises should be strictly discouraged.

The metal casing of a pacemaker tends to align to the longitudinal axis of the external MR magnetic field. This gives rise to magnet-related translational attraction or torque effects. In different studies deflection angles were measured from 9 to 90° for long-bore and from 11 to 90° for short-bore MR systems. Such movement of the pacemaker box may be problematic for patients undergoing MRI, with possible discomfort and the potential for proximal lead fracture.

It is also known that static magnetic fields close the reed switches—tiny electrical relays—of many pacemakers. Reed switch closure has been studied for different orientations and positions relative to the main magnetic field and at different magnetic fields. If reed switches are oriented parallel to the magnetic field, they generally close at 1.0 ± 0.2 mT and open at 0.7 ± 0.2 mT. Different reed switch behavior has been observed at different magnetic field strengths. In low magnetic fields (<50 mT), the reed switches were found to close, while in higher magnetic fields (>200 mT), the reed switches opened in 50% of all tested orientations. Thus, reed switch closure is not predictable with certainty in clinical situations. Despite this unpredictability of the reed switch in these experimental circumstances, tests on isolated pacemakers and in patients with AICDs using continuous monitoring of pacemaker output and temperature at the lead tip at low fields (0.5 T), have shown no pacemaker or AICD dysfunction during MR imaging, and no changes in the programed parameters in any device tested in vivo or in vitro. Furthermore, the only consequence of reed switches closing is that the pacemaker is switched into asynchronous mode, during which a predetermined fixed pacing rate takes over. This effect can be compared to the short period of pacemaker interrogation that takes place in routine pacemaker check-ups.

However, it is not the above effects alone that are responsible for the adverse outcome in patients with pacemakers during MR examinations. More concerning is induction of currents in the pacemaker lead which could cause action potentials in and subsequent contraction of the ventricle. There have indeed been reports in the literature of cardiac pacing occurring at the TR of the sequence.

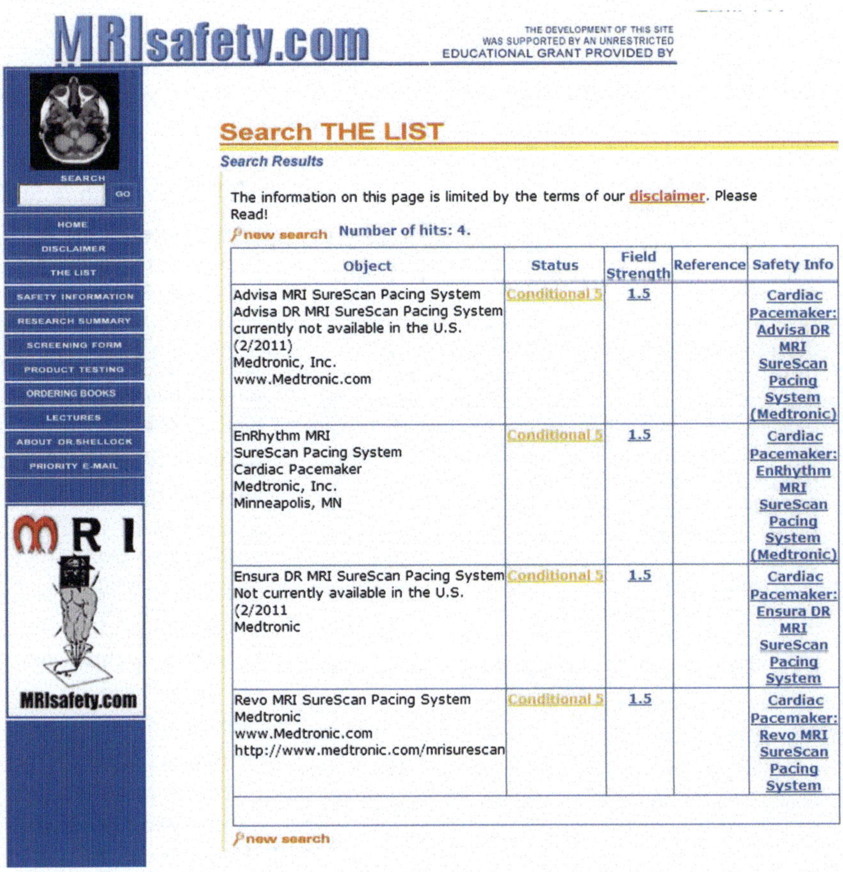

Fig. 6 Screenshot of the website www.mrisafety.com Information about MR compatibility of virtually all medical devices can be found there

Furthermore, temperature increase in the pacemaker lead is a severe and realistic problem. Studies have shown pacemaker electrodes exposed to MR imaging can have temperature increased of up to 63°C after 90 s of scanning. The potential adverse effect of a thermal injury to the myocardial should thus be considered as the main caveat in conduction MRI examinations in these patients, especially if RF power is to be transmitted in the vicinity of the pacemaker and its leads (i.e. MR imaging of the neck, chest and abdomen).

Despite reports in the literature that MR examinations can be performed in patients who are not pacemaker dependent and had the device switched off, it remains inadvisable to perform such examinations considering the potential hazards as stated above. Pacemaker companies advise against it and the American Heart Association issued a statement in that discouraged doctors from performing MRIs on pacemaker patients unless the need for the MRI was compelling enough to warrant the risk of the examination. In the United States, Medicare will not pay for an MRI done on a patient who has a pacemaker. There have been a few reported deaths of pacemaker patients who underwent an MRI and the risks include movement of the pacemaker and re-setting of the pacing pattern. If a patient is somehow accidentally exposed to the MR field, good clinical practise demands that the pacemaker function should to be checked by a trained cardiologist.

The medical company Medtronic developed the Revo MRI Sure scan Pacing System, maybe the first step in allowing a more liberal is of MRI in patients with pacemakers in the future. It is not categorized as 'MRI safe' but rather as 'MR Conditional', meaning that it is designed to allow patients to undergo MRI under the specified conditions for use. A complete system, consisting of a Medtronic Revo MRI Sure Scan IPG implanted with two Cap Sure Fix MRI Sure Scan leads is required for use in the MRI environment. Even then, there are several limitations of this new development (Fig. 6).

To avoid overheating of the metal tips of the leads, RF and gradient exposure of the chest is not allowed, cardiac MR scans are thus forbidden with this first generation model. Other restrictions curtail its randomized use. To quote the senior scientific reviewer for the FDA:

> "In addition to the chest scan exclusion, there is a restriction on how much radio-frequency energy can be deposited into the body by the scanner. MRI scanners have two operating modes for most clinical applications. 'Normal operating mode' is how the scanner is normally programed and that mode restricts the scanner to lower-energy scans (less than 2 Watts per kilogram). This is sufficient energy for most clinical MRI scans. However, for some patients and for certain scans, more power is needed. In those cases, the MRI scanner is placed in 'First level control' mode, which allows for greater energy deposition (up to 4 Watts per kilogram). For patients implanted with the REVO MRI pacemaker, those patients are not allowed to have these higher energy scans" (Knudson 2011).

2.4.2 Temporary External Pacemaker Wires

Often patients are referred early after cardiac surgery with temporary external pacemaker wires still in situ. Usually these are cut off close to the skin before discharge. This condition should not be considered as a contraindication to MRI. In our experience, the external portion of these wires should be contained in plastic, test-tube-like receptacles, taped to the patient's chest. These segments of the wires (the straight wire section) can cause significant susceptibility artifacts on the anterior chest wall. This generally poses no concern for evaluation of left ventricular function for example, though the wires do interfere with image quality in the immediate region of the wire, e.g. if an evaluation of the right coronary artery is to be obtained.

2.4.3 Prosthetic Valves, Surgical Clips and Osteosynthesis Materials

There are standard procedures for testing of prosthetic valves for MRI safety. The term "MRI-safe" is defined by the American Society for Testing and Materials (ASTM) Designation: F 2052. *Standard test method for measurement of magnetically induced displacement force on passive implants in the magnetic resonance environment*. A device is considered to be MRI-safe when this device poses no additional risk to the patient or other individuals in a static magnetic field, but may affect the quality of the diagnostic information.

Prior to the approval of the ASTM, prosthetic valves are tested for translational attraction (average deflection angle measured in magnetic fields up to 3 T), tissue heating in the immediate vicinity of the device, and artifacts.

Most currently used prosthetic valces have been extensively tested in the past and it was found that there is very little interaction between the valves and the magnetic field, i.e. insufficient translational attraction to pose any danger, very little MRI-related heating for these implants, but artifacts characterized for these implants may be problematic if the imaging area of interest is where the implant is located. Therefore, to perform cardiac MRI in patient with artificial valves can be considered safe, but potentially uninteresting seen as limited diagnostic information can be gained from the peri valvular area.

Surgical clips and osteosynthesis material are not considered to be contra-indications for MRI examinations, with the sole exception of cerebral aneurysm clips.

However, in the light of the constant evolution in development of medical devices, the purpose of this chapter is not to provide an exhaustive overview of compatibility of every possible bioprosthetic one may encounter. Several good reference works and pocket guides have been written on this subject and it serves recommendation to keep a copy of such a book in the MRI suite, to be consulted in case of doubt.

3 General Patient Preparation

3.1 Patient Positioning and Coil Placement

Prior to any cardiac MRI, the patient should be briefly interviewed with regards to MR contraindications. We ascertain if the patient has a pacemaker or any other implanted device, retained pacemaker wires or other foreign material inside the body (in particular post-surgical subarachnoid hemorrhage clips). Female patients are best advised to remove any make-up, since small metallic residues in cosmetics may cause artifacts in the images or be potentially hazardous.

In general, it is always recommended to remove jewelry and have the patient disrobe completely and wear a hospital gown (ideally without pockets!). This avoids the accidental retention of materials in pants or shirt pockets, as patients are not always completely aware of exactly which objects pose a potential risk.

For cardiac MR imaging, most systems have specific cardiac or torso coils. These are often multi-element phased-array coils, required for parallel imaging. The number of elements in such dedicated coils ranges from four to eight, and coils with up to 32 channels are currently available. These coils have anterior and posterior elements, which require accurate positioning, critical for adequate signal reception.

The coils should always be centered over the organ of interest. It is important to note that when imaging the heart, the coil placements should be lower than when imaging the aortic arch (e.g. in aortic coarctation). At the beginning of each examination, visual inspection of the localizer or scout images can give an indication as to whether coil placement was performed correctly.

3.2 ECG Monitoring

As already stated in "Cardiac MRI Physics", accurate peak detecting in the ECG is critically important for good quality MR scans. Most MR systems currently use advanced triggering modules based on vectorcardiography (VCG) to improve R-wave detection in the MR environment. They use a three-dimensional and orthogonal lead system. The ECG electrodes should be attached in a cross–shaped or triangular pattern, depending on the number of electrodes of the system. Prior to application of the electrodes, the skin should be cleaned with alcoholic pads or an abrasive gel to improve surface contact. Excess gel should be carefully removed, and if necessary the chest may need to be shaved. Non-metallic, pre-gelled electrodes should be used for optimal result. Note that when the electrodes are removed from their sealed container for a long period, the gel pad tends to dry out and lose good signal transduction.

During positioning, the quality of the ECG trace should be checked, and a constant, high amplitude R-wave and a low T-wave identified. If the tracing is unsatisfactory, re-start and re-position the electrodes.

3.3 Breath-Holding and Free Breathing Scans

Prior to the placement of the cardiac or torso coil and introduction into the magnet bore, the patient should be made properly aware of what is going to happen during the MR examination.

It is essential to explain the breath-hold commands to the patient, and if necessary, to briefly rehearse these instructions. Breath holding can be performed during inspiration or expiration. If measurements are performed during expiration, reproducibility among the different views is higher and the chance of partial volume effects due to slice miss-registration is decreased; though patients generally get the impression they have less 'air' and are likely to give up a breath-hold prematurely. Therefore some investigators prefer to do breath-hold studies in inspiration.

If any sequences using navigator gating are to be used, ask the patient not to move and if possible to breathe as regularly as possible, to avoid deep inspirations and to try to avoid falling asleep.

Lastly provide the patient with headphones so breath-hold commands and other communications can be efficiently conveyed.

The patient is now ready for image acquisition.

4 Specific Patient Preparation

4.1 Stress Testing

As will be demonstrated in the following chapters, cardiac MRI offers several clinically usable approaches for the assessment of ischemic heart disease. Using echocardiography, the analysis of wall motion abnormalities under pharmacological stress with intravenous administration of dobutamine has been established as a sensitive method. It has been shown that using fast cine acquisition techniques, identical incremental stress protocols as used for echocardiography can be applied to cardiac MRI. Other studies have focused on using physiological stress inside the MR scanner, using an MR compatible non-ferromagnetic treadmill or bicycle. It is at present unclear if these devices are really practical to implement on a daily routine clinical basis.

Performing stress MRI studies requires a specific practical approach to address the potential adverse effects during a study, since physical access to the patient is more limited than in echocardiography. Using low dose protocols, side effects are minimal, but at higher doses side effects can occur in 0.25% of patients, including myocardial infarction (0.07%), ventricular fibrillation (0.07%) and sustained ventricular tachycardia (0.1%). The MR unit should be equipped with facilities to allow a rapid extraction of the patient, such as a removable table-top, to enable rapid clinical assessment and treatment in case of adverse events. Resuscitation equipment and medication should be in the immediate vicinity to be administered by experienced staff in case of an emergency.

Physicians performing stress studies should be aware of the patient's medical history and strictly observe the known contraindications. These are: Severe arterial hypertension, unstable angina pectoris, aortic stenosis, severe cardiac arrhythmias, obstructive cardiomyopathy, endocarditis and myocarditis. Patients are asked not to take their beta-blockers and nitrates 24 h prior to the examination.

Before a stress study is initiated, standard ECG leads are applied, as in any other cardiac MR scan. Many experienced users, however, prefer to place electrodes in such a way that permit the acquisition of a standard 12-lead ECG before the MR scan; a policy that can save a considerable amount of time in case of an emergency.

It is important to be aware that ST segment changes indicating ischemia are deemed not to be reliable in the static magnetic field, so the ECG during the scans can only be used for monitoring of the cardiac frequency. Further physiology monitoring requires the use of MR compatible devices. Non-ferromagnetic monitoring devices exist, which can be brought up to a distance of 1–2 m from the entrance of the magnet bore opening. Using such devices, blood pressure can be measured every minute and pulse oximetry continuously monitored.

Furthermore, audiovisual contact with the patient is maintained throughout the MR examination, to be aware of any symptoms that may occur during the dobutamine infusion. At the same time, the acquired images are immediately assessed to detect wall motion abnormalities; the most sensitive sign of a positive stress test.

Indications for termination of a stress studies are: A systolic blood pressure decrease >20 mm Hg below baseline, a systolic blood pressure decrease >40 mm Hg from a previous level, a blood pressure increase >240/120 mm Hg, intractable symptoms and/or new or worsening wall motion abnormalities in at least two adjacent left ventricular segments.

4.2 Pediatric and Neonatal Cardiac MRI

Given the inherent benefits of tissue contrast and resolution in MRI, cardiac studies are frequently used as a complementary technique in children and infants with congenital heart disease to elucidate complex cardiac anatomy. However, the requirement of complete immobility and the ability to follow breathing instructions is often not obtainable in children, due to either age or developmental stage. Therefore general anesthesia or prolonged sedation is often necessary to overcome these limitations and to complete these procedures successfully.

In our own centers, general anesthesia is preferred due to previous experiences with failed sedation or perceived medical risk. The greatest concern during prolonged sedation is respiratory depression and hypoxemia. A study by Lamireau et al. (1998) found an 89% incidence of oxygen desaturation in children who were sedated for endoscopic procedures. For less invasive procedures, a study performed by (Malviya et al. 2000), performed in 922 children undergoing MRI or CT procedures, found a 2.9% incidence of hypoxemia and failure rate of 7% in children who received sedation. In contrast, the procedure was successful in all of the children receiving general anesthesia, with only one incident of laryngospasm (0.7%). Although general anesthesia is a more expensive procedure than sedation, it is an essential aid in successful completion of MRI studies with a minimum of adverse events.

5 Contrast Media-Related Precautions

While allergic reactions to MR contrast media are very rare and usually benign, more serious adverse events linked to the use of these contrast agents were first described in 1997 but only definitively linked to exposure to gadolinium contrast media in 2000. Nephrogenic systemic fibrosis (NSF), previously designated as nephrogenic fibro sing dermopathy, is a rare and serious syndrome that involves fibrosis of skin, joints, eyes and internal organs. Its cause is not fully understood and information about NSF is still being collected. However, there is much evidence to suggest that it is associated with exposure to gadolinium in patients with severe kidney failure. Epidemiological studies suggest that the incidence of NSF is unrelated to gender, race or age and it is not thought to have a genetic basis.

In NSF, patients develop symptoms as early as the day of exposure leading up to 2–3 months after the administration. Usually dermatological symptoms dominate the clinical images, with painful, swollen and itching areas of erythema, usually on the lower limbs. In a more advanced stage, thickened skin and subcutaneous tissues are found with subcutaneous nodules and plaque-like thickening of the epidermis. Further on, NSF can cause painful joint contractures, limitation in range of motion and cachexia. While skin involvement is on the foreground, the process may involve any organ and resembles diffuse scleroderma or systemic sclerosis. In advanced stages, NSF may cause severe systemic fibrosis affecting internal organs including the lungs, heart and liver.

Four contrast agents approved by the U.S. Food and Drug Administration have been principally implicated in NSF, including gadodiamide (Omniscan), gadobenate di meglumine (Multihance), gadopentetate di meglumine (Magnevist) and gadoversetamide (OptiMARK).

Patient with a higher risk are those presenting with chronic kidney disease (CKD) stages 4 and 5, with a glomerular filtration rate (GFR) of less than <30 ml/min, patients on dialysis and patients with reduced renal function who have had or are awaiting liver.

Lower risk cases are patients with CKD 3 (GFR 30–59 ml/min), children under one year of age, because of their immature renal function.

The role of dialysis is sometimes disputed since most patients with NSF have undergone hemodialysis for renal failure, but some have never undergone dialysis while others have received only peritoneal dialysis.

No cases of NSF have ever been reported in patients with GFR values greater than 60 ml/min.

As a general rule, in our institution the guidelines of the European Contrast Media Safety Committee of the European Society of Urogenital Radiology (ESUR) are closely followed. From a practical point of view this means we never use a contrast agent associated with the development of NSF (i.e. avoid gadodiamide, gadopentetate di meglumine or gadoversetamide). In this regard, The European Medicines Agency has classified the gadolinium-containing contrast agents in three groups:

- Least likely (safest) to release free gadolinium ions Gd^{3+} in the body: gadoteric acid (Dotarem), gadobutrol (Gadovist) and gadoteridol (ProHance).
- Intermediate: gadopentetate di meglumine (Magnevist), gadobenate di meglumine (MultiHance), gadoxetate disodium (Primovist -Eovist in the U.S.) and gadofosveset trisodium (Ablavar).
- Most likely to release Gd^{3+}: (gadodiamide) Omniscan and gadoversetamide (OptiMARK).

Especially in at risk patients, always give the lowest dose possible to achieve a diagnostic examination and allow at least one week before giving more contrast material. Systematic measurement of serum creatinine in all patients before an MR examination is not routinely performed since serum creatinine and estimated GFR (eGFR) are not always very accurate indicators of true GFR. In particular, acute renal failure may not be indicated by a single eGFR value. Only in patients with documented renal impairment, eGFR is confirmed before the examination. From a philosophical point of view, strict adherence to these guidelines ensures we do not deny at risk patients with clinically important MR examinations.

6 MRI and Pregnancy

In 2002, the American College of Radiology Blue Ribbon Panel on MR Safety finalized its review of the MR Safe Practice Guidelines as detailed in the so-called White Paper on MR Safety. With regards to safety of MRI procedures in pregnancy, a distinction was made between health care practitioners and patients.

Pregnant health care practitioners are allowed to work in and around the MR unit throughout the entire pregnancy. This includes the positioning of patients, injecting contrast and entering the MR scan room in response to an emergency. Pregnant MR operators are advised not to enter the scanner room during actual data acquisition itself.

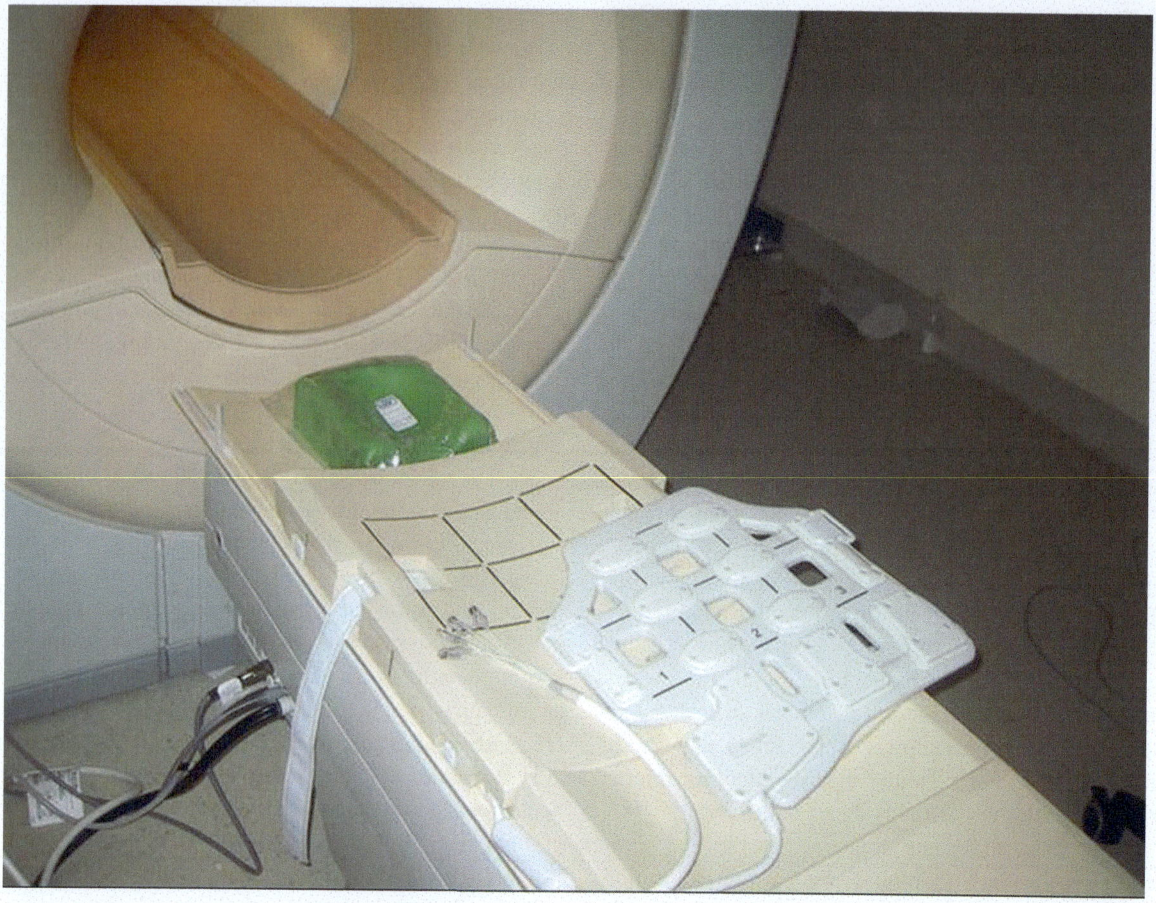

Fig. 7 Six-element cardiac surface coil on a 3T unit

Fig. 8 MR compatible bicycle ergometer with volunteer in place

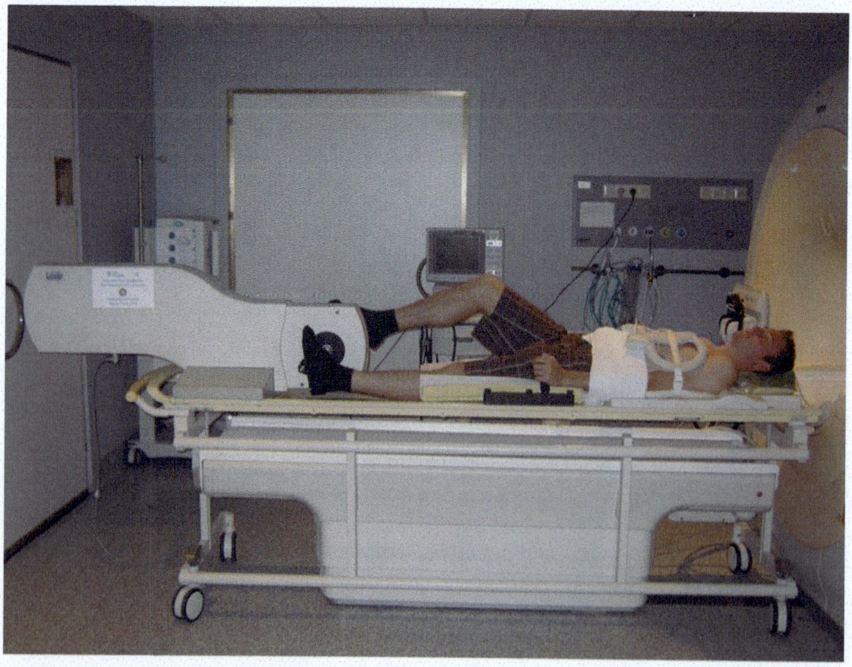

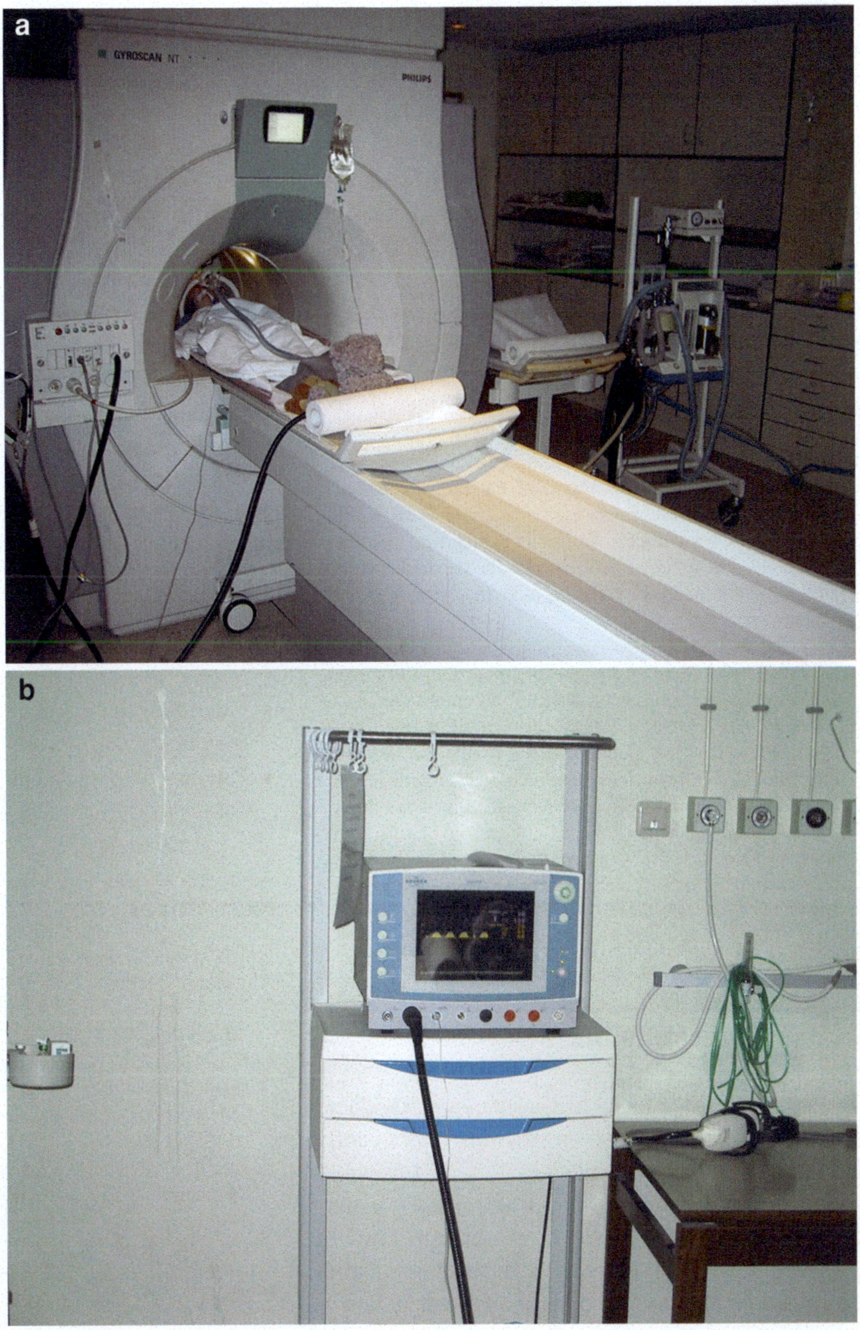

Fig. 9 **a** Patient installation for pediatric MR examination under general anesthesia. The child is mechanically ventilated by a non-ferromagnetic gas-inhalator (*arrow*) and covered with blankets to decrease body temperature loss. **b** Physiological parameters are constantly monitored by use of the MR compatible unit

For pregnant patients, MR scans can be performed if the performing radiologist and the patient's clinician concur that the risk/benefit ratio to the patient warrants that the study be performed. This in practise means that the information provided by the MR examination cannot be acquired by another non-invasive or non-ionizing investigation (e.g. ultrasound). Furthermore, it should be argued that the information derived from the MR scan has therapeutic consequences during the duration of the pregnancy.

Following the guidelines of the ESUR, gadolinium media may be given to the pregnant female if necessary for a definitive diagnosis. Following administration of gadolinium agents to the mother during pregnancy, no neonatal tests are necessary. In the absence of specific information concerning NSF during pregnancy, it seems wise to manage pregnant patients, whatever their renal function, in the same way as children aged under one year to protect the fetus.

Manufacturers of intravenous contrast indicate mothers should not breastfeed their babies for 24–48 h after contrast medium is given. However, both the American College of Radiology (ACR) and the ESUR note that the available data suggest that it is safe to continue breastfeeding after receiving intravenous contrast. The Manual on Contrast Media from the ACR states:

> "Review of the literature shows no evidence to suggest that oral ingestion by an infant of the tiny amount of gadolinium contrast medium excreted into breast milk would cause toxic effects. We believe, therefore, that the available data suggest that it is safe for the mother and infant to continue breastfeeding after receiving such an agent.
>
> If the mother remains concerned about any potential ill effects, she should be given the opportunity to make an informed decision as to whether to continue or temporarily abstain from breastfeeding after receiving a gadolinium contrast medium. If the mother so desires, she may abstain from breastfeeding for 24 h with active expression and discarding of breast milk from both breasts during that period. In anticipation of this, she may wish to use a breast pump to obtain milk before the contrast study to feed the infant during the 24-h period following the examination".

7 Claustrophobia

The enclosed space of an MR scanner can produce a fear of both suffocation and restriction, thus a cardiac MR can often prove difficult for claustrophobic patients. In fact, estimates say that anywhere from 4 to 20% of patients refuse to go through with the scan for precisely this reason. The average cardiac examination takes around 35 min; more than enough time to evoke fear and anxiety in a claustrophobic patient. Careful and empathic guidance of the patient through the process as well as establishment of a comfort zone (controllable air flow within the bore of the magnet, soothing music and lighting) could help reduce claustrophobic reactions, which clearly is a safety concern in MRI.

8 Contraindications to MRI

Any patient with any of the following devices implanted should on a routine basis not be imaged by means of MRI:

- Cardiac pacemaker.
- Automatic implanted cardiac defibrillator.
- Aneurysm clips.
- Carotid artery vascular clamp.
- Neurostimulator.
- Insulin or infusion pump.
- Implanted drug infusion device.
- Bone growth/fusion stimulator.
- Cochlear, otologic or ear implant.

Furthermore, any patients presenting with following medical conditions should also preferentially not be brought into the MRI device: (Figs. 7, 8, 9)

- Patients with severe claustrophobia in which medical sedation is contraindicated or unable to resolve anxiety sufficiently.
- Patients with ocular foreign body (e.g. metal shavings).
- Patients with unstable angina or New York Heart Association functional class IV heart failure.

References

Ahmed S, Shellock FG (2001) Magnetic resonance imaging safety: implications for cardiovascular patients. J Cardiovasc Magn Reson 3:171–182

Collins CM, Liu W, Wang J et al (2004) Temperature and SAR calculations for a human head within volume and surface coils at 64 and 300 MHz. J Magn Reson Imaging 19:650–656

Farling P, McBrien ME, Winder RJ (2003) Magnetic resonance compatible equipment: read the small print!. Anaesthesia 58:86–87

Gimbel JR, Kanal E (2004) Can patients with implantable pacemakers safely undergo magnetic resonance imaging? J Am Coll Cardiol 43:1325–1327

Greatbatch W, Miller V, Shellock FG (2002) Magnetic resonance safety testing of a newly-developed fiber-optic cardiac pacing lead. J Magn Reson Imaging 16:97–103

Grobner T (2006) Gadolinium–a specific trigger for the development of nephrogenic fibro sing dermopathy and nephrogenic systemic fibrosis? Nephrol Dial Transplant 21(4):1104–1108

Kanal E (2002) American college of radiology white paper on MR safety. Am J Roentgenol 178:1335–1347

Kanal E (2004) Clinical utility of the American college of radiology MR safe practice guidelines. J Magn Reson Imaging 19:2–5

Knudson M (2011) New wave of MRI-safe pacemakers set to ship to hospitals. Scientific American, 16 Feb 2011

Lamireau T, Dubreuil M, Daconceicao M (1998) Oxygen saturation during esophagogastroduodenoscopy in children: general anesthesia versus intravenous sedation. J Pediatr Gastroenterol Nutr 27:172–175

Luechinger R, Duru F, Zeijlemaker VA et al (2002) Pacemaker reed switch behavior in 0.5, 1.5, and 3.0 T magnetic resonance imaging units: are reed switches always closed in strong magnetic fields? Pacing Clin Electrophysiol 25: 1419–1423

Malviya S, Voepel-Lewis T, Eldevik OP et al (2000) Sedation and general anaesthesia in children undergoing MRI and CT: adverse events and outcomes. Br J Anaesth 84:743–748

Marckmann P, Skov L, Rossen K et al (2006) Nephrogenic systemic fibrosis: suspected etiological role of gadodiamide used for contrast-enhanced magnetic resonance imaging. J Am Soc Nephrol 17:2359–2362

Martin ET, Coman JA, Shellock FG et al (2004) Magnetic resonance imaging and cardiac pacemaker safety at 1.5 T. J Am Coll Cardiol 43:1315–1324

Nahrendorf M, Hiller KH, Hu K, Zeijlemaker V et al (2004) Pacing in high field cardiac magnetic resonance imaging. Pacing Clin Electrophysiol 27:671–674

Partain CL, Price RR (2004) MR safety. J Magn Reson Imaging 19:1

Pohost GM (2001) Editor's page: is CMR safe? J Cardiovasc Magn Reson 3:9

Shellock FG (2001) Pocket guide to MR procedures and metallic objects. Lippincott, Williams & Wilkins, Philadelphia 0781733537

Shellock FG, Kanal E (1991) Policies, guidelines, and recommendations for MR imaging safety and patient management. SMRI safety committee. J Magn Reson Imaging 1:97–101

Shellock FG, Tkach JA, Ruggieri PM et al (2003) Cardiac pacemakers, ICDs, and loop recorder: evaluation of translational attraction using conventional ("long-bore") and "short-bore" 1.5 and 3.0 T MR systems. J Cardiovasc Magn Reson 5:387–397

Sommer T, Vahlhaus C, Lauck G et al (2000) MR imaging and cardiac pacemakers: in vitro evaluation and in vivo studies in 51 patients at 0.5 T. Radiology 215:869–879

Thomsen HS (2009) Nephrogenic systemic fibrosis: history and epidemiology. Radiol Clin North Am 47(5):827–831

Webb JAW, Thomsen HS, Morcos SK (2005) Members of contrast media safety committee of European society of urogenital radiology (ESUR). The use of iodinated and gadolinium contrast media during pregnancy and lactation. Eur Radiol 15:1234–1240

Cardiac Anatomy

J. Bogaert and A. M. Taylor

Contents

1	**Introduction**	69
2	**Cardiac MRI Techniques**	70
3	**Position of the Heart in the Thorax: Gross Cardiac Anatomy**	70
4	**Cardiac Structures**	71
4.1	Atria	71
4.2	Ventricles	75
4.3	Valves	79
4.4	Coronary Arteries	80
4.5	Pericardium	81
5	**Great Vessels**	82
6	**Key Points**	89
References		90

J. Bogaert (✉)
Department of Radiology and Medical Imaging Research Center (MIRC), University Hospitals Gasthuisberg, Catholic University of Leuven, Herestraat 49, 3000 Leuven, Belgium
e-mail: jan.bogaert@uzleuven.be

A. M. Taylor
Cardiothoracic Unit, Institute of Child Health and Great Ormond Street Hospital for Children, London, UK

Abstract

Magnetic resonance imaging (MRI) is an excellent technique to evaluate cardiac anatomy in normal and pathologic conditions. Using a combination of dark-blood and bright-blood MRI in one or more imaging planes, the different parts of the heart can be studied in detail. This chapter describes the presentation of the different cardiac structures on MRI, as well as the relation of the heart with other structures within the chest. The chapter is extensively illustrated showing the heart and surrounding structures in different image planes, thus allowing to become familiar with the complex cardiac anatomy. Several helpful key points are provided as a guide toward a correct interpretation of cardiac anatomy.

1 Introduction

The first widely accepted, and still one of the most important strengths of MRI is the ability to noninvasively study cardiac morphology and structure. It provides anatomical images of the heart with high spatial contrast resolution, in a fast and reliable fashion. These images can be acquired in every imaginable plane without restrictions in image size, and without need to administer contrast agents (Dinsmore et al. 1984; O'Donovan et al. 1984; Burbank et al. 1988). Whereas the spin-echo (SE) technique was initially applied to study cardiac anatomy, nowadays a variety of MRI sequences are available for this task. For accurate interpretation, a thorough knowledge of cardiac anatomy along

J. Bogaert et al. (eds.), *Clinical Cardiac MRI*, Medical Radiology. Diagnostic Imaging,
DOI: 10.1007/174_2011_334, © Springer-Verlag Berlin Heidelberg 2012

different imaging planes, and on different cardiac MRI techniques, in normal and pathologic conditions is definitely required. Analysis of cardiac anatomy, sometimes, can be very puzzling especially in congenital cardiopathies. A segmental approach, consisting in a careful analysis of the different components (i.e., venous structures, atria, atrioventricular valves, ventricles, ventriculoarterial valves, and great arteries), each with its own typical characteristics, allows to perfectly describe these complex hearts. Radiologists interested in cardiac imaging are often not sufficiently familiar with the cardiac anatomy and have difficulties in dealing with the different intrinsic cardiac axes, while cardiologists often have problems with the tomographic approach and the visualization of cardiac and extracardiac structures on MRI. In this chapter on cardiac anatomy, the specific features of the different cardiac components and their presentation on MRI will be highlighted. A detailed description of the cross-sectional cardiovascular anatomy on MRI along the different body axes (transverse, coronal, sagittal), and the intrinsic cardiac axes (short-axis, horizontal long-axis, vertical long-axis, left ventricular (LV) outflow tract, and right ventricular (RV) outflow tract) is available at the end of this chapter (Figs. 17, 18, 19, 20, 21, 22, 23 and 24). The strategies for cardiac image planning and slice positioning are discussed in "Cardiovascular MR Imaging Planes and Segmentation".

2 Cardiac MRI Techniques

Nowadays, assessment of cardiac anatomy is usually achieved using a combination of dark-blood and bright-blood imaging (Stehling et al. 1996; Simonetti et al. 1996; Winterer et al. 1999; Carr et al. 2001) (see "Cardiac MR Physics"). Historically, the SE-MRI technique was the first available one to study cardiac morphology, providing dark-blood (or black-blood) images (Hawkes et al. 1981; Heneghan et al. 1982; Herfkens et al. 1983; Higgins et al. 1985). Nowadays, the older SE-MRI sequences whereby only one k-line per slice per heartbeat were acquired, have been replaced by fast dark-blood or black-blood T1-weighted SE-MRI techniques providing one or a series of images per breath-hold (Stehling et al. 1996; Simonetti et al. 1996; Winterer et al. 1999) (see "Cardiac MR Physics"). Image quality has become largely independent of the slice direction, slice thickness, and other influencing parameters. Bright-blood imaging, generally regarded as the approach to study cardiac dynamics, such as myocardial contraction patterns, provides excellent morphologic images of the heart, in particular since the advent of the balanced steady-state free precession (SSFP) gradient-echo MRI sequence, combining high contrast between blood and surrounding tissues with high temporal resolution, enabling to visualize subtle anatomical structures, such as valve leaflets, tendinous chords, muscular trabeculations, and pectinate muscles (Higgins et al. 1988; Carr et al. 2001). Besides 2D bright-blood sequences, high spatial resolution 3D bright-blood imaging similar to that used for coronary artery imaging may provide an excellent anatomic detail of the heart (see "Coronary Artery Disease"). Real-time MRI is no longer a research tool, but allows the operator to interactively fly or navigate through the heart, and to fast-determine the cardiac image planes (Castillo and Bluemke 2003). It is quite obvious that this task can only be achieved with an extensive knowledge of the three-dimensional (3D) cardiac anatomy. To summarize, bright-blood and dark-blood techniques should be seen as complementary techniques. For example, differentiation between vascular structures and other anatomical structures devoid of signal such as the air-filled trachea and bronchi, may be challenging by dark-blood imaging, but is usually straightforward using bright-blood imaging. For a similar reason, calcium-containing structures (e.g., calcified valve leaflets) may not be or are hardly detectable using dark-blood imaging.

3 Position of the Heart in the Thorax: Gross Cardiac Anatomy

The heart has a central, ventrobasal location in the thorax and is bordered bilaterally by the lungs, anteriorly by the sternum, and inferiorly by the diaphragm (Fig. 1). It has an oblique position in the thoracic cavity, with the cardiac apex in the left hemithorax ("levocardia"). The long-axis of the heart is rotated about 45° to both the sagittal and the coronal planes. In younger or slender individuals, the heart tends to be more vertical, whereas it tends to be more horizontal in an obese patient. The major part the heart is surrounded by the pericardial sac, and has no physical connections with the surrounding structures except posteriorly and superiorly where the great arteries

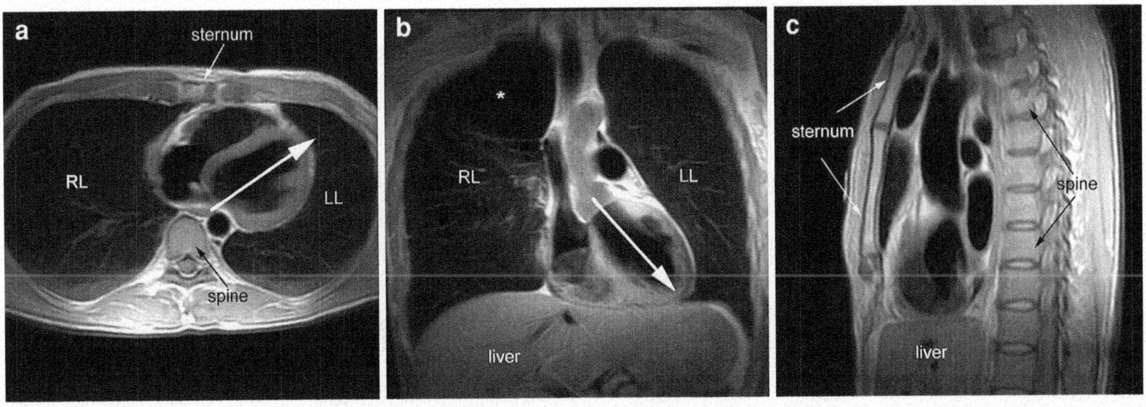

Fig. 1 Position of the heart in the thorax. All images are obtained using dark-blood imaging. **a** Transverse image, **b** coronal image, **c** sagittal image. The *arrow* on the transverse and coronal images indicates the longitudinal axis of the heart. *LL* left lung; *RL* right lung. * bullous emphysema

originate, and the caval and pulmonary veins drain into the atria (Amplatz and Moller 1993).

While the position of the heart in the thorax is relatively constant, the position of the different cardiac components, their intrinsic relationship, as well as their relationship with the great vessels is much more complex, and prone to a large number of congenital variations, isolated or in combination with other extracardiac congenital abnormalities. Knowledge of the gross cardiac anatomy and the specific characteristics of the different cardiac structures enables to describe the most complex congenital cardiopathies (Table 1). The heart is a double two-chambered pump, usually described in terms of "right"-and "left"-sided chambers. In reality, the "right" chambers are more anteriorly positioned within the chest, the "left" chambers more posteriorly, and the ventricles are more inferiorly located than the atria. This is caused by a first important feature of the normal heart, which is that its long axis is not parallel to the long axis of the body. In congenitally malformed hearts, the use of "right" and "left" might be confusing since a "right" may occupy a "left"-sided position, and vice versa. The difficulty is overcome in congenitally malformed hearts by adding the description "morphological" to "right" and "left". The relationship between the "right" and "left" structures of the normal heart are further complicated by the marked twistings of the ventricular outflow tracts. The aorta, although emerging from the left ventricle (and, therefore, a "left" component of the heart) has its valve in the "right"-sided position relative to the pulmonary valve (Anderson 2000).

4 Cardiac Structures

4.1 Atria

4.1.1 Morphological Right Atrium

Both atria, anatomically, can be divided into a venous component, a vestibule of the atrioventricular valve, a septal component, an appendage, and are separated by the atrial septum. The right atrium forms the right heart border (Fig. 2). Embryologically, the right atrium is formed from the sinus venous and the primitive auricle. These two parts of the atrium are separated on the inside by a ridge, the terminal crest or crista terminalis, and on the outside by a groove, the sulcus terminalis. The sinus venosus, forming the posterior part of the right atrium, forms the venous component that has a smooth interior because of its origin as a vessel, while the primitive auricle, having a rough trabeculated interior will form the appendage (Anderson 2000). Pectinate muscles branch from the crest at right angles to run into the appendage. These muscles completely encircle the parietal margin of the vestibule of the atrioventricular valve. The venous component receives the inferior and superior caval veins on its posterior surface, and the coronary sinus at the inferior junction with the septal component. Fibromuscular webs attach to the terminal crest in the regions of the openings of the inferior caval vein and coronary sinus. These are the so-called venous valves, the Eustachian valve in relation to the inferior caval vein, and the Thebesian valve at the coronary sinus.

Table 1 Essentials of the heart

Left atrium	**Right atrium**
Receives pulmonary veins	Receives IVC/SVC-- coronary sinus
Posterosuperior location	Fibromuscular webs
	Eustachian valve (IVC)
	Thebesian valve (coronary sinus)
	Crista terminalis: divides venous component from vestibule
	Prominent pectinate muscles > left atrium
Left atrial appendage	**Right atrial appendage**
Anteriosuperior (over LCx)	Broad triangular
Long/narrow	Wide connection with RA
Small junction	
Left ventricle	**Right ventricle**
Oval or prolate ellipsoid shape	Pyramidal shape
Fine trabeculations	Coarse trabeculations [a]
Inflow and outflow in contact	No connection between inflow and outflow [a]
No infundibulum	Infundibulum [a]
Smooth septal surface	Chordal attachment of septal leaflet of septum [a]
Feeds the aorta	Feeds the pulmonary artery
	Moderator band [a]
	Tricuspid valve more apically positioned than mitral valve [a]

[a] Criteria helpful in differentiating morphological left from right ventricles

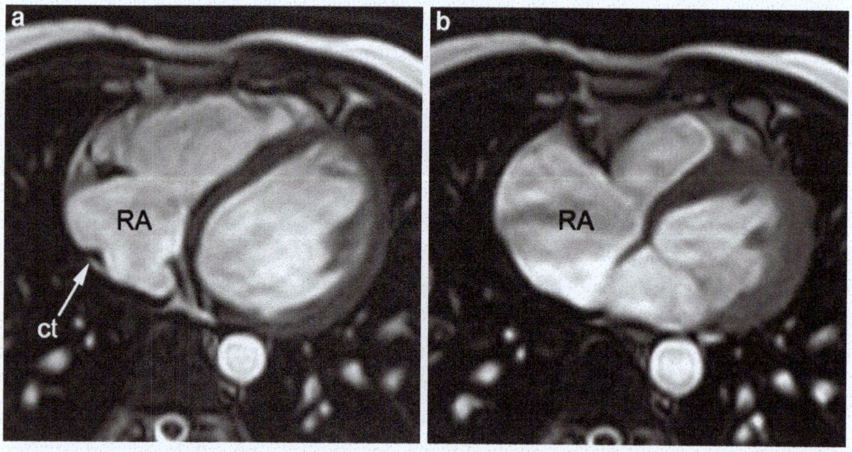

Fig. 2 Right atrium at (**a**) end diastole and (**b**) end systole. The images are obtained in the transverse axis, using bright-blood imaging. The crista terminalis (*ct*) divides the venous component (posteromedially) from the vestibule. Note the important changes in right atrial (*RA*) volume and shape during the cardiac cycle

The coronary sinus running through the left or posterior atrioventricular groove opens into the right atrium above the posteroinferior interventricular groove. Sometimes, the right coronary vein, also draining in the right atrium, is visible in the anterior atrioventricular groove. The junction between the appendage and venous component is particularly wide, and the appendage has a broad, triangular appearance, positioned just ventrally to the entrance of the superior vena cava in the right atrium (Figs. 3, 4). The vestibule is smooth walled and supports the attachments of the leaflets of the tricuspid valve. The different components, as well as the relationship with the caval veins and the coronary sinus can be well

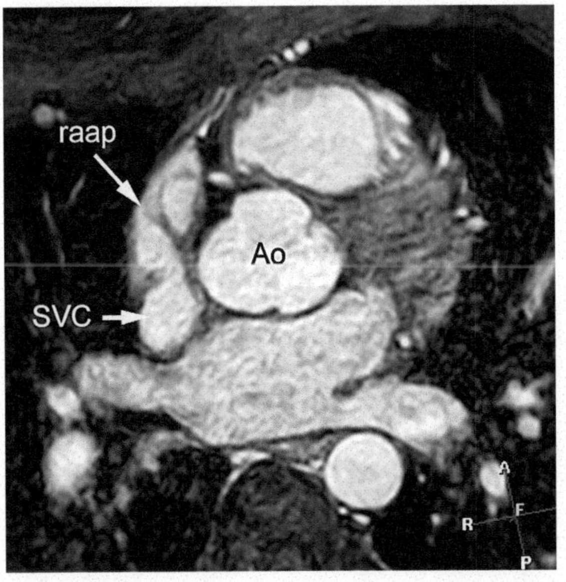

Fig. 3 Right atrial appendage. Transverse image using a 3D bright-blood imaging with submillimeter spatial resolution The right atrial appendage (*raap*) is located ventrally to the superior vena cava (*SVC*) and laterally to the ascending aorta (*Ao*). The high-spatial-contrast resolution enable to depict the pectinate muscles that branch from the crista terminalis and run in right angles to the *raap*

appreciated on several imaging planes, including the transverse, coronal and vertical-long-axis or, sagittal planes (Mohiaddin et al. 1991; Galjee et al. 1995). The terminal crest is routinely visible on dark-blood and bright-blood MRI as a mural nodular or triangular structure adjacent to the lateral wall that connects both the caval veins. This muscular structure may not be misinterpreted as an abnormal intra-atrial mass (Menegus et al. 1992; Meier and Hartnell 1994; Mirowitz and Gutierrez 1992). Bright-blood MRI techniques with submillimeter spatial resolution such as currently used for coronary artery imaging, allow to visualize thinner structures such as the pectinate muscles in the right atrial appendage. Enlargement of the right atrium will easily displace the adjacent lung, while right atrial appendage enlargement encroaches on the upper retro-sternal air space.

4.1.2 Morphological Left Atrium

The morphological left atrium forms the upper posterior heart border with its appendage extending anteromedially. It lies just beneath the carina and anterior to the esophagus. The left atrium extends cranially behind the aortic root and the proximal part of the ascending aorta. The close relationship with the esophagus makes the left atrium very useful as an acoustic window during transesophageal echocardiography. Embryologically, the left atrium also consists of sinus venosus and primitive auricle and they form the same anatomical components such as in the right atrium. The venous component, also posterior located and smooth-walled, receives the four pulmonary veins, one at each corner (Fig. 5). Occasionally five pulmonary veins can be found if the middle pulmonary vein separately drains in the left atrium. The vestibule supports the leaflets of the mitral valve and is also smooth walled. The pectinate muscles, being confined in the appendage, are much less obvious than in the right atrium, and never extend around the atrioventricular junction. The appendage, overlying the left atrioventricular groove and the left circumflex coronary artery (LCx), has a narrow junction with the body of the left atrium and has a long, tubular-shaped appearance (Anderson 2000; Fig. 4). Imaging planes for studying the left atrium are similar to those used to study the right atrium. The relationship of the left atrium with the carina and main stem bronchi is best visible on coronal views. The visualization of the entrance of the pulmonary veins in the left atrium (e.g., to exclude abnormal pulmonary venous return) is best done using a combination of transverse (or four-chamber) and coronal (or short-axis) views. Enlargement of the left atrium displaces the esophagus posteriorly and widens the subcarinal angle. Massive enlargement, exceeding the space in front of the spine, results in encroachment upon the right lung such that the left atrium becomes the border forming on the right and may push the right ventricle forward. Enlargement of the left atrial appendage displaces the adjacent left lung and might be visible as an additional left border on a frontal chest X-ray film.

4.1.3 Atrial Septum

The atrial or interatrial septum separates the left from the right atrium. In the atrial septum is an oval depression, the fossa ovalis. The floor of the fossa ovalis (or oval fossa) is the remains of the septum primum. The septal surface on its right atrial aspect is made up of the floor of the oval fossa and its posteroinferior rim. The superior rim of the fossa

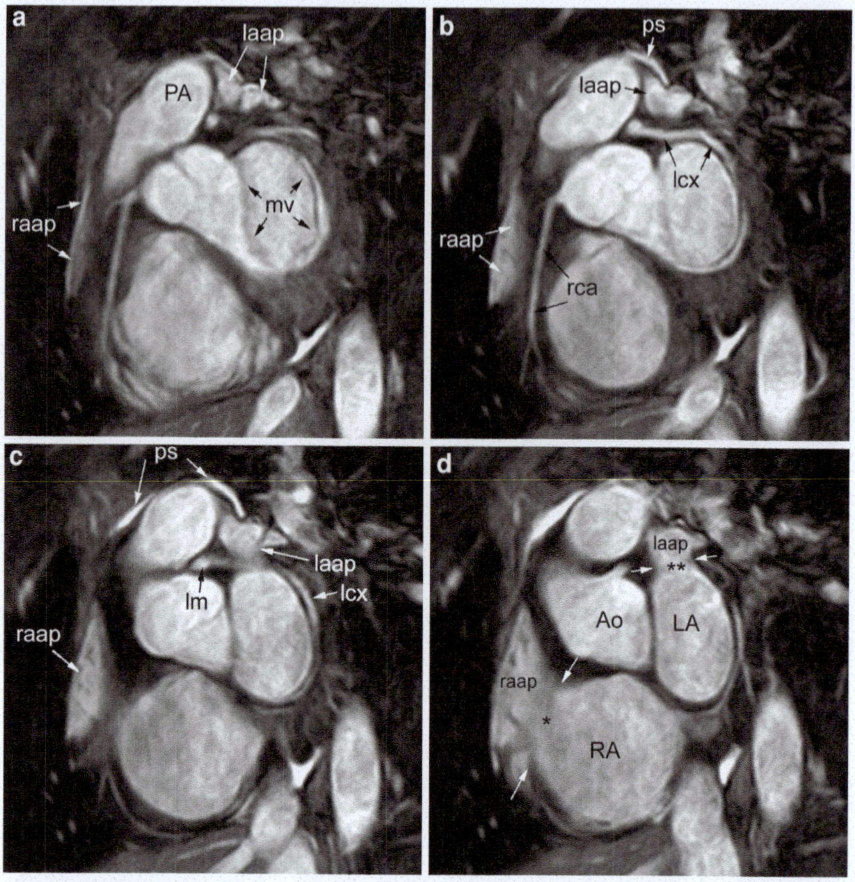

Fig. 4 a–d Right and left atrial appendages. Short-axis images using a 3D bright-blood imaging with submillimeter spatial resolution. While the right atrial appendage (*raap*) has a triangular appearance and a broad communication (*) with the body of the right atrium (*RA*), the left atrial appendage (*laap*) has a narrow junction (**) and a long, tubular appearance. Note the relationship of the appendages with the coronary arteries. The *raap* is dorsally located to the right coronary artery (*rca*), while the *laap* overlies the posterior (or left) atrioventricular groove and the left circumflex coronary artery (*lcx*). Other abbreviations: *Ao* aorta; *LA* left atrium; *lm*, left main stem coronary artery, *PA* pulmonary artery, *ps* pericardial sac

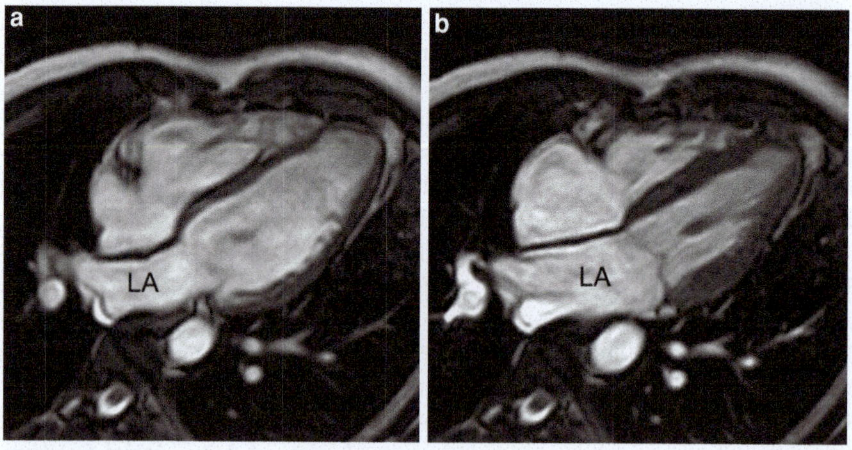

Fig. 5 Left atrium at end diastole (**a**) and end systole (**b**). Horizontal long-axis images using bright-blood imaging. The entrance of the pulmonary vein from the right lower lobe in the left atrium (*LA*) can be well seen

(the so-called septum secundum) is no more than an infolding of the atrial wall between the superior caval vein and the right pulmonary veins. The septal surface is roughened on its left atrial aspect, as is the flap of the oval fossa. The flap valve, superiorly, overlaps the infolded atrial walls (the "septum secundum") so that, even if the two are not fused, there will be no shunting across the septum as long as the left atrial pressure exceeds that in the right atrium. In most cases the atrial septum can be seen on dark-blood imaging as a thin line separating the two atria except at the level of the oval fossa, which is often too thin to

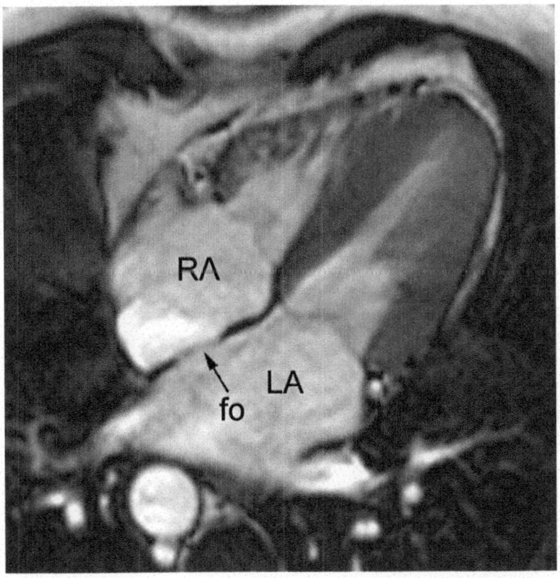

Fig. 6 (Inter)Atrial septum. Horizontal long-axis image using bright blood imaging (end-systolic image)

be seen. This finding might not be misinterpreted as an atrial septal defect. Bright-blood imaging, providing a higher contrast between bright-atrial blood and atrial walls, usually depicts this thin membrane very well (Fig. 6). Sometimes, a fatty infiltration of the atrial septum is observed, which can be easily differentiated from pathological masses by the characteristic signal intensity corresponding to the subcutaneous fat (see "Cardiac Masses"). It is a mostly benign, usually asymptomatic condition, with a low frequency on autopsy series. The atrial septum is best shown in horizontal and longitudinal planes through the heart (e.g., transverse or four-chamber views).

4.2 Ventricles

4.2.1 Morphological Right Ventricle

In a normal heart, the right ventricle sits above the liver and forms the inferior and anterior heart borders with the exception of the apex. The morphological right ventricle can be identified externally by its pyramidal shape, and by its coronary distribution pattern, which is distinctive and typical. The left anterior descending coronary artery (LAD) demarcates the right from the left ventricle. The right ventricles possesses an inlet, an apical trabecular, and an outlet component (Anderson 2000) (Fig. 7). The presentation of the different components is specific for each ventricle and essential to differentiate morphological right from left ventricles. The inlet component (tricuspid valve and atrioventricular septum) surrounds and supports the leaflets and subvalvular apparatus of the tricuspid valve. The leaflets can be divided into septal, anterosuperior, and inferior (or mural) locations within the atrioventricular junction. The most characteristic feature of the tricuspid valve (and thus also of the right ventricle) is the presence of tendinous chords attaching its septal leaflet to the ventricular septum. Chordal attachments to the septal surface are never seen in the morphological left ventricle. The apical trabecular portion of the right ventricle has characteristically coarse trabeculations. The infundibulum is incorporated into the right ventricle, and forms the outflow tract, whereas the right ventricle proper forms the inflow tract. This completely muscular ring supports the three semilunar leaflets of the pulmonary valve. The junction between the infundibulum and the right ventricle is composed of the parietal, septomarginal and moderator bands. The moderator band, a muscular band that contains the continuation of the right bundle branch, passes from the interventricular septum to the anterior wall, and is an essential characteristic of the morphological right ventricle (Fig. 8). The septal and moderator bands are also known as the septomarginal trabeculation. Only a small part of the infundibulum is a truly muscular septum (Fig. 9), while the rest of the posterior margin of the infundibulum, also called supraventricular crest (crista supraventricularis) is caused by an infolding of the roof of the ventricle (also called ventriculoinfundibular fold), and is separated from the aorta by extracardiac space. The separation of the tricuspid and pulmonary valves by the crista supraventricularis is another characteristic of the morphological right ventricle. Additional trabeculations, the septoparietal trabeculations, run round the anterior margin of the infundibulum. The muscular trabeculations are relatively coarse, few, and straight, tending to parallel the right ventriular (RV) inflow and outflow tracts. The papillary muscles of the right ventricle are relatively small (making right ventriculotomy readily possible) and numerous, and they attach both to the septal and free wall surfaces. Because of its numerous attachments to the RV septal surface (mostly to the posteroinferior margin of the septal band), the tricuspid valve may be described as

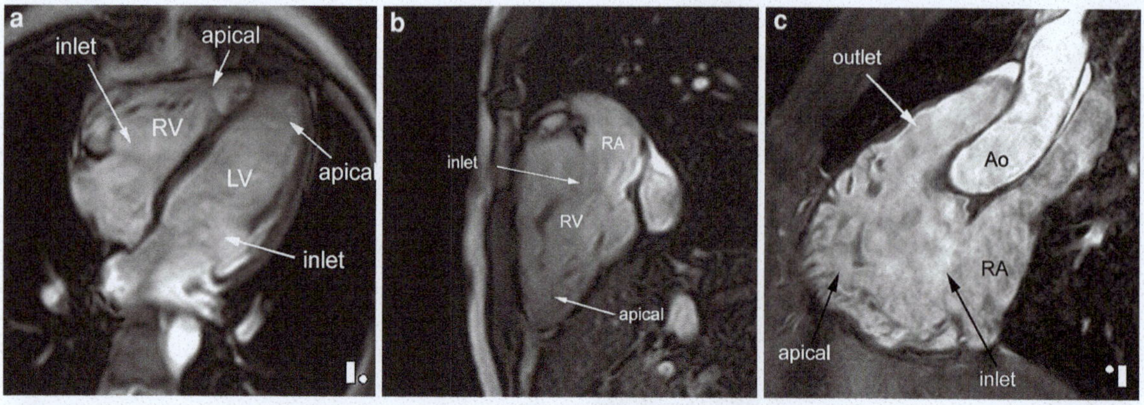

Fig. 7 Components of the right ventricle. Horizontal long-axis image (**a**) *RV* vertical long-axis image (**b**) *RV* inflow and outflow tract image (**c**) using bright-blood imaging. The inlet, apical, and outlet part of the right ventricle are indicated on the different images. *Ao* aorta, *LV* left ventricle, *RA* right atrium, *RV* right ventricle

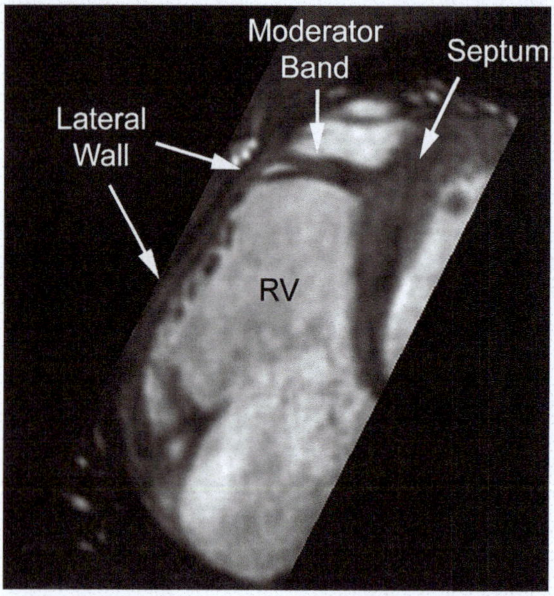

Fig. 8 Moderator band. Horizontal long-axis view, using bright-blood imaging. This muscular structure connects the apical ventricular septum with the apical part of the *RV* free or lateral wall. *RV* right ventricle

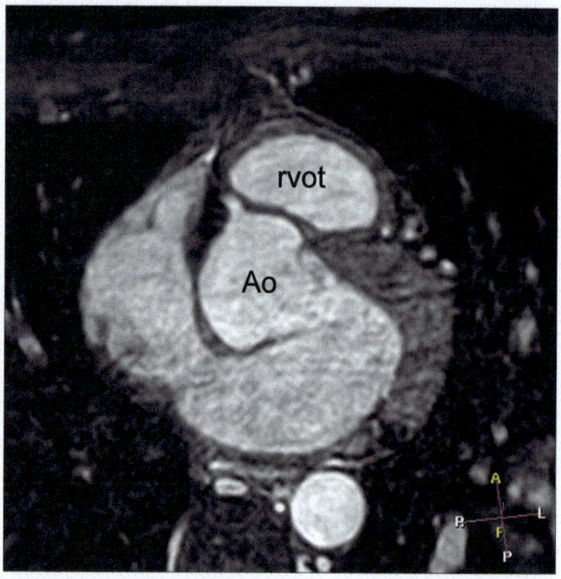

Fig. 9 Infundibulum. Transverse image using 3D bright-blood imaging with submillimeter spatial resolution. The right ventricular outflow tract (*rvot*) is characterized by a complete, thin muscular ring. *Ao* aorta

"septophilic". The lining of the chamber becomes smooth in the infundibulum, a funnel leading to the exit from the chamber, the pulmonary trunk. The normal right ventricle is a relatively thin-walled chamber with an end-diastolic wall thickness of 3–4 mm. Towards the RV apex, there is often a thinning of the free wall which is not to be mistaken for a wall thinning such as found in arrhythmogenic RV cardiomyopathy/dysplasia (see "Heart Muscle Diseases"). Although the RV free wall is considerably thicker than that of the right atrium, it is thinner than the wall of the left ventricle. These relative thicknesses reflect the range of pressures in the chambers. In the right atrium the pressure is usually close to 0 mm Hg, in the right ventricle the pressure rises up to about 25 mm Hg, while in the left ventricle the peak pressure is about 120 mm Hg.

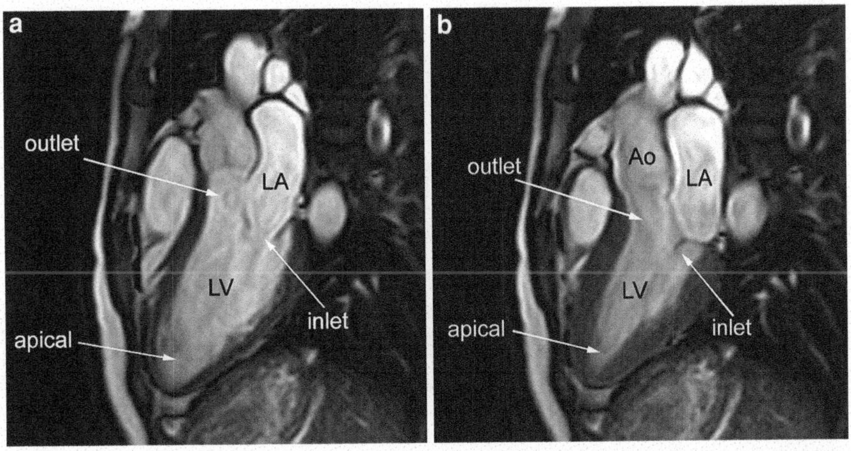

Fig. 10 Components of the left ventricle. Left ventricular inflow–outflow tract flow view at end diastole (**a**) and end systole (**b**), using bright-blood imaging. *Ao* aorta; *LA* left atrium

The complex cardiac anatomy of the morphological right ventricle is best studied using a combination of different imaging planes, i.e., transverse or horizontal long-axis views in combination with short-axis views and/or RV outflow tract views. Other interesting planes to study the right ventricle are described in "Cardiovascular MR Imaging Planes and Segmentation". RV enlargement reduces the retrosternal airspace. Because this space is normally limited, RV enlargement can also displace the left ventricle leftward and posteriorly, and the apex of the heart up and back, lifting the apex of the heart off the hemidiaphragm on the frontal chest radiograph.

4.2.2 Morphological Left Ventricle

The morphological left ventricle in a normal heart is a thick-walled chamber that forms the apex and lower part of the left and posterior heart border. The exterior of the left ventricle is shaped like a cone. Internally, the left ventricle is demarcated by its fine trabeculations, which are numerous, fine muscular projections. Like its morphological right counterpart, the morphological left ventricle also possesses an inlet, an apical trabecular, and an outlet portion. The inlet component contains the mitral valve (or left ventiular (LV) valve) and extends from the atrioventricular junction to the attachments of the prominent papillary muscles (Fig. 10). The most characteristic anatomic feature of the mitral valve is that it has no chordal attachments to the ventricular septum. There are two papillary muscles, the anterior lateral and the posterior medial (Fig. 11). Notably, the papillary muscles do not attach to the septum (Anderson 2000). Since the LV papillary muscles are large and arise only from the free wall surface, this makes left ventriculotomy difficult, except at the apex or at the high paraseptal area. In addition to the anterior descending branch of the left coronary artery (LCA), which externally marks the location of the anterior portion of the ventricular septum, anterior and posterior obtuse marginal branches of the LCA course across the LV free wall. Also known as diagonals, these branches supply the large papillary muscles and the adjacent LV free wall. The apical trabecular portion is the most characteristic feature of the morphological left ventricle which contains the fine characteristic trabeculations. The smooth septal surface also helps in identification, since the morphological left ventricle never possesses a septomarginal trabeculation or a moderator band (Fig. 12). While intracavitary muscular bands are always present on the right as the moderator band, sometimes thin intraventricular strands can be found in the LV apex, known as false tendons. The outlet part, with the aortic valve, is in direct continuity with the inlet part, since normally there is little or no conal musculature beneath the aortic valve, which results in aortic-mitral fibrous continuity. The outlet portion of the left ventricle is distinguished by its abbreviated nature. Two of the three leaflets of the aortic valve have muscular attachments to the outlet component. The remainder of the leaflets take origin from the fibrous tissue of the aortic root, part of this being the extensive area of fibrous continuity with the aortic leaflet of the mitral valve. This fibrous continuity is called mitral-aortic intervalvular fibrosa. It is the posterior aspect of the roof of the outlet,and is therefore particularly short. There is no muscular segment of the

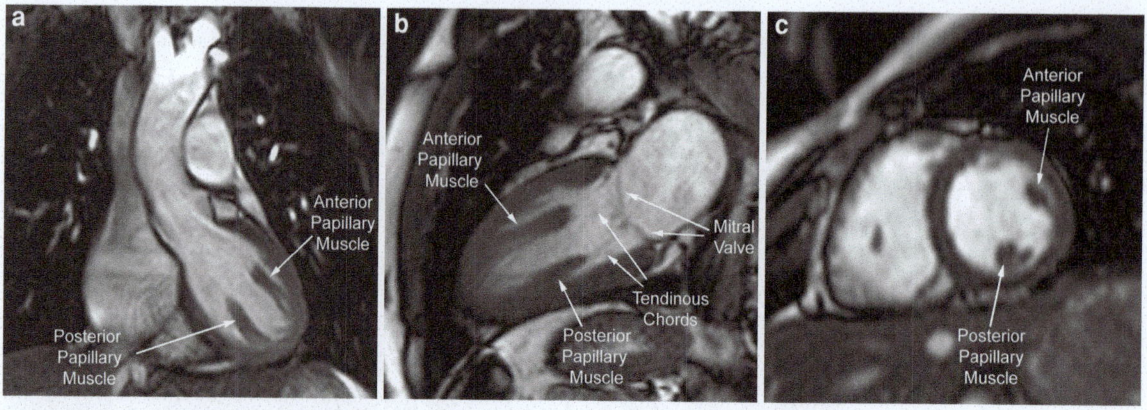

Fig. 11 Left ventricular papillary muscles. Left ventricular outflow tract (**a**) vertical long-axis (**b**) and midventricular short-axis (**c**) view, using bright-blood imaging. The papillary muscles are well depicted as intracavitary structures attached to the posterior(medial) and anterior(lateral) LV wall. Their fibrous extensions, i.e., tendinous chords, towards the mitral valve can be seen on high-quality MR images. Note that the LV septal surface on the short-axis view is free of muscular attachments

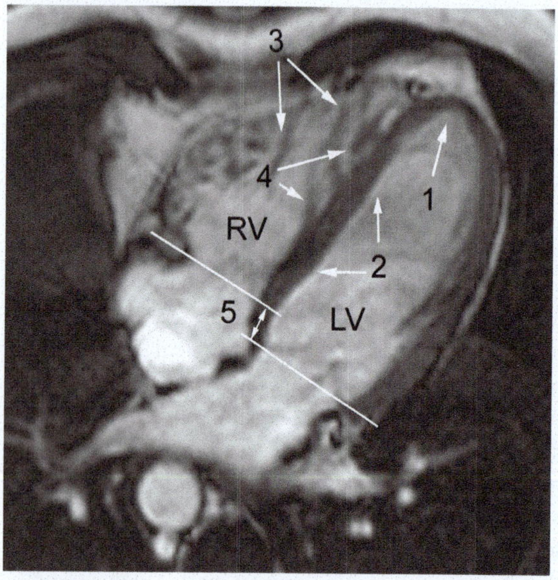

Fig. 12 Essential characteristics of the morphological right and left ventricle. Horizontal long-axis view using bright-blood imaging. Five essential differences can be seen on this image: *1* fine apical trabeculations in LV apex; *2* LV septal surface free of muscular insertions; *3* rough apical trabeculations in RV apex; *4* muscular insertions on RV septal surface; *5* tricuspid valve more apically positioned than mitral valve. *LV* left ventricle; *RV* right ventricle

ventriculoinfundibular fold in the left ventricle separating the arterial and the RV valves. The morphologic left ventricle is usually studied along the three intrinsic cardiac axes, i.e., short-axis, horizontal long-axis, and vertical long-axis views. Other interesting imaging planes are the LV outflow tract view and the LV inflow- and outflow tract view. These imaging planes are particularly interesting in patients with obstructive hypertrophic cardiomyopathy or to depict aortic regurgitation. Wall thicknesses are not uniform throughout the left ventricle. The most pronounced differences are found in the longitudinal direction with a gradual wall thinning toward the LV apex. Compared with the lateral LV wall segments (i.e., end-diastolic wall thickness: 7–8 mm in women, 8–9 mm in men) the LV apex is extremely thin (approximately 3 mm) (see Fig. 10). Less pronounced variations in wall thickness are seen around the LV circumference (Bogaert and Rademakers 2001). LV enlargement enlarges inferiorly and to the left, displacing the left lung.

4.2.3 Ventricular Septum

The ventricular or interventricular septum separates the left from the right ventricle. It is mainly a thick-walled muscular layer, except in the subaortic region where it becomes very thin ("membranous septum"). It contains muscular fibers coming from the LV as well as from the RV free wall. The position and shape of the ventricular septum are determined by the loading conditions. In the unloaded condition the ventricular septum has a flat appearance. In normal loading conditions the septum has a convex shape towards the right ventricle, and this shape is maintained during the cardiac cycle. Enhanced RV filling, as during onset of inspiration, may lead to a slight

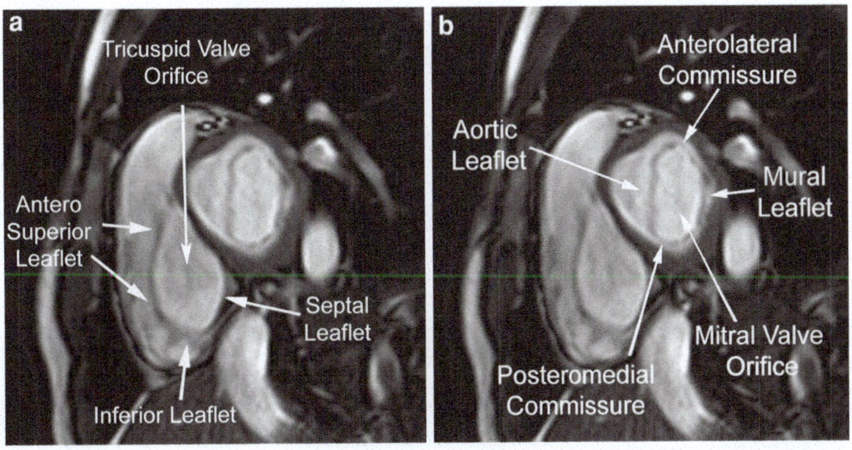

Fig. 13 **a, b** Tricuspid and mitral valve. Short-axis view through atrioventricular valves, using bright-blood imaging during diastole. The leaflets, commissures, and valve orifices can be well appreciated when the valves are opened

flattening of the ventricular septum during early diastolic filling. This phenomenon is called ventricular coupling (see "Cardiac Function" and "Pericardial Disease"). In several cardiac and extracardiac diseases, a pathologic ventricular coupling may occur (e.g., constrictive pericarditis, cor pulmonale, atrial septal defects, severe pulmonary incompetence, pulmonary hypertension). The ventricular septum is best studied in short- and horizontal long-axis views. As with the atrial septum, a diagnosis of septal defect cannot be made on the basis of this morphologic (i.e., black-blood imaging) finding alone and additional bright-blood and flow measurements should be obtained to make a definite diagnosis.

4.3 Valves

Two atrioventricular (AV) (or ventricular) valves connect the atria to the ventricles, a mitral and a tricuspid valve. Embryologically, the mitral valve is always connected to the morphologic left ventricle, while the tricuspid valve is connected to the morphologic right ventricle. There is a difference in positioning along the longitudinal cardiac axis between both valves. The tricuspid valve is always somewhat more apically positioned than the mitral valve, a feature that is very helpful in differentiating the ventricular morphology.

The RV (AV) valve or tricuspid valve, has three leaflets, these being the septal, inferior, and anterosuperior leaflets (Fig. 13). The muscular support of the tricuspid valve is made up of the anterior muscle which is the largest and usually arises from the septomarginal trabeculation. The complex of chords supporting the anteroseptal commissure is dominated by the medial papillary muscle (of Lancisi), a relatively small muscle which arises either as a single band or as a small sprig of chords from the posterior limb of the septomarginal trabeculation (Anderson 2000). The inferior muscle, the smallest of the three, is usually single, and may be represented by several small muscles.

The LV (AV) valve or mitral valve, has aortic and mural leaflets, so named because of their relationship with the leaflets of the aortic valve and the parietal atrioventricular junction, respectively (Fig. 13). The zone of apposition between the two leaflets has anterolateral and posteromedial ends, the so-called commissures, each supported by one of the paired LV papillary muscles embedded in the anterolateral and posteromedial walls of the left ventricle.

The semilunar valves of both great arteries attach across the anatomic ventriculoarterial junction and therefore lack a fibrous supporting annulus such as supports the atrioventricular valves. They have no chordal attachments. The pulmonary artery normally arises from the infundibulum of the right ventricle. The leaflets of the pulmonary and triscupid valves are widely separated by the infundibular musculature. The aortic valve cusps are usually described according to the origin of the coronary arteries—left, right, and noncoronary, although they may also be called anterior, and right and left posterior (Fig. 14). Each valve cusp has a small nodule of connective tissue at its midpoint. When the great arteries are normally related, the noncoronary left coronary commissure of the aortic valve sits directly above the middle of the

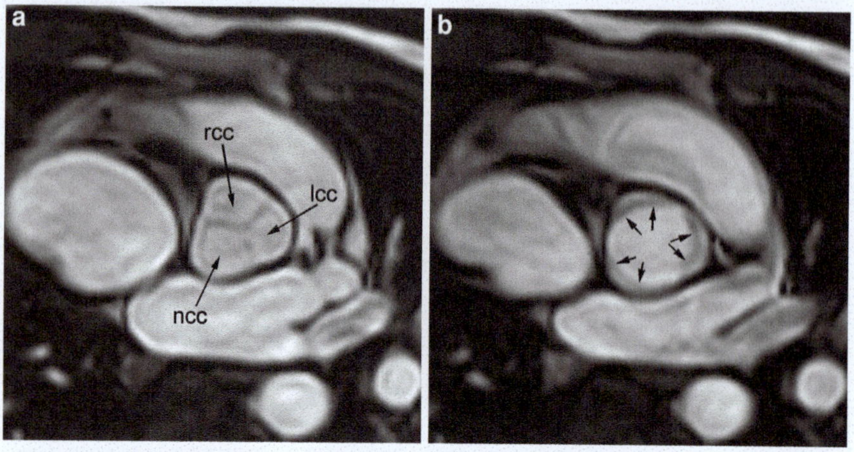

Fig. 14 Aortic valve cusps in closed (**a**) and open (**b**) conditions using bright-blood imaging. The right coronary (*rcc*), left coronary (*lcc*), and noncoronary (*ncc*) cusps in closed condition are similar to a "Mercedes Benz"star. At maximal opening during systole, the cusps are nearly completely apposed to the wall of sinus of Valsalva

anterior mitral leaflet. The noncoronary right coronary commissure sits directly above the membranous septum, which in turn is located directly above the left bundle branch of the conduction system.

Because of their fibrous nature, dark-blood imaging is not ideal to visualize cardiac valves and to study valve pathology. Although they are often seen on dark-blood imaging, especially when in closed position, appreciation of small changes in thickness, structure, and integrity are difficult to appreciate. Bright-blood imaging shows valve leaflet morphology, valve leaflet motion, abnormal valve opening, and valvular flow patterns very well (de Roos et al. 1995). The cardiac valves are best studied in specific imaging planes perpendicular or longitudinally oriented to the valve of interest (see "Cardiovascular MR Imaging Planes and Segmentation").

4.4 Coronary Arteries

Two of the sinuses of Valsalva give rise to coronary arteries. These sinuses are the ones adjacent to the pulmonary truncus.

The right coronary artery (RCA) arises from an ostium located just below the sinotubular junction, in the middle of the right (anterior) sinus of Valsalva (Fig. 15). The RCA courses into the right atrioventricular groove and provides nutrient branches to the infundibulum (infundibular or conal branch) and to the RV free wall (Angelini et al. 1999). The extension, and thus the myocardial perfusion territory of the RCA are highly variable. It may stop proximally in the right atrioventricular groove or may continue into the posterior interventricular groove to the apex or to the left atrioventricular groove ending in the posterolateral LV branch. Occasionally it might extend up to the LAD. In nearly 85–90% of cases, it is normal for the RCA to provide a posterior descending branch that follows the posterior atrioventricular groove as far as the apex of the heart but not beyond (dominant RCA), thus supplying the inferoseptal part of the LV myocardium. In only 5%, the LCx continues as a posterior descending artery (dominant LCx), while in 10% of cases, both the right coronary artery and left circumflex supply the inferior wall (balanced pattern).

The LCA originates from the middle portion of the left anterior sinus of Valsalva, just below the sinotubular junction (Fig. 15). The proximal vessel originating from the left ostium, called the left main stem (LM) or trunk, is only a short conductive arterial segment (± 1 cm) from which the LCx and LAD arteries normally spring. The LAD courses in the anterior interventricular groove, the LCx in the left atrioventricular groove. The LAD gives off branches to both the septum (perforator branches) and the anterolateral wall of the left ventricle (diagonal branches), and the LCx produces branches to the posterolateral wall of the left ventricle, including the posteromedial papillary muscle. The LAD terminates at the cardiac apex, or 1–2 cm before or after the apex. The perforators originate from the LAD at a grossly perpendicular angle and these branches immediately become intramural, coursing within the septum (see "Coronary Artery Disease"). The MRI techniques as well as the ideal imaging planes to study the coronary arteries are described in detail in " Cardiovascular MR Imaging Planesand Segmentation" and "Coronary Artery Disease".

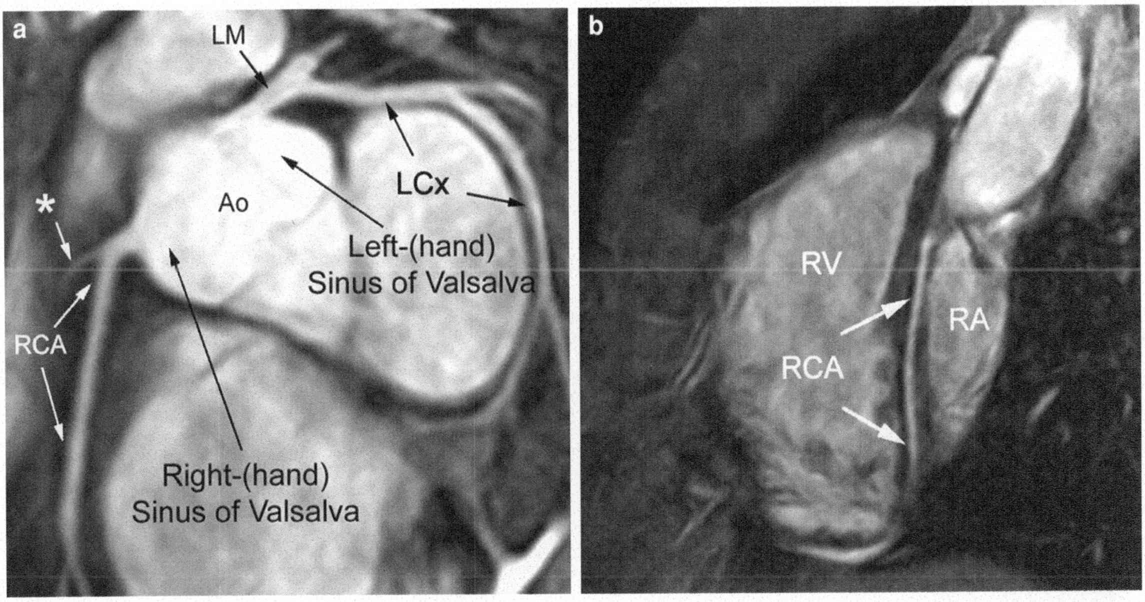

Fig. 15 **a, b** Origin and proximal course of coronary arteries. Short-axis view through the aortic root (**a**) and oblique view through anterior (or right) atrioventricular groove, using 3D bright-blood imaging with submillimeter spatial resolution. (**b**) The right coronary artery (*RCA*) and LCA originate from the right- and left sinus of Valsalva, respectively. The major arteries as well as several branches can be readily depicted. This subject has a *LCx* dominant system. *Ao* aorta; *LM* left main stem coronary artery; *RA* right atrium; *RV* right ventricle; star, conal branch

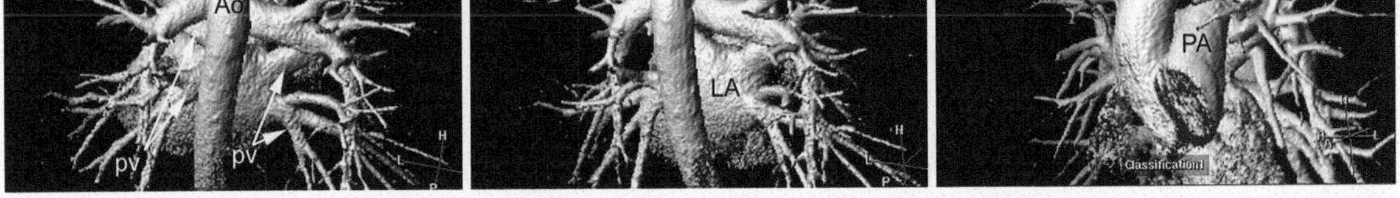

Fig. 16 **a-c** Great vessels of the thorax and neck. 3D ceMRA using maximum intensity projection view, posterior–anterior view (**a**) posterior–anterior view with slightly oblique inclination (**b**) anterior–posterior view (**c**) the aorta (*Ao*), the brachiocephalic vessels (right brachiocephalic trunc (*tbc*), right subclavian artery (*rsa*), right common coronary artery (*rcca*), left common coronary artery (*lcca*), left subclavian artery (*lsa*), and left vertebral artery (*lva*)), the pulmonary artery (*PA*) and its major branches (*pa*) as well as the pulmonary veins (*pv*) entering the left atrium (*LA*) are clearly depicted

4.5 Pericardium

The pericardium envelops the heart and the origin of the great vessels and consists of an outer fibrous layer (the fibrous pericardium) and an inner serous sac (the serous pericardium). This fibrous part is attached to the sternum and diaphragm. The serous pericardium consists of an inner visceral layer (the epicardium), which is intimately connected to the heart and the epicardial fat, and an outer parietal layer, which lines the fibrous pericardium. The visceral layer is reflected from the heart and the root of the great vessels onto the inner surface of the fibrous pericardium to become continuous with the parietal layer. The pericardial cavity lies between these two layers of the serous pericardium. Two serosal tunnels can be identified: the transverse sinus, posterior to the great arteries and anterior to the atria and the superior vena cava, and the oblique sinus, posterior to the left atrium (Groell et al. 1999). The transverse sinus is divided into the following four recesses: the superior aortic recess, inferior aortic recess, left pulmonic recess, and right pulmonic recess. Pericardial sinuses and recesses are frequently depicted on cardiac MR images. Knowledge of their locations is helpful in the differentiation of normal pericardium from pericardial effusions and mediastinal processes such as lymph nodes. Under physiologic conditions, it contains 20–25 ml of serous fluid; however, the amount of fluid may vary considerably among individuals, particularly in children and infants. These differences may explain, at least in part, why in some patients, sinuses or recesses may or may not be seen. Moreover, clinically asymptomatic patients can have large pericardial fluid collections, especially when it accumulates over long periods, and it may be found incidentally. On MR images, the normal pericardial sac is visible as a very thin curvilinear structure of low signal intensity surrounded by the high-intensity mediastinal and (sub)epicardial fat (Sechtem et al. 1986a, 1986b). The pericardium is best visualized over the right heart and cardiac apex, while it is often invisible along the LV free wall, where it is interposed between the myocardium and the low-intensity left lung. In normal subjects, the pericardium has a thickness of 1.2 ± 0.5 mm in diastole and 1.7 ± 0.5 mm in systole (Sechtem et al. 1986a). Similar results (i.e., 1.7 mm, range 1.5–2.0 mm) were found by Bogaert and Duerinckx 1995, evaluating the normal appearance of the pericardium on bright-blood MRI used to visualize coronary arteries. These values exceed the thickness of 0.4–1.0 mm reported for anatomic measurements of pericardial thickness. The layer of normal pericardial fluid present in the pericardial space has also a low intensity, and it likely contributes to the overall pericardial thickness as visualized by MRI. Because MRI is sensitive to the small amount of normal pericardial fluid and depicts its anatomic distribution, it should be valuable in the detection and quantification of even small pericardial effusions (see "Pericardial Disease"). In patients with constrictive pericarditis, Sechtem et al. (1986a) found a pericardial thickness of more than 4 mm. Recent studies, however, have shown that constrictive pericarditis might be present in patients with a normal or near normal pericardial thickness at surgery (Talreja et al. 2003). Thus, in the absence of a thickened pericardium, other diagnostic criteria are needed to differentiate constrictive pericarditis patients from restrictive cardiomyopathy patients. A combination of transverse or long-axis imaging planes and short-axis views ensures the best approach for studying the entirety of the pericardial sac.

Fig. 17 **a–t** Transverse images. *aavg* anterior (or right) atrioventricular groove; *amvl* anterior mitral valve leaflet; *Ao* aorta; *apm* anterior papillary muscle; *av* aortic valve; *azv* azygos vein; c carina; *cs* coronary sinus; *ct* crista terminalis; *Es* esophagus; *ev* Eustachian valve; *ft* false tendon; *gcv* great cardiac vein; hazv hemiazygos vein; *hv* hepatic vein; *ias* interatrial septum; ib intermediate bronchus; *IVC* inferior vena cava; *ivs* interventricular septum; *LA* left atrium; *laap* left atrial appendage; *lcca* left common carotid artery; *liv* left innominate, (or brachiocephalic) vein; *llb* left lower lobe bronchus; *lmb* left main stem bronchus; *lpa* left pulmonary artery; *lsa* left subclavian artery; *LV* left ventricle; *lvot* left ventricular outflow tract; *maif* mitral aortic intervalvular fibrosa; *mb* moderator band; *PA* pulmonary artery (or trunk); *pmvl* posterior mitral valve leaflet; *ppm* posterior papillary muscle; *ps* pericardial sac; *pv* pulmonary vein; *RA* right atrium; *raap* right atrial appendage; *rbca* right brachiocephalic artery; *rca* right coronary artery; *rcv* right cardiac vein; *riv* right innominate (or brachiocephalic) vein; *rmb* right main stem bronchus; *rpa* right pulmonary artery; *RV* right ventricle; *rvap* right ventriular apex; *rvot* right ventricular outflow tract; *SVC* superior vena cava; *T* trachea; *tv* tricuspid valve ▶

5 Great Vessels

The aorta has its origin from the center point of the base of the heart and curves upwards to the aortic arch, where the brachiocephalic vessels have their origin. The junction between the aortic root containing the sinuses of Valsalva and the ascending aorta is called the sinotubular junction. The course of the aortic arch as well as the branching pattern of the brachiocephalic vessels, can be subject to a large number of congenital variations (see "Congenital Heart Disease" and "Great Vessels"). The most frequent presentation is a left-sided aortic arch running over the main stem bronchus with following branching pattern: right brachiocephalic trunk, left common carotid artery, and finally left subclavian artery (Fig. 16). The leaflets of the aortic valve are supported by the three sinuses of Valsalva.

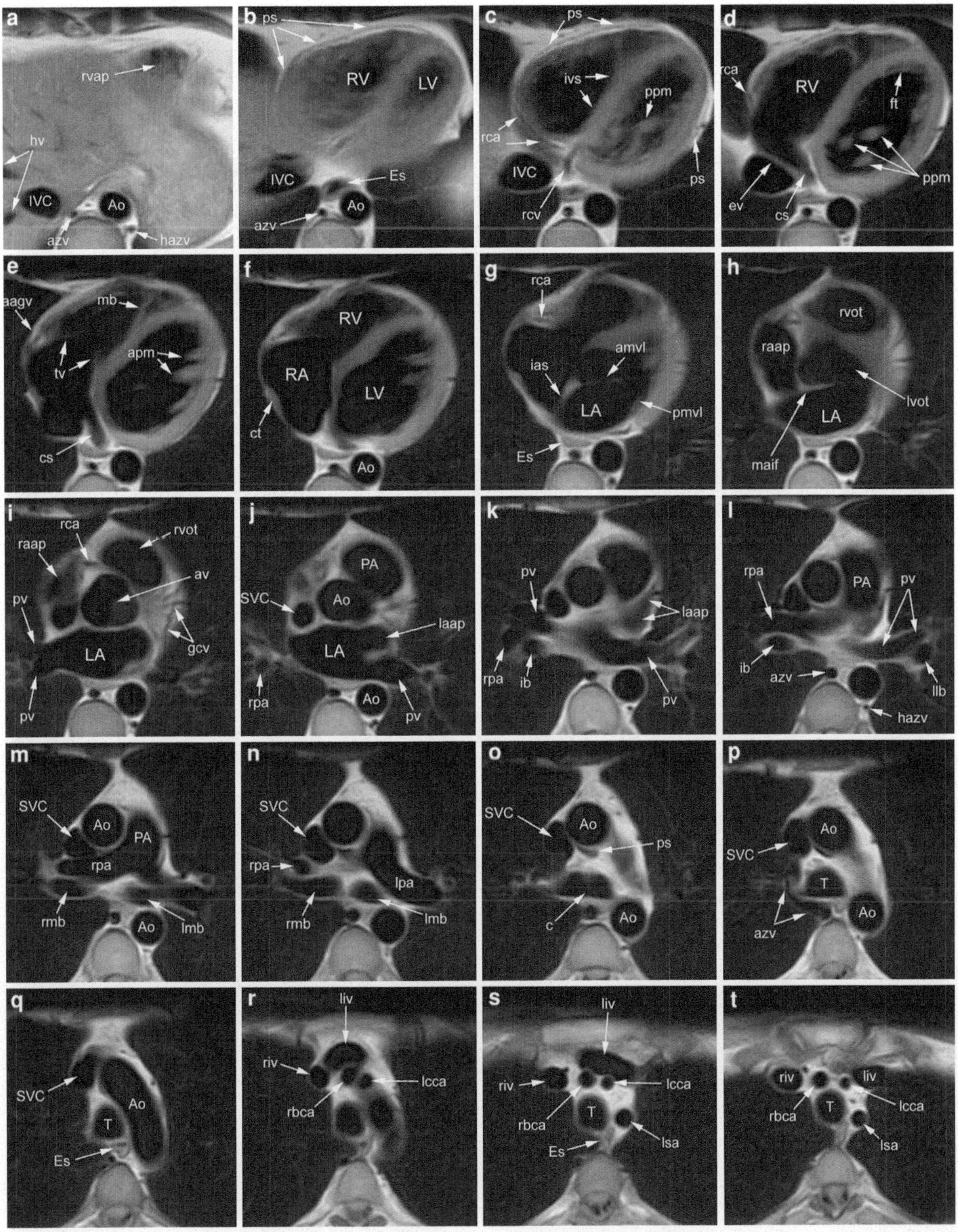
a
rvap
hv
IVC
Ao
azv
hazv
b
ps
RV
LV
IVC
Es
Ao
azv
c
ps
ivs
ppm
rca
IVC
rcv
ps
d
rca
RV
ft
ev
cs
ppm
e
aagv
mb
tv
apm
cs
f
RV
RA
LV
ct
Ao
g
rca
amvl
ias
LA
pmvl
Es
h
rvot
raap
lvot
LA
maif
i
rca
raap
rvot
av
pv
LA
gcv
pv
j
PA
SVC
Ao
laap
LA
rpa
Ao
pv
k
pv
laap
rpa
ib
pv
l
rpa
PA
pv
ib
azv
llb
hazv
m
SVC
Ao
PA
rpa
rmb
Ao
lmb
n
SVC
rpa
lpa
rmb
lmb
o
SVC
Ao
ps
c
Ao
p
Ao
SVC
T
azv
Ao
q
SVC
Ao
T
Es
r
liv
riv
lcca
rbca
s
liv
riv
lcca
rbca
T
Es
lsa
t
riv
liv
rbca
T
lcca
lsa

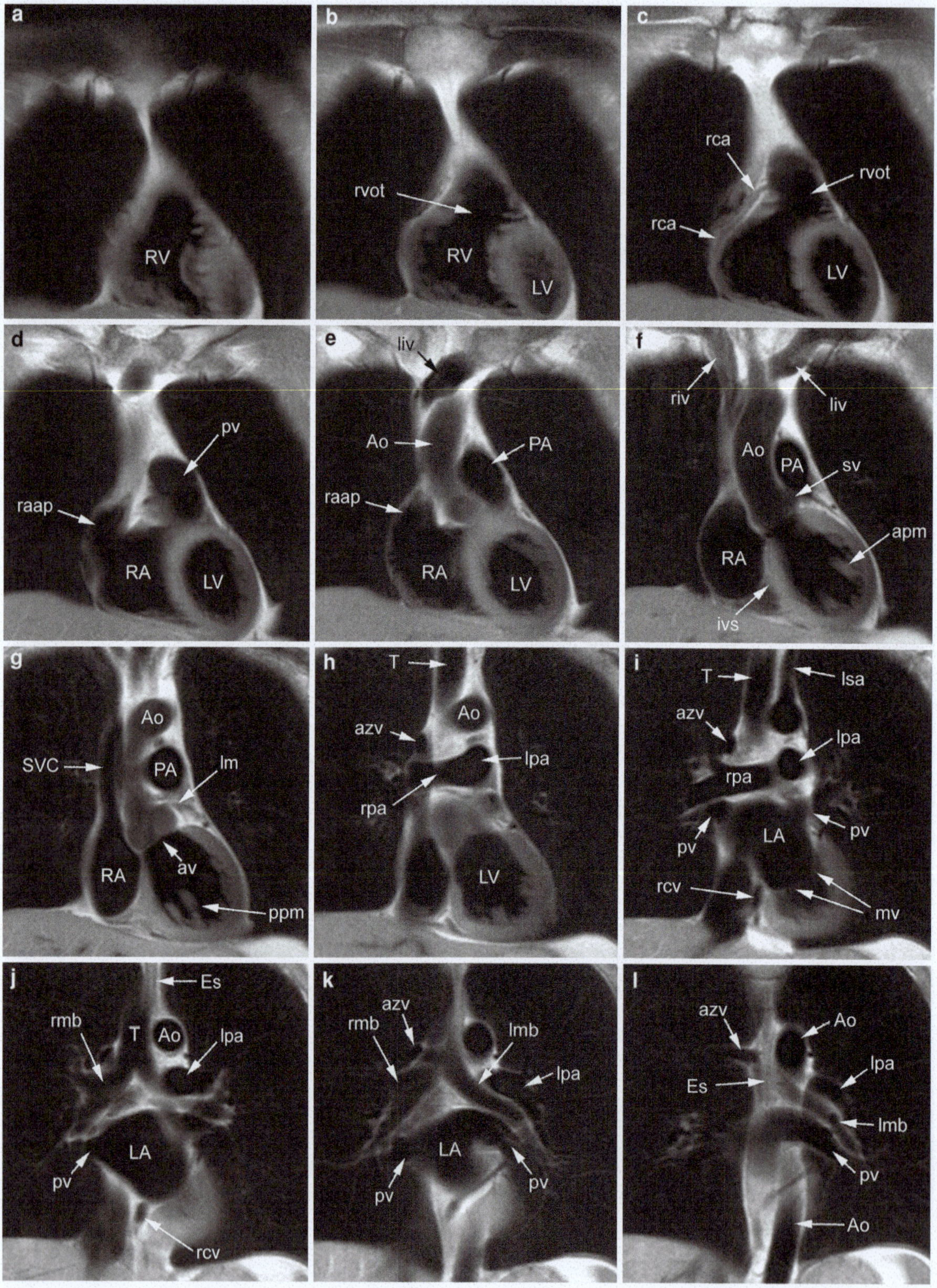

Fig. 18 **a–l** Coronal images. *lm* left main stem coronary artery; *mv* mitral valve; *sv* sinus of valsalva; other abbreviations as in Fig. 17

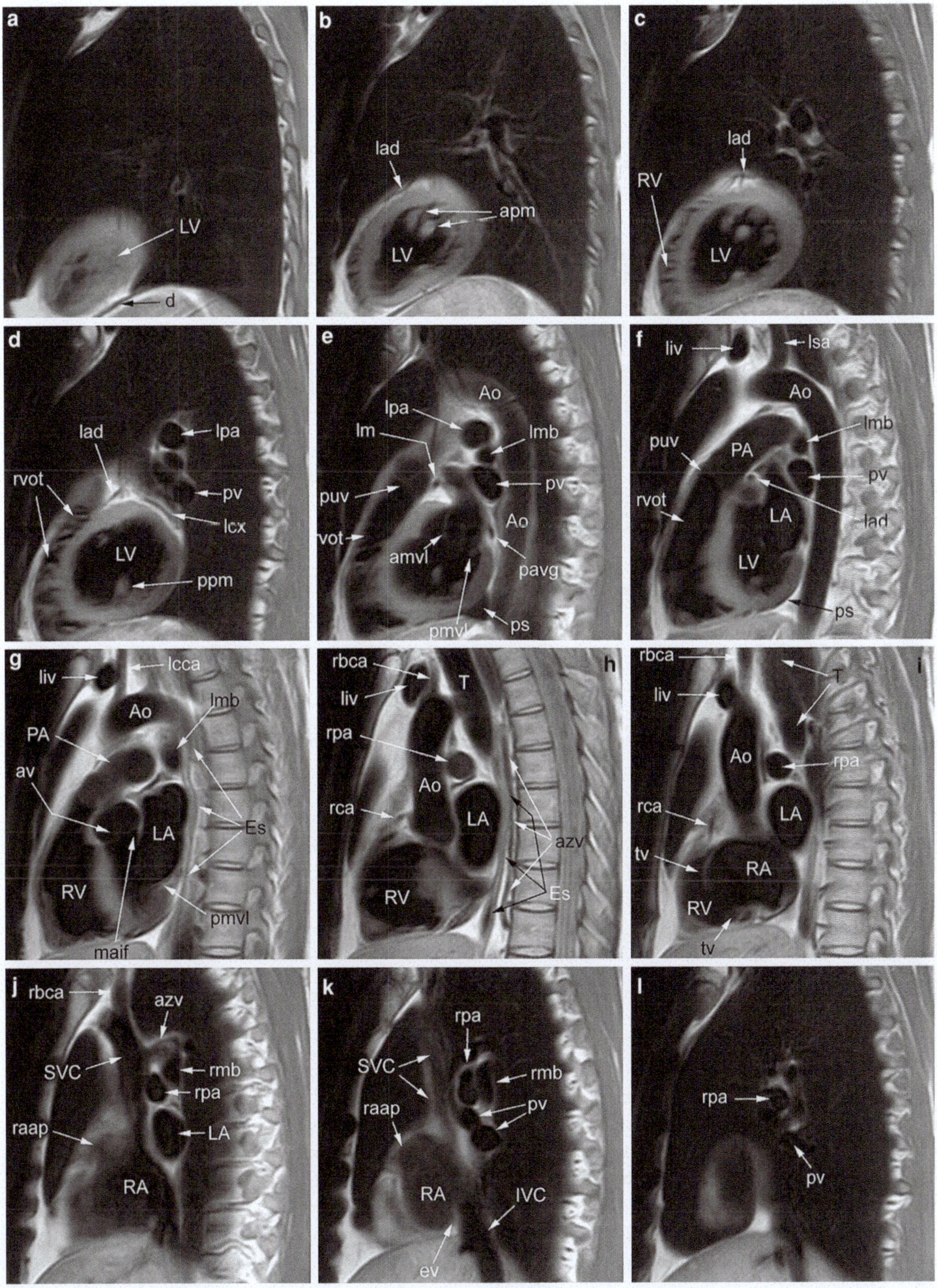

Fig. 19 **a–l** Sagittal images. *lad* left anterior descending coronary artery; *lcx* left circumflex artery; *pavg* posterior (or left) atrioventricular groove; *puv* pulmonary valve; *sv* sinus of valsalva; other abbreviations as in Fig. 17

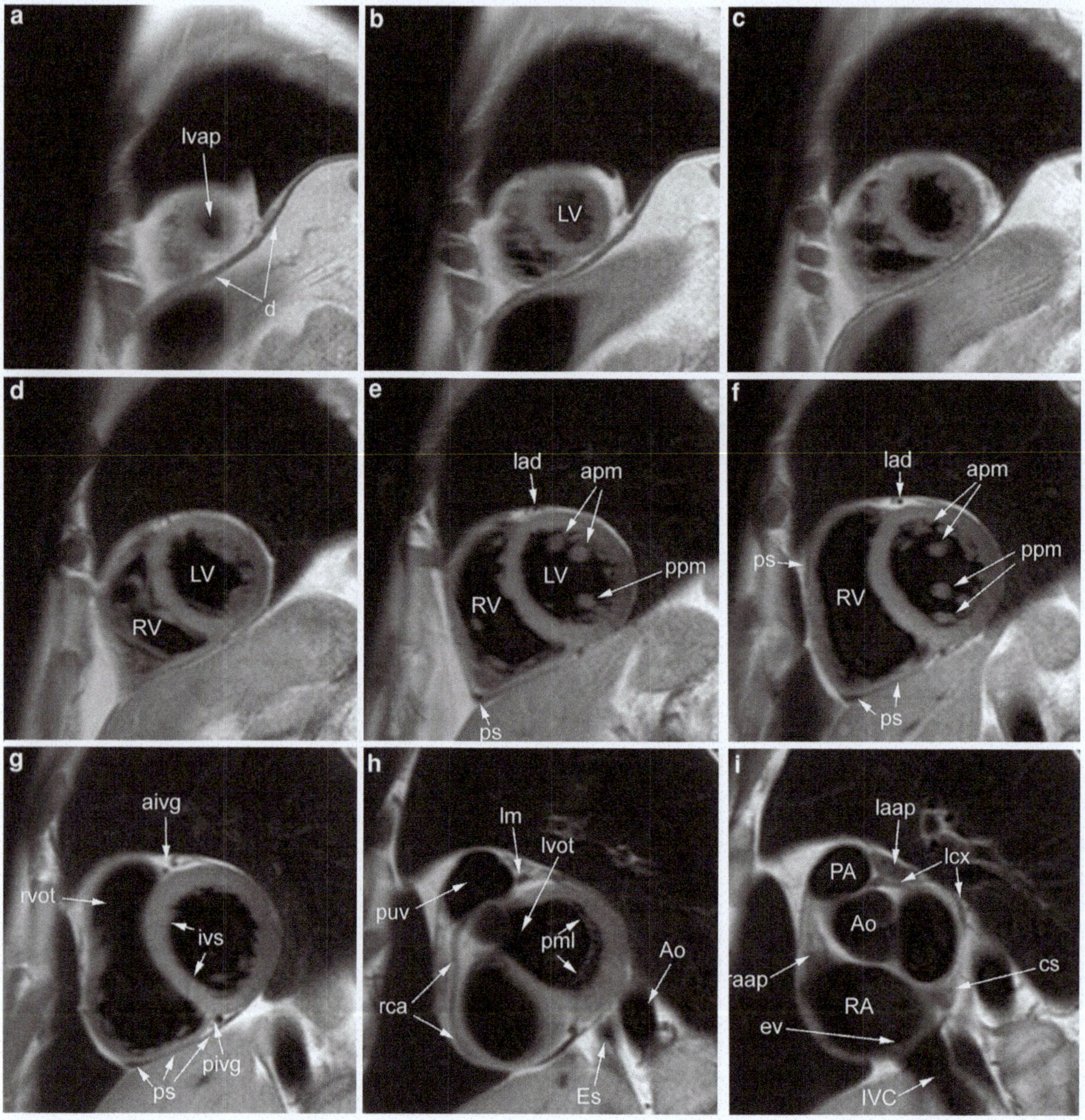

Fig. 20 **a–i** Short-axis images. *aivg* anterior interventricular groove; *d* diaphragm; *lvap* LV apex; *pivg* posterior interventricular groove; other abbreviations as in preceding figures

The pulmonary trunk originates from the muscular pulmonary infundibulum, to its bifurcation into the right and left pulmonary arteries. Two of the sinuses of the pulmonary truncus are always next to the aorta (also called facing sinuses), while the third sinus is non-facing. The ligamentum arteriosus, a fibrous remnant of the arterial duct (or "ductus arteriosus") extends from the pulmonary trunk into the descending aorta. The aortic isthmus is defined as the segment between the site of takeoff of the left subclavian artery and the aorta insertion of the duct. A combination of different imaging planes is recommended to study the thoracic great vessels.

Systemic venous return flow to the heart through the superior and inferior caval veins (venae cavae), which lie on the right side of the spine. The superior caval vein is formed by the confluence of the right and left innominate veins, which lie in front of the brachiocephalic artery. The inferior vena cava has only a small intrathoracic portion. After receiving the hepatic veins

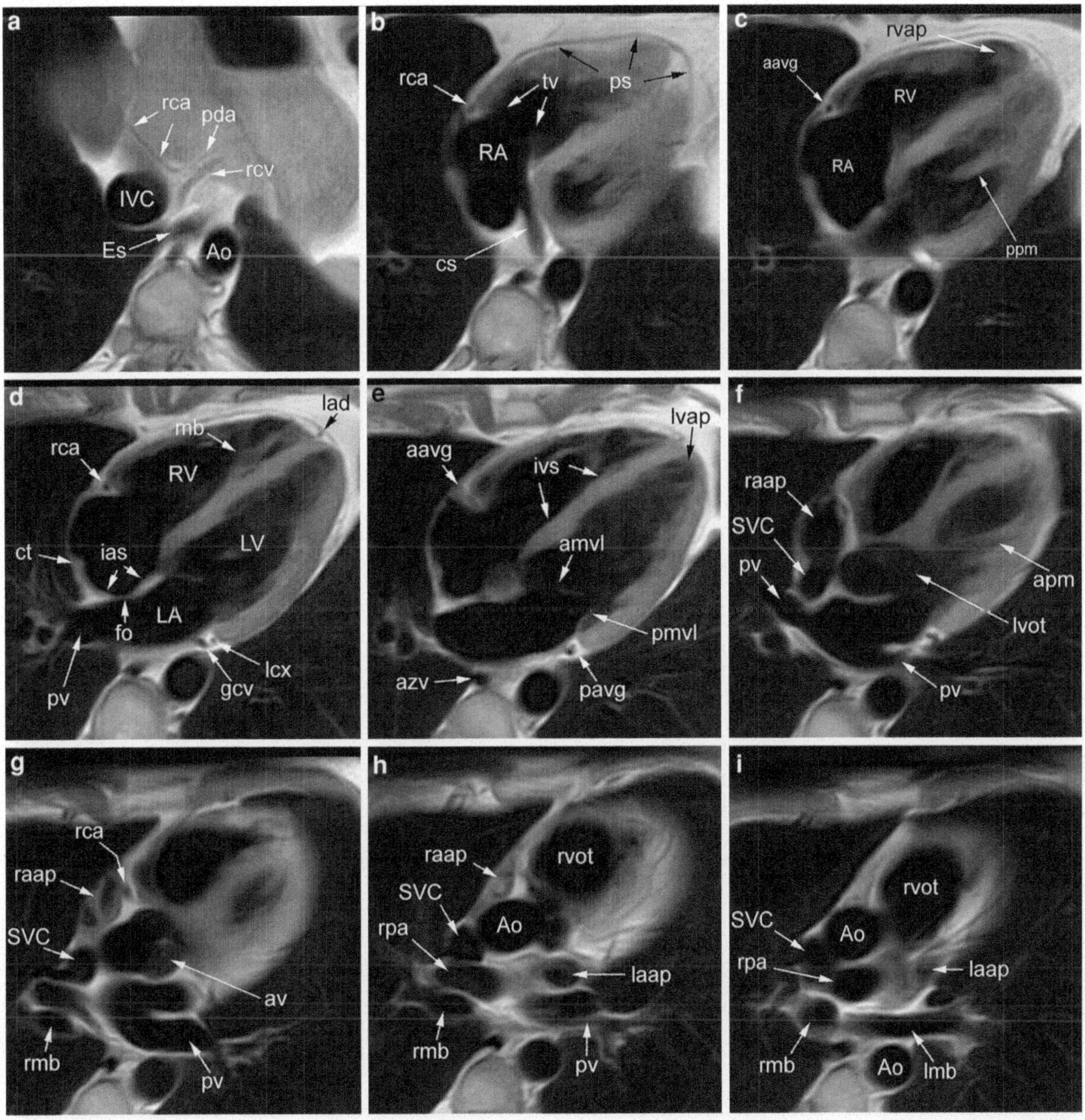

Fig. 21 **a–i** Horizontal long-axis images. *fo* fossa ovalis; *pda* posterior descending artery. Other abbreviations as in preceding figures

it crosses the diaphragm to enter the posterior aspect of the right atrium.

There are two right and left pulmonary veins, joining the posterior aspect of the left atrium (Fig. 16). The right pulmonary veins enter close to the atrial septum. In patients with an atrial septal defect the pulmonary venous blood from the right lung drains preferentially into the right atrium. The two left pulmonary veins frequently join the left atrium as a single trunk. On the other hand, the pulmonary vein draining the right middle lobe may enter separately the left atrium.

The great vessels are usually studied using a combination of dark-blood and bright-blood techniques in different imaging planes. This combination of sequences is the best guarantee to see as well the vessel wall and para-aortic tissues. Often, PC-MRI is used to calculate the flow patterns in blood vessels.

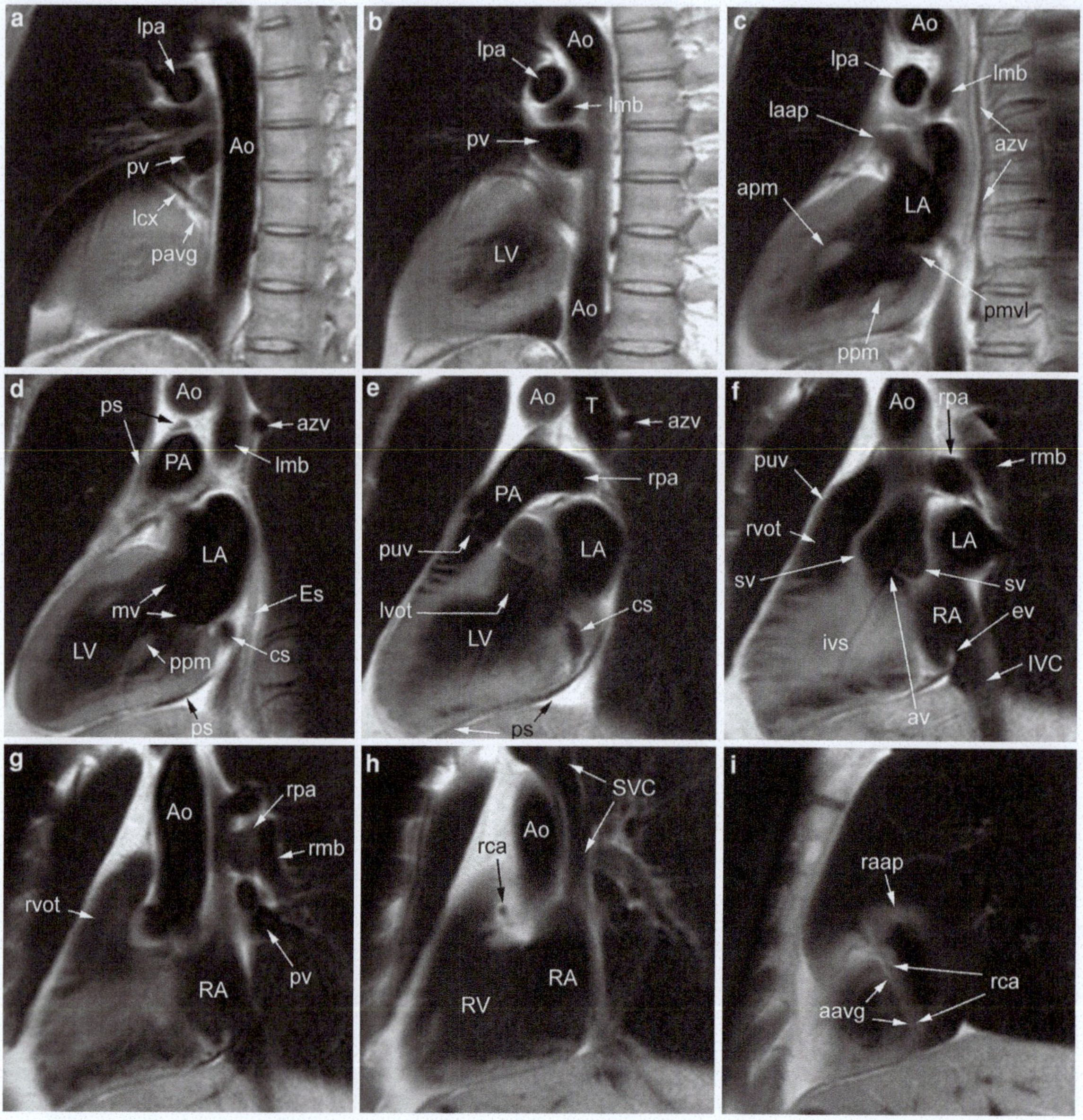

Fig. 22 **a–i** Vertical long-axis images. Abbreviations as in preceding figures

A good imaging plane to start with is the transverse imaging plane. Abnormalities in the course and dimensions of the great vessels are readily depicted in this imaging plane. However, to obtain accurate dimensions, an imaging plane perpendicular to the long-axis of the vessel should be used. Additional imaging in other planes is often necessary to better depict the vascular abnormality (e.g., aortic coarctation) or to better visualize the consequences of valvular pathology on vascular structures (e.g., post-stenotic aortic dilatation). The outflow tract of the right ventricle, the pulmonary trunk, and its bifurcation are well depicted on transverse images, while specific imaging planes in a parasagittal plane through the left and right pulmonary branches can be used for cine imaging and flow measurements (Paz et al. 1993; Murray et al. 1994; Bouchard et al. 1985). Although the thoracic aorta can be visualized over its

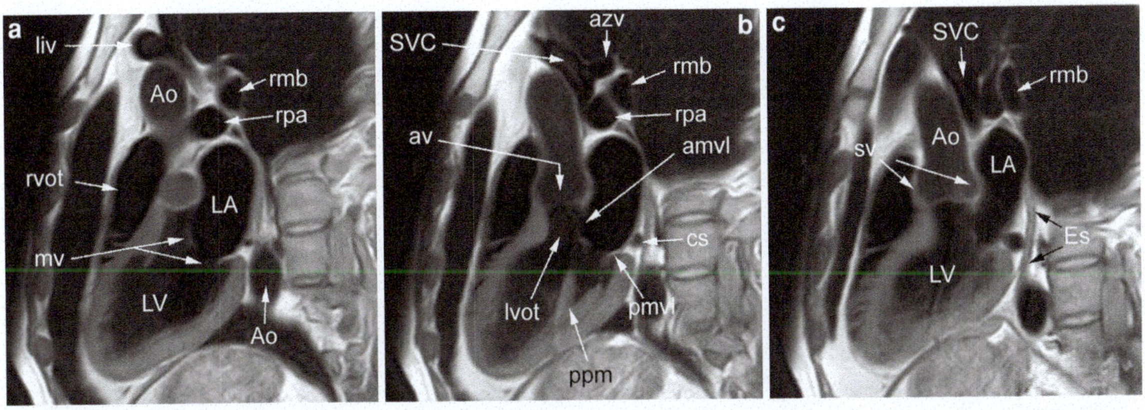

Fig. 23 **a-c** Left ventricular outflow tract images. Abbreviations as in preceding figures

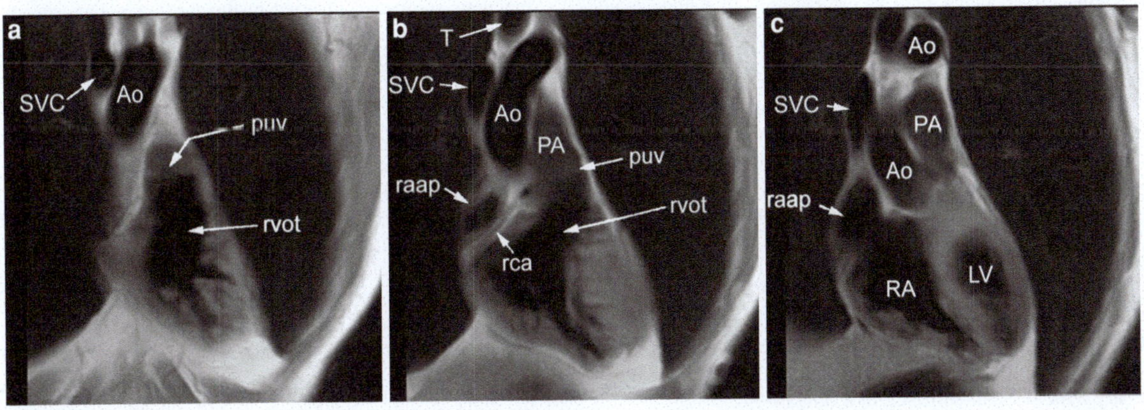

Fig. 24 **a-c** Right ventricular outflow tract images. Abbreviations as in preceding figures

entire course (Friedmann et al. 1985; Byrd et al. 1985; Dinsmore et al. 1986), it is often not possible to achieve this in a single plane, because the aortic arch usually does not fall in the same plane as the ascending and descending aorta. With the advent of 3D ceMRA, depiction of thoracic vessels has been greatly facilitated (Prince 1996).

6 Key Points

- MRI is an excellent technique to evaluate cardiac anatomy, at least if the image acquisition and image interpretation are performed adequately.
- A combination of dark-blood and bright-blood imaging is advisable to appropriately study cardiac anatomy.
- Moreover, a combination of imaging in different cardiac imaging planes is always helpful to better depict cardiac anatomy.
- Always combine morphologic evaluation with functional evaluation of the heart.
- For accurate measurements of dimensions, use imaging planes perpendicular to the structure of interest, e.g., myocardial wall, ventricular cavity, vessel lumen.
- Use of a systematic approach to analyze cardiac anatomy.
- Each of the components of the heart has its specific characteristics, enabling to unravel the most complex congenital cardiopathies.
- The mitral valve is always connected to the morphological left ventricle, while the tricuspid valve is connected to the morphological right ventricle.

The tricuspid valve is more apically positioned than the mitral valve.

- The moderator band always belongs to the morphological right ventricle.
- The septal surface of the LV cavity is smooth, and has no insertions of muscular structures.

References

Amplatz K, Moller JH (eds) (1993) Cardiac anatomy. In: Radiology of congenital heart disease. Mosby Year Book, St-Louis, pp 13–48

Anderson RH (2000) The anatomic structure of the normal heart, and the structure of congenitally malformed hearts. A handbook prepared to support the foundation course in cardiac morphology held at the Institute of Child Health University College London on 10th and 11th Feb 2000, UK pp 2–24

Angelini P, Villason S, Chan AV Jr, Diez JG (1999) Normal and anomalous coronary arteries in humans In: Angelini P (ed) Coronary artery anamalies. A comprehensive approach. Lippincott Williams & Wilkins, Philadelphia, pp 27–79

Bogaert J, Duerinckx AJ (1995) Appearance of the normal pericardium on coronary MR angiograms. J Magn Reson Imaging 5:579–587

Bogaert J, Rademakers FE (2001) Regional nonuniformity of the normal adult human left ventricle. A 3D MR myocardial tagging study. Am J Physiol 280:H610–H620

Bouchard A, Higgins CB, Byrd BF, Amparo EP, Osaki L, Axelrod R (1985) Magnetic resonance imaging in pulmonary hypertension. Am J Cardiol 56:938–942

Burbank F, Parish D, Wexler L (1988) Echocardiographic-like angled views of the heart by MR imaging. J Comput Assist Tomogr 12:181–195

Byrd FB, Schiller NB, Botvinick EH, Higgins CB (1985) Normal cardiac dimensions by magnetic resonance imaging. Am J Cardiol 55:1440–1442

Carr JC, Simonetti O, Bundy J et al (2001) Cine MR angiography of the heart with segmented true fast imaging with steady-state precession. Radiology 219:828–834

Castillo E, Bluemke DA (2003) Cardiac MR imaging. Radiol Clin North Am 41:17–28

de Roos A, Doornbos J, van der Wall EE, van Voorthuisen AE (1995) Magnetic resonance of the heart and great vessels. Nat Med 1:711–713

Dinsmore RE, Wismer GL, Levine RA, Okada RD, Brady TJ (1984) Magnetic resonance imaging of the heart: positioning and gradient angle selection for optimal imaging planes. Am J Roentgenol 143:1135–1142

Dinsmore RE, Liberthson RR, Wismer GL et al (1986) Magnetic resonance imaging of the thoracic aorta in long and short axis planes: comparison with other techniques in patients with aortic aneurysms. Am J Roentgenol 146:309–314

Friedmann BJ, Waters J, Kwan OL, De Maria AN (1985) Comparison of magnetic resonance imaging and echocardiography in determination of cardiac dimensions in normal subjects. J Am Coll Cardiol 5:1369–1376

Galjee MA, Van Rossum AC, van Eenige MJ et al (1995) Magnetic resonance imaging of the pulmonary venous flow pattern in mitral regurgitation. Independence of the investigated vein. Eur Heart J 16:1675–1685

Groell R, Schaffler GJ, Rienmueller R (1999) Pericardial sinuses and recesses: findings at electrocardiographically triggered electron-beam CT. Radiology 212:69–73

Hawkes RC, Holland GN, Moore WS, Roebuck EJ, Worthington BS (1981) Nuclear magnetic resonance (NMR) tomography of the normal heart. J Comput Assist Tomogr 5:605–612

Heneghan MA, Biancaniello TM, Heidelberger E, Peterson SB, Marsh MJ, Lauterbur PC (1982) Nuclear magnetic resonance zeugmatographic imaging of the heart: application to the study of ventricular septal defect. Radiology 143: 183–186

Herfkens RJ, Higgins CB, Hricak H et al (1983) Nuclear magnetic resonance imaging of the cardiovascular system: normal and pathologic findings. Radiology 147:749–759

Higgins CB, Lanzer P, Stark D et al (1985) Assessment of cardiac anatomy using nuclear magnetic resonance imaging. J Am Coll Cardiol 5:77S–81S

Higgins CB, Holt W, Pfugfelder P, Sechtem U (1988) Functional evaluation of the heart with magnetic resonance imaging. Magn Reson Med 6:121–139

Meier RA, Hartnell GG (1994) MRI of right atrial pseudo masses. Is it really a diagnostic problem? J Comput Assist Tomogr 18:398–402

Menegus MA, Greenberg MA, Spindola-Franco H et al (1992) Magnetic resonance imaging of suspected atrial tumors. Am Heart J 123:1260–1268

Mirowitz SA, Gutierrez FR (1992) Fibromuscular elements of the right atrium: pseudomass at MR imaging. Radiology 182:231–233

Mohiaddin RH, Amanuma M, Kilner PJ, Pennell DJ, Manzara C, Longmore DB (1991) MR phase-shift velocity mapping of mitral and pulmonary venous flow. J Comput Assist Tomogr 15:237–243

Murray TI, Boxt LM, Katz J, Reagan K, Barst RJ (1994) Estimation of pulmonary artery pressure in patients with primary pulmonary hypertension by quantitative analysis of magnetic resonance images. J Thorac Imaging 9: 198–203

O'Donovan PB, Ross JS, Sivak ED, O'Donnell JK, Meaney TF (1984) Magnetic resonance imaging of the thorax: the advantages of coronal and sagittal planes. Am J Roentgenol 143:1183–1188

Paz R, Mohiaddin RH, Longmore DB (1993) Magnetic resonance assessment of the pulmonary arterial trunk anatomy, flow, pulsatility and distensibility. Eur Heart J 14: 1524–1530

Prince MR (1996) Body MR angiography with gadolinium contrast agents. Magn Reson Imaging Clin N Am 4:11–24

Sechtem U, Tscholakoff D, Higgins CB (1986a) MRI of the normal pericardium. Am J Roentgenol 147:239–244

Sechtem U, Tscholakoff D, Higgins CB (1986b) MRI of the abnormal pericardium. Am J Roentgenol 147:245–252

Simonetti OP, Finn JP, White RD, Laub G, Henry DA (1996) "Black blood" T2-weighted inversion-recovery MR imaging of the heart. Radiology 199:49–57

Stehling MK, Holzknecht NG, Laub G, Bohm D, von Smekal A, Reiser M (1996) Single-shot T1- and T2-weighted magnetic resonance imaging of the heart with black blood: preliminary experience. Magma 4:231–240

Talreja DR, Edwards WD, Danielson GK et al (2003) Constrictive pericarditis in 26 patients with histologically normal pericardial thickness. Circulation 108:1852–1857

Winterer JT, Lehnhardt S, Schneider B et al (1999) MRI of heart morphology. Comparison of nongradient echo sequences with single-and multislice acquisition. Invest Radiol 34: 516–522

Cardiovascular MR Imaging Planes and Segmentation

A. M. Taylor and J. Bogaert

Contents

1	**Introduction**	93
2	**Imaging Planes for Cardiac Structures**	95
2.1	Body Axes	95
2.2	Cardiac Axes	95
2.3	Left Heart	96
2.4	Right Heart	98
3	**Imaging Planes for Great Vessels**	98
3.1	Aorta	99
3.2	Pulmonary Artery and its Branches	99
4	**Imaging Planes for Coronary Arteries**	102
5	**Interactive Imaging for Definition of Imaging Planes**	103
6	**Segmentation of the LV**	104
7	**Conclusion**	105
	References	106

A. M. Taylor (✉)
Centre for Cardiovascular Imaging,
UCL Institute of Cardiovascular Science
and Great Ormond Street Hospital for Children,
Great Ormond Street, WC1N 3JH, London, UK
e-mail: a.taylor@ich.ucl.ac.uk

J. Bogaert
Department of Radiology and Medical Imaging Research
Center (MIRC), University Hospitals Gasthuisberg,
Catholic University of Leuven, Herestraat 49,
3000 Leuven, Belgium

Abstract

Tomographic imaging of the human body is usually performed along orthogonal image planes (i.e., transverse, coronal, sagittal), but these axes are not well suited for imaging of the heart because of its complex orientation within the thoracic cage with the cardiac apex usually oriented leftward and downward. As a solution, image planes oriented along the long- and short-axis of the heart allow orthogonal imaging within the heart itself. Besides, specific image planes can be selected to appropriately study parts of the heart (e.g., cardiac valves), to evaluate the relation of the heart with the great vessels or to study the great vessels. In this chapter the different image planes to study the heart, coronary arteries and great vessels are explained in detail and a standardized approach is provided how to achieve starting from the body axes, the different image planes currently used in cardiac imaging. In the final section, the segmentation of the left ventricle using the 17-segment frame of reference is discussed.

1 Introduction

In general, structures within the body are described in relation to the "anatomical position" (subject standing upright, facing the observer). Thus, for axial cross-sectional body imaging (MR and CT) the convention is to describe the images as viewed from below as if facing the subject (i.e., subject's right is to the left of the image) (Fig. 1). This principle enables accurate description of the spatial relationship of

J. Bogaert et al. (eds.), *Clinical Cardiac MRI*, Medical Radiology. Diagnostic Imaging,
DOI: 10.1007/174_2011_333, © Springer-Verlag Berlin Heidelberg 2012

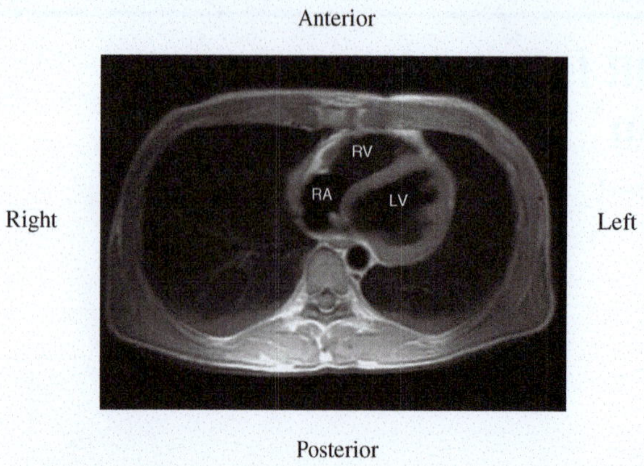

Fig. 1 Axial plane through the mid-thorax. Note that the right ventricle (RV) lies anterior and the left ventricle lies (LV) posterior. The right atrium (RA) is seen in this plane, but the left atrium lies superior and posterior, and is often not seen in the same axial plane as the RA (see "Cardiac Anatomy")

structures within the body in terms of right/left, inferior/superior and medial/lateral, and helps clinicians direct treatment, in particular when surgery is required.

The heart is the exception to this rule, with intracardiac anatomy described according to the axes of the heart, from the pathologist's perspective (heart positioned on its apex, with the atriums above the ventricles)—the so-called "Valentine" approach. Thus, though the ventricles are referred to as right and left, in the majority of subjects they occupy a more anterior and posterior position, respectively, in relation to the body axes on cross-sectional imaging.

Despite this anomaly, the heart will continue to be described in terms of reference to its own axes. In both echocardiography and nuclear scintigraphy the heart is imaged without reference to other structures, and the use of the cardiac axes enables standard points

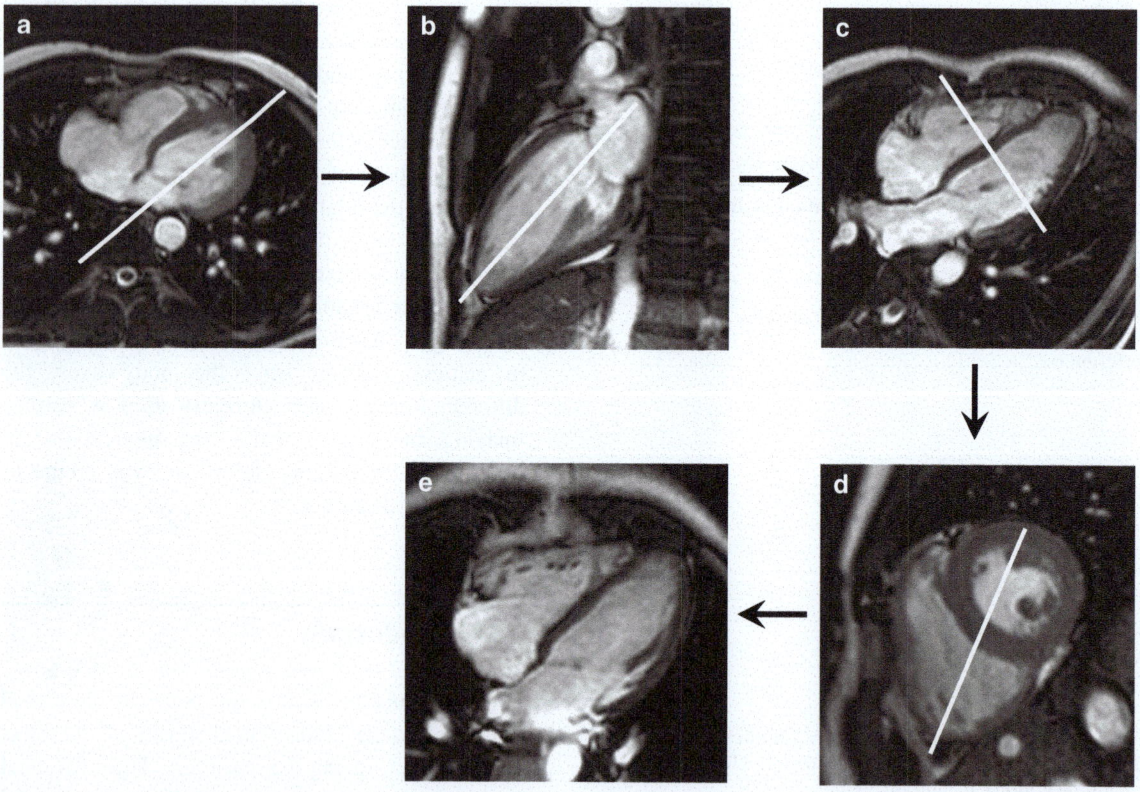

Fig. 2 Cardiac axis imaging planes for the left ventricle, images acquired using a SSFP sequence. The vertical long-axis plane (VLA) (**b**) is aligned from the axial plane (**a**) through the mitral valve and the LV apex, which may be on a separate more inferior slice. The horizontal long-axis plane (HLA) (**c**) is aligned from the VLA through the mitral valve and LV apex. The short-axis plane (SA) (**d**) is aligned from the VLA and HLA planes—perpendicular to both. The 4-chamber plane (**e**) is aligned from the SA through the anterior mitral valve papillary muscle and the apex of the RV

of reference to be maintained in these imaging modalities. Cross-sectional imaging modalities should also describe the heart in terms of this frame of reference (Cerqueira et al. 2002), though more conventional cross-sectional terms of reference can still be used when describing MR and CT images.

2 Imaging Planes for Cardiac Structures

2.1 Body Axes

The transverse or axial plane (Fig. 1) is useful for studying morphology and the relationships of the four cardiac chambers and the pericardium. Sagittal images (see Fig. 4.19) can be used to study the connections between the ventricles and the great vessels, while frontal or coronal images are most useful for investigation of the left ventricular outflow tract (LVOT), the left atrium and the pulmonary veins (see Fig. 4.18). The optimal planes also depend on the global positioning of the heart in the thorax, which is more vertical in young individuals and more diaphragmatic in the elderly. It has to be stressed that while these images are appropriate for evaluation of the overall morphology of the heart, quantitative measurements of wall thickness, cavity dimensions and functional data cannot be obtained accurately since the planes are not perpendicular to the wall or the cavity with the consequence that partial volume effects and obliqueness can introduce a large overestimation of the true dimensions. The cardiac imaging planes are more suitable for this purpose (Longmore et al. 1985).

2.2 Cardiac Axes

To obtain the correct inclinations for imaging in the cardiac axes, a transverse or axial scout view at the level of the left ventricle (LV) is acquired initially (Burbank et al. 1988). On this image, a new plane is chosen running through the apex of the LV and the middle of the left atrioventricular (AV), mitral valve. This yields the vertical long-axis (VLA) plane (Fig. 2b). On this image, a plane chosen to transect the LV apex and the middle of the mitral ring yields the horizontal long-axis (HLA) plane (Fig. 2c). The short-axis (SA) plane can now be prescribed perpendicular to both the VLA and HLA (Fig. 2d). From a SA plane at the level of the mitral valves, the four-chamber view can be acquired (4Ch). The plane for the 4Ch view passes from the most superior mitral valve, "anterolateral" papillary muscle to the inferior angle of the right ventricle (RV) anteriorly, usually through the mid-point of the interventricular septum (Fig. 2e). A true-SA plane can now be prescribed off the 4Ch view perpendicular to the interventricular septum. The inclination of SA slices is not always easy, since the anterior and inferior walls of the LV are not exactly parallel, and no single plane is absolutely perpendicular to both walls. A compromise can be made, by using a SA plane oriented parallel to the mitral valve ring. Furthermore, when a SA stack is being prescribed for ventricular volume calculations, the imaging plane is often best-positioned parallel to the AV valves, between the anterior and posterior AV grooves (Fig. 3).

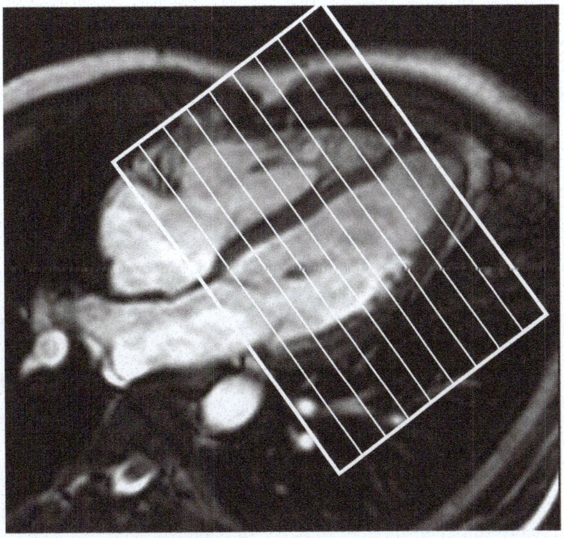

Fig. 3 Alignment of SA stack for analysis of ventricular volumes on the HLA. Note that the basal slice is parallel to the atrioventricular (AV) valves (between the anterior and posterior AV grooves), and almost perpendicular to the interventricular septum, though this can vary between subjects

Beside these standard cardiac imaging planes, specific planes can be chosen depending on the pathology under study. In congenital heart disease it may be necessary to obtain multiple non-classical imaging planes to achieve optimal visualization.

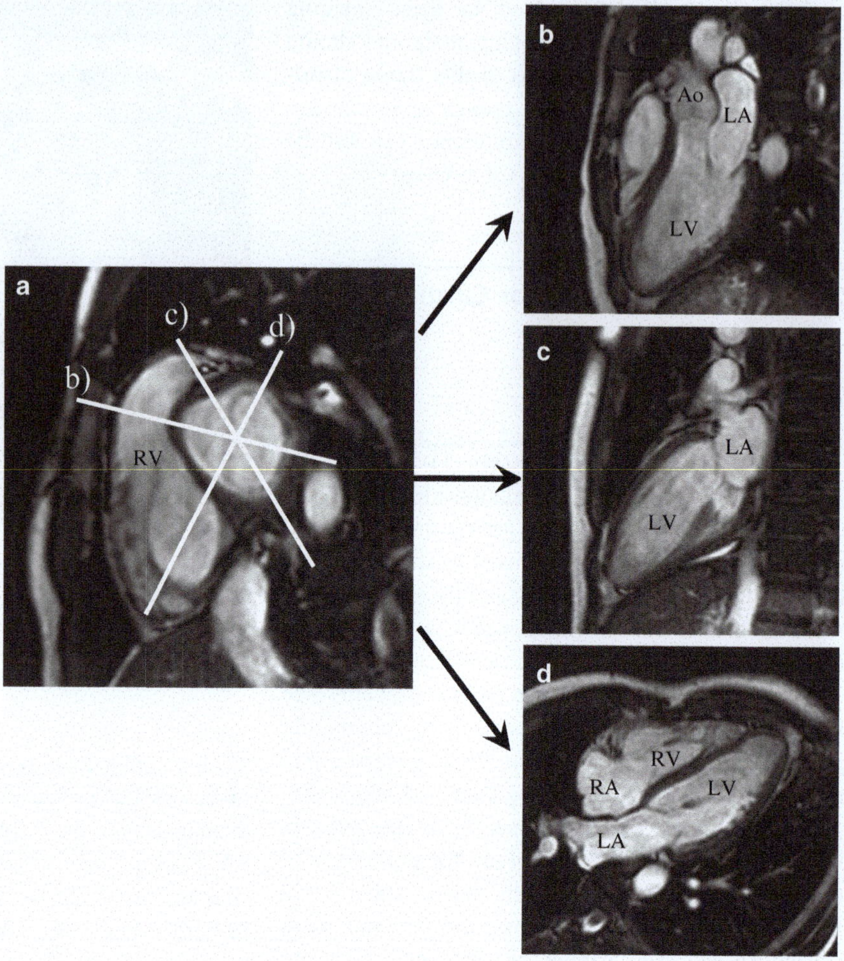

Fig. 4 Imaging planes that can be aligned from the basal SA slice (**a**): The LV inflow (mitral valve)/outflow (aortic valve) view (**b**), the VLA (**c**) and 4-chamber (**d**) views

2.3 Left Heart

From the SA plane the VLA, HLA and LV inflow/outflow (equivalent to the LV two-chamber long-axis view acquired at echocardiography) can be acquired (Fig. 4). This later LV inflow/outflow image is acquired with a plane that passes across the center of the aortic and mitral valves on the basal SA slice, or by performing a three point acquisition with the first point on the LV apex, the second in the center of the mitral valve and the third in the center of the aortic valve. This view is particularly useful for imaging septal hypertrophy and LVOT obstruction in hypertrophic cardiomyopathy. Since this view encompasses the LV inflow, concomitant mitral regurgitation in patients with LVOT obstruction can be easily depicted.

An LVOT view can be acquired by passing an imaging plane through and perpendicular to the aortic valve; oblique coronal orientation (Fig. 5b). This can be easily achieved by indicating on an LV inflow/outflow image a perpendicular imaging plane through the middle of the LVOT and aortic valve. Both the LVOT and LV inflow and outflow planes are well suited for evaluation of aortic valve stenosis and/or regurgitation. A plane through the aortic root ("aortic valve plane"), just above the aortic valve, perpendicular to both the LV inflow/outflow and LVOT views, can be used to assess through-plane aortic flow. This plane is used when quantifying aortic incompetence (Fig. 5). The morphology of the aortic valve (e.g., number of valve leaflets and fusion of leaflets), aortic valve area and orifice can be best studied in this plane using a set of adjacent slices through the aortic valve.

The mitral valve lies in a double oblique plane. Through-plane imaging of the mitral valve to assess

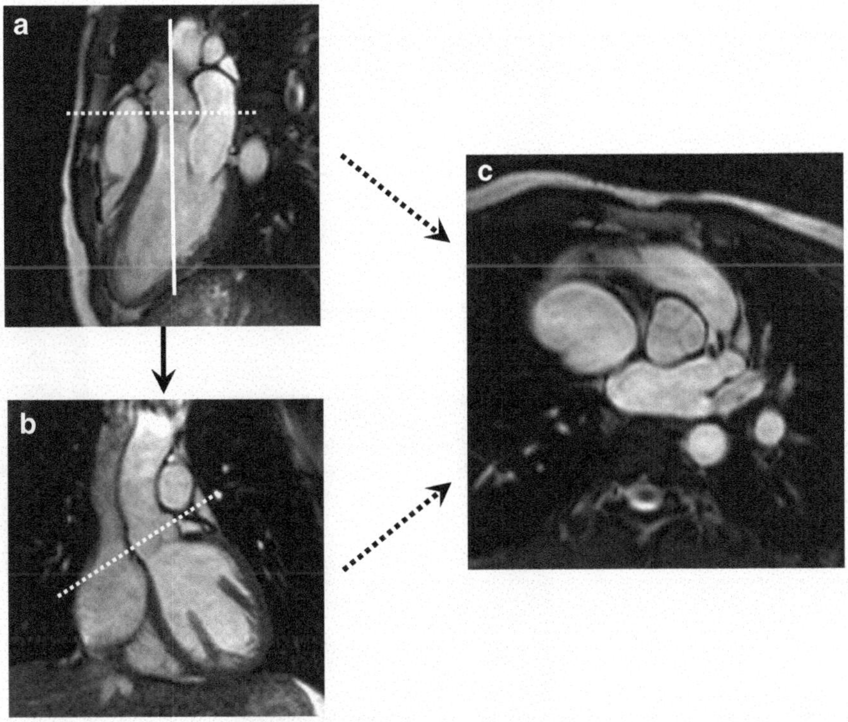

Fig. 5 Alignment of the aortic valve plane (**c**) for aortic flow assessment from the LV inflow/outflow (**a**) and the left ventricular outflow tract (LVOT) (**b**) views (*dotted lines*). The imaging plane should be placed just above the aortic valve, yet just below the origin of the coronary artery origins. The LVOT view is prescribed perpendicular to the LV inflow/outflow view (complete line on (**a**))

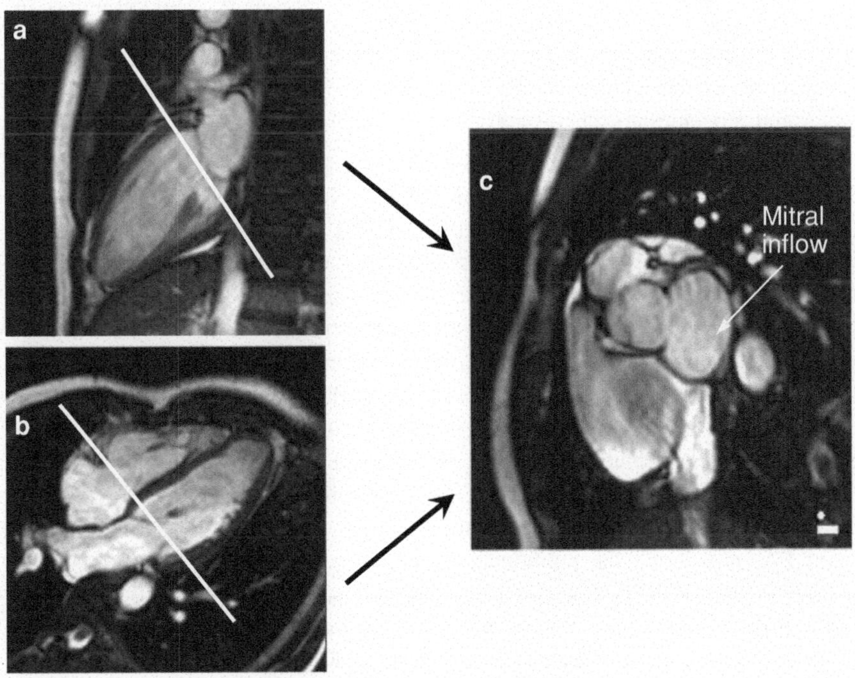

Fig. 6 Alignment of the mitral valve plane (**c**) for LV inflow assessment from the VLA (**a**) and the 4-chamber planes (**b**). The imaging plane should be placed just within the LV

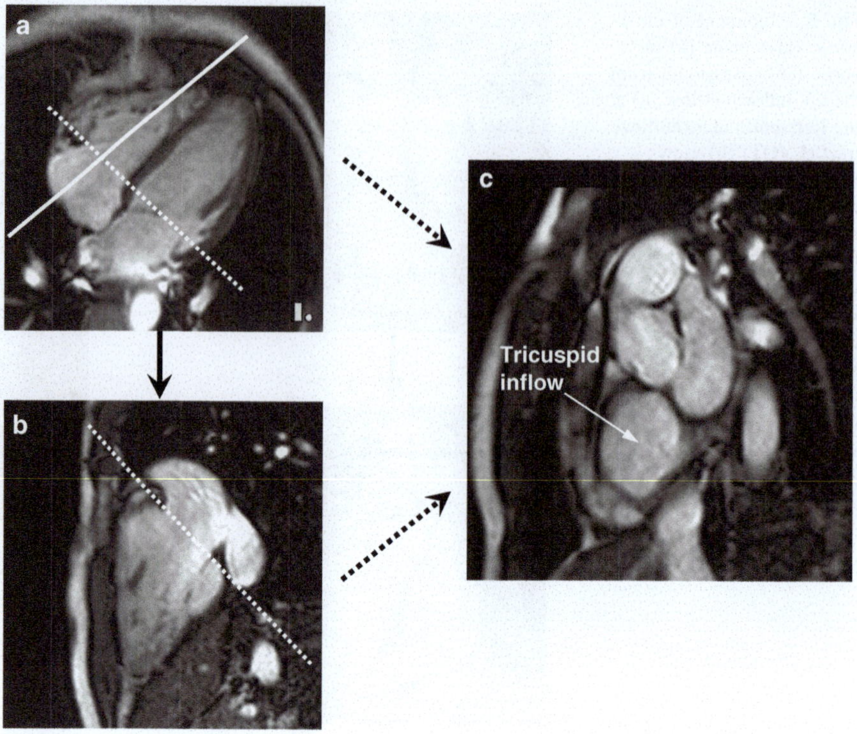

Fig. 7 Alignmentof the tricuspid valve plane (**c**) for RV inflow assessment from the VLA (**a**) and the 4-chamber planes (**b**). The imaging plane should be placed just within the RV

LV inflow curves should therefore be aligned from two views, the VLA and 4Ch (Fig. 6). For flow measurements, the plane should lie just beyond the mitral valve leaflets in the LV.

2.4 Right Heart

A two-chamber view of the right heart can be obtained by placing a plane through the RV apex and the mid-point of the tricuspid valve on the 4Ch view (Fig. 7). The right ventricular outflow tract (RVOT) is visualized by aligning a plane that passes through the main pulmonary artery (PA) and the RV inferiorly from a set of axial images (Fig. 8c). An alternative way to obtain the RVOT view is by aligning a plane that passes through the main PA and descending aorta. This is usually a sagittal or oblique-sagittal plane. A plane perpendicular to this, in an axial or oblique axial orientation, will give a second view through the RVOT (Fig. 8d). A plane through the main PA, just above the pulmonary valve, perpendicular to both RVOT views, can be used to assess through-plane pulmonary flow. This plane is used when quantifying pulmonary incompetence (Fig. 8e).

An inflow/outflow plane of the RV can be acquired using a three-point plan. The first point is placed on the tricuspid valve, the second on the RV apex and the third on the pulmonary valve (Fig. 9).

As with the mitral valve, the tricuspid valve lies in a double oblique plane. Through-plane imaging of the tricuspid valve to assess RV inflow curves should therefore be aligned from two views, the RV 2 chamber view and 4Ch view (Fig. 7c). For flow measurements, the plane should lie just beyond the tricuspid valve leaflets in the RV.

3 Imaging Planes for Great Vessels

When performing 2D imaging through any vessel, it is essential to image in two perpendicular planes to ensure that any narrowings are real and not secondary to partial volume effects.

Furthermore, care must be taken when performing breath-hold 2D acquisitions in the axial plane as varying degrees of breath-hold position may remove small structures from the imaging plane (Taylor et al. 1999).

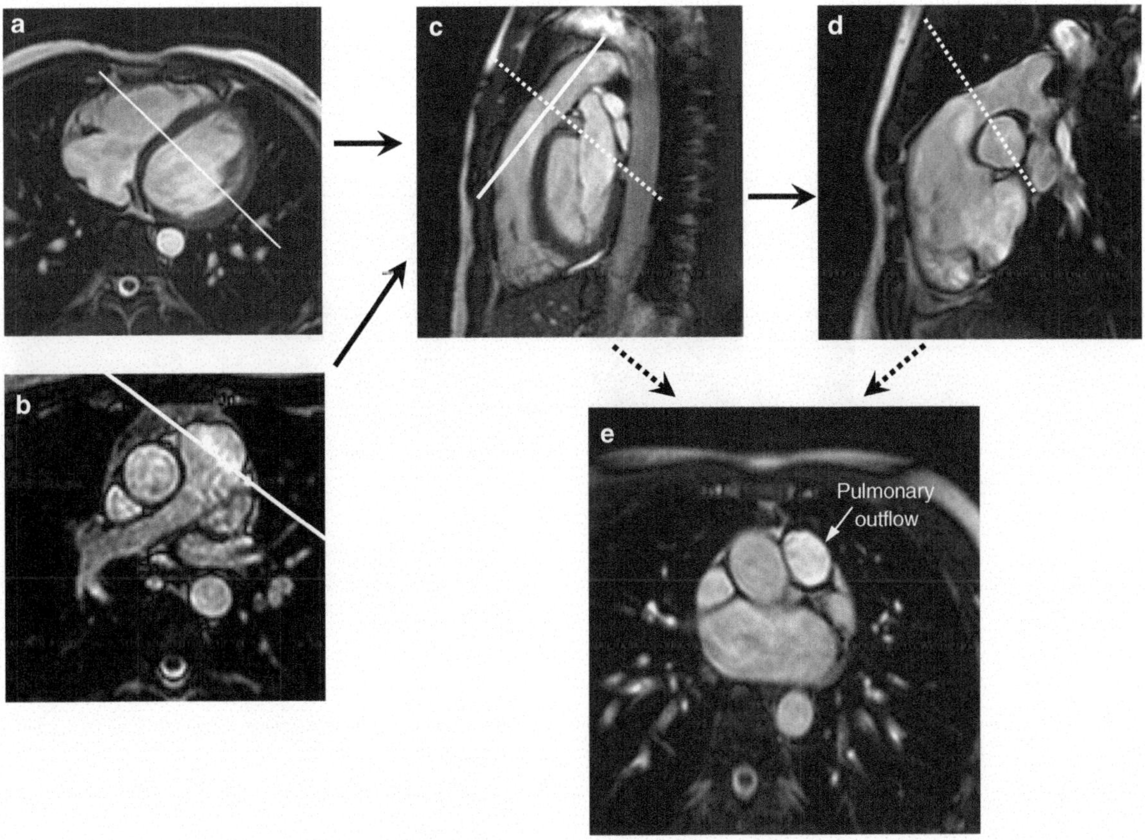

Fig. 8 Alignmentof the pulmonary valve plane (**e**) for pulmonary flow assessment from two perpendicular right ventricular outflow tract (RVOT) (**c** and **d**) views (*dotted lines*). The imaging plane should be placed just above the pulmonary valve. The first RVOT view is prescribed from an oblique plane through the main pulmonary artery and RV on a set of axial images (**a** and **b**). The second RVOT plane is prescribed perpendicular to the first RVOT view (complete line on (**c**))

3.1 Aorta

The aorta can be tortuous in the diseased state, and it can be difficult to align the whole aorta in a single plane. However, large section of the aortic can be aligned in an oblique sagittal plane using a three-point plan (Fig. 10). This is particularly useful for in-plane imaging of aorta jets in aortic coarctation.

When performing a contrast-enhanced 3D MR angiogram (MRA) for aortic pathology, an oblique sagittal volume is the best imaging plane for data acquisition, ensuring that the entire aorta is included in the imaging volume with the shortest acquisition time. If imaging a long section of the head and neck vessels is also required or if pathology of the subclavian arteries (e.g., thoracic outlet syndrome) is suspected, the imaging volume can be placed in the coronal direction, though in-plane image resolution will be reduced (increased field of view) to avoid wrapping in the left-to-right phase encode direction.

3.2 Pulmonary Artery and its Branches

The main PA is usually imaged in the sagittal plane when imaging of the RVOT is performed (Fig. 7b). Imaging in an axial plane, perpendicular to the RVOT view will enable imaging of the PA bifurcation (Fig. 11a).

The right pulmonary artery (RPA) is best imaged in a coronary plane (Fig. 11b) and the left pulmonary artery (LPA) in a sagittal plane (Fig. 11c), both of which can be aligned from the axial images. Branch pulmonary artery flow planes can be prescribed off two perpendicular images for both arteries (axial and coronal for the RPA, axial and sagittal for the LPA),

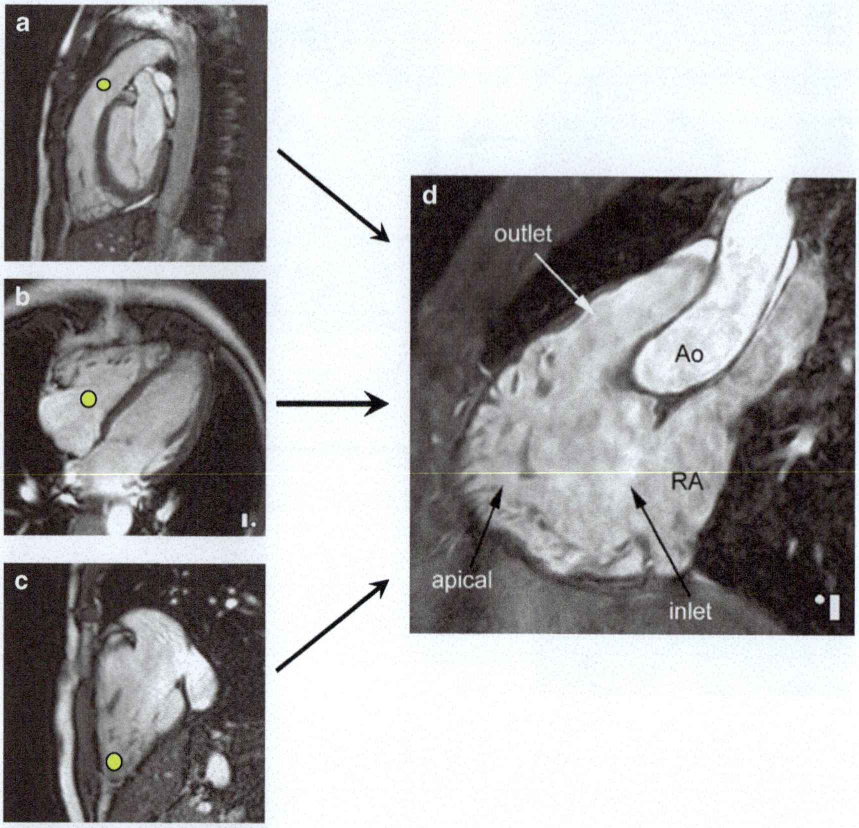

Fig. 9 Alignment of the RV inflow/outflow view (**d**) using a three-point plane: points placed on the pulmonary valve on the RVOT view (**a**), the tricuspid valve on the 4-chamber view (**b**) and the RV apex on the RV 2-chamber view (**c**)

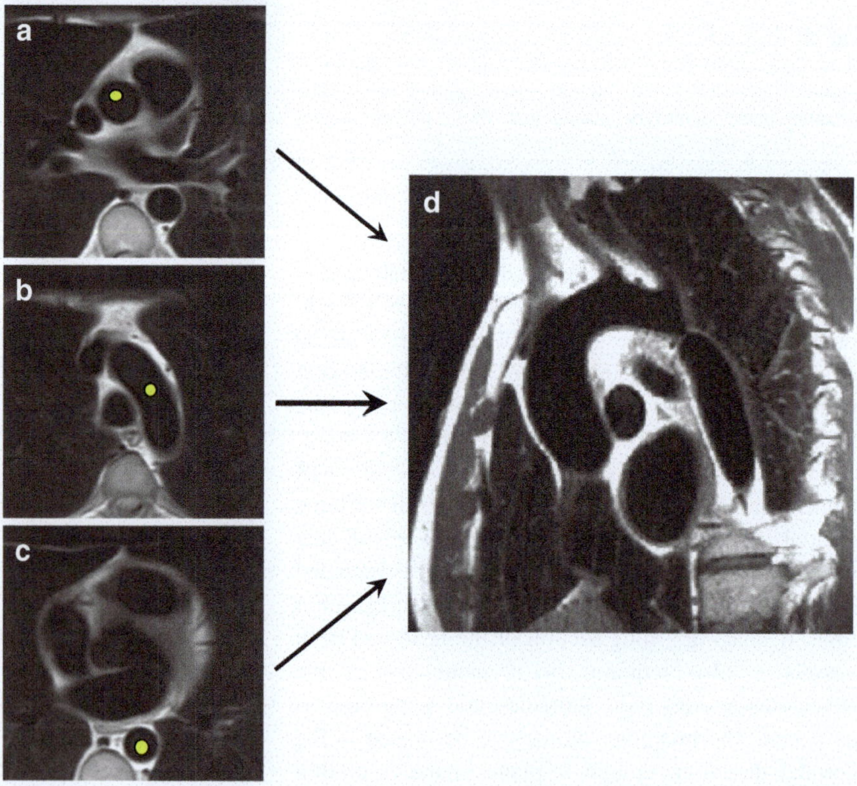

Fig. 10 Alignment of the thoracic aorta using a three-point plane. Points placed on 'black-blood' axial images: **a** ascending aorta; **b** aortic arch and **c** proximal descending aorta. The in-plane image of the thoracic aorta in (**d**) shows a tight aortic coarctation membrane

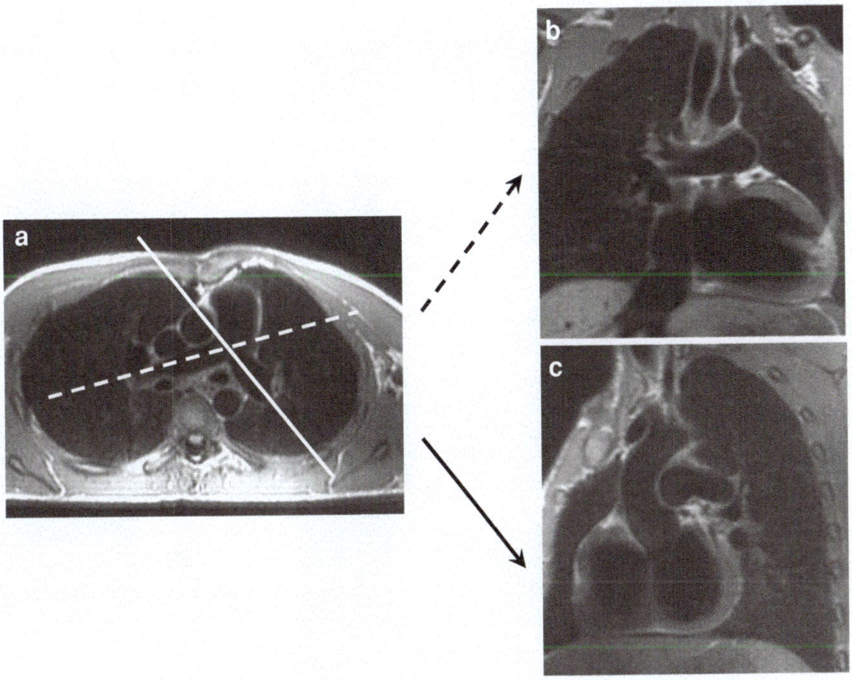

Fig. 11 The right (RPA) and left pulmonary (LPA) arteries do not usually lie in the same axial plane (LPA slightly superior to the RPA). Both arteries can be visualized in an oblique axial plane (**a**). An oblique coronal plane can be used to visualize the RPA (**b**), and an oblique sagittal plane used to visualize the LPA (**c**)

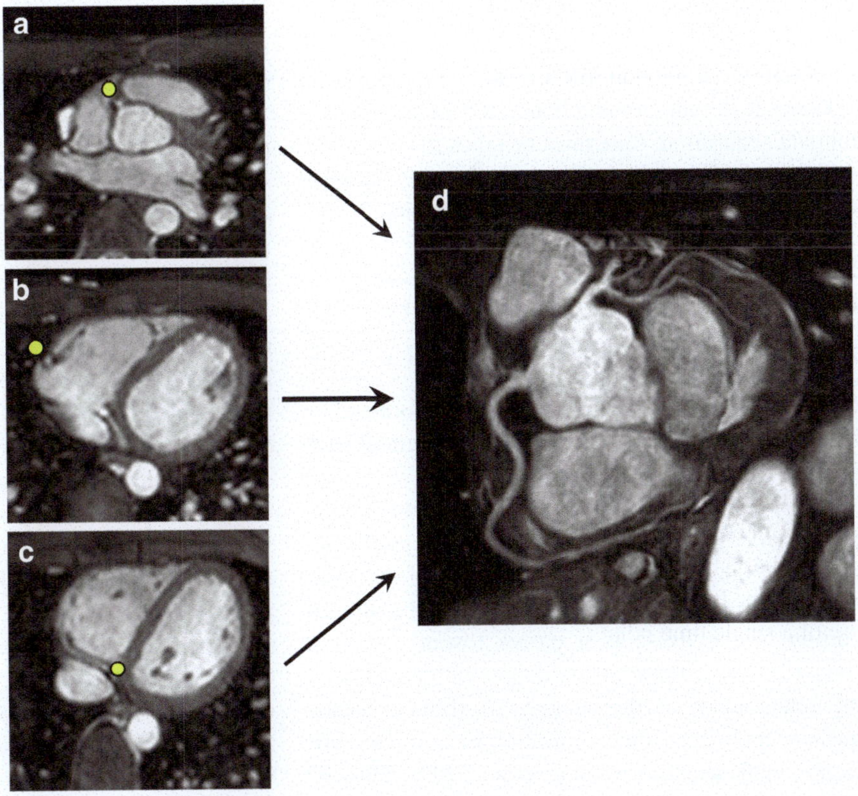

Fig. 12 Alignment of the right coronary artery (RCA) using a three-point plane. Points placed on 'low-spatial resolution' axial images: **a** RCA origin; **b** mid-RCA in the anterior AV groove and **c** distal RCA at the crux of the heart. High-spatial resolution RCA (**d**) is seen anteriorly, the left circumflex (LCx) artery is also seen posteriorly. Note marginal branch of the LCx is seen

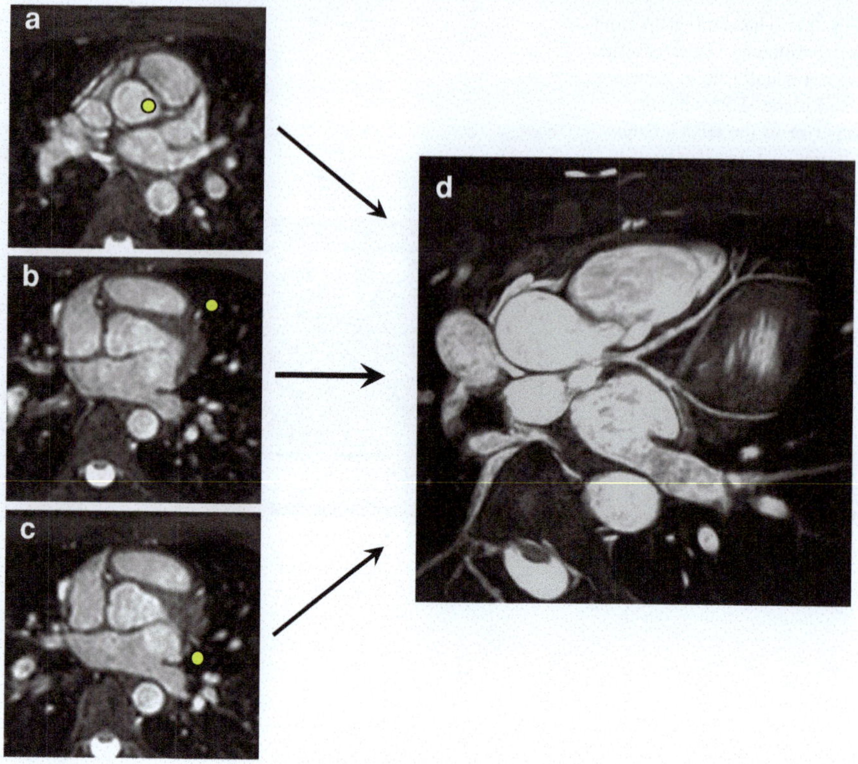

Fig. 13 Alignment of the left coronary artery 'tangential view' using a three-point plane. Points placed on 'low-spatial resolution' axial images: **a** left main stem (LMS) origin; **b** the left anterior descending (LAD) artery as it enters the interventricular groove and **c** the LCx artery as it enters the posterior AV groove. High-spatial resolution image of the proximal left coronary artery visualized (**d**)

to ensure perpendicular velocity vectors for accurate flow mapping.

When performing an MRA of the pulmonary vasculature, a coronal volume is the best imaging plane for data acquisition. Care must be taken to ensure that the right-to-left field of view is sufficiently large to avoid wrapping in the phase encode direction.

4 Imaging Planes for Coronary Arteries

MR coronary angiography can be performed by aligning a narrow 3D volume along the length of each artery.

The RCA plane is aligned using a three-point plan scan, applied on axial images. The points are placed on the RCA origin, the midpoint of the RCA in the anterior AV groove and distally in the inferior portion of the RCA as it passes toward the crux (Fig. 12). These three points define the geometry of the center plane of the imaged 3D volume, subsequently applied for the sub-millimeter coronary MR angiography sequence (Stuber et al. 1999). This 3D volume covers not only the anterior AV groove, but also the posterior AV groove containing the left circumflex artery.

To image the left coronary tree, two scans are performed. The first plane is referred to as the 'tangential view', and images the proximal course of the left main stem (LM), the bifurcation into left anterior descending (LAD) and LCx arteries and their subsequent proximal course. The plane is aligned using a three-point plan scan, using points placed on the LM origin, the mid-point of the LAD and the mid-point of the LCx (Fig. 13). The landmarks on the LAD and LCx should be positioned carefully to assure the longest coverage of the left coronary tree, including the diagonal branching vessels. The second plane is referred to as the 'perpendicular view' and passes through the LM and entire length of the LAD. Three-point planning is again used, with the points placed on the LM origin, the mid LAD and the distal LAD (Fig. 14). On the perpendicular view, the small, septal branches of the LAD are often visualized. In this way, the LM, LCx and LAD (but not the RCA) are scanned in two perpendicular directions. As a result, longer

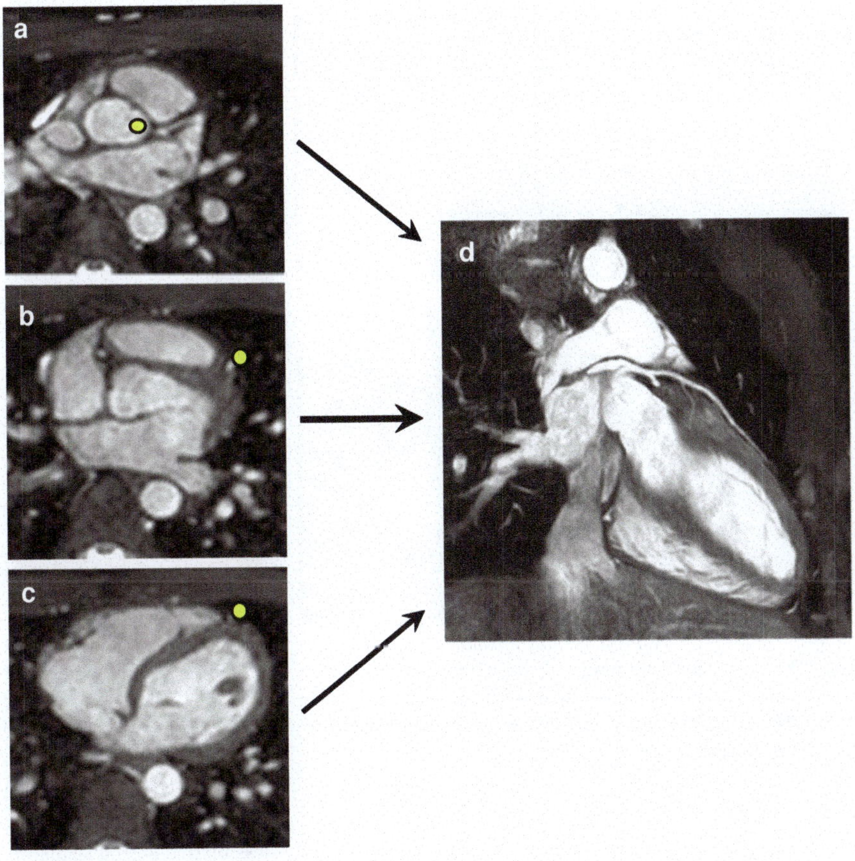

Fig. 14 Alignment of the left coronary artery 'perpendicular view' using a three-point plane. Points placed on 'low-spatial resolution' axial images: **a** LMS origin; **b** the proximal LAD artery as it enters the interventricular groove and **c** the distal LAD artery in the interventricular groove toward the LV apex. High-spatial resolution image of the LMS and LAD visualized (**d**). Note septal branches of the LAD seen

segments of the left coronary artery tree, and more of its branching vessels are visualized. Also, the visualization and description of stenotic lesions benefits from this approach, as lesions are scanned in-plane (better resolution) at least in one direction.

5 Interactive Imaging for Definition of Imaging Planes

Interactive/real-time sequences are increasingly used in cardiac MRI. In real-time imaging, k-space is filled rapidly, and therefore the effects of cardio-respiratory motion on image quality are less pronounced. This imaging can be performed during free breathing and without cardiac gating. Furthermore, because each cine loop is acquired in a single heartbeat, acquisition times are short and the image quality is less susceptible to the effects of an irregular heart rate. However, these benefits come at the cost of lower spatiotemporal resolution, which may affect accuracy (Barkhausen et al. 2002; Lee et al. 2002; Hori et al. 2003; Muthurangu et al. 2004) (Fig 15). However, high spatiotemporal resolution is particularly important for accurate segmentation of the RV, because of its complex trabecular structure. Higher spatiotemporal resolution can be achieved through a combination of k-space under-sampling, and reconstruction algorithms that remove the resultant aliasing. One such technique is k-space and time (k–t) sensitivity encoding (SENSE) imaging. When compared with standard real-time volumetric assessment, radial real-time k–t SENSE imaging accurately quantifies ventricular volumes and function in patients with congenital heart disease, and was superior to standard real-time imaging in terms of image quality and better agreement of volume data with ECG-gated MR. (Fig. 16; Muthurangu et al. 2008). Radial k–t imaging more accurately quantified RV end-diastolic volume than other real-time sequences in this population. Therefore, it is a useful tool in the assessment of congenital heart disease in any

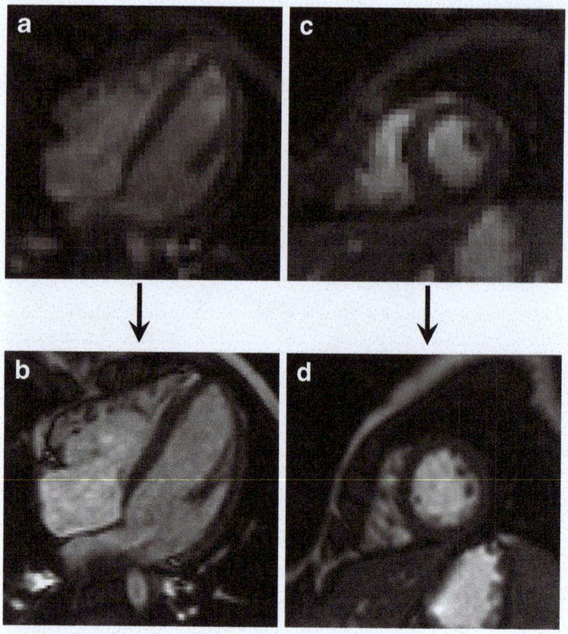

Fig. 15 Low-spatial and temporal resolution real-time, interactive images in the 4-chamber (**a**) and SA planes (**c**) are shown with respective, subsequent high-spatial and temporal resolution SSFP images (**b** and **d**)

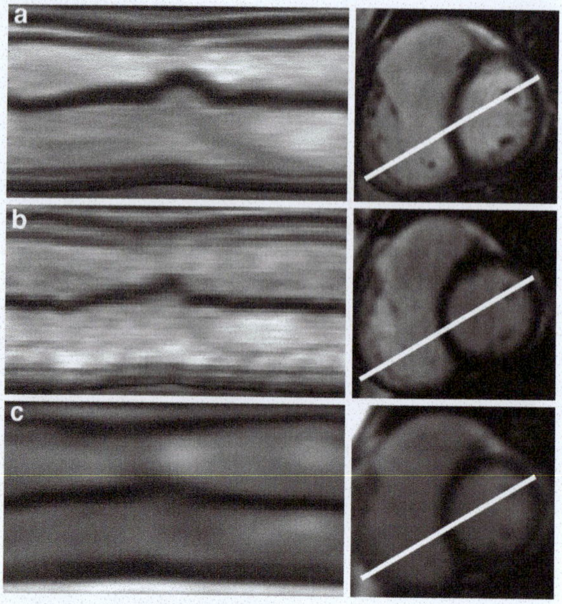

Fig. 16 Pixel profile of a line through both ventricles plotted as a function of time. The geometry of the line is shown on the accompanying short axis image. **a** Cardiac gated profile, (**b**) radial k–t SENSE real-time profile, and (**c**) standard real-time profile. Note the better visualisation of the late systolic septal jump (*marked by arrow*) in the gated and radial k–t—good temporal resolution. The visual quality of the radial k–t images is also better than that of the standard real-time images; less blurred—good spatial resolution

patient who cannot breath-hold, any patient for whom rapid imaging is desirable and in patients with arrhythmia.

6 Segmentation of the LV

For imaging the LV, there is a need for standardization of imaging modalities to assure that accurate intra- and cross-modality comparisons can be made for patient management and research (nuclear cardiology, cardiac ultrasound, cardiovascular MR, cardiovascular CT and cardiac catheterization). Such methods are also important to enable comparison between the various cardiovascular MR techniques. Thus, wall motion abnormalities in one particular segment can be matched with perfusion and/or late-enhancement patterns in the same region of the heart.

A 17-segment frame of reference is used (Cerqueira et al. 2002). The heart is divided into three SA planes along the long axis of the LV: basal, mid-cavity and apical (Fig. 17). These SA planes are then divided radially into six segments for the basal and mid-cavity SA slices, and four segments for the apical slice (Fig. 18); the 17th segment is the apex itself, and is visualized on the long-axis images (VLA, HLA). The radial segments commence at the anterior junction of the LV and RV on the SA image, and are then numbered in an anti-clockwise fashion in equal sized segments around the LV. Thus, the anterior basal segment is segment 1, and the inferior lateral segment is segment 16 (Fig. 18). It should be noted that with a slice thickness of 6–10 mm, the number of SA slices obtained with MRI exceeds the standardized division of the long-axis of the LV in three sections. Thus in practice, the papillary muscles are used as anatomic landmarks to distinguish the mid-cavity SA slices from the apical and basal slices.

The entire 17 segments can be represented in a single image using a Bull's eye plot (Fig. 19) (Post et al. 1999). Furthermore, the segments can be related to the most common distribution of coronary artery anatomy in an attempt to correlate regional wall motion, perfusion and/or late-enhancement abnormalities to specific coronary artery territories (Fig. 20) (Schiller et al. 1989; Post et al. 1999).

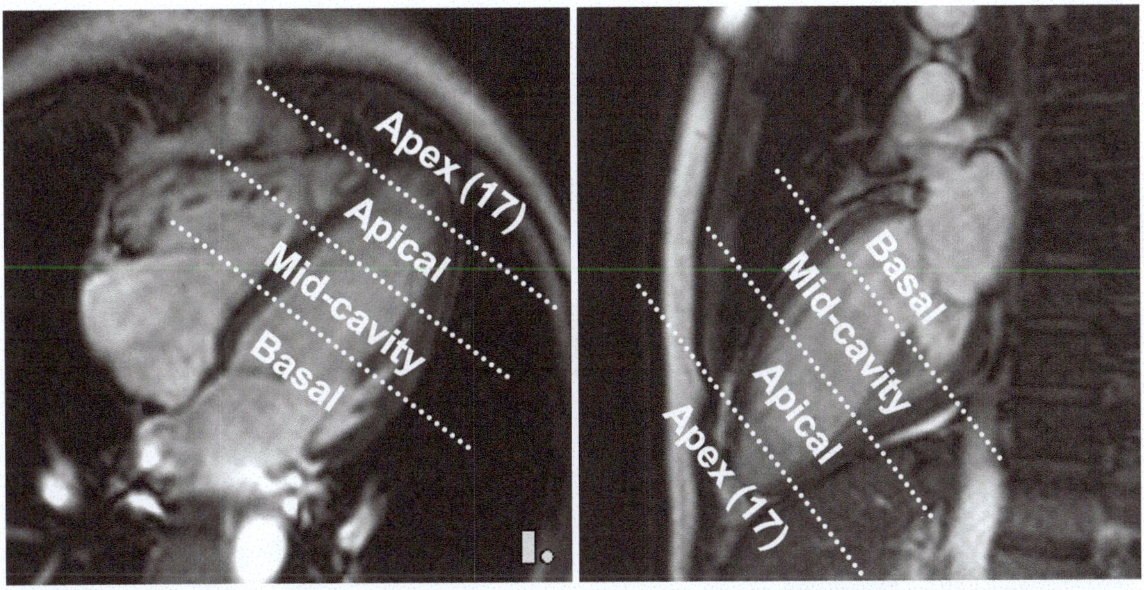

Fig. 17 Division of the LV into basal, mid-cavity and apical SA segments for subsequent segment numbering (see Fig. 18) on 4-chamber and VLA views. Segment 17, the apex, is seen on these long-axis views

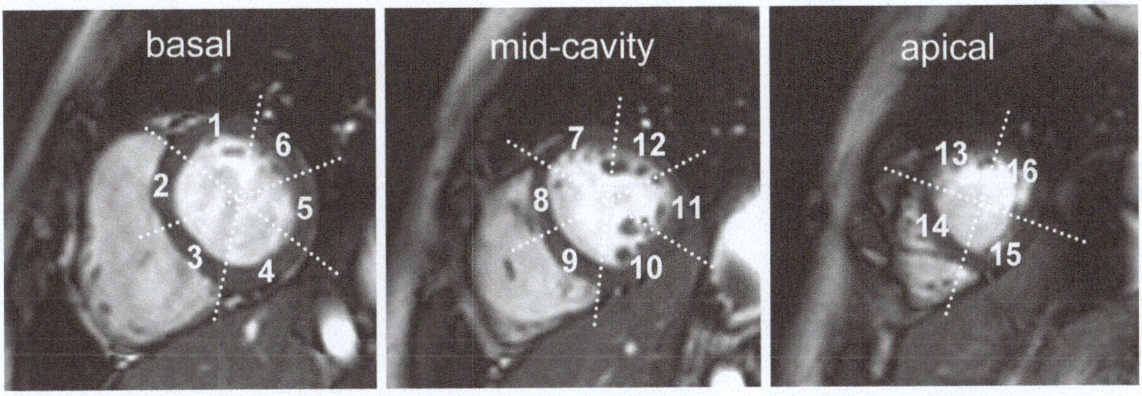

Fig. 18 Subsequent division of SA slices into 6 basal, 6 mid-cavity and 4 apical segments, with segment 17 being the apex seen on the long-axis views (see Fig. 17). Basal: 1—anterior, 2—anteroseptal, 3—inferoseptal, 4—inferior, 5—inferolateral, 6—anterolateral. Mid-cavity: 7—anterior, 8—anteroseptal, 9—inferoseptal, 10—inferior, 11—inferolateral, 12—anterolateral. Apical: 13—anterior, 14—septal, 15—inferior and 16—lateral

Fig. 19 Bull's eye plot representation of all segments of the left ventricle. The segments numbers refer to the same segments as described in Fig. 18

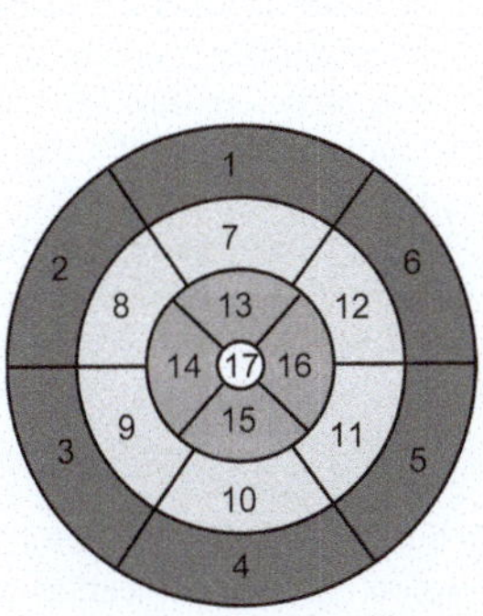

7 Conclusion

An understanding of imaging planes in relation to both the axes of the body and the axes of the heart is necessary when imaging the heart with cardiovascular MR. This enables accurate description of cardiovascular anatomy and reliable standardization between the various cardiovascular imaging modalities.

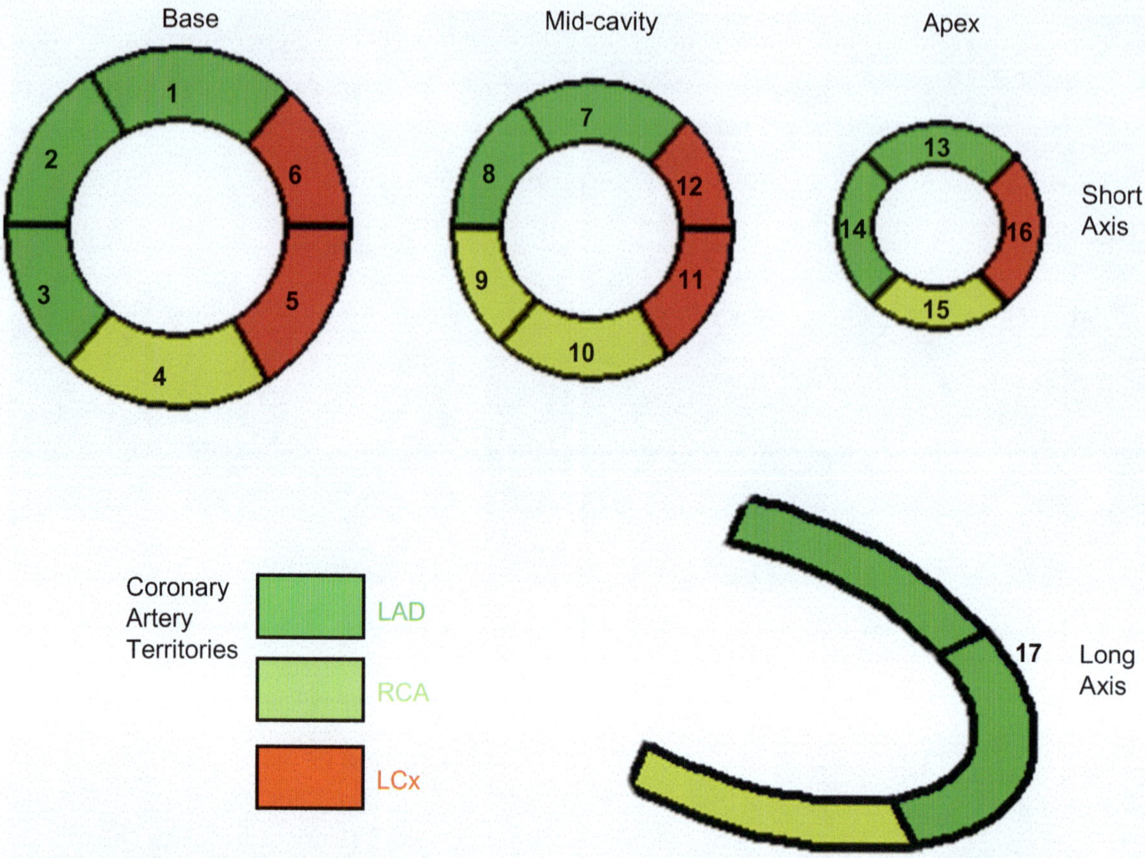

Fig. 20 Correlation between the most common coronary artery distribution pattern and the 17 segments of the left ventricle. Note there is tremendous variability in coronary blood supply to myocardial segments, in particular the apex (segment 17), which depends on right or left dominance

References

Barkhausen J, Goyen M, Ruhm SG, Eggebrecht H, Debatin JF, Ladd ME (2002) Assessment of ventricular function with single breath-hold real-time steady-state free precession cine MR imaging. Am J Roentgenol 178:731–735

Burbank F, Parish D, Wexler L (1988) Echocardiographic-like angled views of the heart by MR imaging. J Comput Assist Tomogr 12:181–195

Cerqueira MD, Weissman NJ, Dilsizian V et al (2002) Standardized myocardial segmentation and nomenclature for tomographic imaging of the heart. Circulation 105:539–542

Hori Y, Yamada N, Higashi M, Hirai N, Nakatani S (2003) Rapid evaluation of right and left ventricular function and mass using real-time true-FISP cine MR imaging without breath-hold: comparison with segmented true-FISP cine MR imaging with breath-hold. J Cardiovasc Magn Reson 5: 439–450

Lee VS, Resnick D, Bundy JM, Simonetti OP, Lee P, Weinreb JC (2002) Cardiac function: MR evaluation in one breath hold with real-time true fast imaging with steady state precession. Radiology 222:835–842

Longmore DB, Underwood SR, Hounsfield GN et al (1985) Dimensional accuracy of magnetic resonance in studies of the heart. Lancet I: 1360–1362

Meier RA, Hartnell GG (1994) MRI of right atrial pseudo masses. Is it really a diagnostic problem? J Comput Assist Tomogr 18:398–402

Muthurangu V, Taylor AM, Andriantsimiavona R et al (2004) A novel method of quantifying pulmonary vascular resistance utilizing simultaneous invasive pressure monitoring and phase contrast MR flow. Circulation 110:826–834

Muthurangu V, Lurz P, Critchely JD, Deanfield JE, Taylor AM, Hansen MS (2008) Real-time assessment of right and left ventricular volumes and function in patients with congenital heart disease by using high spatiotemporal resolution radial k-t SENSE. Radiology 248(3):782–791

Post S, Berman D, Garcia E et al (1999) Imaging guidelines for nuclear cardiology procedures: part 2. J Nucl Cardiol 6:G49–G84

Schiller N, Shah P, Crawford M et al (1989) A recommendation for quantification of the left ventricle by two-dimensional echocardiography. J Am Soc Echocardiogr 5:358–367

Stuber M, Botnar RM, Danias PG et al (1999) Double-oblique free-breathing high resolution three-dimensional coronary magnetic resonance angiography. J Am Coll Cardiol 34: 524–531

Taylor AM, Keegan J, Jhooti P, Gatehouse PD, Firmin DN, Pennell DJ (1999) Differences between normal subjects and patients with coronary artery disease for three different MR coronary angiography respiratory suppression techniques. J Magn Reson Imaging 9:786–793

Cardiac Function

J. Bogaert

Contents

1	**Introduction**	109
2	**Basic Principles of Cardiac Function**	110
3	**Systolic Function**	114
3.1	Ventricular Volumes, Global Function, and Ventricular Mass	114
3.2	Ventricular Stroke Volume Assessment with Phase-Contrast MRI	128
3.3	Regional Ventricular Function	129
4	**Diastolic Function**	141
4.1	Assessment of Diastolic Function and Dysfunction	141
4.2	Ventricular Mass and Volumes	142
4.3	Ventricular Inflow Patterns	142
4.4	Myocardial Tissue Phase Mapping	144
4.5	Atrial Volumes and Function	145
4.6	Ventricular Relaxation	147
4.7	Ventricular Coupling	147
5	**Wall Stress and Myocardial Stress–Strain Relation**	148
6	**Stress Imaging**	149
7	**Postprocessing and Delineation Techniques**	149
8	**Normal Values for Cardiac Function**	152
9	**Key Points**	155
References		156

Abstract

Visualization and quantification of the cardiac pump activity by means of imaging techniques has become an essential part in the diagnosis of many cardiac diseases. This pump activity comprises a repetitive filling and emptying phase whereby one phase or both phases may be impaired by the underlying cardiac disease. Among the different available imaging modalities, MRI has become a preferred one to assess cardiac function because of its noninvasiveness, and the accuracy and reproducibility of the measurements. Moreover, cardiac function assessment by MRI is part of a more comprehensive approach including other facets such as myocardial perfusion imaging and tissue characterization. This chapter is written from the point of view of the imager, starting with a description of the mechanisms of cardiac contraction and relaxation, and how these lead to myocardial deformation and ventricular volume changes throughout the cardiac cycle. Next, it is discussed how imaging techniques can be used to assess these processes at different levels, and what major hurdles need to be passed to achieve reliable estimates of cardiac function parameters. Finally, normal reference values obtained by current MRI sequences are provided at the end of the chapter.

J. Bogaert (✉)
Department of Radiology and Medical Imaging Research Center (MIRC), University Hospitals Gasthuisberg, Catholic University of Leuven, Herestraat 49, 3000 Leuven, Belgium
e-mail: jan.bogaert@uzleuven.be

1 Introduction

As the heart generates the driving force to propagate the blood through the vascular system, assessment of its performance (*cardiac function*) is crucial since

J. Bogaert et al. (eds.), *Clinical Cardiac MRI*, Medical Radiology. Diagnostic Imaging,
DOI: 10.1007/174_2011_335, © Springer-Verlag Berlin Heidelberg 2012

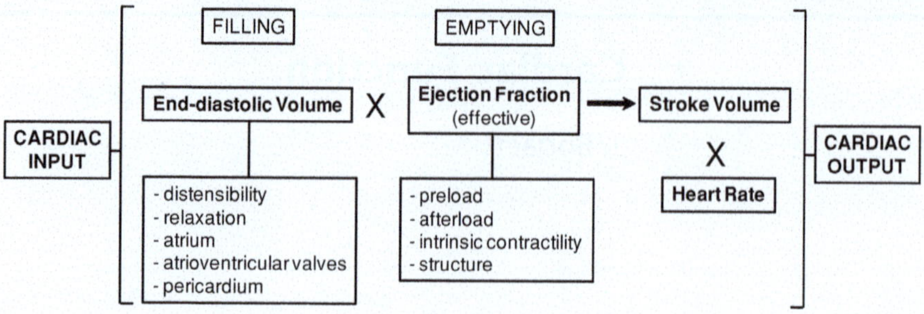

Fig. 1 Determinants of ventricular filling and emptying

many diseases have an impact on the performance of the heart. Although the patient's complaints and clinical examination provide valuable information regarding the functional status of the heart, quantitative measures of cardiac function have been established in the last few decades, and are nowadays routinely used in daily clinical practice. The ease of these measures is that age- and gender-adjusted normalized values can be used as a reference to determine whether a patient's cardiac function is still within normal limits, and thus allow one to assess the severity of dysfunction and to categorize patients. Moreover, functional parameters such as ejection fraction have been shown to yield a prognostic value and are therefore often used as a surrogate for hard end points such as cardiac death in many studies. Although ejection fraction, expressing the relative amount of blood ejected by a ventricle during each cardiac contraction, is definitely the functional parameter with which we are most familiar, it is important to emphasize that cardiac function assessment cannot be reduced or simplified to a single parameter, and that several other parameters need to be considered. It has become clear over the last few decades that unraveling and assessment of cardiac function is extremely complicated. Different pathways and strategies to quantify global and regional cardiac performance have been explored, using a variety of techniques ranging from the injection of dye for determining the cardiac output to assessment of myocardial deformation by implantation of metallic beads. The advent of noninvasive cardiac imaging modalities in particular of echocardiography opened the door toward routine assessment of cardiac function in daily clinical practice. Although assessment of cardiac function with MRI was reported as early as the mid-1980s (Matthaei et al. 1985), it took almost 15 years for it to be introduced into routine cardiac imaging. Despite this long "maturation" phase, we nowadays have the availability of a highly versatile and accurate technique enabling one to study many facets of cardiac function, which can be directly linked with other parameters such as myocardial perfusion, valve function, cardiac morphology, and tissue characteristics. The aim of this chapter is to explain in an understandable way the complexity of cardiac function as well as to provide insight how to use MRI to study this complex issue in an appropriate way.

2 Basic Principles of Cardiac Function

The heart can be considered as a highly sophisticated muscle, conceived to be the central circulatory pump, exhibiting a behavior of well-coordinated repetitive phases of myocardial contraction and ventricular emptying (*systole*) and myocardial relaxation and ventricular filling (*diastole*, Fig. 1). It is a four-chambered organ consisting of a right two-chambered part and left two-chambered part that are anatomically parallel but function serially, and importantly both parts are imbedded within a single pericardial sac, emphasizing an important mutual interaction. Each two-chambered part consists of an atrium, having principally a reservoir function, and a ventricle, creating the driving force to expulse the blood into the systemic and pulmonary vascular system.

Systole is initiated by electrical stimulation of the thick-walled ventricular myocardium, causing an increase in tension and shortening of myocytes, which is translated at the myocardial level into a myocardial deformation or *strain* and myocardial motion, and finally at the ventricular level by a rise in ventricular pressure, and once the transvalvular pressure of the ventriculoarterial valves has been surpassed by ejection of blood in the great vessels and subsequent decrease of the ventricular cavity volumes (Fig. 2).

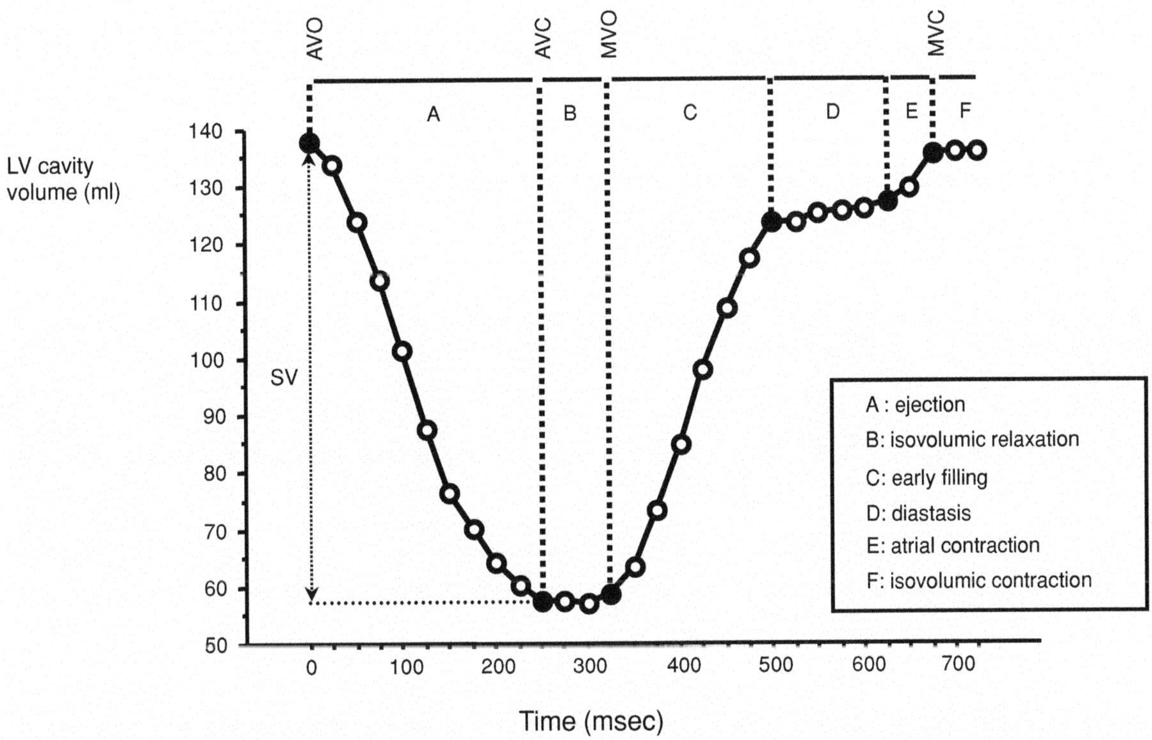

Fig. 2 Volume–time curve of the left ventricle during the cardiac cycle in a 27-year-old normal volunteer. Short-axis cine imaging using contiguous 8-mm-thick slices and 2-mm slice gap. Temporal resolution 24 ms. The different phases of the cardiac cycle (**a–f**) can be well recognized on this volume–time curve. The onset of ejection (**a**) (characterized by a decrease in left ventricular, LV, volume) coincides with the aortic valve opening. On aortic valve closure, the minimal LV volume is obtained. The difference in volume between aortic valve opening and aortic valve closure represents the stroke volume. The time period between aortic valve closure and mitral valve opening is the isovolumic relaxation (**b**). At the moment of mitral valve opening, ventricular filling starts. This is characterized by an early, fast filling phase (**c**), a period with nearly no filling, called "diastasis" (**d**), and a final phase of filling caused by the atrial contraction (**e**). The last part, i.e., isovolumic contraction, starts with mitral valve closure and ends with aortic valve opening (**f**)

Thus, systole consists of a contraction and ejection phase. Contraction starts after electrical stimulation and encompasses mitral valve closure, isovolumic contraction, and ejection as long as the ventricular pressure is higher than the pressure in the receiving vessel. Most fascinating in this cascade of events is the highly efficient design of the heart to function as a pump, allowing it to achieve with a myofiber shortening of only 10–15% a ventricular ejection fraction of 65–70%. The highly complex myofiber anatomy with profound differences in transmural fiber orientation is not at random but in fact represents a powerful mechanism to enhance the efficiency of single-fiber shortening. As we know from anatomical studies and novel techniques such as diffusion MRI (see Sect. 5), left ventricular (LV) midwall fibers have predominantly a circumferential course. Toward the endocardium and epicardium the fiber orientation progressively becomes oblique but in an opposite direction, bringing these fibers into an almost perpendicular orientation to each other (Streeter et al. 1969; Greenbaum et al. 1981). On the other hand, truly longitudinally oriented fibers are, except in the papillary muscles and the endocardial trabeculations, sparse in the LV wall. Fiber contraction leads, because of this complex fiber orientation, to an intricate myocardial and ventricular deformation consisting in a combination of circumferential and longitudinal shortening, radial thickening, and shear motions (e.g., ventricular torsion). Circumferential shortening with centripetal wall motion is primarily caused by midwall fiber contraction, whereas longitudinal LV shortening is largely the result of contraction of the oblique epicardial and endocardial

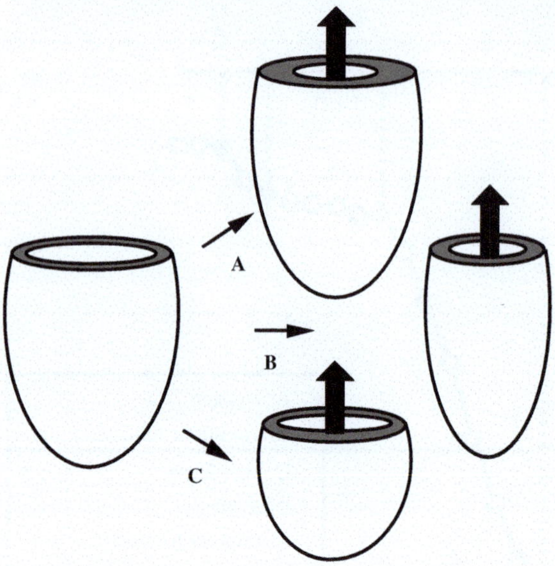

Fig. 3 Mechanisms of (left) ventricular ejection. On the *left* the ventricle at the end of diastole is shown, and on the *right* the ventricle at the end of ejection is shown: **a–c** Three different hypothetical mechanisms of endocardial inward motion: **a** pure wall thickening; **b** circumferential shortening; **c** longitudinal ventricular shortening. The normal ventricular ejection relies on a combination of these three mechanisms

fibers. Myocardial wall thickening ("radial strain"), although in part secondary to circumferential shortening, is mainly caused by a transmural interaction between the oblique epicardial and endocardial fibers, a phenomenon called *myocardial tethering*. Physically, the torque of the epicardial fibers exceeds the endocardial fiber torque, which means that epicardial fiber shortening will largely affect the behavior of the endocardial fiber bundles, and force them to passively rearrange and shorten along the direction of the epicardial fibers, which is nearly perpendicular to the endocardial fiber direction. This passive phenomenon is called *cross-fiber shortening*, and its magnitude exceeds that of the active shortening of endocardial fibers. Taking into account the principle of conservation of mass, shortening of a volume in two directions necessitates lengthening in the third direction, which is radial wall thickening. This tethering is a highly effective mechanism to improve the efficiency of the individual myocardial layers. It has been shown that destruction of the epicardial fibers leads to an abolishment of endocardial cross-fiber shortening and wall thickening. Although myocardial deformation is greatest in the inner part of the myocardium, this deformation is directed by the outer myocardial wall. Myocardial tagging studies have shown in normal human hearts a LV circumferential shortening ranging from 44% in the subendocardial layers and 30% in the midwall layers to 21% in the subepicardial part of the myocardium (Palmon et al. 1994). LV shortening in the longitudinal direction is 17%, and radial wall thickening is approximately 40–50% (Rogers et al. 1991; Bogaert and Rademakers 2001; Figs. 3, 4). The net result on the ventricular level is a volume reduction of approximately 65–70% at the end of systole. If we take into account the complex anatomy, it is understandable that in pathological conditions, such as myocardial ischemia, primarily affecting the subendocardium, functional parameters reflecting subendocardial function such as longitudinal shortening may be a sensitive parameter to early detect ischemia (Brecker 2000).

Diastole represents the filling phase of the ventricles. Although mechanically the filling phase is the period between mitral valve opening and mitral valve closure, filling will be determined by myocardial relaxation, atrial contraction, and the compliance of the ventricle and atrium (Fig. 2). Physiologically and conceptually, diastole encompasses a longer period starting at the time the myocardium loses its ability to generate force and shorten and returns to an unstressed length and force. Thus, ventricular relaxation begins when myofiber tension starts to decline during late ejection, proceeds rapidly as pressure falls during isovolumic relaxation, and continues through the period of early filling. With the onset of myocardial relaxation, the ventricular pressure drops, and continues to drop until a pressure is reached below the pressure of the atrium even after filling has started, caused by the active relaxation process and the presence of restoring forces. It is thought that during contraction and early ejection, energy is stored in the myocardial cytoskeleton or collagen matrix that subsequently during relaxation acts as a restoring force, lowering ventricular pressure and sucking atrial blood into the ventricle. From the moment the ventricular pressure drops under the atrial pressure, the atrioventricular valve opens and ventricular filling starts. Depending also on the ventricular compliance and distensibility, the local gradients across the atrioventricular valve will switch, blood flow will be decelerated, and will only continue through diastasis, dependent on momentum. With atrial contraction a

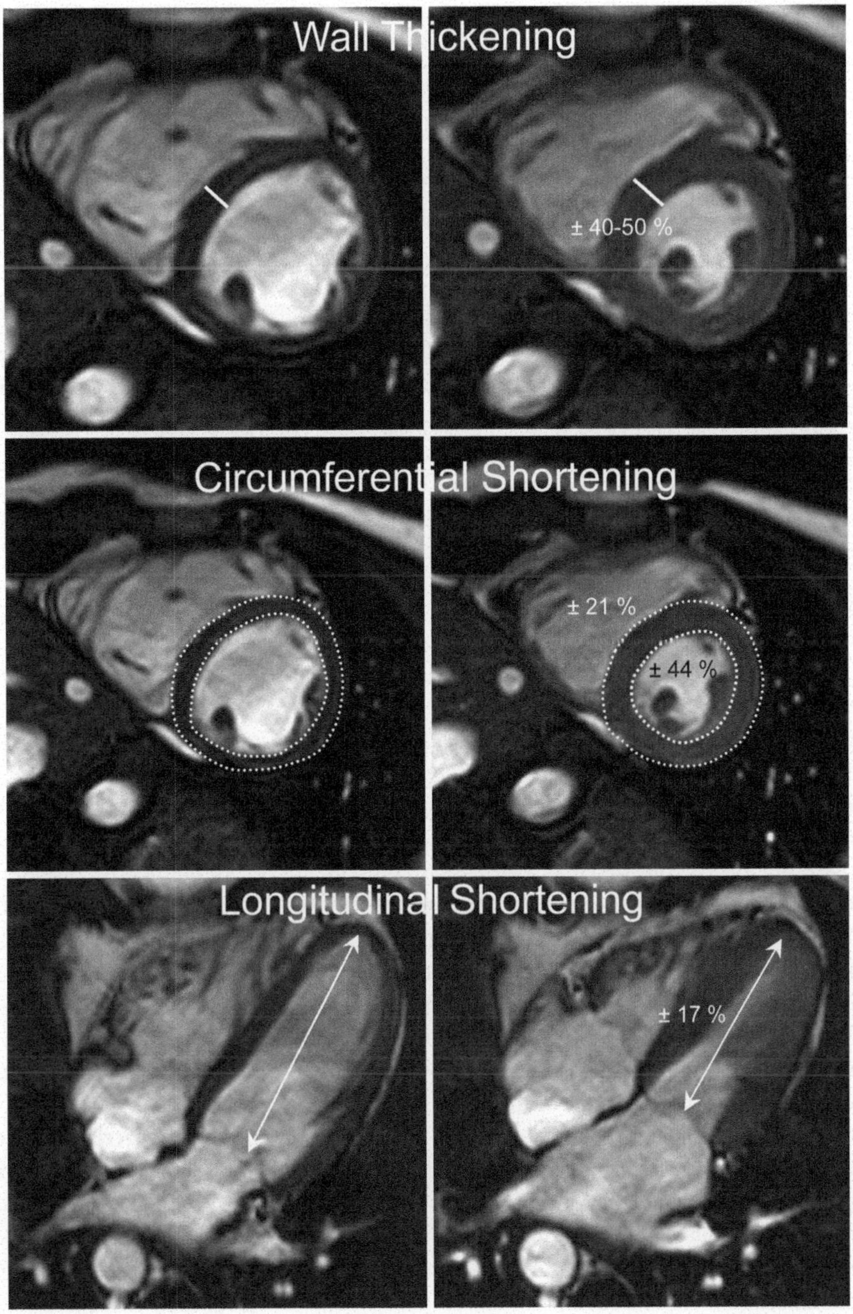

Fig. 4 Mechanisms of (left) ventricular ejection, studied with cine MRI. Cine imaging in the cardiac short axis (*top row* and *middle row*) and the horizontal long axis (*bottom row*) at the end of diastole (*left*) and at the end of systole (*right*). The *top row* represents the mechanism of wall thickening (mean value, approximately 40–50%), the *middle row* shows the mechanism of circumferential shortening, which is larger at the endocardium (mean value approximately 44%) than at the epicardium (mean value approximately 21%), and the *bottom row* shows the mechanism of longitudinal ventricular shortening (mean value approximately 17%)

new gradient and acceleration is created, further filling the ventricle, depending on atrial and ventricular compliance and the force of atrial contraction. Active relaxation is only responsible for the first part of ventricular filling, but its influence can be prolonged in the case of abnormal, prolonged relaxation, for instance, in myocardial ischemia. Compliance, in contrast, is important throughout filling but owing to the shape of the passive pressure–volume relation of the ventricle, it plays its most important role at the end of fast filling and during atrial contraction.

Another characteristic phenomenon in particular of the left ventricle is the torsional or twisting motion, exhibiting a counterclockwise rotation when viewed from the apex (Buchalter et al. 1990, 1994). *Twisting* is an essential component of normal systolic function,

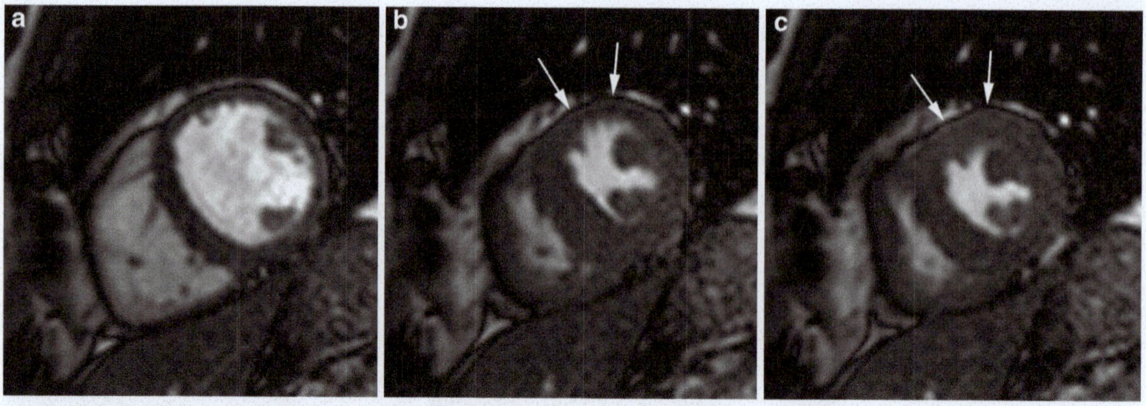

Fig. 5 Postsystolic contraction during a dobutamine–atropine stress MRI study in a patient with significant stenosis in the proximal left anterior descending coronary artery. Cine imaging in the midventricular cardiac short axis at the end of diastole (**a**), at the end of systole (**b**), and on isovolumic relaxation (**c**). During systole (**b**), the ischemic myocardium in the anterior wall is akinetic (*arrows*). However, during isovolumic relaxation (**c**), while the nonischemic regions start to relax, myocardial thickening can be well appreciated in the ischemic anterior LV wall (*arrows*)

whereas untwisting is considered an important determinant of normal myocardial relaxation. Although the exact explanation for this rotational motion is unknown, it is likely related to an imbalance between the obliquely oriented fibers, with dominance of epifibers over endofibers. Torsion likely leads to an increased efficiency of transmural myocardial function by equalizing fiber stress and function, and therefore can be considered as a necessary component of wall thickening and ejection (Arts et al. 1991). Ventricular wringing increases the longer the distance from the base (up to ±28° of rotation) but the spread is fairly homogeneous from the base to the apex. Ventricular untwisting is clearly dissociated from ventricular filling, starting during isovolumic relaxation and sometimes already in the latter part of ejection (Rademakers et al. 1992; Dong et al. 2001). Most likely, ventricular unwringing releases kinetic energy stored in the myocardium during systole as explained in the previous paragraph, and represents a potent mechanism for the suction of blood during early diastole.

Assessment of the ventricular performance also includes assessment of the synchronization of mechanical events between the different parts of the ventricle. In many conditions related to pathological abnormality of the electrical activation or to pathological abnormality of the myocardium itself such as myocardial infarction, ventricular dyssynchrony occurs impeding ventricular performance. Therefore, use of a single time point to look at the end of systole is not sufficient to appreciate well this temporal inhomogeneity or to assess the maximal extent of deformation. Although there is a time point during the cardiac cycle when the ventricle reaches its smallest volume and ejection ends, maximal deformation in different parts of the ventricle does not necessarily coincide with that specific time point. For instance, postsystolic contraction is a well-known phenomenon in ischemically diseased myocardium (Fig. 5). To fully appreciate the dynamic events occurring during the cardiac cycle, therefore, multiple time points should be used.

3 Systolic Function

3.1 Ventricular Volumes, Global Function, and Ventricular Mass

"Global ventricular performance" is generally understood to mean the capability of the ventricles to eject blood into the great vessels. Since the ventricles exhibit a repetitive process of ejection and filling, having a mutual influence on each other, both phenomena should be evaluated together when considering assessment of global ventricular performance. For the sake of simplicity, the diastolic ventricular function is discussed separately (see Sect. 4). Moreover, the condition of the cardiac valves should be taken into account (see "Valvular Heart Disease"). For instance, a leaking valve causes ventricular volume

Table 1 Global functional parameters

EDV − ESV = SV (ml)
SV/EDV = EF (%)
SV × HR = CO (ml/min)
EDVindex = EDV/BSA (ml/m^2)
ESVindex = ESV/BSA (ml/m^2)
CO/BSA = CI (ml/min/m^2)

BSA body surface area, *CI* cardiac index, *CO* cardiac output, *EDV* end-diastolic volume, *EF* ejection fraction, *ESV* end-systolic volume, *HR* heart rate, *SV* stroke volume

overload, whereas ventricular dilatation (e.g., dilated cardiomyopathy) may lead to mitral annulus dilatation and secondary mitral regurgitation.

To achieve a complete analysis of systole, one should describe the temporal changes in ventricular volumes and related velocities throughout systole. In clinical practice, however, systole is usually appreciated considering ventricular volumes at two time points, i.e., maximal filling (end of diastole), and maximal emptying (end of systole). From these, all other global functional parameters can be deduced. Subtracting end-systolic volume from end-diastolic volume yields the stroke volume (Table 1). Dividing stroke volume by end-diastolic volume gives the ejection fraction, whereas multiplying stroke volume and heart rate yields cardiac output. To achieve normalized data, these parameters can be indexed to body parameters, e.g., weight, length, body surface area, and lean body mass. It is obvious that the reliability of the deduced global functional parameters is only as good as the accuracy with which the "raw" ventricular volumes are acquired. Another important parameter of global ventricular performance, and an independent predictor of morbidity and mortality from many cardiac diseases (e.g., coronary artery disease, arterial hypertension), is the ventricular or myocardial mass (Levy et al. 1990).

3.1.1 Strategies for Ventricular Volume, Global Function, and Mass Quantification

Although ventricular volumes and function can be appreciated by visual eyeballing, quantitative measures are largely preferred to achieve a more objective and reproducible assessment. The latter can be achieved by geometric assumptions or by volumetric quantification (Figs. 6, 7, 8, 9). Geometric assumptions compare the ventricular cavity with a geometrical model. Using a (limited) number of standardized measurements of the ventricular cavity, one calculates the corresponding volumes. For the left ventricle, short-axis views (e.g., hemisphere cylinder model and Teichholz model), long-axis views (e.g., biplane ellipsoid model and single-plane ellipsoid model), or a combination of long- and short-axis views can be used for calculations of ventricular models (Dulce et al. 1993; Thiele et al. 2002) (Figs. 6, 7, 8). Geometric assumptions are commonly used in planar imaging techniques, such as contrast ventriculography and radionuclide scintigraphy, as well as in echocardiography (M-mode and two-dimensional). They have the advantage of rapidly providing information regarding ventricular volumes and mass, but they are only reliable as long as the geometrical model corresponds to the true ventricular cavity or myocardial wall, which might not be the case in (focally) diseased ventricles (Bellenger et al. 2000a; Fig. 10). Myerson et al. (2002a) showed that this technique cannot be recommended to assess LV mass, and the volumetric approach is preferable either for a single measurement or to follow up patients.

The advent of tomographic cardiac imaging by means of three-dimensional echocardiography, computed tomography, and MRI opened the door toward true volumetric quantification based on Simpson's rule, i.e., the volume of a complex structure, for instance, the cardiac ventricle, can be accurately assessed by dividing this structure into a set of subvolumes which are quantifiable (Fig. 9). Addition of all subvolumes yields the total volume of the complex structure. In practice, this is done by using a stack of parallel slices entirely encompassing the ventricle (or generally speaking, the cardiac chamber of interest). In the next step, the endocardial border of each slice is delineated, providing a two-dimensional area, and when this multiplied by the distance between two slices (equivalent to the sum of the slice thickness and the interslice distance), a three-dimensional subvolume is obtained. If all three-dimensional subvolumes are summed, the total ventricular volume is obtained. To calculate ventricular mass, epicardial borders need to be delineated as well (Aurigemma et al. 1992; Lima et al. 1993; Forbat et al. 1994; Germain et al. 1992). The area between the endocardial and epicardial border is used to calculate myocardial mass in a similar way as for ventricular volume. The volume

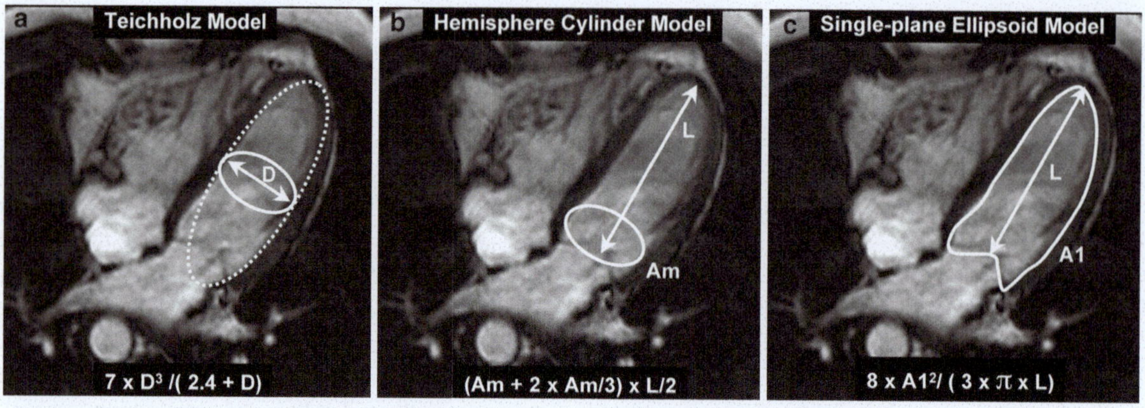

Fig. 6 Geometric assumptions techniques for ventricular quantification; **a** Teichholz method; **b** hemisphere cylinder method; **c** single-plane ellipsoid model. The formula for each of the different techniques is shown. *A* area, *Am* area at mitral level, *D* diameter, *L* length

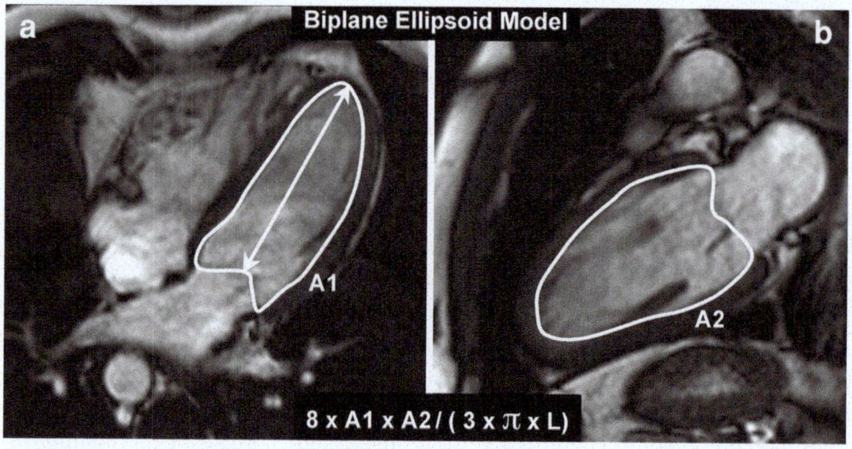

Fig. 7 Biplane ellipsoid model. Horizontal long-axis view (**a**) and vertical long-axis view (**b**). The formula for the calculation is shown . *A* area, *L* length

obtained needs to be multiplied by the specific density of myocardium, i.e., 1.05 g/cm^3, to get myocardial mass. This volumetric approach has superior reproducibility and accuracy in comparison with the geometric assumptions techniques, but has the disadvantage of being more time-consuming for both image acquisition and postprocessing (Grothues et al. 2002, 2004).

To obtain the most reliable estimates of ventricular volumes and masses, several issues, discussed in the following paragraphs, should be taken into consideration. Although volumetric approaches are definitely preferable and should be used as much as possible, a visual estimation of volumes, function, and mass is always recommended because it provides a fast impression about the cardiac condition and should match with the calculated results obtained. Moreover, in clinical practice, geometric assumptions may be of interest, for instance, if the acquired data for volumetric quantification are insufficient for analysis, or if there is a clear mismatch between the observed and calculated results. A simple geometric formula, such as $L_1 \times L_2 \times L_3 \times \pi/6$, where L_1 represent the longitudinal LV diameter (measured on the vertical or horizontal long-axis image) and L_2 and L_3 represent the maximal short-axis LV diameters in two perpendicular views, is very useful for this purpose.

3.1.2 MRI Sequence Design

Nowadays, assessment of ventricular volumes and mass is achieved using bright-blood techniques, which have completely replaced the dark-blood (spin-echo) technique for this purpose. The major

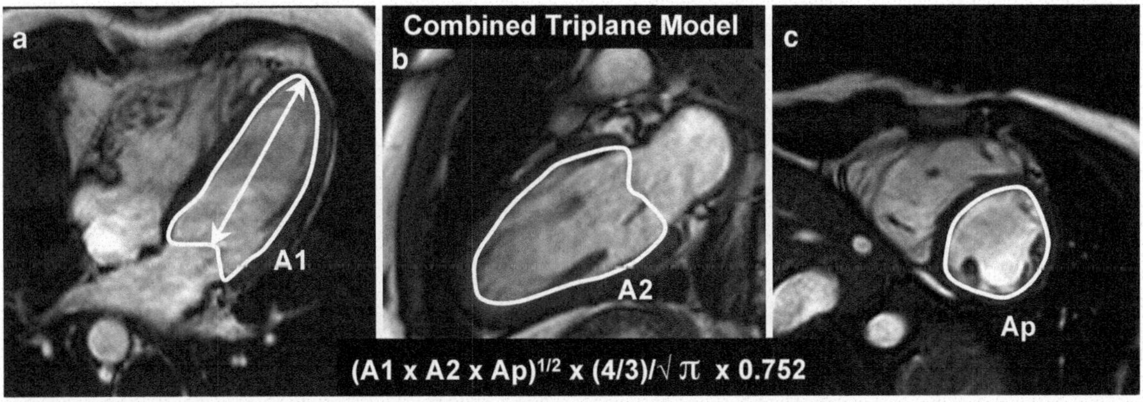

Fig. 8 Combined triplane model. Horizontal long-axis view (**a**), vertical long-axis view (**b**), and midventricular short-axis view (**c**). The formula for the calculation is shown. *A* area, *Ap* area at papillary level

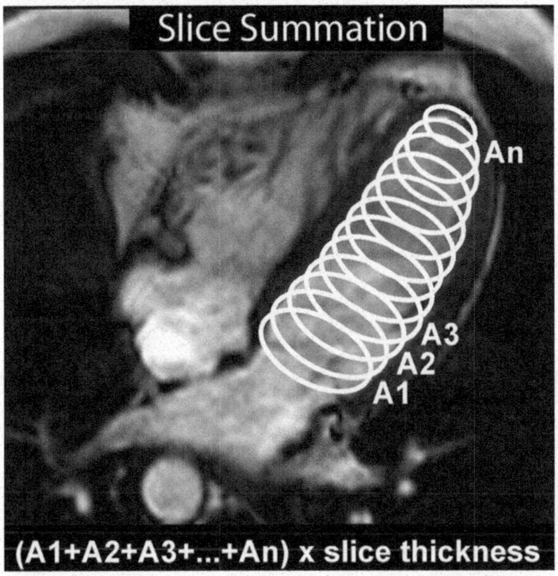

Fig. 9 Slice summation technique for ventricular volume quantification. Horizontal long-axis view. The formula for the calculation is shown. *A* area

shortcoming of the latter technique, even when using the newest developments such as dark-blood turbo spin-echo or half-Fourier single shot turbo spin-echo imaging, is that only a single phase during the cardiac cycle is studied, providing limited information regarding ventricular function, and useful only for assessment of myocardial mass (Caputo et al. 1990; Pattynama et al. 1992; Scharhag et al. 2002). The advantages of the spoiled gradient-echo (GE) technique (i.e., fast low flip angle single shot or fast-field-echo technique) to study ventricular function became evident in the late 1980s (Sechtem et al. 1987; Utz et al. 1987; Buser et al. 1989). If data acquisition is gated or synchronized with the cardiac cycle, time-resolved (*cine*) anatomical images can depict the dynamics of cardiovascular geometry during the cardiac cycle, allowing noninvasive assessment of global and regional cardiac function. This kind of multiphase cardiac imaging is feasible if short repetition times (e.g., 30–40 ms) are used in combination with small flip angles. Although use of segmented spoiled GE sequences was initially very time-consuming, their introduction in the early 1990s allowed the measurement time to be significantly reduced and such sequences to be used in daily routine practice (Atkinson and Edelman 1991; Bloomgarden et al. 1997). By the acquisition of multiple lines of k-space per heart beat (i.e., "segmented k-space approach"), and the use of very short repetition times and low flip angles, the imaging time could be reduced to the length of a breath-hold without compromising temporal resolution when using echo sharing (Sakuma et al. 1993; Bogaert et al. 1995; Schulen et al. 1996). As such, a limited number (e.g., eight to 12) of repeated breath-holds was sufficient to obtain a complete set of short-axis images through the left ventricle. With the advent of the breath-hold segmented spoiled GE technique, MRI became for the first time a competitor to echocardiography, allowing besides morphologic evaluation also accurate functional cardiac evaluation.

The phenomenon of *inflow enhancement* is responsible for the bright-blood appearance when using the spoiled GE technique. During image

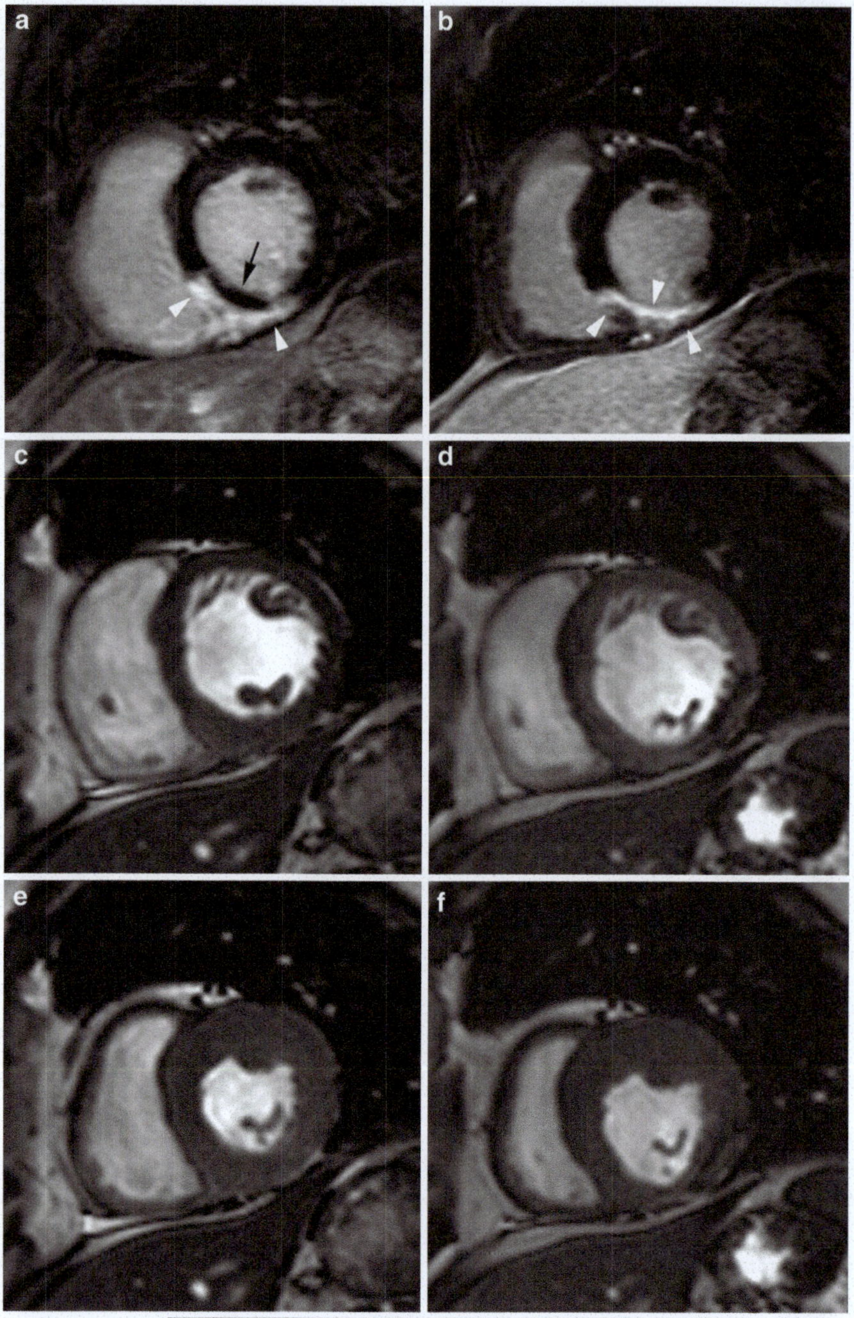

Fig. 10 Important LV remodeling in a patient with acute transmural inferoseptal myocardial infarction. Late Gd MRI at 1 week (**a**) and 4 months (**b**) after infarction. Short-axis cine MRI at 1 week, end-diastolic (**c**) and end-systolic (**e**) time frames; at 4 months end-diastolic (**d**) and end-systolic (**f**) time frames. Late Gd imaging at 1 week shows transmural enhancement inferoseptally in the mid-basal left ventricle (*white arrowheads*), with presence of a no-reflow zone (*black arrow*). The infarct area is edemateously thickened and shows severe hypokinesia on cine MRI (**c–e**). At 4 months, the scarred infarct is visible as a thin hyperintense curvilinear line (*arrowheads*) (**b**), showing akinetic wall motion on cine imaging (**d–f**). Assessment of global LV function using the slice summation volumetric approach shows moderately decreased function in the first week (ejection fraction 54%). However, because of an important remodeling of the ventricle, at 4 months after the acute event, end-diastolic and mainly end-systolic volumes are increased, whereas stroke volume and ejection fraction show an important decrease (ejection fraction 40.5%). Although most of the geometric assumptions techniques show a decrease in global function (ejection fraction), they underestimate the severity of ventricular remodeling (*1W* 1 week; *4M* 4 months)

	EDV (ml)		ESV (ml)		SV (ml)		EF (%)	
	1W	4M	1W	4M	1W	4M	1W	4M
Slice Summation	158	171	73	102	85	69	54.0	40.5
Hemisphere	196	209	99	112	97	97	49.4	46.4
Teichholz	167	173	83	93	84	80	50.2	46.2
Single-plane	202	195	73	83	129	112	63.9	57.4
Biplane	206	200	78	88	128	112	62.1	56.0
Combined Triplane	205	208	81	97	124	111	60.5	53.3

Table 2 Influence of MRI sequence on left ventricular (*LV*) volume and mass calculations in controls and patients

	Spoiled GE	b-SSFP	Difference	*p* value
Controls (n = 10)				
EDV (ml)	133 ± 37	151 ± 37	18 (13%)	<0.001
ESV (ml)	46 ± 14	55 ± 18	9 (17%)	0.001
EF (%)	66 ± 3	64 ± 4	−2 (−3%)	0.19
LV mass (g)	145 ± 46	120 ± 37	−25 (−19%)	<0.001
Patients (n = 10)				
EDV (ml)	202 ± 78	208 ± 69	6 (4%)	0.25
ESV (ml)	116 ± 65	123 ± 65	8 (6%)	0.001
EF (%)	44 ± 14	43 ± 17	−2 (−4%)	0.27
LV mass (g)	202 ± 46	181 ± 51	−21 (−11%)	<0.001

Adapted from Moon et al. (2002)
GE gradient echo, *b-SSFP* balanced steady-state free precession

acquisition, the signal of stationary tissues is progressively suppressed by the repetitive excitation, whereas the blood pool is continuously refreshed by inflow of fully relaxed spins into the image slice. As a consequence, the blood in the cardiac chambers and blood vessels is bright, whereas the surrounding myocardium appears gray. This also explains why imaging in the short-axis direction yields the highest blood–myocardium contrast, whereas imaging in imaging in long-axis planes may suffer from in-plane saturation especially toward the LV apex. The greatest shortcoming of this sequence is the low contrast between blood and myocardium, hampering, for instance, the use of automated edge detection algorithms (Romiger et al. 1999). Several authors, therefore, advocated the use of intravascular contrast agents to increase the blood–myocardium contrast and thus to facilitate endocardial border detection (Stillmann et al. 1997; Alley et al. 1999).

The beginning of this century coincided with the reintroduction and revival of the balanced steady-state free-precession GE sequence, which rapidly became the preferred bright-blood sequence for dynamic cardiac imaging (cine MRI) (Barkhausen et al. 2001; Carr et al. 2001; Thiele et al. 2001; Plein et al. 2001; Moon et al. 2002; Lee et al. 2002; Fieno et al. 2002; Alfakih et al. 2003a; Hori et al. 2003; Spuentrup et al. 2003). Use of this sequence, introduced in the early 1980s, was hampered for a long time because of issues such as main field nonuniformity, eddy currents, and inhomogeneous magnetic susceptibility, which have been solved with the newest-generation scanners. The steady-state signal is largely independent of inflow but is dependent on the T2-to-T1 ratio. The benefits are not only a higher contrast between cardiac cavities (high signal) and adjacent myocardium (low signal), but also a significant improvement in endocardial border detection (Barkhausen et al. 2001). Endocardial trabeculations and papillary muscles are sharply defined independent of slice orientation. A first consequence is that automated algorithms should benefit from the increased blood-myocardium contrast, but otherwise the increased anatomic detail may pose new challenges to these algorithms. Second, the differences in endocardial border visualization between sequences will have a significant impact on calculations of myocardial thickness and mass, and ventricular volumes. Practically, the novel sequence yields consistently a significantly thinner myocardial wall and lower myocardial mass but conversely a higher ventricular volume than the old spoiled GE sequences (Moon et al. 2002; Alfakih et al. 2003a; Table 2). Similar consistent differences between both sequences were reported for cine imaging at high field (3 T) (Hudsmith et al. 2006; Grothues et al. 2007). Moreover, it is obvious that new reference values are needed, although some suggest that existing databases can be converted (Malayeri et al. 2008; Cain et al. 2009). At the end of this chapter a summary of normal values is provided (Maceira et al. 2006a, b, 2010).

3.1.3 Spatiotemporal Resolution, Acquisition Time, and Acquisition Window Length

Cine imaging is constrained by several issues, and one should strive to find the best compromise between parameters, which are hardware-, software-, and patient-related. Patient-related issues (e.g., patient safety, comfort) are primordial but only to a small extent modifiable. For instance, one can endeavor to increase the temporal resolution but if this is at the expense of unacceptable long breath-hold periods this will negatively impact patient comfort and cooperation, and ultimately impair image quality. On the other hand, progress in hardware and software design has been that impressive in the last three decades that imaging can be pushed nowadays toward its limits, with high spatial and temporal resolution real-time free breathing and four-dimensional breath-hold imaging as the newest developments (Jahnke et al. 2006; Muthurangu et al. 2008).

Parameters that are important to consider for cine imaging are acquisition window length, total acquisition time, and spatial and temporal resolution. These parameters are not independent but have a mutual influence on each other. Changing one parameter will have an immediate impact on the other parameters. As discussed before, with the implementation of the segmented k-space technique, the total imaging time could be reduced to the length of a breath-hold period. Hereby, the total acquisition time can be traded for temporal resolution, and vice versa. To illustrate this, if one uses 128 phase-encoding steps and a repetition time of 9 ms, an increase of the number of k-lines acquired per heart beat of 2 (from seven to nine) decreases the breath-hold length by four heart beats (from 18 to 14) but obligatorily prolongs the acquisition window length by 18 ms (from 63 to 81 ms). Thus, faster imaging is possible, hereby increasing patient comfort, but these benefits are opposed by increased motion blurring caused by the longer acquisition length. Increasing acquisition length (e.g., 100 ms) also signifies a lower number of image frames per cardiac cycle, making dynamic views shaky and resulting in a temporal resolution that may be too low to accurately study the different events occurring during the cardiac cycle, which may be worsened, for instance, during stress imaging with high heart rates (Setser et al. 2000). Incorrect determination of the end of systole (which lasts only for 40–50 ms) leads to an overestimation of end-systolic volumes and underestimation of stroke volumes and ejection fractions (Barkhausen et al. 2002; Miller et al. 2002).

Several approaches have been developed to modify one of the above-mentioned parameters (e.g., temporal resolution) without influencing the others. One is echo sharing or view sharing, which allows one to double the effective temporal resolution without changing the true temporal resolution or acquisition time (number of k-lines × repetition time—Foo et al. 1995). It is based on reconstructing an intermediate image with a timing exactly between two original images, which is achieved by using the second half of the k-lines from the original image immediately before and the first half of the k-lines from the original image just after the newly reconstructed image. A second way to increase temporal resolution is by using echo-planar readout schemes, shortening acquisition times (Lamb et al. 1996; Bornstedt et al. 2001). A third and highly versatile approach is parallel imaging (see "Cardiac MR Physics"; Sodickson and Manning 1997; Griswold et al. 1999; Weiger et al. 2000; van den Brink et al. 2003). Parallel imaging offers a spectrum of flexibility that can be used to shorten scan times in patients with limited breath-hold capacity, or to increase the temporal or spatial resolution (Kacere et al. 2005). One of the major strengths of MRI is its high spatial resolution. Normally, an in-plane pixel size of 1–2 mm can be achieved in a reasonable breath-hold period while maintaining high temporal resolution. Further increase in spatial resolution would imply longer acquisition times extending beyond the limits of acceptable breath-hold periods. If the pixel size increases, the accuracy of measurements, primarily of ventricular volumes, decreases (Miller et al. 2002). Slice thickness and slice spacing are two other important parameters to consider, since they are a main determinant of the total measurement time and have an impact on assessment of global and regional function. Use of thinner slices may be beneficial to obtain sharper depiction of the myocardial borders, and to reduce partial volume effects, in particular in the LV apex, but the downside is that more slices (and thus more breath-holds) are required to encompass the ventricle, which increases the time for both acquisition and postprocessing. Moreover, the thinner the slice, the lower the signal-to-noise ratio, although this is partially counteracted by the high intrinsic contrast-to-noise ratios achieved with current cine imaging sequences. In practice, a slice thickness of 6–10 mm in adults and 5–8 mm in children can be recommended. Slices do not necessarily need to be contiguous, and a small slice gap (e.g., 2–4 mm) is acceptable to reduce the measurement and postprocessing time without influencing the accuracy of measurements (Debatin et al. 1992a; Cottin et al. 1999).

3.1.4 Ultrafast and Real-Time Cine Imaging

The acquisition length of "regular" cine imaging has been reduced to the duration of one breath-hold period, during which up to three image slices can be obtained. To cover completely the ventricle, a number of repeated breath-holds is required. Although this is sufficient to scan most patients in resting conditions, there are a number of occasions where accelerated imaging with further reduction in acquisition length is absolutely required, allowing one to acquire data in real time without the need for breath-holding. These include patients with severe cardiac arrhythmias, patients unable to cooperate with or having difficulties in breath-holding such as young children with congenital heart disease and elderly patients having difficulties to understand the operator's instructions, and examinations during stress conditions. Although regular cine sequences can be modified into real-time sequences, this is at the cost of lower spatiotemporal resolution, which may affect diagnostic accuracy and impair image quality. This has urged several groups to develop clinically useful ultrafast and real-time sequences with an acceptable temporal resolution (below 50 ms) and in-plane spatial resolution (below 2.5 mm) (Kramer et al. 2008). In addition to use of techniques such as view or echo sharing and parallel imaging, a substantial reduction in measurement time can be achieved by developing novel strategies to fill the k-space (e.g., partial k-space filling, radial or spiral k-space filling), and by exploiting correlations in k-space and time (k-t) such as k-t BLAST and k-t SENSE techniques (see "Cardiac MR Physics"; Setser et al. 2000; Nagel et al. 2000; Kaji et al. 2001; Barkhausen et al. 2002; Lee et al. 2002; Spuentrup et al. 2003; Hori et al. 2003; Kühl et al. 2004; Taylor et al. 2005; Jahnke et al. 2006, 2007; Muthurangu et al. 2008; Lurz et al. 2009). Other groups have explored the use of novel multichannel technology to speed up the acquisition time for real-time two-dimensional and segmented three-dimensional cine imaging (Parish et al. 2010; Davarpanah et al. 2010). The results are promising, showing good correlations between regular and accelerated cine imaging and applicable for both ventricles. As an alternative to standard ECG-triggered cine imaging, prospective cardiac–respiratory self-gated cine imaging has recently been proposed (Manka et al. 2010). Particularly for patients who are unable to hold their breath for a long period and for patients who show ECG signal disturbances, this sequence may be a valuable alternative.

3.1.5 Correction for Through-Plane Motion

Through-plane motion represents a major challenge to achieve accurate volume measurements of the ventricular cavities during the cardiac cycle. The currently used two-dimensional tomographic MRI techniques with fixed imaging planes encounter problems in the study of organs such as the heart exhibiting a three-dimensional deformation pattern. The position of the heart with regard to a (fixed) imaging plane constantly changes during the cardiac cycle, and thus the heart will move forward and backward through the slice of interest, a phenomenon called "through-plane motion." Thus, besides the in-plane deformation and motion, one should take into account the effect of through-plane motion as well. The latter is most obvious at the atrioventricular interface, when the heart is imaged in the short-axis direction. Owing to the longitudinal systolic shortening of the ventricles (approximately 15% in normal ventricles), the base of the heart moves toward the cardiac apex (Rogers et al. 1991). As a direct consequence, a short-axis slice positioned at the end of diastole in the ventricular base will move during systole into the atrium, and then return to its original position during diastole (Fig. 11). Without correction for through-plane motion, end-systolic ventricular volumes are significantly overestimated, and stroke volumes are underestimated (Marcus et al. 1999a). Although slice-tracking techniques whereby the position of the image slice is corrected for the through-plane motion have been presented, they have not yet become clinically available (Kozerke et al. 1999, 2001). Thus, correction techniques need to be applied during image postprocessing, or alternative

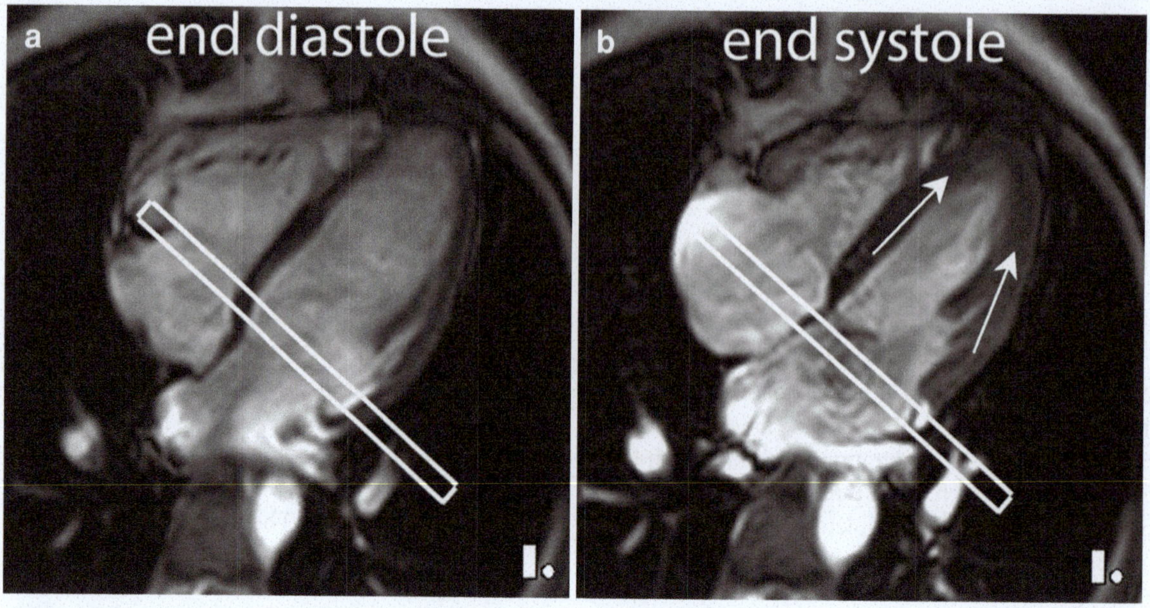

Fig. 11 Effect of through-plane motion. Horizontal long-axis cine imaging with end-diastolic (**a**) and end-systolic (**b**) time frames. As a consequence of longitudinal shortening (*arrows*) of the ventricle during systole, a slice through the basal part of the left ventricle at the end of diastole will be positioned in the left atrium at the end of systole

approaches need to be used where the effects of through-plane motion have a less important influence on the volumetric measurements (see Sect. 3.1.6). A first approach is the slice-omission technique, omitting slicing that are atrially located at the end of systole. This can be achieved taking into account ventricular morphology, which is straightforward for the left ventricle but more cumbersome for the right ventricle. Short-axis slices with a complete LV muscular ring are considered as ventricular, whereas incomplete muscular rings with less than 50 or 75% myocardium or thin-walled rings are considered as atrial and are not taken into account. Although this approach is easy to apply, it is not entirely correct since the LV outflow tract is not taken into account. Moreover, for instance, in patients with an inferobasal LV infarct the normal myocardium may be replaced by a thin fibrous scar and thus mistaken for an atrial slice. This approach is much more difficult to apply to the right ventricle because of the thin tight ventricular free wall. A second approach is to use information regarding the magnitude of long-axis shortening. This can be achieved by measuring the longitudinal shortening on a vertical or horizontal long axis and in a next step by determining the number of short-axis slices that need to be omitted at the end of systole, or preferably by determining the position of the atrioventricular valve on long-axis views and projecting this information onto short-axis images. A third approach is to use anatomical information specific for the ventricles/atria to define the position of the atrioventricular valve. This approach is more difficult since it assumes appropriate knowledge of cardiac morphology. Finally, it is important to emphasize that because through-plane motion has a major impact on calculated ventricular volumes, a consistent approach is definitely necessary for repeated studies.

3.1.6 Cardiac Image Plane

Another important issue in assessing ventricular volumes and function is the choice of imaging plane. It is of interest to discuss and compare the advantages and limitations of the different cardiac imaging planes for both global and regional functional assessment. The short-axis image plane is the most commonly used. The left ventricle is shown as a doughnut with the thin-walled right ventricle ventrally attached to it. On these short-axis slices 16 of the 17 standardized wall segments are well visible (except the LV apex or segment 17, see "Cardiovascular MR Imaging Planes and Segmentation"; Cerqueira et al. 2002). Contouring of the endocardial and epicardial borders poses no problem and myocardial contraction patterns are well evaluable. However, it is not well suited to evaluate the apical region of the ventricles, as well as the atrioventricular interface, and no information regarding longitudinal shortening is available. As discussed in the previous section, correction for through-plane motion is of utmost importance to achieve correct estimates of ventricular volumes. A simple calculation underscores the magnitude of potential errors. The most basal short-axis slice (using a thickness of 1 cm) has a volume of 17 ± 9 ml at the end of diastole and 9 ± 4 ml at the end of systole, (normal volunteers, unpublished data). For LV end-diastolic and end-systolic volumes of 130 ml and 45 ml, respectively, including or excluding this slice leads to a volume change of 13% and 20%, respectively.

The horizontal long-axis image plane (and also the transverse image plane) has the intrinsic advantage that the atrioventricular valves and their motion during the cardiac cycle, as well as the ventricular apices, are well visible. Moreover, in this plane the effects of through-plane motion, for instance, at the region of the aortic or pulmonary valve, are far less pronounced than the through-plane motion occurring at the basal part of the ventricles in short-axis views. Redoing our simple calculation, the subaortic image slice has a volume of 6 ± 1 ml at the end of diastole and 5 ± 1 ml at the end of systole (unpublished data). Any inaccuracies will have a much smaller impact on LV volume calculations than the short-axis image plane. However, this image plane focuses also shortcomings. Because the image plane is nearly perpendicular to the direction of diaphragmatic motion, inconsistencies in breath-hold depth between the consecutive breath-holds may lead to erroneous volume measurements. Moreover, the risk of partial volume effects is greater than in the short-axis direction, in particular along the anterior and inferior LV wall, and in the neighborhood of the papillary muscles.

A combination of imaging planes may potentially overcome some of the inaccuracies related to the use of a single image plane approach. A combination of long-axis and short-axis images, for instance, whereby short-axis information is used for the main, central part of the left ventricle and the long-axis information is used for assessment of the apical and basal part of the left ventricle, may be a good alternative. Fusion of short- and long-axis information, however, is still quite challenging. Another intrinsically highly appealing approach, described by Bloomer et al. (2001) is a radial approach with long-axis views, whereby the image plane is oriented radially around the long-axis centerline of the left ventricle (Clay et al. 2006). This approach has several intrinsic advantages. The aortic valve, mitral valve, and LV apex are well visible; the effects of through-plane motion and partial volume effects are minimal, and interobserver variability is low (variability less than 2.3%). The greatest shortcoming is that the sequence is designed to study the left ventricle, and therefore no information regarding right ventricular (RV) volumes and function is provided.

3.1.7 Endocardial and Epicardial Borders, Myocardial Trabeculations, and Papillary Muscles

As discussed in Sect. 3.1.2, the design of the bright-blood sequence significantly influences endocardial border visualization and thus has a nonnegligible impact on ventricular volume and mass values. Moreover, visualization of the external myocardial border on bright-blood imaging may be impeded at the heart–lung or heart–diaphragm interface because of lack of contrast between these structures. Black-blood cine imaging has recently been proposed as an alternative for improved epicardial border depiction (Basha et al. 2009). In our experience, border delineation may be improved by using the dynamics of cine imaging, i.e., using the forward and backward button allows one to easily discriminate contractile myocardial tissue from surrounding tissues.

Although anatomical structures such as the papillary muscles and endocardial muscular trabeculations represent only a small part of the myocardium, their weight is nonnegligible and it should be decided during image analysis whether they belong to the myocardium or whether they are included in the ventricular cavity, and it is obvious that for repeated studies a consistent approach is obligatory (Papavassiliu et al. 2005; Janik et al. 2008; Weinsaft et al. 2008; Table 3; Fig. 12). The approach to be used will be influenced by the underlying pathological abnormality. For instance, if the question is assessment of myocardial mass such as in patients with arterial hypertension, aortic stenosis, hypertrophic cardiomyopathy, or myocardial storage diseases, it is advisable to include papillary muscle volumes because they are

Table 3 Inclusion or exclusion of papillary muscles and trabeculations into the LV cavity and the influence on global functional parameters and LV mass

	Papillary muscles and trabeculations included	Papillary muscles excluded	Trabeculations excluded
EDV (ml)	130.8 ± 33.4	120.8 ± 31.7	101.1 ± 27.8*
ESV (ml)	51.2 ± 15.5	42.4 ± 14.3	32.6 ± 11.1*
EF (%)	60.9 ± 3.7	65.2 ± 4.4	68.2 ± 4.8*
Mass (g)	110.6 ± 23.1	118.7 ± 23.0	129.7 ± 25.1*

$^*p < 0.001$

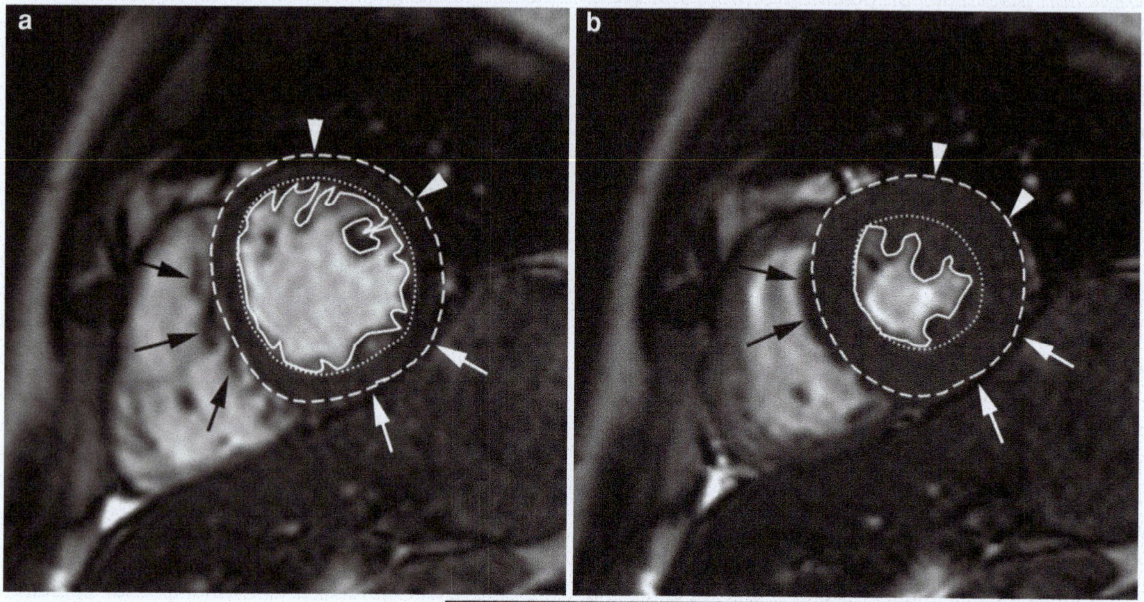

	EDV (ml)	ESV (ml)	SV (ml)	EF (%)	Mass (g)
Papillary muscles / trabeculations included in myocardium	134	39	95	71	138
Papillary muscles / trabeculations included in LV cavity	161	59	102	63	114

Fig. 12 Impact of endocardial trabeculations and papillary muscles on calculations of LV volumes, mass, and function. Midventricular short-axis cine imaging at the end of diastole (**a**) and at the end of systole (**b**). The *continuous line* shows the endocardial border including the papillary muscles and trabeculations into the myocardium. The *fine dashed line* shows the endocardial border, excluding the aforementioned structures from the myocardium. The *coarse dashed line* shows the epicardial LV border. Note that the interface with the adjacent lung (*white arrowheads*) and infradiaphragmatic structures (*white arrows*) impedes the visualization of the epicardial contours. Compaction of the endocardial trabeculations in the right ventricle to the ventricular septum at the end of systole (*black arrows*) may lead to an overestimation of the true septal wall thickness and thus of the LV mass

usually pathologically remodeled or involved. In most other conditions, however, it may be recommendable to consider the papillary muscles and myocardial trabeculations as part of the ventricular cavity. For instance, to achieve homogeneous regional data on systolic LV wall thickening, the papillary muscles and trabeculations located principally along the lateral LV wall can be best excluded both at the end of diastole and at the end of systole. This approach yields data regarding the thickness and systolic thickening of the compact myocardial layer (see Table 13; Dawson et al. 2011). Regarding the right ventricle, which usually more trabeculated than its left counterpart, it is nearly impossible to delineate all individual trabeculations.

3.1.8 Recommendations for Right Ventricular Volume, Function, and Mass Assessment

Quantification of RV volume, mass, and function is important in numerous congenital and acquired cardiac diseases primarily or concomitantly affecting the right ventricle (Katz et al. 1993; Tardivon et al. 1994; Casalino et al. 1996; Marcus et al. 1998; Kroft et al. 2000; Hoeper et al. 2001). Because of the complex anatomy and form, the thin wall with coarse trabeculations, and the anterior position within the chest of the right ventricle, accurate imaging of RV function is challenging with traditional imaging modalities such as echocardiography (Mertens and Friedberg 2010). Although MRI can tackle these challenges much more easily, and therefore can be considered presently as the reference technique, recommendations for appropriate image acquisition and analysis are needed (Sugeng et al. 2010; Haber et al. 2005). It is obvious that because of the complex shape of the right ventricle, volumetric quantification is preferred above geometric assumptions (Markiewicz et al. 1987a). The influence of the image plane on ventricular volume calculations was discussed in Sect. 3.1.6. Whereas for the left ventricle the short-axis plane is the standard image plane, the transverse or horizontal long-axis plane is probably more appropriate to quantify RV volumes and function (Jauhiainen et al. 2002; Alfakih et al. 2003b). In patients with primary RV disease (e.g., arrhythmogenic RV dysplasia/cardiomyopathy–pulmonary hypertension–tetralogy of Fallot), most likely a combination of imaging in two perpendicular directions, e.g., short-axis and horizontal long-axis imaging, is the most appropriate because it yields the advantage that regional function can be well assessed throughout the right ventricle. Accurate quantification of RV mass remains problematic in patients with normal RV wall thickness, and even in patients with wall hypertrophy it remains challenging and time-consuming to delineate the individual trabeculations (Winter et al. 2008). For RV wall mass calculations the ventricular septum is usually excluded. Normal values for RV volumes, function, and mass are provided at the end of this chapter (see Table 7).

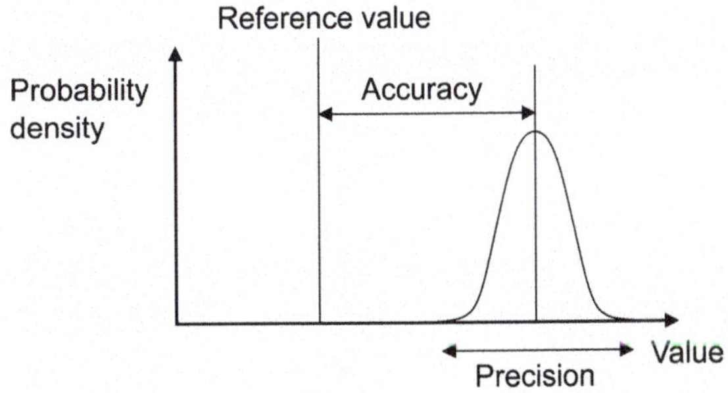

Fig. 13 Accuracy and precision of cine imaging measurements. "Accuracy" indicates the proximity of the measurement result to the true value, and "precision" indicates the degree of reproducibility of the measurement. (From http://en.wikipedia.org/wiki/Accuracy_and_precision)

3.1.9 Accuracy and Precision of Measurements

A measurement, for example, of LV ejection fraction, is valid if it is both accurate and precise. It is important to be familiar with the difference between the terms "accuracy" and "precision" (Fig. 13). "Accuracy" is the degree of veracity, whereas "precision" is the degree of reproducibility or repeatability. Ideally a measurement device, such as cardiac MRI, should be both accurate and precise, with measurements all close to and tightly clustered around a single value, representing the truth. To determine the accuracy of a technique, comparison with a reference standard (e.g., phantom model) (Debatin et al. 1992a, b; Verberne et al. 2006) is the most established method, and the question to be answered is how close does the estimate approach the reference.

However, when estimates are repeated by same observer in the same person over a short period of time under the same conditions using the same instrument, most likely different values will be obtained (Semelka et al. 1990a, b; Yamaoka et al. 1993; Pattynama et al. 1993, 1995; Bogaert et al. 1995). The size of the data cluster determines how precise the technique is, or how reproducible the measurements are. Knowledge of the precision is crucial to determine whether a change in a measured parameter is due to a real change or due to a lack of precision, and it has to take into account the relative contribution of interstudy, interobserver, and intraobserver error (or variability). For instance, a 5% gain in LV ejection fraction after myocardial infarction may reflect a true functional improvement (e.g., recovery of stunned myocardium) when using one imaging

Table 4 Variability of LV measurements obtained with cine MRI

	Mean value	Within-subject variance	Within-subject SD	95% range for change
EDV (ml)	187	20.2	4.5	12.5
ESV (ml)	68	15.9	4.0	11.0
SV (ml)	119	14.0	3.7	10.4
EF (%)	63.6	2.97	1.7	4.8
CO (l/min)	6.86	0.13	0.36	0.99
MM (g)	119.4	16.9	4.1	11.4

The 95% range for change is also called the "repeatability coefficient." Data were calculated by performing ten repeated MRI studies in two controls over a period of five consecutive days. Imaging was performed in the short-axis direction using b-SSFP cine MRI
SD standard deviation, *MM* myocardial mass

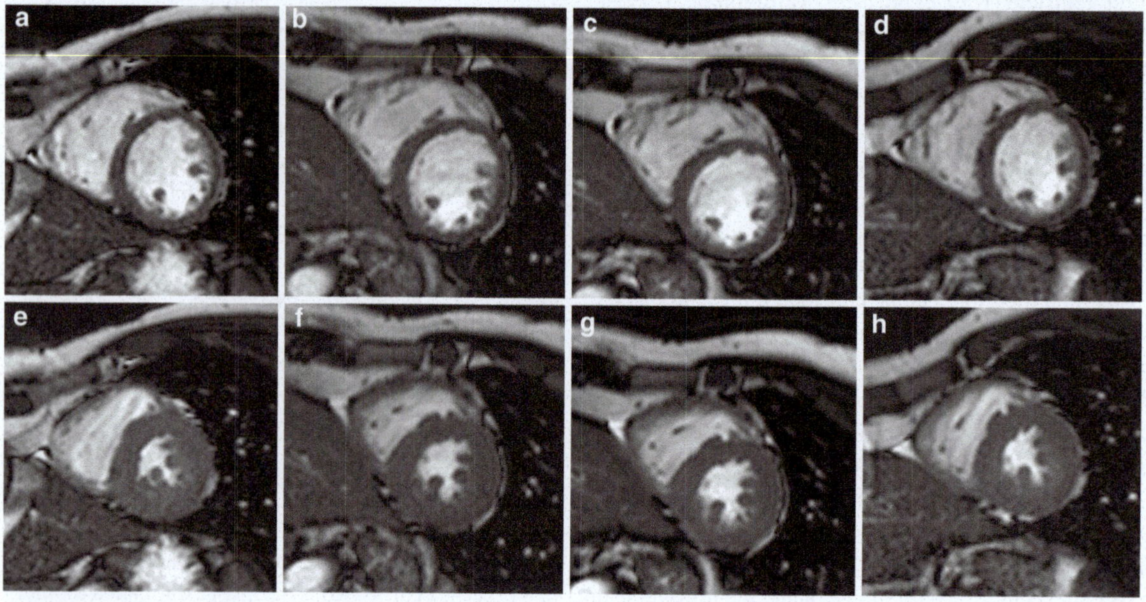

Fig. 14 End-diastolic (*top*) and end-systolic (*bottom*) short-axis cine images at the midventricular level from four different studies obtained in a control subject (see Table 4). Note slight differences in respiratory depth between studies

modality but lack of precision when using another. Precision is usually characterized in terms of the standard deviation (SD) of the measurements. The spread of measured values around the expected value, reflecting the statistical dispersion, is also known the *variance* (Fig. 13). The square root of the variance, or the *within-subject SD*, is often used as a summary of dispersion. This parameter indicates the limits around a single measurement that must be regarded as possible values for the true measurement. To determine whether in a patient a change in the value between repeated measurements reflects a true change, the *95% range for change* or *repeatability coefficient* is used, which is defined as $2\sqrt{2} \times$ within-subject SD. In analogy to a previous study by Pattynama et al. (1993), the above values were recalculated for the novel steady-state free-precession cine MRI sequence by performing ten repeated studies in two normal controls (Table 4, Figs. 14, 15).

The precision of an imaging technique determines the sample size required to demonstrate a clinical change, which is a major cost in pharmaceutical trials (Bottini et al. 1995; Bellenger et al. 2000b). Compared with echocardiography using geometric models to quantify LV volumes and mass, breath-hold cine MRI with volumetric ventricular quantification has a much higher reproducibility, thus requiring smaller sample sizes than echocardiography to detect changes in volumes, mass, and function (Myerson et al. 2002b;

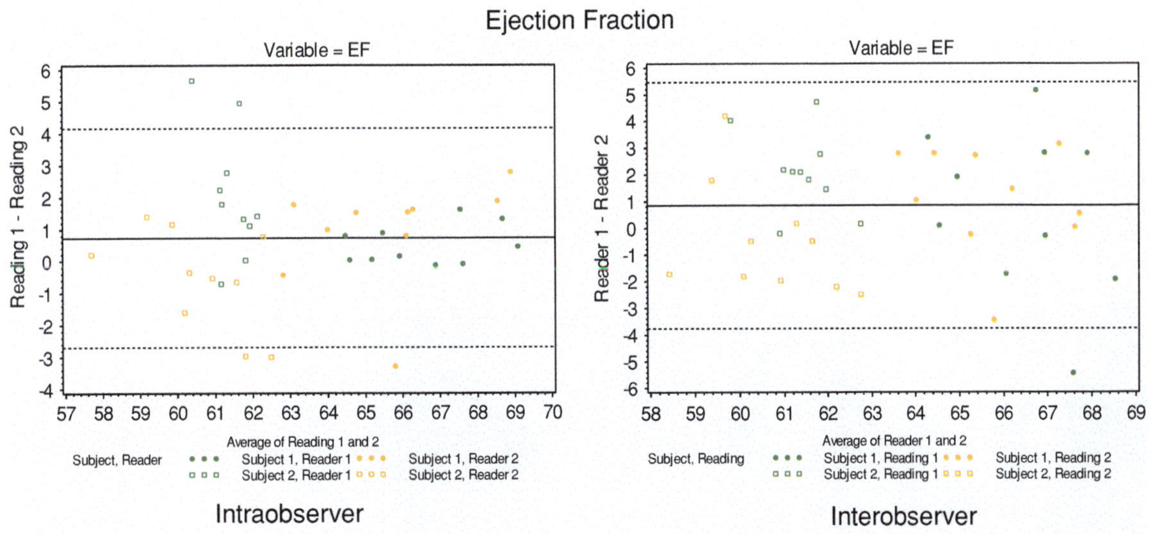

Fig. 15 Bland–Altman plots showing mean the interobserver and intraobserver difference, and the upper and lower limits of agreement for LV ejection fraction. The range of values for the ejection fraction obtained in ten repeated cine imaging studies in two healthy controls can be well appreciated. The *open circles* represents one control, and the *filled circles* represent the other control. All studies were read twice by one observer, as well as independently by a second observer, allowing the intraobserver and interobserver variability to be calculated

Table 5 Sample size required to detect the same change in LV mass and function by echocardiography and MRI with a power of 90% and $p < 0.05$

Clinical change	Echocardiography		MRI		Reduction in sample size (%)
	SD	*n*	SD	*n*	
EDV, 10 ml	23.8	121	7.4	12	90
ESV, 10 ml	15.8	53	6.5	10	81
EF, 3% (abs)	6.6	102	2.5	15	85
Mass, 10 g	36.4	273	6.4	9	97

Adapted from Bellenger et al. (2000a, b, c)

Table 5). In a study by Grothues et al. (2004) evaluating the interstudy reproducibility of MRI, they reported lower reproducibility values for the right ventricle, indicating that the sample sizes for this ventricle need to be larger than those for the left ventricle.

3.1.10 Comparison with Other Cardiac Imaging Techniques

Since the first publications on the use of MRI for quantification of cardiac volumes, function, and mass, results have been compared with those obtained with other "established" techniques, such as contrast ventriculography, echocardiography, radionuclide imaging, and indicator dilution or thermodilution techniques (Longmore et al. 1985; Stratemeier et al. 1986; Kaul et al. 1986; Mogelvang et al. 1986; Dilworth et al. 1987; Markiewicz et al. 1987b; van Rossum et al. 1988a, b; Culham and Vince 1988; Debatin et al. 1992b; Gopal et al. 1993; Herregods et al. 1994; Bavelaar-Croon et al. 2000; Chuang et al. 2000; Bellenger et al. 2000a, 2002; Chuang et al. 2000; Myerson et al. 2002a; Rajappan et al. 2002; Sierra-Galan et al. 2003; Ichikawa et al. 2003). Nowadays, we notice the opposite phenomenon, i.e., MRI is increasingly used to validate other (novel) quantification approaches, emphasizing that MRI has become a front player when it comes to assessment of cardiac functional performance (Sugeng et al. 2006; Niemann et al. 2007; Nesser et al. 2007, 2009). Another important issue is whether results are interchangeable

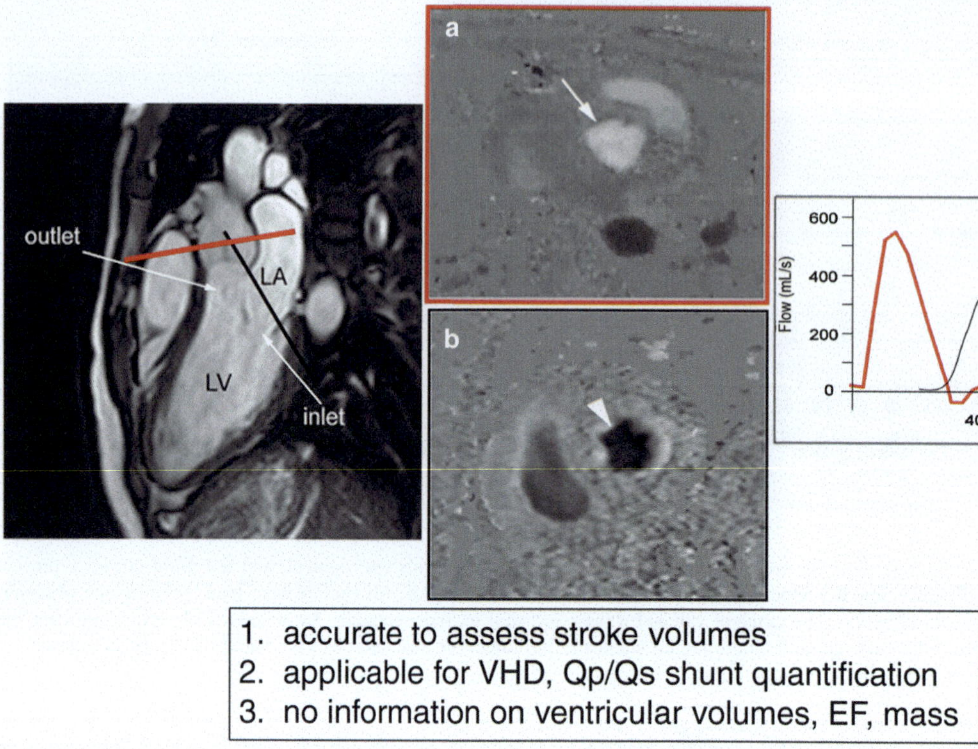

Fig. 16 Ventricular stroke volume assessment with phase-contrast MRI. The *left panel* shows a LV inflow–outflow tract view. Phase-contrast velocity imaging through the aortic root (*red line*) or the mitral valve (*black line*) allows one to visualize and quantify the amount of blood that passes through the aortic root (*arrow*, **a**) and the mitral valve (*arrowhead*, **b**), and allows one to calculate the stroke volume curves (*right panel*). Although this technique is accurate for measurement of stroke volume, no information is provided on ventricular volumes, ejection fraction, or mass. This technique is routinely used for valvular heart disease assessment and for shunt calculation

among imaging modalities. The literature often shows poor to moderate agreement between imaging techniques, and points out that one has to be careful when extrapolating data (Bellenger et al. 2000a, 2002; Bavelaar-Croon et al. 2000; Chuang et al. 2000; Rajappan et al. 2002). This is not surprising if we realize that with a single imaging technique differences of up to 15% in ejection fraction were found in 39 participating centers that tested their performance to assess LV ejection fraction with a gated single-photon-emission computed tomography phantom (Verberne et al. 2006).

3.2 Ventricular Stroke Volume Assessment with Phase-Contrast MRI

Phase-contrast imaging does not provide information on ventricular volumes, ejection fraction, or mass, but it is still a very attractive, fast sequence that is very often used in daily routine practice to assess cardiac performance (Kondo et al. 1991; Fig. 16). It can be seen as an adjunct to the previously described volumetric approaches to assess the cardiac ventricles. Although volumetric approaches deduce the ventricular stroke volume by measuring the difference between end-diastolic and end-systolic volume, similar information can be obtained by performing a flow measurement through the atrioventricular ("inflow") or the ventriculoarterial ("outflow") valve of the ventricle of interest. In normal circumstances, volumetric stroke volumes and inflow and outflow stroke volumes should be identical. This combined approach is the method to quantify leaking cardiac valves and determine the degree of secondary ventricular remodeling (see "Valvular Heart Disease"). By measuring stroke volumes in the ascending aorta and pulmonary artery, one can noninvasively quantify

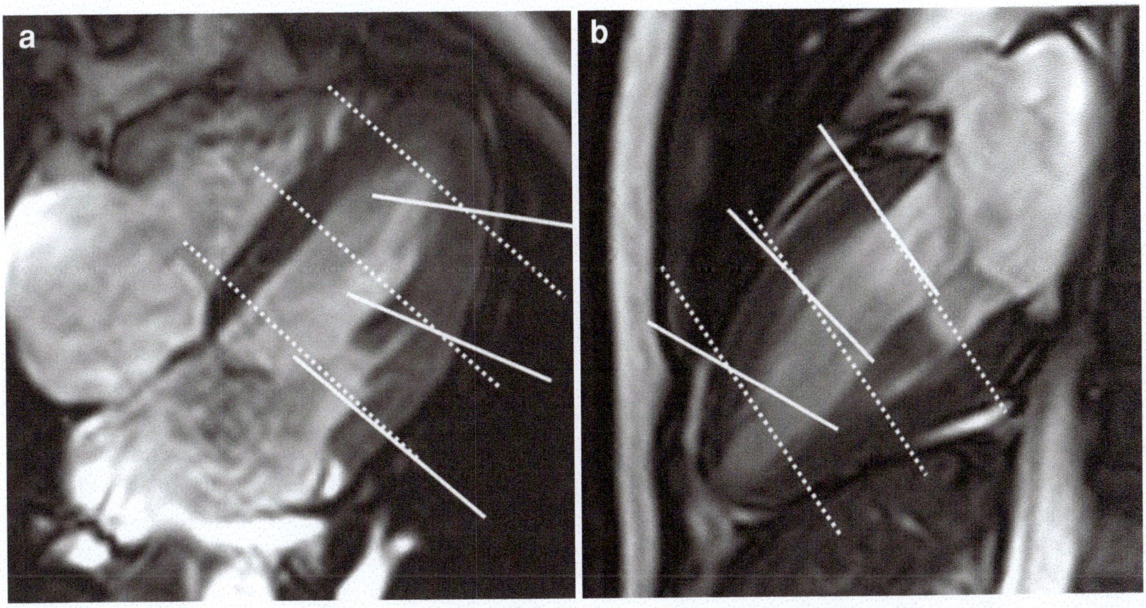

Fig. 17 Overestimation of true myocardial wall thickness using nonperpendicular imaging. Horizontal (**a**) and vertical (**b**) cine imaging showing the end-systolic time frame. The short-axis image direction is shown by the *dashed lines*. Although the risk of overestimation of true myocardial wall thickness (ideal slice cut for correct measurement shown by the *full lines*) is minimal at the LV base, because of its curved nature, the wall thickness is significantly overestimated approaching the LV apex

the presence and severity of a cardiac shunt (Arheden et al. 1999; Beerbaum et al. 2001; Powell et al. 2003; see "Congenital Heart Disease").

3.3 Regional Ventricular Function

A comprehensive evaluation of ventricular performance should extend beyond the level of assessment of global ventricular performance (see Sect. 3.1) and should also include evaluation of regional performance. This is crucial since many cardiac diseases focally affect the heart, causing functional impairment in the diseased region. The net effect on global performance depends on the extent of regional dysfunction, and the impact on the remote myocardium. In the following sections, first the routinely used parameters to express regional ventricular function are highlighted, followed by a discussion on myocardial tagging and how this technique can be used to measure myocardial strain.

3.3.1 Myocardial Wall Motion and Wall Thickening

As mentioned in Sect. 2, the left ventricle exhibits a complex contraction, causing longitudinal and circumferential shortening, and myocardial wall thickening. These can be evaluated to express regional performance. For instance, preserved myocardial wall thickness is a good indicator of the presence of viable myocardium in the setting of chronic myocardial ischemia (Baer et al. 1994), whereas systolic wall thickening provides a powerful measure of regional performance, which is independent of any external reference point and can be used for assessment during pharmacological stress. Wall motion and wall thickening can be visually assessed using a grading system or can be quantified. A useful visual grading system for systolic wall thickening is normal wall thickening, diminished or absent wall thickening, systolic wall thinning, and conversely increased wall thickening. Delineating endocardial and epicardial borders at the end of diastole and at the end of systole, usually on short-axis cine images, enables one to calculate absolute and relative wall thickening. The results can be averaged and expressed per region, using, for instance, the standardized 17-segment approach, or a modified centerline technique running through the middle of the myocardium on which 100 chords are defined and the systolic changes in chord length quantified (see Fig. 40). Although both methods represent an accurate way to express wall thickening, some comments are necessary. To achieve a correct estimate of wall thickness, one should perform perpendicular measurements through the wall. However, as shown in Fig. 17, short-axis images cut the myocardium not perpendicularly but obliquely in the LV apex, leading to some degree of partial volume effect and overestimation. Three-dimensional reconstructions can completely compensate for this deviation and provide an exact wall thickness (Aurigemma et al. 1992; Lima et al. 1993; Forbat et al. 1994). Second, because of through-plane motion, one should correct for this motion to achieve correct measurements of wall thickening (Pattynama et al. 1992). Third, as mentioned in Sect. 3.1.7, the papillary muscles as well as trabeculations may significantly influence (i.e., overestimate) wall thickness values, especially at the end of systole. Therefore, it is advisable to exclude during delineation both structures from the myocardium (Dawson et al. 2011; Fig. 12).

For regional wall motion analysis, a semiquantitative visual analysis is often used clinically. Different grades for wall motion are used: normokinesia (i.e., normal wall motion toward the center of the ventricle), hypokinesia (i.e., decreased wall motion), akinesia (i.e., absent wall motion), dyskinesia (i.e., outward wall motion), and hyperkinesia (i.e., increased wall motion) (Fig. 18). Hypokinetic wall motion can be furthermore subdivided according to the severity (e.g., mild, moderate, severe). As for systolic wall thickening, contouring of the endocardial and epicardial border may help to quantify motion, e.g., the amount of centripetal motion of the endocardial border during systole. Again some comments are needed. First, circumferential wall motion is expressed using a reference point, which is usually the center point of the LV cavity. Use of a fixed center point may be preferable to use of a floating center point (i.e., center point redefined at the end of systole), in particular in patients with focal disease (e.g., myocardial infarction), because the latter tends to overestimate the wall motion in the diseased regions at the cost of wall motion in the remote regions (Masci et al. 2009). Second, endocardial circumferential wall motion is heavily influenced by wall thickness and systolic wall thickening (see Sect. 2). Therefore, Ugander et al. (2010) argued that epicardial wall motion and related changes in epicardial volume are a better measure of short-axis function than endocardial motion. Third, to accurately quantify wall motion patterns, myocardial markers are needed enabling one to trace the motion throughout the cardiac cycle. Although this can be achieved to a limited extent using anatomical landmarks (RV insertions, papillary muscles), MRI myocardial tagging and related techniques are ideal for this purpose. Finally, in contrast to the three-layered configuration of the LV wall (i.e., oblique endocardial and epicardial layer, circumferential midwall), the RV wall has a two-layered appearance with oblique epicardial and longitudinally oriented endocardial fibers, whereby the latter follow the direction of the inflow and outflow tract. As a consequence, the kinetics of the RV wall differs from that of its left counterpart, exhibiting a similar twisting pattern, but more longitudinal strain and a greater amount of displacement.

3.3.2 Myocardial Strain and Motion Imaging

Myocardial *strain* can be defined as the relative two-dimensional or three-dimensional deformation of myocardium by an internal or external force, whereas *strain rate* is the rate of this deformation (Abraham and Nishimura 2001). Before the era of MRI, implantation of metallic beads, strain gauges, or coils was indispensable to study myocardial strain and motion patterns (Hansen et al. 1988; Waldman et al. 1985, 1988), evidently limiting this kind of research to animal models or posttransplant patients. In the late 1980s, two landmark articles opened the door toward noninvasive myocardial strain assessment using an MRI technique called *myocardial tagging* (Zerhouni et al. 1988; Axel and Dougherty 1989a, b). Briefly, tagging consists in creating markers on the myocardium that can be used as internal landmarks to depict the myocardial deformation. Spatially selective destruction of the myocardial magnetization occurs if in one or more planes orthogonal to the imaging plane radio-frequency pulses are applied prior to the imaging process (Fig. 19). As a consequence, at the intersection of the tagging plane(s) and the imaging plane, local magnetization is destroyed and this will be visible as hypointense or black line(s) on the image plane in clear contrast with the nontagged gray myocardium. If subsequent myocardial deformation occurs, these tag line(s) will deform, and this deformation and displacement can be used for strain analysis (Young and Axel 1992; Young et al. 1993). Depending on the T1 relaxation time of myocardium, the tags slowly fade away but normally persist for

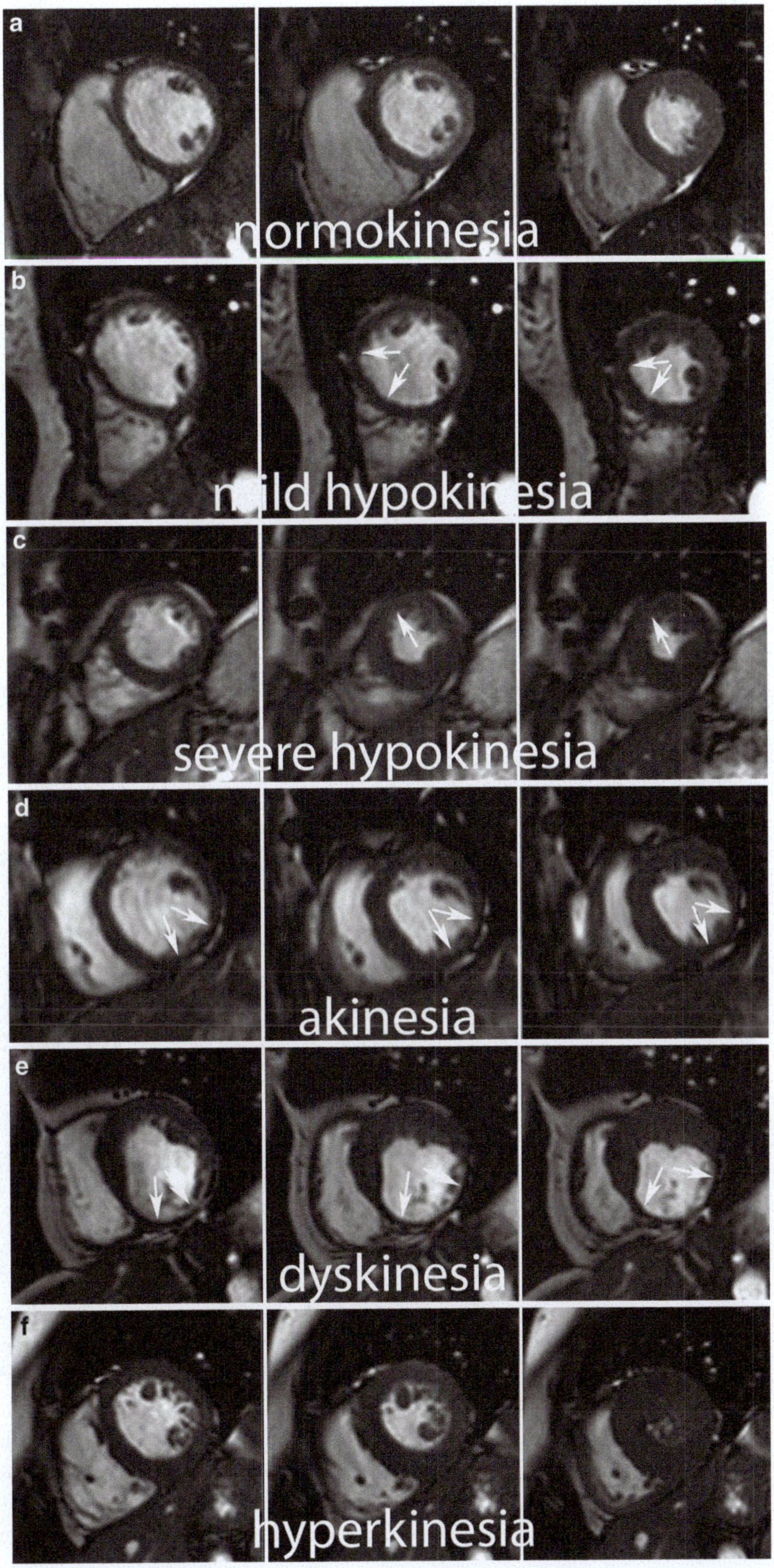

Fig. 18 Examples of the different wall motion patterns on short-axis cine imaging. Each row shows an end-diastolic (*left*), a mid-systolic (*middle*), and an end-systolic (*right*) image.
a Normokinesia, **b** minor hypokinesia in ventricular septum (*arrows*), **c** focal severe hypokinesia in anterior LV wall (*arrows*), **d** akinesia of the inferolateral LV wall in an old transmural myocardial infarction (*arrows*), **e** dyskinesia of the inferior wall in a patient with an old transmural myocardial infarction with aneurysm formation (*arrows*), and **f** hyperkinesia of the entire LV wall in a patient with a severe congenital aortic stenosis. Careful analysis of endocardial and epicardial border motion during cardiac contraction allows one to express the wall motion pattern. Dynamic assessment using the viewing mode is very helpful for visual analysis. Note the outward motion of the aneurysm in the patient with the dyskinetic wall motion pattern (**e**), and the subtotal occlusion of the LV cavity in the patient with the hyperkinetic wall motion pattern (**f**). Moreover, focal hypokinesia (**b**) may be masked if the contractility of the surrounding myocardium is well preserved

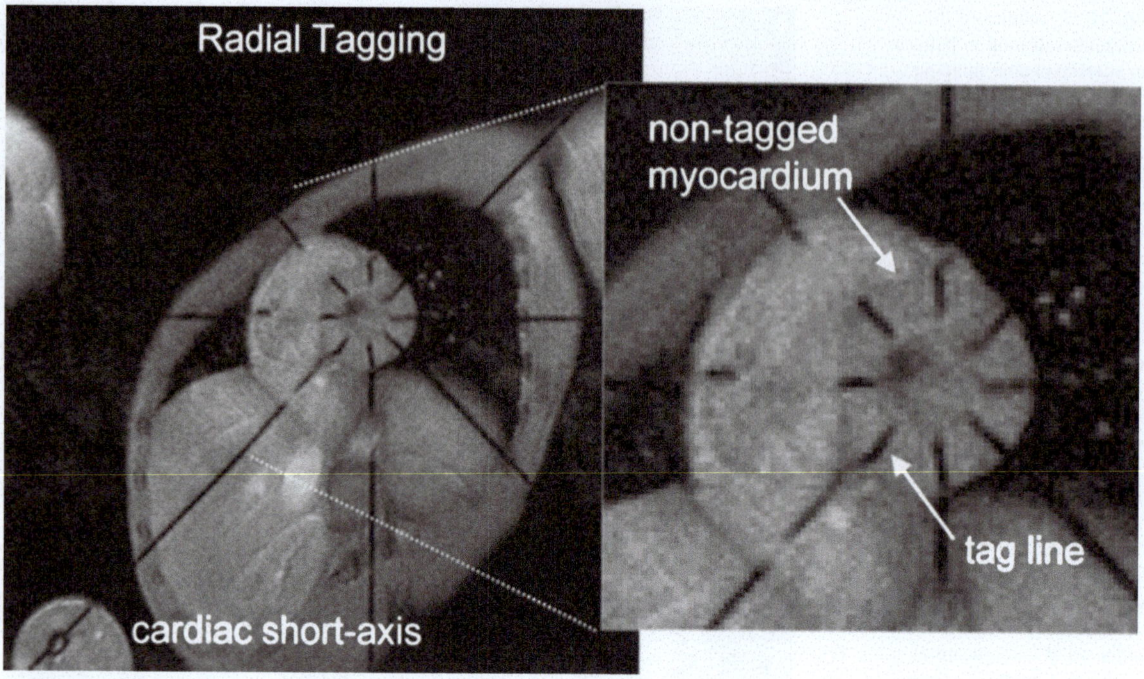

Fig. 19 Principles of creating myocardial tags using radial MRI tagging. Short-axis view (*left*) and enlarged view (*right*) using the spoiled gradient-echo technique. Tag prepulses, in four tag planes perpendicular on the short-axis plane crossing in the center of the left ventricle, create eight tag lines on the myocardium. These tag lines are in contrast with the nontagged myocardium, and allow one to analyze the myocardial deformation during the cardiac cycle

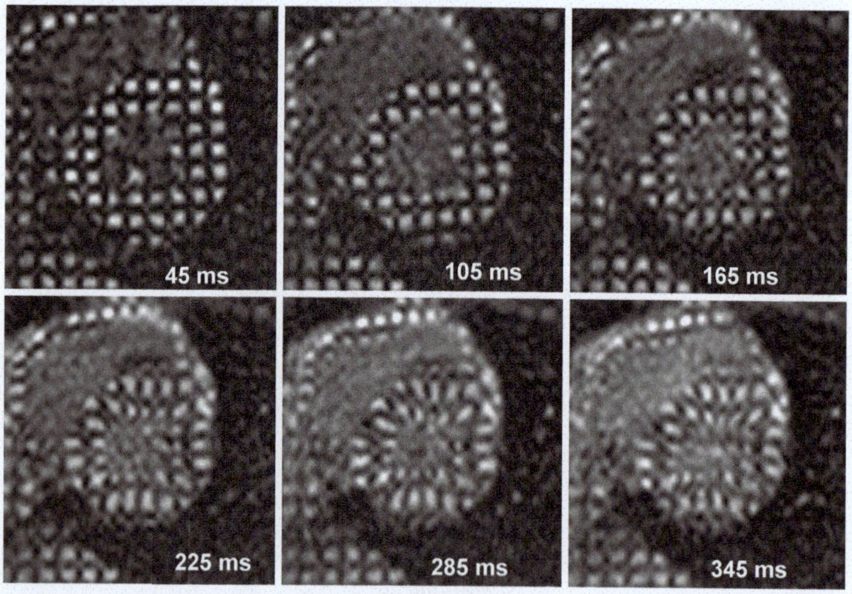

Fig. 20 Spatial modulation of magnetization (SPAMM) tagging creates a grid on the myocardium. Example of short-axis SPAMM tagging. Six time points are shown during cardiac systole (45–345 ms). The original grid at the end of diastole is rapidly deformed by the myocardial deformation. Note that in the inner myocardial layers, deformation is larger than in the outer layers

several hundred milliseconds, and if they are implemented at the time of the end of diastole, a large portion of the cardiac cycle can be studied. Different types of tagging sequences are currently available (Axel et al. 2005). Spatial modulation of magnetization (SPAMM) tagging is likely the most frequently used tagging technique (Axel and Dougherty 1989a, b; Fig. 20). The tagging sequence modulates the magnetization, and

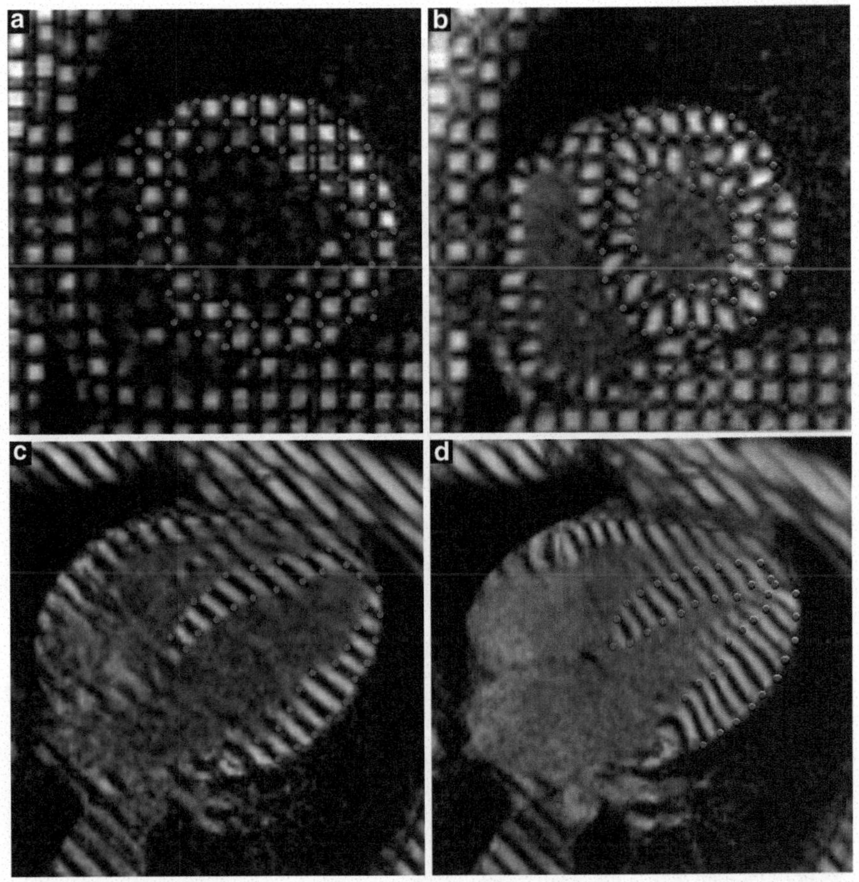

Fig. 21 Two-dimensional tagging analysis. Tagging in the cardiac short-axis view (**a**, **b**) and horizontal long-axis view (**c**, **d**) and end-diastolic (*right*) and end-systolic (*left*) time frames. Tracking of the grid intersections (indicated in *red*) on the short-axis views and the intersections of the tags with the endocardial and epicardial border (indicated in *red*) on the long-axis views allows one to analyze the local myocardial deformation

thus the magnetic resonance signal, with a sinusoid line profile in one direction or in two perpendicular directions, creating a set of parallel line tags or a grid on the myocardium. It is basically a two-dimensional approach, although three-dimensional approaches have been proposed (Kuijer et al. 2002; Ryf et al. 2002). The other approach is to use precise definition of the tag lines, enabling one to study a ventricle in different geometric patterns (Zerhouni et al. 1988). Because of the helical configuration, an elegant approach to study the left ventricle is the use of a radial geometric pattern with the tag lines crossing each other in the center of the LV cavity, whereas in the long-axis direction, parallel oriented tags are used (see Fig. 21). Both approaches have advantages and disadvantages. Radial tagging has the advantage of easier merging of short-axis and long-axis images in a truly three-dimensional data set (Fig. 14). The markers or tagging points are more homogeneously distributed over the myocardium, and the endocardial and epicardial borders are more easily delineated than on SPAMM tagged images. However, implementation of these tags is not straightforward and no postprocessing packages are commercially available. Prolonged tag persistence can be achieved when scanning with high-field (3-T) magnets (i.e., longer T1 relaxation time), and by using optimized sequences such as complementary SPAMM tagging (Fischer et al. 1993). Several further improvements of the tagging technique have been proposed, but an extensive description is beyond the scope of this chapter (Bolster et al. 1990; Pipe et al. 1991; Rogers et al. 1991; McVeigh and Zerhouni 1991; McVeigh and Atalar 1992; Hendrich et al. 1994; Moore et al. 1994; O'Dell et al. 1995; Perman et al. 1995; Bosmans et al. 1996; Spiegel et al. 2003). It should be added that tagging can be perfectly applied to the right ventricle as well (Naito et al. 1995), but the thin RV wall and complex RV geometry makes tagging technically more challenging. For completeness, tagging techniques are not exclusively designed to study the myocardium, but can also be applied to evaluate inflammatory fusion of pericardial layers, to distinguish slow flow from thrombus, or

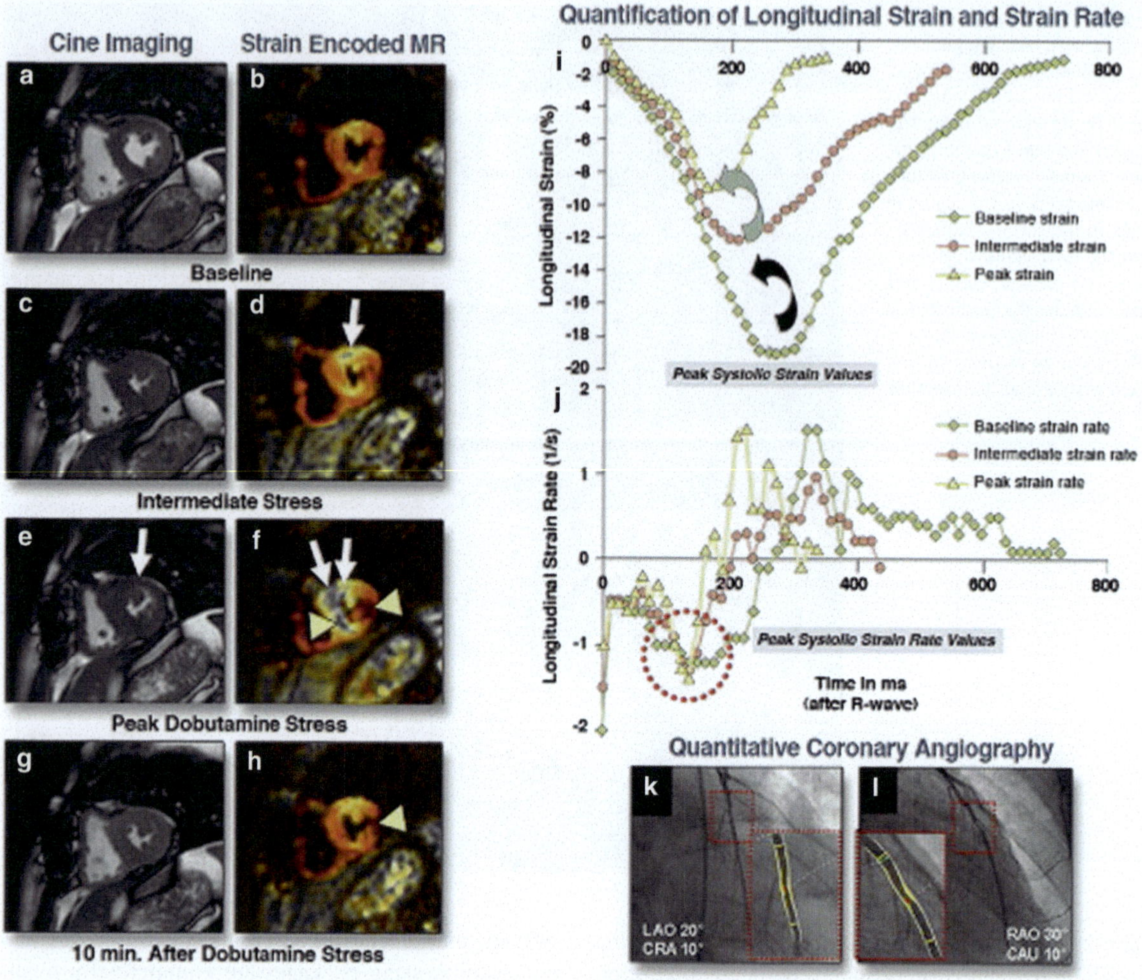

Fig. 22 Strain-encoded (SENC) MRI in a patient with CAD. Mid-short-axis SENC and cine images are shown (**a–h**). With cine images, inducible ischemia is detected only during peak stress in the midanterior left ventricular wall (**e**, *white arrow*). Conversely, with SENC images, a subtle, albeit clearly detectable, strain defect is already observed during intermediate stages (**e**, *white arrow*). Quantification analysis showed that peak systolic strain decreased stepwise during inotropic stimulation (as indicated by *black arrows* and *green arrows* in **i**), whereas the peak systolic strain rate remained unchanged (**j**, *dotted circle*). The presence of a 68% diameter lesion in the left distal anterior descending artery was confirmed by angiography (**k**, **l**). *Arrowheads* indicate signal voids on SENC images due to low signal-to-noise ratio. (Reprinted from Korosoglou et al. 2010b)

to differentiate solid structures (e.g., differentiate muscular tissue from tumor) (Hatabu et al. 1994; Kojima et al. 1999). A major shortcoming to clinically implement myocardial tagging is the tedious and time-consuming analysis, necessitating operator interaction. To overcome this problem, the harmonic phase (HARP) method, measuring the spectral peaks in k-space, was proposed, providing automatic and rapid analysis of tagged images, thus opening the door toward strain imaging in stress conditions (Osman et al. 1999; Sampath et al. 2003). In 2001, Osman et al. (2001) proposed the strain-encoded (SENC) MRI method, based on the principle of HARP-MRI. Instead of planning the tag surfaces orthogonal to the image plane, positioning tag planes parallel to the image plane provides information regarding through-plane motion and strain. This is achieved by applying the tagging (modulation) gradient in the slice-selection direction. In this way short-axis SENC-MRI provides information regarding the longitudinal cardiac strain.

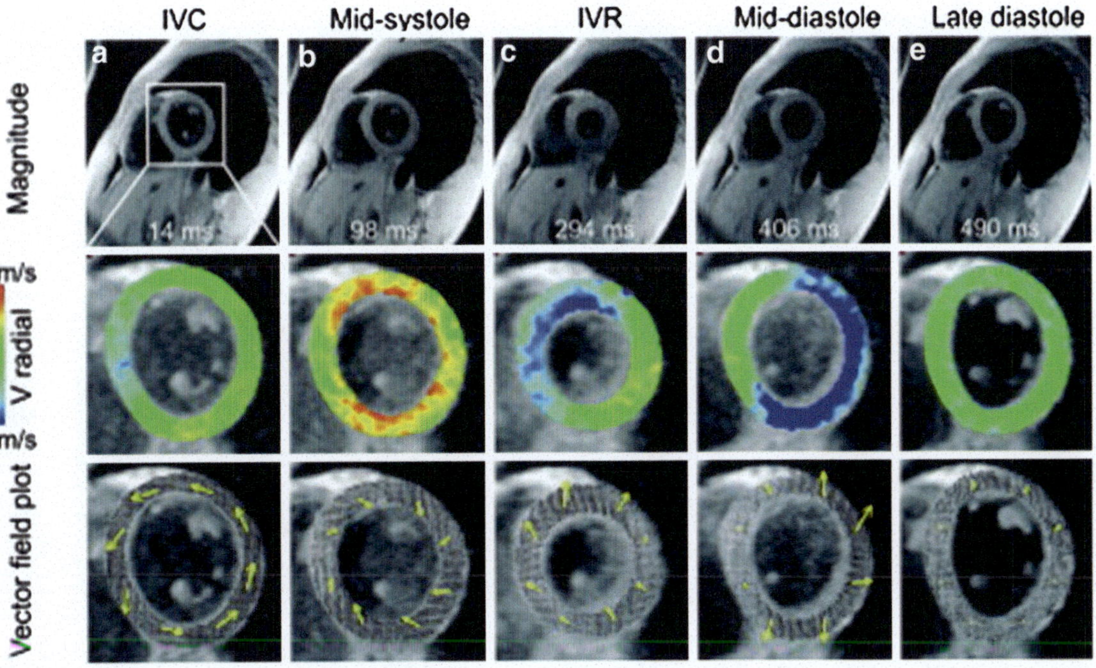

Fig. 23 Magnitude images (*top row*), color-coded maps of radial velocities (*middle row*), and pixelwise arrow plots of in-plane velocity vector fields (*bottom row*) in a basal slice for five cardiac frames (isovolumetric contraction/relaxation). The data set of a healthy volunteer was acquired during free breathing with a temporal resolution of 13.8 ms. (Reprinted from Jung et al. 2006b)

To compute a SENC strain map, two SENC images with different tuning frequencies (low and high tuning) are acquired. This strain map is subsequently overlaid on the anatomical image, and is presented as a color-coded functional image. Pan et al. (2006) developed a real-time FastSENC variant with an in-plane resolution of 4 mm $\times$ 4 mm, a temporal resolution of 37 ms, and complete coverage of the cardiac cycle. This technique has the major advantage over conventional tagging techniques that strains are directly visualized. Promising results have been reported by single centers, awaiting a more widespread use of the FastSENC technique (Fig. 22) (Korosoglou et al. 2008, 2009a, 2010a, b; Neizel et al. 2009).

A second approach to measure myocardial motion is phase-contrast velocity imaging (Constable et al. 1994; Lingamneni et al. 1995). Since each pixel contains velocity data, this intrinsic information can be used to measure myocardial velocities and displacement. Displacement encoding with stimulated echoes (DENSE) imaging represents a phase-contrast imaging sequence that is optimized to measure myocardial displacement and enable two- or three-dimensional tissue tracking (Aletras et al. 1999a, b; Kim et al. 2004; Spottiswoode et al. 2008; Hess et al. 2009). Recently, the DENSE technique showed that the highest contractility inside the LV myocardium has the form of an open figure eight, suggesting the existing of a functional helical myocardial band (Nasiraei-Moghaddam and Gharib 2009). Tissue phase mapping is another optimized phase-contrast imaging sequence with three-dimensional velocity encoding, sensitivity for low velocities, and black-blood preparation to directly measure myocardial velocities with high spatial and temporal resolution (as short as 14 ms) (Petersen et al. 2006; Jung et al. 2006a; Föll et al. 2009, 2010; Lutz et al. 2011; Figs. 23, 24). Although the temporal resolution is excellent, making it competitive with tissue-Doppler imaging, the data acquisition and image processing times remain long, limiting its use in daily practice (Föll et al. 2009).

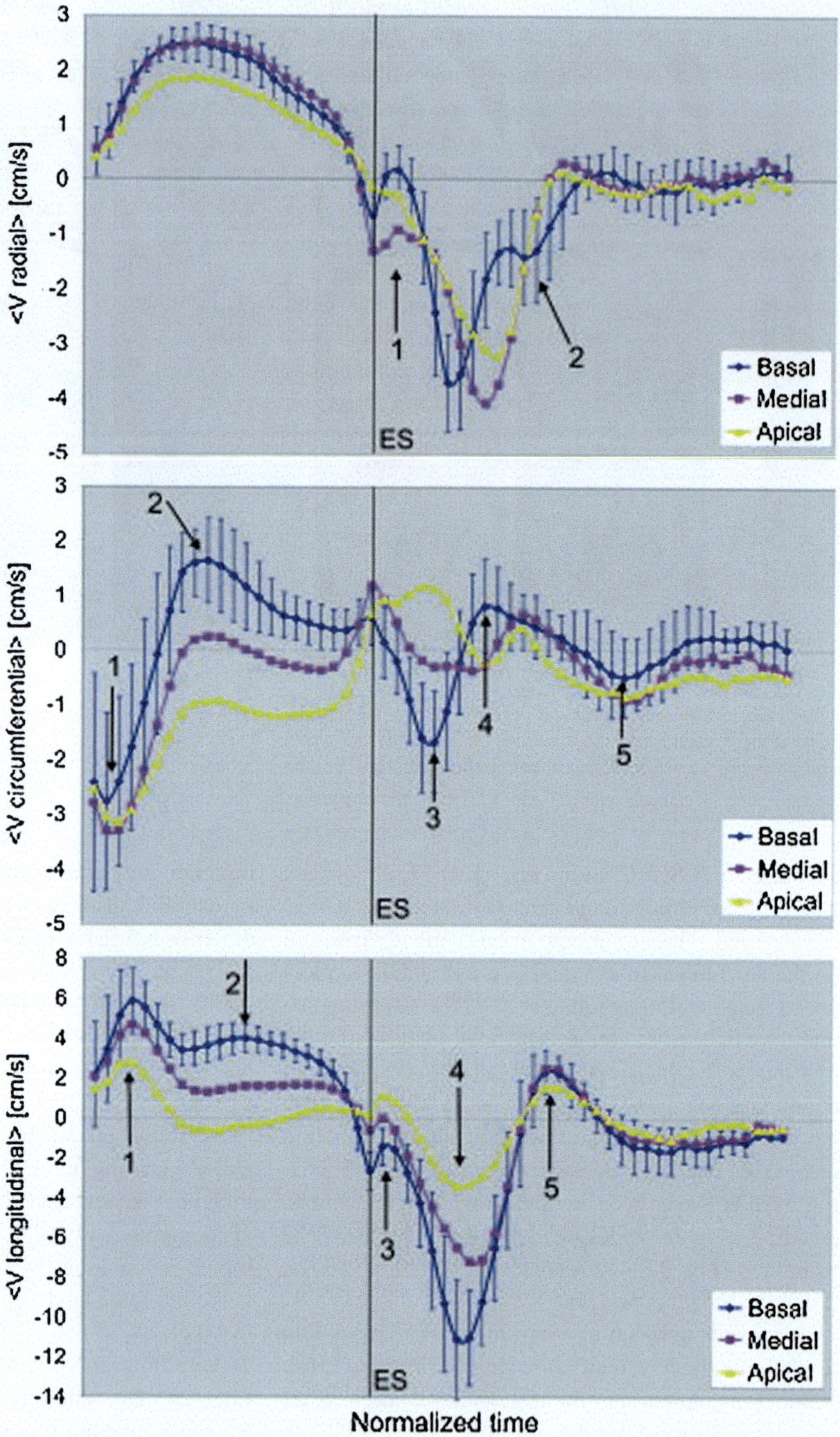

Fig. 24 Time courses of radial (*top*), circumferential (*middle*), and longitudinal (*bottom*) velocities with high temporal resolution averaged over all volunteers. Each graph shows a comparison of data for basal, midventricular, and apical slice location. *ES* end of systole. (Reprinted from Jung et al. 2006b)

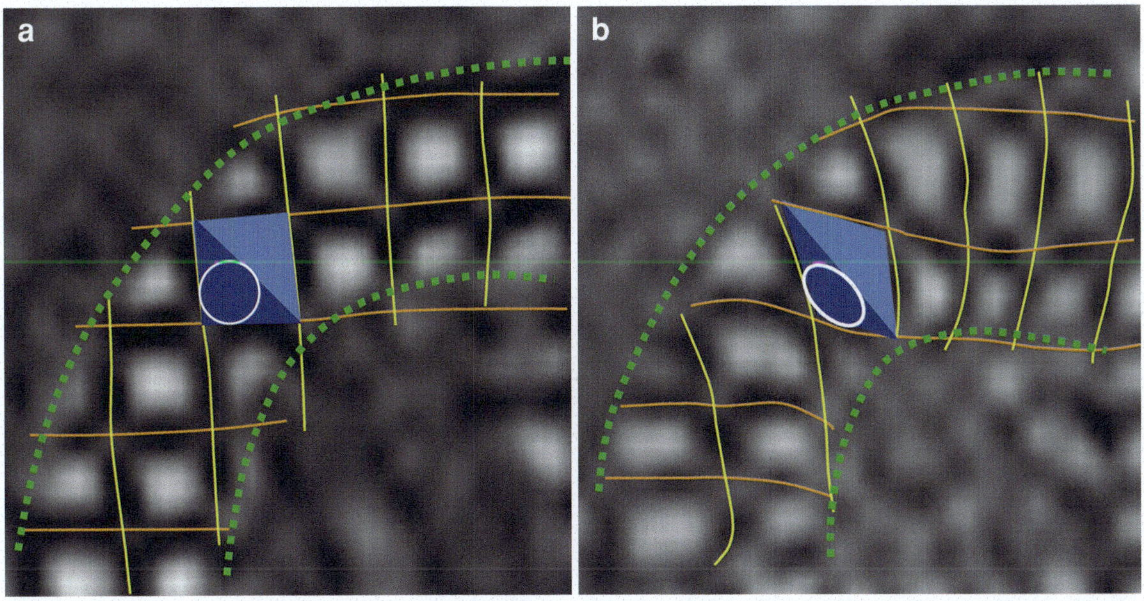

Fig. 25 Two-dimensional principal strain analysis ("Moore's principle"). Short-axis SPAMM tagging at the end of diastole (**a**) and at the end of systole (**b**). The circle that fits in the equiangular triangle at the end of diastole is transformed by the underlying myocardial deformation into an oval at the end of systole. This oval is defined by two axes. The short axis corresponds with the first principal strain. This is a shortening strain and corresponds with the circumferential shortening. The long axis of the oval represents the third principal strain. This strain is a positive strain and corresponds with the radial strain (systolic wall thickening). The principal axes reflect the direction of the principal strains. The axes of shortening and lengthening correspond closely with the direction of circumferential shortening and wall thickening, respectively. The *dashed lines* represent the endocardial and epicardial borders

3.3.3 Principles of Myocardial Strain Analysis

To properly describe and decompose the complex three-dimensional myocardial strain during the cardiac cycle, one can use a Cartesian coordinate system, or describe strain independently of a coordinate system (Waldman et al. 1985, 1988; Figs. 25, 26, 27). It is obvious that a local cardiac coordinate system is much more practical to describe and understand myocardial strain than the *XYZ* coordinate used by the magnet (Fig. 26). This local coordinate system consists of three orthogonal axes, radial–circumferential–longitudinal (RCL), the first two, i.e., circumferential and longitudinal, are oriented tangential to the LV wall, whereas the third one, i.e., radial, is perpendicular to the LV wall. Deformation is then described in three normal strains and three shear strains (Moore et al. 1992; Pipe et al. 1991; Young and Axel 1992; Young et al. 1993, 1994; Bogaert 1997; Götte et al. 2006). Normal strains quantify displacements or changes in length along a coordinate system. They can be positive or negative, for example, positive radial strains represent wall thickening, whereas negative strains represent segment shortening for longitudinal shortening. Shear strains quantify forces acting in two opposite directions. These will typically deform a square into a parallelogram (Fig. 27). For the RCL coordinate system, the shear strains are radial–circumferential, longitudinal–radial, and circumferential–longitudinal. The best known shear strain is the circumferential–longitudinal shear strain, describing the LV (un)twisting. Quantification of the shear strain is a parameter of ventricular torsion (Buchalter et al. 1990; Lorenz et al. 2000). In Fig. 26 shows how with the use of merging of tagging at short-axis and long-axis levels (using the planes both for imaging and for tagging) the left ventricle can be divided into 32 small myocardial pieces (*cuboids*) (Goshtasby and Turner 1996; see Fig. 26). Each of these cuboids is defined by eight node points, obtained from the crossing of tag lines with endocardial and epicardial borders, allowing a four-dimensional analysis of this cuboid based on the three-dimensional displacement of the node points

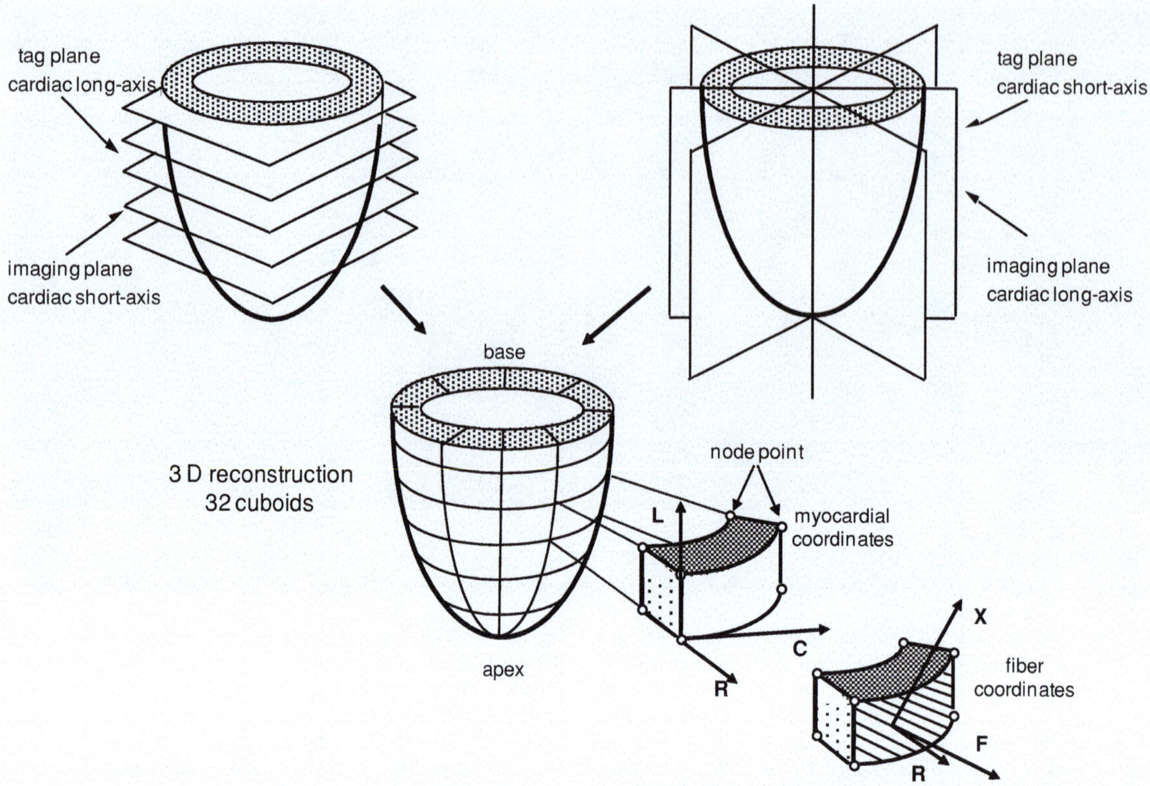

Fig. 26 Merging of long-axis and short-axis radial tagging into a three-dimensional myocardial deformation scheme. Using a combination of long-axis and short-axis tagging, one can divide the LV myocardium into small blocks of myocardial tissue (*cuboids*) defined by the node points in three-dimensional space. Their coordinates can be expressed in a local cardiac radial–circumferential–longitudinal coordinate system or in a fiber radial–fiber–cross-fiber coordinate system. This approach allows a three-dimensional strain calculation during the cardiac cycle

during the cardiac cycle. To increase our understanding of how the basic action of fiber shortening and lengthening relates to the regional myocardial and global ventricular deformation, the RCL coordinate system can be transformed into a local fiber coordinate system (radial–fiber–cross-fiber), using standard fiber angle orientations obtained from autopsy studies (ideally these data should be measured in vivo using, for instance, diffusion tensor imaging). The fiber direction represents the oblique direction of the endocardial or epicardial fibers, whereas the cross-fiber is oriented orthogonally in the endocardial or epicardial surface, and the radial axis remains the same as in the RCL coordinate system.

If no coordinate system is used, one can describe myocardial strain in three principal strains and and with three principal angles or axes of deformation (Waldman et al. 1985; Azhari et al. 1993; Croisille et al. 1999; Fig. 25). The (end-systolic) principal strains are ranked according to the magnitude of deformation starting with the (most) negative. Thus, the first principal strain is a shortening strain. The second is often negligible but sometimes shows a substantial shortening, especially near the endocardium, whereas the third principal strain is usually a positive (or thickening) strain, corresponding to the radial strain. The principle axes reflect the direction of the three principal strains. Whereas at the subepicardium the principal axis of shortening corresponds to the direction of the obliquely oriented subepicardial fibers, at the subendocardium this axis is nearly perpendicular to the endocardial fiber direction, suggesting substantial transmural fiber interaction, leading to the so-called phenomenon of cross-fiber shortening (Waldman et al. 1985, 1988; Rademakers et al. 1994).

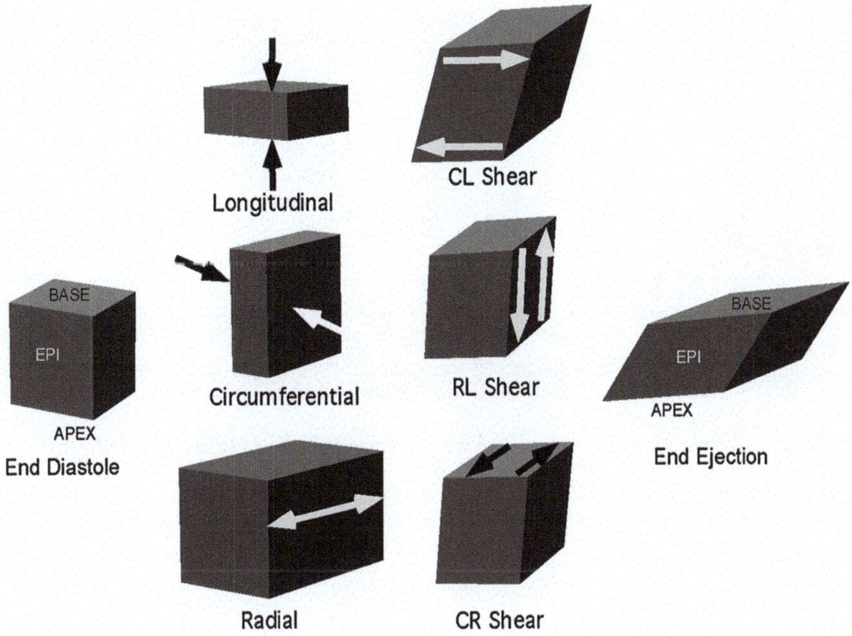

Fig. 27 Decomposition of the complex deformation of the myocardial cuboid during systole into three normal strains (*middle left*) and three shear strains (*middle right*). Nondeformed myocardial cuboid at the of end diastole (*left*) and the same cuboid at the end of systole (*right*)

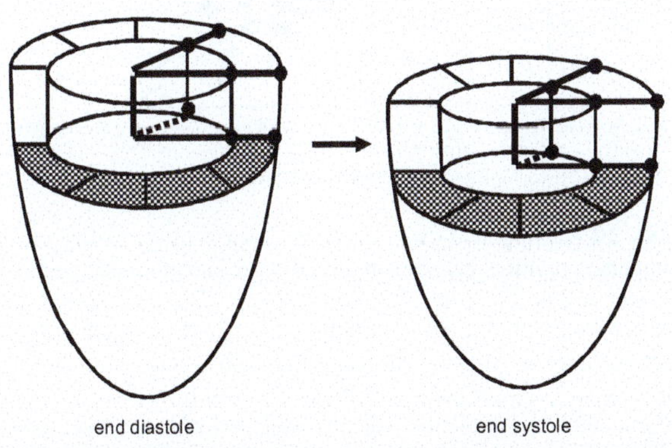

Fig. 28 Regional ejection fraction. Two adjacent radial tag lines on two adjacent levels describe an intracavitary triangle with the apex in the center of the left ventricle and the base on the endocardial surface. In this way, one cuboid describes a triangular volume, which permits calculation and quantification of the regional ejection fraction for this cuboid

3.3.4 Regional Ejection Fraction

Defining a simple-to-use parameter that expresses regional performance, i.e., regional ejection fraction, remains challenging. Such a parameter would be most welcome to better appreciate the contribution of the different parts of the ventricular wall to the global ventricular performance. As mentioned earlier, tagging can be used to divide the myocardium into small cuboids. Since each cuboid describes a triangular volume of blood, the changes in this blood volume over the cardiac cycle can be used to calculate a regional ejection fraction (Bogaert et al. 1999, 2000; Bogaert and Rademakers 2001; Rademakers et al. 2003; Fig. 28). This parameter can be seen as a composite measure reflecting the effects of circumferential and longitudinal shortening and radial thickening occurring in the cuboid. It is a relative measure, and therefore, for example, near the ventricular apex, the triangular blood volumes are somewhat smaller and a larger regional ejection fraction could still represent a smaller absolute volume change than at the base. Another approach to achieve an estimate of regional ejection fraction particularly in patients with focal myocardial disease, such as patients with a myocardial infarction, is the merging of late Gd MRI and cine MRI.

The infarct area can be determined on the late Gd images, whereas the functionality of this area, preferably using a fixed-center system, can be determined on the cine images (Fig. 29; Masci et al. 2009).

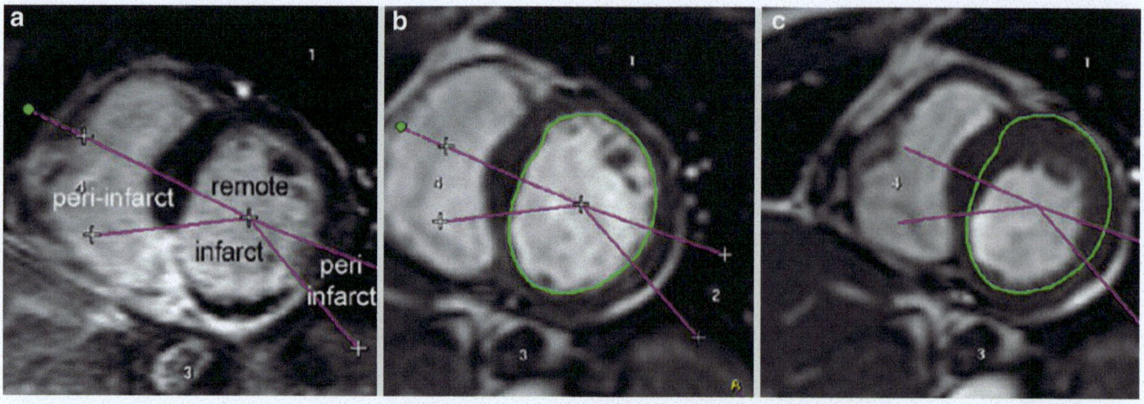

Fig. 29 Regional ejection fraction assessment by merging cine imaging and late Gd imaging in a patient with an acute inferior LV infarct. Late Gd imaging (**a**) and cine imaging at the end of diastole (**b**) and at the end of systole (**c**). The extent of enhancement on late Gd imaging can be used to determine the infarct area, and next to define periinfarct border zones as well as the remote myocardium on cine images. This approach allows one to calculate a regional ejection fraction in the infarcted area, i.e., 16.5%, and remote myocardium, i.e., 66.2%. (Adapted from Masci et al. 2009)

3.3.5 Intrinsic Myocardial Contractility

All parameters used clinically to express ventricular performance such as stroke volume, ejection fraction, fractional shortening or rate of ejection, and circumferential or fiber shortening are not only determined by the intrinsic myocardial contractility but are also significantly influenced by the ventricular loading (preloading and afterloading) conditions (Streeter et al. 1970; Mirsky et al. 1988; Legget 1999; Abraham and Nishimura 2001). A load-free estimate of the intrinsic myocardial contractility would be welcome in many cardiac diseases, for example, in patients with dilated cardiomyopathies. This can be achieved by evaluating the influence of a progressive increase of ventricular afterload (e.g., by leg lifting, pharmacologic interventions, or static exercise, handgrip) on ventricular functional parameters such as fractional shortening and shortening velocities. The inverse linear relation between both of these reflects the intrinsic myocardial contractility (Mirsky et al. 1988). In patients with aortic stenosis presenting with reduced ejection fraction, it may be of value to distinguish between reduced myocardial shortening due to excessive afterload and that due to depressed myocardial contractility (Borow et al. 1992; Legget 1999). Rather than varying the end-systolic LV wall stress to determine the myocardial contractility, Rademakers et al. (Rademakers et al. 2003) used the regional differences in wall stress to determine a stress–strain relation, reflecting myocardial contractility at a single load level. A close inverse linear relationship was found between regional wall stress (or load) and regional ejection fraction (Fig. 30). This implies that regions with higher (end-systolic) load contribute relatively less to the ventricular ejection than regions with lower load (Fujita et al. 1993). Moreover, the tight link between regional stress and strain suggests that myocardial contractility is highly uniform throughout the left ventricle. Although the afterload is similar for the entire ventricle, because of

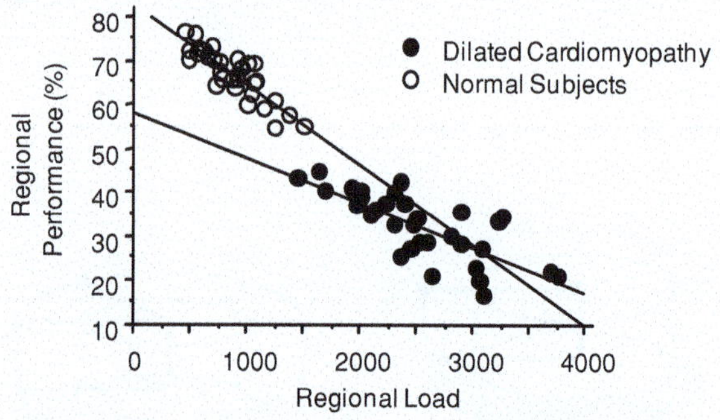

Fig. 30 Assessment of intrinsic contractility using the (inverse) relation between regional load and regional performance in a group of healthy controls ($n = 87$) and patients with idiopathic dilated cardiomyopathy ($n = 12$). The regional load (or wall stress) is obtained using the radii of curvature in the long-axis and short-axis directions, the wall thickness, and the intraventricular pressure. The regional performance represents the regional ejection fraction (see Fig. 28). R^2 of the correlation in controls is 0.76 and in patients with dilated cardiomyopathy is 0.58. (Partially adapted from Bogaert 1997; Rademakers et al. 2003)

important differences in regional morphology (wall thickness, circumferential and longitudinal radii of curvatures), local loading conditions differ significantly, and consequently the regional functional response differs too (Bogaert and Rademakers 2001).

3.3.6 Myocardial Tagging and Ventricular Morphology

MRI myocardial tagging techniques, especially radial tagging and to a lesser extent SPAMM tagging, provide information about local ventricular morphology, in particular myocardial wall thickness and the radii of curvature. For instance, adjusting the tag length for longitudinal wall curvature provides more reliable estimates of true myocardial wall thickness especially in the apical half of the left ventricle (Lima et al. 1993) (see also Table 12). The circumferential radius of curvature and the longitudinal radius of curvature are calculated in each cuboid using the chord and arch lengths fitting a model. A small radius of curvature denotes a curved surface, whereas a large radius of curvature is representative of a flat surface. Changes in the radii of curvature during the cardiac cycle denote regional shape changes of the ventricle and can be used together with wall thickness to calculate wall stresses (Beyar et al. 1993).

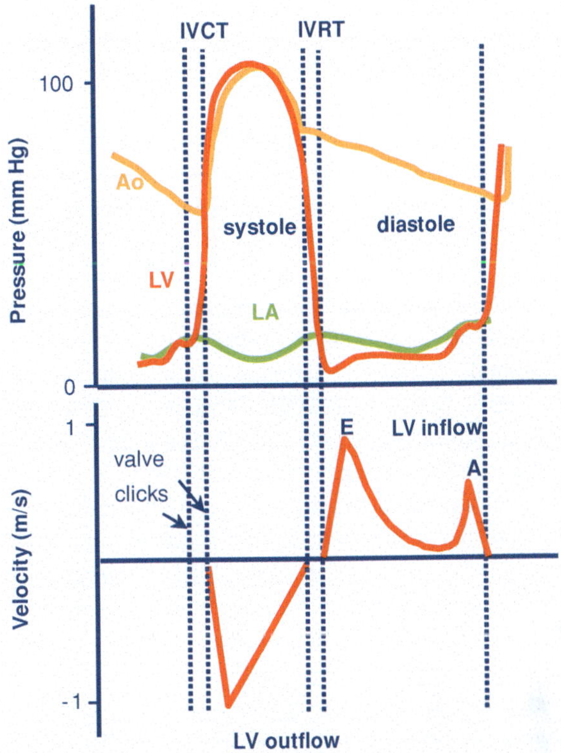

Fig. 31 Pressure and velocity changes in the left atrium, left ventricle, and aorta during the cardiac cycle. *Ao* aorta, *IVCT* isovolumic contraction time, *IVRT* isovolumic relaxation time

4 Diastolic Function

Heart failure caused by a predominant abnormality in diastolic function (i.e., *diastolic heart failure*) is considered to be responsible for at least one third of all patients with congestive heart failure (Paelinck et al. 2002; Rademakers and Bogaert 2006; Caudron et al. 2011; see also "Heart Failure and Heart Transplantation"). However, the diagnosis of diastolic dysfunction and diastolic heart failure is still challenging because of controversy concerning the definition of diastolic dysfunction and the criteria for diastolic heart failure. "Diastolic dysfunction" refers to a condition in which abnormalities in mechanical function are present during diastole. Abnormalities in diastolic function can occur in the presence or absence of a clinical syndrome of heart failure and with normal or abnormal systolic function. "Diastolic dysfunction" describes an abnormal mechanical property; "diastolic heart failure" describes a clinical syndrome (Zile and Brutsaert 2002). Noninvasive imaging plays a central role in the diagnosis of heart failure, assessment of prognosis, and monitoring of therapy, and the role of MRI is rapidly emerging in this field (Karamitsos et al. 2009).

4.1 Assessment of Diastolic Function and Dysfunction

For several reasons, assessment of diastolic (dys)function is definitely more challenging and complicated than evaluation of systolic (dys)function. Since different physiological mechanisms contribute to ventricular filling, the study of diastolic (dys)function is hampered by the absence of an easily obtained global parameter such as ejection fraction used to express global systolic function. The ventricular relaxation process is difficult to assess by noninvasive means, because imaging methods cannot directly measure cavity pressure changes (Fig. 31).

Echocardiographic, Doppler, and radionuclide parameters of diastolic function are derived from rates of inflow of blood or outward movement of the myocardium (Lester et al. 2008). However, the process of relaxation occurs mostly during the diastolic isovolumic period of the cardiac cycle, before blood flow or wall motion begins. Indexes measured later in the cycle examine only the final stages of relaxation. Furthermore, these parameters are subject to "pseudonormalization" because the variation in atrial pressure profoundly affects filling dynamics and thus confounds attempts to indirectly estimate the relaxation rate (Dong et al. 2001; Hees et al. 2004). In normal subjects, aging has a significant impact on RV and LV filling patterns (Iwase et al. 1993). Although Doppler echocardiography is currently the most used noninvasive imaging technique to assess diastolic function (Mandinov et al. 2000), MRI is emerging as a valuable alternative, having the unique potential of three-dimensional function analysis with great accuracy and reproducibility (Bellenger et al. 2000a; Paelinck et al. 2002; Daneshvar et al. 2010; Caudron et al. 2011). Another unique advantage of MRI is that information regarding diastolic (dys)function can be linked to morphologic and tissue characteristics, allowing, for example, not only patients with cardiac amyloidosis or myocardial iron deposition to be diagnosed but also the functional consequences to be evaluated (see "Heart Muscle Diseases"). It was recently shown that the degree of myocardial fibrosis depicted with late Gd MRI significantly correlates with the degree of diastolic dysfunction in a broad range of cardiac conditions (Moreo et al. 2009).

4.2 Ventricular Mass and Volumes

As ventricular mass is a major determinant of diastolic function and filling, precise and accurate quantification is crucial. As discussed earlier, MRI is not dependent on assumptions about the shape and geometry, but its volumetric approach provides highly accurate values with very good intraobserver and interobserver variability (see Sect. 3.1.9). The current cine imaging sequences in combination with parallel imaging allow dynamic cardiac imaging with temporal resolutions as short as 10 ms. This should allow one to accurately follow the changes in ventricular volumes throughout the cardiac cycle, and to obtain the ventricular filling curves, and their derivative with peak rates and time to peak rate (Fujita et al. 1993; Soldo et al. 1994; Kudelka et al. 1997; Fig. 2). Moreover, MRI can potentially provide interesting information with regard to the timing and rate of wall thinning. This interesting (but underused) parameter is very helpful to differentiate normal from pseudonormal inflow patterns, but necessitates a tedious and often time-consuming delineation of the epicardial and endocardial borders. Finally, MRI allows one to quantify atrial volumes, providing information on atrial filling and emptying curves in normal, diseased, and transplanted hearts (Jarvinen et al. 1994a, b; Lauerma et al. 1996).

4.3 Ventricular Inflow Patterns

Doppler echocardiography has emerged clinically as the most important tool to obtain reliable and useful data on diastolic performance. It consists of an assessment of mitral flow and pulmonary venous flow patterns for the left side of the heart, and tricuspid flow and hepatic of inferior vena cava flow patterns for the right side of the heart, thereby measuring peak velocities, acceleration and deceleration times, and the duration of isovolumic relaxation (Fig. 32). Similar measurements can be performed by phase-contrast MRI (Mohiaddin et al. 1990, 1991; Mostbeck et al. 1993; Galjee et al. 1995; Kroft and de Roos 1999). An advantage of MRI over Doppler echocardiography is that MRI can quantify the flow through the entire valve area or vessel, in contrast to Doppler imaging, where flow and flow velocity are measured in a relatively small area of interest. Since flow is not necessary homogeneously spread, a change in positioning of the Doppler sample volume can yield different values, with possible impact on the interpretation (Fyrenius et al. 1999). With the advent of real-time MRI, also available for phase-contrast imaging, it has become feasible to quantify in real time ventricular inflow, as well as venous flow patterns (van den Hout et al. 2003). This allows evaluation of respiratory-related beat-to-beat variation, and should help to differentiate patients with restrictive cardiomyopathy from those with constrictive pericarditis (Giorgi et al. 2003; see "Pericardial Disease"). Improvements in the design of the two-dimensional

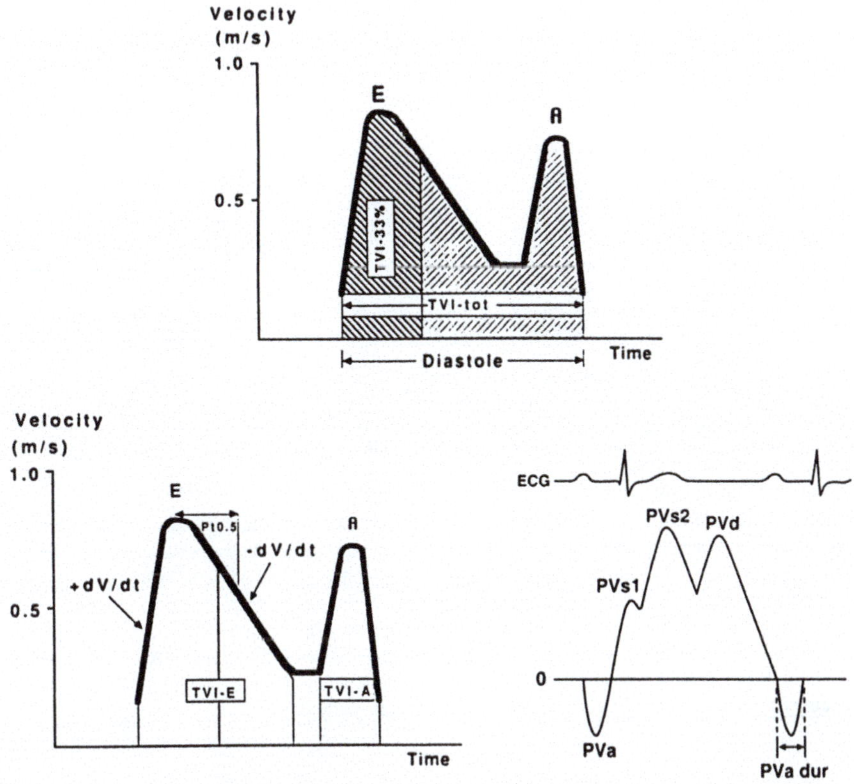

Fig. 32 Transmitral and pulmonary venous flow pattern. The *upper panel* shows early diastolic (E) and atrial (A) filling velocity. The pressure half time ($PT_{0.5}$), the total time–velocity integral ($t_{VI\text{-}tot}$), and the first–third filling fraction ($t_{VI\text{-}33\%}$) are shown in the *left panel*. The *right panel* shows the pulmonary vein flow pattern (PV): atrial flow reversal (PV_a), early systolic flow velocity (PV_{s1}), and mid-systolic flow velocity(PV_{s2}) as well as diastolic flow velocity (PVd). PVa_{dur} represents the duration of atrial flow reversal. (Reprinted from Mandinov et al. 2000)

phase-contrast imaging sequence have been presented, such as three-dimensional three-directional phase-contrast imaging with retrospective tracking adapted to the continuously changing position and angulation of the mitral or tricuspid valve (Westenberg et al. 2008; Brandts et al. 2011).

The transmitral (or transtricuspid) velocity pattern is easy to acquire and can rapidly categorize patients with normal or abnormal diastolic function by the E/A ratio (ratio of early to late filling velocity—Fig. 32). The acquisition plane is placed perpendicular to the LV (or RV) inflow at the top of the mitral (tricuspid) valve opening. In healthy, young individuals, most of the ventricular filling occurs in early diastole, so the $E/A > 1$ (Figs. 32, 34). When there is an impairment in myocardial relaxation (e.g., myocardial hypertrophy, ischemia), early diastolic filling decreases progressively, and a vigorous compensatory atrial contraction ("atrial kick") occurs. This results in a reversed E/A ratio ($E/A < 1$, corresponding to a "delayed relaxation" pattern), increased deceleration time, and increased isovolumic relaxation time (Figs. 33, 35). However, with increasing age, myocardial relaxation is prolonged, and myocardial stiffness and chamber stiffness increase, also resulting in a decrease of the E/A ratio. If ventricular compliance is reduced (e.g., restrictive cardiomyopathy), the filling pressures increase, leading to a compensatory augmentation of the atrial pressure with an increase in early filling despite a concomitant impaired relaxation. As a consequence, this filling pattern resembles a normal filling pattern ("pseudonormalization" pattern, $E/A > 1$). This pattern, however, represents abnormalities of both relaxation and compliance and is distinguished from normal filling by a shortened early deceleration time. In patients with a severe decrease in ventricular compliance, atrial pressures are markedly elevated and are compensate for with vigorous early diastolic filling for impaired relaxation. This "restrictive" filling pattern ($E/A \gg 1$) is consistent with an abnormal rise in ventricular pressure and an abrupt deceleration of flow with little additional deceleration during mid-diastole and atrial contraction (Fig. 33; Mandinov et al. 2000).

Analysis of the venous flow patterns in the pulmonary veins or caval veins also provides valuable

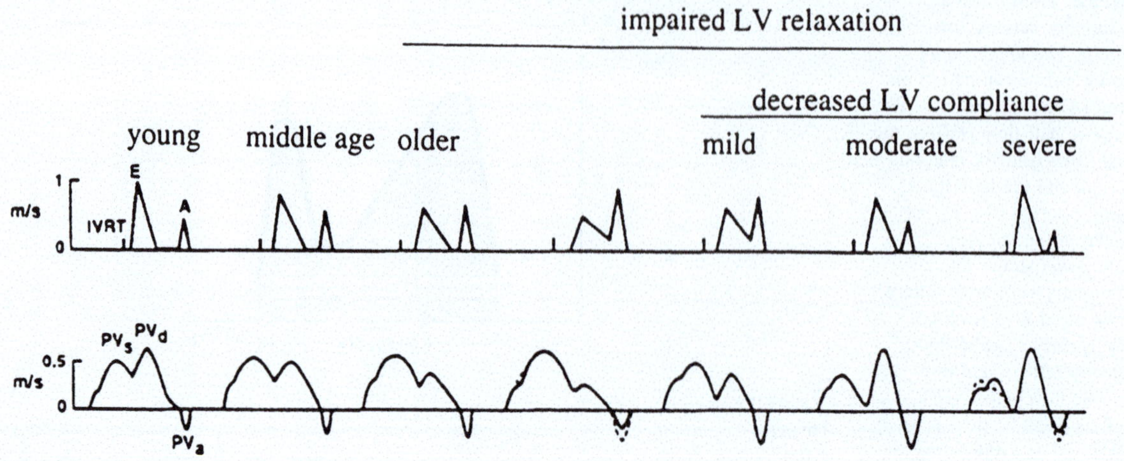

Fig. 33 Transmitral and pulmonary venous flow pattern according to Appelton and Hatle. With increasing age the *E*/*A* ratio decreases. In elderly patients the ratio is less than 1 ("impaired relaxation" pattern), and the pulmonary venous flow shows a decrease in diastolic flow. In subjects with impaired LV relaxation (e.g., myocardial hypertrophy, ischemia), the filling pattern shows a further decrease in the E-wave, whereas with a decrease in LV compliance the filling pattern changes toward normal ("pseudonormalization") and even shows enhanced early diastolic filling with an *E*/*A* ratio greater than 2 ("restrictive filling" pattern). With the progressive decrease in LV compliance, pulmonary venous flow shows a diminution of systolic flow with an enhanced early diastolic flow and a reversal of atrial flow. (Reprinted from Mandinov et al. 2000)

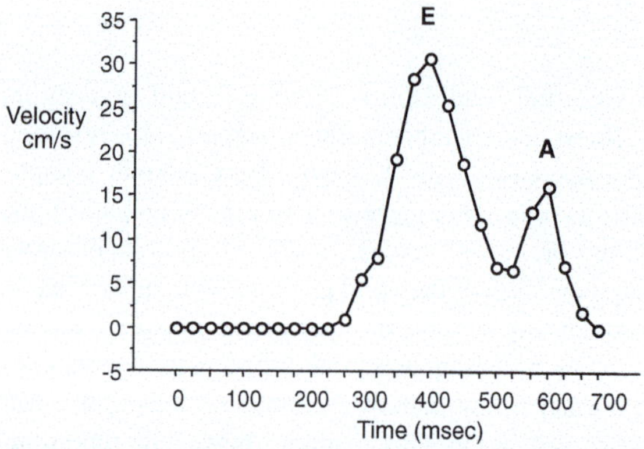

Fig. 34 Mitral inflow pattern in a 24-year-old normal subject. The fast, early filling velocity (*E*) is almost twice as large the flow velocity during atrial contraction (*A*)

information regarding LV or RV diastolic (dys)function, respectively (Fig. 32). The S wave represents the forward venous flow occurring during ventricular systole. It is determined by atrial relaxation, and by the atrioventricular valve annulus motion due to longitudinal ventricular shortening. The D wave represents the forward diastolic venous flow and reflects ventricular filling. Finally, the A wave, which has a direction opposite to that of the S and D waves, occurs during atrial contraction, and reflects ventricular compliance. Whereas in younger subjects, the D-wave velocity is larger than the S-wave velocity, with aging the D-wave velocity decreases as a result of an age-related prolonged and impaired myocardial relaxation and the A wave increases in magnitude (Figs. 33, 36). In patients with decreased ventricular compliance, the systolic venous flow is diminished, the early diastolic flow is enhanced, and flow during atrial contraction is reversed. The latter is the result of contraction against increased afterload caused by elevated diastolic filling pressure and increased ventricular stiffness. Accordingly, reversed flow into the pulmonary or caval veins occurs, resulting in a venous A wave that is high in magnitude and long in duration.

4.4 Myocardial Tissue Phase Mapping

As discussed already, the flow through the mitral (tricuspid) valve results from the instantaneous atrioventricular pressure gradient. It is a dynamic phenomenon determined by several parameters, such

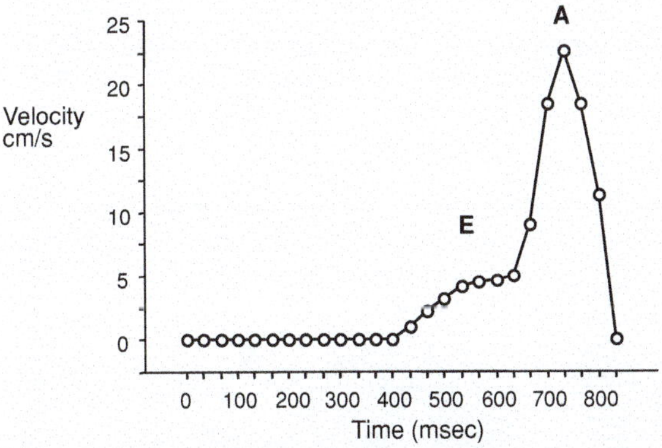

Fig. 35 Severe myocardial relaxation disturbance leading to a reversal of the *E*/*A* ratio. The early filling velocities are strongly decreased (*E*), whereas the late filling velocities are increased (*A*)

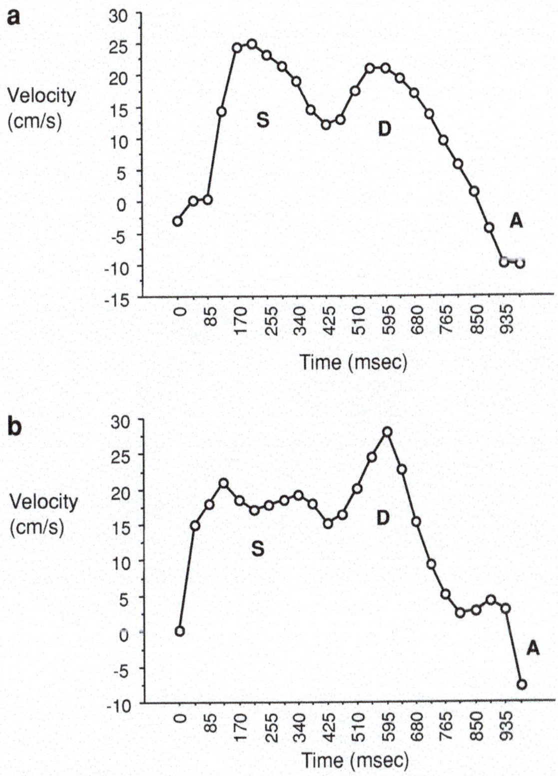

Fig. 36 Venous flow patterns in a 39-year-old normal subject through the inferior vena cava (**a**) and pulmonary vein (**b**). In the inferior vena cava, the systolic forward flow velocity (*S*) is slightly larger than the diastolic forward flow velocity (*D*). *A* represents the reversed flow caused by the atrial contraction. In the pulmonary vein (**a**), diastolic forward flow velocities slightly exceed systolic forward velocities

as atrial pressure, elastic recoil of the ventricle, myocardial relaxation, and chamber compliance. Use of this parameter to differentiate patients with impaired myocardial relaxation (e.g., LV hypertrophy) may be challenging, because inflow curves may be very similar. Similarly to Doppler tissue imaging, myocardial tissue phase mapping can be used to measure myocardial velocities and thus to obtain data regarding myocardial relaxation (Paelinck et al. 2005). So, normalizing early mitral velocity for the influence of myocardial relaxation by combining *E* with the early myocardial tissue velocity (Ea) provides a more accurate estimate of filling pressure. To measure myocardial velocities, short-axis phase-contrast velocity imaging with a low velocity encoding (e.g., 30 cm/s) and that is slightly more apical than the plane for measuring the mitral flow is chosen. Similar to Doppler measurements, the inferior septal basal level is the best localization to optimally measure myocardial velocities (Caudron et al. 2011). The myocardial tissue phase mapping curve is composed of three waves: Sa, corresponding with the longitudinal systolic LV shortening, and the diastolic velocities (Ea and Aa) that are markers of myocardial relaxation (Fig. 37). The ratio *E*/Ea provides information regarding filling pressures: if the *E*/Ea < 8, the filling pressures are considered to be low; if *E*/Ea > 15, the filling pressures are considered to be increased; if the *E*/Ea ratio is between 8 and 15, additional investigation is necessary, such as analysis of the pulmonary venous flow. Other techniques such as myocardial tagging and magnetic resonance elastography have been proposed to study diastolic function, but currently their role in daily clinical practice is limited (Edvardsen et al. 2002; Elgeti et al. 2009).

4.5 Atrial Volumes and Function

Assessment of atrial volumes is becoming increasingly important because an increased atrial volume is an independent predictor of adverse cardiovascular events, including stroke and congestive heart failure (Whitlock et al. 2010). In patients with diastolic dysfunction, atrial size is considered a reliable

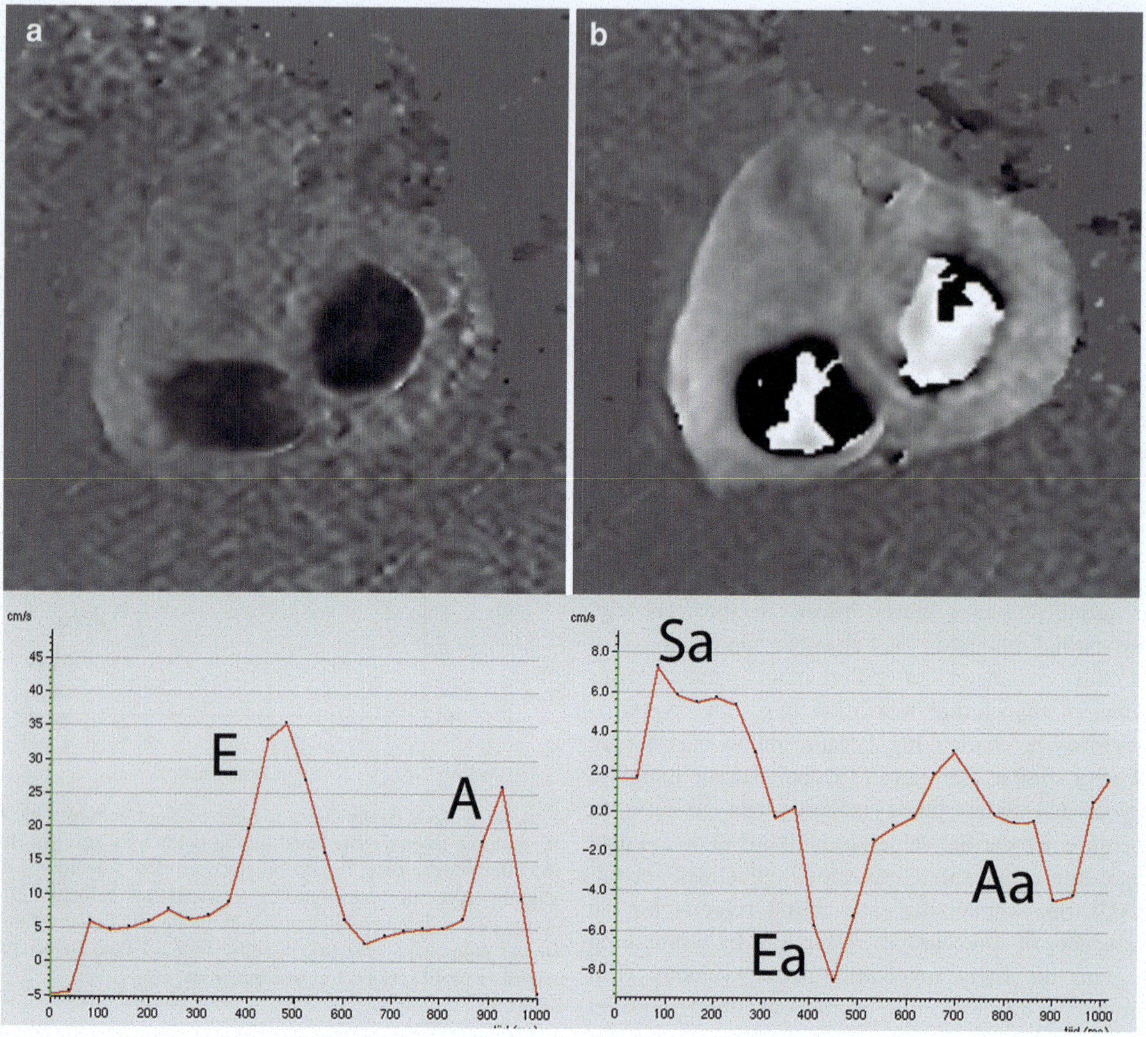

Fig. 37 Phase-contrast velocity imaging to assess mitral inflow and myocardial velocities in a 47-year old man. Short-axis imaging at the level of the mitral valve (**a**) and 1 cm toward the LV apex (**b**) using a velocity encoding of 1 m/s (**a**) and 30 cm/s (**b**). The mitral inflow (**a**) shows $E > A$. Myocardial tissue phase mapping allows one to appreciate longitudinal velocities throughout the cardiac cycle, with systolic shortening (*Sa*), early diastolic lengthening (*Ea*), and late diastolic lengthening due to the atrial contraction (*Aa*). From the ratio of *E*/Ea, i.e., 35 cm/s/8 cm/s (i.e., 4.4), diastolic dysfunction can be excluded

indicator of the duration and severity of dysfunction, regardless of the loading conditions at the time of the examination (Maceira et al. 2010). The atria have primarily a reservoir function, modulating ventricular filling. If ventricular filling pressure increases, the atria will consequently dilate. However, other causes of atrial dilatation, such as atrial fibrillation, mitral/tricuspid valve stenosis, and regurgitation, have to be excluded (Caudron et al. 2011). To achieve the maximal atrial size, measurements should be performed at the end of systole. Different methods are currently available, e.g., one-dimensional measurements (transverse and/or longitudinal diameters), planimetry performed on a four-chamber view, biplane area-length methods using a four-chamber and vertical two-chamber view, and a volumetric method using a set of short-axis images from the base of the atrium to the atrioventricular junction (Anderson et al. 2005; Hudsmith et al. 2005, 2007). Others prefer the use of the vertical long-axis because of a better definition of the atrioventricular borders (Jarvinen et al. 1994a, b). For the volumetric approach of the left atrium, the appendage is usually included, whereas the pulmonary veins are excluded from the left atrial volume. At the end of this chapter a summary of normal values for atrial dimensions, areas, and volumes is given based on a recent study by Maceira et al. (2010) of 120 healthy subjects covering six decades. For a more extensive overview including indexed age- and gender-specific values, we refer to specific literature (Jarvinen et al. 1994a, b; Anderson et al. 2005; Sievers et al. 2005; Hudsmith et al. 2005, 2007; Tsao et al. 2008). Besides a reservoir function, the atrium also has a conduit function, and has an active contractile function. To obtain data regarding the phasic changes in atrial volumes and function, volumetric imaging of the atria enable one to measure maximal and minimal atrial volume, atrial volume just before atrial contraction, atrial reservoir volume, atrial ejection fraction, and passive atrial emptying volume (Jarvinen et al. 1994a, b; Lauerma et al. 1996; Wen et al. 2010).

4.6 Ventricular Relaxation

Cardiac catheterization with simultaneous pressure and volume measurements is the gold standard for assessing ventricular relaxation and ventricular compliance. The myocardial or ventricular relaxation can be quantified by calculation of the time constant (τ) of myocardial relaxation. High-fidelity manometer-tipped catheters measure the intraventricular pressure changes. The pressure from the time of aortic valve closure to mitral valve opening is fitted to a monoexponential equation. In normal humans, τ is 30–40 ms, and relaxation is considered to be "complete" after three time constants (90–120 ms). Assessment of ventricular relaxation by noninvasive means, e.g., Doppler echocardiography and radionuclide methods, is difficult because imaging methods cannot directly measure cavity pressure. The measured indexes such as rates of inflow of blood and outward movement of the myocardium reflect only the final stages of relaxation. MRI myocardial tagging, however, allows accurate and noninvasive measurement of the global and regional deformation and shape of the heart and its cavities throughout the cardiac cycle, enabling the calculation of strains (normal and shear). One shear strain parameter that has particular importance for diastolic function is the circumferential–longitudinal shear or torsion, expressing wringing motion of the left ventricle (Rademakers et al. 1992; Dong et al. 1999). Counterclockwise torsion develops during ejection, but the clockwise recoil of torsion, or untwisting, is a deformation that occurs largely during isovolumic relaxation, before mitral valve opening. This recoil is associated with the release of restoring forces that have been accumulated during systole and is thought to contribute to diastolic suction (Robinson et al. 1986). The extent of torsion is correlated with cavity pressure, and its recoil rate is closely related to the rate of pressure fall and the relaxation time constant (τ) (Dong et al. 2001). Recently, Hees et al. (2004), studying changes in recoil rate with aging using myocardial tagging, remarkably found that the decrease in early filling velocities with aging was rather related to changes in left atrial pressure than to changes in myocardial relaxation behavior. Untwisting may be abnormal in timing and extent in several diseases, including heart failure from various causes, myocardial infarction, hypertrophy due to hypertension, and aortic disease (Matter et al. 1996; Stuber et al. 1999).

4.7 Ventricular Coupling

Although the left and right ventricles are physically separate in humans, both ventricles are anatomically and functionally bound together in many ways. They share a common ventricular septum and ventricular, myocardial bundles and are enclosed and bound together by the common pericardium. In addition, the left ventricle is indirectly connected with the right ventricle via the pulmonary circulation (so-called series interaction). There is a close functional interaction between the right and left ventricles, not only in diastole but also in systole. This ventricular interaction is reflected by the position and configuration of the ventricular septum, which is determined by the pressure difference between the left and right ventricles, i.e., the transseptal pressure gradient. In normal loading conditions the septum has a concave shape toward the left ventricle because of a left-to-right positive transseptal pressure gradient, and this shape is maintained during the cardiac cycle (Weyman et al. 1976, Brinker et al. 1980; Guzman et al. 1981; Lima et al. 1986). The phenomenon whereby the function of one ventricle is altered by changes in the filling of the other is called *ventricular coupling* or *interventricular dependence*. Pathologic ventricular coupling

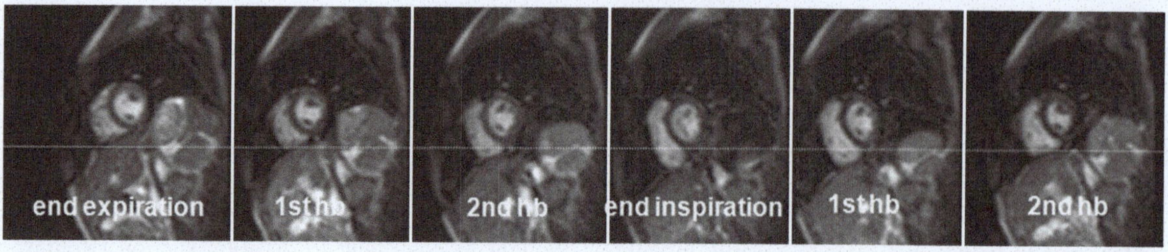

Fig. 38 Real-time cine imaging to assess the influence of respiration on ventricular filling. Cardiac short-axis cine imaging showing six images obtained at early diastolic filling at six points of respiration. The end-expiratory time frame is shown on the *left*. The *horizontal dashed line* shows the position of the diaphragm at the end of inspiration. Eventual inspiratory septal flattening/inversion and total septal excursion can be easily assessed using real-time cine imaging. (Partially adapted from Francone et al. 2005)

occurs when there is an acute or chronic imbalance between the LV and RV loading conditions, e.g., constrictive pericarditis, mitral stenosis, and cor pulmonale (Weyman et al. 1977; Jessup et al. 1987; Giorgi et al. 2003). In these circumstances, this imbalance will lead to an abnormal motion and configuration of the ventricular septum. Ventricular coupling is moreover significantly influenced by respiration (Hatle et al. 1989; Klein et al. 1993; Hurrell et al. 1996). During inspiration, the intrathoracic pressure decreases, leading to a diminished pulmonary venous return and a decreased LV filling and an increased systemic venous return and RV filling, whereas the opposite phenomenon is found during expiration. Assessment of the impact of respiration on ventricular coupling is, for instance, crucial to differentiate patients with constrictive pericarditis from those with restrictive cardiomyopathy.

Presently, Doppler echocardiography is the image modality of choice to assess the influence of respiration on ventricular inflow and septal motion (Hatle et al. 1989). With the advent of MRI systems with stronger gradient systems, faster gradient switching capabilities, and new cine MRI sequences in combination with parallel imaging, the time required for data acquisition has shortened considerably, enabling real-time dynamic evaluation of ventricular septal motion and configuration throughout the cardiac cycle. This has opened up new perspectives for cardiac MRI to become competitive with echocardiography. Real-time cine imaging allows one to evaluate the impact of respiration on ventricular filling such as in patients with restrictive inflow patterns (Fig. 38) (Francone et al. 2005, 2006), or in patients with chronic cor pulmonale (Iino et al. 2008). In patients with constrictive pericarditis, a ventricular septal flattening or inversion was found on real-time MRI during early ventricular filling (see "Pericardial Disease"). The intensity of the abnormalities was most pronounced for the first heart beat after onset of inspiration, and rapidly decreased for the next heart beats, and completely disappeared during expiration. This pattern was absent in patients with restrictive cardiomyopathy.

5 Wall Stress and Myocardial Stress–Strain Relation

Wall stress, or the force generated by the intraventricular cavity pressure on the surrounding myocardial wall, is a major determinant of the systolic myocardial deformation and ventricular ejection. Moreover, myocardial oxygen consumption is closely related to wall stress. Since wall stress cannot be measured, it has to be assumed (Arts et al. 1991). Several assumptions for wall stress have been proposed, the one more complex than the other, but most of them are based on the measurable parameters, i.e., wall thickness, radii of curvature, and systolic blood pressure, whereas parameters such as the influence of the fiber direction and anisotropy are usually ignored (Wong and Rautaharju 1968; Streeter et al. 1970; Janz 1982). For a similar cavity pressure, wall stress decreases if the wall becomes more curved, or if the wall thickness increases. This explains why the LV apex, which is highly curved, can sustain high systolic pressures without bulging or rupturing. Because of the lower wall stress in the LV apex, the systolic strains and thus the contribution to the ventricular ejection is proportionally larger in the apex than in other segments of the left ventricle (Bogaert and Rademakers 2001). The transmural spread of wall stress is inhomogeneous, with the highest wall stresses in the subendocardium, making this area especially vulnerable to ischemia. Wall stress gradually decreases toward the subepicardium.

With the advent of MRI, in particular of myocardial tagging and related techniques, accurate information can be obtained on regional morphology, i.e., wall thickness and circumferential and longitudinal radii of curvature, and regional myocardial strain data can also be obtained. MRI diffusion techniques have been shown to noninvasively depict myocardial fiber directions, and even to quantify myocardial fiber shortening (Hsu et al. 1998; Scollan et al. 1998; Tseng et al. 2000; Buckberg et al. 2006; Sosnovik et al. 2009; Nasiraei-Moghaddam and Gharib 2009). This should allow more accurate estimates of regional wall stresses, and should allow the regional stress–strain relationship to be determined (Rademakers et al. 2003). Using a simple formula for wall stress estimations, based on wall thickness (corrected for angulation), circumferential and longitudinal radii of curvature, and systolic blood pressure, rather than the true measured intraventricular pressure, Rademakers et al. (2003) found a close, inverse relation between the regional systolic wall stress and the corresponding amount of deformation. Since systolic wall stress is also a major determinant of myocardial relaxation, quantification may be helpful in unraveling the regional pattern in myocardial relaxation. The same principles are also valid for assessment of RV wall stress, which is even more difficult to estimate, mainly because of the complex shape of the right ventricle (Naito et al. 1995; Yim et al. 1998). As mentioned already, improved insight into wall stress would also help us to better understand the mechanism of ventricular coupling and the impact on ventricular filling.

6 Stress Imaging

In patients with obstructive coronary artery disease, myocardial function at rest is often within normal limits. However, during periods of increased oxygen consumption, e.g., during physical exercise, the oxygen supply through a stenotic coronary artery might be insufficient to cover the increased needs, leading to regional or more global myocardial ischemia (see "Myocardial Perfusion, Ischemic Heart Disease"). A series of events, i.e., the ischemic cascade, occurs after the onset of disturbances in myocardial blood flow, starting with diastolic and systolic functional abnormalities, followed by changes in the ECG and later symptoms of angina. With the new imaging modalities, earlier manifestations of ischemia could be used as a marker of significant coronary artery disease. Although clinically still underused, MRI likely has the greatest potential as a stress imaging technique. For this purpose, stress perfusion, stress cine MRI, stress myocardial tagging, and strain encoding and FastSENC, and even stress aortic flow measurements have been applied (Pennell et al. 1990, 1992; 1995; Baer et al. 1992, 1993, 1994; Cigarroa et al. 1993; van Rugge et al. 1993a, b, 1994; Hartnell et al. 1994; Croisille et al. 1999; Jahnke et al. 2006; Korosoglou et al. 2009a, b). This issue is discussed extensively in "Ischemic Heart Disease".

7 Postprocessing and Delineation Techniques

Fast and accurate analysis of image data is a prerequisite for each imaging modality to be implemented in clinical routine. The success of other imaging techniques, such as radionuclide imaging, depends on the availability of postprocessing techniques with fast, automated extraction of ventricular volumes, function, and mass. Although MRI has all the intrinsic qualities to be considered a reference technique for assessment of global and regional cardiac function, mainly the lack of easy-to-use postprocessing and delineation techniques still hampers a thorough clinical use (Young et al. 2000). One of the major strengths of MRI, i.e., the superb depiction of cardiac morphology, is unfortunately the greatest challenge for most automated delineation techniques. Another impediment is the discrimination between atria and ventricles because of difficulties in defining the atrioventricular valve position. Different methods have been reported for automatic segmentation of the endocardial border, including region growing, edge detection, adaptive thresholding, fuzzy logic, volumetric surface detection, and three-dimensional information for contour detection (Singelton and Pohost 1997; Furber et al. 1998; Baldy

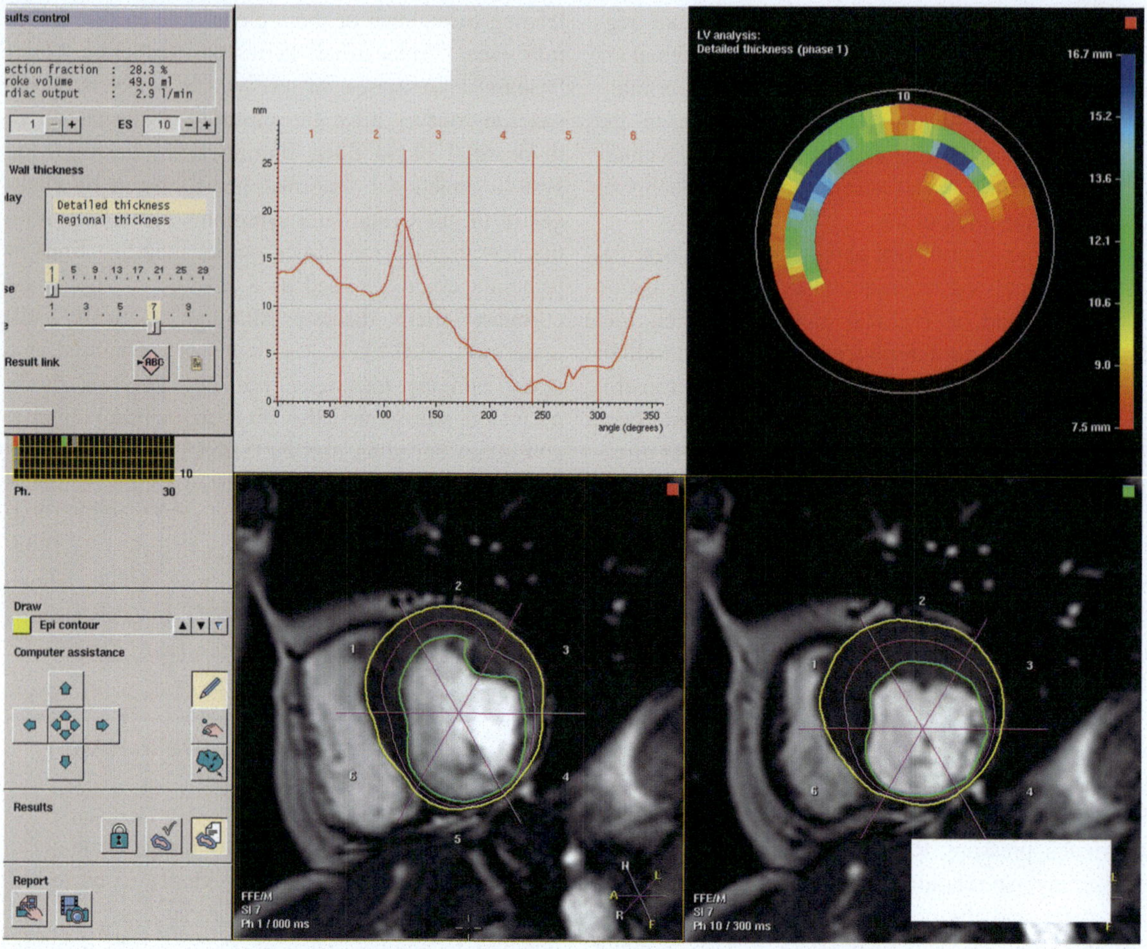

Fig. 39 Assessment of regional cardiac function on a commercially available workstation (Easy-Vision, Philips Medical Systems, Best, The Netherlands) in a patient with a large, inferior aneurysm following a transmural myocardial infarction. After epicardial and endocardial contours have been contoured, several parameters such as wall thickness, absolute and relative systolic wall thickening, and endocardial wall motion can be assessed. The results can be shown numerically, graphically (*top left*), or as a bull's eye (*top right*), better allowing one to appreciate the spread of data throughout the left ventricle

et al. 1994; Lalande et al. 1999; Santaralli et al. 2003; Corsi et al. 2005; van Geuns et al. 2006; Codella et al. 2008). Results have been ambiguous. Van der Geest et al. (1997) concluded that LV functional parameters can be obtained with a high degree of accuracy with semiautomatic contour detection, Romiger et al. (1999) reported that semiautomatic evaluation is erroneous and manual correction of the contours took more time than manual contour tracing. Use of the same software in the balanced steady-state free-precession technique provided, in contrast, accurate cardiodynamic measurements (Barkhausen et al. 2001). Currently, most vendors of MRI instruments have dedicated postprocessing packages available (Fig. 39). Besides, other companies have specialized in commercial software for analysis of cardiac MRI studies, including analysis of myocardial tagging studies. Because of the growing interest in cardiac MRI, postprocessing tools will certainly improve soon (Fig. 40). One way to accomplish this task is by using a priori knowledge of the ventricular anatomy and function patterns (preferably of both ventricles) in normal subjects and a series of different cardiac disease states. This approach would likely be very useful in improving the reliability of a (semi)automated delineation technique.

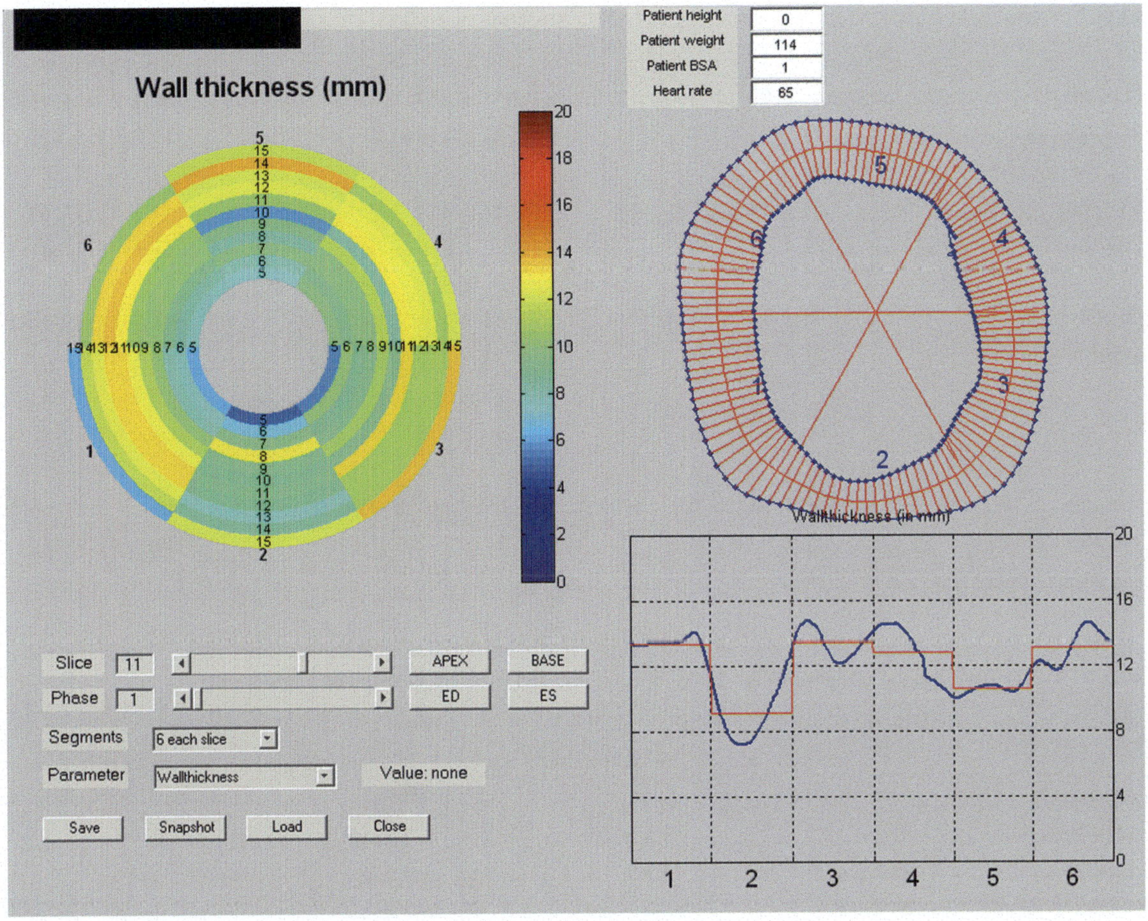

Fig. 40 Modified centerline technique to express regional morphology (wall thickness) and function (systolic wall thickening and motion) using changes in chord length

Table 6 Normal left ventricular values (mean, SD, and 95% confidence interval)

	All (n = 120)	Males (n = 60)	Females (n = 60)
EDV (ml)	142 ± 21 (102, 183)	156 ± 21 (115, 198)	128 ± 21 (88, 168)
EDV/BSA (ml/m^2)	78 ± 9 (60, 95)	80 ± 9 (63, 98)	75 ± 9 (57, 92)
ESV (ml)	47 ± 10 (27, 68)	53 ± 11 (30, 75)	42 ± 10 (23, 60)
ESV/BSA (ml/m^2)	26 ± 5 (16, 36)	27 ± 6 (16, 38)	24 ± 5 (15, 34)
SV (ml)	95 ± 14 (67, 123)	104 ± 14 (76, 132)	86 ± 14 (58, 114)
SV/BSA (ml/m^2)	52 ± 6 (40, 64)	53 ± 6 (41, 65)	50 ± 6 (38, 63)
EF (%)	67 ± 5 (58, 76)	67 ± 5 (58, 75)	67 ± 5 (58, 76)
Mass (g)	127 ± 19 (90, 164)	146 ± 20 (108, 184)	108 ± 18 (72, 144)
Mass/BSA (g/m^2)	69 ± 8 (53, 84)	74 ± 9 (58, 91)	63 ± 8 (48, 77)

Data adapted from Maceira et al. (2006a)

BSA body surface area, *EDV* end-diastolic volume, *EF* ejection fraction, *ESV* end-systolic volume, *SV* stroke volume

Table 7 Normal right ventricular values (mean, SD, and 95% confidence interval)

	All (n = 120)	Males (n = 60)	Females (n = 60)
EDV (ml)	144 ± 23 (98, 190)	163 ± 25 (113, 213)	126 ± 21 (84, 168)
EDV/BSA (ml/m^2)	78 ± 11 (57, 99)	83 ± 12 (60, 106)	73 ± 9 (55, 92)
ESV (ml)	50 ± 14 (22, 78)	57 ± 15 (27, 86)	43 ± 13 (17, 69)
ESV/BSA (ml/m^2)	27 ± 7 (13, 41)	29 ± 7 (14,43)	25 ± 7 (12, 38)
SV (ml)	94 ± 15 (64, 124)	106 ± 17 (72, 140)	83 ± 13 (57, 108)
SV/BSA (ml/m^2)	51 ± 7 (37, 65)	54 ± 8 (38, 70)	48 ± 6 (36, 60)
EF (%)	66 ± 6 (54, 78)	66 ± 6 (53, 78)	66 ± 6 (54, 78)
Mass (g)	48 ± 13 (23, 73)	66 ± 14 (38, 94)	48 ± 11 (27, 69)
Mass/BSA (g/m^2)	31 ± 6 (19, 43)	34 ± 7 (20, 47)	28 ± 5 (18, 38)

Data adapted from Maceira et al. (2006b)

Table 8 Sex- and age-specific pediatric values for ventricular size and mass indexed for BSA (mean, SD)

	Boys		Girls	
	8–15 years (n = 35)	16–20 years (n = 35)	8–15 years (n = 16)	16–20 years (n = 13)
Left ventricle				
EDV/BSA (ml/m^2)	81.9 ± 12.9	93.5 ± 10.9	78.7 ± 10.7	80.7 ± 9.5
ESV/BSA (ml/m^2)	28.2 ± 6.7	35.9 ± 7.1	28.9 ± 6.1	29.0 ± 7.5
SV/BSA (ml/m^2)	53.7 ± 8.5	57.6 ± 5.9	49.7 ± 8.3	51.7 ± 6.8
EF (%)	65.7 ± 4.9	61.8 ± 4.3	63.2 ± 6.3	65.7 ± 4.9
CO/BSA (l/min/m^2)	4.42 ± 0.85	4.02 ± 0.79	3.94 ± 0.62	3.85 ± 0.86
Mass/BSA (g/m^2)	52.1 ± 10.6	67.6 ± 7.7	48.2 ± 8.2	51.2 ± 7.3
Right ventricle				
EDV/BSA (ml/m^2)	82.9 ± 12.6	90.2 ± 10.9	78.3 ± 9.7	79.7 ± 10.3
ESV/BSA (ml/m^2)	31.3 ± 6.1	36.1 ± 6.3	29.2 ± 4.6	30.4 ± 6.9
SV/BSA (ml/m^2)	51.6 ± 8.4	54.1 ± 7.3	49.1 ± 6.8	49.3 ± 6.3
EF (%)	62.3 ± 4.3	60.0 ± 4.4	62.6 ± 3.6	62.1 ± 6.0
Mass/BSA (g/m^2)	18.3 ± 5.5	26.9 ± 7.9	17.3 ± 4.7	20.4 ± 5.5

Data adapted from Sarikouch et al. (2010)

8 Normal Values for Cardiac Function

Before the cardiac performance in a patient can be defined as abnormal, the normal values for ventricular volumes, function, and mass as well as their physiological ranges (95% confidence intervals) need to be known (Lorenz et al. 1999; Lorenz 2000; Marcus et al. 1999b). Normal values are not only influenced by body constitution, age, sex, and level of training or fitness, but also by technical issues such as MRI sequence design, use of imaging plane and image analysis. A compilation of the currently available literature data is provided is provided in several tables. To improve the convenience of these tables for routine clinical use, normalized data (i.e., indexed to

Table 9 LV and right ventricular morphologic and functional parameters of triathletes and control subjects

	Triathletes (n = 26)	Control subjects (n = 27)
Left ventricle		
EDV/BSA (ml/m^2)	115 ± 12	91 ± 11
ESV/BSA (ml/m^2)	46 ± 10	37 ± 8
SV/BSA (ml/m^2)	69 ± 7	54 ± 8
Mass/BSA (g/m^2)	83 ± 8	64 ± 7
EF (%)	60.2 ± 5.6	59.5 ± 6.0
CO/BSA (l/min/m^2)	4.0 ± 0.6	3.7 ± 0.8
Wall thickness (mm)	9.8 ± 1.0	8.5 ± 0.9
Right ventricle		
EDV/BSA (ml/m^2)	124 ± 13	97 ± 13
ESV/BSA (ml/m^2)	56 ± 8	44 ± 8
SV/BSA (ml/m^2)	69 ± 10	54 ± 7
Mass/BSA (g/m^2)	28 ± 2	21 ± 3
EF (%)	55.2 ± 4.8	55.3 ± 4.5

Data adapted from Scharf et al. (2010)

Table 10 Normal left atrial values (mean, 95% confidence interval)

	All (n = 120)	Males (n = 60)	Females (n = 60)
Longitudinal diameter—4-ch (cm) SD 0.7[a]	5.7	5.9	5.5
	(4.3, 7.0)	(4.5, 7.2)	(4.1, 6.9)
Longitudinal diameter/BSA—4-ch (cm/m^2) SD 0.4[a]	3.1	3.0	3.2
	(2.3, 3.9)	(2.3, 3.7)	(2.4, 4.1)
Transverse diameter—4ch (cm) SD 0.5	4.1	4.1	4.1
	(3.0, 5.1)	(3.0, 5.2)	(3.0, 5.1)
Transverse diameter/BSA—4-ch (cm/m^2) SD 0.3[a]	2.2	2.1	2.4
	(1.6, 2.8)	(1.5, 2.8)	(1.8, 3.0)
Area—4-ch (cm^2) SD 3.7[a]	21	22	20
	(14, 28)	(14, 30)	(14, 27)
Area/BSA—4-ch (cm^2/m^2) SD 1.8[a]	12	11	12
	(8, 15)	(7, 15)	(8, 15)
Volume (ml) SD 14.9[a]	73	77	68
	(44, 102)	(48, 107)	(42, 95)
Volume/BSA (ml/m^2) SD 6.7	40	39	40
	(27, 53)	(26, 53)	(27, 52)

Data adapted from Maceira et al. (2010)
4-ch four-chamber view
[a] Significant differences ($p < 0.05$) between males and females on multivariable analysis. Atrial appendages were included in the analysis

Table 11 Normal values of LV wall thickness and chamber dimensions

Study	*n*	Sequence	PWT	IVS	EDD	2-chl	4-chl
			mm (mm/m^2)	mm (mm/m^2)	mm (mm/m^2)	mm (mm/m^2)	mm (mm/m^2)
Salton et al. (2002)	63 males	Spoiled GE	9.9 (5.0)	10.1 (5.1)	50.2 (25.3)	82.3 (41.3)	81.9 (41.5)
	(95% upper limit)		11.2 (6.0)	11.7 (6.2)	58.5 (29.7)	93.8 (46.8)	93.0 (47.7)
	79 females	Spoiled GE	8.7 (5.2)	8.9 (5.3)	45.6 (27.1)	73.2 (43.5)	71.7 (42.7)
	(95% upper limit)		9.8 (6.3)	10.1 (6.4)	51.1 (31.8)	83.7 (48.4)	81.5 (47.8)

The values normalized to body surface area are given in *parentheses*. All results are shown at the end of diastole
2-chl two-chamber length, *4-chl* four-chamber length, *EDD* end-diastolic diameter, *IVS* interventricular septum thickness, *PWT* posterior wall thickness

Table 12 Regional variation in LV wall thickness and myocardial strains in a normal population, using three-dimensional MRI myocardial tagging

	Basal	Mid	Apical
End-diastolic wall thickness (mm)			
Septum	9.1	9.3	8.0
Inferior	9.3	9.3	8.1
Lateral	9.6	9.6	8.2
Anterior	9.6	9.2	7.6
Radial thickening (%)			
Septum	32	38	40
Inferior	36	37	38
Lateral	36	35	44
Anterior	35	45	53
Circumferential shortening (%)			
Septum	28	34	39
Inferior	36	40	43
Lateral	36	42	46
Anterior	28	38	42
Longitudinal shortening (%)			
Septum	14	17	18
Inferior	21	18	20
Lateral	21	19	21
Anterior	18	15	17
Circumferential–longitudinal shear strain (%)			
Septum	10	11	12
Inferior	14	6	6
Lateral	12	6	5
Anterior	11	11	11

Data from Bogaert (1997). The study group consisted of 87 normal subjects (31 females), ranging from 21 to 75 years. Data were obtained using a radial tagging technique, dividing the LV myocardium into 32 cuboids. These data are the means for 12 regions, i.e., four segments (septum, inferior, lateral, anterior) per level (basal, mid, apical). The longitudinal and circumferential shortening strains represent the endocardial strain. The circumferential–longitudinal shear strain quantifies LV torsion

Table 13 End-diastolic wall thickness of myocardial wall per segment using the 16-segment frame of reference

Segment	Males (n = 60)	Females (n = 60)
Basal		
1	8.6 ± 0.2	7.1 ± 02
2	10.5 ± 0.3	8.6 ± 0.3
3	9.6 ± 0.2	7.8 ± 0.2
4	8.5 ± 0.2	6.9 ± 0.2
5	7.7 ± 0.2	6.3 ± 0.2
6	7.7 ± 0.2	6.3 ± 0.1
Mid		
7	7.2 ± 0.2	6.1 ± 0.2
8	8.6 ± 0.2	7.1 ± 0.2
9	8.8 ± 0.2	7.4 ± 0.2
10	7.7 ± 0.1	6.5 ± 0.2
11	6.8 ± 0.1	5.7 ± 0.1
12	6.9 ± 0.1	5.6 ± 0.2
Apical		
13	6.5 ± 0.2	6.0 ± 0.2
14	7.9 ± 0.2	6.6 ± 0.2
15	6.6 ± 0.2	5.7 ± 0.2
16	6.4 ± 0.2	5.9 ± 0.2

Adapted from Dawson et al. (2011). The data are expressed in millimeters, and were obtained exclusively using the thickness of the compacted myocardial layer

body surface area), confidence limits, separate data for females and males, or different age groups, and the type of MRI sequence are given (Tables 6, 7). Normal MRI values in children are shown in Table 8. Values for triathletes are shown in Table 9. Normal left atrial values are given in Table 10. Normal values for LV wall thickness, and chamber dimensions are shown in Table 11. Table 12 shows the regional variation in myocardial wall thickness and myocardial strains in a normal population group (Bogaert 1997). Table 13 shows the end-diastolic thickness of the myocardial wall per segment using only the myocardial compacta, thus excluding the trabeculated part.

9 Key Points

- Assessment of cardiac function involves evaluation of both systolic and diastolic function.
- The efficiency of the myofiber shortening is strongly enhanced by the complex fiber anatomy, leading to a phenomenon of transmural fiber interaction. As a result, the left ventricle undergoes a circumferential and longitudinal ventricular shortening, and extensive wall thickening during systole, allowing an ejection fraction of 65–70% to be obtained with a fiber shortening of only 10–15%.
- MRI can be considered together with echocardiography as the primary imaging modality to assess cardiac function.
- Cine MRI is likely the reference technique to quantify ventricular volumes, function, and mass.
- One should be aware of different parameters, such as through-plane motion, anatomical structures, and temporal and spatial resolution, that have a major impact on the results. One should therefore use a consistent approach when assessing cardiac function with MRI.
- The volumetric quantification approach is superior to geometric assumptions, but is more time-consuming for data acquisition and analysis.
- One should use a combination of short-axis and long-axis (horizontal and vertical) views to study

the regional LV function. Because of its complex shape, the right ventricle can be best studied using a combination of short-axis and longitudinal (axial or horizontal long-axis) views.

- Myocardial tagging is an ideal technique to analyze myocardial deformation but requires time-consuming postprocessing. Novel approaches such as SENC-MRI provide direct strain information and are highly appealing as a useful clinical alternative.
- MRI has an arsenal of techniques to accurately assess cardiac diastolic function.
- There is still need for more sophisticated automated analysis packages for functional cardiac evaluation.

References

Abraham TP, Nishimura RA (2001) Myocardial strain: can we finally measure contractility? J Am Coll Cardiol 37:731–734

Aletras AH, Ding S, Balaban RS, Wen H (1999a) DENSE: displacement encoding with stimulated echoes in cardiac functional MRI. J Magn Reson 137:247–252

Aletras AH, Balaban RS, Wen H (1999b) High-resolution strain analysis of the human heart with fast-DENSE. J Magn Reson 140:41–57

Alfakih K, Plein S, Thiele H et al (2003a) Normal human left and right ventricular dimensions for MRI as assessed by turbo gradient echo and steady-state free precession imaging sequences. J Magn Reson Imaging 17:323–329

Alfakih K, Plein S, Bloomer T, Jones T, Ridgway J, Sivananthan M (2003b) Comparison of right ventricular volume measurements between axial and short axis orientation using steady-state free precession magnetic resonance imaging. J Magn Reson Imaging 18:25–32

Alley MT, Napel S, Amano Y et al (1999) Fast 3D cardiac cine MR imaging. J Magn Reson Imaging 9:751–755

Anderson JL, Horne BD, Pennell DJ (2005) Atrial dimensions in health and left ventricular disease using cardiovascular magnetic resonance. J Cardiovasc Magn Reson 7:671–675

Arheden H, Holmqvist C, Thilen U et al (1999) Left-to-right shunts: comparison of measurement obtained with MR velocity mapping and with radionuclide angiography. Radiology 211:453–458

Arts T, Bovendeerd PHM, Prinzen FW, Reneman RS (1991) Relation between left ventricular cavity pressure and volume and systolic fiber stress and strain in the wall. Biophys J 59:93–102

Atkinson DJ, Edelman RR (1991) Cineangiography of the heart in a single breath hold with a segmented turboflash sequence. Radiology 178:357–360

Aurigemma G, Davidoff A, Silver K, Boehmer J (1992) Left ventricular mass quantitation using single-phase cardiac magnetic resonance imaging. Am J Cardiol 70:259–262

Axel L, Dougherty L (1989a) Heart wall motion: improved method for spatial modulation of magnetization for MR imaging. Radiology 172:349–350

Axel L, Dougherty L (1989b) MR imaging of motion with spatial modulation of magnetization. Radiology 171:841–845

Axel L, Montillo A, Kim D (2005) Tagged magnetic resonance imaging of the heart: a survey. Med Image Analysis 9:376–393

Azhari H, Weiss JL, Rogers WJ, Siu CO, Zerhouni EA, Shapiro EP (1993) Noninvasive quantification of principal strains in normal canine hearts using tagged MRI images in 3D. Am J Physiol Heart Circ Physiol 264:33–41

Baer FM, Smolarz R, Jungehulsing M et al (1992) Feasibility of high-dose dipyridamole MRI for detection of coronary artery disease and comparison with coronary angiography. Am J Cardiol 69:51–56

Baer FM, Theissen P, Smolarz K et al (1993) Dobutamine versus dipyridamole-magnetic resonance imaging: safety and sensitivity for the diagnosis of coronary artery stenoses. Z Kardiol 82:494–503

Baer FM, Theissen P, Schneider CA, Voth E, Schicha H, Sechtem U (1994) Magnetic resonance imaging techniques for the assessment of residual myocardial viability. Herz 19:51–64

Baldy C, Duke P, Crossville P, Magnum IE, Revel D, Amyl M (1994) Automated myocardial edge detection from breath-hold cine MR images: evaluation of left ventricular volumes and mass. Magn Reson Imaging 12:589–598

Barkhausen J, Ruehm SG, Goyen M, Buck T, Laub G, Debatin J (2001) MR evaluation of ventricular function: true fast imaging with steady-state precession versus fast low-angle shot cine MR imaging: feasibility study. Radiology 219: 264–269

Barkhausen J, Goyen M, Rühm SG et al (2002) Assessment of ventricular function with single breath-hold real-time steady-state free precession cine MR imaging. Am J Roentgenol 178:731–735

Basha TA, Ibrahim EH, Weiss RG, Osman NF (2009) Cine cardiac imaging using black-blood steady-state free precession (BB-SSFP) at 3T. J Magn Reson Imaging 30:94–103

Bavelaar-Croon CDL, Kayser HWM, van der Wall EE et al (2000) Left ventricular function: correlation of quantitative gated SPECT and MR imaging over a wide range of values. Radiology 217:572–575

Beerbaum P, Köperich H, Barth P, Esdorn H, Gieseke J, Meyer H (2001) Noninvasive quantification of left-to-right shunts in pediatric patients: phase-contrast cine magnetic resonance imaging compared with invasive oxymetry. Circulation 103: 2476–2482

Bellenger NG, Burgess MI, Ray SG et al (2000a) Comparison of left ventricular ejection fraction and volumes in heart failure by echocardiography, radionuclide ventriculography and cardiovascular magnetic resonance. Are they interchangeable? Eur Heart J 21:1387–1396

Bellenger NG, Davies LV, Francis JM, Coats AJS, Pennell DJ (2000b) Reduction of sample size for studies of remodeling of heart failure by the use of cardiovascular magnetic resonance. J Cardiovasc Magn Reson 2:271–278

Bellenger NG, Francis JM, Davies CL, Coats AJ, Pennell DJ (2000c) Establishment and performance of a magnetic resonance cardiac function clinic. J Cardiovasc Magn Reson 2:271–278

Bellenger NG, Marcus NJ, Rajappan K, Yacoub M, Banner NR, Pennell DJ (2002) Comparison of techniques for the measurement of left ventricular function following cardiac transplantation. J Cardiovasc Magn Reson 4:255–263

Beyar R, Weiss JL, Shapiro EP, Graves WL, Rogers WJ, Weisfeldt ML (1993) Small apex-to-base heterogeneity in radius-to-thickness ratio by three-dimensional magnetic resonance imaging. Am J Physiol 264:H133–H140

Bloomer TN, Plein S, Radjenovic A et al (2001) Cine MRI using steady state free precession in the radial long axis orientation is a fast and accurate method for obtaining volumetric data of the left ventricle. J Magn Reson Imaging 14:685–692

Bloomgarden DC, Fayad ZA, Ferrari VA, Chin B, Sutton MGA (1997) Global cardiac function using fast breath-hold MRI: validation of new acquisition and analysis techniques. Magn Reson Med 37:683–692

Bogaert J (1997) Three-dimensional strain analysis of the human left ventricle. PhD dissertation, Catholic University, Leuven

Bogaert J, Rademakers FE (2001) Regional nonuniformity of the normal adult human left ventricle. A 3D MR myocardial tagging study. Am J Physiol 280:H610–H620

Bogaert JG, Bosmans H, Rademakers F et al (1995) Left ventricular quantification with breath-hold MR imaging: comparison with echocardiography. MAGMA 3:5–12

Bogaert J, Maes A, Van de Werf F et al (1999) Functional recovery of subepicardial myocardial tissue in transmural myocardial infarction after successful reperfusion. Circulation 99:36–43

Bogaert J, Bosmans H, Maes A, Suetens P, Marchal G, Rademakers FE (2000) Remote myocardial dysfunction following acute anterior myocardial infarction. Impact of LV shape on regional function. J Am Coll Cardiol 35: 1525–1534

Bolster BJ, McVeigh ER, Zerhouni EA (1990) Myocardial tagging in polar coordinates with use of striped tags. Radiology 177:769–772

Bornstedt A, Nagel E, Schalla S, Schnackenburg B, Klein C, Fleck E (2001) Multi-slice dynamic imaging: complete functional cardiac MR examination within 15 seconds. J Magn Reson Imaging 14:300–305

Borow KM, Neumann A, Marcus RH, Sareli P, Lang RM (1992) Effects of simultaneous alterations in preload and afterload on measurements of left ventricular contractility in patients with dilated cardiomyopathy: comparisons of ejection phase, isovolumetric and end-systolic force-velocity indexes. J Am Coll Cardiol 20:787–795

Bosmans H, Bogaert J, Rademakers FE et al (1996) Left ventricular radial tagging acquisition using gradient-recalled-echo techniques: sequence optimization. MAGMA 4:123–133

Bottini PB, Carr AA, Prisant M, Flickinger FM, Allison JD, Gottdiener JS (1995) Magnetic resonance imaging compared to echocardiography to assess left ventricular mass in the hypertensive patient. Am J Hypertens 8:221–228

Brandts A, Bertini M, van Dijk E-J et al (2011) Left ventricular diastolic function assessment from three-dimensional three-directional velocity-encoded MRI with retrospective valve tracking. J Magn Reson Imaging 33:312–319

Brecker SJD (2000) The importance of long axis ventricular function. Heart 84:577–579

Brinker JA, Weiss JL, Lappe DL et al (1980) Leftward septal displacement during right ventricular loading in man. Circulation 61:626–633

Buchalter MB, Weiss JL, Rogers WJ (1990) Noninvasive quantification of left ventricular rotational deformation in normal humans using magnetic resonance imaging myocardial tagging. Circulation 81:1236–1244

Buchalter MB, Rademakers FE, Weiss JL, Rogers WJ, Weisfelt ML, Shapiro EP (1994) Rotational deformation of the canine left ventricle measured by magnetic resonance tagging: effects of catecholamines, ischaemia, and pacing. Cardiovasc Res 28:629–635

Buckberg GD, Mahajan A, Jung B, Markl M, Hennig J, Ballester-Rodes M (2006) MRI myocardial motion and fiber tracking: a confirmation of knowledge from different imaging modalities. Eur J Cardio-Thorac Surg 295: S165–S177

Buser PT, Auffermann W, Holt WW et al (1989) Noninvasive evaluation of global left ventricular function with use of cine nuclear magnetic resonance. J Am Coll Cardiol 13:1294–1300

Cain PA, Ahl R, Hedstrom E et al (2009) Age and gender specific normal values of left ventricular mass, volume and function for gradient echo magnetic resonance imaging: a cross sectional study. BMC Med Imaging 9:1–10

Caputo GR, Suzuki JI, Kondo C et al (1990) Determination of left ventricular volume and mass with use of biphasic spin-echo MR imaging: comparison with cine MR. Radiology 177:773–777

Carr JC, Simonetti O, Bundy J et al (2001) Cine MR angiography of the heart with segmented true fast imaging with steady-state precession. Radiology 219:828–834

Casalino E, Laissy JP, Soyer P, Bouvet E, Vachon F (1996) Assessment of right ventricle function and pulmonary artery circulation by cine MRI in patients with AIDS. Chest 110: 1243–1247

Caudron J, Fares J, Bauer F, Dacher JN (2011) Evaluation of left ventricular diastolic function with cardiac MR imaging. Radiographics 31:239–261

Cerqueira MD, Weissman NJ, Dilsizian V et al (2002) Standardized myocardial segmentation and nomenclature for tomographic imaging of the heart. J Cardiovasc Magn Reson 4:203–210

Chuang ML, Hibberd MG, Salton CJ (2000) Importance of imaging method over imaging modality in noninvasive determination of left ventricular volumes and ejection fraction. J Am Coll Cardiol 35:477–484

Cigarroa CG, de Filippi C, Brickner ME, Alvarez LG, Wait MA, Grayburn PA (1993) Dobutamine stress echocardiography identifies hibernating myocardium and predicts recovery of left ventricular function after coronary revascularization. Circulation 88:430–436

Clay SR, Alfakih K, Radjenovic A et al (2006) Normal range of human left ventricular volumes and mass using steady state free precession MRI in the radial long-axis orientation. Magn Reson Mater Phys 19:41–45

Codella NCF, Weinsaft JW, Cham MD, Janik M, Prince MR, Wang Y (2008) Left ventricle: automated segmentation by using myocardial effusion threshold reduction and intravoxel computation at MR imaging. Radiology 248:1004–1012

Constable RT, Rath KM, Sinusas AJ, Gore JC (1994) Development and evaluation of tracking algorithms for cardiac wall motion analysis using phase velocity MR imaging. Magn Reson Med 32:33–42
Corsi C, Lamberti C, Catalano O et al (2005) Improved quantification of left ventricular volumes and mass based on endocardial and epicardial surface detection from cardiac MR images using level set models. J Cardiovasc Magn Reson 7:595–602
Cottin Y, Touzery C, Guy F et al (1999) MR imaging of the heart in patients after myocardial infarction: effect of increasing intersection gap on measurements of left ventricular volume, ejection fraction and wall thickness. Radiology 213:513–520
Croisille P, Moore CC, Judd RM et al (1999) Differentiation of viable and nonviable myocardium by the use of three-dimensional tagged MRI in 2-day old reperfused canine infarcts. Circulation 99:284–291
Culham J, Vince DJ (1988) Cardiac output by MR imaging: an experimental study comparing right ventricle and left ventricle with thermodilution. J Can Assoc Radiol 39: 247–249
Daneshvar D, Wei J, Tolstrup K, Thomson LEJ, Shufelt C, Merz CNB (2010) Diastolic dysfunction: improved understanding using emerging imaging techniques. Am Heart J 160:394–404
Davarpanah AH, Chen Y-P, Kino A et al (2010) Accelerated two- and three-dimensional cine MR imaging of the heart by using a 32-channel coil. Radiology 254:98–108
Dawson DK, Maceira AM, Ray VJ et al (2011) Regional thicknesses and thickening of compacted and trabeculated myocardial layers of the normal left ventricle studied by cardiovascular magnetic resonance. Circ Cardiovasc Imaging 4:139–146
Debatin JF, Nadel SN, Sostman HD, Spritzer CE, Evans AJ, Grist TM (1992a) Magnetic resonance imaging-cardiac ejection fraction measurements: phantom study comparing four different methods. Invest Radiol 27:198–204
Debatin JF, Nadel SN, Paolini JF et al (1992b) Cardiac ejection fraction: phantom study comparing cine MR imaging, radionuclide blood pool imaging and ventriculography. J Magn Reson Imaging 2:135–142
Dilworth LR, Aisen AM, Mancini J, Lande I, Buda AJ (1987) Determination of left ventricular volumes and ejection fraction by nuclear magnetic resonance imaging. Am Heart J 113:24–32
Dong SJ, Hees PS, Huang WM, Buffer SA, Weiss JL Jr, Shapiro EP (1999) Independent effects of preload, afterload, and contractility on left ventricular torsion. Am J Physiol 277:H1053–H1060
Dong SJ, Hees PS, Siu CO, Weiss JL, Shapiro EP (2001) MRI assessment of LV relaxation by untwisting rate: a new isovolumic phase measure of τ. J Cardiovasc Magn Reson 281:H2002–H2009
Dulce MC, Mostbeck GH, Friese KK, Caputo GR, Higgins CB (1993) Quantification of the left ventricular volumes and function with cine MR imaging: comparison of geometric models with three-dimensional data. Radiology 188: 371–376
Edvardsen T, Gerber BL, Garot J, Bluemke DA, Lima JAC, Smiseth OA (2002) Quantitative assessment of regional myocardial deformation by Doppler strain rate echocardiography in humans. Validation against three-dimensional tagged magnetic resonance imaging. Circulation 160:50–56
Elgeti T, Laule M, Kaufels N et al (2009) Cardiac MR elastography: comparison with left ventricular pressure measurement. J Cardiovasc Magn Reson 11:44
Fieno DS, Jaffe WC, Simonetti OP, Judd RM, Finn JP (2002) TrueFISP: assessment of accuracy for measurement of left ventricular mass in an animal model. J Magn Reson Imaging 15:526–531
Fischer SE, McKinnon GC, Maier SE, Boesiger P (1993) Improved myocardial tagging contrast. Magn Reson Med 30:191–200
Föll D, Jung B, Staehle F et al (2009) Visualization of multidirectional regional left ventricular dynamics by high-temporal-resolution tissue phase mapping. J Magn Reson Imaging 29:1043–1052
Föll D, Jung B, Elfried S et al (2010) Magnetic resonance tissue phase mapping of myocardial motion. New insight in age and gender. Circ Cardiovasc Imaging 3:54–64
Foo TK, Bernstein MA, Aisen AM, Hernandez RJ, Collick BD, Bernstein T (1995) Improved ejection fraction and flow velocity estimates with use of view sharing and uniform repetition time excitation with fast cardiac techniques. Radiology 195:471–478
Forbat SM, Karwatowski SP, Gatehouse PD, Firmin DN, Longmore DB, Underwood SR (1994) Technical note: rapid measurement of left ventricular mass by spin echo magnetic resonance imaging. Br J Radiol 67:86–90
Francone M, Dymarkowski S, Kalantzi M, Bogaert J (2005) Real-time MRI of ventricular septal motion: a novel approach to assess ventricular coupling. J Magn Reson Imaging 21:305–309
Francone M, Dymarkowski S, Kalantzi M, Rademakers FE, Bogaert J (2006) Assessment of ventricular coupling with real-time cine MRI and its value to differentiate constrictive pericarditis from restrictive cardiomyopathy. Eur Radiol 16:944–951
Fujita N, Duerinckx AJ, Higgins CB (1993) Variation in left ventricular regional wall stress with cine magnetic resonance imaging: normal subjects versus dilated cardiomyopathy. Am Heart J 125:1337–1345
Furber A, Balzer P, Cavaro-Menard C et al (1998) Experimental validation of an automated edge-detection method for a simultaneous determination of the endocardial and epicardial borders in short-axis cardiac MR images: application in normal volunteers. J Magn Reson Imaging 8:1006–1014
Fyrenius A, Wigstrom L, Bolger AF et al (1999) Pitfalls in Doppler evaluation of diastolic function: insights from 3-dimensional magnetic resonance imaging. J Am Soc Echocardiogr 12:817–826
Galjee MA, van Rossum AC, van Eenige MJ, Visser FC, Kamp O, Falke TH, Visser CA (1995) Magnetic resonance imaging of the pulmonary venous flow pattern in mitral regurgitation. Independence of the investigated vein. Eur Heart J 16:1675–1685
Germain P, Roul G, Kastler B, Mossard JM, Bareiss P, Sacrez A (1992) Inter-study variability in left ventricular mass measurement. Comparison between M-mode echography and MRI. Eur Heart J 13:1011–1019

Giorgi B, Matton N, Dymarkowski S, Rademakers FE, Bogaert J (2003) Assessment of ventricular septal motion in patients clinically suspected of constrictive pericarditis, using magnetic resonance imaging. Radiology 228:417–424
Gopal AS, Keller AM, Rigling R, King DL, King DK Jr (1993) Left ventricular volume and endocardial surface area by three-dimensional echocardiography: comparison with two-dimensional echocardiography and nuclear magnetic resonance imaging in normal subjects. J Am Coll Cardiol 22:258–270
Goshtasby AA, Turner DA (1996) Fusion of short-axis and long-axis cardiac MR images. Comput Med Imaging Graph 20:77–87
Götte MJW, Germans T, Rüssel IK et al (2006) Myocardial strain and torsion quantified by cardiovascular magnetic resonance tissue tagging. Studies in normal and impaired left ventricular function. J Am Coll Cardiol 48:2002–2011
Greenbaum RA, Ho SY, Gibson DG, Becker AE, Anderson RH (1981) Left ventricular fibre architecture in man. Br Heart J 45:248–263
Griswold MA, Jakob PM, Chen Q et al (1999) Resolution enhancement in single-shot imaging using simultaneous acquisition of spatial harmonics (SMASH). Magn Reson Med 41:1236–1245
Grothues F, Smith GC, Moon JCC et al (2002) Comparison of interstudy reproducibility of cardiovascular magnetic resonance with two-dimensional echocardiography in normal subjects and in patients with heart failure or left ventricular hypertrophy. Am J Cardiol 90:29–34
Grothues F, Moon JC, Bellenger NG, Smith GS, Klein HU, Pennell DJ (2004) Interstudy reproducibility of right ventricular volumes, function, and mass with cardiovascular magnetic resonance. Am Heart J 147:218–223
Grothues F, Boenigk H, Graessner J, Kanowski M, Klein HU (2007) Balanced steady-state free precession versus segmented fast low-angle shot for the evaluation of ventricular volumes, mass, and function at 3 Tesla. J Magn Reson Imaging 26:392–400
Guzman PA, Maughan WL, Yin FC et al (1981) Transseptal pressure gradient with leftward septal displacement during the Mueller manoeuvre in man. Br Heart J 46:657–662
Haber I, Metaxas DN, Geva T, Axel L (2005) Three-dimensional systolic kinematics of the right ventricle. Am J Physiol Heart Circ Physiol 289:H1826–H1833
Hansen DE, Daughters G, Alderman EL, Ingels NJ, Miller DC (1988) Torsional deformation of the left ventricular midwall in human hearts with intramyocardial markers: regional heterogeneity and sensitivity to the inotropic effects of abrupt rate changes. Circ Res 62:941–952
Hartnell G, Cerel A, Kamalesh M et al (1994) Detection of myocardial ischemia, value of combined myocardial perfusion and cineangiographic MR imaging. Am J Roentgenol 163:1061–1067
Hatabu H, Gefter WB, Axel L (1994) MR imaging with spatial modulation of magnetization in the evaluation of chronic central pulmonary thromboemboli. Radiology 190:791–796
Hatle LK, Appleton CP, Popp RL (1989) Differentiation of constrictive pericarditis and restrictive cardiomyopathy by Doppler echocardiography. Circulation 79:357–370
Hees PS, Fleg JL, Dong SJ, Shapiro EP (2004) MRI and echocardiographic assessment of the diastolic dysfunction of normal aging: altered LV pressure decline or load? Am J Physiol 286:H782–H788
Hendrich K, Xu Y, Kim S, Ugurbil K (1994) Surface coil cardiac tagging and (31)P spectroscopic localization with B-1-insensitive adiabatic pulses. Magn Reson Med 31:541–545
Herregods M, De Paep G, Bijnens B et al (1994) Determination of left ventricular volume by two-dimensional echocardiography: comparison with magnetic resonance imaging. Eur Heart J 15:1070–1073
Hess AT, Zhong X, Spottiswoode BS, Epstein FH, Meintjes EM (2009) Myocardial 3D strain calculation by combining cine displacement encoding with stimulated echoes (DENSE) and cine strain encoding (SENC) imaging. Magn Reson Med 62:77–84
Hoeper MM, Tongers J, Leppert A, Baus S, Maier R, Lotz J (2001) Evaluation of right ventricular performance with a right ventricular ejection fraction thermodilution catheter and MRI in patients with pulmonary hypertension. Chest 102:502–507
Hori Y, Yamada N, Higashi M, Hirai N, Nakatani S (2003) Rapid evaluation of right and left ventricular function and mass using real-time true-FISP cine MR imaging without breath-hold: comparison with segmented true-FISP cine MR imaging with breath-hold. J Cardiovasc Magn Reson 5:439–450
Hsu EW, Muzikant AL, Matulevicius SA, Penland RC, Henriquez CS (1998) Magnetic resonance myocardial fiber-orientation mapping with direct histologic correlation. Am J Physiol 274:H1627–H1634
Hudsmith LE, Petersen SE, Francis JM, Robson MD, Neubauer S (2005) Normal human left and right ventricular and left atrial dimensions using steady state free precession magnetic resonance imaging. J Cardiovasc Magn Reson 7: 775–782
Hudsmith LE, Petersen SE, Tyler DJ et al (2006) Determination of cardiac volumes and mass with FLASH and SSFP cine sequences at 1.5 and 3 Tesla: a validation study. J Magn Reson Imaging 24:312–318
Hudsmith LE, Cheng AS, Tyler DJ et al (2007) Assessment of left atrial volumes at 1.5 Tesla and 3 Tesla using FLASH and SSFP cine imaging. J Cardiovasc Magn Reson 9: 673–679
Hurrell DG, Nishimura RA, Higano ST et al (1996) Value of dynamic respiratory changes in left and right ventricular pressures for the diagnosis of constrictive pericarditis. Circulation 93:2007–2013
Ichikawa Y, Sakuma H, Kitagawa K et al (2003) Evaluation of left ventricular volumes and ejection fraction using fast steady-state cine MR imaging: comparison with left ventricular angiography. J Cardiovasc Magn Reson 5: 333–342
Iino M, Dymarkowski S, Chaothawee L, Delcroix M, Bogaert J (2008) Time course of reversed cardiac remodeling after pulmonary endarterectomy in patients with chronic pulmonary thromboembolism. Eur Radiol 18:792–799
Iwase M, Nagata K, Izawa H (1993) Age-related changes in left and right ventricular filling velocity profiles and their relationship in normal subjects. Am Heart J 126: 419–426
Jahnke C, Paetsch I, Gebker R, Bornstedt A, Fleck E, Nagel E (2006) Accelerated 4D dobutamine stress MR imaging with

k-t BLAST: feasibility and diagnostic performance. Radiology 241:718–728
Jahnke C, Nagel E, Gebker R et al (2007) Four-dimensional single breath-hold magnetic resonance imaging using kt-BLAST enables reliable assessment of left- and right-ventricular volumes and mass. J Magn Reson Imaging 25:737–742
Janik M, Cham MD, Ross MI et al (2008) Effects if papillary muscles and trabeculae on left ventricular quantification: increased impact of methodological variability in patients with left ventricular hypertrophy. J Hypertens 26:1677–1685
Janz RF (1982) Estimation of local myocardial stress. Am J Physiol 242:H875–H881
Jarvinen VM, Kupari MM, Hekali PE, Poutanen VP (1994a) Assessment of left atrial volumes and phasic function using cine magnetic resonance imaging in normal subjects. Am J Cardiol 73:1135–1137
Jarvinen VM, Kupari MM, Hekali PE, Poutanen VP (1994b) Right atrial MR imaging studies of cadaveric atrial casts and comparisons with right and left atrial volumes and function in healthy subjects. Radiology 191:137–142
Jauhiainen T, Järvinen VM, Hekali PE (2002) Evaluation of methods for MR imaging of human right ventricular heart volumes and mass. Acta Radiol 43:587–592
Jessup M, Sutton MS, Weber KT, Janicki JS (1987) The effect of chronic pulmonary hypertension on left ventricular size, function, and interventricular septal motion. Am Heart J 113:1114–1122
Jung B, Markl M, Föll D, Hennig J (2006a) Investigating myocardial motion by MRI using tissue phase mapping. Eur J Cardiothorac Surg 29S:S150–S157
Jung B, Föll D, Böttler P et al (2006b) J Magn Reson Imaging 24:1033–1039
Kacere RD, Pereyra M, Nemeth MA, Muthupillai R, Flamm SD (2005) Quantitative assessment of left ventricular function: steady-state free precession MR imaging with or without sensitivity encoding. Radiology 235:1031–1305
Kaji S, Yang PC, Kerr AB et al (2001) Rapid evaluation of left ventricular volume and mass without breath-holding using real-time interactive cardiac magnetic resonance imaging system. J Am Coll Cardiol 38:527–533
Karamitsos TD, Francis JM, Myerson S, Selvanayagam JB, Neubauer S (2009) The role of cardiovascular magnetic resonance imaging in heart failure. J Am Coll Cardiol 54:1407–1424
Katz J, Whang J, Boxt LM et al (1993) Estimation of right ventricular mass in normal subjects and in patients with primary pulmonary hypertension by nuclear magnetic resonance imaging. J Am Coll Cardiol 21:1475–1481
Kaul S, Wismer GL, Brady TJ (1986) Measurement of normal left heart dimensions using optimally oriented MR images. Am J Roentgenol 146:75–79
Kim D, Gilson WD, Kramer CM, Epstein FH (2004) Myocardial tissue tracking with two-dimensional cine displacement-encoded MR imaging: development and initial evaluation. Radiology 230:862–871
Klein AL, Cohen GI, Pietrolungo JF et al (1993) Differentiation of constrictive pericarditis from restrictive cardiomyopathy by Doppler transesophageal echocardiographic measurements of respiratory variations in pulmonary venous flow. J Am Coll Cardiol 22:1935–1943
Kojima S, Yamada N, Goto Y (1999) Diagnosis of constrictive pericarditis by tagged cine magnetic resonance imaging. N Engl J Med 341:373–374
Kondo C, Caputo GR, Semelka R, Foster E, Shimakawa A, Higgins CB (1991) Right and left ventricular stroke volume measurements with velocity-encoded cine MR imaging: in vitro and in vivo validation. Am J Roentgenol 157:9–16
Korosoglou G, Youssel AA, Bilchick KC et al (2008) Real-time fast strain-encoded magnetic resonance imaging to evaluate regional myocardial function at 3.0 Tesla: comparison to conventional tagging. J Magn Reson Imaging 27:1012–1018
Korosoglou G, Futterer S, Humpert PM et al (2009a) Strain-encoded cardiac MR during high-dose dobutamine stress testing: comparison to cine imaging and to myocardial tagging. J Magn Reson Imaging 29:1053–1061
Korosoglou G, Lossnitzer D, Schellberg D et al (2009b) Strain-encoded cardiac magnetic resonance imaging as an adjunct for dobutamine stress testing. Incremental value to conventional wall motion analysis. Circ Cardiovasc Imaging 2:132–140
Korosoglou G, Elhmidi Y, Steen H et al (2010a) Prognostic value of high-dose dobutamine stress magnetic resonance imaging in 1, 493 consecutive patients. Assessment of myocardial wall motion and perfusion. J Am Coll Cardiol 56:1225–1234
Korosoglou G, Lehrke S, Wochele A et al (2010b) Strain-encoded CMR for the detection of inducible ischemia during intermediate stress. J Am Coll Cardiol Imaging 3:361–371
Kozerke S, Scheidegger MB, Pedersen EM, Boesiger P (1999) Heart motion adapted cine phase-contrast flow measurements through the aortic valve. Magn Reson Med 42: 970–978
Kozerke S, Schwitter J, Pedersen EM, Boesiger P (2001) Aortic and mitral regurgitation: quantification using moving slice velocity mapping. J Magn Reson Imaging 14:106–112
Kramer CM, Barkhausen J, Flamm SD, Kim R, Nagel E (2008) Society for cardiovascular magnetic resonance board of trustees task force on standardized protocols standardized cardiovascular magnetic resonance imaging (CMR) protocols. J Cardiovasc Magn Reson 10:35
Kroft LJ, de Roos A (1999) Biventricular diastolic cardiac function assessed by MR flow imaging using a single angulation. Acta Radiol 40:563–568
Kroft LJM, Simons P, Van Laar JM, de Roos A (2000) Patients with pulmonary fibrosis: cardiac function assessed with MR imaging. Radiology 216:464–471
Kudelka AM, Turner DA, Liebson PR, Macioch JE, Wang JZ, Barron JT (1997) Comparison of cine magnetic resonance imaging and Doppler echocardiography for evaluation of left ventricular diastolic function. Am J Cardiol 80:384–386
Kühl HP, Spuentrup E, Wall A et al (2004) Assessment of myocardial function with interactive non-breath-hold real-time MR imaging: comparison with echocardiography and breath-hold cine MR imaging. Radiology 231:198–207
Kuijer JPA, Marcus JT, Götte MJW, van Rossum AC, Heethaar RM (2002) Three-dimensional myocardial strains at end-systole and during diastole in the left ventricle of normal humans. J Cardiovasc Magn Reson 4:341–351
Lalande A, Legrand L, Walker PM et al (1999) Automatic detection of left ventricular contours from cine magnetic resonance imaging using fuzzy logic. Invest Radiol 34: 211–217

Lamb HJ, Doornbos J, Van der Velde EA, Kruit MC, Reiber JH, de Roos A (1996) Echo planar MRI of the heart on a standard system: validation of measurements of left ventricular function and mass. J Comput Assist Tomogr 20:942–949
Lauerma K, Harjula A, Jarvinen V, Kupari M, Keto P (1996) Assessment of right and left atrial function in patients with transplanted hearts with the use of magnetic resonance imaging. J Heart Lung Transplant 15:360–367
Lee VS, Resnick D, Bundy JM, Simonetti OP, Lee P, Weinreb JC (2002) Cardiac function: MR evaluation in one breath hold with real-time true fast imaging with steady-state precession. Radiology 222:835–842
Legget ME (1999) Usefulness of parameters of left ventricular wall stress and systolic function in the evaluation of patients with aortic stenosis. Echocardiography 16:701–710
Lester SJ, Tajik AJ, Nishimura RA, Kandheria BK, Seward JB (2008) Unlocking the mysteries of diastolic function. Deciphering the Rosetta stone 10 years later. J Am Coll Cardiol 51:679–689
Levy D, Garrison RJ, Savage DD, Kannel WB, Castelli WP (1990) Prognostic implications of echocardiographically determined left ventricular mass in the Framingham heart study. N Engl J Med 322:1561–1566
Lima JA, Guzman PA, Yin FC et al (1986) Septal geometry in the unloaded living human heart. Circulation 74:463–468
Lima JAC, Jeremy R, Guier W et al (1993) Accurate systolic wall thickening by nuclear magnetic resonance imaging with tissue ragging: correlation with sonomicrometers in normal and ischemic myocardium. J Am Coll Cardiol 21:1741–1751
Lingamneni A, Hardy PA, Powell KA, Pelc NJ, White RD (1995) Validation of cine-phase-contrast MR imaging for motion analysis. J Magn Reson Imaging 5:331–338
Longmore DB, Underwood SR, Hounsfield GN (1985) Dimensional accuracy of magnetic resonance in studies of the heart. Lancet 15:1360–1362
Lorenz CH (2000) The range of normal values of cardiovascular structures in infants, children and adolescents measured by magnetic resonance imaging. Pediatr Cardiol 21:37–46
Lorenz CH, Walker ES, Morgan VL, Klein SS, Graham TP Jr (1999) Normal human right and left ventricular mass, systolic function, and gender differences by cine magnetic resonance imaging. J Cardiovasc Magn Reson 1:7–21
Lorenz CH, Pastorek JS, Bundy JM (2000) Delineation of normal human left ventricular twist throughout systole by tagged cine magnetic resonance imaging. J Cardiovasc Magn Reson 2:97–108
Lurz P, Muthurangu V, Schievano S et al (2009) Feasibility and reproducibility of biventricular volumetric assessment of cardiac function during exercise using real-time radial k-t SENSE magnetic resonance imaging. J Magn Reson Imaging 29:1062–1070
Lutz A, Bornstedt A, Manzke R, Etyngier P et al (2011) Acceleration of tissue phase mapping by k-t BLAST: a detailed analysis of the influence of k-t BLAST for the quantification of myocardial motion at 35. J Cardiovasc Magn Reson 13:5
Maceira AM, Prasad SK, Khan M, Pennell DJ (2006a) Normalized left ventricular systolic and diastolic function by steady state free precession cardiovascular magnetic resonance. J Cardiovasc Magn Reson 8:417–426
Maceira AM, Prasad SK, Khan M, Pennell DJ (2006b) Reference right ventricular systolic and diastolic function normalized to age, gender and body surface area from steady-state free precession cardiovascular magnetic resonance. Eur Heart J 27:2879–2888
Maceira AM, Cosín-Sales J, Roughton M, Prasad SK, Pennell DJ (2010) Reference left atrial dimensions and volumes by steady state free precession cardiovascular magnetic resonance. J Cardiovasc Magn Reson 12:65
Malayeri AA, Johnson WC, Macedo R, Bathon J, Lima JAC, Bluemke DA (2008) Cardiac cine MRI: quantification of the relationship between fast gradient echo and steady-state free precession for determination of myocardial mass and volumes. J Magn Reson Imaging 28:60–66
Mandinov L, Eberli FR, Seiler C, Hess OM (2000) Diastolic heart failure. Cardiovasc Res 45:813–825
Manka R, Buehrer M, Boesiger P, Fleck E, Kozerke S (2010) Performance of simultaneous cardiac-respiratory self-gated three-dimensional MR imaging of the heart: initial experience. Radiology 255:909–916
Marcus JT, Vonk Noordegraaf A, De Vries PM et al (1998) MRI evaluation of right ventricular pressure overload in chronic pulmonary disease. J Magn Reson Imaging 8:999–1005
Marcus JT, Götte MJW, DeWaal LK et al (1999a) The influence of through-plane motion on left ventricular volumes measured by magnetic resonance imaging: implications for image acquisition and analysis. J Cardiovasc Magn Reson 1:1–6
Marcus JT, DeWaal LK, Götte MJ, van der Geest RJ, Heethaar RM, Van Rossum AC (1999b) MRI-derived left ventricular function parameters and mass in healthy young adults: relation with gender and body size. Int J Card Imaging 15:411–419
Markiewicz W, Sechtem U, Higgins CB (1987a) Evaluation of the right ventricle by magnetic resonance imaging. Am Heart J 113:8–15
Markiewicz W, Sechtem U, Kirby R, Derugin N, Caputo GC, Higgins CB (1987b) Measurement of ventricular volumes in the dog by nuclear magnetic resonance imaging. J Am Coll Cardiol 10:170–177
Masci PG, Dymarkowski S, Rademakers FE, Bogaert J (2009) Determination of regional ejection fraction in patients with myocardial infarction by using merged late gadolinium enhancement and cine MR: feasibility study. Radiology 250:50–60
Matter C, Nagel E, Stuber M, Boesiger P, Hess OM (1996) Assessment of systolic and diastolic LV function by MR myocardial tagging. Basic Res Cardiol 91(Suppl 2):23–28
Matthaei D, Frahm J, Haase A, Hanicke W (1985) Regional physiological functions depicted by sequences of rapid magnetic resonance images. Lancet 19:893
McVeigh ER, Atalar E (1992) Cardiac tagging with breath-hold cine MRI. Magn Reson Med 28:318–327
McVeigh ER, Zerhouni EA (1991) Noninvasive measurement of transmural gradients in myocardial strain with MR imaging. Radiology 180:677–683
Mertens LL, Friedberg MK (2010) Imaging of the right ventricle—current state of the art. Nat Rev Cardiol 7:551–563

Miller S, Simonetti OP, Carr J, Kramer U, Finn JP (2002) MR imaging of the heart with cine true fast imaging with steady-state precession: influence of spatial and temporal resolutions on left ventricular functional parameters. Radiology 223:263–269

Mirsky I, Corin WJ, Murakami T, Grimm J, Hess OM, Krayenbuehl HP (1988) Correction for preload in assessment of myocardial contractility in aortic and mitral valve disease. Application of the concept of systolic myocardial stiffness. Circulation 78:68–80

Mogelvang J, Thomsen C, Mehlsen J, Bräckle G, Stubgaard M, Henriksen O (1986) Evaluation of left ventricular volumes measured by magnetic resonance imaging. Eur Heart J 7:1016–1021

Mohiaddin RH, Wann SL, Underwood R, Firmin DN, Rees S, Longmore DB (1990) Vena caval flow: assessment with cine MR velocity mapping. Radiology 177:537–541

Mohiaddin RH, Amanuma M, Kilner PJ, Pennell DJ, Manzara C, Longmore DB (1991) MR phase-shift velocity mapping of mitral and pulmonary venous flow. J Comput Assist Tomogr 15:237–243

Moon JCC, Lorenz CH, Francis JM, Smith GC, Pennell DJ (2002) Breath-hold FLASH and FISP cardiovascular MR imaging: left ventricular volume differences and reproducibility. Radiology 223:789–797

Moore CC, O'Dell WG, McVeigh ER, Zerhouni EA (1992) Calculation of three-dimensional left ventricular strains from biplanar tagged MR images. J Magn Reson Imaging 2:165–175

Moore CC, Reeder SB, McVeigh ER (1994) Tagged MR imaging in a deforming phantom: photographic validation. Radiology 190:765–769

Moreo A, Ambrosio G, De Chiara B et al (2009) Influence of myocardial fibrosis on left ventricular diastolic function. Noninvasive assessment by cardiac magnetic resonance and echo. Circ Cardiovasc Imaging 2:437–443

Mostbeck GH, Hartiala JJ, Foster E, Fujita N, Dulce MC, Higgins CB (1993) Right ventricular diastolic filling: evaluation with velocity-encoded cine MRI. J Comput Assist Tomogr 17:245–252

Muthurangu V, Lurz P, Critchely JD, Deanfield JE, Taylor AM, Hansen MS (2008) Real-time assessment of right and left ventricular volumes and function in patients with congenital heart disease by using high spatiotemporal resolution radial k-t SENSE. Radiology 248:782–791

Myerson SG, Montgomery HE, World MJ, Pennell DJ (2002a) Left ventricular mass. Reliability of M-mode and 2-dimensional echocardiographic formulas. Hypertension 40:673–678

Myerson SG, Bellenger NG, Pennell DJ (2002b) Assessment of left ventricular mass by cardiovascular magnetic resonance. Hypertension 39:750–755

Nagel E, Schneider U, Schalla S et al (2000) Magnetic resonance real-time imaging for the evaluation of left ventricular function. J Cardiovasc Magn Reson 2:7–14

Naito H, Arisawa J, Harada K, Yamagami H, Kozuka T, Tamura S (1995) Assessment of right ventricular regional contraction and comparison with the left ventricle in normal humans: a cine magnetic resonance study with presaturation myocardial tagging. Br Heart J 74:186–191

Nasiraei-Moghaddam A, Gharib M (2009) Evidence for the existence of a functional helical myocardial band. Am J Physiol Heart Circ Physiol 296:H127–H131

Neizel M, Lossnitzer D, Korosoglou G et al (2009) Strain-encoded MRI for evaluation of left ventricular function and transmurality in acute myocardial infarction. Circ Cardiovasc Imaging 2:116–122

Nesser HJ, Sugeng L, Corsi C et al (2007) Volumetric analysis of regional left ventricular function with real-time three-dimensional echocardiography: validation by magnetic resonance and clinical utility testing. Heart 93:572–578

Nesser HJ, Mor-Avi V, Gorissen W et al (2009) Quantification of left ventricular volumes using three-dimensional echocardiographic speckle tracking: comparison with MRI. Eur Heart J 30:1565–1573

Niemann PS, Pinho L, Balbach T et al (2007) Anatomically oriented right ventricular volume measurements with dynamic three-dimensional echocardiography validated by 3-Tesla magnetic resonance imaging. J Am Coll Cardiol 50:1668–1676

O'Dell WG, Moore CC, Hunter WC, Zerhouni EA, McVeigh ER (1995) Three-dimensional myocardial deformations: calculation with displacement field fitting to tagged MR images. Radiology 195:829–835

Osman NF, Kerwin WS, McVeigh ER, Prince JL (1999) Cardiac motion tracking using CINE harmonic phase (HARP) magnetic resonance imaging. Magn Reson Med 42:1048–1060

Osman NF, Sampath S, Atalar E, Prince JL (2001) Imaging longitudinal cardiac strain on short-axis images using strain-encoded MRI. Magn Reson Med 46:324–334

Paelinck BP, Lamb HJ, Bax JJ, Van der Wall EE, de Roos A (2002) Assessment of diastolic function by cardiovascular magnetic resonance. Am Heart J 144:198–205

Paelinck BP, de Roos A, Bax JJ et al (2005) Feasibility of tissue magnetic resonance imaging: a pilot study in comparison with tissue Doppler imaging and invasive measurement. J Am Coll Cardiol 45:1109–1116

Palmon LC, Reichek N, Yeon SB et al (1994) Intramural myocardial shortening in hypertensive left ventricular hypertrophy with normal pump function. Circulation 89:122–131

Pan L, Stuber M, Kraitchman DL, Fritzges DL, Gilson WD, Osman NF (2006) Real-time imaging of regional functional using FastSENC. Magn Reson Med 55:386–395

Papavassiliu T, Kühl HP, Schröder M et al (2005) Effect of endocardial trabeculae on left ventricular measurements and measurement reproducibility at cardiovascular MR imaging. Radiology 236:57–64

Parish V, Hussain T, Beerbaum P et al (2010) Single breath-hold assessment of ventricular volumes using 32-channel coil technology and an extracellular contrast agent. J Magn Reson Imaging 31:838–844

Pattynama PM, Doornbos J, Hermans J, van der Wall EE, de Roos A (1992) Magnetic resonance evaluation of regional left ventricular function. Effect of through-plane motion. Invest Radiol 27:681–685

Pattynama PM, Lamb HJ, van der Velde EA, van der Wall EE, de Roos A (1993) Left ventricular measurements with cine and spin-echo MR imaging: a study of reproducibility with variance component analysis. Radiology 187:261–268

Pattynama PM, Lamb HJ, van der Velde EA, van der Geest RJ, van der Wall EE, De Roos A (1995) Reproducibility of MRI-derived measurements of right ventricular volumes and myocardial mass. Magn Reson Imaging 13:53–63

Pennell DJ, Underwood SR, Ell PJ, Swanton RH, Walker JM, Longmore DB (1990) Dipyridamole magnetic resonance imaging: a comparison with thallium-201 emission tomography. Br Heart J 64:362–369

Pennell DJ, Underwood SR, Manzara CC et al (1992) Magnetic resonance imaging during dobutamine stress in coronary artery disease. Am J Cardiol 70:34–40

Pennell DJ, Firmin DN, Burger P et al (1995) Assessment of magnetic resonance velocity mapping of global ventricular function during dobutamine infusion in coronary artery disease. Br Heart J 74:163–170

Perman WH, Creswell LL, Wyers SG, Moulton MJ, Pasque MK (1995) Magnetic resonance imaging during dobutamine stress in coronary artery disease. Am J Cardiol 70:34–40

Petersen SE, Jung BA, Wiesmann F et al (2006) Myocardial tissue phase mapping with cine phase-contrast MR imaging: regional wall motion analysis in healthy volunteers. Radiology 238:816–826

Pipe JG, Boes JL, Chenevert TL (1991) Method for measuring three-dimensional motion with tagged MR imaging. Radiology 181:591–595

Plein S, Bloomer TN, Ridgway JP, Jones TR, Bainbridge GJ, Sivananthan MU (2001) Steady-state free precession magnetic resonance imaging of the heart: comparison with segmented k-space gradient-echo imaging. J Magn Reson Imaging 14:230–236

Powell AJ, Tsai-Goodman B, Prakash A, Greil GF, Geva T (2003) Comparison between phase-velocity cine magnetic resonance imaging and invasive oxymetry for quantification of atrial shunts. Am J Cardiol 91:1523–1525

Rademakers FE, Bogaert J (2006) Cardiac dysfunction in heart failure with normal ejection fraction: MRI measurements. Prog Cardiovasc Dis 49:215–227

Rademakers FE, Buchalter MB, Rogers WJ et al (1992) Dissociation between left ventricular untwisting and filling: accentuation by catecholamines. Circulation 85:1572–1581

Rademakers FE, Rogers WJ, Guier WH et al (1994) Relation of regional cross-fiber shortening to wall thickening in the intact heart. Three-dimensional strain analysis by NMR tagging. Circulation 89:1174–1182

Rademakers FE, Marchal G, Mortelmans L, Van de Werf F, Bogaert J (2003) Evolution of regional performance after an acute anterior myocardial infarction in humans using magnetic resonance tagging. J Physiol 546:777–787

Rajappan K, Livieratos L, Camici PG, Pennell DJ (2002) Measurement of ventricular volumes and function: a comparison of gated PET and cardiovascular magnetic resonance. J Nucl Med 43:806–810

Robinson TF, Factor SM, Sonnenblick EH (1986) The heart as a suction pump. Sci Am 254:84–91

Rogers WJ, Shapiro EP, Weiss JL et al (1991) Quantification of and correction for left ventricular systolic long-axis shortening by magnetic resonance tissue tagging and slice isolation. Circulation 84:721–731

Romiger MB, Bachmann GF, Geuer M et al (1999) Accuracy of right and left ventricular heart volume and left ventricular muscle mass determination with cine MRI in breath holding technique. Rofo Fortschr Geb Rontgenstr Neuen Bildgeb Verfahr 170:54–60

Ryf S, Spiegel MA, Gerber M, Boesiger P (2002) Myocardial tagging with 3D CSPAMM. J Magn Reson Imaging 16:320–325

Sakuma H, Fujita N, Foo TK et al (1993) Evaluation of left ventricular volume and mass with breath-hold cine MR imaging. Radiology 188:377–380

Salton CJ, Chuang ML, O'Donnell CJ et al (2002) Gender differences and normal left ventricular anatomy in an adult population free of hypertension. J Am Coll Cardiol 39:1055–1060

Sampath S, Derbyshire A, Atalar E, Osman NF, Prince JL (2003) Real-time imaging of two-dimensional cardiac strain using a harmonic phase magnetic resonance imaging (HARP-MRI) pulse technique. Magn Reson Med 50: 154–163

Santaralli MF, Positano V, Michelassi C, Lombardi M, Landini L (2003) Automated cardiac MR image segmentation: theory and measurement segmentation. Med Eng Phys 25:149–159

Sarikouch S, Peters B, Gutberlet M et al (2010) Sex-specific pediatric percentiles for ventricular size and mass as reference values for cardiac MRI. Assessment by steady-state free-precession and phase-contrast MRI flow. Circ Cardiovasc Imaging 3:65–76

Scharf M, Brem MH, Wilhelm M, Schoepf UJ, Uder M, Lell MM (2010) Atrial and ventricular functional and structural adaptations of the heart in elite triathletes assessed with cardiac MR imaging. Radiology 257:71–79

Scharhag J, Schneider G, Urhausen A, Rochette V, Kramann B, Kindermann W (2002) Athlete's Heart. Right and left ventricular mass and function in male endurance athletes and untrained individuals determined by magnetic resonance imaging. J Am Coll Cardiol 40:1856–1863

Schulen V, Schick F, Loichat J et al (1996) Evaluation of k-space segmented cine sequences for fast functional cardiac imaging. Invest Radiol 31:512–522

Scollan DF, Holmes A, Winslow R, Forder J (1998) Histological validation of myocardial microstructure obtained from diffusion tensor magnetic resonance imaging. Am J Physiol 275:H2308–H2318

Sechtem U, Pflugfelder PW, Gould RG et al (1987) Measurement of right and left ventricular volumes in healthy individuals with cine MR imaging. Radiology 163:697–702

Semelka RC, Tomei E, Wagner S et al (1990a) Interstudy reproducibility of dimensional and functional measurements between cine magnetic resonance studies in the morphologically abnormal left ventricle. Am Heart J 119: 1367–1373

Semelka RC, Tomei E, Wagner S et al (1990b) Normal left ventricular dimensions and function: interstudy reproducibility of measurements with cine MR imaging. Radiology 174:763–768

Setser RM, Fischer SE, Lorenz CH (2000) Quantification of left ventricular function with magnetic resonance images acquired in real-time. J Magn Reson Imaging 12:430–438

Sierra-Galan LM, Ingkanisorn WP, Rhoads KL, Agyeman KO, Arai AE (2003) Qualitative assessment of regional left ventricular can predict MRI or radionuclide ejection fraction: an objective alternative to eyeball estimates. J Cardiovasc Magn Reson 5:451–463

Sievers B, Addo M, Kirchberg S et al (2005) How much are atrial volumes and ejection fraction assessed by cardiac magnetic resonance imaging influenced by the ECG gating method? J Cardiovasc Magn Reson 7:587–593

Singelton HR, Pohost GM (1997) Automatic cardiac MR image segmentation using edge detection by tissue classification in pixel neighborhoods. Magn Reson Med 37:418–424

Sodickson DK, Manning WJ (1997) Simultaneous acquisition of spatial harmonics (SMASH): fast imaging with radiofrequency coil arrays. Magn Reson Med 38:591–603

Soldo SJ, Norris SL, Gober JR, Haywood LJ, Colletti PM, Terk M (1994) MRI-derived ventricular volume curves for the assessment of left ventricular function. Magn Reson Imaging 12:711–717

Sosnovik DE, Wang R, Dai G, Reese TG, Wedeen WJ (2009) Diffusion MR tractography of the heart. J Cardiovasc Magn Reson 11:47

Spiegel MA, Luechinger R, Schwitter J, Boesiger P (2003) Ring Tag: ring-shaped tagging for myocardial centerline assessment. Invest Radiol 38:669–678

Spottiswoode BS, Zhong X, Lorenz CH, Mayosi BM, Meintjes EM, Epstein FH (2008) 3D myocardial tissue tracking with slice followed cine DENSE MRI. J Magn Reson Imaging 27:1019–1027

Spuentrup E, Schroeder J, Mahnken AH et al (2003) Quantitative assessment of left ventricular function with interactive real-time spiral and radial MR imaging. Radiology 227:870–876

Stillmann AE, Wilke N, Jerosch-Herold M (1997) Use of an intravascular T1 contrast agent to improve MR cine myocardial-blood pool definition in man. J Magn Reson Imaging 7:765–767

Stratemeier EJ, Thompson R, Brady TJ (1986) Ejection fraction determination by MR imaging: comparison with left ventricular angiography. Radiology 158:775–777

Streeter DD, Spotnitz HM, Patel DP, Ross J, Sonnenblick EH (1969) Fiber orientation in the canine left ventricle during diastole and systole. Circ Res 24:339–347

Streeter DD, Vaishnav RN, Patel DJ, Spotniz HM, Ross J, Sonnenblick EH Jr (1970) Stress distribution in the canine left ventricle during diastole and systole. Biophys J 10:343–363

Stuber M, Scheidegger MB, Fischer SE et al (1999) Alterations in the local myocardial motion pattern in patients suffering from pressure overload due to aortic stenosis. Circulation 27:361–368

Sugeng L, Mor-Avi V, Weinert L et al (2006) Quantitative assessment of left ventricular size and function: side-by-side comparison of real-time three-dimensional echocardiography and computed tomography with magnetic resonance reference. Circulation 114:654–661

Sugeng L, Mor-Avi V, Weinert L et al (2010) Multimodality comparison of quantitative volumetric analysis of the right ventricle. J Am Coll Cardiol Imaging 3:10–18

Tardivon AA, Mousseaux E, Brenot F et al (1994) Quantification of hemodynamics in primary pulmonary hypertension with magnetic resonance imaging. Am J Respir Crit Care Med 150:1075–1080

Taylor AM, Dymarkowski S, De Meerleer K et al (2005) Validation and application of single breath-hold cine cardiac MR for ventricular function assessment in children with congenital heart disease at rest and during adenosine stress. J Cardiovasc Magn Reson 7:743–751

Thiele H, Nagel E, Paetsch I et al (2001) Functional cardiac MR imaging with steady-state free precession (SSFP) significantly improves endocardial border delineation without contrast agents. J Magn Reson Imaging 14:362–367

Thiele H, Paetsch I, Schnackenburg B et al (2002) Improved accuracy of quantitative assessment of left ventricular volume and ejection fraction by geometric models with steady-state free precession. J Cardiovasc Magn Reson 4:327–339

Tsao CW, Josephson ME, Hauser TH et al (2008) Accuracy of electrocardiographic criteria for atrial enlargement: validation with cardiovascular magnetic resonance. J Cardiovasc Magn Reson 10:7–14

Tseng W-YI, Reese TG, Weisskoff RM, Brady TJ, Wedeen VJ (2000) Myocardial fiber shortening in humans: initial results of MR imaging. Radiology 216:128–139

Ugander M, Carlsson M, Arheden H (2010) Short-axis epicardial volume change is a measure of cardiac left ventricular short-axis function, which is independent of myocardial wall thickness. Am J Physiol Heart Circ Physiol 298:H530–H535

Utz JA, Herfkens RJ, Heinsimer JA et al (1987) Cine MR determination of left ventricular ejection fraction. Am J Roentgenol 148:839–843

van den Brink JS, Watanabe Y, Kuhl CK et al (2003) Implications of SENSE MR in routine clinical practice. Eur J Radiol 46:3–27

van den Hout RJ, Lamb HJ, van den Aardweg JG et al (2003) Real-time MR imaging of aortic flow: influence of breathing on left ventricular stroke volume in chronic obstructive pulmonary disease. Radiology 229:513–519

van der Geest RJ, Buller VG, Jansen E et al (1997) Comparison between manual and semiautomated analysis of left ventricular volume parameters from short-axis MR images. J Comput Assist Tomogr 21:756–765

van Geuns RJM, Baks T, Gronenschild EHBM et al (2006) Automatic quantitative left ventricular analysis of cine MR images by using three-dimensional information for contour detection. Radiology 240:215–221

van Rossum AC, Visser FC, Sprenger M, Van Eenige MJ, Valk J, Roos JP (1988a) Evaluation of magnetic resonance imaging for determination of left ventricular ejection fraction and comparison with angiography. Am J Cardiol 15:628–633

van Rossum AC, Visser FC, van Eenige MJ, Valk J, Roos JP (1988b) Magnetic resonance imaging of the heart for determination of ejection fraction. Int J Cardiol 18:53–63

van Rugge FP, Holman ER, van der Wall EE, De Roos A, van der Laarse A, Bruschke AVG (1993a) Quantitation of global and regional left ventricular function by cine magnetic resonance imaging during dobutamine stress in normal human subjects. Eur Heart J 14:456–463

van Rugge FP, Van der Wall EE, de Roos A, Bruschke AVG (1993b) Dobutamine stress magnetic resonance imaging for detection of coronary artery disease. J Am Coll Cardiol 22:431–439 van Rugge FP, Van der Wall EE, Spanjersberg SJ et al (1994) Magnetic resonance imaging during dobutamine stress for detection and localization of coronary artery disease: quantitative wall motion analysis using a modification of the centerline method. Circulation 90:127–138

Verberne HJ, Dibbets-Schneider P, Spijkerboer A et al (2006) Multicenter intercomparison assessment of consistency of left ventricular function from a gated cardiac SPECT phantom. J Nucl Cardiol 13:801–810

Waldman LK, Fung YC, Covell JW (1985) Transmural myocardial deformation in the canine left ventricle. Normal in vivo three-dimensional finite strains. Circ Res 57: 152–163

Waldman LK, Nosan D, Villarreal F, Covell JW (1988) Relation between transmural deformation and local myofiber direction in canine left ventricle. Circ Res 63:550–562

Weiger M, Pruessmann KP, Boesiger P (2000) Cardiac real-time imaging using SENSE: sensitivity encoding scheme. Magn Reson Med 43:177–184

Weinsaft JW, Cham MD, Janik M et al (2008) Left ventricular papillary muscles and trabeculae are significant determinants of cardiac MRI volumetric measurements: effects on clinical standards in patients with advanced systolic dysfunction. Int J Cardiol 126:359–365

Wen Z, Zhang Z, Yu W, Fan Z, Du J, Lv B (2010) Assessing the left atrial phasic volume and function with dual-source CT: comparison with 3T MRI. Int J Cardiovasc Imaging 26:83–92

Westenberg JJM, Roes SD, Marsan SD et al (2008) Mitral valve and tricuspid valve blood flow: accurate quantification with 3D velocity-encoded MR imaging with retrospective valve tracking. Radiology 249:792–800

Weyman AE, Wann S, Feigenbaum H, Dillon JC (1976) Mechanism of abnormal septal motion in patients with right ventricular volume overload: a cross-sectional echocardiographic study. Circulation 54:179–186

Weyman AE, Heger JJ, Kronik TG, Wann LS, Dillon JC, Feigenbaum H (1977) Mechanism of paradoxical early diastolic septal motion in patients with mitral stenosis: a cross-sectional echocardiographic study. Am J Cardiol 40:691–699

Whitlock M, Garg A, Gelow J, Jacobson T, Broberg C (2010) Comparison of left and right atrial volume by echocardiography versus cardiac magnetic resonance imaging using the area-length method. Am J Cardiol 106:1345–1350

Winter MM, Bernink FJP, Groenink M et al (2008) Evaluating the systemic right ventricle by CMR: the importance of consistent and reproducible delination of the cavity. J Cardiovasc Magn Reson 10:40–47

Wong AYK, Rautaharju PM (1968) Stress distribution within the left ventricular wall approximated as a thick ellipsoidal shell. Am Heart J 75:649–662

Yamaoka O, Yabe T, Okada M et al (1993) Evaluation of left ventricular mass: comparison of ultrafast computed tomography, magnetic resonance imaging, and contrast left ventriculography. Am Heart J 126:1372–1379

Yim PJ, Ha B, Ferreiro JI et al (1998) Diastolic shape of the right ventricle of the heart. Anat Rec 250:316–324

Young AA, Axel L (1992) Three-dimensional motion and deformation of the heart wall: estimation with spatial modulation of magnetization—a model-based approach. Radiology 185:241–247

Young AA, Axel L, Dougherty L, Bogen DK, Parenteau CS (1993) Validation of tagging with MR imaging to estimate material deformation. Radiology 188:101–108

Young AA, Kramer CM, Ferrari VA, Axel L, Reichek N (1994) Three-dimensional left ventricular deformation in hypertrophic cardiomyopathy. Circulation 90:854–867

Young AA, Cowan BR, Thrupp SF, Hedley WJ, Dell'Italia LJ (2000) Left ventricular mass and volume: fast point calculation with guide-point modeling on MR images. Radiology 216:597–602

Zerhouni EA, Parish DM, Rogers WJ, Yang A, Shapiro EP (1988) Human heart: tagging with MR imaging—a new method for noninvasive assessment of myocardial motion. Radiology 169:59–63

Zile MR, Brutsaert DL (2002) New concepts in diastolic dysfunction and diastolic heart failure: part 1. Diagnosis, prognosis and measurements of diastolic function. Circulation 105:1387–1393

Myocardial Perfusion

J. Bogaert and K. Goetschalckx

Contents

1 Introduction 167

2 Pathophysiology of Myocardial Perfusion 168

3 Modalities to Assess Myocardial Perfusion 169
3.1 Nuclear Medicine 169
3.2 Myocardial Contrast Echocardiography 170
3.3 Magnetic Resonance Imaging 170

4 Techniques for MR Myocardial Perfusion Imaging 171
4.1 Principles and Assumptions 171
4.2 Challenges and Approaches for Ultrafast Imaging 174
4.3 Myocardial Signal Nulling 176
4.4 Coverage of the Entire Ventricle 177
4.5 Compensation for Respiratory Motion 177
4.6 Contrast Media for MR Myocardial Perfusion 178
4.7 Magnetic Field Strength 181

5 Stress Imaging 183

6 Myocardial Perfusion Analysis 185
6.1 Visual Analysis 185
6.2 Semiquantitative MPI Analysis 188
6.3 Quantification of Myocardial Blood Flow 189

7 Clinical Applications of MR-MPI 192

8 Key Points 195

References 196

Abstract

Coronary plaque formation impeding myocardial perfusion is the most frequent cause of myocardial ischemia. Myocardial perfusion imaging by MRI is rapidly gaining acceptance as a useful clinical tool to assess the hemodynamic significance of coronary artery stenoses, and to depict myocardial ischemia. MRI techniques have significantly advanced over the last years, enabling to accurately study first-pass myocardial perfusion providing visual, semiquantitative or quantitative data on myocardial blood flow patterns. This chapter focuses on how imaging techniques, in particular MRI, can be used to study myocardial perfusion. The main emphasis of this chapter is on the challenges MRI faces to appropriately study the first-pass of a contrast agent through the heart, and on the solutions and approaches that have been developed to tackle the issues. In a second part, the approaches for image interpretation and to deduct (semi-)quantitative measures of myocardial perfusion are highlighted, and the clinical use and relevance of MRI in daily practice is discussed.

1 Introduction

Myocardial perfusion imaging (MPI) is a vital part of the assessment of patients with ischemic heart disease (IHD). In normal circumstances myocardial oxygen

J. Bogaert (✉)
Department of Radiology and Medical Imaging Research Center (MIRC), University Hospitals Gasthuisberg, Catholic University of Leuven, Herestraat 49, 3000 Leuven, Belgium
e-mail: jan.bogaert@uz.kuleuven.ac.be

K. Goetschalckx
Department of Cardiovascular Diseases, University Hospitals Gasthuisberg, Catholic University of Leuven, Herestraat 49, 3000 Leuven, Belgium

J. Bogaert et al. (eds.), *Clinical Cardiac MRI*, Medical Radiology. Diagnostic Imaging,
DOI: 10.1007/174_2011_359, © Springer-Verlag Berlin Heidelberg 2012

supply is well balanced to the continuous changing myocardial oxygen needs. An imbalance may cause myocardial ischemia, which is usually due to atheromatous plaque formation in one or more epicardial coronary arteries, and/or due to a disturbance of the microvascular circulation. It is well known from literature that anatomic assessment of coronary artery (CA) stenosis severity provides limited, often misleading information regarding the impact on myocardial perfusion distally to the culprit lesion, potentially influencing patient outcome (Schuijf et al. 2006; Gould 2009; Tonino et al. 2009). To depict hemodynamic significant stenoses, stress testing revealing stress-induced myocardial ischemia has become a well-established method for evaluating the presence and pathological severity of coronary artery disease (CAD). In clinical practice, exercise or pharmacological stress nuclear imaging are the most widely used techniques for this purpose. Since the early 1990s, thanks to the advent of faster magnetic resonance (MR) imaging techniques, MPI in rest and stress conditions by means of MRI (MR-MPI) has become feasible (Atkinson et al. 1990), has been well validated, and can be considered a preferred tool to investigate myocardial ischemia in particular because other valuable information regarding function, flow, viability and tissue characteristics can be obtained with the same tool without substantial prolongation of the study duration (Hamon et al. 2010; Schwitter and Arai 2011). However, it is crucial to emphasize that myocardial perfusion is highly complex and the evaluation remains difficult. Also MR-MPI focus serious challenges, some of them have been appropriately tackled while others remain more difficult to solve.

2 Pathophysiology of Myocardial Perfusion

A unique feature of the myocardium is its oxidative metabolism with a limited and short-lived capacity for anaerobic metabolism. Therefore, any consideration of myocardial perfusion needs to stress the pivotal relationship between myocardial oxygen requirements and coronary blood flow. In normal conditions, there is a balance between oxygen demand and oxygen supply. Oxygen demand is primarily influenced by wall stress, heart rate, and contractility, while oxygen supply is determined by the coronary blood flow and the oxygen extraction. The oxygen extraction in the myocardial microcirculation is high under basal conditions (i.e., with an oxygen saturation of coronary sinus blood of only 20–30%). Therefore, it is mandatory that changes in myocardial oxygen demand result from similar changes in coronary flow.

The increase in coronary blood flow primarily relies on vasodilation. A normal coronary circulation may increase its flow in resting conditions by a factor of 4–6. Quantitative perfusion measurements performed by positron emission tomography (PET) studies show a baseline myocardial blood flow (MBF) of 0.7–1.2 ml/min/g while the flow in the hyperemic myocardium was 3.7–6.7 ml/min/g. The capacity to increase the coronary flow or the *coronary flow reserve* is defined by the ratio of flow during maximum vasodilation to flow under resting conditions and is normally in the range of 3.5–5 (Araujo et al. 1991; Uren et al. 1994). There are also transmural differences with a greater oxygen demand as well as flow and oxygen extraction in the inner myocardial layers. For that reason, and because the oxygenated blood supply enters the myocardium from the subepicardium, the inner layers are much more vulnerable to ischemia, which explains why myocardial necrosis starts in the inner layers with a variable transmural spread of necrosis (Reimer and Jennings 1979).

Conditions with an imbalance between oxygen demand and oxygen supply are predominantly the result of coronary atheromatosis with one or several stenoses on the coronary arteries. This imbalance causes myocardial ischemia, and, if prolonged, myocardial necrosis. Perturbations in the myocardial microcirculation with angiographically normal coronary arteries may also cause myocardial ischemia but are much less frequent. The flow profile across a stenosis has a close relation with the degree of stenosis. A narrowing <70% of the luminal diameter has only a minimal influence on the flow resistance, while above 70%, flow resistance sharply increases and leads to a significant pressure drop across the stenosis (Gould et al. 1990; Uren et al. 1994). However, in resting conditions, the myocardial perfusion is not altered until the CA has an 85–90% diameter stenosis. This is the result of progressive arteriolar vasodilation, which allows coronary flow to be maintained even in the presence of a high-grade stenosis and to guarantee a normal myocardial perfusion (Klocke 1990). However, as the *coronary vasodilator reserve* is used to compensate for the impaired flow, this mechanism gets partially or completely exhausted and flow cannot be increased adequately during stress conditions. Under these circumstances, the myocardium distal to less severe coronary stenosis (i.e., between 50 and 85%) may become ischemic and the stenosis is hemodynamically significant, even if resting perfusion is preserved (Gould 1978, 1990). The coronary reserve is reduced or diminished and cannot be induced by vasodilatory stimulus. This explains why stress testing is crucial for assessment of the hemodynamic impact of a CA stenosis, and why information regarding absolute MBF as well flow reserve are necessary to fully understand the hemodynamic consequences (Gould 2009).

3 Modalities to Assess Myocardial Perfusion

Numerous techniques have been developed for measuring coronary flow and myocardial perfusion in experimental and clinical settings; these include electromagnetic flowmeters, coronary sinus indicator-dilution techniques, velocity probes, inert gas washout analysis, labeled particles administered into the coronary arteries or the left ventricle (radioactive microspheres), and radionuclides trapped in the myocardium. In the clinical setting, only radionuclide imaging is routinely used to assess myocardial perfusion. More recently, new clinically useful techniques such as contrast echocardiography and MR-MPI have become available.

3.1 Nuclear Medicine

Nuclear medicine is still a cornerstone in the assessment of myocardial perfusion in CAD patients. Most cardiologists are well aware of the possibilities of this technique. Nuclear medicine techniques are well validated and their role in risk stratification for major adverse cardiac events is well-established (Iskandrian and Iskandrian 1999). Most often the single-photon emission computed tomography (SPECT) technique is used to diagnose and evaluate the severity of CAD (Shaw and Iskandrian 2004), while PET is more accurate but also more expensive and less available (Bacharach et al. 2004).

3.1.1 Single-Photon Emission Computed Tomography

Following intravenous administration of radionuclides [such as thallium201(^{201}Tl), technetium 99 m (^{99m}Tc) sestamibi (MIBI), and ^{99m}Tc Teboroxime] the relative myocardial distribution of these radionuclides is measured. Different protocols are used for ^{201}Tl and ^{99m}Tc-MIBI because in contrast to ^{201}Tl, ^{99m}Tc-MIBI exhibits little or no redistribution within the first 1–2 h after administration. ^{201}Tl is injected during stress, while redistribution of the tracer is measured at rest after a delay (e.g., 4 h). MIBI SPECT is performed by means of an injection of tracer during stress and a second injection at rest (or vice versa). In regions with an impaired myocardial perfusion this will result in a lower number of counts (i.e., a defect) compared with normally perfused regions. To detect hemodynamically significant stenoses (see 2), stress protocols are used. The latter cause *reversible* defects, i.e., defect is present on stress but absent at rest (i.e., redistribution on ^{201}Tl SPECT), while *fixed* defects (i.e., no redistribution at rest) are interpreted as myocardial necrosis. The severity of the defect (i.e., reduction in counts) is related to stenosis severity while the extent of the defect is related to the myocardium supplied by the stenotic artery (Patterson et al. 1994).

Although SPECT is widely used in clinical practice yielding good sensitivity, i.e., 89%, (95% CI, 84–93%) and moderate specificity i.e., 65% (95% CI, 54–74%) (Kim et al. 2001), certain pitfalls need to be mentioned. An important issue is the radiation of the injected isotopes, with an exposure ranging between 8 and 20 mSv depending on the protocol used. In patients with severe CA stenosis ^{201}Tl scintigraphy can fail to distinguish viable from nonviable myocardium, and this technique may not be sensitive enough for the detection of low-range collateral flow to the ischemic myocardium (Hadjimiltiades et al. 1989). In a study by Wagner et al. comparing SPECT with delayed gadolinium MRI subendocardial infarcts were systematically missed by SPECT because of the lack in spatial resolution, while MRI matched very well with histology (Wagner et al. 2003). Furthermore, interpretation of ^{201}Tl scintigraphy scans requires experience (Henkin et al. 1994).

False-positive studies are common as thallium depends very much on body habitus. It is not uncommon for the female breast shadow to be interpreted as a septal defect. Imprecise selection of LV long axis during reconstruction may erroneously result in areas of decreased activity (Henkin et al. 1994). The use of attenuation correction methods and analysis of wall motion from gated studies reduces the rate of false-positive results and improves the specificity of the test (Blankstein and Di Carli 2010). In patients with multivessel CAD, hypoperfusion of the entire myocardium may mask regional abnormalities (Lima et al. 2003).

3.1.2 Positron Emission Tomography

PET is very useful for assessing myocardial perfusion and metabolism (Gould 1990). Assessment of myocardial perfusion with PET can be performed with nitrogen-13 ammonia, oxygen-15 H20, rubidium-82, or carbon-11 acetate. PET has several advantages over SPECT, such as a higher spatial resolution and the possibility to measure absolute MBF expressed in ml min^{-1} g^{-1} (Schweiger 1994; Kivelitz et al. 1997a, b; Klocke 1983; Kloner et al. 1992; Kraitchman et al. 1996; Bacharach et al. 2004). This is advantageous in patients with balanced ischemia caused by left main or three-vessel CAD in which maximal MBF is reduced in all regions of the left ventricle, or in patients in whom the myocardial ischemia is caused by microvascular dysfunction. The value of PET in the evaluation of myocardial ischemia and viability has been reported in several studies (Tillisch et al. 1986; Araujo et al. 1991; Demer et al. 1989; Schweiger 1994; Muzik et al. 1998). The reported sensitivity of PET for detecting angiographic stenosis $\geq$50% is 91% (range 83–100%) and the specificity is 89% (range 73–100%) (Blankstein and Di Carli 2010). Drawbacks of PET are patient exposure to radiation, availability and limited half-life of PET tracers, cost and availability of PET scanners, and the limited spatial resolution when compared to MRI. Misregistration of attenuation and emission images, due to diaphragmatic displacement, body mass index, and heart size, is common in cardiac PET imaging and may cause artifactual, false-positive myocardial perfusion defects (Loghin et al. 2004). Finally it should be said that for myocardial ischemia and viability assessment MRI has become a strong competitor to PET (see 6.1 in "Ischemic Heart Disease").

3.2 Myocardial Contrast Echocardiography

Another means to study myocardial perfusion is myocardial contrast echocardiography (MCE). Intravenous or intracoronary injection of microbubbles provides good estimates of coronary blood flow and can be used to detect CAD (Meza et al. 1996; Wei et al. 1998). Advantages of MCE are the real-time mode, the absence of injection of radioactive tracers, and the good spatial resolution. Its role in the clinical setting, however, needs to be further established. In patients with known or suspected CAD, is the information obtained by MCE on the location of perfusion abnormalities and their physiologic relevance (reversible or irreversible) similar to that provided by SPECT (Kaul et al. 1997). Determination of endocardial-to-epicardial blood flow ratios during myocardial ischemia, however, is problematic with MCE (Vatner 1980). Different semiquantitative parameters have been proposed for the assessment of perfusion with MCE (Unger et al. 1994; Wei et al. 1998). Both triggered, high mechanical-index (second harmonic) imaging and real-time, low mechanical-index approaches have led to improvements in this respect (Porter et al. 2001; Masugata et al. 2001), but it has not been demonstrated that capturing an adequate arterial input function (AIF) for modeling is feasible. The role in routine clinical practice is yet not established (Sicari et al. 2008).

3.3 Magnetic Resonance Imaging

MPI with MRI has become possible since the early 1990s. Over the years the procedure used for clinical MR-MPI has not changed substantially. Following intravenous injection of a contrast agent, the *first-pass* of the agent through the heart is imaged using fast MRI techniques, and the changes in myocardial signal-intensity (SI) during the first-pass are used to visually, semiquantitatively or quantitatively evaluate the myocardial perfusion in resting or during stress conditions (Fig. 1) (Table 1). However, it was obvious from the very beginning that MR-MPI is technically highly demanding, obligating to push the MR physical possibilities to its limits, hereby trying to find an optimal compromise between imaging speed and image quality, and to reduce unwanted side

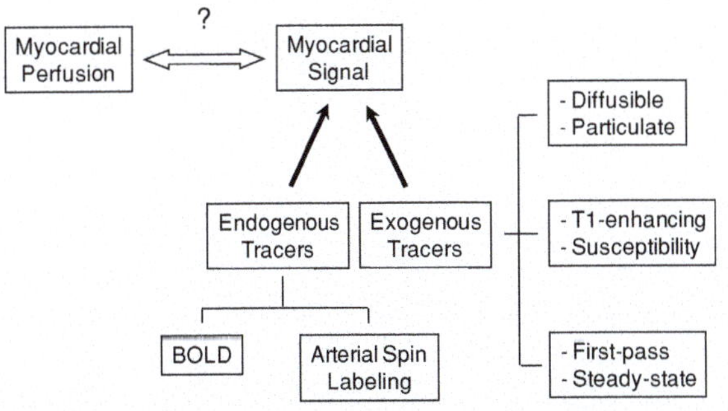

Fig. 1 Different strategies for myocardial MR perfusion imaging. Myocardial MR perfusion is based on changes in myocardial signal intensity caused by use of endogenous or exogenous tracers. These changes are assumed to reflect myocardial perfusion. Abbreviations: BOLD, blood oxygenation level-dependent

effects as much as possible (Tsao 2010). In the following sections, the complexity to study and to quantify myocardial perfusion, and the contribution of technical innovations over the last two decades that helped to facilitate and to increase the robustness of MR-MPI will be explained in detail.

4 Techniques for MR Myocardial Perfusion Imaging

4.1 Principles and Assumptions

Although hypoperfused myocardium may be easily identified by visual analysis and yield sufficient diagnostic accuracy in experienced readers, this simple approach is not always sufficient and subtle differences may escape the eye as might be needed for follow-up examination or to evaluate therapeutic effects on myocardial perfusion. Furthermore, quantitative evaluation will be more objective than subjective assessment by eye. More quantitative information can be obtained from SI-versus-time (SI-time) curves generated from data obtained during early passage of contrast agent. In normally perfused myocardium, the curve starts from a baseline SI level and increases to maximum during the passage of contrast agent through the myocardium. The downslope of the curve is interpolated by a new upslope corresponding to recirculation of the contrast agent (Fig. 2).

In general, quantification of myocardial perfusion is done in two steps. First, a concentration-versus-time curve has to be obtained from the SI-time curve. The second step of quantification is to extract parameters of myocardial perfusion from the concentration–time curve. Quantification of myocardial perfusion using first-pass MR-MPI faces a lot of challenges that have to be overcome. A straightforward quantification needs some general requirements: (a) a nondiffusable tracer, (b) a complete washout of the tracer from the myocardium, (c) a single-spike (point-shaped) input function, and (d) a linear correlation between the tracer and the SI. These requirements are not fulfilled with gadolinium (Gd)-DTPA: (1) the contrast agent diffuses rapidly from the intravascular space into the interstitial space and remains there until complete clearance. The diffusion is flow-dependent. While in normally perfused myocardium the extraction fraction varies from 40 to 60%, it can decrease to only 20% with increasing flow (Tong et al. 1993b); (2) the injection of the contrast agent in a peripheral vein leads to a dilution of contrast agent with a slow and spread input curve (Keijer et al. 2000); (3) a linear correlation between tracer and SI is not maintained in all contrast agent concentrations (Burstein et al. 1991; Manning et al. 1991; Schwitter et al. 1997; Fritz-Hansen et al. 1996). Thus, to attempt myocardial perfusion quantification from dynamic tomographic MR images the kinetics of the tracer in the tissue must be known and described with an appropriate model of distribution. Furthermore, the blood-pool input function must be correctly defined. It has to be kept in mind that with MR the effects of Gd-DTPA on proton relaxivity rather than the concentration of gadolinium-DTPA in the myocardium is detected. This makes the acquired signal dependent on water exchange rates between the different components (Judd et al. 1995a; Donahue et al. 1997; Larsson et al. 2001) and leads to SIs which are not necessarily proportional to the concentration of the agent (Mauss et al. 1985; Burstein et al. 1991; Wendland et al. 1994; Donahue et al. 1994; Judd et al. 1995a). Thus, MR perfusion techniques do not measure the absolute quantity of contrast medium either in the myocardium or in the blood. Wedeking and coworkers have noted that at low contrast agent concentration, the concentration of the agent can be calculated from the SI (Wedeking et al. 1992). Increasing the dose leads to a saturation of signal enhancement and extravasation of the contrast agent, which obscures the clearance phase of the first-pass (Wendland et al. 1994). In practice, at

Table 1 Requirements for Myocardial first-pass perfusion MRI

Temporal resolution (i.e., one image per heartbeat)
Acquisition window as short as possible (i.e., less than 100 ms)
Constant magnetization/image/slice
Spatial resolution (transmural discrimination)
Coverage of the left ventricle
Relationship between signal intensity and contrast dose (i.e., input function) that is quantifiable (linear)
Contrast- and signal-to-noise ratios that are sufficiently high to allow discrimination between normal and ischemic regions of the myocardium
Correction for respiration (total measurement time 45–60 s)

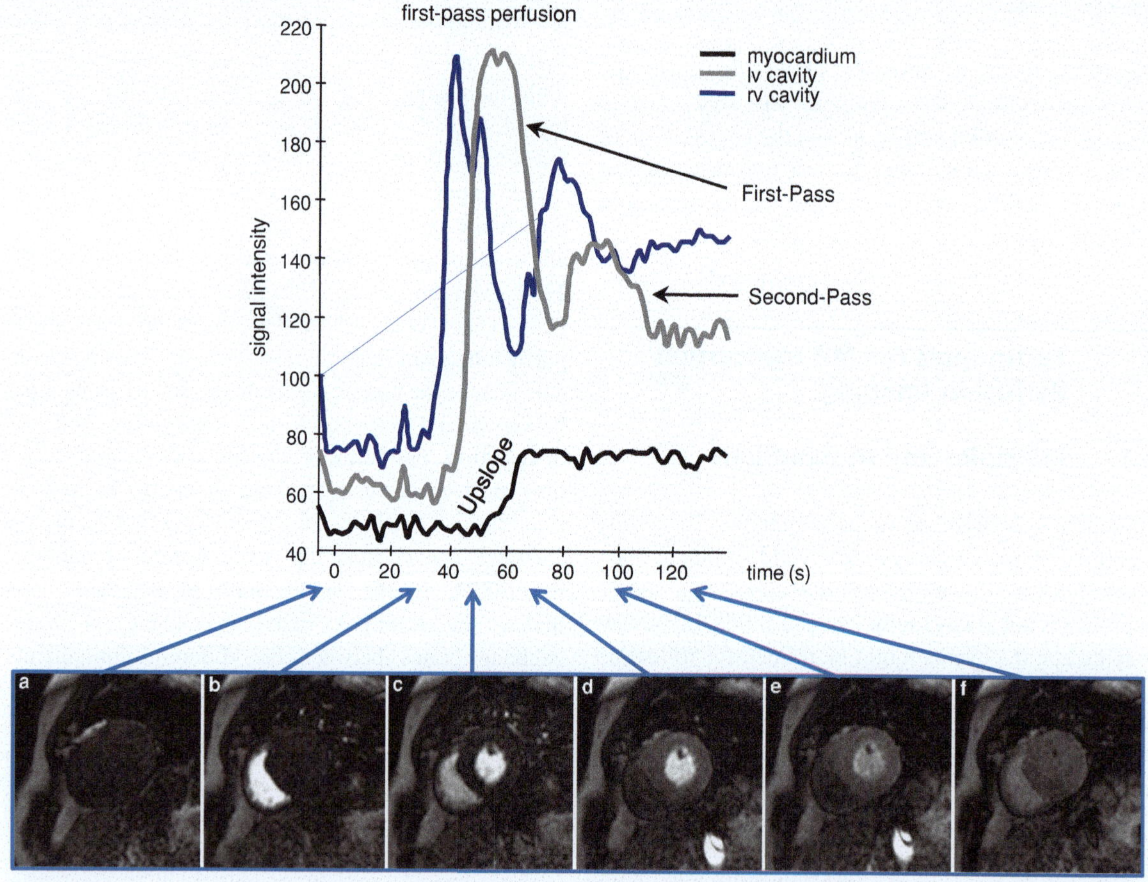

Fig. 2 First-pass signal intensity-time curves of the RV cavity, LV cavity, and the myocardium with corresponding 6 short-axis MR-MPI perfusion images showing the different phases of the first-pass. Before contrast arrival, the signal of the heart is suppressed by a saturation-recovery or inversion-recovery pulse (**a**). At the moment of arrival of the contrast bolus in the heart the RV cavity enhances with rise in SI (**b**). This temporary enhancement is followed by enhancement of the LV cavity (**c**), followed by enhancement of the myocardium (**d**). Approximately 20 s later, a smaller second peak is visible, representing the second pass (**e**). The enhancement in the myocardium is much less pronounced and characterized by the absence of a sharp decline in SI and the presence of a second peak. The latter phenomena are caused by rapid extravasation of gadolinium into the interstitium, which is responsible for a slow washout

concentrations between 0.2 and 1.2 mmol/l, the SI displays a linear progression compared with the Gd-DTPA concentrations. Above this limit, the signal increase becomes nonlinear as full relaxation Is approached due to ever-decreasing T1 and due to signal loss induced by the T2* effect. Above 5.0 mmol/l, increasing Gd-DTPA concentrations result in a drop in SI as the signal losses induced by the T2* effect become dominant (Burstein et al. 1991; Canet et al. 1995; Manning et al. 1991; Schwitter et al. 1997; Wendland et al. 1994; Keijer et al. 2000; Tong et al. 1993a, b).

At the present time, myocardial MR perfusion research makes several, in part hypothetical, simplified assumptions that are incorporated into models for quantification of myocardial perfusion: (a) myocardial water is freely diffusible between the different compartments (intravascular, interstitial, and intracellular); (b) extravascular gadolinium contrast agents enhance myocardial signal monoexponentially (i.e., the regional SI time courses change linearly with the amount of contrast agent injected); (c) MR contrast media behave as a blood component of physiologic interest in its flow patterns; (d) MR contrast agents do not perturb the physiologic parameters being measured; (e) the measured parameters are constant in the MR images used for calculation (Saeed et al. 1995). Two models have been used for quantification of myocardial perfusion by MR by intra- and extravascular contrast agents, i.e., the central volume model and the modified Kety model. Both models are highlighted in detail in Sect. 6.3.

Quantification has been attempted by several groups and also validated in animals and small number of patients (Burstein et al. 1991; Tong et al. 1993a; Diesbourg et al. 1992; Fritz-hansen et al. 1998; Jerosch-Herold and Wilke 1997; Larsson et al. 1996, Larsson et al. 1996; Vallee et al. 1997; Wilke et al. 1994; Jerosch-Herold et al. 2002; Köstler et al. 2004; Christian et al. 2004; Hsu et al. 2006; Ritter et al. 2006; Utz et al. 2008; Groothuis et al. 2010). Nevertheless, quantification of MR myocardial perfusion is still based on many assumptions and simplified models, giving rather an estimate that correlates to MBF than a true quantitative measure of MBF.

To circumvent the problems associated with quantitative analysis of myocardial perfusion, semiquantitative parameters have been used such as the upslope (Al-Saadi et al. 2000a), mean transit time, maximal SI (Schaefer et al. 1992), and time to 50% maximal SI (Taylor et al. 2004). Semiquantitative parameters should mainly be derived from the early wash-in phase of the contrast agent, because Gd-DTPA is an extracellular agent that leaks out the vascular bed rapidly (approximately 30–50% during the first-pass) (Tong et al. 1993a, b). Thus, the early part of the SI-time curve is mainly influenced by perfusion and to a lesser extent by diffusion; whereas the later parts are increasingly influenced by diffusion (Al-Saadi et al. 2000a, 2001). Compared with other semiquantitative parameters of the first-pass SI-time curve, a linear fit of the upslope has been shown to be the most reliable parameter for evaluating myocardial perfusion (Al-Saadi et al. 2001) and seems to be a very sensitive semiquantitative parameter for alterations of myocardial perfusion (Kroll et al. 1996; Judd et al. 1999; Jerosch-Herold et al. 2003). The upslope is easy to determine, is highly reproducible, with low inter- and intra-observer variability (Al-Saadi et al. 2000a), and has been evaluated and validated by several groups (Al-Saadi et al. 2000a, b, 2001; Giang et al. 2004; Ibrahim et al. 2002; Schwitter et al. 2001; Thiele et al. 2003). Since such a fit does not depend on the downslope of the SI-time curve, it can be determined from a peripheral injection of Gd-DTPA. Whereas the upslope or the maximal SI may be sufficient for the detection of severe CA stenosis (>85% diameter stenosis) with a rest perfusion study, the differences between normal and ischemic segments are small and a great overlap is found, necessitating to perform a similar study during stress conditions (Al-Saadi et al. 2000a; Lauerma et al. 1997). This approach allows calculation of the myocardial perfusion reserve (MPR), which is defined as the ratio of perfusion before and after vasodilatation with dipyridamole or adenosine (Matheijssen et al. 1996; Lauerma et al. 1997; Wilke et al. 1997; Cullen et al. 1999) (Fig. 3). Others have used semiquantitative parameters, which were derived only from a stress perfusion study without the need of a rest study (Schwitter et al. 2001). All semiquantitative parameters and the calculated MPR indices show an underestimation of perfusion estimates that seems to be less when evaluating the upslope (Ibrahim et al. 2002; Jerosch-Herold et al. 2003). The degree of underestimation is dependent on the dose of contrast agent and the type of sequence used.

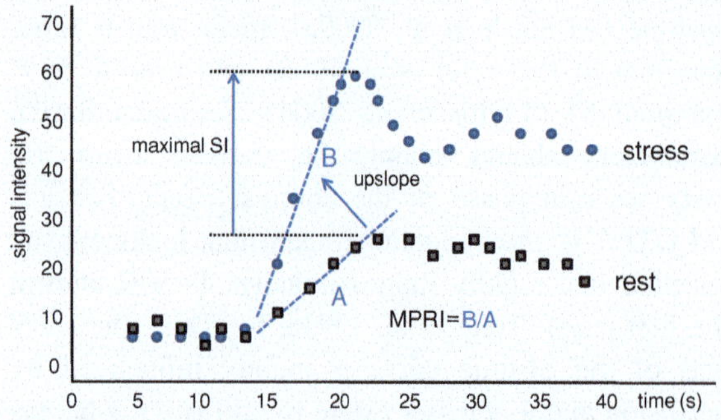

Fig. 3 Alterations of the SI-time curves after stress testing. The figure show first-pass curves of the same myocardial segment at rest (*gray dots*) and after vasodilation with adenosine (*blue dots*). After vasodilation maximal signal intensity increases and the upslope becomes steeper. A myocardial perfusion reserve index (MPRI) can be calculated from these alterations by dividing the parameter at stress through the same parameter at rest. Abbreviations: SI, signal intensity

For all kinds of perfusion analysis, an accurate delineation of the AIF is required. Evaluated parameters and estimates of myocardial perfusion need a correction for the input function to adjust for different hemodynamic conditions and different kinetics of bolus applications. This allows for inter- and intraindividual comparisons and the calculation of MPR. However, at commonly used doses, contrast agent concentrations in the blood-pool are very high. The signal loses linearity to contrast agent concentration and T2* effects may become dominant. This makes an adequate evaluation of the blood-pool SI curve very inexact. Since the input function is a main obstacle in quantitative and semiquantitative evaluation of MR myocardial perfusion, a low-dose prebolus (*dual-bolus approach*) has been proposed to calculate the AIF. Using a small prebolus the signal saturation effects are limited, while the subsequent large bolus is used to determine the myocardial response providing adequate signal-to-noise ratio (Fig. 4) (Christian et al. 2004; Köstler et al. 2004; Groothuis et al. 2010) (see also Sect. 4.6.5).

4.2 Challenges and Approaches for Ultrafast Imaging

Any myocardial MR perfusion sequence designed to monitor the first-pass of a contrast medium must meet several requirements (Table 1). It must: (a) simultaneously collect data of the entire heart, (b) provide sufficient temporal coverage to characterize wash-in and washout kinetics of the contrast agent bolus with a multislice acquisition every or at least every other heartbeat, (c) render sufficient spatial resolution for accurate localization of small perfusion deficits, (d) be sensitive to the signal changes brought about by the bolus with a signal and contrast-to-noise ratios that are sufficient to allow discrimination between normal and ischemic myocardium, (f) provide a relationship between SI and contrast concentration that is quantifiable and is preferably linear. A compact bolus of MR contrast media is necessary for perfusion studies to obtain pure first-pass transit of contrast through the myocardium. This is currently achieved using ultrafast imaging techniques. However, ultrafast imaging poses several practical challenges, and it is easy to push imaging speed too far, resulting in images of non-diagnostic quality (Tsao 2010). Thus, it important to balance the trade-off between speed and image quality. Historically, imaging speed was increased primarily through improvements in gradient performance. At present, gradient switching rate has reached regulated safety limits, which were established to reduce the risk for peripheral nerve stimulation (Budinger et al. 1991). Increased efficiency in imaging time can be obtained in the 3 key components of image formation in MRI, i.e., (1) pulse sequence, (2) *k*-space, and (3) reconstruction (see Chapter on Cardiac MR Physics).

For MR-MPI, fast spoiled gradient-echo (GE), echo planar imaging (EPI) techniques, and balanced steady-state-free-precession (b-SSFP) techniques are used. Fast spoiled-GE technique sequences use small flip angles with very short repetition times and a magnetization preparatory pulse. The latter can be an inversion-recovery, saturation-recovery, or partial saturation-recovery pulse. The objective of this preparatory pulse is to suppress the myocardium at the moment of contrast arrival, thus enlarge the range of SI's of the myocardium before and after administration of contrast agents, and to provide T1-weighted images. Magnetization preparation with an inversion (180°) pulse needs an inversion time of approximately 400 ms to initially zero SI of the myocardium. Thus the myocardium is initially dark, which enlarges the range of signal intensities of the myocardium before and after applying contrast agents. Since a certain number of *k*-lines (e.g., 64,128) are needed to fill the

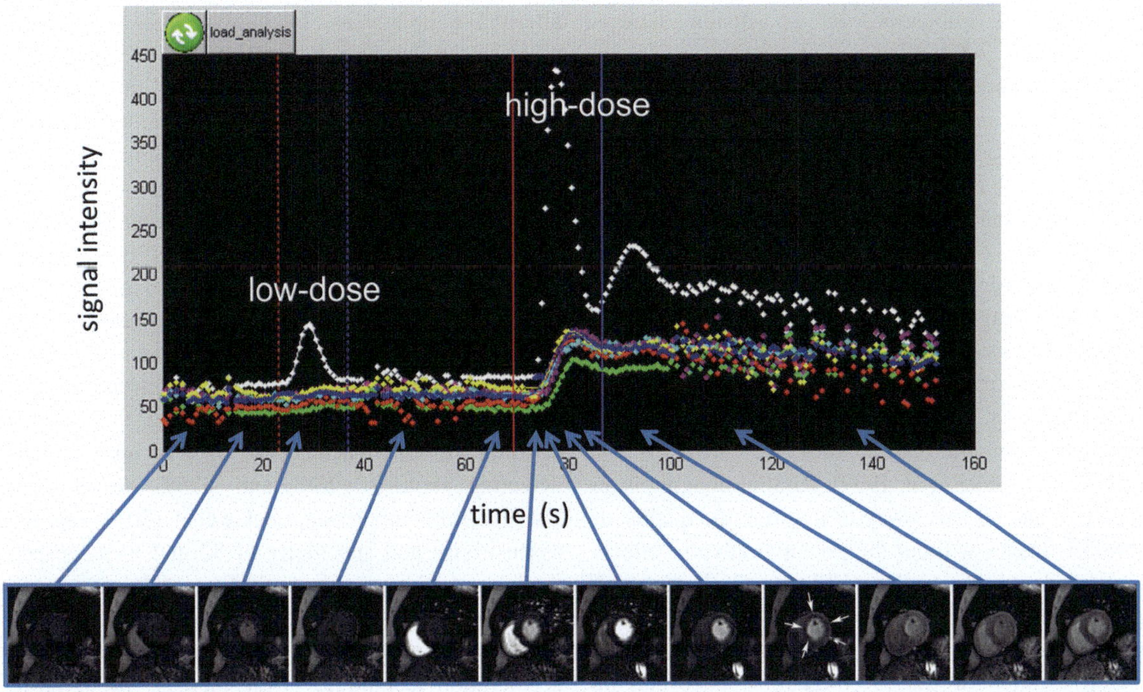

Fig. 4 MR-MPI in a patient with 3-vessel disease using double-bolus regimen during adenosine stress. First pass of low-dose (0.0027 mmol/kg body weight) followed 40 s later by high-dose (0.05 mmol/kg body weight) bolus gadolinium-DOTA (Dotarem®). Twelve short-axis MR-MPI frames are shown (left to right) representing the first-pass of the low- and high-dose bolus; and corresponding SI-time curve. The first-pass of the low-dose bolus is characterized by faint enhancement of the LV cavity (shown by moderate changes in SI-time curves (*white curve*), while the changes in myocardial enhancement are not detectable (*colored curves*). First pass of the high-dose bolus is characterized by strong enhancement of the LV cavity followed by myocardial enhancement. Presence of extensive perfusion defects in the 3 coronary perfusion territories (*white arrows*). Absolute MBF quantification enables to estimate the severity of the perfusion defects

k-space, the total acquisition time may be too long to obtain motion-free images during the cardiac cycle resulting in blurred images by cardiac motion. The latter can be reduced by spreading the data acquisition over two or three heartbeats (segmented *k*-space approach), but this approach reduces the number of data points allowing to appreciate the myocardial first-pass. The prototype sequence of ultrafast imaging is EPI. This sequence uses ultrafast gradient switching to acquire multiple gradient echoes and to entirely fill the *k*-space after a single excitation pulse, hereby reducing acquisition time to less than 100 ms for each image (Mansfield 1977). EPI can be T2*-weighted or T1w-weighted when using a magnetization preparation pulse (mostly saturation pulse) (Edelman and Li 1994). Though EPI has the potential to image the heart with sufficient temporal resolution and is therefore perfectly suited to study fast and dynamic phenomena such as the myocardial perfusion following bolus injection of contrast media, it is prone to image artifacts (e.g., geometric distortion, lower spatial resolution). Spatial resolution can be improved, and spatial distortion reduced, by using a multishot data acquisition (Wetter et al. 1995). Moreover, imaging speed using fast spoiled-GE techniques can be boosted combining it with EPI readout. For example, using a TR of 8 ms and an EPI-factor of 11, acquisition time per image can be reduced to less than 100 ms. The third fast sequence for MPI is the b-SSFP technique (Schreiber et al. 2002; Hunold et al. 2004; Lee et al. 2004). Although image contrast depends on T2/T1 tissue properties, an inversion/saturation magnetization prepulse results in predominantly T1-weighted images. Compared with spoiled-GE imaging, this sequence yields higher signal-to-noise and contrast-to-noise ratios. Though the image quality is improved, this sequence is more susceptible to artifacts at the border of myocardium and contrast enhanced ventricular cavity than spoiled-GE sequences, which may significantly impede evaluation of subendocardial perfusion defects (Fenchel et al. 2004; Weber et al. 2007).

The acquired data are arranged into a data matrix called *k*-space and once the data matrix is filled up the data area converted into an image by a mathematical process known as reconstruction. As discussed above, image speed can be increased by acquiring more than data line per excitation (EPI or spiral approach). Another approach for reduction in acquisition time is "keyhole" imaging whereby only a limited part of *k*-space corresponding to the low spatial frequencies is sampled during first-pass, thus significantly reducing acquisition time, but images show rather low signal-to-noise and contrast-to noise ratios (Walsh et al. 1995; Reeder et al. 1999). Parallel imaging is an attractive and effective way to improve the quality of ultrafast images without the potential adverse effects associated with using a long EPI train (Kellman et al. 2004; Plein et al. 2005; Tsao 2010). Since each coil of a multiarray coil provides information about the spatial location of the MR signal, *k*-space can be undersampled during first-pass, and afterwards converted into a fully acquired *k*-space through reconstruction. The improvement in image quality is analogous to that obtained with multishot approach. Thus, acceleration up to approximately a three-fold can be achieved with parallel imaging, and these advantages can be traded for an improved spatial coverage or increased number of image slices. Moreover, it has been shown that parallel imaging extends linearity between SI and contrast medium concentration with a direct benefit for semiquantitative analysis (Weber et al. 2007). To further improve imaging speed, one can take advantage of the inherent redundancy within the data. Data acquisition can be shortened exploiting correlations in *k*-space and time (*k*-t), e.g. *k*-t sensitivity encoding (SENSE), by undersampling along the spatial frequency (*k*) and temporal (*t*) encoding axes which leads to signal aliasing in the reciprocal spatiotemporal frequency. To unfold signal aliasing from the data undersampling, one uses an estimate of the signal distribution in the spatiotemporal frequency that is obtained from a fully-sampled low-resolution training matrix (Tsao et al. 2003; Plein et al. 2007). By using a 5 × k-t SENSE and 11 training profiles, Plein et al. (2008a) performed MR-MPI with a spatial resolution of $1.4 \times 1.4 \times 10\ \text{mm}^3$, a temporal resolution of 120 ms, and four short-axis slices acquired at alternative heartbeats. Because of the high spatial resolution right ventricular (RV) MPI was performed as well. Gebker et al. (2007) proposed the *k*-t broad-use linear acquisition speed-up technique (BLAST), as an alternative to the *k*-t SENSE technique. Further improvement can be achieved by combining *k*-t SENSE with parallel imaging to double the (low) resolution of the training images (*k*-t SENSE + method) (Manka et al. 2010). Using a 3.0T system for MPI, a net acceleration up to 6.15 and in-plane resolution of 1.1×1.1 to $1.4\ \text{mm}^2$ was achieved. In a small group of patients (n = 20) high diagnostic accuracy was achieved, as reflected by the areas under the receiver-operating characteristic curve of 0.94 and 0.82 for detecting stenosis >50% and >75%, respectively. Using a similar approach, Lockie et al. (2011) reported a sensitivity and specificity of 82 and 94%, respectively, to depict hemodynamically significant stenoses in 43 patients using invasively determined FFR as reference. An additional advantage of the above acceleration techniques is the increase in signal-to-noise ratio (Plein et al. 2007; Gebker et al. 2007). Since *k*-t SENSE can be used to improve spatial resolution, temporal resolution, and slice coverage, it was recently reported that dark-rim artifact could be reduced when maximizing spatial resolution by *k*-t SENSE acceleration (Maredia et al. 2010).

4.3 Myocardial Signal Nulling

The better the signal of myocardium can be suppressed at the moment of contrast arrival, the better the range of myocardial SI changes can be appreciated during the first-pass phase, and the better the T1-weighting. Different types of magnetization preparation pulses are available to achieve these goals. Probably best known is the *inversion-recovery* (180°) preparation pulse with a subsequent delay of 300–400 ms to null the myocardial signal. This pulse works well in patients with a regular heart rhythm because the extent of T1 relaxation is between images is constant. However, in patients with arrhythmias, the change in R–R interval causes a difference in T1 relaxation between images. As a consequence, the SI changes over time are modulated by sources other than the passage of the contrast agent leading to a decrease in quality and diagnostic accuracy. Moreover, the need of a long inversion time interferes with the acquisition of multiple slices per heartbeat, and thus with the coverage of the heart. To overcome these problems, Tsekos et al. (1995) proposed an arrhythmia-insensitive contrast enhancement technique to produce T1 weighting that is independent of the magnitude of longitudinal magnetization at the moment of the ECG trigger pulse. It exists in a non-section-selective 90° RF pulse (*saturation-recovery*) that nulls the longitudinal magnetization, and a gradient crusher pulse that dephases the transverse magnetization. Although the degree of T1-weighting is less than inversion-recovery preparation, saturation-recovery is much less vulnerable to artifacts and is currently the most commonly used approach. Another plus is the shorter prepulse delay (e.g., 150 ms) which is advantageous for multislice scanning and improved ventricular coverage. When performing multislice MPI, one should realize that use of a single inversion-recovery or saturation-recovery pulse for all slices results in a different T1 relaxation, and different signal-to-noise and contrast-to-noise ratios for each slice. The notch pulse saturation technique, with a 90° preparation pulse for each slice, is an appealing solution for this problem (Ding et al. 1998; Slavin et al. 2001). It uses the "dead" inversion time for imaging in adjacent slice positions, leading to improved coverage and signal-to-noise ratios. Judd et al. (1995b) replaced the inversion-recovery pulse in the inversion-recovery turbo-FLASH sequence by a train of preparatory RF pulses. These nonselective preparatory RF pulses drive the magnetization to a steady-state prior to the image acquisition. To obtain T2-weighted imaging, the same type of acquisitions can be used with other preparation pulses, such as 90°–180°–90° triplets (Anderson and Brown 1993).

4.4 Coverage of the Entire Ventricle

Another major challenge for MR-MPI is to track the first-pass of contrast agent throughout the entire myocardium without sacrificing temporal or spatial resolution. Thanks to the advances in ultrafast imaging (see 4.2) and myocardial signal nulling (see 4.3), multislice imaging is feasible on most clinical scanners. From a clinical point of view 3 short-axis slices covering the basal, mid and apical part of the LV are a strict minimum to appropriately evaluate regional myocardial perfusion. Further increasing the number of slices is only beneficial if the diagnostic accuracy does not drop (Nagel et al. 2003). This depends on the type of sequence and preparatory pulse chosen for MPI. Regardless of the type of preparation used, the magnetization recovery time plays a major role in determining contrast, signal-to-noise ratio, and the maximum number of slices that can be acquired. More slices per cardiac cycle can be acquired when using a short recovery time, at the expense however, of a lower signal-to-noise ratio. A longer recovery time yields higher signal-to-noise ratio and better contrast, but at the sacrifice of the number of slices that can be acquired. As discussed above, the notched saturation pulse allows long magnetization recovery times without sacrificing slice coverage (Slavin et al. 2001). Although spatial coverage can be improved by acquiring images not only during diastole (preferable) but also during systole, it is more appropriate to acquire all image slices during one phase of the cardiac cycle, because it was recently shown that while resting MBF is independent of the cardiac phase, adenosine-induced hyperemia yields significantly higher MBF and MPR in diastole than in systole (Radjenovic et al. 2010). Recently, thanks to the above-described improvements in ultrafast imaging (e.g., *k*-t SENSE) in combination with 3.0T imaging a fully 3D MR-MPI sequence was presented (Manka et al. 2011; Vitanis et al. 2011). Complete coverage of the left ventricle was achieved with 16 slices, a reconstructed voxel size of $2.3 \times 2.3 \times 5.0$ mm^3 and an acquisition time of 200 ms per image slice and one image acquired every heartbeat (Manka et al. 2011).

4.5 Compensation for Respiratory Motion

Suppression of gross cardiac motion due to respiration is strongly recommended during first-pass perfusion imaging. Because it is unfeasible for most patients to hold their breath for 45 s to 1 min, alternative strategies are needed. A first approach yielding good clinical results, is to ask the patients to deeply breath-in and breath-out just before the start of and during the first seconds after the injection of contrast agent in a cubital vein. Just before the arrival of contrast in the heart, the patient is asked to stop breathing as long as possible. If the patient is no longer able to stop breathing, he is allowed to breathe shallow till the end of the measurement. As an alternative shallow breathing during the entire examination can be used. Although this is more patient-friendly it may impede visual as well as quantitative analysis. Elastic matching techniques and model-based registration are helpful to automatically correct for respiratory-induced cardiac motion (Adluru et al. 2006). Recently, prospective slice-tracking and free-breathing MR-MPI has become available and may be of interest in incooperative patients unable to hold their breath (Pedersen et al. 2009).

4.6 Contrast Media for MR Myocardial Perfusion

In daily routine clinical practice, MR-MPI is most commonly performed using the first-pass of commercially available gadolinium chelates. The value of other paramagnetic contrast agents, such as manganese gluconate, iron oxide particles, deuterium, or magnetic susceptibility agents, such as dysprosium, has been investigated but yet not entered the clinical arena (Schaefer et al. 1989; Atkinson et al. 1990; Mitchell and Osbakken 1991; Canet et al. 1993; Kantor et al. 1994). Contrast agents are usually classified according to their distribution pattern, i.e., extracellular and intravascular contrast media (Table 2) or to their effects on longitudinal (T1-enhancing contrast agents) or transverse relaxation (magnetic susceptibility agents or T2* contrast agents). Alternatively, the blood level-dependent (BOLD) technique uses the paramagnetic properties of deoxyhemoglobin as endogenous contrast agent to measure myocardial oxygenation, and to depict hemodynamic significant CAD (Atalay et al. 1993; Wright et al. 2001; Friedrich et al. 2003; Jahnke et al. 2010; McCommis et al. 2010).

4.6.1 Extracellular Contrast Media

Extracellular contrast agents, such as Gd-DTPA (Magnevist®), Gd-DTPA-BMA (Omiscan®), Gd-BOPTA (Multihance®), and Gd-DOTA (Dotarem®), are low molecular weight contrast agents (<1000 Da) that rapidly diffuse through the capillary walls into the interstitium (Weinmann et al. 1983). Their kinetic modeling is complex and has to take into account various flow- and tissue-dependent variables, such as extraction fraction and partition coefficient (Burstein et al. 1991; Diesbourg et al. 1992; Wendland et al. 1994). Because of their rapid extravasation and redistribution, ultrafast imaging techniques are obligatory to image the inflow of contrast agent following bolus injection (Schaefer et al. 1992). A typical first-pass of a contrast bolus through the heart starts with a sudden increase of RV blood-pool SI at the moment of contrast arrival, followed by an increase of LV blood-pool SI, and subsequently a smaller myocardial SI increase of the myocardium. While the signal rapidly drops in the ventricular cavities, the myocardial SI slowly decreases because of the extravasation of contrast agent through the capillary bed (Wendland et al. 1994). During first-pass approximately 50% of the contrast agent extravasates, but the magnitude is flow-dependent (Brasch 1992; Tong et al. 1993a, b). Regarding the optimal contrast dose for MR-MPI, results from several single- and multicenter studies, using a wide range of contrast doses (i.e. 0.01–0.15 mmol/kg), have shown that the optimum contrast dose is most likely 0.05–0.1 mmol/kg, using an injection rate of 4–5 ml/s followed by a 20 ml saline flush administered at the same rate (Schaefer et al. 1992; Matheijssen et al. 1996; Schwitter et al. 1997;Al-Saadi et al. 2000a; Wolf et al. 2004; Giang et al. 2004; Schwitter et al. 2008). Most studies show that higher doses of contrast yield greater myocardial enhancement but do not increase diagnostic accuracy. In particular at higher doses susceptibility artifacts become more prominent, and may be mistaken for real perfusion defects thereby increasing the number of false-positives (Wolf et al. 2004). Moreover, at higher doses, the maximal relative increase in SI begins to saturate, thus hindering quantitative evaluation (Schwitter et al. 1997). At lower contrast doses, lower myocardial enhancement occurs with decrease in signal- and contrast- to noise ratios, potentially hampering visual detection of perfusion defects (see also Sect. 4.6.5).

4.6.2 Intravascular Contrast Media

The role of intravascular or blood-pool contrast agents for MPI has been investigated by several groups in animals and humans (Canet et al. 1993; Revel et al. 1996; Kraitchman et al. 1996; Johansson et al. 1998; Panting et al. 1999; Bjerner et al. 2001; Gerber et al. 2002; Reimer et al. 2004; Dewey et al. 2004). A first type of intravascular contrast agents are macromolecular MR contrast media, or nondiffusible

Table 2 Extracellular versus intravascular contrast agents

	Extracellular	Intravascular
Examples		
T1-enhancing	Gd-DTPA	Dextran-(Gd-DTPA)
	Gd-DOTA	Albumin-(Gd-DTPA)
	Gd-BOPTA	Polylysine-(Gd-DTPA)
		USPIO
Magnetic susceptibility (T2*)	Dy-DTPA	Albumin-(Dy-DTPA)
		MION
		SPIO
		USPIO
Molecular weight (daltons)	<1,000	>50,000
Distribution	Intravascular Interstitial	Intravascular
Distribution volume	30–40%	5–10%
Intravascular Half-life	20 min	180 min (MION)
Excretion	Renal	Renal/MPS*
Application(s)		
T1-enhancing CM	Most widely and clinically used	Blood volume
	MR contrast agent	Tissue perfusion
		Capillary integrity
		MR angiography
T2* CM	Detection of ischemia and early infarction and differentiation between occlusive and reperfused myocardial infarction	See T1-enhancing CM
MR perfusion imaging	First-pass imaging	First-pass imaging
		Steady-state imaging

CM Contrast media, *DTPA* diethylene-triamine penta-acetic acid, *Dy* dysprosium, *Gd* gadolinium, *MION* monocrystalline iron oxides, *MPS* mononuclear phagocytic system, *SPIO* superparamagnetic iron oxides, *USPIO* ultrasmall superparamagnetic iron oxides, * iron oxide molecules are accumulated into the MPS system

agents, which are typically gadolinium molecules bound to large molecules such as albumin, polylysine, and dextrans (>50,000 Da). The relatively large size of these molecules confines them to the intravascular space for a significant period. A second type are molecules that are removed from the vascular space by the mononuclear phagocytic system, such as superparamagnetic iron oxide particles (Canet et al. 1993; Revel et al. 1996; Johansson et al. 1998; Panting et al. 1999; Reimer et al. 2004). Blood-pool agents have several intrinsic advantages for MPI. Since they remain in the vascular space for a considerable time, first-pass imaging is not hampered by the rapid diffusion of the contrast agent to the interstitial space, and thus the changes in SI better reflect the true myocardial perfusion. Another advantage of the prolonged intravascular half-life, is that first-pass is not strictly required to assess myocardial perfusion allowing to perform MPI at steady-state (Rosen et al. 1990; Weiskoff et al. 1993; Tong et al. 1993a, b; Wendland et al. 1994; Arteaga et al. 1994; Gerber et al. 2002; Dewey et al. 2004). However, since the blood-pool agents remain confined to the vascular space, counting for only 10% of the tissue volume, signal-to-noise ratios will be significantly lower than with the diffusible (extracellular) contrast media (see Fig. 6). Increasing the dose may increase signal-to-noise ratio in the myocardium, but results in strong susceptibility and T2* artifacts in the LV cavity. Moreover, detection of myocardial infarction and scar tissue in CAD patients is unsure with intravascular contrast media. At the present time, most of these intravascular contrast agents are not available for clinical use.

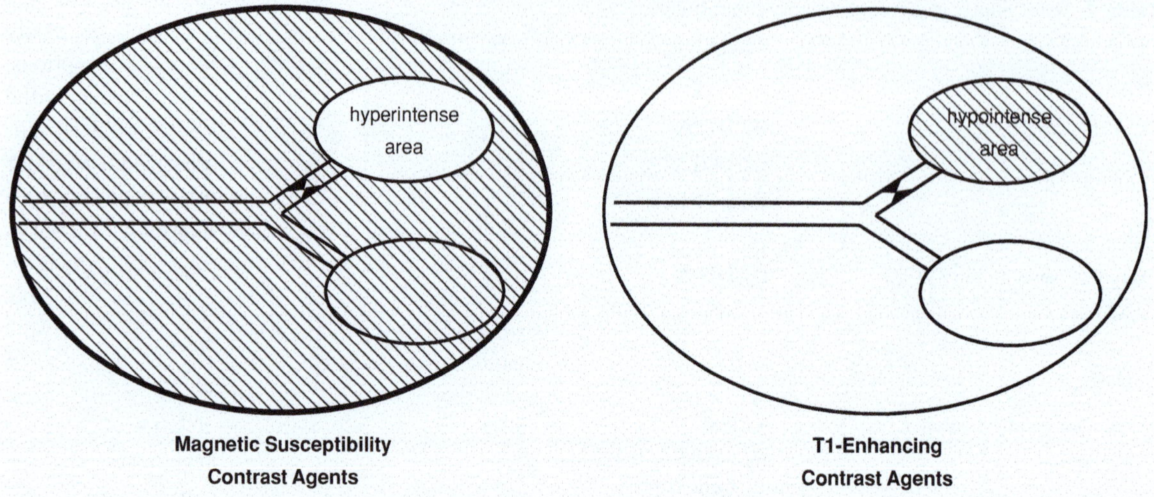

Fig. 5 T1-enhancing versus magnetic susceptibility contrast agents. This figure shows the differences in myocardial signal intensity after administration of magnetic susceptibility contrast agents *(left)* and T1-enhancing contrast agents *(right)*. Following bolus injection of magnetic susceptibility MR contrast agents, such as dysprosium or iron oxide particles, the normally perfused myocardium *(below)* will show a drop in signal intensity; this is not the case for the hypoperfused myocardium *(above)*, which therefore appears as a hyperintense area. In contrast, T1-enhancing contrast agents (e.g., gadolinium) show an enhancement of the normal myocardium that is absent in hypoperfused myocardial regions; the latter thus appear as a "cold" spot

4.6.3 T1-Enhancing and Magnetic Susceptibility MR Contrast Media

MR contrast media act by influencing the relaxation times of the neighboring resonating protons. Several magnetic materials, such as manganese, gadolinium, dysprosium, and iron, are used for this purpose. Their effect can be either a shortening of the longitudinal relaxation (i.e., T1 enhancing), a shortening of the transversal relaxation (i.e., magnetic susceptibility), or a combination of both. For example, at low gadolinium doses, T1 effects prevail while at higher doses susceptibility effects become dominant causing signal loss on T2*/T2 sensitive sequences (Saeed et al. 1995). Thus, using T1-enhancing contrast agents, hypoperfused myocardium is visible as a dark region while it appears bright using magnetic susceptibility agents (Yu et al. 1993) (Fig. 5). While gadolinium is most frequently used as a T1-enhancing contrast agent, dysprosium is a typical magnetic susceptibility contrast agent (Wendland et al. 1993). Ultra-small superparamagnetic iron oxide particles (USPIO) can be used for both T1-weighted and T2*-weighted MR-MPI (Panting et al. 1999; Reimer et al. 2004).

4.6.4 Endogenous Contrast Media

The BOLD technique exploits the paramagnetic properties of deoxyglobin to be used as endogenous contrast agent to measure myocardial oxygenation, and thus to depict hemodynamic significant CAD (Atalay et al. 1993; Wright et al. 2001; Friedrich et al. 2003; Fieno et al. 2004; Shea et al. 2005; Jahnke et al. 2010; McCommis et al. 2010). An increased oxyhemoglobin and decreased deoxyhemoglobin myocardial content result in higher T2* and T2 values, leading to a corresponding signal enhancement on T2*- or T2-weighted imaging, respectively. The latter sequences can be spin-echo (McCommis et al. 2010) or gradient-echo based (Jahnke et al. 2010), and can be easily integrated in stress/rest MR-MPI studies. Good agreement was found between BOLD SI increase and MPR index, PET, and microspheres for the detection of myocardial ischemia.

4.6.5 Single Versus Dual-Bolus Approach

For semiquantitative, and in particular for quantitative MPI analysis, the AIF is needed, which is usually obtained by defining a region of interest in the LV cavity, that is used to track the SI changes during

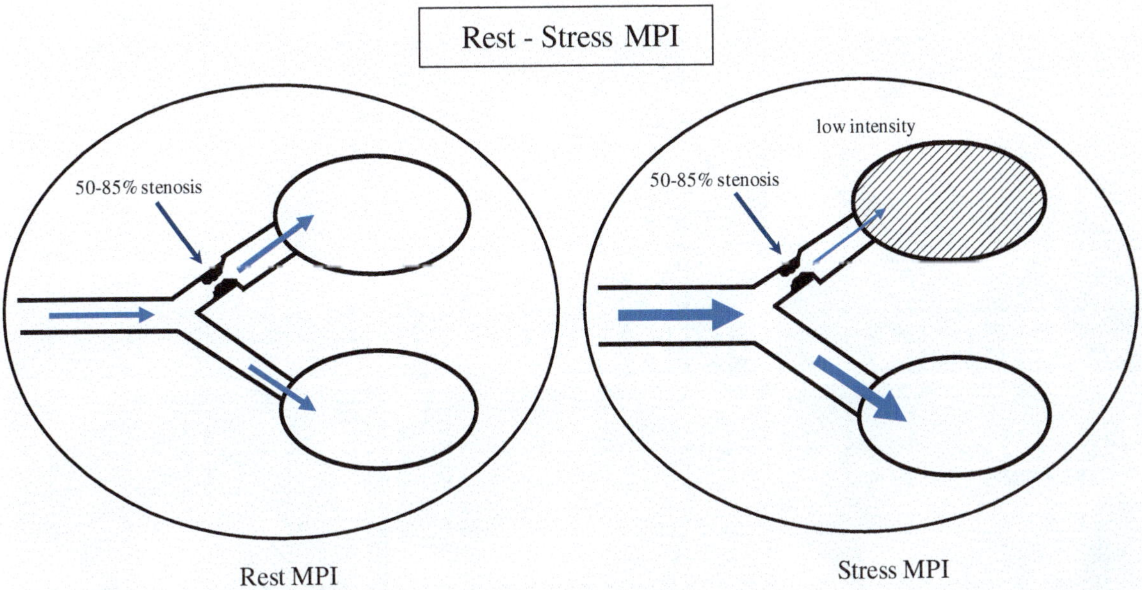

Fig. 6 Principle of rest-stress myocardial perfusion imaging. A hemodynamic significant stenosis (50–85% lumen narrowing) may be undetected during resting conditions because compensatory vasodilatation maintains normal resting blood flows (*left*). During stress conditions (*right*), such as after the administration of dipyridamole or adenosine, the myocardium supplied by the stenotic coronary artery becomes hypoperfused and will be visible as a low intensity area using T1-enhancing contrast agents

first-pass of contrast. To extract quantitative data on myocardial perfusion for instance using the Fermi-model deconvolution (see 6.3), a linear relation between concentration of contrast and SI is assumed, an assumption that is clearly violated using 'normal' contrast doses, i.e., 0.05–0.1 mmol/kg. These doses are needed to provide a myocardial response with adequate signal-to-noise ratio, but signal saturation occurs in the LV cavity rendering the AIF unreliable. On the other hand lowering the contrast dose immediately affect signal to noise ratio. Therefore, a dual-bolus regimen has been proposed starting with a low-dose prebolus, e.g., one tenth of the normal dose, followed by second normal contrast dose, whereby the low-dose prebolus is used to correct the AIF (Ibrahim et al. 2002; Köstler et al. 2004; Christian et al. 2004, 2008; Hsu et al. 2006; Utz et al. 2008; Kurita et al. 2009; Patel et al. 2010) (Fig. 4). A direct comparison between single and dual-bolus approach showed that semiquantitative measures as MPR are not heavily influenced by T1-induced saturation effects (maximum bias of 10%), though it is important to keep in mind that the single bolus approach considerably overestimates both rest and hyperemic blood flow (Utz et al. 2008). Christian et al. (2008) found that the dual-bolus technique provided more accurate estimates of MBF than the single bolus technique when smaller regions were assessed, while Groothuis et al. (2010) reported no incremental value of the dual-bolus technique over single bolus technique for the detection of significant CAD.

4.7 Magnetic Field Strength

Several clinical and simulation studies have shown that MR-MPI is not only feasible on high-field (i.e., 3.0 T) MR units but offers several advantages compared to 1.5 T scanners (Meyer et al. 2008; Christian et al. 2008). In particular when equipped with the novel features, such as parallel imaging, and *k-t* SENSE imaging (see 4.2), image quality can be improved and artifacts reduced, offering similar or improved diagnostic accuracy compared to 1.5 T MR-MPI for the detection of CAD (Cheng et al. 2007; Theisen et al. 2007; Plein et al. 2008b; Christian et al. 2009). Three Tesla might become the preferred field strength for MR-MPI in the near future, allowing high

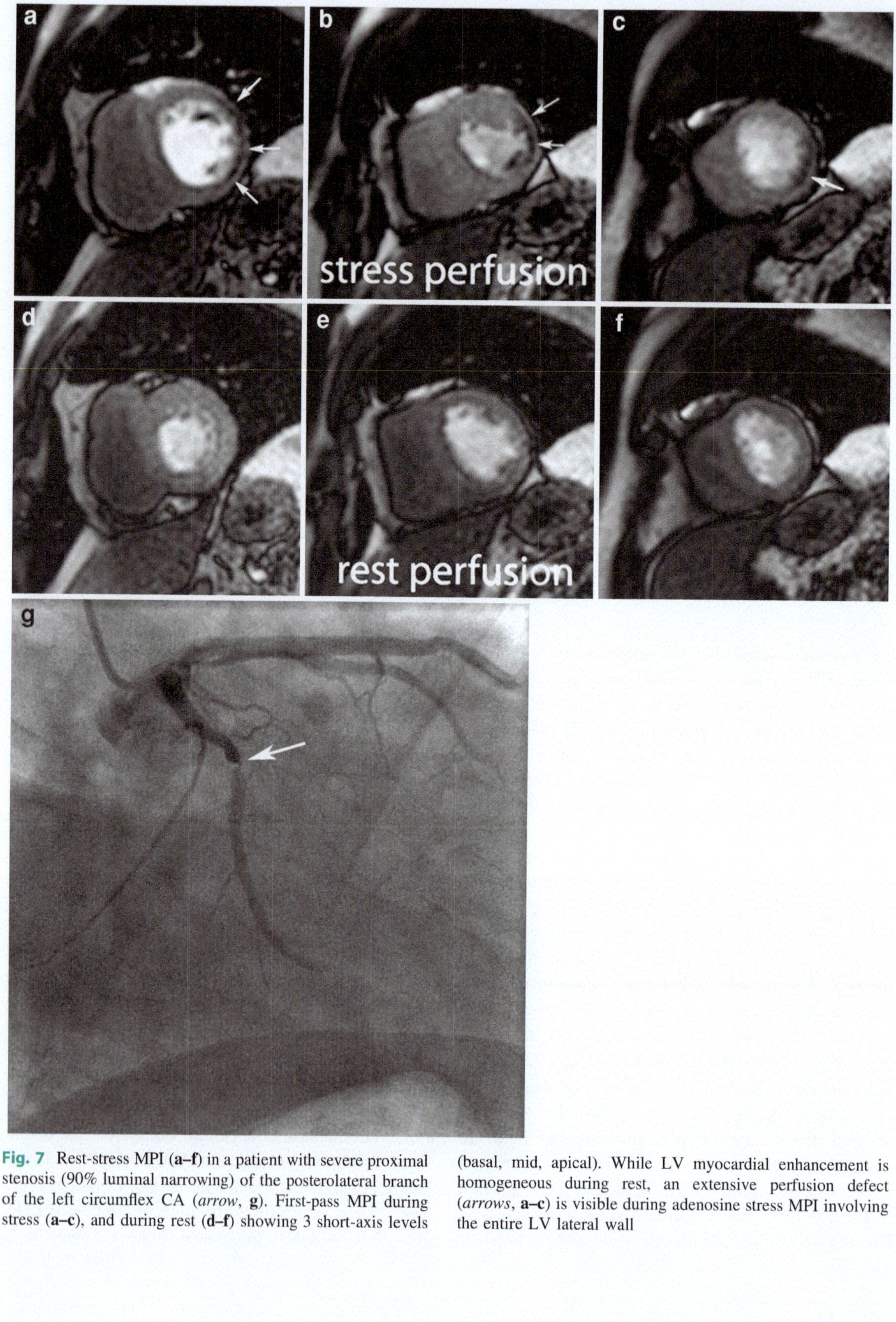

Fig. 7 Rest-stress MPI (**a–f**) in a patient with severe proximal stenosis (90% luminal narrowing) of the posterolateral branch of the left circumflex CA (*arrow*, **g**). First-pass MPI during stress (**a–c**), and during rest (**d–f**) showing 3 short-axis levels (basal, mid, apical). While LV myocardial enhancement is homogeneous during rest, an extensive perfusion defect (*arrows*, **a–c**) is visible during adenosine stress MPI involving the entire LV lateral wall

spatial resolution multi 2D and 3D imaging with subsequent reduction of dark-rim artifacts (Plein et al. 2007; Manka et al. 2010; Lockie et al. 2011; Vitanis et al. 2011).

5 Stress Imaging

Myocardial ischemia at rest, such as in hibernating myocardium due to high-grade CA stenosis, is much less frequently found than exercise-induced ischemia. Therefore, stress imaging is essential in detecting hemodynamically significant CAD. A stenosis is considered *hemodynamically significant* if the coronary blood flow at stress is insufficient to cover myocardial oxygen demand, resulting in a reduced coronary flow reserve, wall motion abnormalities or a perfusion defect at stress, according to the detection modality used (Fig. 6). Stress can be induced by physical exercise or by the intravenous administration of pharmacological agents such as dipyridamole, adenosine or dobutamine/atropine. *Physical exercise*, e.g. using an MR compatible bike, is possible in an MRI environment, but has its particular technical difficulties due to the increased body and cardiac motion and high heart rate. The major issues in exercise MR imaging relate to the temporal resolution constraints of the technique which are usually overcome by combining data from multiple triggered or gated cardiac cycles. This presents two significant limitations during exercise: firstly obtaining a good ECG signal during exercise is difficult and, secondly, even when this is possible gated exercise images are prone to considerable artifacts due to the cardiac translation resulting from body and respiratory movements. *Pharmacological agents*, instead, have been shown to be safe, well tolerated, and to reproducibly induce myocardial ischemia. *Dobutamine/atropine* is known to increase myocardial oxygen demand, thereby provoking wall motion abnormalities. An advantage of dobutamine is its rapid onset of action and short half-life (120 s), allowing for gradual titration. In hibernating myocardium, a biphasic response occurs, with an increase in contractility at low-dose (5–10–15 μg/kg/min) indicating contractile reserve and viability, and hypokinesia at high-dose (20–40 μg/kg/min combined with fractionated atropine 250 μg bolus up to a maximal dose of 1.0 mg) (Senior and Lahiri 1995). Its vasodilatory capacity can also be used to evaluate perfusion, but this is less established (Gebker et al. 2011). Severe complications (sustained ventricular tachycardia, ventricular fibrillation, myocardial infarction, cardiogenic shock) are rare but may be expected in 0.1–0.3% of patients (Wahl et al. 2004). After stress termination, dobutamine side effects can be reversed by beta-blocker administration (e.g. esmolol 0.5 mg/kg slowly intravenously). To increase sensitivity of the test, it is recommended to stop beta-blocker treatment 24–48 h prior to examination.

In clinical practice, *adenosine* and *dipyridamole* are the most commonly used pharmacological vasodilators. A drawback is the higher cost of adenosine. Adenosine and dipyridamole seem to be equally effective in producing myocardial ischemia. In healthy subjects, coronary blood flow increases four- to fivefold over the baseline value of approximately 0.8–1.2 ml min^{-1} g^{-1} (Wilson et al. 1990). Vasodilators induce ischemia by the so-called "steal-phenomenon". Vasodilation mainly occurs in the non-stenotic coronary arteries resulting in a redistribution of blood towards the non-stenotic regions by stealing it from the stenotic regions. When coronary flow is challenged by infusion of a vasodilator, the area in jeopardy becomes visible during first-pass of contrast agent (Schwitter et al. 2001; Saeed et al. 1994) (Figs. 6, 7). Both agents have been studied extensively and are widely applied for myocardial perfusion evaluation by SPECT and PET, and are approved by the US FDA for inducing coronary hyperemia (Cerqueira et al. 1994; Siebert et al. 1998). Adenosine induces endothelial-independent vasodilation at the so-called resistance vessels (arterioles, precapillary sphincters) by activating the alpha-2 receptors leading to smooth muscle cell relaxation. Dipyridamole indirectly does the same, by inhibiting the adenosine reuptake in the endothelial and smooth muscle cells, thereby increasing the interstitial adenosine concentration. Hemodynamic effects of both vasodilators are comparable with a reduction in systolic and diastolic blood pressure and an increase in heart rate. The reduction in blood pressure is more pronounced with adenosine, whereas the increase in heart rate is stronger with dipyridamole. Dipyridamole induces a significant increase in rate-pressure product (systolic blood pressure multiplied by heart rate), which can be considered a parameter of myocardial oxygen demand, whereas adenosine does not (own

Table 3 Myocardial perfusion imaging protocol using adenosine infusion dosage of 0.14 mg/kg body weight/min during 3–6 min

Adenosine dose 5 mg/ml			
Patient weight (kg)	Dose/Rate (mg/min)	Total volume (pure adenosine (ml/u) 5 mg/ml for 6 min)	Injection rate
40	5.6	6.7	67
45	6.3	7.6	76
50	7.0	8.4	84
55	7.7	9.2	92
60	8.4	10.1	101
65	9.1	11	109
70	9.8	12	118
75	10.5	12.6	126
80	11.2	13.4	134
85	11.9	14.3	143
90	12.6	15.1	151
95	13.3	16	160
100	14.0	16.8	168

Table 4 Myocardial perfusion imaging protocol using dipyridamole infusion dosage of 0.14 mg/kg body weight/min during 6 min

Dipyridamole dose 5 mg/ml			
Patient Weight (kg)	Dose/ Rate (mg/ min)	Total volume (pure dipyridamole (ml/u) 5 mg/ml for 6 min)	Injection Rate
40	5.6	6.7	67
45	6.3	7.6	76
50	7.0	8.4	84
55	7.7	9.2	92
60	8.4	10.1	101
65	9.1	11	109
70	9.8	12	118
75	10.5	12.6	126
80	11.2	13.4	134
85	11.9	14.3	143
90	12.6	15.1	151
95	13.3	16	160
100	14.0	16.8	168

unpublished data). Generally, vasodilators are considered not to increase cardiac work load significantly (Pennell 1994), but in high-grade CA stenosis, adenosine and dipyridamole are known to also induce wall motion abnormalities (Paetsch et al. 2004; Galbazzi et al. 2010). Adenosine is administered by an infusion of 140 µg/kg/min and the maximal vasodilative effect to start imaging is usually reached after 3–4 min (Table 3). The infusion must continue until all images are taken, because of the very short half-life (<10 s) of adenosine. A MPI protocol with dipyridamole uses an infusion dosage of 0.14mg/kg/body weight/minute during 6 minutes, with the peak of vasodilation reached at about 2 minafter finishing the infusion (Table 4). The half-life of dipyridamole is about 30 min, so there is more time for imaging. All effects of dipyridamole can be reversed more quickly by administration of aminophylline (0.250 mg intravenously over 5 min). Mild side effects for dipyridamole are headache, dizziness, nausea and chest pain (due to stimulation of nociceptors, mostly not due to ischemia) and occur relatively frequent, but less in diabetics (own unpublished data). Severe side effects such as AV-block, bronchospasm or myocardial infarction are very rare, and can be treated by administration of aminophylline (Picano et al. 1997). For persistent chest pain, nitroglycerine can be given. For adenosine, side effects are similar but often more pronounced: flushing, warmth, headaches, dizziness, nausea and chest pain. The same severe side effects as with dipyridamole can occur, but usually resolve after termination of the adenosine infusion, with exeption of the bronchospasms (Cerqueira et al. 1994). For people above 75 years of age and heart transplantation patients, dipyridamole is preferred above adenosine, because of the increased risk for asystole with the latter (Toft et al. 1998). Contra-indications for adenosine and dipyridamole are high degree AV-block, asthma bronchialc, severe COPD or patients taking carbamazepine or dipyridamole. Care has to be taken that patients have refrained from beverages or food containing caffeine before a dipyridamole or adenosine test, because these reduce the sensitivity of the test. In patients showing an inadequate hemodynamic response to standard adenosine protocol, i.e., heart rate increase <10 bmp or systolic blood pressure decrease <10 mm Hg, Karamitsos et al. (2010), proposed a high-dose adenosine protocol up to 0.210 µg kg–1 min–1. This was well tolerated and safe, and led to an adequate hemodynamic response in 16/18 patients with an initial inadequate hemodynamic response. Finally, although the risk of adverse side effects is small, emergency precautions, such as trained evacuation procedures and trained personal for resuscitation should be present.

6 Myocardial Perfusion Analysis

6.1 Visual Analysis

Visual assessment of first-pass MPI allows qualitative evaluation of regional myocardial perfusion in resting and stress conditions. When performed by experienced readers, acceptable diagnostic accuracies can be achieved (see 7 and 4.1 in "Ischemic Heart Disease"). As such, visual analysis is a valuable alternative to the tedious and often time-consuming (semi)-quantitative approaches. A true stress-induced myocardial perfusion defect usually has typical features that help to distinguish it e.g. from dark-rim artifacts, diffuse microvascular ischemia, fixed defects or true ischemia at an infarct border, and thus reduce the number of false-positive readings (Fig. 8). Thorough analysis allows to depict, to locate and to grade severity of defects. The onset of a myocardial perfusion defect coincides with the start of myocardial enhancement, which is later than the contrast arrival in the LV cavity and later than the occurrence of a dark-rim artifact. The defect, visible as a non- or slow-enhancing part of the myocardium, is most pronounced in the subendocardium (as is the dark-rim artifact) and the transmural extent is variable. Depending on the severity of the CA stenosis, as well as the presence of collateral vessels, the duration of the defect ranges from brief (i.e., a few heartbeats) to prolonged (i.e., persistent till the second pass), while it resolves from the edge to the center of the perfusion defect, thus from subepi- to subendo-cardium. Moreover, the defect obeys anatomic borders as well as the boundaries of the CA perfusion territories, whereas the dark-rim artifact does not. The size is determined by the position of the stenosis along the CA (Figs. 9, 10). The presentation of the defect differs according the CA involved, i.e., to our own experience (a) defects caused by left anterior descending (LAD) CA stenosis are usually stripe-like and typically involve one or more of LV anteroseptal, anterior, or anterolateral segments; (b) right coronary artery (RCA) lesions cause crescent shaped inferobasal perfusion defects; (c) left circumflex (LCx) lesions involve the lateral LV wall and not infrequently have a speckled appearance. Since perfusion defects respect vascular territories, significant CAD in two or more coronary arteries will be visible as separate or contiguous perfusion defects (see Fig. 8.21). Microvascular disease, instead, presents as a circular subendocardial defect not respecting perfusion territories. Since susceptibility artifacts may present in a similar way, differentiation between both conditions may be challenging.

Though some centers perform only stress MPI (Lubbers et al. 2011), adding a rest MPI study is not only needed for MPR calculation, but it has also a benefit for visual analysis. Perfusion defects, caused by hemodynamically significant stenoses, are usually only visible during stress perfusion imaging, or should be more pronounced during stress than in rest. Moreover, perfusion-like defects may occur in chronic, scarred infarcts in the absence of a CA stenosis. This is due to the low capillary density in the scar compared to normal myocardium, simulating a perfusion defect on MPI. Typically these defects are present also at rest (therefore called "fixed defects"), and the extent matches well with the findings on late gadolinium imaging. If, however, a larger perfusion defect is encountered, in particular during stress, this is suspect of concomitant CAD, causing residual ischemia in the borders of an infarct territory. In patients with a successfully reperfused acute myocardial infarction, MPI shows in approximately 50% of patients a perfusion-like defect in the core of the infarct territory. This is caused by severe microvascular damage in the infarct core, a phenomenon also called *no-reflow* (Taylor et al. 2004; Bogaert et al. 2007) (see 5.2.3 in "Ischemic Heart Disease"). If stress MPI is needed in a patient with a history of myocardial infarction, it is advisable to start first with the stress study, because subsequent enhancement of the infarct may impede detection of perfusion defects on stress MPI.

When performing stress-rest MPI studies, the best is to analyze stress and rest studies simultaneously in a standardized way, assessing the 3 main perfusion territories one by one, for the presence of perfusion defects (Fig. 7). Perfusion abnormalities can be best described using a segmental approach, for example using a modified AHA 16-segment model

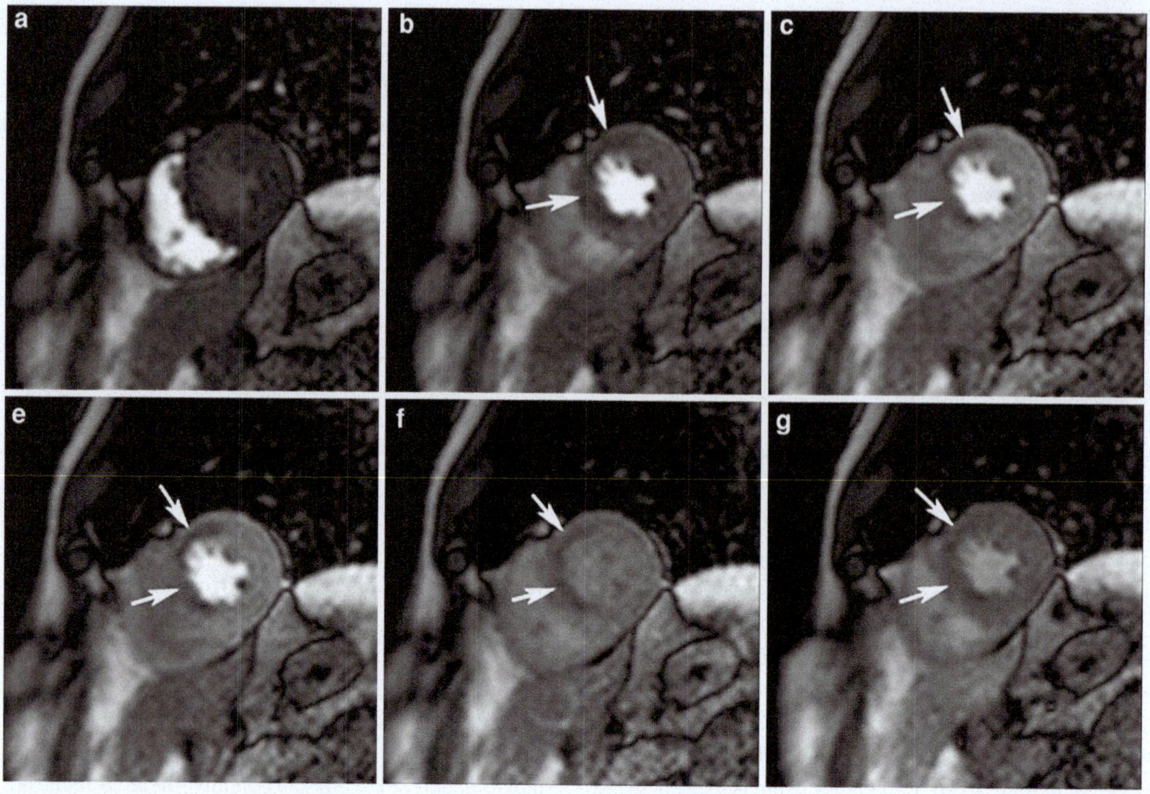

Fig. 8 Typical pattern of hemodynamically significant stenosis on MR-MPI during adenosine stress. Six time frames of midventricular short-axis MR-MPI, starting from arrival of contrast in RV cavity (**a**) to the time of second pass (**f**). A perfusion defect in the anteroseptal LV wall with approximately 50% transmurality becomes visible at the moment the remainder of the myocardium normally enhances (*arrows*, **b, c**). The perfusion defect remains present during the washout phase (*arrows*, **e**) till the second pass (*arrows*, **f**). At coronary angiography, a 75% stenosis was shown in the mid left anterior descending CA

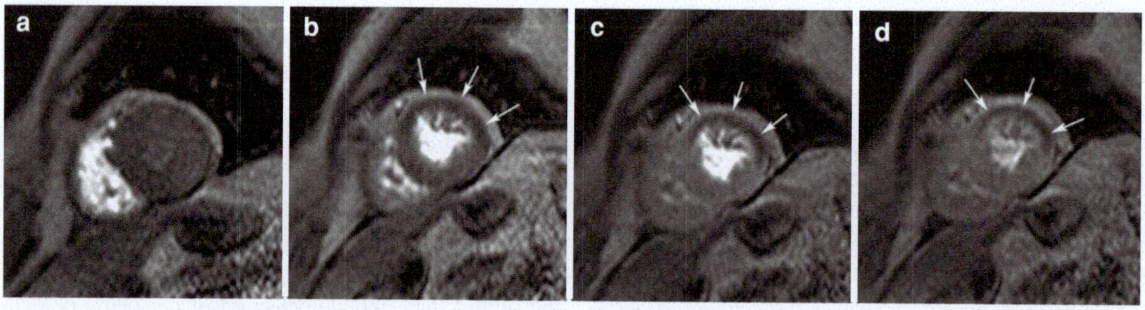

Fig. 9 Example of an extensive perfusion defect in the LV anterolateral wall during adenosine stress MR-MPI. Four time frames of midventricular short-axis MR-MPI. A nearly transmural defect involving the LV anteroseptal, anterior, and anterolateral wall is well visible (*arrows*)

(see "Cardiovascular MR Imaging Planes and Segmentation" and "Ischemic Heart Disease"). Though a good quality MPI study is an essential prerequisite, even in experienced hands, artifacts such as dark-rim artifacts, stripe artifacts, infolding artifacts, blurring, and artifacts due to respiratory motion

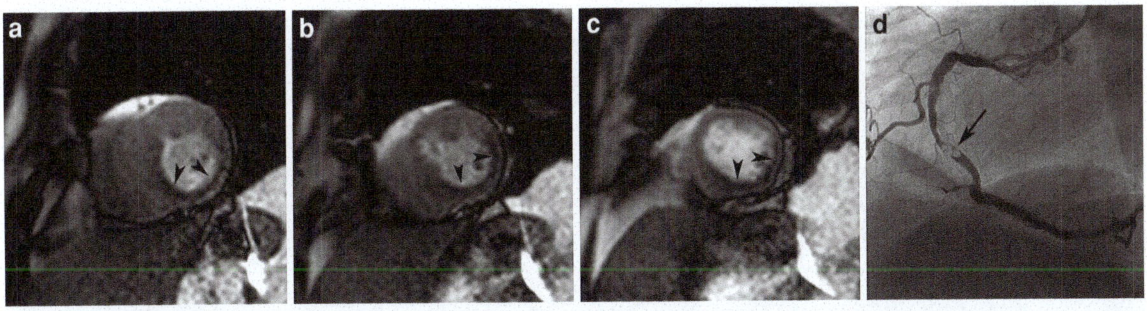

Fig. 10 Example of an extensive perfusion defect in LV inferolateral wall during adenosine stress MR-MPI (**a–c**) in a patient with high-grade stenosis of mid right CA (*arrow*, **d**). First-pass MR-MPI at 3 short-axis levels (basal (**a**), mid (**b**), and apical (**c**) level). Presence of an extensive area of hypo-enhancement (50–75% transmural extent) in the entire LV inferolateral wall (*black arrowheads*, **a–c**). Note the concomitant lack of wall thickening (most remarkable in the basal slice) due to myocardial ischemia

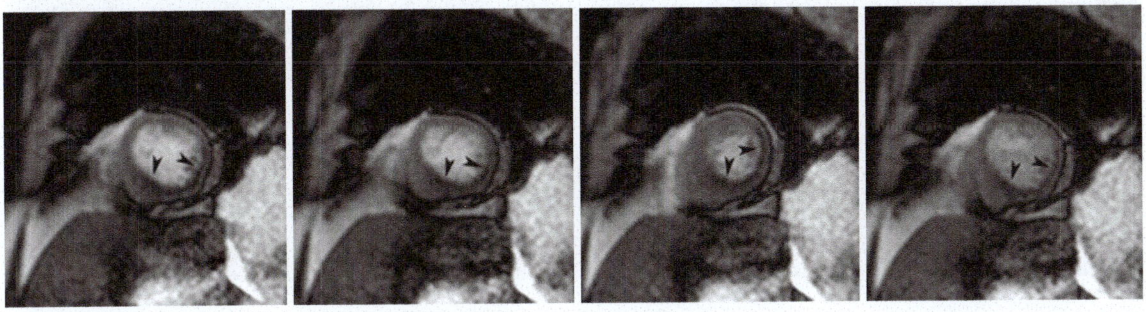

Fig. 11 Example of cardiac motion artifacts due to triggering problems at the moment of first-pass of contrast through the heart. Four consecutive time frames showing apical short-axis slice during adenosine stress. Note the deformation of the cardiac contour between consecutive images. Presence of an inferolateral perfusion defect in a patient with a mid RCA stenosis

or mistriggering, are not infrequently present, and when severe may hamper or make interpretation impossible (Fig. 11). Probably the most annoying are the dark-rim artifacts (Fig. 12). They typically occur at the interface between blood-pool and myocardium, and appear as soon as the contrast arrives in the LV cavity thus before the start of the myocardial enhancement. The exact origin of this artifact is unclear and several causes are suggested: motion artifacts, Gibbs truncation, nonuniform *k*-space weighting, and susceptibility caused by the difference in relaxivity between enhanced blood-pool and non-enhanced myocardium, explaining why these artifacts get worse when a higher contrast dose is used (Wolf et al. 2004), as well as why some sequences such as the balanced SSFP sequence are more sensitive for this kind of artifacts (Fenchel et al. 2004; Di Bella et al. 2005; Weber et al. 2007; Meyer et al. 2008; Ferreira et al. 2008). They preferably occur in the basal half of the left ventricle, along the septal border and around the papillary muscles. Since they are not true perfusion defects, they often appear darker than the non-enhanced myocardium, and thus darker than a true perfusion defect. They tend to rapidly decrease in severity and disappear during the washout phase of contrast, but may reoccur during the second pass, albeit with a lower intensity. What makes these artifacts annoying is firstly that they are usually more pronounced during hyperemia, thus falsely yielding the impression of true perfusion defect, and secondly that a true perfusion defect may underlie a susceptibility artifact. The newest MR-MPI sequences with improved spatial resolution (see 4.2) enable improved differentiation between subendocardial perfusion defect and dark-rim artifact (Manka et al. 2010; Lockie et al. 2011). Other artifacts, such as stripe or infolding artifacts, are usually easier to differentiate from true perfusion defects, but when severe may

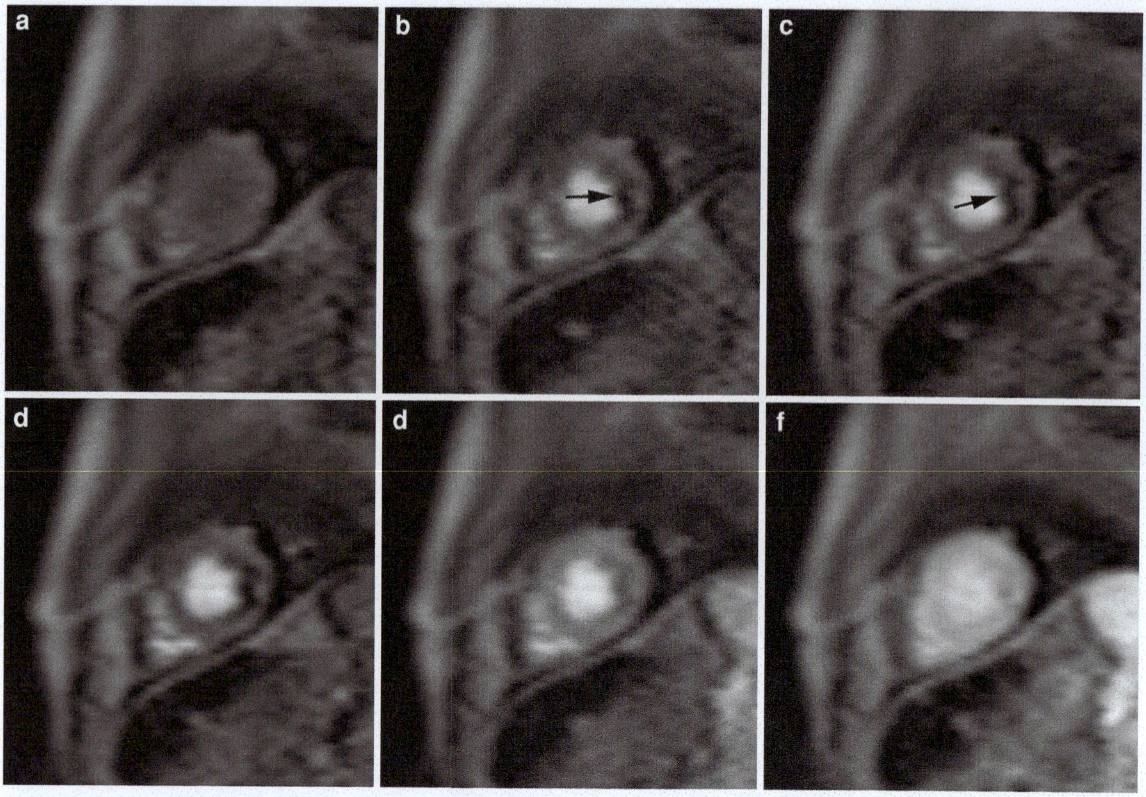

Fig. 12 Example of dark-rim artifact. Six time frames showing first-pass of contrast in apical cardiac short-axis (**a–f**). At the moment of contrast arrival in the LV cavity, occurrence of dark-rim in LV lateral border at the blood-myocardial interface, persisting for several heart beats (*arrows*, **b–c**). Typically a dark-rim artifact has a lower signal intensity than the surrounding suppressed myocardium, and starts before onset of myocardial enhancement

make interpretation impossible. Inappropriate triggering leads to images acquired at different time points during the cardiac cycle, which often makes interpretation impossible. Respiration artifacts are often annoying, especially for (semi)quantitative analysis, and as discussed above, it is advisable to suspend breathing at least for the relatively short period that covers the wash-in of contrast agents (Al-Saadi et al. 2000a; Jerosch-Herold et al. 2004).

6.2 Semiquantitative MPI Analysis

For semiquantitative analysis of myocardial perfusion, usually the changes in SI in the myocardium during first-pass of contrast agent through the heart are used enabling to make SI-time curves (Fig. 2). This is achieved by contouring endo- and epi-cardial borders excluding the papillary muscles, a task that may be tedious and time-consuming to perform in ten to hundreds of images (Kurita et al. 2009). Though automated tracking software to correct cardiac position for respiratory-induced shift is available (Bidaut and Vallée 2001), it still hampers routine use in a clinical setting. Following contouring, the LV wall can be divided in several segments, and each segment can be assessed as a single unit, or can be divided in different layers (e.g. endocardial and epicardial layer). The analysis of SI-time curves can be performed in different ways. The SI's before injection of the agent at the time *T*null are averaged and used as offset (Fig. 13). The following parameters can easily be calculated: (a) the rate of increase in SI after the bolus injection of contrast agent, using a linear fit; (b) the maximum SI increase; (c) the time from *T*null to the maximum SI increase; (d) the time from appearance of contrast agent in the LV cavity to appearance of contrast agent in the myocardium (contrast appearance time); (e) time to 50% of maximal SI; (f) the SI decrease after the peak SI (downslope); or (g) the

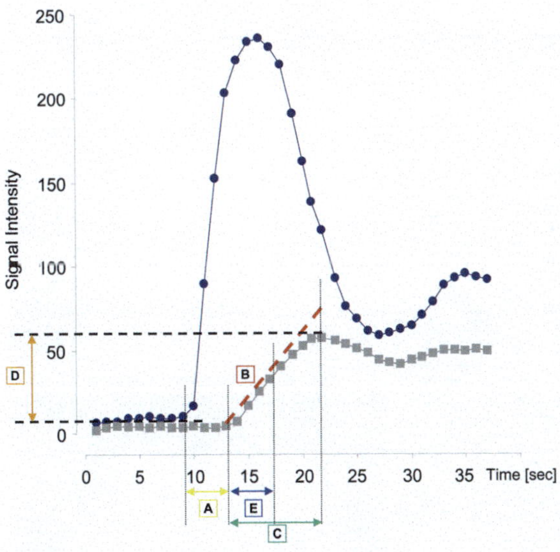

Fig. 13 Analysis of the signal intensity-time curve. After a series of precontrast-images to acquire baseline signal intensity, the signal intensity increases in the LV cavity and, with a delay called "contrast appearance time" (*A*), in the myocardium. The rate of increase in signal intensity is measured by the upslope (*B*). After 5–10 s (time to peak; *C*) the signal intensity peaks (maximal signal intensity; *D*). Another semiquantitative parameter is the time to 50% maximal signal intensity (time to 50%; *E*)

mean transit time using an exponential fit (Al-Saadi et al. 2000a, b; Schwitter et al. 2001; Ibrahim et al. 2002; Manning et al. 1991; Matheijssen et al. 1996). Some approaches require the application of more complex fitting procedures, such as the gamma-variate fit. Such fit procedures, are, however, sensitive to noise, sampling rate, and maximal signal achieved, and may result in an additional source of error when extracting semiquantitative parameters out of the fitted curve (Benner et al. 1997). As the upslope and maximum SI increase are accepted parameters describing myocardial perfusion (Manning et al. 1991; Wilke et al. 1993; Al-Saadi et al. 2000a; Nagel et al. 2003; Christian et al. 2004; Rieber et al. 2006), the sampling rate, i.e., the number of time points on the upslope or from onset of signal enhancement to maximum SI increase, is of paramount importance. The time of inflow of contrast medium is typically in the range of 7–12 s. If the sampling rate is too low, it will result in an unreliable assessment of both upslope and maximum signal enhancement. For a reliable assessment of the upslope, a linear fit of 4 consecutive data points obtained is recommended. Since the SI-time curve flattens when approaching maximal SI, it is advisable not to include the latter time points; otherwise the upslope will be underestimated. It is obvious that a reliable assessment is only achievable when sufficient data are acquired, thus preferably every heartbeat. As discussed above, because of the fast extravasation of contrast media to the extracellular space, the process of myocardial perfusion and diffusion occurs almost simultaneously. It is generally believed that the upslope best reflects the wash-in or true perfusion phase of contrast in the myocardium. The different parameters can be shown using parametric myocardial perfusion maps (Germain et al. 2001; Panting et al. 2001) (Fig. 14).

During myocardial hyperemia there is a shortening of the rise time to peak SI, a higher peak SI, and a clear descending limb after the peak signal, reflecting the higher perfusion rate due to stress-induced vasodilation and hyperemia. In analogy to the coronary flow reserve, the MPR can also be determined, being defined as the ratio of regional MBF during hyperemia to that during resting conditions. This ratio, however, may deviate from the coronary flow reserve, depending on the level of collateral blood flow (Gould et al. 1990). The differences in regional perfusion can be quantified by defining a relative myocardial perfusion index as the ratio of the myocardial perfusion in the territory of the stenosed CA to the myocardial perfusion in a remote normal zone (Gould et al. 1990). Such an approach is not preferred, because patients with even severe multiterritorial ischemia may have a normal ratio and thus their ischemia would go undetected (*balanced ischemia*).

6.3 Quantification of Myocardial Blood Flow

Absolute MBF quantification might be of interest for several reasons. First, increase in diagnostic accuracy compared to semi- or full-quantitative approaches, in particular in patients with three-vessel disease. Second, increased knowledge of true myocardial hemodynamics. Semi-quantitative measures, using MPR, provide no information regarding resting (nor hyperemic) MBF but only tell something about how both are related. As stated by Gould (1978), a stenosis is considered hemodynamic significant if the coronary or myocardial reserve cannot be induced by vasodilatory stimulus. In case of decreased MPR, it is

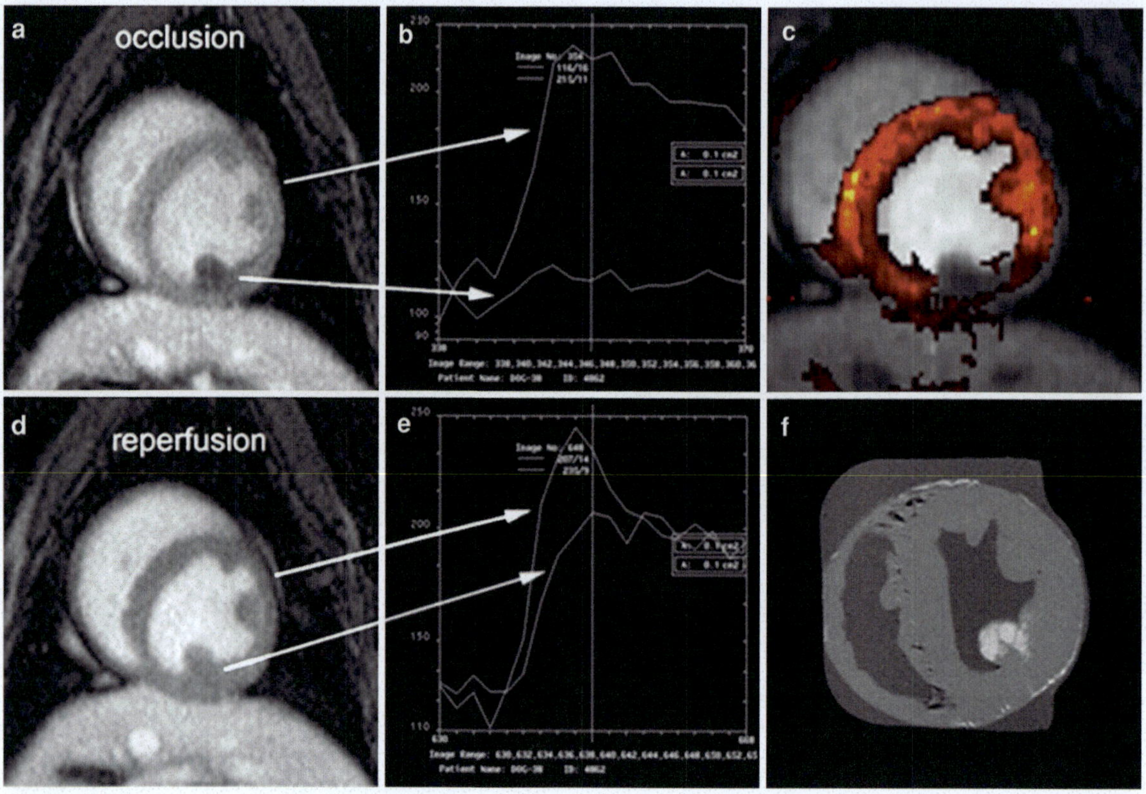

Fig. 14 First-pass perfusion images of an experimental occlusion (**a**) and after reperfusion (**d**) with the corresponding signal intensity-time curves of an ischemic segment compared with a normally perfused segment in the same slice (**b**, **e**). Note the very flat appearance of the signal intensity in the ischemic segment during occlusion (**b**) and the improvement after reperfusion (**e**) when compared with normal signal intensity curves. Even improved after reperfusion, the upslope and the maximal signal intensity remain lower than the normally perfused control segment (**e**). The parametric display (**c**) shows a spared area of color, reflecting the hypoperfused segment that matches the necrosis as shown by delayed enhancement imaging (**f**). Courtesy of Prof. Dr. Y. Ni, UZ Leuven,Leuven, Belgium

impossible to say whether this is due to an increased resting MBF, whether the hyperemic response is impaired, or whether both phenomena come into play. Thirdly, rest MBF increases with age, whereas hyperemic MBF seems to have a quadrangular relationship. Finally, gender dependency or independency is still a matter of debate.

Analysis of SI-time curves provides relative but no absolute values on myocardial perfusion. A normal blood flow zone is required for comparison, obviously limiting the use of relative parameters (e.g. upslope integral) in the setting of multivessel disease. Current strategies to quantify myocardial perfusion are based on two different models, i.e., the *central volume principle*, and the *modified Kety model*. The central volume principle (Zierler 1962) has been derived from the indicator-dilution theory as described by W.F. Hamilton and colleagues, in 1932, with the assumption that the indicator does not move into the tissue, a condition that is clearly not fulfilled by extracellular contrast media. The Stewart-Hamilton equation relates the flow (F) through an organ with the total amount of injected tracer (M) and the tracer concentration as measured in the draining veins $c_\mathrm{d}(t)$:

$$F = \frac{M}{\int_0^\infty c\mathrm{d}(t)\mathrm{d}t} \tag{1}$$

A number of assumptions are, however, necessary:

1. the tracer is not extracted from the blood-pool
2. the flow should not be affected by the tracer
3. the tracer must be thoroughly mixed with the blood
4. it must be corrected for recirculation of the tracer

Additional information is obtained from the mean transit time (*MTT*), which represents the time the contrast agent needs to pass the myocardium, which is calculated as follows (Meier and zierler 1954):

$$MTT = \frac{\int_0^\infty t.cd(t)d}{\int_0^\infty cd(t)d} \qquad (2)$$

Here it is presumed that the tracer is injected as a bolus, but corrections can be made for a longer injection. Equation 3 further relates this *MTT* with the volume *V* occupied by the tracer in the myocardium (myocardial blood volume) and the flow (Block et al. 1995):

$$MTT = \frac{V}{F} \qquad (3)$$

Thus, the theory states that the *MTT* (which is the normalized first moment of the output concentration curve) is the ratio of the tissue blood volume to its blood flow. Assuming tissue blood volume remains constant, *MTT* will be directly correlated to MBF and, thus, presents a semi-quantitative parameter that correlates better to myocardial perfusion than the previously discussed parameters.

$$\mathrm{MTT} \sim \frac{1}{\mathrm{F}} \qquad (4)$$

If myocardial blood volume could be calculated in absolute numbers, quantification of MBF would be possible. However, only a relative value of myocardial blood volume can be derived from the first-pass curve by determining the area under the curve, which is proportional to myocardial blood volume for blood-pool agents (Le Bihan and Turner 1992).

However, it has to be borne in mind that the central volume principle applies to the output concentration curve. MR can measure flow in the coronary sinus but these measurements provide only data regarding global and not regional myocardial flow. Therefore, the residue detection method is used (Lassen and Perl 1979). In that method, the myocardial contrast concentration, derived from if the SI-time curves, is converted to an output function. However, this condition needs an instantaneous contrast agent injection. The decrease in contrast agent concentration should be equal to the amount of contrast agent leaving the system. Therefore, the input function should be shorter than the transfer function through the myocardium. Such an instantaneous injection of contrast cannot be achieved noninvasively. For that reason calculation of the MTT cannot be easily determined without making several assumptions. Therefore, use of MTT for evaluation of myocardial perfusion by MR, as proposed by several groups (Wilke et al. 1993), has been criticized (Weiskoff et al. 1993). Models for calculation are required, such as the multiple pathway, axillary distributed model of blood tissue exchange that integrates the effects of the myocardial vascular architecture and the flow distribution (Kroll et al. 1996). Jerosch-Herold and colleagues have described the converted tissue SI curve to be represented as convolution of the tissue impulse response with the arterial input. The initial amplitude of the tissue impulse response equals the tissue blood flow. However, deconvolution is very sensitive to noise and constraints need to be applied to stabilize the mathematical process of deconvolution. The susceptibility to noise can be reduced by constraining the deconvolution with a parameterized model for probability distribution of tracer residence times in a region of interest. The Fermi function has been applied as an empirical model for the impulse response (Fermi constrained deconvolution) (Jerosch-Herold et al. 1998). Subsequently the same group has introduced a model-independent approach (Jerosch-Herold et al. 2002). Both approaches could show sufficient correlation to microsphere measurements.

The second approach to quantify myocardial perfusion is derived from the Kety model (Kety 1951), which applies, in contrast to the central volume principle, only for extravascular contrast agents. These contrast agents distribute in two compartments: the intravascular and the extracellular space. A two-model compartment with necessary derivations of equations applied for MR have used the term "modified Kety model" or "single capillary model" (Diesbourg et al. 1992; Larsson et al. 1996; Ishida et al. 2011). This model assumes that the capillary bed can be seen as a tube with uniform distribution and permeability of contrast agent. The lateral diffusion of the contrast agent is not considered in this model (Kety 1951). The axial diffusion is proportional to the difference of concentration across capillary membrane and to a coefficient *E* that describes nonequilibrium effects, the extraction efficiency. The equation describes the relation between MBF and local myocardial contrast agent concentration (CM), the myocardial extraction efficiency of the contrast agent (*E*), the arterial blood concentration of the contrast agent (Ca), and the partition coefficient between the vascular bed and the extracellular volume of distribution of the contrast agent (λ) which is equivalent to the interstitial space volume fraction (Larsson et al. 1996; Diesbourg et al. 1992).

$$\mathrm{CM} = \mathrm{MBF}.E.\mu\,\mathrm{Ca.e}^{-[\mathrm{MBF}.E/\lambda]}$$

The concentration can be expressed as deconvolution of the AIF with the residual impulse function:

$$\mathrm{MBF}.E.e^{-[\mathrm{MBF}.E/\lambda]}$$

The residual function depends on 3 parameters: MBF, extraction efficiency, and the partition coefficient. Whereas *E* is defined as (according to Kety):

$$E = 1 - \exp(-\mathrm{PS}/\mathrm{MBF})$$

Where PS is the permeability surface area product that describes the diffusion of the contrast agent through the capillary membrane. Because *E* and MBF present a product with two variables that depend on each other in a way to vary generally in opposite direction, it is very difficult to extract MBF from the equation. In general the product *E*.MBF is measured (Ishida et al. 2011). This product is called the unidirectional transfer constant (K_i).

$$K_i = F.E$$

For low flow, *E* will be high. The transport across the capillaries is more flow limited than diffusion limited and the product $E{\cdot}F$ is more sensitive to flow. Severe ischemia is one exception in which *E* and *F* change in the same direction. For high-flow conditions, the transport of the contrast agent will be more diffusion limited than flow limited (Vallee et al. 1997). However, the product $E{\cdot}F$ increased with high-flow but tends to plateau for very high flows. In conclusion, the determined parameters describe not only myocardial perfusion, but also mainly the first-order transfer constant from the blood to the myocardium and the distribution volume of contrast agent in the myocardium.

Quite often, an assessment of quantitative parameters over a particular organ shows regional heterogeneities that provide clinically useful information. For a thorough quantitative evaluation of perfusion from currently available MR images, the following corrections have to be considered:

1. Tracer concentrations have to be calculated from signal intensities in MR images. The relation between concentration of Gd and SI is usually not known. In practice, a calibration is necessary for all sequences with their applied parameters (TR/TE/flip angle/time delays, etc.).
2. Most contrast agents used in clinical practice diffuse rapidly from the intravascular to the extravascular space. This effect can be incorporated in more difficult models that prescribe an organ as consisting of different compartments that mutually interact.
3. Correction for recirculation is usually performed using a gamma-variate fit of the AIF.
4. The effects of a finite contrast agent injection can be corrected using deconvolution based on the same AIF.

7 Clinical Applications of MR-MPI

From a clinical point of view MR-MPI is increasingly used in daily routine practice. Cardiologists are rapidly becoming aware of the value of this technique to study CAD patients, in particular when combined with cine imaging and late Gd imaging (see "Ischemic Heart Disease"). This comprehensive exam provides essential information regarding the presence or absence of hemodynamically significant CA stenosis, evidence of previous (unknown or unrecognized) myocardial infarction, and global/regional ventricular function in a 45 min exam. In times of limited financial resources, these types of comprehensive exams will rapidly gain importance in clinical decision-making, and in predicting patient outcome. To summarize, MR-MPI exams are usually performed during first-pass of a bolus of extracellular contrast media through the heart (i.e., 0.05–0.1 mmol/kg), using fast sequences (i.e., spoiled gradient-echo or balanced SSFP) equipped with techniques to speed up data acquisition or reconstruction (e.g., EPI read-out, parallel imaging, *k-t* SENSE or *k-t* BLAST techniques), on a 1.5T or 3.0T system. Saturation prepulses are most often used to suppress myocardial signal and to obtain T1-weighting. Imaging is performed in at least 3 short-axis slices, and images are obtained during cardiac diastole, preferably one image/heartbeat for each slice. Myocardial hyperemia is usually achieved using dipyridamole or adenosine infusion. Image analysis can be performed visually, semiquantitatively or quantitatively. A dual-bolus approach enables to avoid saturation effects in the AIF, and is used for both semiquantitative as quantitative purposes (Fig. 4).

For the most part MR-MPI has been used to study myocardial perfusion in CAD patients (see 4.1 in "Ischemic Heart Disease"), though this technique is useful in many other cardiac diseases as well, such as e.g. hypertrophic cardiomyopathy (see 4.1.1 in "Heart Muscle Diseases"). This accuracy of MR-MPI in clinical routine has been compared to other techniques, such as coronary angiography ± CFR/FFR, SPECT, PET. The value of qualitative, visual analysis in the detection of CA stenosis has been shown to achieve good diagnostic accuracy as compared to coronary angiography and SPECT (Sensky et al. 2002; Nagel et al. 2003; Schwitter et al. 2008). Besides, several groups have measured (semiquantitative) MPR index values in normal subjects and CAD patients and established cut-off values for MPR index values to differentiate between flow-limiting and non-flow limiting stenoses (Cullen et al. 1999; Al-Saadi et al. 2000a, b; Ibrahim et al. 2002; Kurita et al. 2009; Watkins et al. 2009). In a study by Al-Saadi et al. (2000a) a MPR index could be determined from the upslope in normal myocardial segments of 2.33 ± 0.41 versus 1.08 ± 0.23 in ischemic segments ($p < 0.001$). A cut-off value of 1.5 (mean minus 2 SD of normal segments) allowed discrimination of normal from ischemic segments with good sensitivity and specificity (90 and 83% respectively). The usefulness of this approach has been confirmed and applied in several studies (Rieber et al. 2006; Costa et al. 2007) (see 4.1 in "Ischemic Heart Disease"). A growing number of centers have used MR-MPI to quantify absolute myocardial perfusion, using both the single and dual-bolus approach. Cullen et al. (1999) have calculated the MPR index based on a more quantitative approach by measuring the unidirectional transfer constant (K_i) and found in normal subjects an MPR index of 4.21 ± 1.16 versus 2.02 ± 0.7 in patients with angiographically proven CAD ($p < 0.02$). The MPRI index was inversely related to the severity of the CA stenosis. Remarkably, MPRI index was also lower in non-flow limiting stenosis (<40% diameter) than in volunteers. Taking ^{15}O-water PET as the in vivo standard of reference, Chareonthaitawee et al. (2001) reported rest and stress perfusion values of 1.0 ± 0.2 and 3.5 ± 1.0 ml/g/min in normal volunteers. Hsu et al. (2006) using dual-bolus MR-MPI found similar values, i.e., 1.0 ± 0.2 and 3.4 ± 0.6 ml/g/min while other groups reported smaller values, i.e., 0.52 ± 0.11 and 1.8 ± 0.5 ml/g/min, and an MPR of 3.6 ± 1.3 (Ritter et al. 2006). Compared to the single bolus approach, the dual-bolus approach yielded smaller values for absolute myocardial perfusion (Groothuis et al. 2010), i.e., for rest perfusion 0.5 ± 0.2 versus 2.2 ± 0.9 ml/g/min, and for stress perfusion 1.4 ± 0.6 versus 4.1 ± 1.1 ml/g/min; but otherwise a higher MPR, i.e., 3.1 ± 1.3 versus 2.0 ± 0.5.

Other studies have reported improved accuracy when combining myocardial perfusion with cine MRI to detect associated wall motion abnormalities (Hartnell et al. 1994; Penzkofer et al. 1999), or with myocardial tagging enabling to assess concomitant changes in regional myocardial function and principal strains (Kraitchman et al. 1996), and by adding late Gd MRI (Kellman et al. 2006; Cury et al. 2006). Several studies have stressed the advantages of MR-MPI compared to radionuclide imaging for obtaining information on the heterogeneous transmural enhancement (subepi-, mid-, and subendocardium), which may reflect the variability in myocardial perfusion across the wall (Wilke et al. 1993; Edelman and Li 1994; Lee et al. 2004; Keijer et al. 2000). In a study by Lee et al., MR-MPI identified better than 201Tl and 99 mTc SPECT imaging regional reductions in full-thickness MBF during global coronary vasodilation over the full-range of vasodilation (using microspheres as gold standard). Moreover, transmural flow gradients can be identified, and their magnitude increases progressively as flow limitations become more severe and endocardial flow is increasingly compromised (Lee et al. 2004).

Besides assessment of "primary" CAD, MR-MPI studies have been performed in patients receiving balloon angioplasty or stenting (Al-Saadi et al. 2000b; Fenchel et al. 2005; Bernhardt et al. 2009; Manka et al. 2011), coronary artery bypass graft (CABG) surgery (Bernhardt et al. 2009; Kelle et al. 2010; Arnold et al. 2011), treatment with angiogenesis (Laham et al. 2002), and have been performed in patients after transplantation (Muehling et al. 2003). In CABG patients, Kelle et al. (2010 reported a (short) delay in contrast arrival but similar wash-in

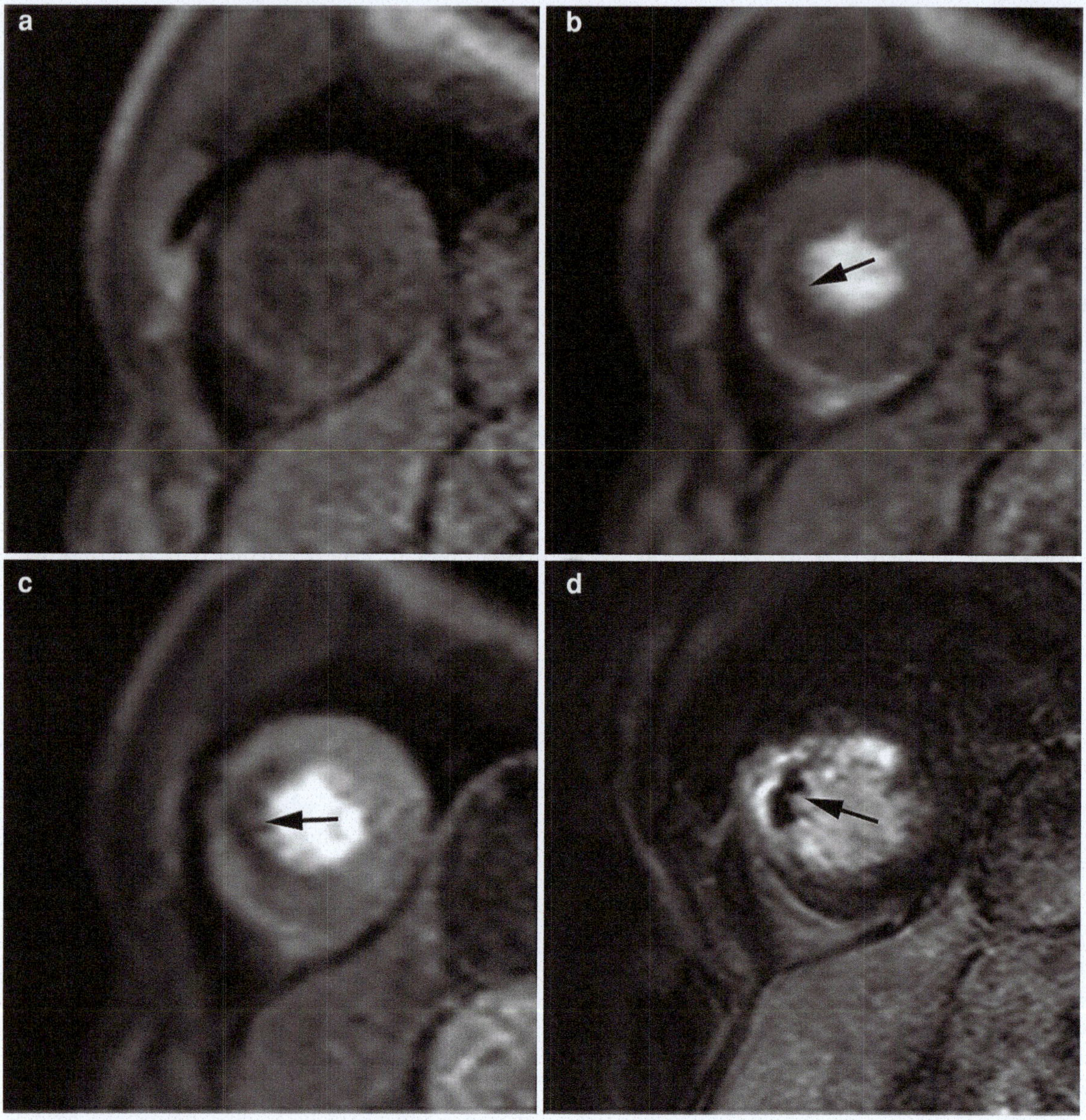

Fig. 15 First pass MR-MPI study in a patient with an anteroseptal myocardial infarction. Baseline image before contrast arrival (**a**). Due to the prepulse, which nulls the signal in the myocardium, very little contrast is usually present in these images. A clear differentiation between myocardium and LV cavity is difficult. Wash-in of the contrast agent in the myocardium showing a subendocardial perfusion defect in the anteroseptal segment (*arrow*, **b**). The perfusion defect persists even after the wash-in period, a sign for severe hypoperfusion (*arrow*, **c**). Late Gd imaging shows the necrotic area with a nonenhanced core, reflecting microvascular obstruction (*arrow*, **d**). Note the match between the size of the perfusion defect during first-pass and the necrosis as determined by delayed enhancement

and peak enhancement in the bypassed myocardium, while Bernhardt et al. (2009) reported reduced diagnostic accuracy that could be due to altered flow and perfusion kinetics. In patients with a reperfused acute myocardial infarction, MR-MPI is helpful to assess the patency of the infarct-related artery and to assess the presence of microvascular obstruction ("no-reflow" area) in the infarct territory (Lima et al. 1995; Taylor et al. 2004; Bogaert et al. 2007) (Fig. 15) (see "Ischemic Heart Disease").

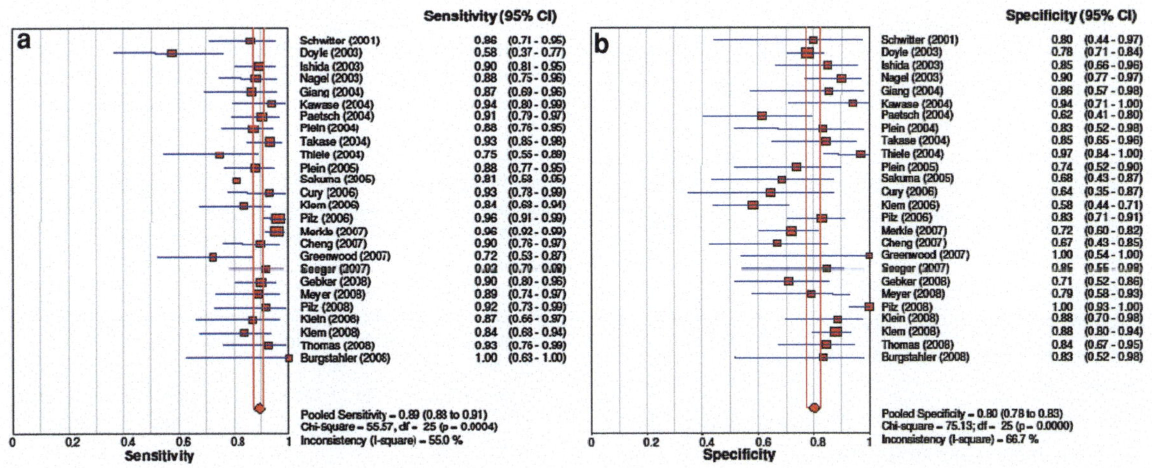

Fig. 16 Forest plot of patient-level sensitivity (**a**) and specificity (**b**) of stress perfusion MR-MPI, compared with coronary angiography. Reprinted from Hamon et al. (2010) with permission

Finally, in a recent meta-analysis by Nandalur et al. including 14 studies (1,516 patients), perfusion imaging demonstrated a sensitivity of 91% (CI 88–94%) and a specificity of 81% (CI 77–85%) (Nandalur et al. 2007). Similar results were shown in another, recent meta-analysis by Hamon et al. (2010) including 26 studies (2,125 patients), i.e., a high specificity (89%), and a moderate specificity (80%) (Fig. 16). Explanations for the moderate specificity of MR-MPI are the presence of dark-rim artifacts and the presence of microvascular disease. Also the value of the reference technique, i.e., coronary angiography, can be questioned. As discussed above, invasively determined FFR most likely is a better reference standard than coronary angiography alone (Rieber et al. 2006; Watkins et al. 2009). Interestingly, adenosine stress MPI yielded a higher sensitivity than with dipyridamole (i.e., 90% vs. 86%, $p = 0.022$), and a tendency to a better specificity (i.e., 81% vs. 77%, $p = 0.065$). In the meta-analysis by Hamon et al. (2010), visual analysis provided a higher sensitivity but a lower specificity than semiquantitative analysis. It should be emphasized that most MR-MPI studies, so far, were performed in populations with high disease prevalence, questioning its value in populations with intermediate or low disease prevalence (Nandalur et al. 2007; Hamon et al. 2010) (Fig. 17).

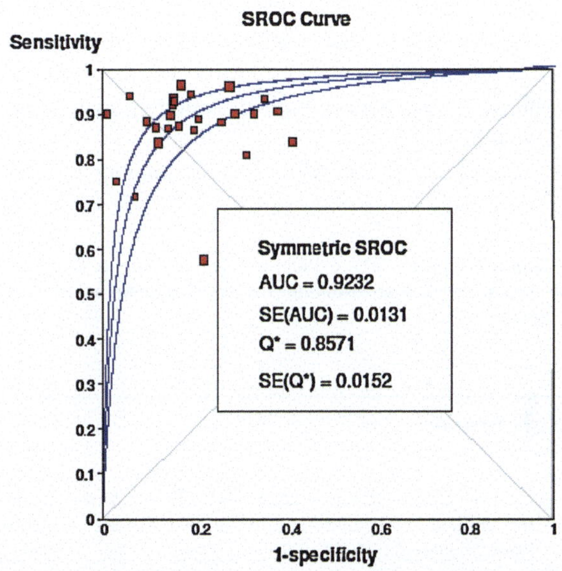

Fig. 17 Plot of receiver operator characteristic curve of stress perfusion MR-MPI, compared with coronary angiography. Reprinted from Hamon et al. (2010) with permission

8 Key Points

- The advent of rapid MR imaging techniques has made it possible to study in real-time physiologic events such as myocardial perfusion.
- Myocardial MR perfusion imaging is or can be part of a more comprehensive approach to study IHD patients.

- The ideal MR perfusion sequence is an ultrafast sequence, that entirely covers the heart during the first-pass of contrast, yielding high contrast between normal and hypoperfused myocardium.
- The ideal contrast agent for myocardial perfusion assessment is not yet available. Extracellular contrast agents are hampered by their rapid diffusion into the interstitial space. Intravascular contrast agents are intrinsically appealing but yield lower signal-to-noise ratios because of the smaller distribution volume and are yet not commercially available.
- Although semiquantitative and quantitative perfusion analysis is possible, visual assessment remains clinically the most often used analysis tool.
- Use a systematic approach for visual perfusion analysis. Start by ruling out and grading the influence of artifacts on the perfusion study. Perfusion defects caused by CAD have typical appearances.
- Semiquantitative and quantitative evaluation needs further improvement of postprocessing tools to allow for an automated self-detection of myocardial contours.
- Assessment of the MPR is a promising tool to detect and assess the severity of CAD.

Acknowledgments The authors would like to thank Dr Nidal Al-Saadi for his contribution to the first edition of this chapter.

References

Adluru G, Dibella EV, Schabel MC (2006) Model-based registration for dynamic cardiac perfusion MRI. J Magn Reson Imaging 24:1062–1070

Al-Saadi N, Nagel E, Gross M et al (2000a) Noninvasive detection of myocardial ischemia from perfusion reserve based on cardiovascular magnetic resonance. Circulation 101:1379–1383

Al-Saadi N, Nagel E, Gross M et al (2000b) Improvement of myocardial perfusion reserve early after coronary intervention: assessment with cardiac magnetic resonance imaging. J Am Coll Cardiol 36:1557–1564

Al-Saadi N, Gross M, Bornstedt A et al (2001) Comparison of various parameters for determining an index of myocardial perfusion reserve in detecting coronary stenosis with cardiovascular magnetic resonance tomography. Z Kardiol 90:824–834

Anderson CM, Brown JJ (1993) Cardiovascular magnetic resonance imaging: evaluation of myocardial perfusion. Coron Artery Dis 4:354–360

Araujo LI, Lammertsma AA, Rhodes CG et al (1991) Noninvasive quantification of regional myocardial blood flow in CA disease with oxygen 15 labeled carbon dioxide inhalation and positron emission tomography. Circulation 93:857–885

Arnold JR, Francis JM, Karamitsos TD et al (2011) Myocardial perfusion imaging following coronary artery bypass surgery using cardiovascular magnetic resonance: a validation study. Circ Cardiovasc Imaging (electronic press)

Arteaga C, Canet E, Ovize M, Janier M, Revel D (1994) Myocardial perfusion assessed by subsecond magnetic resonance imaging with a paramagnetic macromolecular contrast agent. Invest Radiol 29:S54–S57

Atalay MK, Forder JR, Chacko VP, Kawamoto S, Zerhouni EA (1993) Oxygenation in the rabbit myocardium: assessment with susceptibility-dependent MR imaging. Radiology 189: 759–764

Atkinson DJ, Burstein D, Edelman RR (1990) First-pass cardiac perfusion: evaluation with ultrafast MR imaging. Radiology 174:757–762

Bacharach SL, Bax JJ, Case J et al (2004) PET myocardial glucose metabolism and perfusion imaging: part 1—guidelines for patient preparation and data acquisition. J Nucl Cardiol 10:543–554

Bernhardt P, Spiess J, Levenson B et al. (2009) Combined assessment of myocardial perfusion and late gadolinium enhancement in patients after percutaneous coronary intervention or bypass grafts. A multicenter study of an integrated cardiovascular magnetic resonance protocol. J Am Coll Cardiol Img 2:1292-1300

Benner T, Heiland S, Erb G, Forsting M, Sartor K (1997) Accuracy of gamma-variate fits to concentration–time curves from dynamic susceptibility-contrast enhanced MRI: influence of time resolution, maximal signal drop and signal-to-noise. Magn Reson Imaging 15:307–317

Bidaut LM, Vallée JP (2001) Automated registration of dynamic MR images for the quantification of myocardial perfusion. J Magn Reson Imaging 13:648–655

Bjerner T, Johansson L, Ericsson A, Wikström G, Hemmingsson A, Ahlström (2001) First-pass myocardial perfusion MR imaging with outer-volume suppression and the intravascular contrast agent NC100150 injection: preliminary results in eight patients. Radiology 221:822–826

Blankstein R, Di Carli MF (2010) Integration of coronary anatomy and myocardial perfusion imaging. Nat Rev Cardiol 7:226–236

Block JC, Henrikson O, Gotze AH et al (1995) Magnetic resonance perfusion imaging with gadolinium-DTPA. A quantitative approach for the kinetic analysis of first-pass residue curves. Invest Radiol 30:393–699

Bogaert J, Kalantzi M, Rademakers FE, Dymarkowski S, Janssens S (2007) Determinants and impact of microvascular obstruction in successfully reperfused ST-segment elevation myocardial infarction. Assessment by magnetic resonance imaging. Eur Radiol 17:2572–2580

Brasch RC (1992) New directions in the development of MR imaging contrast media. Radiology 183:1–11

Budinger TF, Fischer H, Hentschel D, Reinfelder HE, Schmitt F (1991) Physiological effects of fast oscillating magnetic field gradients. J Comput Assist Tomogr 15:909–914

Burstein D, Taratuta E, Manning WJ (1991) Factors in myocardial "perfusion" imaging with ultrafast MRI and Gd-DTPA administration. Magn Reson Med 20:299–305

Canet E, Revel D, Forrat R et al (1993) Superparamagnetic iron oxide particles and positive enhancement for myocardial perfusion studies assessed by subsecond T-1-weighted MRI. Magn Reson Imaging 11:1139–1145

Canet E, Doulk P, Janier M et al (1995) Influence of bolus volume and dose of gadolinium chelate for first-pass myocardial perfusion MR imaging studies. J Magn Reson Imaging 5:411–415

Cerqueira MD, Verani MS, Schwaiger M, Heo J, Iskandrian AS (1994) Safety profile of adenosine stress perfusion imaging: results from the Adenoscan Multicenter Trial Registry. J Am Coll Cardiol 23:384–389

Chareonthaitawee P, Kaufmann PA, Rimoldi O, Camici PG (2001) Heterogeneity of resting and hyperemic myocardial blood flow in healthy humans. Cardiovasc Res 50:151–161

Cheng ASH, Pegg TJ, Karamitsos TD et al (2007) Cardiovascular magnetic resonance perfusion imaging at 3-tesla for the detection of coronary artery disease: a comparison with 1.5-tesla. J Am Coll Cardiol 49:2440–2449

Christian TF, Rettmann DW, Aletras AH et al (2004) Absolute myocardial perfusion in canines measured by using dual-bolus first-pass MR imaging. Radiology 232:677–684

Christian TF, Aletras AH, Arai AE (2008) Estimation of absolute myocardial blood flow during first-pass MR perfusion imaging using a dual-bolus injection technique: comparison to single-bolus injection method. J Magn Reson Imaging 27:1271–1277

Christian TF, Bell SP, Whitesell L, Jerosch-Herold M (2009) Accuracy of cardiac magnetic resonance of absolute myocardial blood flow with a high-field system: comparison with conventional field strength. J Am Coll Cardiol Img 2:1103–1110

Costa MA, Shoemaker S, Futamatsu H et al (2007) Quantitative magnetic resonance perfusion imaging detects anatomic and physiologic coronary artery disease as measured by coronary angiography and fractional flow reserve. J Am Coll Cardiol 50:514–522

Cullen JHS, Horsfield MA, Reek CR, Cherryman GR, Barnett DB, Samani NJ (1999) A myocardial perfusion reserve index in humans using first-pass contrast-enhanced magnetic resonance imaging. J Am Coll Cardiol 33:1386–1394

Cury RC, Cattini CAM, Gabure LAG et al (2006) Diagnostic performance of stress perfusion and delayed enhancement MR imaging in patients with coronary artery disease. Radiology 240:39–45

Demer LL, Gould KL, Goldstein RA et al (1989) Assessment of coronary artery disease severity by positron emission tomography. Comparison with quantitative arteriography in 193 patients. Circulation 79:825–835

Dewey M, Kaufels N, Laule M et al (2004) Magnetic resonance imaging of myocardial perfusion and viability using a blood pool contrast agent. Invest Radiol 39:498–505

Di Bella EVR, Parker DL, Sinusas AJ (2005) On the dark rim artifact in dynamic contrast-enhanced MRI myocardial perfusion studies. Magn Reson Med 54:1295–1299

Diesbourg LD, Prato FS, Wisenberg G et al (1992) Quantification of myocardial blood flow and extracellular volumes using a bolus injection of Gd-DTPA: kinetic modeling in canine ischemic disease. Magn Reson Med 23:239–253

Ding S, Wolff SD, Epstein FH (1998) Improved coverage in dynamic contrast-enhanced cardiac MRI using interleaved gradient-echo EPI. Magn Reson Med 39:514–519

Donahue K, Burstein D, Manning W, Gary M (1994) Studies of Gd-DTPA relaxivity and proton exchange rates in tissue. Magn Reson Med 32:66–76

Donahue KM, Weiskoff RM, Burstein D (1997) Water diffusion and exchange as they influence contrast enhancement. J Magn Reson Imaging 7:102–110

Edelman RR, Li W (1994) Contrast-enhanced echo-planar MR imaging of myocardial perfusion: preliminary study in humans. Radiology 190:771–777

Fenchel M, Franow A, Stauder NI et al. (2005) Myocardial perfusion after angioplasty in patients suspected of having single-vessel coronary artery disease: improvement detected at rest-stress first-pass perfusion MR imaging – initial experience. Radiology 237:67-74

Fenchel M, Helber U, Simonetti OP et al (2004) Multislice first-pass myocardial perfusion imaging: comparison of saturation recovery (SR)-TrueFISP-two-dimensional (2D) and SR-TurboFLASH-2D pulse sequences. J Magn Reson Imaging 36:225–231

Ferreira P, Gatehouse P, Bucciarelli-Ducci C, Wage R, Firmin D (2008) Measurement of myocardial frequency offsets during first-pass of a gadolinium-based contrast agent in perfusion studies. Magn Reson Med 60: 860–870

Fieno DS, Shea SM, Li Y, Harris KR, Finn JP, Debiao L (2004) Myocardial perfusion imaging based on the blood oxygen level-dependent effect using T2-prepared steady-state free-precession magnetic resonance imaging. Circulation 110: 1284–1290

Friedrich MG, Niendorf T, Schulz-Menger J, Gross CM, Dietz R (2003) Blood-oxygen level-dependent magnetic resonance imaging in patients with stress-induced angina. Circulation 108:2219–2223

Fritz-Hansen T, Rostrup E, Larsson HB et al (1996) Measurement of the arterial concentration of Gd-DTPA using MRI: a step toward quantitative perfusion imaging. Magn Reson Med 36:225–231

Fritz-Hansen T, Rostrup E, Ring P, Larsson H (1998) Quantification of gadolinium-DTPA concentrations for different inversion times using an IR-turbo flash pulse sequence: a study on optimizing multislice perfusion imaging. Magn Reson Imaging 16:893–799

Galbazzi N, Rigo F, Reverberi C (2010) Detection of coronary artery disease by combined assessment of wall motion, myocardial perfusion and coronary flow reserve: a multiparametric contrast stress-echocardiography study. J Am Soc Ec hocardiogr 23:1242–1250

Gebker R, Jahnke C, Paetsch I et al (2007) MR imaging perfusion imaging with k-space and time broad-use linear acquisition speed-up technique: feasibility study. Radiology 245:863–871

Gebker R, Jahnke C, Manka R et al (2011) High spatial resolution myocardial perfusion imaging during high-dose dobutamine/atropine stress magnetic resonance using *k-t* SENSE. Int J Cardiol (electronic press)

Gerber BL, Bluemke DA, Chin BB et al (2002) Single-vessel coronary artery stenosis: myocardial perfusion imaging with Gadomer-17 first-pass MR imaging in a swine model of comparison with gadopentetate dimeglumine. Radiology 225:104–112

Germain P, Roul G, Baruthio J et al (2001) Myocardial flow reserve parametric map, assessed by first-pass MRI compartmental analysis at the chronic stage of infarction. J Magn Reson Imaging 13:352–360

Giang TH, Nanz D, Coulden R et al (2004) Detection of coronary artery disease by magnetic resonance perfusion imaging with various contrast medium doses: first European multi-centre experience. Eur Heart J 25:1657–1665

Gould K (1978) Noninvasive assessment of coronary stenosis by myocardial perfusion imaging during pharmacologic coronary vasodilatation. I. Physiologic basis and experimental validation. Am J Cardiol 41:267–278

Gould KL (1990) Positron emission tomography and interventional cardiology. Am J Cardiol 66:51F–58F

Gould KL (2009) Does coronary flow trump coronary anatomy? J Am Coll Cardiol Img 2:1009–1023

Gould KL, Kirkeeide RL, Buchi M (1990) Coronary flow reserve as a physiologic measure of stenosis severity. J Am Coll Cardiol 15:459–474

Groothuis JGJ, Kremers FPPJ, Beek AM et al (2010) Comparison of dual and single bolus magnetic resonance myocardial perfusion imaging for detection of significant coronary artery disease. J Magn Reson Imaging 32:88–93

Hadjimiltiades S, Watson R, Hakki AH, Heo J, Iskandrian AS (1989) Relation between myocardial thallium-201 kinetics during exercise and quantitative coronary angiography in patients with one vessel coronary artery disease. J Am Coll Cardiol 13:1301–1308

Hamon M, Fau G, Née G, Ehtisham J, Morello R, Hamon M (2010) Meta-analysis of the diagnostic performance of stress perfusion cardiovascular magnetic resonance for detection of coronary artery disease. J Cardiovasc Magn Reson 12:29

Hartnell G, Cerel A, Kamalesh M et al (1994) Detection of myocardial ischemia: value of combined myocardial perfusion and cineangiographic MR imaging. Am J Roentgenol 163:1061–1067

Henkin RE, Kalousdian S, Kikkawa RM, Kemel A (1994) 201-Thallium myocardial perfusion imaging utilizing single-photon emission computed tomography (SPECT). American Medical Association

Hsu L-U, Rhoads KL, Holly JE, Kellman P, Aletras AH, Arai AE (2006) Quantitative myocardial perfusion analysis with a dual-bolus contrast-enhanced first-pass MRI technique in humans. J Magn Reson Imaging 23: 315–322

Hunold P, Maderwald S, Eggebrecht H, Vogt FM, Barkhausen J (2004) Steady-state free precession sequences in myocardial first-pass perfusion MR imaging: comparison with turboFLASH imaging. Eur Radiol 14:409–416

Ibrahim T, Nekolla SG, Schreiber K et al (2002) Assessment of coronary flow reserve: comparision between contrast-enhanced magnetic resonance imaging and positron emission tomography. J Am Coll Cardiol 39:864–870

Ishida M, Ichihara T, Nagata M et al (2011) Quantification of myocardial blood flow using model based analysis of first-pass perfusion MRI: extraction fraction of Gd-DTPA varies with myocardial blood flow in human myocardium. Magn Reson Med (electronic press)

Iskandrian S, Iskandrian AE (1999) Risk assessment using single-photon emission computed tomographic technetium-99 m sestamibi imaging. J Am Coll Cardiol 32:57–62

Jahnke C, Gekber R, Manka R, Schnackenburg B, Fleck E, Paetsch I (2010) Navigator-gated 3D blood oxygen-level dependent CMR at 3.0-T for detection of stress-induced myocardial ischemic reactions. J Am Coll Cardiol Img 3:375–384

Jerosch-Herold M, Wilke N (1997) MR first-pass imaging: quantitative assessment of transmural perfusion and collateral flow. Int J Card Imaging 13:205–218

Jerosch-Herold M, Wilke N, Stillman AE (1998) Magnetic resonance quantification of the myocardial perfusion reserve with a Fermi function model for constrained deconvolution. Med Phys 25:73–84

Jerosch-Herold M, Swingen C, Seethamraju RT (2002) Myocardial blood flow quantification with MRI by modeled-independent deconvolution. Med Phys 25:73–84

Jerosch-Herold M, Hu X, Murthy NS, Rickers C, Stillman AE (2003) Magnetic resonance imaging of myocardial contrast enhancement with MS-325 and its relation to myocardial blood flow and the perfusion reserve. J Magn Reson Imaging 18:544–554

Jerosch-Herold M, Seethamraju RT, Swingen CM, Wilke NM, Stillman AE (2004) Analysis of myocardial perfusion MRI. J Magn Reson Imaging 19:758–770

Johansson LO, Akenson P, Ragnarsson A, Ahlström H (1998) Myocardial perfusion using a new ultra small paramagnetic iron oxide, enabling T2* perfusion with very short echo-times: first trials in humans. In: Proceedings of international society for magnetic resonance in medicine, sixth scientific meeting and exhibition, Sydney, Australia, 18–24 April 1998, p 903

Judd RM, Ataly MK, Rottman GA, Zerhouni EA (1995a) Effects of myocardial water exchange on T1 enhancement during bolus administration of MR contrast agents. Magn Reson Med 33:215–223

Judd RM, Reeder SB, Atalar E, McVeigh ER, Zerhouni EA (1995b) A magnetization-driven gradient echo pulse sequence for the study of myocardial perfusion. Magn Reson Med 34:276–282

Judd RM, Reeder SB, May-Newman K (1999) Effects of water exchange on the measurement of myocardial perfusion using paramagnetic contrast agents. Magn Reson Med 34: 276–282

Kantor HL, Rzedzian RR, Buxton R et al (1994) Contrast induced myocardial signal reduction: effect of lanthanide chelates on ultra high speed MR images. Magn Reson Imaging 12:51–59

Karamitsos TD, Ntusi NAB, Francis JM, Holloway CJ, Myerson SG, Neubauer S (2010) Feasibility and safety of high-dose adenosine perfusion cardiovascular magnetic resonance. J Cardiovasc Magn Reson 12:66

Kaul S, Senior R, Dittrich H, Raval U, Khattar R, Lahiri A (1997) Detection of coronary artery disease with myocardial contrast echocardiography: comparison with 99mTc-sestamibi single-photon emission tomography. Circulation 96:785–792

Keijer JT, van Rossum AC, van Eenige MJ et al (2000) Magnetic resonance imaging of regional myocardial perfusion in patients with single-vessel coronary artery disease:

quantitative comparison with (201)thallium-SPECT and coronary angiography. J Magn Reson Imaging 11: 607–615

Kelle S, Graf K, Dreysse S, Schnackenburg B, Fleck E, Klein C (2010) Evaluation of contrast wash-in and peak enhancement in adenosine first-pass perfusion CMR in patients post bypass surgery. J Cardiovasc Magn Reson 12:28

Kellman P, Derbyshire JA, Agyeman KO, McVeigh ER, Arai AE (2004) Extended coverage first-pass perfusion imaging using slice-interleaved TSENSE. Magn Reson Med 51: 200–204

Kellman P, Aletras AH, Hsu L-Y, McVeigh ER, Arai AE (2006) T_2* Measurement during first-pass contrast-enhanced cardiac perfusion imaging. Magn Reson Med 56: 1132–1134

Kety SS (1951) The theory and applications of the exchange of inert gas at the lungs and tissues. Pharmacol Rev 3:1

Kim C, Kwok YS, Heagerty P, Redberg R (2001) Pharmacologic stress testing for coronary disease diagnosis: a meta-analysis. Am Heart J 142:934–944

Kivelitz DE, Bis KG, Wilke NM, Jerosch-Herold M, Juni JE, Hamm BK (1997a) Quantitative MR first-pass perfusion imaging demonstrates coronary artery patency post interventions. Radiology 205(Suppl):254

Kivelitz DE, Wilke NM, Bis KG, Jerosch-Herold M, Juni JE, Hamm BK (1997b) Quantitative MR first-pass versus N13-ammonia PET perfusion imaging in coronary artery disease. Radiology 205(Suppl):253

Klocke F (1983) Measurements of coronary blood flow and degree of stenosis: current clinical implications and continuing uncertainties. J Am Coll Cardiol 1:31–36

Klocke FJ (1990) Cognition in the era of technology: "seeing the shades of gray". J Am Coll Cardiol 16:763–769

Kloner RA, Przyklenk K, Rahimtoola SH, Braunwald E (1992) In: Opie LH (ed) Stunning, hibernation and calcium in myocardial ischemia and reperfusion. Kluwer, Dordrecht, pp 251–280

Köstler H, Ritter C, Lipp C, Hahn D, Sandstede J (2004) Prebolus quantitative MR heart perfusion imaging. Magn Reson Med 52:296–299

Kraitchman DL, Wilke N, Hexeberg E et al (1996) Myocardial perfusion and function in dogs with moderate coronary stenosis. Mag Reson Med 35:771–780

Kroll K, Wilke N, Jerosch-Herold M et al (1996) Accuracy of modeling of regional myocardial flows from residue functions of an intravascular indicator. Am J Physiol (Heart Circ Physiol) 40:H1643–H1655

Kurita T, Sakuma H, Onishi K et al (2009) Regional myocardial perfusion reserve determined using myocardial perfusion magnetic resonance imaging showed a direct correlation with coronary flow velocity reserve by Doppler flow wire. Eur Heart J 30:444–452

Laham RJ, Simons M, Pearlman JD, Ho KK, Baim DS (2002) Magnetic resonance imaging demonstrates improved regional systolic wall motion and thickening and myocardial perfusion of myocardial territories treated by laser myocardial revascularization. J Am Coll Cardiol 39:1–8

Larsson HB, Fritz-Hansen T, Rostrup E et al (1996) Myocardial perfusion modeling using MRI. Magn Reson Med 35: 716–726

Larsson HB, Rosenbaum S, Fritz-Hansen T (2001) Quantification of the effect of water exchange in dynamic contrast MRI perfusion measurements in the brain and the heart. Magn Reson Med 46:272–281

Lassen NA, Perl W (1979) Tracer kinetic methods in medical physiology. Raven Press, New York

Lauerma K, Virtanen KS, Sipila LM, Hekali P, Aronen HJ (1997) Multislice MRI in assessment of myocardial perfusion in patients with single vessel proximal left anterior descending coronary artery disease before and after revascularization. Circulation 96:2859–2867

Le Bihan D, Turner R (1992) The capillary network: a link between IVIM and classical perfusion. Magn Reson Med 27:171–178

Lee DC, Simonetti OP, Harris KR et al (2004) Magnetic resonance versus radionuclide pharmacological stress perfusion imaging for flow-limiting stenoses of varying severity. Circulation 110:58–65

Lima JAC, Judd RM, Bazille A, Schulman SP, Atalar E, Zerhouni EA (1995) Regional heterogeneity of human myocardial infarcts demonstrated by contrast-enhanced MRI. Potential mechanisms. Circulation 92:1117–1125

Lima RS, Watson DD, Goode AR, Siadaty MS, Ragosta M, Beller GA, Samady H (2003) Incremental value of combined perfusion and function over perfusion alone by gated SPECT myocardial perfusion imaging for detection of severe three-vessel coronary artery disease. J Am Coll Cardiol 42:64–70

Lockie T, Ishida M, Perera D et al (2011) High-resolution magnetic resonance myocardial perfusion imaging at 3.0-tesla to detect hemodynamically significant coronary stenoses as determined by fractional flow reserve. J Am Coll Cardiol 57:70–75

Loghin C, Sdringola S, Gould KL (2004) Common artifacts in PET myocardial perfusion images due to attenuation-emission misregistration: clinical significance, causes, and solutions. J Nucl Med 45:1029–1039

Lubbers DD, Rijlaarsdam-Hermsen D, Kuijpers D et al (2011) Performance of adenosine "stress-only" perfusion MRI in patients without a history of myocardial infarction: a clinical outcome study. Int J Cardiovasc Imaging (Electronic press)

Manka R, Vitanis V, Boesiger P, Flammer AJ, Plein S, Kozerke S (2010) Clinical feasibility of accelerated, high spatial resolution myocardial perfusion imaging. J Am Coll Cardiol Img 3:710–717

Manka R, Jahnke C, Kozerke S et al (2011) Dynamic 3-dimensional stress cardiac magnetic resonance perfusion imaging. Detection of coronary artery disease and volumetry of myocardial hypoenhancement before and after cornary stenting. J Am Coll Cardiol 57:437–444

Manning WJ, Atkinson DJ, Grossman W, Paulin S, Edelman RR (1991) First-pass nuclear magnetic resonance imaging studies using gadolinium-DTPA in patients with coronary artery disease. J Am Coll Cardiol 18:959–965

Mansfield P (1977) Multiplanar image formation using NMR spin echoes. J Physiol (Lond) 10:L55–L58

Maredia N, Radjenovic A, Kozerke S, Larghat A, Greenwood JP, Plein S (2010) Effect of improving spatial or temporal resolution on image quality and quantitative perfusion assessment with k-t SENSE acceleration on first-pass CMR myocardial perfusion imaging. Magn Reson Med 64:1616–1624

Masugata H, Lafitte S, Peters B, Strachan GM, DeMaria AN (2001) Comparison of real-time and intermittent triggered myocardial contrast echocardiography for quantification of coronary stenosis severity and transmural perfusion gradient. Circulation 104:1550–1556

Matheijssen NA, Louwerenburg HW, van Rugge FP et al (1996) Comparison of ultrafast dipyridamole magnetic resonance imaging with dipyridamole SestaMIBI SPECT for detection of perfusion abnormalities in patients with one-vessel coronary artery disease: assessment by quantitative model fitting. Magn Reson Med 35:221–228

Mauss Y, Grucker D, Fornasiero D, Chambron J (1985) NMR compartmentalization of free water in the perfused rat heart. Magn Reson Med 2:187–194

McCommis KS, Goldstein TA, Abendschein DR et al (2010) Quantification of regional myocardial oxygenation by magnetic resonance imaging: validation with positron emission tomography. Circ Cardiovasc Imaging 3:41–46

Meier P, Zierler KL (1954) On the theory of the indicator-dilution method for measurement of blood flow and volume. J Appl Physiol 6:731–744

Meyer C, Strach K, Thomas D et al (2008) High-resolution myocardial stress perfusion at 3T in patients with suspected coronary artery disease. Eur Radiol 18:226–233

Meza MF, Mobarek S, Sonnemaker R et al (1996) Myocardial contrast echocardiography in human beings: correlation of resting defects to sestamibi single photon emission computed tomography. Am Heart J 132:528–535

Mitchell MD, Osbakken M (1991) Estimation of myocardial perfusion using deuterium nuclear magnetic resonance. Magn Reson Imaging 9:545–552

Muehling OM, Wilke NM, Panse P et al (2003) Reduced myocardial perfusion reserve and transmural pressure gradient in heart transplant arteriopathy assessed by magnetic resonance imaging. J Am Coll Cardiol 42:1054–1060

Muzik O, Duvernoy C, Beanlands RS et al (1998) Assessment of diagnostic performance of quantitative flow measurements in normal subjects and patients with angiographically documented coronary artery disease by means of nitrogen 13 ammonia and positron emission tomography. J Am Coll Cardiol 31:534–540

Nagel E, Klein C, Paetsch I et al (2003) Magnetic resonance perfusion measurements for the noninvasive detection of coronary artery disease. Circulation 108:432–437

Nandalur KR, Dwamena BA, Choudhri AF, Nandalur MR, Carlos RC (2007) Diagnostic performance of stress cardiac magnetic resonance imaging in the detection of coronary artery disease. J Am Coll Cardiol 50:1343–1353

Paetsch I, Jahnke C, Wahl A, Gebker R, Neuss M, Fleck E, Nagel E (2004) Comparison of dobutamine stress magnetic resonance, adenosine stress magnetic resonance, and adenosine stress magnetic resonance perfusion. Circulation 110:835–842

Panting JR, Taylor AM, Gatehouse PD et al (1999) First-pass myocardial perfusion imaging and equilibrium signal changes using the intravascular contrast agent NC100150 injection. J Magn Reson Imaging 10:404–410

Panting JR, Gatehouse PD, Yang GZ (2001) Echo-planar magnetic resonance myocardial perfusion imaging: parametric map analysis and comparison with Thallium SPECT. J Magn Reson Imaging 13:192–200

Patel AR, Antkowiak PF, Nandalur KR et al (2010) Assessment of advanced coronary artery disease: advantages of quantitative cardiac magnetic resonance perfusion analysis. J Am Coll Cardiol 56:561–569

Patterson RE, Horowitz SF, Eisner RL (1994) Comparison of modalities to diagnose coronary artery disease. Semin Nucl Med 24:286–310

Pedersen H, Kelle S, Ringgaard S et al (2009) Quantification of myocardial perfusion using free-breathing MRI and prospective slice tracking. Magn Reson Med 61:734–738

Pennell DJ (1994) Pharmacological cardiac stress: when and how? Nucl Med Commun 15:578–585

Penzkofer H, Wintersperger BJ, Knez A, Weber J, Reiser M (1999) Assessment of myocardial perfusion using multisection first-pass MRI and color-coded parameter maps: a comparison to 99mTc Sesta MIBI SPECT and systolic myocardial wall thickening analysis. Magn Reson Imging 17:161–170

Picano E, Ostojic M, Sicari R, Baroni M, Cortigiani L, Pingitore A on behalf of the EPIC (Echo Persantin International Cooperative) study group (1997) Dipyridamole stress echocardiography: state of the art 1996. Eur Heart J 18 (Suppl D):D16-D23

Plein S, Radjenovic A, Ridgway JP et al (2005) Coronary artery disease: myocardial perfusion MR imaging with sensitivity encodign versus conventional angiography. Radiology 235:423–430

Plein S, Ryf S, Schwitter J, Radjenovic A, Boesiger P, Kozerke S (2007) Dynamic contrast-enhanced myocardial perfusion MRI accelerated with *k-t* SENSE. Magn Reson Med 58:777–785

Plein S, Kozerke S, Suerder D et al (2008a) High spatial resolution myocardial perfusion cardiac magnetic resonance for the detection of coronary artery disease. Eur Heart J 29:2148–2155

Plein S, Schwitter J, Suerder D, Greenwood JP, Boesiger P, Kozerke S (2008b) k-Space and time sensitivity encoding-accelerated myocardial perfusion MR imaging at 3.0T: comparison with 1.5T. Radiology 249:493–500

Porter TR, Xie F, Silver M, Kricsfield D, Oleary E (2001) Real-time perfusion imaging with low mechanical index pulse inversion Doppler imaging. J Am Coll Cardiol 37:748–753

Radjenovic A, Biglands JD, Larghat A et al (2010) Estimates of systolic and diastolic myocardial blood flow by dynamic contrast-enhanced MRI. Magn Reson Med 64:1696–1703

Reeder SB, Atalar E, Faranesh AZ, McVeigh ER (1999) Multi-echo segmented k-space imaging: an optimized hybrid sequence for ultrafast imaging. Magn Reson Med 41: 375–385

Reimer KA, Jennings RB (1979) The wavefront progression of myocardial ischemic cell death. II: transmural progression of necrosis within the framework of ischemic bed size (myocardium at risk) and collateral flow. Lab Invest 40:633–644

Reimer P, Bremer C, Allkemper T, Engelhardt M, Mahler M, Ebert W, Tombach B (2004) Myocardial perfusion and MR angiography of chest with SHU 555C: results of placebo-controlled clinical phase I study. Radiology 231:474–481

Revel D, Canet E, Sebbag L et al (1996) First-pass and delayed magnetic resonance imaging studies of reperfused myocardial infarction with iron oxide particles. Acad Radiol 3:S398–S401

Rieber J, Huner A, Erhard I et al (2006) Cardiac magnetic resonance perfusion imaging for the functional assessment of coronary artery disease: a comparison with coronary angiography and fractional flow reserve. Eur Heart J 27: 1465–1471

Ritter C, Brackertz A, Sandstede J, Beer M, Hahn D, Köstler H (2006) Absolute quantification of myocardial perfusion under adenosine stress. Magn Reson Med 56:844–849

Rosen BR, Belliveau JW, Vevea JM, Brady TJ (1990) Perfusion with NMR contrast agents. Magn Reson Med 14: 249–265

Saeed M, Wendland MF, Higgins CB (1994) Contrast media for MR imaging of the heart. J Magn Reson Imaging 4: 269–279

Saeed M, Wendland MF, Higgins CB (1995) The developing role of magnetic resonance contrast media in the detection of ischemic heart disease. Proc Soc Exp Biol Med 208: 238–254

Schaefer S, Lange RA, Kulkarni PV et al (1989) In vivo nuclear magnetic resonance imaging of myocardial perfusion using the paramagnetic contrast agent manganese gluconate. J Am Coll Cardiol 14:472–480

Schaefer S, van Tyen R, Saloner D (1992) Evaluation of myocardial perfusion abnormalities with gadolinium-enhanced snapshot MR imaging in humans (Work in progress). Radiology 185:795–801

Schreiber WG, Schmitt M, Kalden P, Mohrs OK, Kreitner KF, Thelen M (2002) Dynamic contrast-enhanced myocardial perfusion imaging using saturation-prepared TrueFISP. J Magn Reson Imaging 16:641–652

Schuijf JD, Wijns W, Jukema JW et al (2006) Relationship between noninvasive coronary angiography with multi-slice computed tomography and myocardial perfusion imaging. J Am Coll Cardiol 48:2508–2514

Schweiger M (1994) Myocardial perfusion imaging with PET. J Nucl Med 35:693–698

Schwitter J, Arai EA (2011) Assessment of cardiac ischaemia and viability: role of cardiovascular magnetic resonance. Eur Heart J 32:799–809

Schwitter J, Debatin JF, von Schulthess GK, McKinnon GC (1997) Normal myocardial perfusion assessed with multi-shot echo-planar imaging. Magn Reson Med 37:140–147

Schwitter J, Nanz D, Kneifel S et al (2001) Assessment of myocardial perfusion in coronary artery disease by magnetic resonance: a comparison with positron emission tomography and coronary angiography. Circulation 103: 2230–2235

Schwitter J, Wacker CM, van Rossum AC et al (2008) MR-IMPACT: comparison of perfusion-cardiac magnetic resonance with single-photon emission computed tomography for the detection of coronary artery disease in a multicentre, multivendor, randomized trial. Eur Heart J 29:480–489

Senior R, Lahiri A (1995) Enhanced detection of myocardial ischemia by stress dobutamine echocardiography utilizing the "biphasic" response of wall thickening during low and high dose dobutamine infusion. J Am Coll Cardiol 26:26–32

Sensky PR, Samani NJ, Reek C, Cherryman GR (2002) Magnetic resonance perfusion imaging in patients with coronary artery disease: a qualitative approach. Int J Cardiovasc Imaging 18:373–383

Shaw LJ, Iskandrian AE (2004) Prognostic value of gated myocardial perfusion SPECT. J Nucl Cardiol 11:171–185

Shea SM, Fieno DS, Schirf BE et al (2005) T2-prepared steady-state free precession blood oxygen level-dependent MR imaging of myocardial perfusion in a dog stenosis model. Radiology 236:503–509

Sicari R, Nihoyannopoulos P, Evangelista A et al (2008) Eur J Echocardiogr 9:415–437

Siebert JE, Eisenberg JD, Pernicone JR, Cooper TG (1998) Practical myocardial perfusion studies via adenosine pharmacologic stress. In: Proceedings of international society for magnetic resonance in medicine, sixth scientific meeting and exhibition, Sydney, Australia, 18–24 April 1998, p 902

Slavin GS, Wolff SD, Gupta SN, Foo TK (2001) First-pass myocardial perfusion MR imaging with interleaved notched saturation: feasibility study. Radiology 219:258–263

Taylor AJ, Al-Saadi N, Abdel-Aty H et al (2004) Detection of acutely impaired microvascular reperfusion after infarct angioplasty with magnetic resonance imaging. Circulation 109:2080–2085

Theisen D, Wintersperger BJ, Huber A, Dietrich O, Reiser MF, Schönberg SO (2007) Myocardial perfusion imaging with Gadobutrol: a comparison between 3 and 1.5 Tesla with an identical sequence design. Invest Radiol 42:499–506

Thiele H, Plein S, Ridway JP et al (2003) Effects of missing dynamic images in myocardial perfusion reserve index calculation: comparison between an every heartbeat and an alternate heartbeat acquisition. J Cardiovasc Magn Reson 5:343-352

Tillisch J, Brunken R, Marshall R et al (1986) Reversibility of cardiac wall-motion abnormalities predicted by positron tomography. N Engl J Med 3:884–888

Toft J, Mortensen J, Hesse B (1998) Risk of atrioventricular block during adenosine pharmacologic stress testing in heart transplant recipients. Am J Cardiol 82:696–697

Tong CY, Prato FS, Wisenberg G et al (1993a) Techniques for the measurement of the local myocardial extraction efficiency for inert diffusible contrast agents such as gadopentate dimeglumine. Magn Reson Med 30:332–336

Tong CY, Prato FS, Wisenberg G et al (1993b) Measurement of the extraction efficiency and distribution volume for Gd DTPA in normal and diseased canine myocardium. Magn Reson Med 30:337–346

Tonino PA, De Bruyne B, Pijls NH et al (2009) FAME study investigators. Fractional flow reserve versus angiography for guiding percutaneous coronary intervention. N Engl J Med 360:213–224

Tsao J (2010) Ultrafast imaging: principles, pitfalls, solutions, and applications. J Magn Reson Imaging 32:262–266

Tsao J, Boesiger P, Pruessmann KP (2003) k-t BLAST and k-t SENSE: dynamic MRI with high frame rate exploiting spatiotemporal correlations. Magn Reson Med 50: 1031–1042

Tsekos NV, Zhang Y, Merkle H et al (1995) Fast anatomical imaging of the heart and assessment of myocardial perfusion with arrhythmia insensitive magnetization preparation. Magn Reson Med 34:530–536

Unger EF, Banai S, Shou M et al (1994) Basic fibroblast growth factor enhances myocardial collateral flow in a canine model. Am J Physiol 266:H1588–H1595

Uren NG, Melin JA, De Bruyne B et al (1994) Relation between myocardial blood flow and the severity of coronary artery stenosis. N Engl J Med 330:1782–1788

Utz W, Gresier A, Niendorf T, Dietz R, Schulz-Menger J (2008) Single- or dual-bolus approach for the assessment of myocardial perfusion reserve in quantitative MR perfusion imaging. Magn Reson Med 59:1373–1377

Vallee JP, Sostman HD, MacFall JR et al (1997) MRI quantitative myocardial perfusion with compartment analysis: a rest and stress study. Magn Reson Med 38:981–989

Vatner SF (1980) Correlation between acute reductions in myocardial blood flow and function in conscious dogs. Circ Res 47:201

Vitanis V, Manka R, Giese D et al (2011) High resolution three-dimensional cardiac perfusion imaging using compartment-based k-t prinicipal component analysis. Magn Reson Med 65:575–587

Wagner A, Mahrholdt H, Holly TA et al (2003) Contrast-enhanced MRI and routine single photon emission computed tomography (SPECT) perfusion imaging for detection of subendocardial myocardial infarcts: an imaging study. Lancet 361:374–379

Wahl A, Paetsch I, Gollesch A, Roethemeyer S, Foell D, Gebker R, Langreck H, Klein C, Fleck E, Nagel E (2004) Safety and feasibility of high-dose dobutamine-atropine stress cardiovascular magnetic resonance for diagnosis of myocardial ischaemia: experience in 1000 consecutive cases. Eur Heart J; 25:1230–1236

Walsh EG, Doyle M, Lawson MA, Blackwell GG, Pohost GM (1995) Multislice first-pass myocardial perfusion imaging on a conventional clinical scanner. Magn Reson Med 34:39–47

Watkins S, McGeoh R, Lyne J (2009) Validation of magnetic resonance myocardial perfusion imaging with fractional flow reserve for the detection of significant coronary heart disease. Circulation 120:2207–2213

Weber S, Kronfeld A, Kunz P et al (2007) Comparison of three accelerated pulse sequences for semiquantitative myocardial perfusion imaging using sensitivity encoding incorporating temporal filtering (TSENSE). J Magn Reson Imaging 26:569–579

Wedeking P, Sotak CH, Telser J, Kumar K, Chang CA, Tweedle MF (1992) Quantitative dependence of MR signal intensity on tissue concentration of Gd(HP-DO3A) in the nephrectomized rat. Magn Reson Imaging 10:97–108

Wei K, Jayaweera AR, Firoozan S et al (1998) Quantification of myocardial blood flow with ultrasound-induced destruction of microbubbles administered as a constant venous infusion. Circulation 97:473–483

Weinmann HJ, Brasch RC, Press WR, Wesbey GE (1983) Characteristics of gadolinium-DTPA complex: a potential NMR contrast agent. AJR 142:619–624

Weiskoff RM, Chesler D, Boxerman JL, Rosen BR (1993) Pitfalls in MR measurement of tissue blood flow with intravascular tracers: which mean transit time? Magn Reson Med 29:553–558

Wendland MF, Saeed M, Masui T, Derugin N, Higgins CB (1993) First pass of an MR susceptibility contrast agent through normal and ischemic heart: gradient-recalled echo-planar imaging. J Magn Reson Imaging 3:755–760

Wendland MF, Saeed M, Yu KK et al (1994) Inversion recovery EPI of bolus transit in rat myocardium using intravascular and extravascular gadolinium-based MR contrast media: dose effects on peak signal enhancement. Magn Reson Med 32:319–329

Wetter DR, McKinnon GC, Debatin JF, von Schulthess G (1995) Cardiac echo-planar MR imaging: comparison of single- and multiple-shot techniques. Radiology 194:765–770

Wilke N, Simm C, Zhang J et al (1993) Contrast-enhanced first-pass myocardial perfusion imaging: correlation between myocardial blood flow in dogs at rest and during hyperemia. Magn Reson Med 29:485–497

Wilke N, Jerosch-Herold M, Stillman AE et al (1994) Concepts of myocardial perfusion imaging in magnetic resonanceimaging. Magn Reson Q 10:249–286

Wilke N, Jerosch-Herold M, Wang Y et al (1997) Myocardial perfusion reserve: assessment with multisection, quantitative, first-pass MR imaging. Radiology 204:373–384

Wilson RF, Wyche K, Christensen BV, Zimmer S, Laxson DD (1990) Effects of adenosine on human coronary arterial circulation. Circulation 82:1595–1606

Wolf SD, Schwitter J, Coulden R et al (2004) Myocardial first-pass perfusion magnetic resonance imaging. A dose-ranging study. Circulation 110:732–737

Wright KB, Klocke FJ, Deshpande V et al (2001) Assessment of regional differences in myocardial blood flow using T2-weighted 3D BOLD imaging. Magn Reson Med 46: 573–578

Yu KK, Saeed M, Wendland MF et al (1993) Comparison of T1-enhancing and magnetic susceptibility magnetic resonance contrast agents for demarcation of the jeopardy area in experimental myocardial infarction. Invest Radiol 28:1015–1023

Zierler K (1962) Indicator dilution methods for measuring blood flow, volume, and other properties of biological systems: a brief history and memoir. Ann Biomed Eng 28:836–848

Ischemic Heart Disease

J. Bogaert and S. Dymarkowski

Contents

1	**Epidemiology**	203
2	**Pathophysiology**	204
3	**Imaging Strategies**	207
3.1	Functional Imaging	207
3.2	Myocardial Perfusion Imaging	210
3.3	Edema Imaging	211
3.4	Contrast Enhanced MRI	213
3.5	Myocardial Fat Imaging	223
4	**Stable Coronary Artery Disease**	223
4.1	Stress Perfusion Imaging	224
4.2	Stress Function Imaging	225
5	**Acute Coronary Syndrome**	228
5.1	Characterization of the Jeopardized Myocardium	229
5.2	Assessment of Myocardial Infarction Severity	232
5.3	Patterns of Enhancement Depending on Infarct Location	241
5.4	Infarct-Related Complications	243
5.5	Infarct Healing and Ventricular Remodeling	247
5.6	Peri-Procedural Necrosis	248
5.7	Role of MRI in Patients with Acute Chest Pain	249
6	**Chronic Ischemic Cardiomyopathy**	250
6.1	Ischemic Heart Disease and Heart Failure	250
6.2	Myocardial Viability Assessment	251
6.3	Cardiac Resynchronization Therapy	255
7	**Prognosis Assessment**	255
8	**Clinical Imaging Strategies: Practical Recipes**	256
9	**Key Points**	258
References		259

J. Bogaert (✉) · S. Dymarkowski
Department of Radiology and Medical Imaging Research Center (MIRC), University Hospitals Gasthuisberg, Catholic University of Leuven, Herestraat 49, 3000 Leuven, Belgium
e-mail: jan.bogaert@uzleuven.be

Abstract

Ischemic heart disease (IHD) is the leading cause of morbidity and mortality in industrialized countries and poses an enormous financial burden on our society. As a consequence rational, evidence-based use of diagnostic and therapeutic means will be needed to prevent financial lapses and to guarantee an affordable medicine in the coming years. Magnetic resonance imaging is rapidly gaining widespread acceptance to investigate the full spectrum of patients presenting with symptoms of myocardial ischemia, ranging from stable coronary artery disease, over acute coronary syndrome, to the prediction of functional recovery post-revascularization in patients with chronic ischemic cardiomyopathy. In this chapter the MRI strategies to investigate IHD patients are discussed in detail, emphasizing the comprehensive approach converging information regarding myocardial perfusion, function and tissue characterization. Besides extensive illustration about the use of MRI, timelines for comprehensive MRI are provided for each IHD subgroup including standard and optional sequences.

1 Epidemiology

Although the mortality associated with ischemic heart disease (IHD) has declined in the recent decades, due to therapeutic improvements (e.g., thrombolytic agents, early revascularization, ACE inhibitors and beta-blockers) and to prevention campaigns reducing the incidence of myocardial infarction (MI), IHD

J. Bogaert et al. (eds.), *Clinical Cardiac MRI*, Medical Radiology. Diagnostic Imaging,
DOI: 10.1007/174_2011_336, © Springer-Verlag Berlin Heidelberg 2012

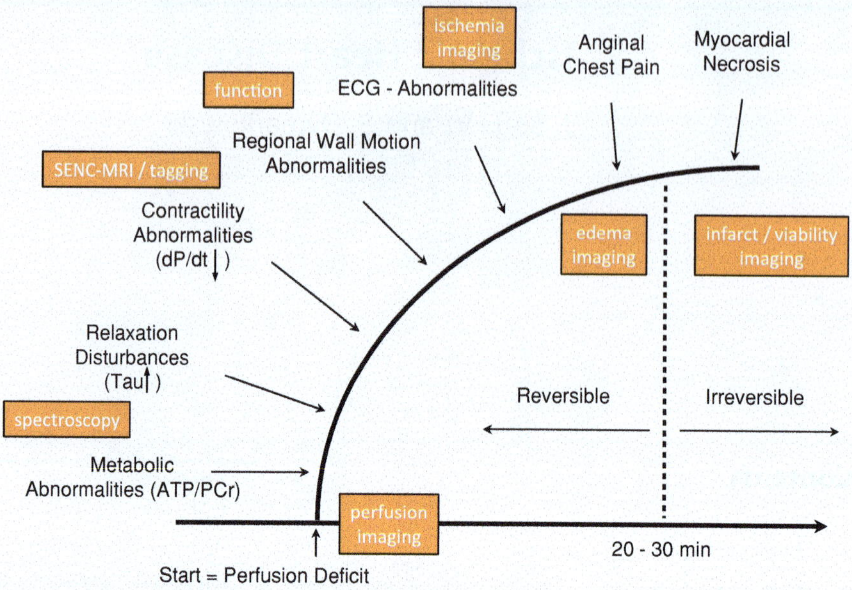

Fig. 1 Diagram of the Ischemic Cascade and the role of SENC-MRI (strain-encoded-MRI) Techniques. MRI is of value to assess the ischemic cascade at different levels such as shown in the colored boxes

remains the leading cause of in adults in developed countries and the prevalence will continue to increase (Beller 2001; Lloyd-Jones et al. 2010; Yeh et al. 2010). Worldwide, it is estimated that IHD will become the number one cause of death by 2020 (Fuster 1999). Survivors of a first acute MI are thought to die of IHD at later ages due to heart failure and late cardiac deaths. Moreover, the increased life span will contribute to the increased incidence of cardiovascular disease and increased number of deaths from heart disease. Other contributing factors to an increased prevalence of IHD are an increasing prevalence of type II diabetes, physical inactivity and obesity. In times of constrained financial budgets (Escolano 2010), the increasing prevalence of IHD will urge for the rational use of diagnostic and therapeutic means. One of the challenges is to define regularly updated appropriateness criteria for cardiac imaging techniques (Hendel et al. 2006; Hundley et al. 2010). In the last two decades MRI has emerged as the prime player in the clinical and preclinical detection of IHD as well in prognosis assessment (Lockie et al. 2009; Kim et al. 2010; Bingham and Hachamovitch 2011). The aims of this chapter are to provide the reader with a state-of-the art of how the newest cardiac MRI techniques can be used to study IHD patients and to enlarge our knowledge of the complex pathophysiology, in particular, in the detection of obstructive coronary artery disease (CAD), in acute coronary syndromes and in chronic ischemic cardiomyopathy.

2 Pathophysiology

The heart is provided with its own nutrient vessels, i.e. the coronary arteries, which are unfortunately particularly vulnerable to the systemic disorder of atherosclerosis. This is known as coronary artery disease (CAD), which is the main cause of IHD. Broadly speaking, an atherosclerotic plaque may impinge on the coronary artery lumen slowly and progressively (*chronic stable plaque*), and/or may suddenly impair coronary flow due to a combination of plaque rupture and thrombosis (*acute coronary syndrome*). Ultimately these events lead to dysfunction and/or death of the myocardium. Taking into account the short-lived capacity of the myocardium to sustain ischemia, coronary artery occlusion triggers an "*ischemic cascade*" in the perfusion territory distal to the occluded coronary artery (defined as the *jeopardized myocardium* or *myocardium at risk*), starting with metabolic disturbances shifting aerobic oxidative metabolisms almost immediately to anaerobic glycolysis, followed by diastolic and later systolic dysfunction and finally ECG changes and symptoms of angina (Fig. 1). The time frame of events is short, for instance systolic contraction will cease within seconds after coronary occlusion

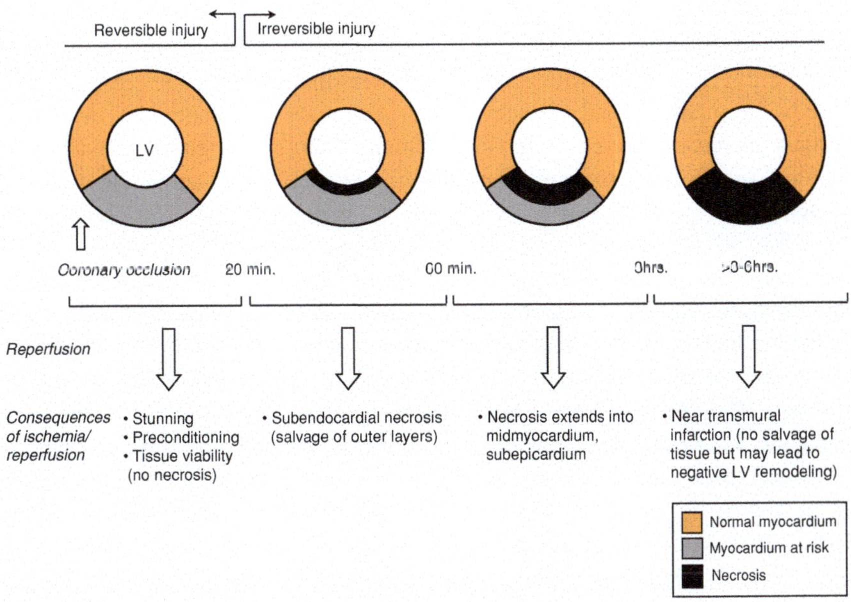

Fig. 2 Effects of ischemia and reperfusion on myocardial tissue viability and necrosis. Studies in anesthetized canine model of proximal coronary artery occlusion. Adapted from Kloner and Jennings 2001

(Jennings et al. 1978). After approximately 20–30 min of sustained ischemia, the metabolic changes become irreversible causing intracellular edema together with accumulation of toxic metabolites, myocardial cell apoptosis, ultimately leading to myocyte necrosis. As the systolic wall stress and the resulting oxygen consumption are greater in the inner part of the myocardium, necrosis initiates in this part of the myocardium whereby the lateral boundaries of infarction closely correspond to the myocardium at risk. If ischemia persists, necrosis progresses in a transmural wave front taking 3–6 h to reach the subepicardium (Reimer and Jennings 1970, 1979) (Fig. 2). Whereas the initial extent of necrosis is determined by the extent of the myocardium at risk, the final extent of necrosis is largely determined by the degree of transmural progression (Lee et al. 1981). Viable tissue, mainly in the subepicardium, may survive the acute injury, and show an improvement in the metabolism and function following reperfusion (Gropler et al. 1992; Bogaert et al. 1999). The extent of myocardial necrosis depends on many factors: (1) myocardium of risk, (2) residual blood flow to the ischemic territory, (3) myocardial oxygen consumption during ischemia and (4) duration of ischemia (Reimer et al. 1985). The presence of a small fraction of perfusion to the infarct bed, from either antegrade or collateral flow, can significantly delay necrosis and limit the infarct size (Rivas et al. 1976). However, collateral circulation usually takes time to become functional (Patterson et al. 1993), and is often insufficiently developed in acute coronary syndrome patients because of rupture of non- or minimally stenotic coronary plaques.

Current therapeutic strategies are focused on urgent restoration of epicardial flow using mechanical or thrombolytic approaches. The aim is to salvage the jeopardized but viable myocardium in the myocardium at risk distal to the culprit lesion, to reduce adverse infarct and ventricular remodeling, and to improve patient outcome. The faster the restoration of myocardial perfusion, the lesser the transmural extent of necrosis, and the more the ischemically, jeopardized myocardium will be salvaged (Hochman and Choo 1987; Francone et al. 2009). In fact, the amount of myocardial salvage drastically decreases after the first 90 min and at 6 h myocardial salvage is nearly zero. Thus, the beneficial effects (in terms of short- and long-term survival) of myocardial reperfusion in the golden hour(s) are largely due to myocardial salvage but any benefit obtained after the sixth hour is likely independent from the myocardial salvage (*'open artery-theory'*). Despite the beneficial effects of reperfusion, it has been shown that the process of cell death may continue during the first hours of reperfusion, a phenomenon called "*myocardial reperfusion injury*" (Matsumura et al. 1998; Becker et al. 1999; Gerber et al. 2000; Yellon and Hausenloy 2007). This is a complex and not completely understood phenomenon that is typically found in the core of the infarct and occurs frequently despite successful recanalization with restoration of a normal flow in the infarct-related coronary artery. Although primary percutaneous coronary intervention (PCI) enables an effective recanalization of the infarct-related artery in the vast majority of patients, nonetheless, in a consistent number of patients myocardial reperfusion is hampered by microvascular obstruction (MVO) with a complete lack of tissue perfusion. The main determinants of MVO are (1) reperfusion injury, (2) severity of ischemia and (3) extent of myocardial necrosis. The presence of MVO is an independent predictor of death and adverse LV remodeling (see Sects. 5.2.3 and 7).

According to the Joint ESC/ACCF/AHA/WHF Task Force for the Redefinition of Myocardial Infarction, myocardial infarctions are usually classified by (a) location, (b) size (focal necrosis, small (<10%), moderate (10–30%) and large (>30% of LV myocardium), and (c) temporally as evolving (<6 h), acute (6 h–7 days), healing (7–28 days) and healed (>28 days) (Thygesen et al. 2007). *Post-infarction LV remodeling* is the process of changes in ventricular size, shape, and function that occurs in the days, weeks and months following the acute event (Sutton and Sharpe 2000). In an early phase (within 72 h), the remodelling involves the infarct zone with an expansion of the infarct size due to tissue edema, hemorrhage, and acute inflammation (Reimer and Jennings 1979). The latter changes cause an overestimation of infarct size when the data are referred either to tissue wet or dry weight. In severe cases acute dilation and thinning of the necrotic wall without new tissue necrosis may occur, and eventually result in early ventricular rupture or evolve toward aneurysm formation. The acute loss in myocardium results in an abrupt increase in loading conditions in the infarcted border zone and remote non-infarcted myocardium, leading to an early LV dilatation. Especially large transmural infarctions, infarctions related to lesions in the distribution of the left anterior descending coronary artery, and infarctions with severe MVO, are prone to "*infarct expansion*". During the infarct healing phase an opposite phenomenon occurs whereby the necrotic tissue is progressively replaced by a dense fibrotic scar, causing a significant reduction in the initial infarct size (Reimer and Jennings 1979). Late adverse remodeling involves the LV globally and is associated with a time-dependent dilatation, alterations in ventricular architecture, and mural hypertrophy to distribute the increased wall stresses more evenly throughout the damaged LV. Adverse LV remodeling is an important trigger for the evolution of a post-infarct ventricle toward an ischemic cardiomyopathy and heart failure.

If the duration of occlusion is less than 15 min, myocyte injury may be reversible, with prolonged but reversible contractile dysfunction—"stunned myocardium" (Braunwald and Kloner 1982), defined as "prolonged post-ischemic contractile dysfunction of myocardium salvaged by reperfusion". This may take days to weeks to normalize, although it can be reversed with inotropic agents. The clinical counterparts of brief periods of transient ischemia include angina, unstable angina, coronary vasospasm, and transient ischemia induced by inflation of an angioplasty balloon in the coronary arteries (Kloner and Jennings 2001). Very brief episodes of ischemia as short as 5 min, followed by reperfusion, protect the heart from a subsequent longer coronary artery occlusion by markedly reducing the amount of necrosis that results from the test episode of ischemia. This phenomenon, called "*ischemic preconditioning*" is a powerful cardioprotective effect, and might be an effective means to clinically minimize the stunning phenomenon (Kloner and Jennings 2001).

When a milder degree of ischemia is persistent for weeks, months or years, myocytes become dysfunctional by down-regulation of energy consumption through a lower level of aerobic and/or anaerobic metabolism (Maes et al. 1994). If perfusion is restored to these dysfunctional areas prior to irreversible ultra structural changes occurring, these segments may functionally return to normal, although the recovery is typically slow taking up to more than one year in severe forms (Bax et al. 2001; Bondarenko et al. 2008). This type of ischemia associated with a chronic and reversible LV dysfunction has been termed "*hibernating myocardium*" (Rahimtoola 1989) and is used to describe viable myocardium in a state of persistent but potentially reversible dysfunction secondary to a chronic coronary artery stenosis with impaired myocardial blood flow (Selvanayagam et al. 2005a, b). It is considered an adaptive mechanism to preserve the structural integrity of the myocardium and to prevent myocyte death. In patients with severe chronic LV dysfunction due to CAD, it is important to distinguish dysfunctional but viable myocardium from necrotic tissue in order to determine preoperatively the benefit of the revascularisation procedure (Kim et al. 2000). Although the simplistic classification of stunning and hibernating myocardium is derived from clinical observations and imperfect animal experiments with many exceptions and overlaps (Bashour and Mason 1990; Neill et al. 1986; Nienaber et al. 1991), it is at least conceptually of clinical significance. For therapeutic decision-making, e.g., to choose for PCI or coronary bypass grafting (CABG) procedure, it is important to discern between viable and nonviable myocardium (Wu et al. 2011).

3 Imaging Strategies

Basically the role of imaging in IHD patients is threefold: first, visualization of CAD, second, evaluation of the consequences of CAD on the heart, in particular the impact on myocardial perfusion and function, and third depiction of (ir)-reversible myocardial damage (Beller 2000). Although cardiac MRI could not fulfill its promises to reliable image coronary arteries (this role is currently claimed by cardiac computed tomography), this technique has become a preferred imaging modality to study the ischemic consequences of CAD on myocardial perfusion, function and myocardial integrity (Dall'Armellina et al. 2010; Morton et al. 2010a). In clinical practice, using a comprehensive MRI approach, the above information can be obtained within a single exam taking not more than 30–45 min. Although technical challenges presently limit a more routine clinical use of magnetic resonance spectroscopy (MRS), this technique has become a standard method in experimental cardiology for studying many aspects of cardiac metabolism, including for instance cardiac high-energy phosphate metabolites ATP and phosphocreatine in IHD patients (Neubauer 2007; Bottomley et al. 2009).

3.1 Functional Imaging

A direct consequence of IHD is a temporary or permanent impairment of myocardial contractility not only in the ischemic zone but affecting a large part of one or both ventricles, leading to a reduced ventricular performance. Cine MRI (see "Cardiac Function") provides a noninvasive, accurate and reproducible means to visualize regional wall motion and contraction patterns and to calculate ventricular volumes and function, making it appealing as imaging modality to use not only in daily clinical routine, but also for example for evaluating novel therapies, and to study long-term effects such as ventricular remodeling (Thiele et al. 2001; Janssens et al. 2006; Ganame et al. 2011) (Fig. 3). Although noninvasive functional cardiac evaluation is often automatically linked to echocardiography, cine MRI should be considered as a fast, robust and probably more accurate alternative. Even in ill cardiac patients unable to hold their breath or in patients with atrial fibrillation, real-time non-gated cine imaging can be a valuable alternative to estimate the degree of ventricular dilation and dysfunction, to visualize focal aneurysm formation or to image concomitant valve pathology.

For functional analysis, the heart is best studied along different imaging planes. Ventricular volumes, mass and function can be quantified using a contiguous set of image slices completely encompassing the ventricles (for this purpose usually the cardiac short-axis is used). In addition, these images can be used to assess circumferential or longitudinal wall motion patterns, and the amount of (systolic) wall thickening. Functional impairment can be expressed qualitatively, e.g., hypokinetic, akinetic or dyskinetic wall motion, or quantitatively using the relative or absolute wall thickening. To achieve consensus between readers and between imaging modalities, it is recommended to use the standardized 17-segment model as initially proposed by the American Society for Echocardiography (Cerqueira 2002) (see "Cardiovascular MR Imaging Planes and Segmentation"). It should be noted that although the coronary artery distribution can be attributed per segment, there is an important variability in coronary blood supply in a large number of segments (see Fig. 19 in Chapter "Cardiovascular MR Imaging Planes and Segmentation") (Ortiz-Pérez et al. 2008). A limitation of the above model is that the extent of myocardial ischemia/infarction does not necessarily respect segment borders, thus leading to segments with mixed tissue characteristics. Use of a merged late Gd—cine imaging approach, in contrast, enables to define regions with similar tissue

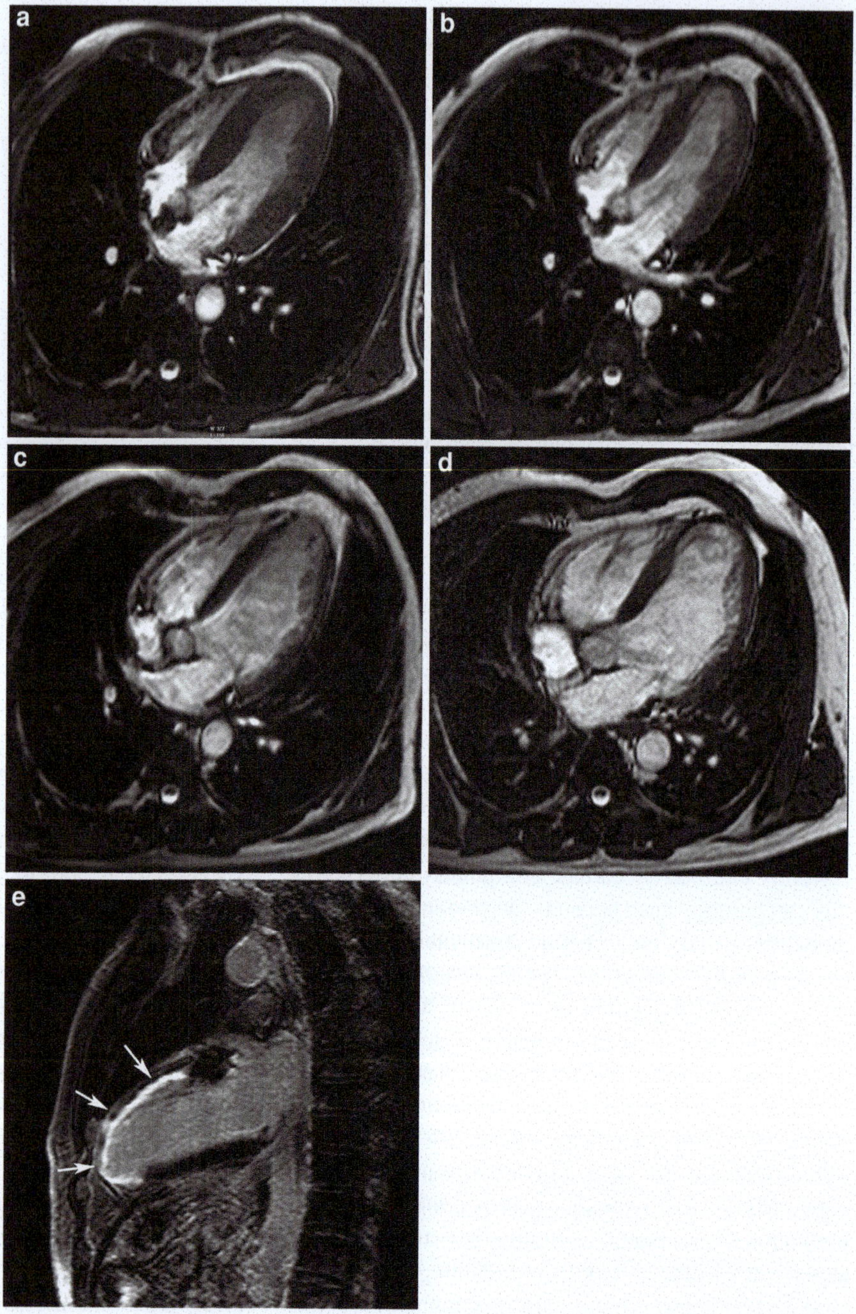

Fig. 3 Use of MRI for long-term follow-up of ventricular remodeling post-myocardial infarction. Horizontal long-axis cine imaging at 1 week (**a**), 4 months (**b**), 1 year (**c**), and 5 years (**d**) after the acute event (end-diastolic time frames). Vertical long-axis late Gd imaging (**e**). Late Gd imaging shows extensive anteroapical myocardial infarction (*arrows*, **e**). Cine imaging allows to appreciate the infarct healing with thinning of the LV apex, and the progressive LV dilatation over time (**a–d**). The LV end-diastolic volumes at 1 week, 4 months, 1 year and 5 years are 167, 180, 230, 257 ml respectively

characteristics (e.g., infarct, peri-infarct and remote myocardium) facilitating the evaluation of complex processes such as infarct or ventricular remodeling (Masci et al. 2009) (Fig. 4).

Although evaluation of cardiac function in resting conditions provides valuable information regarding myocardial contractility, in CAD patients it is often necessary to evaluate myocardial contractility patterns under stress conditions using either physical or pharmacological stress. The goal is basically to detect (or exclude) the presence of hemodynamic significant stenoses ('flow-limiting') (*ischemia testing*) (Fig. 5), and/or to evaluate whether during stress conditions dysfunctional myocardium improves contractility (*viability testing*) (see Sect. 6). Because the available imaging time per stress level is limited, fast

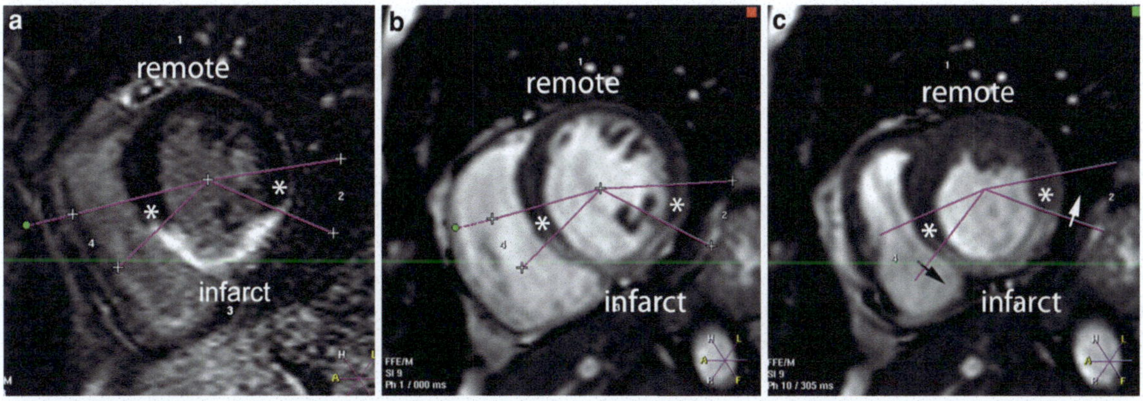

Fig. 4 Merging of late Gd imaging and cine imaging. Short-axis late Gd imaging (**a**), and cine imaging post-contrast administration at end diastole (**b**) and end systole (**c**). Late Gd imaging provides detailed information regarding the presence, location and extent of myocardial necrosis/scarring (**a**). This information can be used to define regions with similar tissue characteristics, such as infarct, peri-infarct (*) or remote myocardium, and to subsequently analyze regional function in these areas. An alternative approach is to perform cine imaging post-contrast administration. The advantage of the latter approach is that it intrinsically corrects for ventricular torsion (*arrows*, **c**). Adapted from Masci et al. 2009

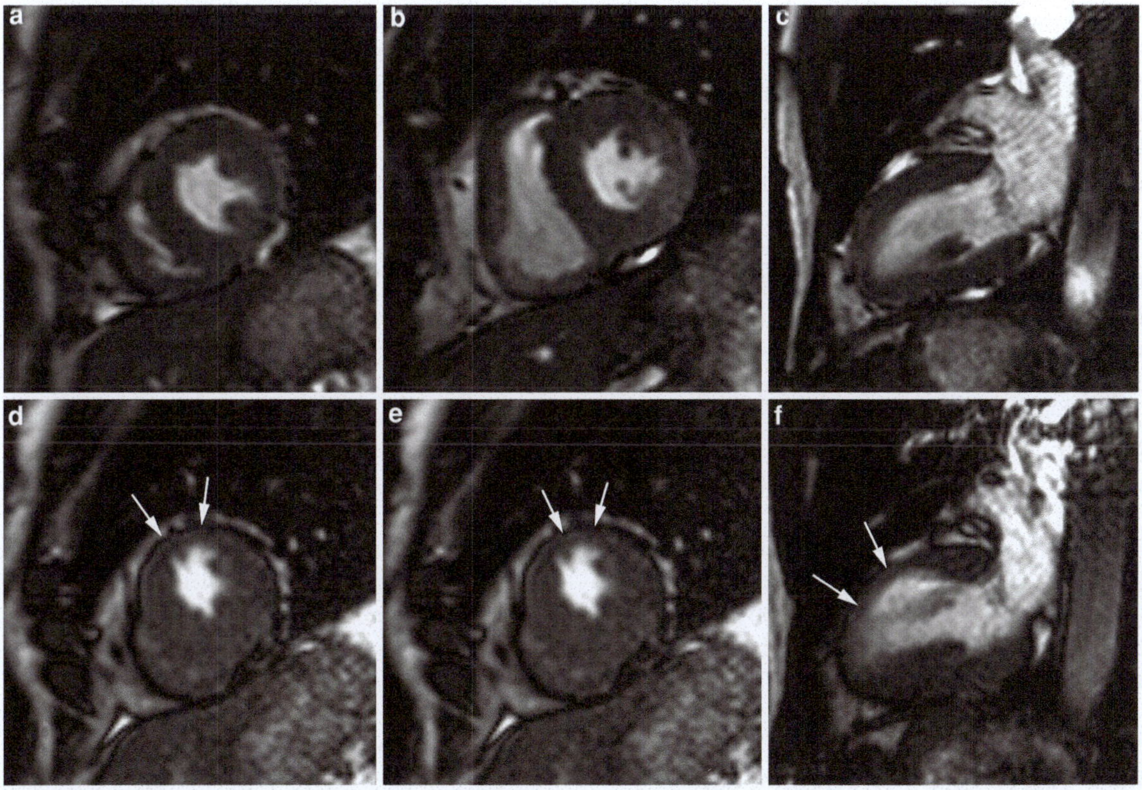

Fig. 5 Stress-inducible ischemic wall motion abnormalities (WMA) in a 60-year old patient with recurrent ischemia after PTCA. Cine imaging at rest (*above*) and during high-dose stress (40 µg/kg/min + 0.25 mg atropine) (*below*). End-systolic cine image frames in 2 cardiac short-axis (**a**, **b**, **d**, **e**) and vertical long-axis (**c**, **f**). While normal contraction is present at rest (**a**, **b**, **c**), at high-dose stress, stress-induced WMA occurs in the LV anterior wall (segment 7, 13), shown by focal akinesia (*arrows*, **d**, **e**, **f**). Note the increased contractility and wall thickening in the non-ischemic segments. The ischemic segment showed some post-systolic wall thickening (not shown). The cardiac catheterization confirmed the presence of a 60% stenosis in the proximal LAD

cine imaging sequences are needed (Jahnke et al. 2006). Functional (stress) imaging in IHD patients is usually part of a more comprehensive approach, established to determine the different ischemic substrates of dysfunctional myocardium. In particular, complementary information is achieved by adding late Gd imaging enabling to depict acute and/or healed myocardial infarction. For example dysfunctional myocardium showing no or only limited myocardial scarring at late Gd imaging has a high likelihood of being viable, whereas extensive scarring suggests non-viable tissue with low likelihood of functional recovery post-revascularization (Kim et al. 1999, 2000; Hillenbrand et al. 2000).

The mechanisms of myocardial contraction are complex and the observed ventricular wall motion and thickening patterns observed with routine cine imaging do not allow to appreciate the underlying mechanisms. Myocardial tagging MRI techniques in contrast (see "Cardiac Function") allow to create non-invasive tag or grid lines on the myocardium, allowing to analyze the myocardial deformation 2 or 3 dimensionally throughout the cardiac cycle, and to calculate myocardial strains, shear strains and principal strains (Bogaert and Rademakers 2001). These tagging techniques have shown to be extremely helpful to elucidate in IHD patients the complex interaction between reversible/irreversible morphologic alterations and myocardial contractility and loading, not only in the damaged area but throughout the entire ventricle (Kramer et al. 1993 and 1996a, b; Croisille et al. 1999; Bogaert et al. 1999, 2000; Garot et al. 2002; Rademakers et al. 2003). Due to the elaborative post-processing, the clinical use of myocardial tagging is currently limited. Recently, Korosoglou et al. proposed a fast direct color-coded strain visualization using SENC (i.e., strain-encoded) MRI obviating the need for post-processing (Korosoglou et al. 2009a). In particular, this novel technique is appealing in stress functional studies (see Sect. 4.2).

3.2 Myocardial Perfusion Imaging

Any consideration about myocardial perfusion needs to address the pivotal relationship between myocardial oxygen requirements and coronary blood flow (see "Myocardial Perfusion"). In normal conditions, there is a balance between myocardial oxygen demand and oxygen supply. Since oxygen extraction in the myocardium is already high under basal conditions, the changes in oxygen demand result in proportional variations of myocardial blood flow. The imbalance between oxygen demand and supply is primarily the result of coronary atheromatosis leading to one or several stenoses in the coronary arteries. In resting conditions, the myocardial perfusion is not altered until the coronary artery has a 85–90% stenosis. This is the result of the coronary vasodilator reserve, which compensates for the effects of coronary stenoses under basal conditions. However, during stress conditions the coronary reserve cannot be induced by a further vasodilatory stimulus. Under these circumstances, the myocardium distal to less severe coronary stenosis (i.e. between 50 and 85%) may become ischemic and the coronary artery stenosis can be considered as hemodynamically significant (Gould 1978, 2009).

The most frequently used approach to assess myocardial perfusion imaging (MPI) with MRI (MR-MPI) is monitoring of the first-pass of contrast medium through the heart, using a bolus injection of MR contrast media in combination with fast MR sequences (see "Myocardial Perfusion"). Perfusion studies can be performed during resting conditions and/or during administration of a vasodilating agent (e.g., adenosine—dipyridamole). Whereas normally perfused myocardium enhances homogeneously during first-pass, hypo-or non perfused regions appear dark for a variable amount of time during/after first-pass, are most intense in the subendocardial part of the myocardium and typically respect coronary artery perfusion territories (Fig. 6). Image analysis can be qualitative, semi-quantitative or quantitative. Visual (i.e. qualitative) analysis is often used clinically, and is a fast and accurate approach at least in experienced hands. Semi-quantitative measurements, may be of use for instance to calculate the myocardial perfusion reserve (MPR) index in patients with suspected CAD, while quantitative measures aim to determine the myocardial blood supply similar to what is achieved with positron-emission-tomography (PET) (Al-Saadi et al. 2000a; Gerber et al. 2008).

In patients with a reperfused acute MI, MPI studies at rest frequently show a "perfusion deficit" in the infarct territory. These defects correspond to no-reflow zones also defined as microvascular obstruction (MVO), and are typically subendocar-

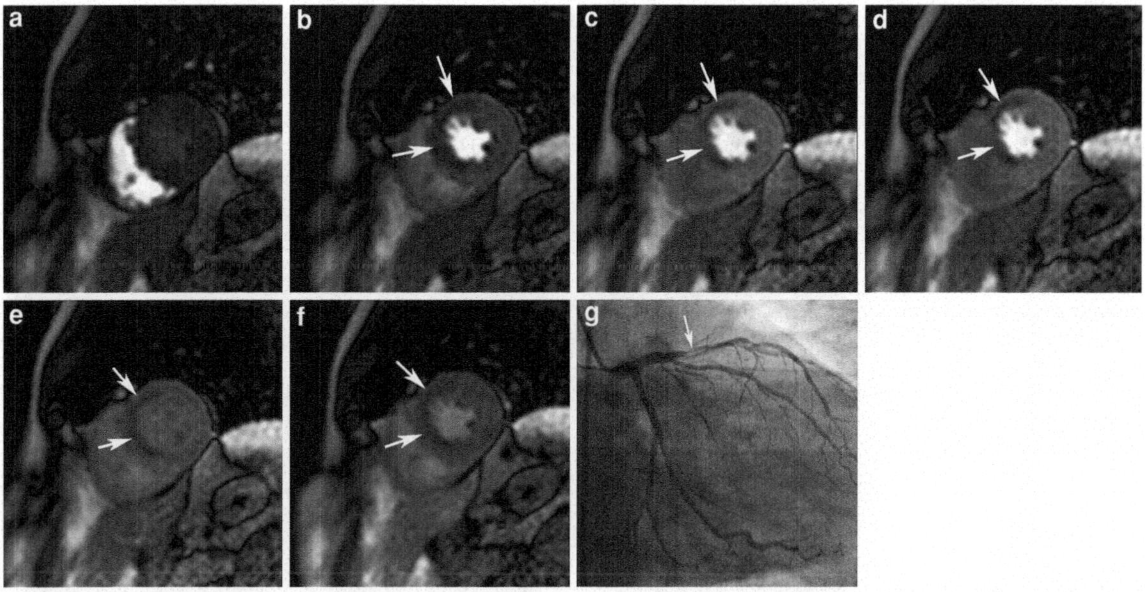

Fig. 6 Adenosine-induced stress perfusion defect in the LV anteroseptal wall due to in-stent restenosis. Short-axis MPI-MR (midventricular level) showing six time frames during first pass of contrast through the heart (**a–f**). The defect in the LV anteroseptal wall becomes visible when the myocardium starts to enhance (*arrows*, **b**). Both the transmural and circumferential extents of the perfusion defect are well visible (*arrows*, **c–d**). There is a long persistence of the defect which is still present during the second pass of contrast through the heart (*arrows*, **f**). Confirmation of in-stent restenosis by coronary angiography (*arrow*, **g**)

dially or centrally located (see Sect. 5.2.3) (Taylor et al. 2004; Bogaert et al. 2007). In cases of occlusive infarcts extensive perfusion defects can be found. In patients with a healed MI, often a faint perfusion defect or delay can be found in the scarred region, and should not be mistaken as a true perfusion defect. Because of the lower capillary density in fibrotic tissue compared to normal myocardium, this region may appear hypo-intense. In patients with suspected CAD, MPI is performed during vasodilatatory stress to depict hemodynamically significant coronary artery stenoses (see Sect. 4.1).

3.3 Edema Imaging

Since proton relaxation times are tissue specific, differences in relaxation times can be exploited to differentiate normal from pathological tissue. Increased free water in the infarcted myocardium prolongs T1- and T2-relaxation, and this prolongation is related to the duration of ischemia (Williams et al. 1980; Higgins et al. 1983; Johnston et al. 1985). Differences in T1-relaxation have shown not to be clinically useful for infarct detection unless paramagnetic contrast agents are administered (see Sect. 3.4). T2-relaxation time, in contrast, is linearly correlated to the percentage of free water, and infarcted myocardium is visible on T2-weighted MR sequences (T2w-imaging) as areas of increased signal intensity (Higgins et al. 1983; McNamara et al. 1985). Although used by many groups to detect and quantify MI (Rokey et al. 1986; Matheijssen et al. 1991; Dulce et al. 1993), the relation between changes in T2-relaxation times and MI is complex (Canby et al. 1987; Wisenberg et al. 1988). In the setting of acute ischemia, the amount of free water may increase not only in the irreversible but also in the reversible injured myocardium, leading to an overestimation of the true extent of myocardial necrosis. This is related to reversible cell swelling, increased capillary permeability in the surrounding ischemic rim and occurrence of myocardial edema (Wisenberg et al. 1988; Schaefer et al. 1988; Ni et al. 1998; Pislaru et al. 1999; Choi et al. 2000; Dymarkowski et al. 2002). Currently, it is accepted that the hyperintense myocardium on T2w-imaging reflects the myocardium at risk, i.e. the myocardium that is ischemically jeopardized and at risk to become necrotic (Aletras et al. 2006; Friedrich 2010) (see Sect. 5.1.1).

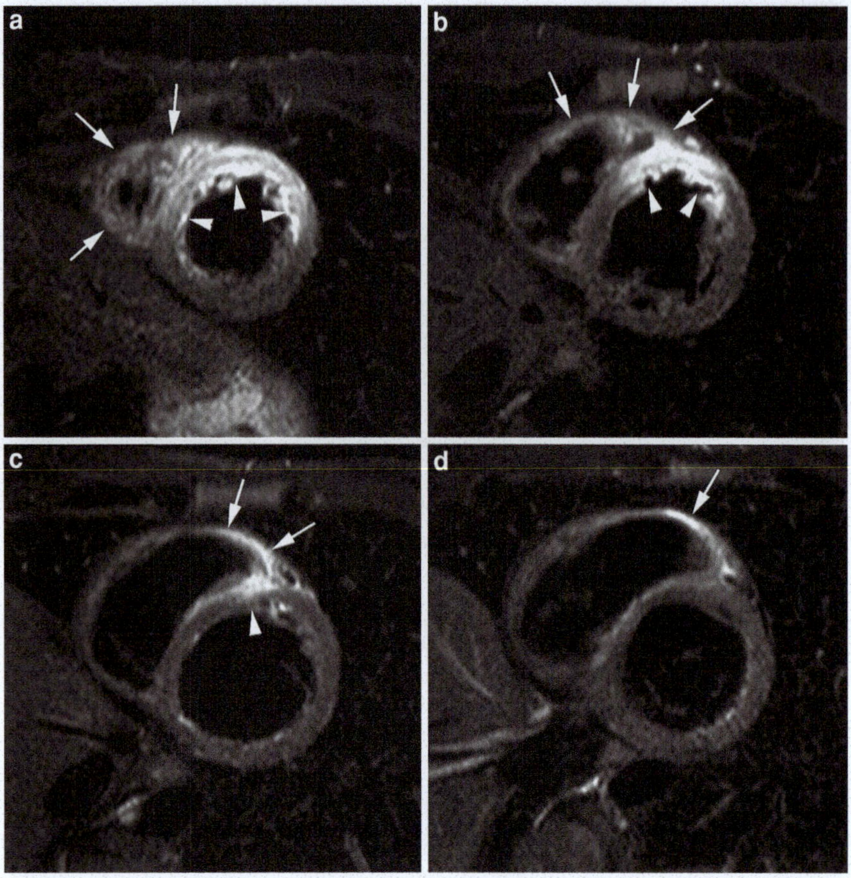

Fig. 7 Edema imaging in a patient with a reperfused acute anteroseptal myocardial infarction (day 3 post MI). Short-axis T2w-imaging at 4 levels (**a–d**). The jeopardized, edematous myocardium is visible as the myocardium showing increased signal intensity (*arrowheads*, **a–c**). Note the extension of the edema towards the adjacent RV anterior wall (*arrows*, **a–d**)

Abnormalities are most evident in the acute and subacute phases of infarction and slowly fade away due to processes of infarct healing with scar formation and resorption of infarct-related myocardial edema and inflammation (Carlson et al. 2009). Healed infarcts, because of the lower water content in the fibrotic scar may have decreased signal intensity compared with adjacent normal myocardium (McNamara et al. 1986). Thus, in addition T2w-imaging distinguishes between a recent and a healed MI (Abdel-Aty et al. 2004, 2009). It should be emphasized, however, that other conditions such as acute myocarditis or transplant rejection may present equally focal or diffuse myocardial edema (Marie et al. 2001; Yelgec et al. 2007).

Currently, segmented T2-weighted fast spin-echo sequences, equipped with inversion pulses to null the signal of fat and blood (T2-weighted short-inversion-time inversion-recovery (T2w-STIR) MRI) ("*triple inversion-recovery sequences*"), are most commonly used for this purpose, and have dramatically improved image quality compared to the older non-breath hold T2-weighted SE sequences (Simonetti et al. 1996) (Fig. 7). T2w-imaging, however, is prone to several problems, including variability in signal intensity caused by phased array coils, improper timing issues causing signal loss in the posterior wall, high signal from slow flowing blood adjacent to the jeopardized myocardium that can mimic and mask adjacent myocardial edema in the subendocardium, motion artifacts, and subjective nature of image interpretation of T2w sequences (Aletras et al. 2008; Giri et al. 2009). Surface coil correction algorithms are important to correct signal intensity for distance to surface coil. To reduce interpretation bias, a lower limit of signal intensity 2SD > signal intensity of remote myocardium is generally used to define myocardial edema. Novel, more robust sequences for edema imaging of the heart using the T2 prepared SSFP or hybrid TSE-SSFP sequence approach have been recently proposed (Kellman et al. 2007; Aletras et al. 2008), but are yet not widely available. An alternative approach to T2w-imaging is to directly quantify the T2 of the myocardium (Huang et al. 2007; Giri et al. 2009). Advantages of using a quantitative T2-mapping are the minimization of artifacts associated with T2w-imaging, image contrast less dependent on user-defined parameter setting, and a less subjective interpretation (Giri et al. 2009). Moreover, subtle T2 differences may be more easily detected. Blume et al. proposed an interleaved T1 and T2 relaxation time mapping for necrosis and edema detection (Blume et al. 2009). T2-values for normal myocardium typically range between 50 and 55 ms on a 1.5T scanner (Giri et al. 2009).

Finally, it was found that a considerable number of acute MI patients does not show homogeneous bright signal on T2w-imaging in the jeopardized myocardium, but instead show a central hypo-intense zone. The latter is related to the breakdown of hemoglobin into deoxy-hemoglobin causing shortening of T2-relaxation times (Lotan et al. 1990, 1992; Basso et al. 2007). Thus, besides depiction of myocardial edema, T2w-imaging can be used to noninvasively visualize the presence of post-reperfusion myocardial hemorrhage (see 5.2.4).

3.4 Contrast Enhanced MRI

3.4.1 MRI Contrast Agents for IHD Imaging

Over the past 30 years, many groups have focused on the development and use of MRI contrast agents for MI detection. Historically, the first agent evaluated for this purpose was manganese (Mn^{2+}) (Lauterbur et al. 1978; Brady et al. 1982). Manganese is taken up only in viable myocardial cells and thus has characteristics similar to those of thallium. It shortens T1 relaxation time (and to a much lesser extent also T2 relaxation time). Using T1-weighted sequences normal myocardium appears bright, while signal in infarcted myocardium remains nearly unchanged, and therefore appears dark relative to the viable myocardium. Manganese-DPDP can be used to delineate the jeopardized, ischemic myocardium during coronary artery occlusion, to differentiate between occlusive and reperfused infarcts, and to improve infarct detection (Pomeroy et al. 1989; Saeed et al. 1989; Bremerich et al. 2000, Flacke et al. 2003). However, due to unacceptable cardiotoxic effects, manganese is not yet approved for clinical cardiac imaging (Wolf and Baum 1983).

Since the mid 1980s, the paramagnetic gadolinium-chelated contrast agents, mainly Gd-diethylenetriamine pentaacetic acid (DPTA), useful for examination of brain tumors, have extensively been evaluated for MI imaging in both the acute and chronic setting (Wesbey et al. 1984; McNamara et al. 1986; de Roos et al. 1988, 1989) (see "MR Contrast Agents for Cardiac Imaging" for an extensive reading). This relatively small molecule with predominant T1-shortening features at low doses, rapidly diffuses from the intravascular into the interstitial space following intravenous injection, and is rapidly eliminated by renal clearance. Due to differences in pharmacokinetics and distribution volume between normal and infarcted/scarred myocardium, the latter appears bright (Fig. 8). It is currently the only group of paramagnetic contrast agents that is routinely used for cardiac imaging (licensed/FDA approved). Although a vast number of scientific studies have convincingly shown the added value of contrast-enhanced MRI to study a variety of cardiac diseases, gadolinium contrast agents are not infarct-specific. As such, myocardial enhancement is aspecific, but the location and pattern enhancement add important information regarding the underlying etiology (Mahrholdt et al. 2005). Information obtained with other MRI sequences, e.g., edema imaging, may add in the diagnosis and differential diagnosis. Because of lack of specificity of gadolinium contrast agents, several groups have sought for infarct-specific contrast agents. Phosphonate-modified gadolinium (Gd)-DTPA with high affinity for calcium-rich tissues, and antimyosin-antibody labeled contrast agents have been proposed (Weissleder et al. 1992; Adzamli et al. 1993), but have been excluded for clinical use to date because of unacceptable side effects. Porphyrin-based contrast agents, initially developed as "tumor-seeking" agents, have been extensively validated for acute infarct imaging (Ni et al. 1995, 1997, 1998; Herijgers et al. 1997; Pislaru et al. 1999; Saeed et al. 1999, 2001). Although the precise mechanism is unclear, strong and prolonged accumulation is found in necrotic myocardial tissue, showing a perfect match with histochemical TTC staining (Figs. 9 and 10). Unfortunately because of the inherent photosensitizing properties, neurotoxic and hepatotoxic side effects, these agents have currently found no access yet toward clinical applications.

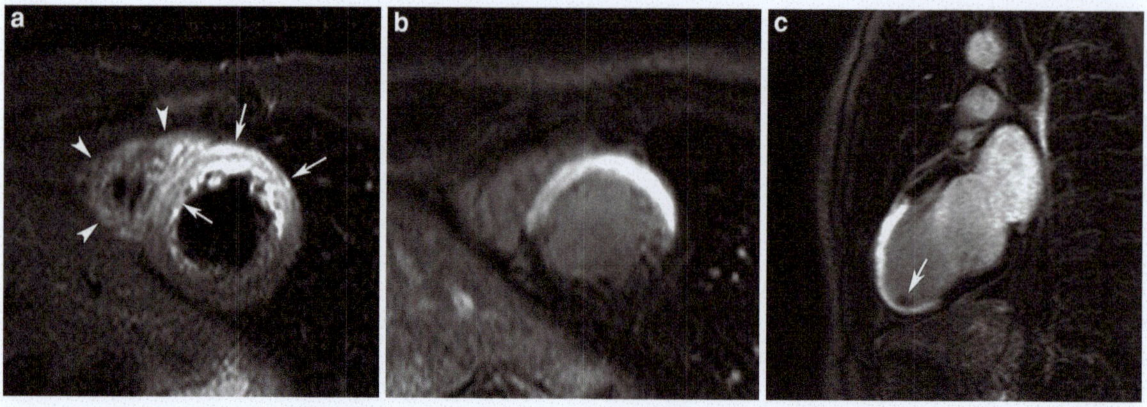

Fig. 8 Combined edema imaging and late Gd imaging in a patient with a reperfused anteroseptal myocardial infarction (same patient as in Fig. 7). Short-axis T2w-imaging (**a**), and late Gd imaging in short-axis (**b**) and vertical long-axis plane (**c**). While the extent of edema can be well appreciated on T2w-imaging (*arrows/arrowheads*, **a**), there is strong transmural enhancement on late Gd imaging (**b**) of the LV anteroseptal wall nicely corresponding to the area of edema. The involvement of the LV apex can be well appreciated on the vertical long-axis view (**c**). Note the presence of a small thrombus in the LV apex (*arrow*, **c**). In contrast to the extent of edema toward the right ventricle (*arrowheads*, **a**), there is no evidence of late enhancement of the RV free wall

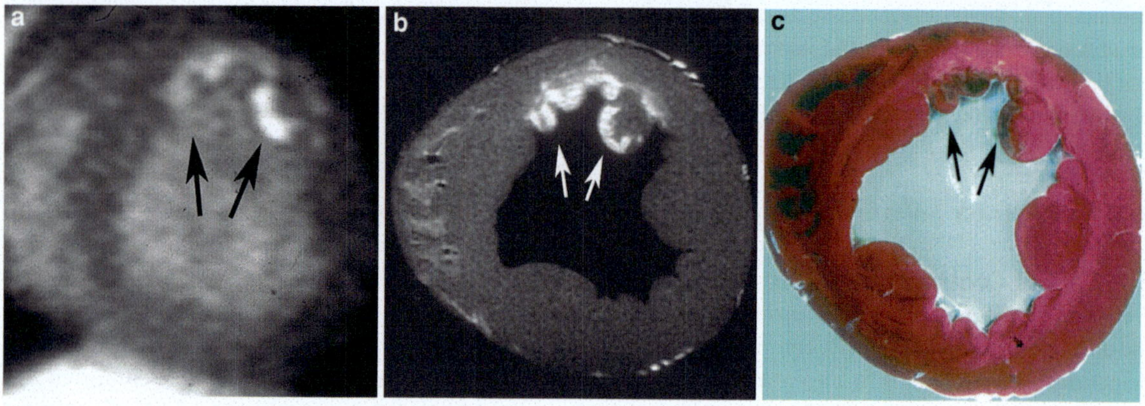

Fig. 9 Infarct specificity of a necrosis-avid contrast agent in an experimental animal model. In this model, the LAD coronary artery was reperfused after 90 min of occlusion. In vivo T1-weighted gradient echo image (**a**) showing subendocardial enhancement in the anterior LV wall and the anterior papillary muscle after intravenous administration of 0.05 mmol/kg gadolinium-bis-mesoporphyrin (*arrows*, **a**). The corresponding ex vivo T1-weighted spin-echo image (**b**) and the post-mortem TTC-stained specimen (**c**) shows clear correlation towards infarct size and necrosis distribution (*arrows*, **b**, **c**). Courtesy of Prof. Dr. Y. Ni. UZ Leuven, Leuven, Belgium

3.4.2 Contrast Enhanced MRI in Acute Myocardial Infarction

Any discussion regarding imaging of MI (and related issues such as quantification of infarct size, transmurality, etc.), should be made taking into account the complexity of events in evolving and established myocardial infarctions intermingled with reparative mechanisms that initiate very early after onset of MI and ultimately finish with a completely healed, stiff fibrotic scar (Reimer and Jennings 1979; Thygesen et al. 2007). These dynamic, ongoing processes of necrosis, edema, inflammation and tissue repair are difficult to control, and may explain some discrepancies in reported study findings.

There is irrefutable evidence that administration of extracellular Gd-based contrast agents in acute MI results in a time-varying infarct enhancement, which is different from normal myocardium (Fig. 11). Several factors, however, contribute to the "observed" myocardial enhancement. Basically, these can be divided into infarct-related (pathophysiological and histopathological) factors, contrast

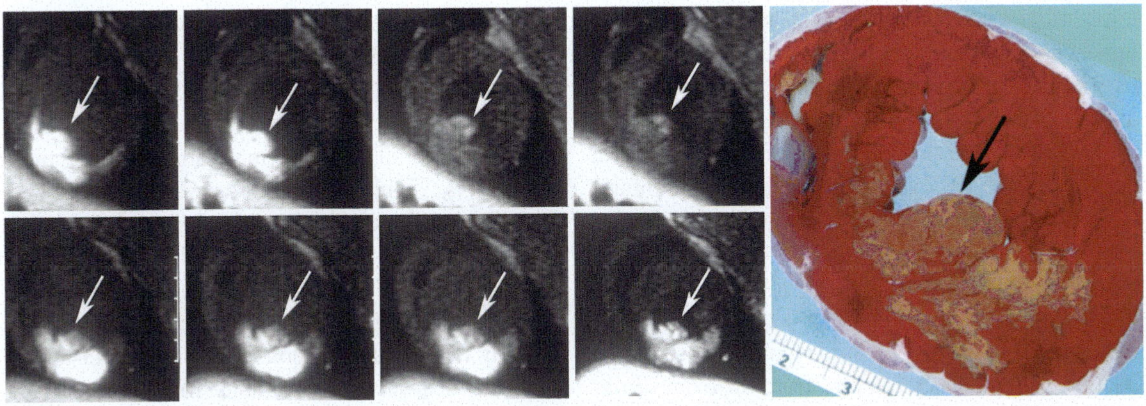

Fig. 10 Comparison of non-specific (*top row*) and an infarct-specific contrast agent (*bottom row*) in an animal model with large induced inferior wall infarction including the posterior papillary muscle. *Top row* from *left* to *right*: short-axis late Gd images taken 30 min, 1, 2, and 3 h after administration of Gd-DTPA (0.1 mmol/kg) show progressive wash-out of the agent from the infarction. *Bottom row*: corresponding images at identical time points after injection of 0.05 mmol/kg gadolinium-bis-mesoporphyrin show constant appearance of the enhanced infarction volume. Postmortem TTC-stained specimen confirms the presence of an inferior infarction (*arrow*, *right panel*). Courtesy of Prof. Dr. Y. Ni. UZ Leuven, Leuven, Belgium

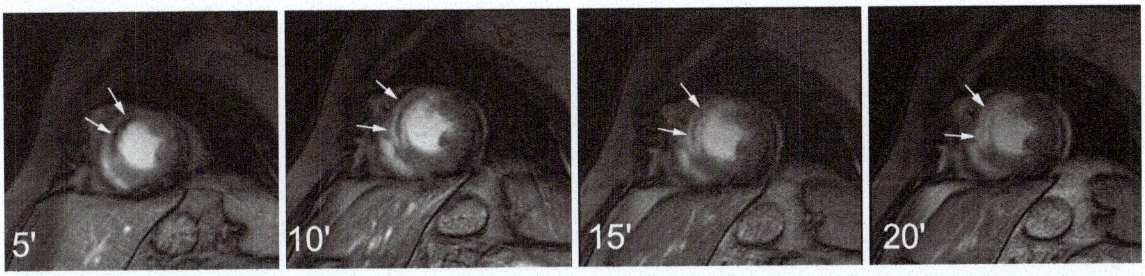

Fig. 11 Changes over time in the infarcted myocardium in a patient with an acute transmural anteroseptal myocardial infarction using contrast-enhanced MRI (early/late Gd imaging). At 5 min post-contrast administration an area of microvascular obstruction (*arrows*) is well visible. Fill-in of the no-reflow zone at later imaging with sharp demarcation of the infarcted myocardium (*arrows*)

agent-related, and MR sequence-related issues. The condition of the blood supply toward the infarcted region, patency of the microvasculature, distribution volume, impaired or delayed clearance in the infarcted area, and size and depth of the myocardial infarction can be considered as infarct-related factors (Kim et al. 1996). The above factors may either increase and/or decrease Gd-concentration in the infarcted myocardium. Early after reperfusion, the hyperemic response in the reperfused myocardium results in an increased delivery toward and thus in higher gadolinium concentrations in the jeopardized myocardium as compared to normal myocardium (Schaefer et al. 1988). The supply of contrast agent to the infarcted region is dependent on the patency of the infarct-related artery, presence of collaterals to the jeopardized myocardium and patency of the microcirculation in the infarcted myocardium. The myocardial distribution volume may increase due to interstitial edema (increased capillary permeability—inflammatory repair) and/or disruption of the myocyte membrane after prolonged ischemia, allowing intracellular diffusion of the contrast agent (Arheden et al. 1999; Flacke et al. 2001; Klein et al. 2007; Ibrahim et al. 2010).

An unresolved issue still causing a lot of controversy, is whether myocardial enhancement within the jeopardized myocardium exclusively reflects irreversible damaged myocardium, or whether ischemically injured but potentially viable myocardium in the peripheral rim of the infarct or in ischemic myocardium without infarction may enhance as well on post-contrast administration. One group of experts advocates the first hypothesis (Kim et al. 1999; Rehwald et al. 2002), while others are in favor of a slight but significant overestimation of the true infarct size (Schaefer et al. 1988, 1999; Judd et al. 1995b; Arheden et al. 1999; Saeed et al. 2001; Engblom et al. 2009; Ibrahim et al. 2010). Since wash-in and wash-out of contrast are dynamic processes, timing of imaging post-contrast administration is crucial (Oshinski et al. 2001), ranging from an overestimation immediately (i.e, first 5 min post-contrast administration), to an underestimation at late imaging. The optimal time window for infarct imaging should be somewhere between 10 and 25 min post-contrast administration. Because of the delayed or late period of imaging, this kind of imaging is called in the literature: delayed (gadolinium) (DE/DGE) or late (gadolinium) enhancement (LE/LGE). For simplicity we use *late Gd MRI* (or *late Gd imaging*) in contrast to *early Gd imaging* which is generally used to depict MVO (see Fig. 12). In addition, optimal time of imaging seems to vary with length of occlusion. Moreover, the extent of enhancement is significantly influenced by the time between onset of infarct and the time of imaging. Kim et al demonstrated an overestimation of infarct size at 3 days post-infarction, disappearing when studies were repeated at 8 weeks (Kim et al. 1999). Although this can be explained by volume loss due to infarct shrinkage (up to four-fold decrease between 4 days and 6 weeks post-infarction (Reimer and Jennings 1979) two recent studies showed a significant decrease in the extent of enhancement between day 1 and day 7 post-infarction, suggesting an overestimation of the extent of irreversible damage at very early imaging (day 1), and emphasizing the need to underscore the impact of timing of imaging on infarct sizing early after acute MI (Engblom et al. 2009; Ibrahim et al. 2010). Finally, as mentioned above myocardial enhancement is aspecific but the pattern and location of enhancement add important information regarding the underlying etiology, enabling to differentiate acute MI from other entities such as acute myocarditis. In addition information obtained with other MRI sequences, e.g., edema imaging, are helpful in further refining the diagnosis, for instance to differentiate between an acute and chronic nature of an infarction.

To summarize, contrast-enhanced imaging (for MRI sequences details see Sect. 3.4.4) is a robust, well-validated and accurate tool to depict myocardial necrosis in the acute setting of MI. Following administration of contrast material, infarcted myocardium is visible as a time-varying enhancement distinguishable from normal myocardium. One should, however, comprehend that extracellular contrast agents are aspecific and non-avid for myocardial necrosis. Moreover, contrast-enhanced imaging is also advantageous to depict infarct-related abnormalities such as thrombus formation or pericarditis (Mollet et al. 2002; Taylor et al. 2006).

3.4.3 Contrast Enhanced MRI in Healed Myocardial Infarction

Although initially a few studies claimed that chronic or healed myocardial infarcts did not enhance post contrast administration (Eichstaedt et al. 1986; Nishimura et al. 1989; van Dijkman et al. 1991), these findings have been contradicted by several other studies, invariably showing that in patients with stable CAD, myocardial enhancement in areas of dysfunctional myocardium corresponds closely to fixed defects on thallium SPECT, and areas of flow-metabolism matched defects on FDG-PET scans, histologically representing scarred or fibrotic tissue (Fedele et al. 1994; Ramani et al. 1998; Klein et al. 2002; Wagner et al. 2003; Kühl et al. 2003; Knuesel et al. 2003) (Fig. 13). Moreover, the reproducibility of late Gd MRI in patients with healed myocardial infarctions is excellent (Mahrholdt et al. 2002) (Fig. 14). This technique is nowadays routinely used to depict infarct-related myocardial scarring, is helpful to differentiate dilated cardiomyopathy from LV dysfunction related to CAD (McCrohon et al. 2003), to predict functional recovery post-coronary revascularization (Kim et al. 2000) and has prognostic significance (Cheong et al. 2009)

The exact mechanism of increased myocardial enhancement in chronic myocardial scar remains incompletely understood. Likely explanations are differences in wash-in and wash-out contrast kinetics, differences in distribution volume between scarred and normal myocardium. In healed MI, fibrotic scar tissue, mainly consisting of collagen, increases the interstitial space per unit volume, causing gadolinium agents to diffuse rapidly into the interstitial, but not the intracellular space (Lima et al. 1995).

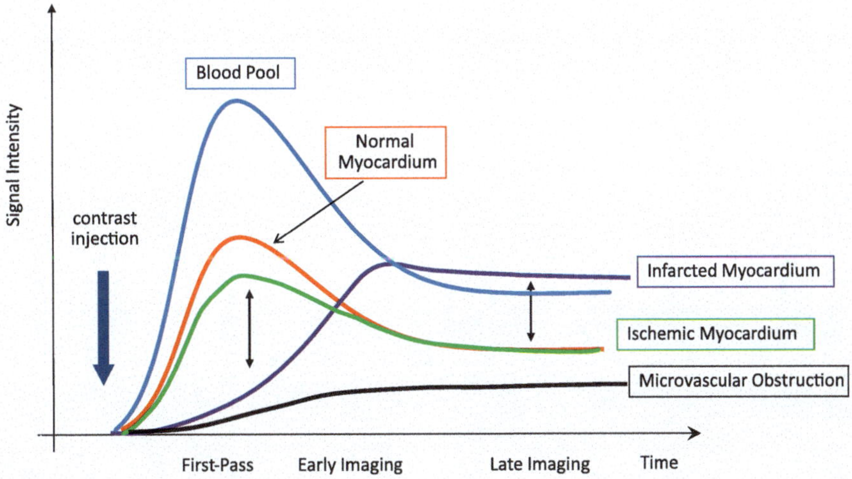

Fig. 12 Time-varying signal intensity changes in the blood pool, and in the normal and pathological myocardium following contrast administration in a patient with acute myocardial infarction. Normal myocardium is characterized by a rapid wash-in and wash-out of contrast, while signal intensity infarcted myocardium progressively increases. Microvascular obstruction is characterized by lack of signal and slow decrease in extent over time

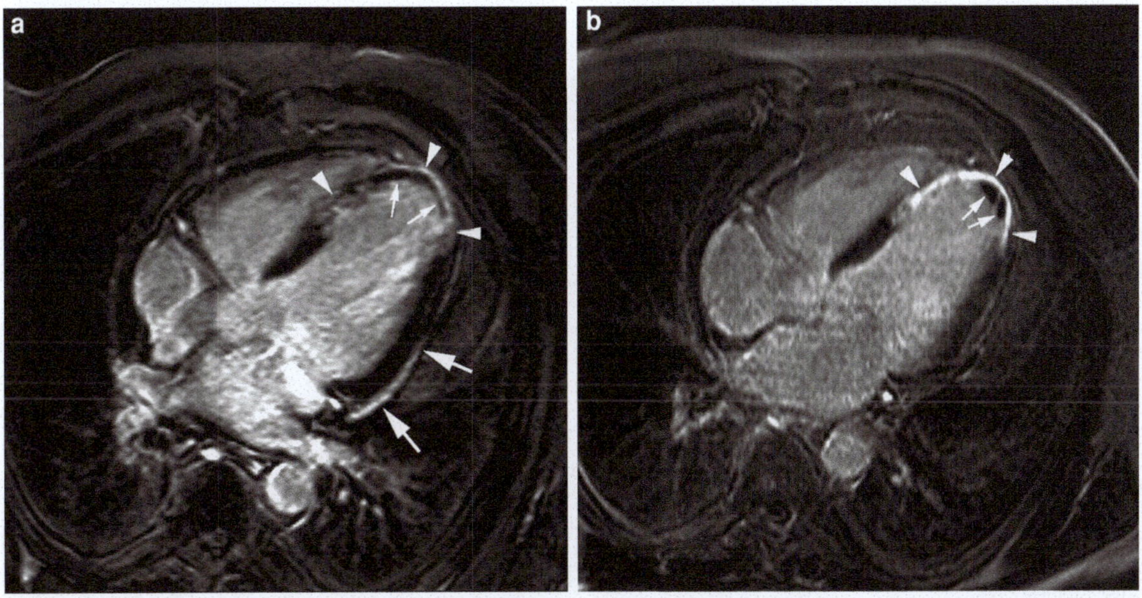

Fig. 13 Evolution of an acute towards a healed myocardial infarction in a 52-year-old patient with anteroapical infarction. Late Gd imaging in horizontal image plane at 1 week (**a**) and 4 months (**b**) after the acute event. At 1 week, presence of diffuse enhancement of the apical part of the ventricular septum and LV apex (*arrowheads*, **a**) with large area of microvascular obstruction (*small arrows*, **a**). Note the presence of some pericardial enhancement over the laterobasal part of the LV (*arrows*, **a**). At 4-month follow-up, the infarct has thinned and strongly enhances (*arrowheads*, **b**). Note the presence of a small mural thrombus in LV apex (*arrows*, **b**)

3.4.4 Choosing the Ideal Approach for Contrast Enhanced MRI

Since the initial observations that ischemically injured myocardium could be differentiated from normal myocardial tissue with MRI, numerous studies have been performed using a variety of pulse sequences (Rehr et al. 1986; Tscholakoff et al. 1986; Lima et al. 1995; Judd et al. 1995a, b; de Roos et al. 1989). Although in these studies, significant differences between the increased signal intensity of infarcted

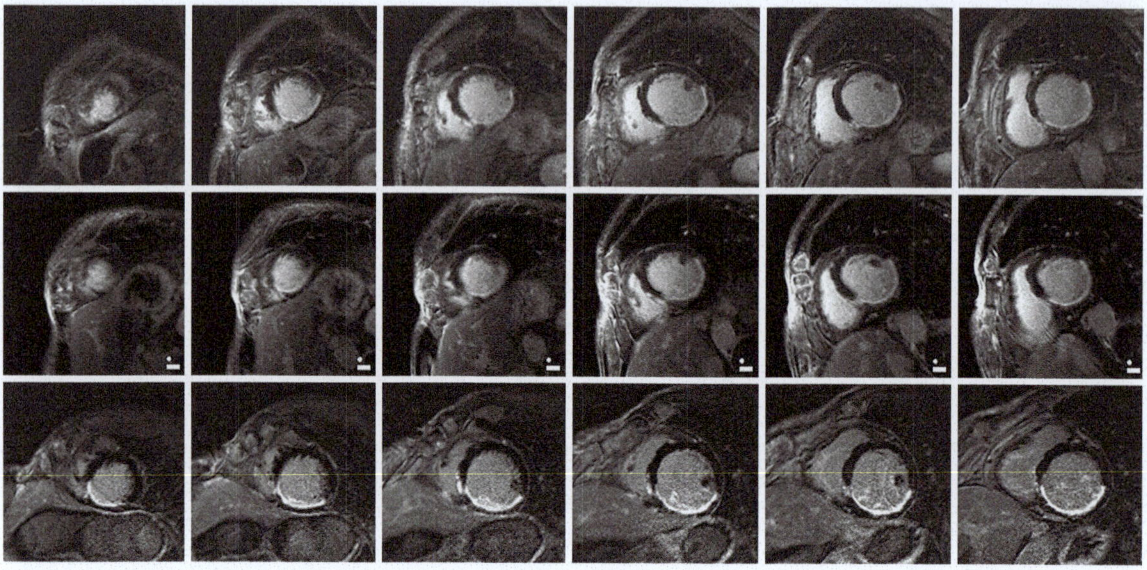

Fig. 14 Reproducibility of late Gd imaging. Three series of short-axis late Gd images obtained in a 63-year-old patient with known healed myocardial infarction. The first study (*top row*) shows a large transmural inferolateral infarction. Follow-up studies performed 3 and 5 months later (*middle* and *bottom row*, respectively) show near identical findings

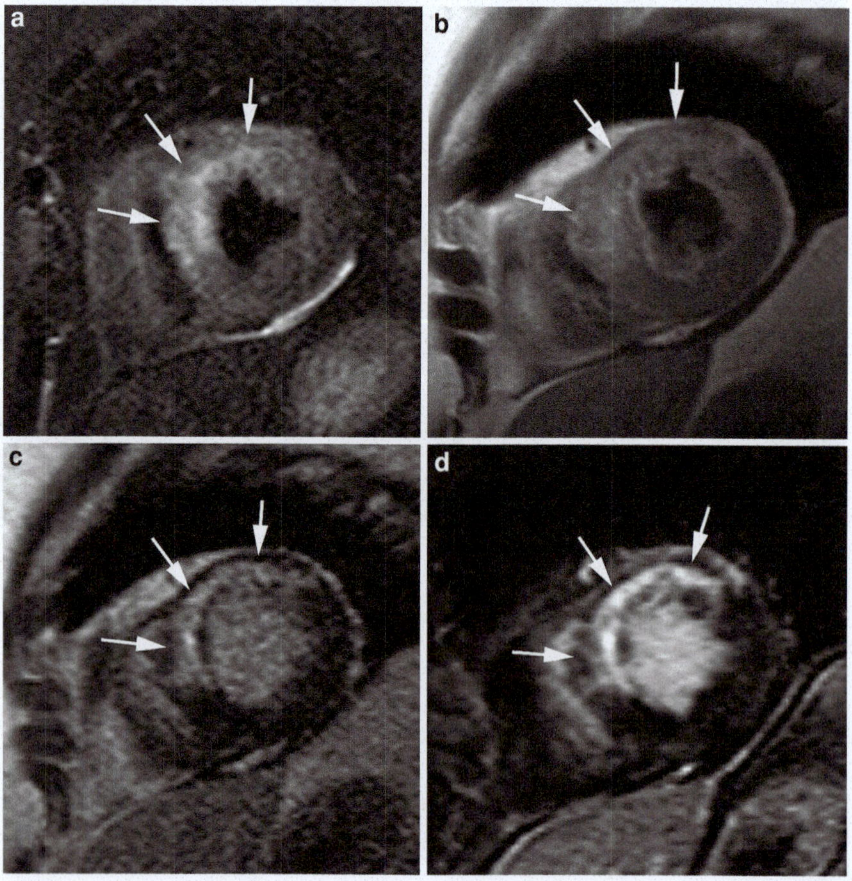

Fig. 15 Choice of imaging sequence for infarct imaging. 59-year-old patient with acute anteroseptal myocardial infarction (*arrows*) imaged by T2w-imaging (**a**), T1w-imaging using fast spin-echo (**b**), two-dimensional late Gd imaging (**c**) and three-dimensional late Gd imaging (**d**). Note the huge increase in contrast difference between normal and infarcted myocardium stepping over from T1w-imaging using fast spin-echo to late Gd imaging. Furthermore, 3D has the benefit over 2D techniques of the intrinisic higher signal-to-noise ratio

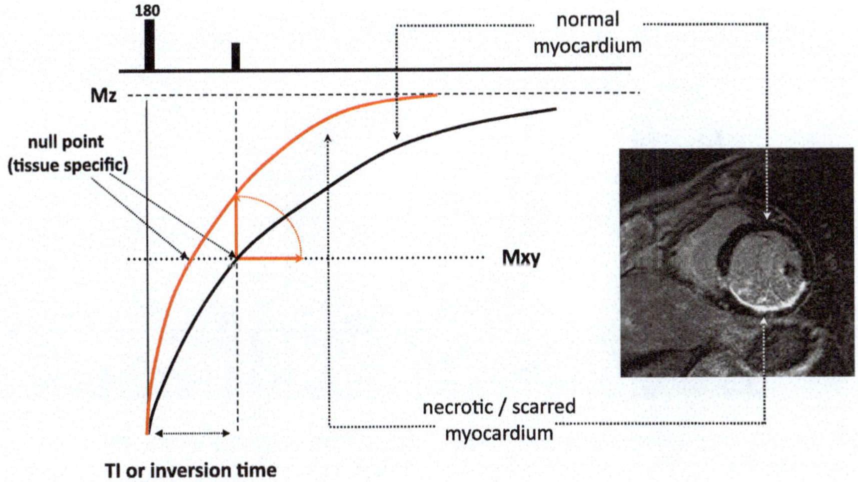

Fig. 16 Inversion-recovery gradient-echo sequence providing strong T1-weighting. By adding an inversion pulse (180°) and use of an appropriate inversion time (TI), the contrast between normal (*shown in dark*) and necrotic/fibrotic myocardium (*shown in white*) can be substantially increased compared to conventional MRI sequences (see also 15)

myocardium and normal myocardium were reported, more robust techniques with improved differential contrast between normal and pathological tissue were needed for routine use in the clinical setting (Fig. 15).

Over the previous years, the scales have tipped in favor of using gradient-echo sequences, a trend that was probably initiated by a paper from Edelman et al., describing a segmented T1-weighted gradient echo sequence, originally intended to be used for liver imaging without contrast agents (Edelman et al. 1990). This sequence produces strongly T1-weighted images owing to the use of an inversion pulse before image acquisition (Fig. 16). Segmentation of the acquisition generates images that are more strongly dependent on the inversion recovery of magnetization than are single-shot sequences. This technique was further optimized by Simonetti et al. for use in cardiac imaging, synchronizing the acquisition to mid-diastole for motion free imaging, and using gradient-moment refocusing to reduce motion artifacts (Simonetti et al. 2001). Most importantly, choosing the appropriate length of the inversion time (TI), the signal of normal myocardium could be nullified, resulting in a ten-fold improvement in contrast between infarcted and normal myocardium in comparison to previously used techniques. This sequence has rapidly become the standard sequence for both early and late Gd imaging. A major benefit is the high spatial resolution (e.g., 1.4 × 1.9 × 6.0 mm), which is up to 60 times greater than what is currently achievable with SPECT. As a result, late Gd MRI has been shown to be superior in detecting subendocardial infarcts that are systemically missed by SPECT (Wagner et al. 2003; Ibrahim et al. 2007). The lower limit for depicting infarcted myocardial tissue by late Gd imaging is estimated at 1 g versus 10 g for SPECT imaging, thus allowing to depict minimal myocardial damage for example, papillary muscle necrosis or peri-procedural myocardial damage (Porto et al. 2006; Larose 2006; Di Bella et al. 2008) (Fig. 17).

Since administration of a contrast agent is essential for appropriate infarct imaging, a crucial issue is dose ranging (Kim et al. 2003). In most animal and patient studies, a dose of 0.2 mmol of contrast agent per kilogram of body weight has been used. Moreover, in a recent multicenter study including 566 patients with acute or healed MI, a dose ≥0.2 mmol of gadoversetamide/kg yielded the highest sensitivity for infarct detection (Kim et al. 2008). Although it is clear that too low doses (<0.1 mmol/kg) result in a brief and insufficient infarct enhancement, the above results should be put in perspective. Increasing the dose of contrast agent not only increases the cost and the risk for rare side effects such as nephrogenic systemic fibrosis in those with severe renal impairment, but also the brighter blood pool using higher contrast doses may obscure subendocardial infarcts. Therefore, there is a trend towards use of a lower dose (e.g., 0.15 mmol/kg of body weight), which may be a better compromise for clinical use on a 1.5 T MR

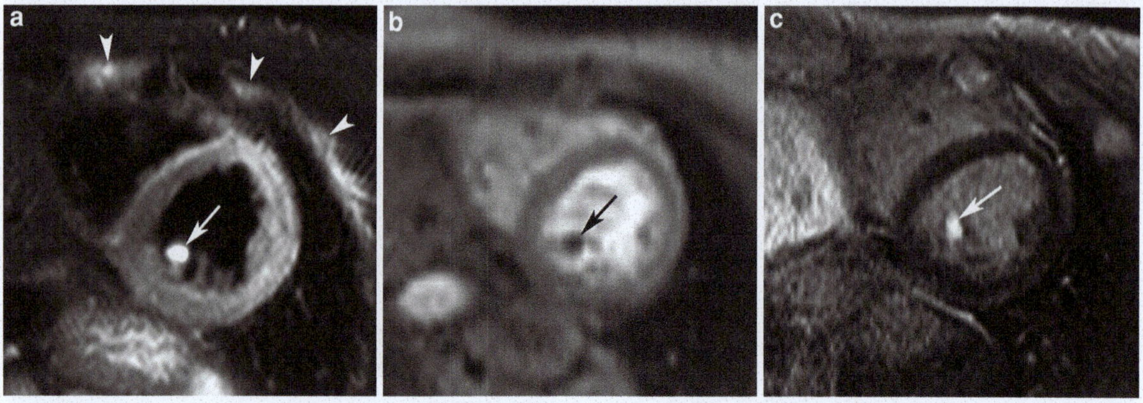

Fig. 17 Infarction of the inferior papillary muscle in a patient who received cardiac resuscitation following sudden cardiac arrest. Short-axis T2w-imaging (**a**), first pass perfusion MRI (**b**) and late Gd imaging (**c**). T2w-imaging shows edema of the inferior papillary muscle (*arrow*, **a**) and edema in the anterior chest wall due to cardiac massage. MPI-MR shows perfusion defect of the inferior papillary muscle while strong enhancement is found at late Gd imaging (*arrow*, **b**, **c**). This example nicely shows the capability of current MRI techniques to depict subtle myocardial abnormalities. (Adapted from Di Bella et al. 2008)

unit. Use of contrast agents with higher T1-relaxivity (e.g Gd-BOPTA) at 0.1 mmol/kg or with higher osmolarity (e.g., gadobutrol) are other appealing alternatives (Tumkosit et al. 2009).

For MI imaging, the goal is to maximize the signal intensity ratio between normal and infarcted myocardium, which can be achieved by choosing the inversion delay that exactly nullifies the signal of normal myocardium (or in other words the time at which the magnetization of normal myocardium crosses the line of zero longitudinal magnetization). This optimal inversion time (TI) is, however, not a fixed value, but is determined by several factors, including amount of contrast administered, time between contrast administration and imaging, infarct characteristics, cardiac output, renal clearance, patient's size etc. As a consequence of renal clearance, the Gd-concentration of blood and myocardium gradually decreases (and vice versa the T1-relaxation increases) necessitating constant adjustment (i.e., prolongation) of the TI in order to keep the normal myocardium optimally suppressed. This can be achieved by using a TI scout or Look-Locker sequence (Look and Locker 1970; Scheffler and Hennig 2001), whereby a series of images with varying TIs are obtained, easily allowing to choose the optimal TI for subsequent infarct imaging. Although an experienced user can estimate the TI-value reasonably well on the basis of the patient's size, the amount of contrast agent administered, and the time after contrast agent injection, the technique still leaves quite a large margin for error. For images acquired 5–20 min after administration of 0.2 mmol/kg contrast material, TI values typically vary between 200 and 250 ms for early images, to 250–300 ms for late images (Fig. 18). An inappropriate choice of TI results in loss of contrast between normal and infarcted myocardium, which can cause an underestimation of the extent of infarction, and may introduce specific image artifacts (Kim et al. 2003; Stuber et al. 2005) (see Sect. 3.4.5). Since the early reports on the use of contrast enhanced MRI for imaging acute MI, it was shown that a considerable number of patients showed a central dark core in the enhanced myocardium corresponding to an area of MVO (de Roos et al. 1989) (see Sect. 5.2.3). For an optimal evaluation of the incidence and extent of MVO, imaging should be performed as soon as possible following myocardial contrast enhancement, i.e., early Gd imaging is required. Use of a long TI, in the order of 550–600 ms, may furthermore improve MVO visualization, because with these long inversion times differentiation between normal myocardium and MVO is facilitated (Bekkers et al. 2009, 2010). Nowadays 2D or 3D late Gd imaging sequences are available for MI imaging. Whereas 3D volumes offer the obvious advantage of acquiring the complete cardiac volume in a single breath-hold, 2D sequences seem to suffer less from motion blurring and partial volume effects (Kühl et al. 2004).

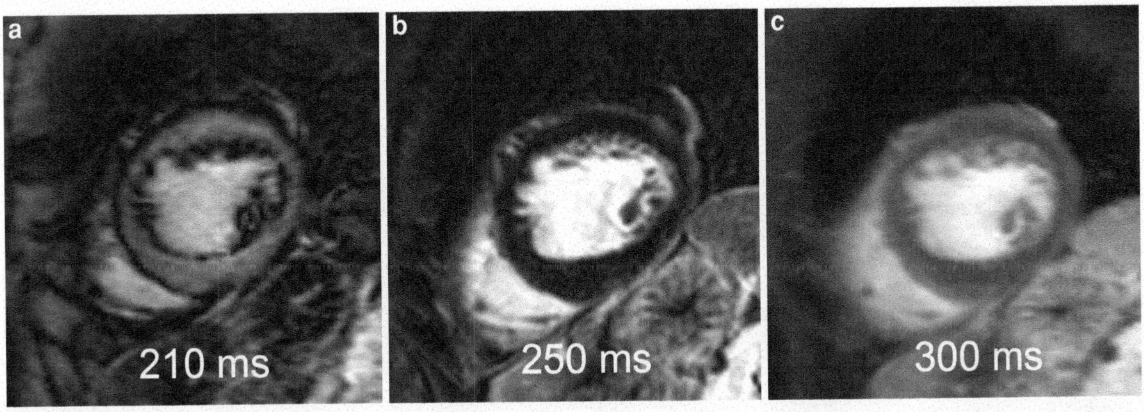

Fig. 18 Impact of inversion time on late Gd image quality. Short-axis images obtained 12–14 min after injection of 0.2 mmol/kg Gd-DTPA using a variable inversion time, i.e. 210 ms (**a**), 250 ms (**b**), and 300 ms (**c**). Using a too short inversion time (**a**), typically yields a myocardium presenting gray in the mid-wall section with hypointense epi- and endocardial borders. Using a too long inversion time produces prolonged recovery of magnetization with contrast loss, resulting in gray myocardium (**c**). A correctly chosen inversion time provides images with homogeneous dark myocardium (**b**)

An elegant approach, proposed by Kellman et al., to reduce the need to continuously adjust the TI in order to achieve a good signal intensity suppression of normal myocardium, is the 'phase sensitive image reconstruction' (PSIR) technique (Kellman et al. 2002) (Fig. 19). The PSIR sequence acquires a background phase map during the same acquisition of the image. This phase map is used to make a pixel map of the polarities inside the image after magnetization recovery and to provide background noise reduction (Kellman et al. 2004). This is in fact a measure on how the different tissues regain magnetization after inversion and can be used through complex reconstruction to obtain intensity normalized images in which the image level and window, and not the TI is used to maximize the contrast ratio. Therefore the inversion delay can be more arbitrarily chosen to a default or 'mean' value. Magnitude IR images underestimate infarct sizes using TI shorter than the optimum TI, PSIR images provide consistent image quality and infarct size determination independent of TI (Huber et al. 2005; Setser et al. 2005). Currently, multi-2D single breath-hold and respiratory-gated 3D PSIR late Gd MRI sequences have become available, significantly the reducing the acquisition time compared to the original 2D single plane PSIR sequence (Huber et al. 2007; Kino et al. 2009) (Fig. 19). This 3D sequence with a 1.9 × 1.9 × 2.0 mm^3 seemed particularly useful for detecting small atypical scars compared to the 2D approach.

Infarct imaging on 3.0 Tesla MR scanners is feasible, providing superior image quality compared with 1.5 Tesla. Using identical contrast doses, increased SNR and CNR values are found (Klumpp et al. 2006; Bauner et al. 2007). The PSIR technique is also available for 3.0 Tesla imaging providing higher CNR values than at 1.5T (Huber et al. 2006).

Another important issue is quantification of the extent of myocardial late enhancement in order to accurately determine the infarct size. In clinical practice, visual contouring the enhanced myocardium on the late Gd images is commonly used but tends to slightly overestimate the infarct volume and spatial extent (Hsu et al. 2006a). Semi-automated approaches such as using a number (e.g., 5–6) of standard deviations above the mean signal intensity of remote myocardium, or using the full-width at half maximum method, and computer algorithms provide a more objective approach for accurate and reproducible infarct sizing (Amado et al. 2004; Hsu et al. 2006a, b; Beek et al. 2009).

3.4.5 Optimizing Image Quality

In patient studies, image quality of late Gd MRI may be compromised by several factors. Since most sequences are acquired in breath-hold, duration and number of breath-hold periods may be at the upper limit of the patient's capability so that motion artifacts occur especially at the end of the study. On late Gd images, for example, motion-related

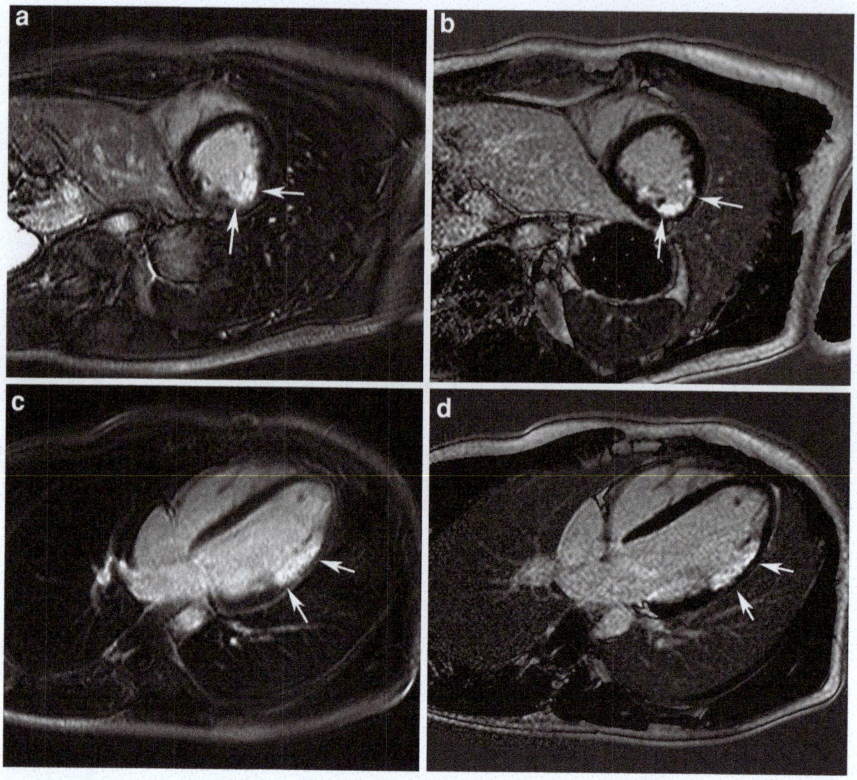

Fig. 19 Phase-sensitive image reconstruction (PSIR) technique in a patient with a healed myocardial infarction in mid lateral LV wall. Short-axis imaging (**a**, **b**), and horizontal long-axis (**c**, **d**) imaging using conventional three-dimensional late Gd imaging (**a**, **c**) and two-dimensional late Gd imaging using PSIR technique (**b**, **d**). The location as well as the transmural extent of late myocardial enhancement (*arrows*) and differentiation with non-enhanced myocardium is improved using the PSIR technique

hyperintense lines, may hamper differentiation with true myocardial enhancement. Following a few simple rules it is usually possible to determine whether they are artifact-related or not. Motion-related artifacts occur generally in phase-encoding direction. Thus, changing phase-encoding direction may be used to see whether it reoccurs. The most problematic are artifacts related to movement of the heart, for example, if the patient starts to breathe out at the end of the acquisition. This can create a cardiac-shaped overlay on the actual image and may hamper proper image analysis. If uncertainty exists about the nature of such an artifact, it is useful to realize that an artifact never respects anatomical borders and usually a contour can be found outside the heart, revealing the nature of this imaging finding. Long breath-holds can be avoided by performing measurements during free breathing using navigator gradients, or by decreasing the total acquisition time. This can be performed by decreasing the rectangular field of view, if the patient's size permits. Another valid alternative is the use of parallel imaging to decrease total acquisition time. Motion-related artifacts may also be caused by cardiac motion itself. Ideally, late Gd imaging should be performed during periods of low cardiac motion such as cardiac diastasis. However, in patients with high heart rates this period may be too short for 3D sequences obtained in a single breath-hold. In these cases it is advisable to use 2D sequences that have a shorter acquisition window, or use the free-breathing navigator approach.

As discussed above, determining the optimal TI for nulling of normal myocardium can be difficult. It must be done for each patient and for each time point after injection individually. Errors in selecting correct inversion delays may result in loss of contrast between normal and abnormal myocardium and introduce specific artifacts. Although PSIR techniques have become a valuable alternative, routine late Gd imaging is still frequently used in daily practice. Therefore, some practical guidelines may be of help in determining whether or not a late enhancement image can be considered as adequate (Fig. 18). If a correct inversion time is chosen, signal of normal myocardium should be close to zero and thus appear very dark on the late Gd images, the LV blood pool should be intermediately intense (white to gray-white) and a myocardial infarction or scar should be the most intense structure in the image. If this is not the case, the TI is likely not set correctly. The following artefacts may occur:

- If the blood pool appears too dark, the TI is likely too short and needs to be increased significantly to allow sufficient recovery. An increase of up to 50 ms may be necessary.
- If the TI is very close to the optimal inversion delay, but still too short, a speckled appearance (suppressed myocardium interspersed with non-suppressed white spots or lines) may occur, or the endo- and epicardial borders may appear dark with gray myocardium in between. Small increments in TI in steps of 10 ms, until optimal suppression of normal myocardium is attained, are advisable.
- If the area of late enhancement is gray and only slightly more intense than the myocardium or the blood, the TI is too long. A decrease in steps of 10 ms is advisable.
- On the other side of the spectrum, if there is no contrast between blood, myocardium and infarcted tissue (if present) and all structures appear to be too dark, this indicates either that the contrast has already washed out or an insufficient amount of contrast agent was injected.

An artifact that is often seen, especially in dilated ventricles resembles subendocardial enhancement in a ring-shaped distribution, and may cover the entire endocardial surface. Usually this 'pseudo-enhancement' is not confined to a coronary artery territory and can be a distant from the infarcted tissue. This artifact is most likely caused by slow flow in dilated ventricles or aneurysms or by trapping of contrast in between trabeculations. Very little can be done to avoid it, although it is less pronounced on images acquired later, e.g., 25 min, after contrast administration. Knowledge about the exact wall thickness, such as can be obtained from cine MRI may be of help to differentiate between true or pseudo-enhancement.

3.5 Myocardial Fat Imaging

Lipomatous metaplasia is a common finding occurring during infarct healing. It is found at autopsy in up to 84% of patients with LV myocardial scars associated with chronic IHD (Baroldi et al. 1997; Goldfarb et al. 2009). Contrast enhanced MRI permits to depict myocardial scar tissue but fails to depict lipomatous metaplasia. The multi-echo Dixon approach to water and fat suppression is currently likely the most appealing technique to depict lipomatous metaplasia in healed MI (Kellman et al. 2009; Goldfarb et al. 2009). Alternatively, the chemical shift occurring at the border zone between fat- and water-containing tissue using b-SSFP sequences (cine imaging) can be used to detect fat within the myocardium (Fig. 20) (Lücke et al. 2010).

4 Stable Coronary Artery Disease

Since in the majority of patients with presumptive symptoms of myocardial ischemia, CAD is the underlying cause, noninvasive imaging of obstructive CAD has become the topic of extensive research in the last decades. Imaging can be focused either on detection (or exclusion) of coronary artery plaques (and determination of plaque stenosis severity) (*'anatomic imaging'*), and/or assessment of the consequences of CAD on myocardial perfusion and function (*'ischemia imaging'*). It remains an issue of intense debate which one of the above approaches is to be recommended in decision making, a thorough description of the pros and cons is, therefore, beyond the scope of this chapter (Tonino et al. 2009; Gould 2009; Pfisterer et al. 2010). In brief, the value of several non or minimally invasive imaging techniques has been explored as substitute for catheter-based coronary angiography. Although in the 1990s, MRI was highly appealing for non invasive CAD detection, lengthy acquisition times and lack of robustness still hamper routine acquisition (see "Coronary Artery Disease"). In contrast, fast and accurate depiction of coronary artery plaques can be achieved nowadays with the newest generation of multi-detector computed tomography scanners with low to modest irradiation doses (Achenbach and Raggi 2010). Further reduction in radiation dose can be achieved with iterative reconstruction algorithms (Singh et al. 2011). Despite the current limited clinical value of MRI in coronary plaque detection, substantial progress has been made in myocardial ischemia assessment, making this technique an attractive and valuable alternative to stress echocardiography and radionuclide pharmacological stress perfusion imaging (e.g., SPECT imaging) for studying CAD patients. MRI has several advantages compared to the above techniques. No radioactive marker has to be injected

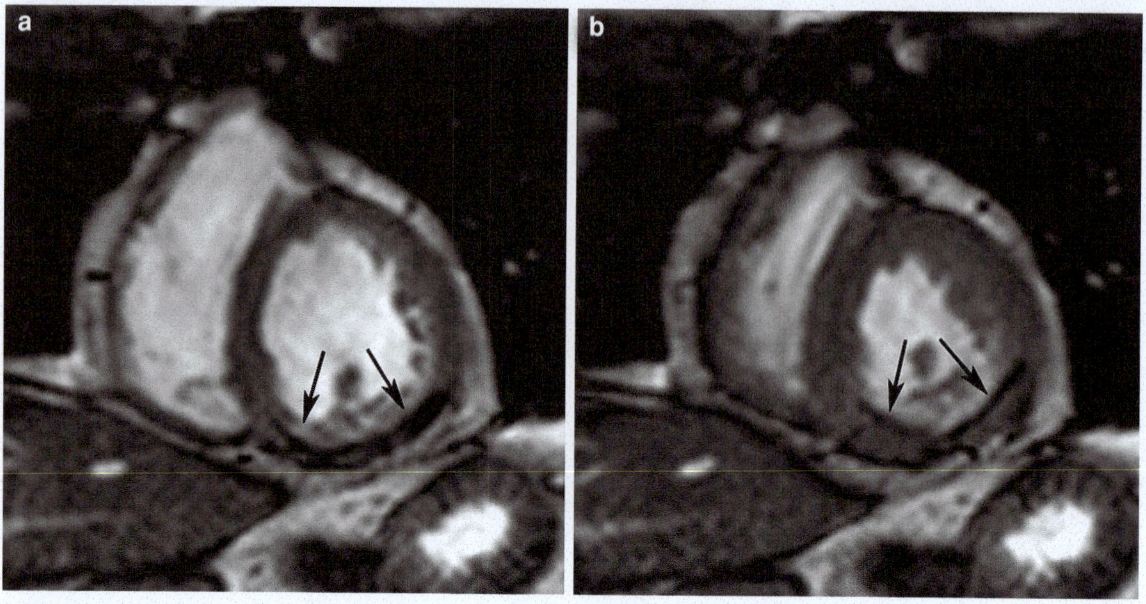

Fig. 20 Lipomatous metaplasia in a patient with a subendocardial inferior infarct. Short-axis cine imaging at end diastole (**a**) and end systole (**b**). Chemical shift occurs at the border between the fat- and water-containing tissue (*arrows*, **a**, **b**). Note the impaired contractility of the infarcted myocardium

to achieve similar information regarding myocardial perfusion defects, and the information can be obtained in a single exam not taking longer than 30–45 min. The superior spatial resolution of MRI permits to visualize smaller, subendocardially located, perfusion defects not infrequently missed by SPECT (Lee et al. 2004). The newest high-resolution perfusion MRI sequences with in-plane pixel resolution up to 1.1×1.1 mm^2 not only improve diagnostic accuracy but also allow assessment of RV perfusion (Plein et al. 2008a; Manka et al. 2010). Moreover, this technique is not hampered by soft-tissue and attenuation artifacts. Similar to PET scanning, quantitative data on myocardial blood supply can be achieved with myocardial perfusion MRI (Hsu et al. 2006c). Compared to stress echocardiography, MRI provides reliable image quality not limited by the adequacy of the acoustic window. Per stress level, images can be easily acquired in standardized (repeatable) planes, and easily compared on an offline workstation reducing operator-dependency. An added value of MRI is its comprehensive approach, meaning that stress imaging is part of a broader assessment of the CAD spectrum, for instance including edema imaging—necrosis/scar imaging—coronary artery imaging and functional imaging (Sensky et al. 2000; Plein et al. 2002, 2004; Foo et al. 2005; Bodi et al. 2005; Cury et al. 2006; Klem et al. 2006; Bingham and Hachamovitch 2011).

4.1 Stress Perfusion Imaging

Basically, rather than injecting a radioactive tracer to study the uptake in myocardial cells during rest and stress, MRI uses the first pass of an intravenously injected paramagnetic contrast agent during administration of a vasodilator (i.e. dipyridamole or adenosine) to depict hemodynamically significant coronary artery stenosis (Fig. 6) (see "Myocardial Perfusion"). At present this technique has been well validated (Wilke et al. 1997; Al-Saadi et al. 2000a, b; Schwitter et al. 2001; Nagel et al. 2003; Lee et al. 2004), showing similar or even better accuracy as compared to routinely used techniques such as SPECT imaging (Schwitter et al. 2008). In a meta-analysis by Nandalur et al. including 14 studies (1,516 patients), perfusion imaging demonstrated a sensitivity of 91% (CI 88–94%) and a specificity of 81% (CI 77–85%) (Nandalur et al. 2007). Although the disease prevalence was high (57.4%), questioning its value in populations with lower disease prevalence, it should be mentioned that also studies performed before 2000 using older MRI sequences were included in this meta-analysis. Whereas in daily clinical practice, stress-induced perfusion defects are usually visually assessed looking at the presence of subendocardial or transmural hypo-intense rim during the first-pass of contrast in one or more coronary artery perfusion territories semi-quantitative or quantitative approaches have become available slowly finding their way into the clinical practice. A relatively simple semi-quantitative method, used by several groups, is the assessment of the myocardial perfusion reserve (MPR) or MPR index in patients with CAD, which is defined as the ratio of regional myocardial blood flow under hyperemic conditions to that under resting conditions, and has been validated against other techniques such as coronary fractional flow reserve measurements (Wilke et al. 1997; Cullen et al. 1999; Al-Saadi et al., 2000a; Kurita et al. 2009; Watkins et al. 2009). Since it also takes into account the collateral flow, it may be a more accurate parameter than the coronary flow reserve to assess the impact of CAD on myocardial perfusion. Al-Saadi et al. found a significant difference in myocardial perfusion reserve between ischemic and normal myocardial segments (1.08 ± 0.23 and 2.33 ± 0.41, $P<0.001$, Fig. 10) (Al-Saadi et al. 2000a). Using a cut-off value of 1.5, the diagnostic sensitivity, specificity and diagnostic accuracy for the detection of coronary artery stenosis (≥75%) were 90, 83, and 87% respectively. In a similar study by Cullen et al., a negative correlation was found between the MPR index and percent coronary artery stenosis ($r = -0.81$, $P<0.01$) (Cullen et al. 1999). Using fractional flow reserve in addition to the degree of stenosis on coronary angiography as reference modality, an MPR index cut-off value of 1.5 was able to distinguish hemodynamically relevant from non-relevant coronary lesions with a sensitivity of 88% (CI 74–100%) and specificity of 90% (CI 84–96%) (Rieber et al. 2006). Watkins et al. using a similar study protocol reported a sensitivity and specificity of 91 and 94% respectively (Watkins et al. 2009). A somewhat higher MPR cut-off value to differentiate between flow and non-flow limiting stenosis was found by (Costa et al. 2007). After PCI with stent implantation or CABG surgery, a significant improvement in MPR index was reported, thus providing information about the success of interventional procedures in stenosed coronary arteries (Al-Saadi et al. 2000b; Fenchel et al. 2005). This improvement was more pronounced after stenting (Fig. 21). Klem et al. showed in patients without known obstructive CAD or prior MI that adding late Gd MRI for scar imaging to stress perfusion imaging, increases the test specificity and accuracy (Klem et al. 2006). Diagnostic accuracy of this combined protocol is lower in CABG patients compared to patients with suspected CAD or PCI patients (Bernhardt et al. 2009). Although most stress perfusion studies are performed at 1.5T, perfusion imaging at 3T is clinically feasible and intrinsically appealing because of the increase in signal to noise ratio (Cheng et al. 2007; Meyer et al. 2008). Finally, alternatives to first-pass perfusion imaging, such as use of myocardial blood oxygen level-dependent (BOLD) MRI, has recently shown to reliably detect stress-induced myocardial ischemia (Jahnke et al. 2010).

In patients with microvascular dysfunction ("cardiac syndrome X"), the exact role of stress perfusion MRI is not yet established. These patients present with typical anginal chest pain, and not infrequently have classic ST-segment depression on exercise testing but do show normal coronary arteries. Panting et al. reported typical subendocardial perfusion defects not respecting coronary artery perfusion territories in patients suspected of syndrome X during adenosine stress MRI, and the perfusion abnormalities were in the majority of patients associated with chest pain (Panting et al. 2002). These above findings were contradicted by a study by Vermeltfoort et al. (2007), while two more recent studies favored again stress-induced subendocardial ischemia in syndrome X patients (Lanza et al. 2008; Cook et al. 2009). Since first-pass perfusion is prone to dark-rim artifacts occurring at the subendocardial border, it is yet unclear to what extent these artifacts may interfere with depiction subendocardial ischemia (Camici 2007).

4.2 Stress Function Imaging

Although it is possible to perform exercise testing in an MR environment using a specific MR-compatible cycle ergometer (Tops et al. 2005), functional stress testing is usually performed during dobutamine (± atropine) administration. Dobutamine, as a ß-agonist, stimulates the β-receptors of myocytes and increases contractility, heart rate and stroke volume through increased ATP- and oxygen consumption and

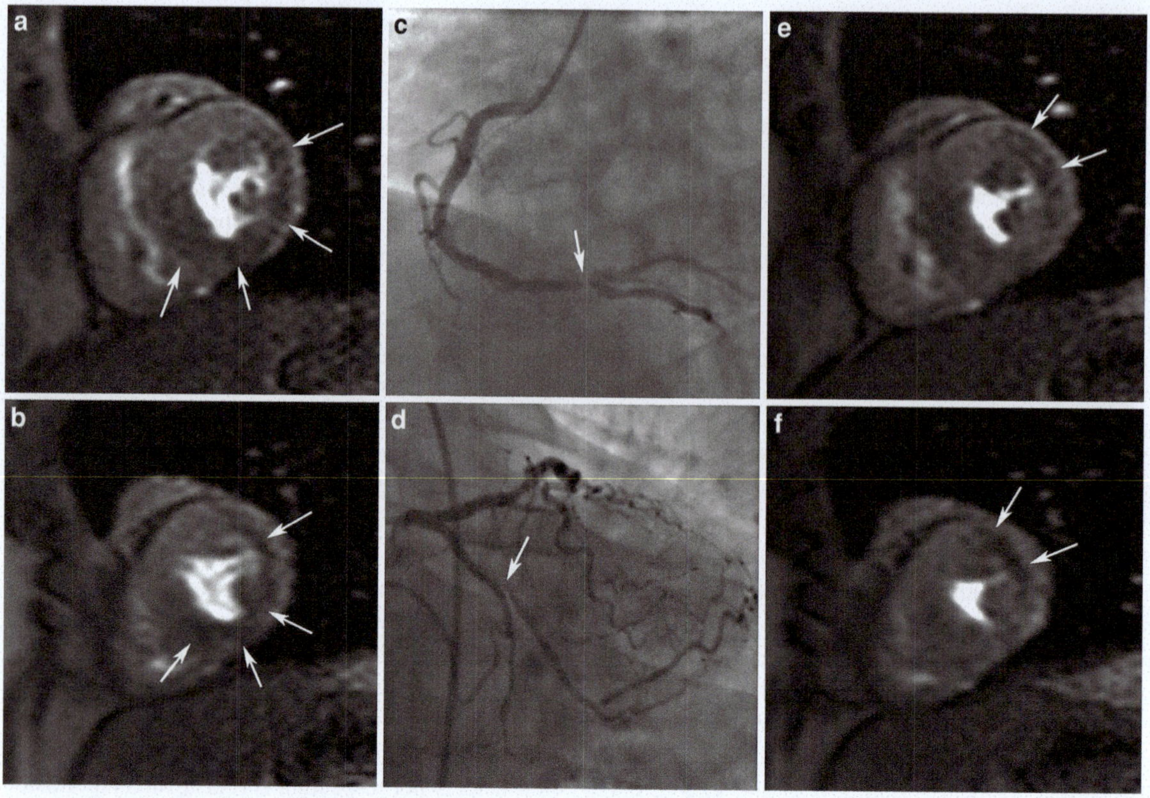

Fig. 21 First pass MPI–MR during adenosine stress before (**a**, **b**) and after (**e**, **f**) PCI. First-pass imaging before PCI shows extensive stress-induced perfusion defect in the inferolateral LV wall (*arrows*, **a**, **b**). Subsequent coronary angiography shows high-grade stenosis (95%) in distal right coronary artery and proximal high-grade (90%) stenosis in first lateral branch of left circumflex coronary artery (*arrow*, **d**). Following PCI with stent placement of the high-grade stenosis in distal right coronary artery, adenosine stress MPI–MR shows normalization of the perfusion in inferior LV wall while the myocardial perfusion defect in the LV lateral wall persists (*arrows*, **e**, **f**)

resembles physical exercise (Ruffolo 1987). Using a stepwise dose increment of dobutamine, the precise nature of the ischemic substrate can be further differentiated, e.g., stunned, ischemic, hibernated, necrotic/scarred myocardium, and can be used to discriminate ischemic myocardium from the functional border zone (Buda et al. 1987; Cigarroa et al. 1993; Van Rugge et al. 1993, 1994; Wu et al. 2011).

During stress testing, myocardium supplied by a normal coronary artery will show progressive increase in myocardial contractility. In contrast, myocardium supplied by a flow-limiting coronary stenosis will become ischemic when the compensatory increase in coronary blood supply is insufficient to match the increased demand in oxygen, i.e. when the coronary flow reserve is superseded. This in turn will cause a decrease in regional contractility and lead to new wall motion abnormalities (WMA) (Fig. 5). Besides detection of flow-limiting coronary stenoses in patients suspected of obstructive CAD, two other applications for stress function imaging are the differentiation between viable and non-viable dysfunctional myocardium in patients with chronic CAD (see Sect. 6), and differentiation between stunned and irreversibly damaged myocardium in patients with a recent myocardial infarction. In contrast to the detection of flow-limiting stenoses where a high-dose regimen is used, the latter indications are typically performed with low-dose regimen ($\leq$20 µg/kg dobutamine) (Baer et al. 1994; Dendale et al. 1997).

Practically, stress function imaging for detecting flow-limiting stenoses is started in resting conditions acquiring cine MR images in a set of standardized imaging planes through the ventricles. In our center we acquire four short-axis planes and a horizontal and vertical long-axis image, achieved in 3 consecutive

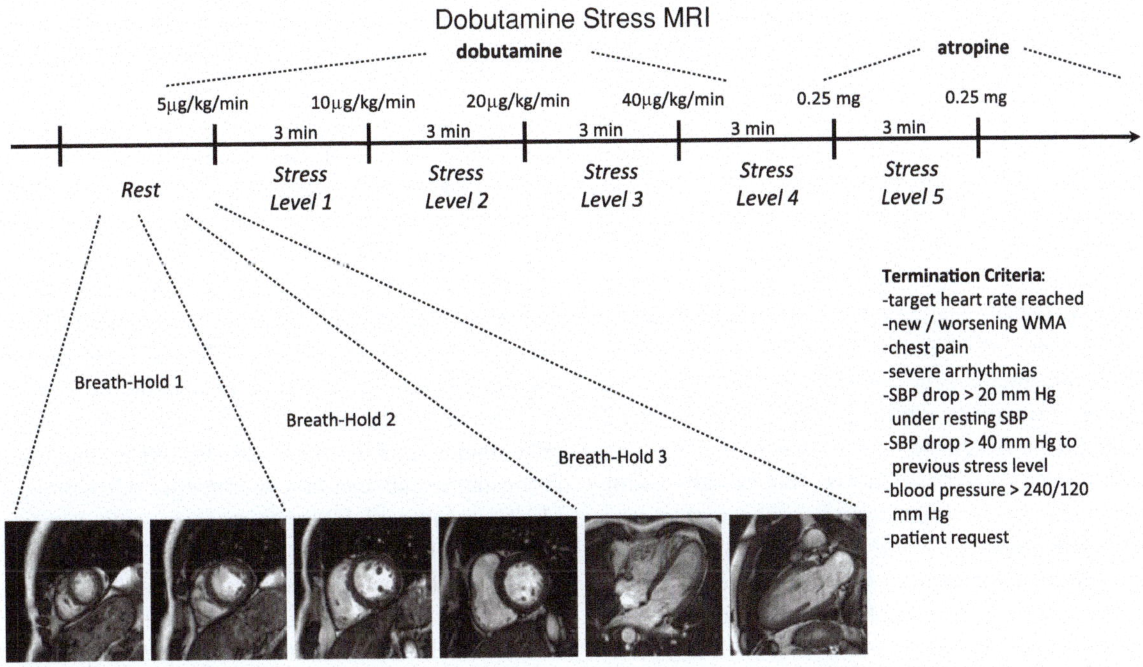

Fig. 22 Practical schematic for dobutamine stress MRI. For each stress level, 4 short-axis and two long axis cine studies are obtained in 3 consecutive breath-hold periods. If termination criteria are not met at the highest dobutamine dose, atropine can be additionally administered

breath-holds (Fig. 22). This approach allows to evaluate regional contractility in all segments of the left ventricle. In addition, we perform a single breath-hold 3D cine MRI sequence encompassing the entire left ventricle, allowing to calculate LV volumes and ejection fraction (Jahnke et al. 2006). Other centers use similar acquisition schemes, for instance adding a 3-chamber view. Next, dobutamine infusion is started at low dose (5 μg/kg body weight per minute) and after 3 min the above cine MRI sequences are repeated. The images are immediately transferred to an off-line workstation and analyzed for new or worsening WMA. If normal, the dose of dobutamine is increased to the next stress level, and the above approach is repeated. For high-dose stress imaging we use rest, 5, 10, 20, 40 μg/kg dobutamine as consecutive stress levels. When WMAs develop or worsen, or when the patient develops chest pain at a certain stress level, the test is considered positive for hemodynamically significant CAD and the infusion is terminated. If the target heart rate of the patient, i.e, (220 age) × 0.85, is not reached at 40 μg/kg dobutamine, intravenous atropine as a chronotropic agent can be additionally administered at up to 2 mg using fractionate doses of 0.25 mg every minute (Korosoglou et al. 2010a, b). Dobutamine administration needs to be stopped on patient request, and is also discontinued if: the systolic blood pressure decreases >20 mmHg below the baseline systolic blood pressure; or the systolic blood pressure decreases >40 mmHg from a previous level; or the blood pressure increases to above 240/120 mmHg; or when severe arrhythmias occur. Additionally, at peak stress a first pass myocardial perfusion study can be performed to simultaneously assess perfusion patterns (Gebker et al. 2008). Moreover, in case of a positive stress study, the above MRI sequences can be repeated 5 min after stopping dobutamine administration to evaluate the function recovery of dysfunctional segments. Since the physical access to the patient in an MR scanner is much more limited than in echocardiography, and 12-lead ECG monitoring is not reliable in an MR environment, a specific approach to address the potential adverse effects is required during functional stress imaging (for details, see "Practical Set-Up"). Hemodynamic parameters such as heart rate and blood pressure should be closely monitored. Stress function imaging teams should be equipped with cardiac resuscitation material and be trained in case of cardiac complications for fast patient evacuation from the magnet to a resuscitation save environment. Using low-dose stress protocols, side effects are minimal, but the risk for adverse effects increases at higher doses. The German Heart Institute, however, has shown that in a large unselected patient group of over 1,000 patients, referred for high-dose dobutamine-atropine stress MRI, side effects were minimal (Wahl et al. 2003). This and other studies have shown that high-dose functional stress imaging in an MR environment can be considered as safe and feasible in patients with suspected or known CAD (Kuijpers et al. 2004a).

Although functional stress studies are usually performed by echocardiography, image quality is often suboptimal (>15% of studies), and the inter- and intra-observer agreement is low. In contrast, stress function MRI offers reliable image quality with high spatial and temporal resolution, showing good agreement between readers (Paetsch et al. 2006). Two studies have demonstrated the superiority of high-dose stress dobutamine MRI to high-dose dobutamine stress echocardiography in detecting patients with significant CAD (≥50% diameter stenosis) (Nagel et al. 1999; Hundley et al. 1999). In particular, patients with poor echocardiogeneity benefit from MRI stress testing. The better MR image quality was deemed responsible for the higher accuracy (86.0 vs. 72.7%). Currently, the most commonly used approach for evaluating functional stress studies is visual analysis of new or worsening WMAs using a high-dose dobutamine/atropine regimen using a 16 (or 17) segment classification system by the AHA, yielding good sensitivity (83–96%) and specificity (80–100%) for detection of significant CAD (Strach et al. 2006), and the diagnostic accuracy is not influenced by gender (Gebker et al. 2010a). However, visual analysis is prone to subjective interpretation, and thick-walled ventricles especially in combination with small ventricular cavities may obscure underlying wall motion abnormalities. To increase diagnostic accuracy, myocardial tagging techniques are an interesting alternative (Kuijpers et al. 2003). Since they allow assessment of myocardial deformation patterns, more subtle parameters of ischemia can be detected at lower stress levels, thereby reducing the need for high-dose stress regimen (Paetsch et al. 2005). A routine application is, however, hampered by the need for time-consuming image tagging analysis (Kraitchman et al. 2003; Kramer and Hundley 2010). As an alternative Korosoglou et al. recently presented a fast direct color-coded strain visualization using SENC (i.e. strain-encoded MRI) not only providing incremental value for the detection of CAD compared to conventional wall motion readings, but moreover enabling to detect CAD at intermediate stress levels with similar accuracy to that provided by cine MR imaging. The rationale is that these SENC techniques enable to detect subtle wall deformation abnormalities in the ischemic myocardium earlier in the ischemic cascade than the onset of WMA's (Korosoglou et al. 2009a, b; 2010b). When the above promising results can be confirmed by other groups, SENC imaging yields promise to become a major player in ischemia testing. Another interesting issue is whether addition of a first pass myocardial imaging sequence at peak dose dobutamine adds diagnostic value in CAD detection. In a relatively small group of patients, Lubbers et al. found this additional sequence helpful to decide whether a new WMA was due to inducible left bundle branch block (no perfusion defect) rather than due to significant CAD (Lubbers et al. 2008). In a study involving 455 consecutive patients the addition of perfusion imaging at peak stress increased sensitivity at the expense of specificity, resulting in an identical overall diagnostic accuracy (Gebker et al. 2008). However, in patients with concentric LV hypertrophy and concentric remodeling diagnostic accuracy can be increased adding first pass perfusion imaging, because wall motion analysis is impeded in these thick-walled ventricles (Gebker et al. 2010b). The added value of performing functional stress imaging at 3T in CAD patients is not yet clarified. It has been shown that high-dose stress imaging at 3T is feasible yielding similar diagnostic values compared to 1.5T (Kelle et al. 2008).

5 Acute Coronary Syndrome

Acute coronary syndrome (ACS) occurs in the setting of sudden plaque erosion or rupture with intracoronary thrombosis and partial to complete cessation of the downstream myocardial perfusion. The available diagnostic tools at the moment of presentation, i.e, blood biomarkers, electrocardiography and ultrasonography, only provide a partial insight into the complex, evolving processes in the jeopardized myocardium. MRI, as a clinical tool, allows accurate appraisal of the myocardium in the first hours after the onset of chest pain providing substantial supporting information to standard imaging tools.

5.1 Characterization of the Jeopardized Myocardium

5.1.1 Myocardium at Risk

The myocardium (or area) at risk can be defined as that part of the myocardium that will become ischemic and ultimately necrotic when coronary blood supply ceases, or in other words, the myocardium in the anatomical distribution of the involved vessel(s) distal to the critical lesion(s) (Lee et al. 1981). The myocardium at risk is a major determinant of infarct size, because it predicts the maximal area of myocardium at risk for necrosis. In autopsied hearts, the lateral edge of necrosis closely approximated the lateral extent of the area at risk, independently of infarct size, while the transmural extent of necrosis was largely variable. It is important to stress that the anatomical site of occlusion of the coronary artery does not reliably predict the size of the area at risk (Feiring et al. 1987). Although angiographic criteria were assessed to estimate more accurately the myocardium at risk using the Bypass Angioplasty Revascularization Investigation Myocardial Salvage Index (BARI) (Alderman and Stadius 1992; Ortiz-Pérez et al. 2007; Wright et al. 2009), there is a need for imaging techniques directly and accurately depicting the area at risk.

There is cumulating evidence that T2w-imaging (see Sect. 3.3) is at present one of the most appealing techniques to non invasively assess the area at risk (Aletras et al. 2006; Tilak et al. 2008; Abdel-Aty et al. 2009; Berry et al. 2010). Whereas late Gd imaging in acute infarct patients provides information about the amount of myocardium that is irreversibly injured (Fieno et al. 2000), T2w-imaging visualizes the myocardium that is at risk and can be potentially salvaged using appropriate reperfusion treatment (Fig. 23) (see Sect. 5.1.3). T2w-imaging has, besides its non invasive nature, the advantage over other techniques such as microspheres (animal models), SPECT imaging (humans) or manganese-enhanced MRI (animal models), that the area at risk can be determined retrospectively, i.e., post-reperfusion, as abnormalities that last at least one week after the acute event (Sinusas et al. 1990; Schulz-Menger et al. 2003; Natanzon et al. 2005; Wright et al. 2009; Carlson et al. 2009). Since development of myocardial edema (i.e., ischemia causes dysfunction of ATP-dependent sodium–potassium channels, altering transmembrane sodium gradients causing intracellular edema) is an early feature in ACS, adding T2w-imaging to the MRI exam in an ACS patient enables to identify myocardium at risk and may serve as a very useful diagnostic marker in patients with unstable angina or evolving myocardial infarction in the emergency department (Curry et al. 2008; Raman et al. 2010). Abdel-Aty et al. recently showed that edema imaging depicts acute ischemic injury within the first 30 min after onset of ischemia, before the onset of irreversible myocardial injury (i.e. troponin elevation, late gadolinium enhancement) (Abdel–Aty et al. 2009). The presentation of myocardial edema on T2w-imaging is not necessarily homogeneously hyperintense, especially in patients with intramyocardial hemorrhage where the center of the myocardium at risk may become hypointense due to the paramagnetic effects of the breakdown products of hemogloblin (Foltz et al. 2006; Ganame et al. 2009) (see Sect. 5.2.4). Moreover, readers should realize that in the acute setting of cardiac-related chest pain, patients with Tako-Tsubo cardiomyopathy and acute myocarditis may show also myocardial edema (see "Heart Muscle Diseases"). Thus, T2w-imaging is a sensitive technique for depicting myocardial edema, but is not infarct specific.

5.1.2 Infarct Imaging

Contrast enhanced MRI, using the late Gd imaging technique, is an accurate, well-validated tool to visualize the presence of MI both in the acute and chronic settings. Infarct imaging is mainly based on the differential and time-varying effect of the contrast agent on the relaxation times of normal and infarcted myocardium, whereby contrast ratios can be substantially increased using the abovementioned late Gd imaging sequence. Although the optimal time point for infarct imaging is deemed to be 10–20 min after the injection of the contrast agent, it is important to understand what happens after injection on the myocardial tissue level (Oshinski et al. 2001). Immediately after contrast administration, there is a

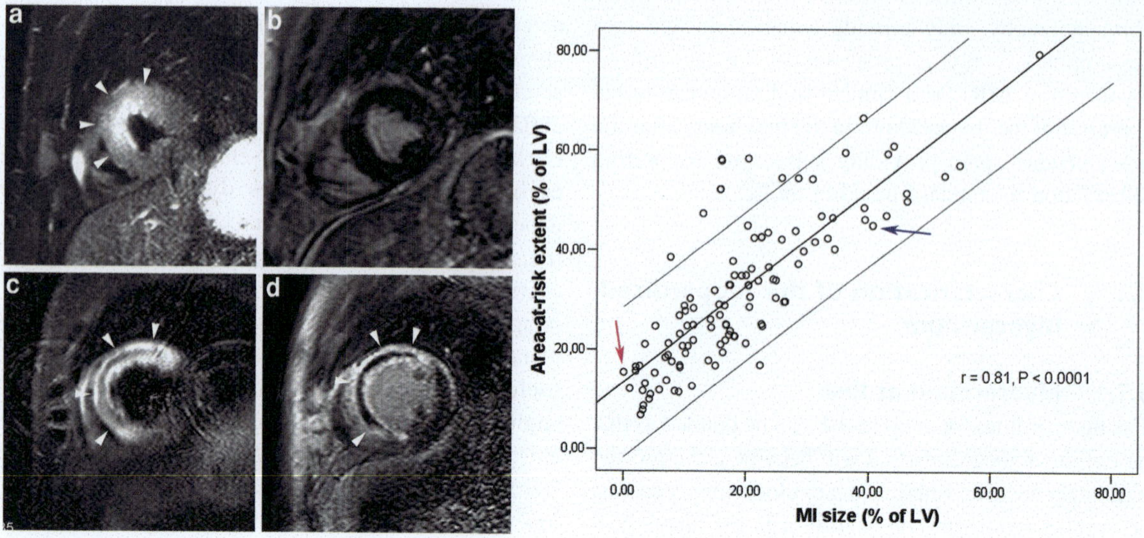

Fig. 23 Complementary value of T2w-imaging (**a**, **c**) and late Gd imaging (**b**, **d**) in acute infarct imaging. A first patient shows a large area of myocardial edema in the anteroseptal LV wall (*arrowheads*, **a**) but not late enhancement (**b**), corresponding to an aborted infarction. The second patient equally shows an extensive area of myocardial edema in the anteroseptal LV wall (*arrowheads*, **c**). Following contrast administration, strong enhancement occurs in the anteroseptal LV wall (*arrowheads*, **d**). The extent of enhancement nearly equals the extent of myocardial edema, leaving no or at most a minimal amount of myocardial salvage. In addition, this patient shows a large central hypo-intense zone within the edematous myocardium corresponding to myocardial hemorrhage (**c**), and an extensive area of microvascular obstruction (**d**). The relationship between extent of myocardial edema (i.e., area-at-risk) and extent of late enhancement (i.e., MI size), obtained in 137 patients, is shown in the graph. Adapted from Masci et al. (2010a). On the graph, patient one is shown by the *red arrow*, patient two by the *blue arrow*

brief enhancement of the normal myocardium (wash-in phase) but due to the rapid wash-out of contrast, the enhancement of normal myocardium is already substantially decreased 5 min after contrast administration. An opposite phenomenon is observed in infarcted myocardium. At 5 min, T1-relaxation time is significantly shorter than early after contrast injection, making the infarct area bright relative to the viable myocardium, thus substantially improving the visualization of the infarct area and increasing the accuracy of infarct quantification (McNamara et al. 1986; Eichstaedt et al. 1989). Somewhere between 5 and 30 min after contrast administration T1-relaxation of the infarcted or scarred myocardium is shortest and thus optimal for imaging with late Gd imaging (Fig. 12), while after 30 min due to substantial wash-out of contrast in the infarcted myocardium T1-relaxation times again increase impeding visualization of the infarct area (Dymarkowski et al. 2002). Depending on the location, depth and severity of infarction, several patterns of enhancement have been described, yielding important information regarding infarct severity and prognosis assessment (see 5.2).

5.1.3 Myocardial Salvage

The myocardium supplied by an acutely occluded artery defines the anatomical area at risk for infarction (see Sect. 5.1.1). Since the limited capacity of myocytes to sustain prolonged ischemia, the earlier the perfusion can be restored more myocardium can be salvaged ('*time is myocardium*'). In this perspective, determination of myocardial salvage relating extent of necrosis to extent of myocardium at risk, provides valuable information helpful, to assess the efficacy of reperfusion therapy. Myocardial salvage can be determined with SPECT imaging, and although this technique has been used in several clinical trials, it suffers from several limitations, such as low spatial resolution, need for isotope injection in the acute setting of coronary occlusion potentially interfering with patient care, and requirement of 2 separate perfusion studies leading to additional radiation exposure (Eitel et al. 2010). As a non invasive alternative,

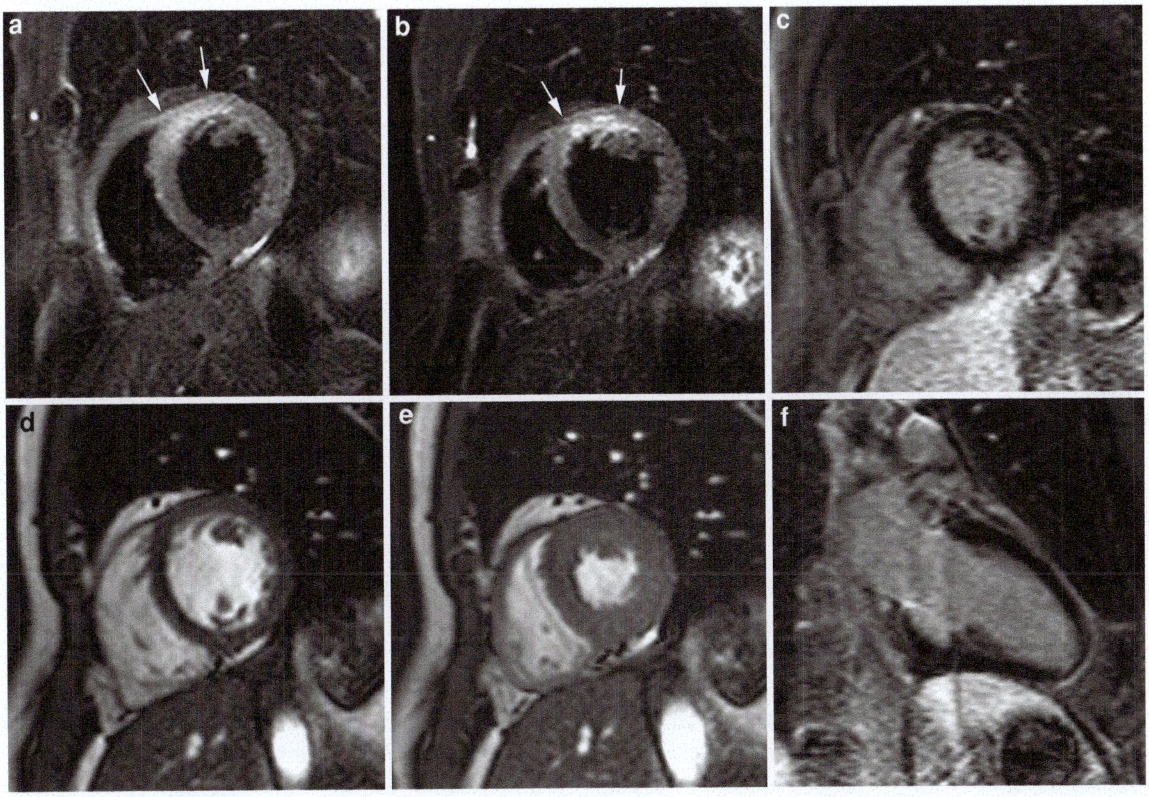

Fig. 24 Reversible ischemic injury ('aborted myocardial infarction') without tissue necrosis in a 54-year-old patient with angina-like symptoms, acute ischemic changes on ECG and mildly elevated troponin levels. Short-axis T2w-imaging (**a**, **b**) shows edema in the anteroseptal LV wall (*arrows*, **a**, **b**). Short-axis cine imaging at end diastole (**d**) and end systole (**e**) show normal wall motion, while no abnormal myocardial enhancement is shown on late Gd imaging (**e**, **f**), ruling out macroscopic tissue infarction

similar information can be obtained using a combination of edema imaging and late Gd imaging (Dymarkowski et al. 2002) (Fig. 23). Using this approach, Ibanez et al. (2007) showed in a pig model the beneficial effects of metoprolol administration pre-reperfusion on myocardial salvage and post-reperfusion functional improvement (Ibanez et al. 2007). Although the myocardium at risk exceeds the irreversible damaged myocardium (Friedrich et al. 2008; Wright et al. 2009), both are closely related (Masci et al. 2010a; Berry et al. 2010). Usually, edema involves the entire width of the myocardial wall, whereas the transmural spread of necrosis is variable. Interestingly in an MRI study by Francone et al., it was shown that increasing ischemia time does not affect the extent of myocardium at risk but results in an increasing infarct size and subsequently decreased myocardial salvage (Francone et al. 2009). In particular, salvaged myocardium was markedly reduced after 90 min of coronary occlusion. Early mechanical reperfusion and maintenance of antegrade or collateral flow independently preserves myocardial salvage primarily through a reduction of infarct transmurality (Ortiz-Pérez et al. 2010). Myocardial salvage is independently associated with early ST-segment resolution (Friedrich et al. 2008; Masci et al. 2010a), and is an independent predictor of adverse LV remodeling and major cardiac events (i.e, cardiac deaths, nonfatal myocardial infarction) (MACE) at intermediate follow-up (Eitel et al. 2010; Masci et al. 2010a). Early reperfusion can result in *aborted infarction*, thus achieving the ultimate myocardial salvage (Lamfers et al. 2003). Although the diagnosis of aborted MI is based on major ST-segment resolution of the ST-segment elevation on the initial ECG and lack of significant increase of myocardial enzyme release, a combined edema imaging and late Gd imaging approach may be appealing in visualizing aborted MI (Figs. 23 and 24).

5.2 Assessment of Myocardial Infarction Severity

5.2.1 Infarct Size

A key characteristic of myocardial tissue is its low regenerative capacity, i.e. myocytes are terminally differentiated cells having lost the capacity to renew damaged myocardium. Although progenitor cells residing in the heart have been found, their reparative role in infarct healing seems very limited. Instead, ischemically irreversibly damaged myocardium is replaced in the weeks and months following the acute event by an afunctional, fibrotic scar. As a consequence, the amount of contractile tissue lost, or the infarct size, is a crucial determinant of adverse LV remodeling. To cause heart failure 25% of the ventricle should be lost, while infarction of 40% results in cardiogenic shock (Murry et al. 2006). Estimation of the amount of irreversibly lost myocardium is thus imperative to assess infarct severity and because it is the prognosticator to determine adverse ventricular remodeling and patient outcome (Sobel et al. 1972; Roes et al. 2007; Wu et al. 2008). Moreover, infarct size is often used as a surrogate end point to assess the efficacy of novel treatments (Gibbons et al. 2004; Fuster et al. 2006). Late Gd imaging is a well-validated, accurate and reproducible tool for sizing acute, healing and healed infarcts (Rehwald et al. 2002; Mahrholdt et al. 2002; Hendel et al. 2006; Thiele et al. 2006; Hundley et al. 2010), and because of its high spatial resolution enabling depiction of small MIs should be considered the reference imaging modality for infarct sizing (Wagner et al. 2003; Ibrahim et al. 2007). MRI is increasingly being used to determine the relationship among infarct size, ventricular remodeling and patient outcome (Orn et al. 2007; Roes et al. 2007; Wu et al. 2008). Also, in patients with healed or unrecognized myocardial infarctions (see Sect. 5.2.6), the presence and extent of scarred tissue on late Gd MRI shows strong, and independent association with MACE and cardiac mortality (Kwong et al. 2006, 2008; Cheong et al. 2009; Steel et al. 2009; Kelle et al. 2009).

5.2.2 Transmural Infarct Extent

Besides infarct size, several other parameters should be taken into consideration when assessing infarct severity. Amongst them, there is the transmural extent of necrosis. Early restoration of myocardial perfusion might stop the transmural progress of necrosis and salvage the jeopardized, but still viable in the outer myocardium (Thiele et al. 2007; Francone et al. 2009). The combination of a superior in-plane spatial resolution, and high contrast between normal and damaged myocardium on late Gd imaging, enables accurate determination of the transmural infarct extent, and makes this technique superior to other techniques such as SPECT imaging (Wagner et al. 2003; Schuijf et al. 2004; Hayat et al. 2006; Ibrahim et al. 2007). Infarct transmurality can be expressed using a semi-quantitative score and dividing the myocardial wall into 4 equidistant segments (Wu et al. 2001; Wagner et al. 2003; Ibrahim et al. 2007) or using an automated quantification approach (Berbari et al. 2009). In 1989, de Roos et al., described 4 different patterns of enhancement in MI on contrast enhanced spin-echo imaging (de Roos et al. 1989) (Fig. 25). The patterns mirror the severity of infarction, are linked to other parameters reflecting infarct severity such as cardiac enzymes, loss in regional function and are of prognostic importance (Holman et al. 1993; Lima et al. 1995; Kim et al. 1996; Rogers et al. 1999; Gerber et al. 2000; Ingkanisorn et al. 2004). Patterns 1 (*subendocardial infarct*) and 2 (*transmural infarct*) reflect the severity of transmural extent of necrosis, pattern 3 the presence of microvascular obstruction (*no-reflow*) (see Sect. 5.2.3), and pattern 4 epicardial coronary artery obstruction (*occlusive infarct*). Since then, several contrast enhanced MRI based studies have shown that increasing infarct transmurality is related with lack of inotropic reserve and impaired recovery of contractile function, and in addition is associated with more pronounced post-infarct wall thinning, aneurysm formation and adverse ventricular remodeling (Jugdutt and Khan 1992; Hillenbrand et al. 2000; Gerber et al. 2001; Taylor et al. 2004; Tarantini et al. 2006a, b; Engblom et al. 2009). Also in patients with healed infarcts and ventricular dysfunction, scar transmurality as determined by late Gd imaging predicts functional recovery post-revascularization and patient survival (Kim et al. 2000; Beek et al. 2003; Cheong et al. 2009) (Fig. 48).

5.2.3 Microvascular Obstruction or No-Reflow

In patients with an ST-segment elevation MI, the current treatment is primarily focused to achieve early and sustained restoration of the coronary flow in the

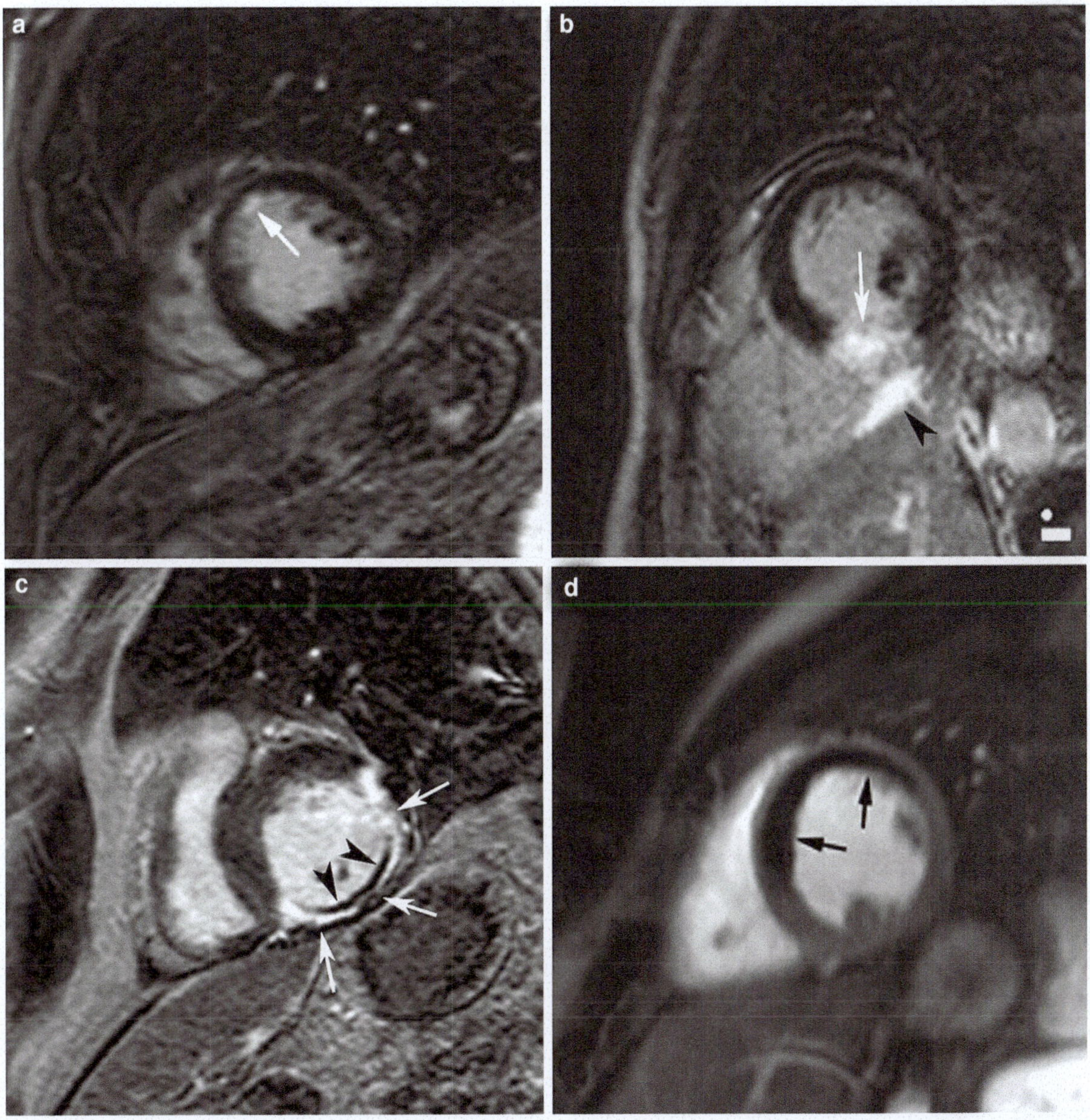

Fig. 25 Four patterns of enhancement on late Gd imaging reflecting different grades of infarct severity. Short-axis late Gd imaging obtained in 4 different patients. Panel a shows **a** limited subendocardial enhancement in the anteroseptal LV wall (*arrow*). Panel **b** shows a transmural enhancement inferoseptally (*arrow*) with extension towards the RV inferior wall (*arrowhead*). Panel **c** shows extensive transmural enhancement in inferolateral LV wall (*arrows*) with presence of subendocardial region of microvascular obstruction (*arrowhead*). Panel **d** shows extensive zone of non-enhancement in the anteroseptal LV wall (*arrows*), corresponding with occlusive infarct, though differentiation with extensive zone of microvascular obstruction is not straightforward

culprit coronary artery by means of primary percutaneous coronary intervention (PCI) or thrombolytic therapy. However, the process of myocardial reperfusion itself, can harm the jeopardized myocardium, thereby reducing the beneficial effects of reperfusion, a phenomenon called *myocardial reperfusion injury* (Yellon and Hausenloy 2007; Camici and Crea 2007) (Fig. 26). A considerable number of patients, ranging between 5 and 50% according to the methods used, and the population under study, shows lack of restoration of blood flow at myocardial level despite a successful procedure (Niccoli et al. 2009). This

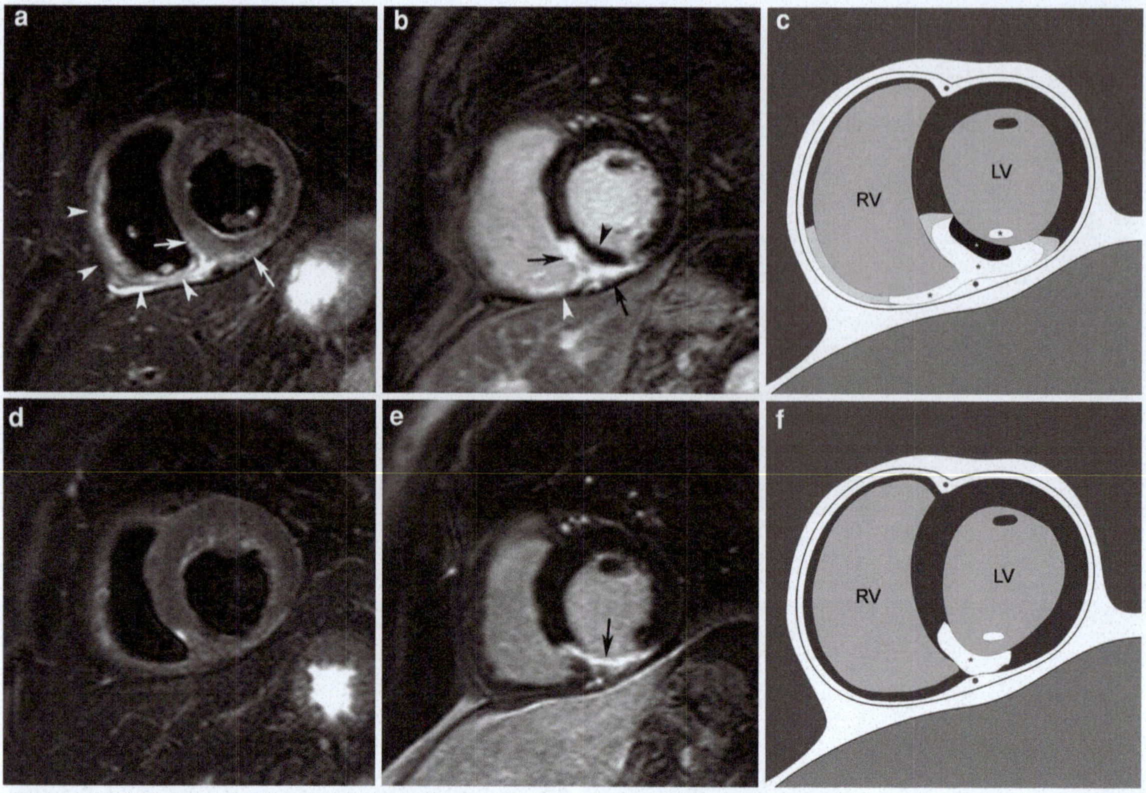

Fig. 26 Patient with inferior myocardial infarction studied in the acute phase (i.e., first week) (*top row*) and at 4 months after the acute event (*bottom row*). Short-axis T2w-imaging (**a**, **d**), late Gd imaging (**b**, **e**) and schematic drawing of the different components of the damaged myocardium in the acute (**c**) and healed (**f**) phase using a short-axis view. The presence and extent of myocardial edema in the LV inferoseptal wall (*arrows*, **a**) in the acute phase can be well appreciated on T2w-imaging. Note the important extent of edema towards the RV wall (*arrowheads*, **a**). The latter needs to be differentiated from the pericardial fluid along the inferior RV wall exhibiting a very high signal intensity. Late Gd imaging (**b**) shows presence of a transmural enhancement of the inferoseptal LV wall (*arrows*), presence of an important zone of microvascular obstruction (*black arrowhead*), and extension of enhancement towards the RV inferior wall (*white arrowhead*). At follow-up the myocardial edema has completely resolved (**d**) while late Gd imaging shows thinning of the infarcted myocardial wall (*arrow*, **e**). Note that the RV inferior wall does not show residual enhancement. Schematic drawing: normal myocardium: *dark-gray*; edematous myocardium: *light-gray*; infarcted/scarred myocardium: *bright*; microvascular obstruction: *dark*. Note the concomitant infarction of the inferior papillary muscle (*, **c**)

phenomenon is called *no-reflow* and is due to MVO. Since the initial description in a dog model by Kloner et al. (Kloner et al. 1974), the no-reflow phenomenon has been extensively evaluated. No-reflow is related to more severe myocardial damage (Bogaert et al. 2007) (Fig. 27), increases with the duration of ischemia time (Tarantini et al. 2005; Francone et al. 2009) and is independently associated with lack of functional recovery, adverse ventricular remodeling and worse patient outcome (Ito et al. 1992, Wu et al. 1998a; Rogers et al. 1999; Kramer et al. 2000; Gerber et al. 2000; Taylor et al. 2004; Hombach et al. 2005; Baks et al. 2006; Funaro et al. 2009; Nijveldt et al. 2008; Orn et al. 2009; Weir et al. 2010a). MVO has a complex and multifactorial pathogenesis including: distal embolization, ischemia–reperfusion injury and individual predisposition of coronary microcirculation to injury (Yellon and Hausenloy 2007; Niccoli et al. 2009; Bekkers et al. 2010). The coronary microcirculation in the infarct core is obstructed by endothelial disruption, microvascular compression due to myocardial cell swelling and associated interstitial edema, massive infiltration of coronary microcirculation by neutrophils and platelets occurring at the time of reperfusion and dislodgment of microemboli from the epicardial coronary thrombus and from

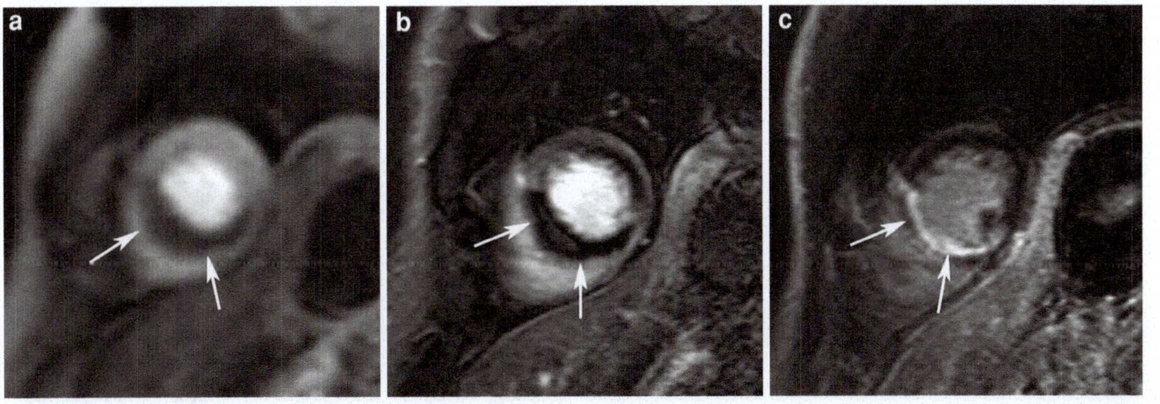

Fig. 27 Imaging of microvascular obstruction. First pass perfusion imaging (**a**), early Gd imaging early post-infarction (**b**), and late Gd imaging at 4-month follow-up (**c**) in a patient with a large septal infarct. First pass imaging shows a large septal perfusion defect (*arrows*, **a**) corresponding to a large microvascular obstruction on early Gd imaging (*arrows*, **b**). Note the important thinning of the infarcted myocardium at follow-up (*arrows*, **c**)

fissured plaques in particular during primary PCI (Niccoli et al. 2009). To further optimize reperfusion therapies and achieve an open-microvessel environment, treatment strategies are nowadays targeted at the main pathogenetic mechanisms of no-reflow (Liu et al. 2007; Sardella et al. 2009; Desmet et al. 2011). Although most no-reflows are sustained due to irreversible changes, some may spontaneous improve and should be regarded as reversible (microvascular "stunning") (Galiuto et al. 2003). In a study by Rochitte et al. (1998) a three-fold increase in the central hypoenhanced region was found by contrast enhanced MRI during the first 48 h after reperfusion, suggestive of progressive microvascular damage after reperfusion. These results are consistent with progressive microvascular and myocardial injury after reperfusion. Beyond 2 days, the progress causing no-reflow expansion most likely stabilizes and persists at least till 9 days post-infarction (Wu et al. 1998b). Since MVO is composed of several degrees of severity, the microvascular damage is most severe in the infarct core, causing a complete occlusion (no-reflow), while in the peripheral layers less severe damage causing subobstruction presents as low-reflow. This might explain the observed differences in spatial extent between myocardial contrast echocardiography and contrast enhanced MRI (Wu et al. 1998b). The presence of no-reflow is not limited to ST-segment elevation MI but is frequently found in non-ST-segment elevation MI as well (Mewton et al. 2009).

No-reflow can be assessed during primary PCI with Thrombolysis In Myocardial Infarction (TIMI) flow grade and myocardial blush grade (MBG) post-reperfusion, the ST-segment resolution early post-reperfusion, and can be better quantified by noninvasive imaging techniques such as myocardial contrast echocardiography and late Gd imaging (Niccoli et al. 2009). Angiographic no-reflow is defined as a TIMI flow grade <3 or a grade 3 with a MBG 0 to 1 (range 0–3 with higher scores indicating better perfusion). Lack of ST-resolution <50 or 70%, 1 h post-reperfusion is considered as no-reflow. On myocardial contrast echocardiography, no-reflow is defined as lack of intramyocardial contrast opacification following peripheral injection of microbubbles. Contrast enhanced MRI has become without any doubt the preferential technique for MVO depiction. Although the novel late Gd imaging techniques have greatly facilitated the detection, MVO was already described and recognized by de Roos et al. in 1989 as a separate pattern ('type 3') (Fig. 25), yielding a less favorable outcome (de Roos et al. 1989). MVO typically presents on late Gd imaging as a subendocardially located hypointense area within the enhanced myocardium, and is clearly distinguishable from completely reperfused infarcts presenting as homogeneous enhancement (Lima et al. 1995). Judd et al. validated the MRI findings of no-reflow using thioflavin-S to demarcate no-reflow regions (Judd et al. 1995a, b).

To fully appreciate the extent of MVO, imaging should be performed as soon as possible, i.e., the first

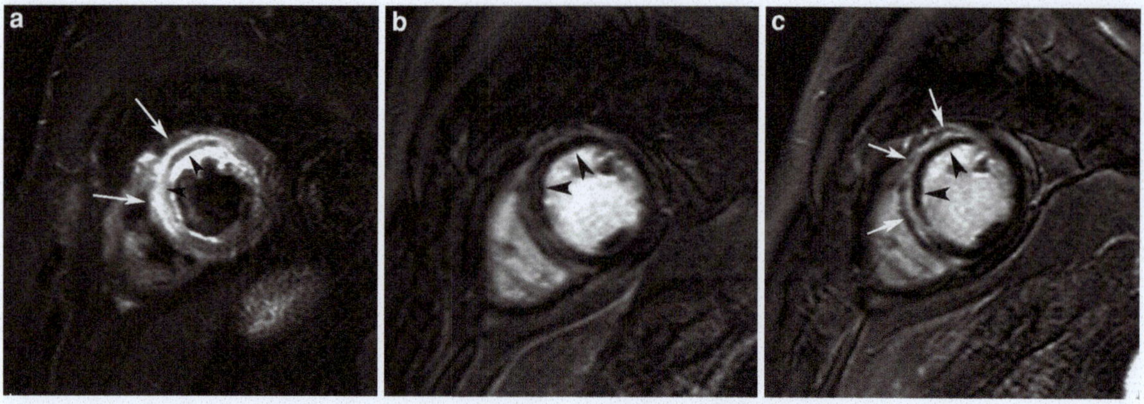

Fig. 28 Imaging of microvascular obstruction. Short-axis T2w-imaging (**a**), early Gd imaging (**b**) and late Gd imaging (**c**) in a patient with an extensive reperfused acute anteroseptal myocardial infarction. Presence of an extensive zone of myocardial edema in the LV anteroseptal wall (*arrows*, **a**) with evidence of concomitant myocardial hemorrhage (*arrowheads*, **a**). On early Gd imaging, a large zone of microvascular obstruction is present (*arrowheads*, **b**). At late imaging, a significant shrinkage of the microvascular obstruction has occurred (*arrowheads*, **c**) while the infarct has substantially become enhanced (*arrows*, **c**)

minutes following intravenous contrast administration (Lima et al. 1995; Wu et al. 1998a, b). Due to diffusion of Gd-molecules into the no-reflow zone, the size of MVO progressively decreases over time (Fig. 28). In 52 reperfused ST-elevation MIs, we found a reduction in the number (32 vs. 27 of patients) and spatial extent of no-reflow ($36 \pm 25\%$ vs. $16 \pm 14\%$ of late enhancement extent) between early and late Gd imaging (Bogaert et al. 2007). Currently, either first pass perfusion imaging or early Gd imaging is used for MVO imaging. Taylor et al. used the increase in time to 50% maximum myocardial enhancement during first pass perfusion to express impaired microvascular reperfusion (delay ≥ 2 s) (Taylor et al. 2004). However, this sequence may not be ideal to evaluate the extent of no-reflow because of the limited number of image slices (usually 3), the lower spatial resolution and the dynamic nature of first pass. Newer techniques, such as k-t SENSE, can be used to improve spatial resolution and ventricular coverage of first pass imaging, thereby largely overcoming the above limitations (Mather et al. 2009). With first pass perfusion imaging, sensitivity may be increased, however, at the expense of specificity, since central hypo-enhancement may also appear in the setting of significant coronary artery stenosis. As an appealing alternative, early Gd imaging (1–4 min) can be recommended since it allows full coverage of the left ventricle with better spatial resolution images. Whereas initially, early imaging was usually performed with inversion times optimized to nullify myocardium, Bekkers et al proposed the use of a longer inversion time (e.g., 500–600 ms) rendering the normal myocardium brighter and thus improving visualization of no-reflow zones (Bekkers et al. 2009) (Fig. 29). Several groups have recently reported that hypoenhancement on late Gd imaging is a better prognostic marker of LV remodeling than early Gd imaging (Nijveldt et al. 2008, 2009; de Waha et al. 2010). A likely explanation for the stronger predictive value in their studies, is that at the time of late Gd imaging, infarcts with small no-reflow zones and infarcts with large low-reflow zones have become homogeneously enhanced by wash-in of contrast in the low/no reflow areas, so that only the infarcts with severe microvascular damage were considered as true no-reflow infarcts. Because of this discrepancy regarding timing further research is required to define the optimal time point for no-reflow imaging.

5.2.4 Post-Reperfusion Myocardial Hemorrhage

Whereas non-reperfused infarcts are typically anemic, restoration of myocardial perfusion is frequently associated with significant interstitial extravasation of red blood cells caused by severe microvascular damage (Bresnahan et al. 1974; Higginson et al. 1982; Garcia-Dorado et al. 1990). Since the latter represents a later event in the course of myocardial infarction than myocardial cell necrosis (i.e, endothelial cells are

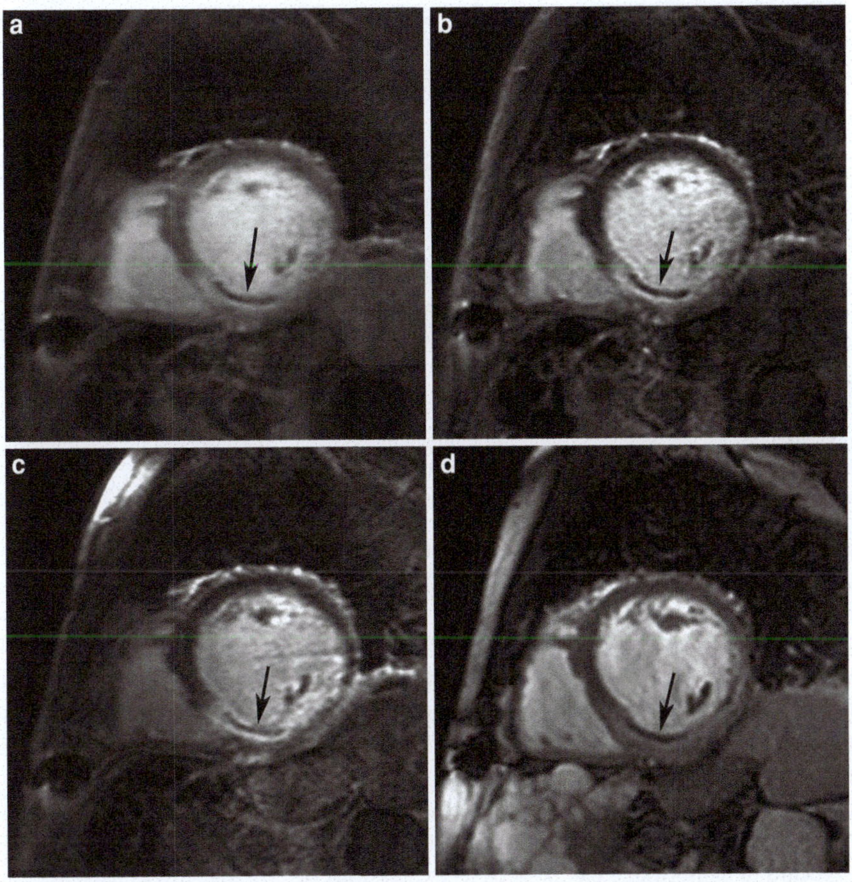

Fig. 29 Comparison of techniques for visualizing microvascular obstruction. Early Gd imaging using long (i.e., 550 ms) (**a**) versus short (i.e., 250 ms) (**b**) inversion time. Late Gd imaging (**c**) and cine imaging post contrast administration (**d**). A zone area of microvascular obstruction is visible as a hypointense subendocardial line in the LV inferoseptal wall (*arrow*)

more resistant to ischemia than myocytes), intramyocardial hemorrhage is a phenomenon that reflects severe microvascular injury and thus can be used as a marker for reperfusion injury (Fishbein et al. 1980; Asanuma et al. 1997). Several studies, both in vivo and in cadaver hearts, have shown the potential of T2w-imaging to depict intramyocardial hemorrhage, using the paramagnetic properties of hemoglobin breakdown products (Lotan et al. 1990; 1992; Basso et al. 2007; Ochiai et al. 1999). Deoxyhemoglobin in the hemorrhagic myocardium causes shortening of T2-relaxation times, and thus may provide a non invasive approach to detect and quantify myocardial hemorrhage. Lotan et al. found an excellent correlation ($r = 0.96$) between the zones of decreased signal intensity on T2-weighted MRI and the size of hemorrhage from ^{51}Cr red blood cell labeling (Lotan et al. 1992). Thus, on edema imaging (see Sect. 3.3) hemorrhagic infarcts will have a heterogeneous appearance typically presenting with a hypo-intense core and a peripheral hyperintense rim (Basso et al. 2007), and can easily be differentiated from non-hemorrhagic infarct presenting homogeneously increased signal intensity in the myocardium at risk (Figs. 23–30) (Ganame et al. 2009). It should be noted that the low signal intensity from the hemorrhage may have an impact on the determination of the area at risk (O'regan et al. 2009; Mikami et al. 2009). Quantification of the T2* relaxation values of the hemorrhagic component is more difficult, because of fluctuations in the relaxation behavior in acute reperfused hemorrhagic infarcts due to breakdown of hemoglobin, decompartmentalization due to red cell lysis and subsequent iron compartmentalization in macrophages, and because of opposing effects of edema and hemorrhage on T2-values (Lotan et al. 1992; Foltz et al. 2006). In a study of 98 patients with reperfused ST-segment myocardial infarction, we found intramyocardial hemorrhage in 25% of patients (Ganame et al. 2009). Patients with hemorrhagic infarcts had a lower pre-TIMI flow, higher cardiac enzymes, larger infarct size and greater infarct transmurality, larger no-reflow zone and a lower myocardial

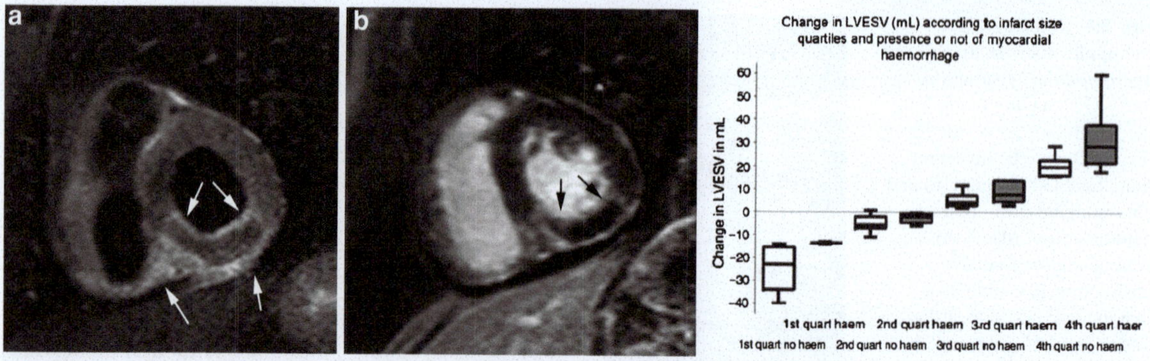

Fig. 30 Hemorrhagic myocardial infarction. Short-axis T2w-imaging (**a**) and late Gd imaging (**b**). The jeopardized myocardium in the inferior LV wall is hypointense with hyperintense edematous rim extending toward the inferior RV wall (*arrows*, **a**). Late Gd imaging shows important microvascular obstruction in the infarcted myocardium (*arrows*, **b**). The figure (*right*) shows that the incidence of hemorrhagic myocardial infarction (*dark boxes*) increases with increasing infarct size (4 quartiles of infarct size shown). However, hemorrhagic infarcts show more adverse remodeling at 4 month follow-up (i.e., increase in LV end-systolic volume) than non-hemorrhagic infarcts, independent of the infarct size. Adapted from Ganame et al. (2009)

salvage index. This and other recent studies have shown that intramyocardial hemorrhage is an independent predictor of adverse LV remodeling regardless of the initial infarct size, and a strong univariable predictor of MACE (Ganame et al. 2009; Mather et al. 2010; Eitel et al. 2011) (Fig. 30). Since intramyocardial hemorrhage has a close and intricate relation with microvascular injury, MVO as well as myocardial hemorrhage can be seen as expressions of severe tissue damage. Thus it is questionable whether the extravasation of red blood cells with subsequent cell lysis increases tissue turgor and microvascular compression, and thus contributes to an aggravation of MVO severity and extent.

5.2.5 Infarct Tissue Heterogeneity

Accurate risk stratification is essential for effective treatment planning after MI. As shown in Sects. 5.2.3 and 5.2.4 infarct tissue characterization with MRI has herein an increasingly important role. Additionally, there is substantial evidence that the peri-infarct border may be an important arrhythmogenic substrate leading to ventricular arrhythmias and sudden cardiac death. Whereas dense, fibrous scars in the infarcted myocardium incapable of depolarization cannot cause arrhythmias, the infarct border zone, containing a mixture of non-viable and viable myocardium may be an arrhythmogenic substrate. There might be an important role for late Gd imaging to quantify this 'gray' myocardium. Yan et al. found that characterization of the peri-infarct zone with MRI provided incremental predictive value for survival beyond LV volumes and LV ejection fraction (Yan et al. 2006). The heterogeneity of signal intensities within the infarct after gadolinium administration corresponds to different infarct zones with variable amounts of fibrosis and myocytes. To define the gray area, the authors used intermediate signal intensity (between 2SDs and 3SDs above remote regions, opposed to 5SDs as is used to define myocardial necrosis). Of note, the gray myocardium was not necessarily confined to the border of the infarct, but was also found in more central locations. Schmidt et al. used the full-width at half-maximum approach for infarct definition, and to provide an index of tissue heterogeneity (Schmidt et al. 2007). Several other groups confirmed the above findings (Roes et al. 2009; Heidary et al. 2010). Peters et al. proposed a higher spatial resolution 3D late Gd imaging technique to improve visualization of the peri-infarct region and to depict small areas of fibrosis such as heterogeneously scarred papillary muscles, which may be the site of ventricular arrhythmias post-infarction (Peters et al. 2009). Furthermore, Detsky et al. proposed multi-contrast late Gd imaging with automated analysis, yielding a more reproducible measurement of infarct core and gray zones (Detsky et al. 2009).

5.2.6 Right Ventricular Infarction

Right ventricular (RV) infarction is usually an expression of a biventricular acute MI, whereas isolated forms of RV infarctions are rare (i.e. <3% of all cases of RV acute MI) (Andersen et al. 1987)

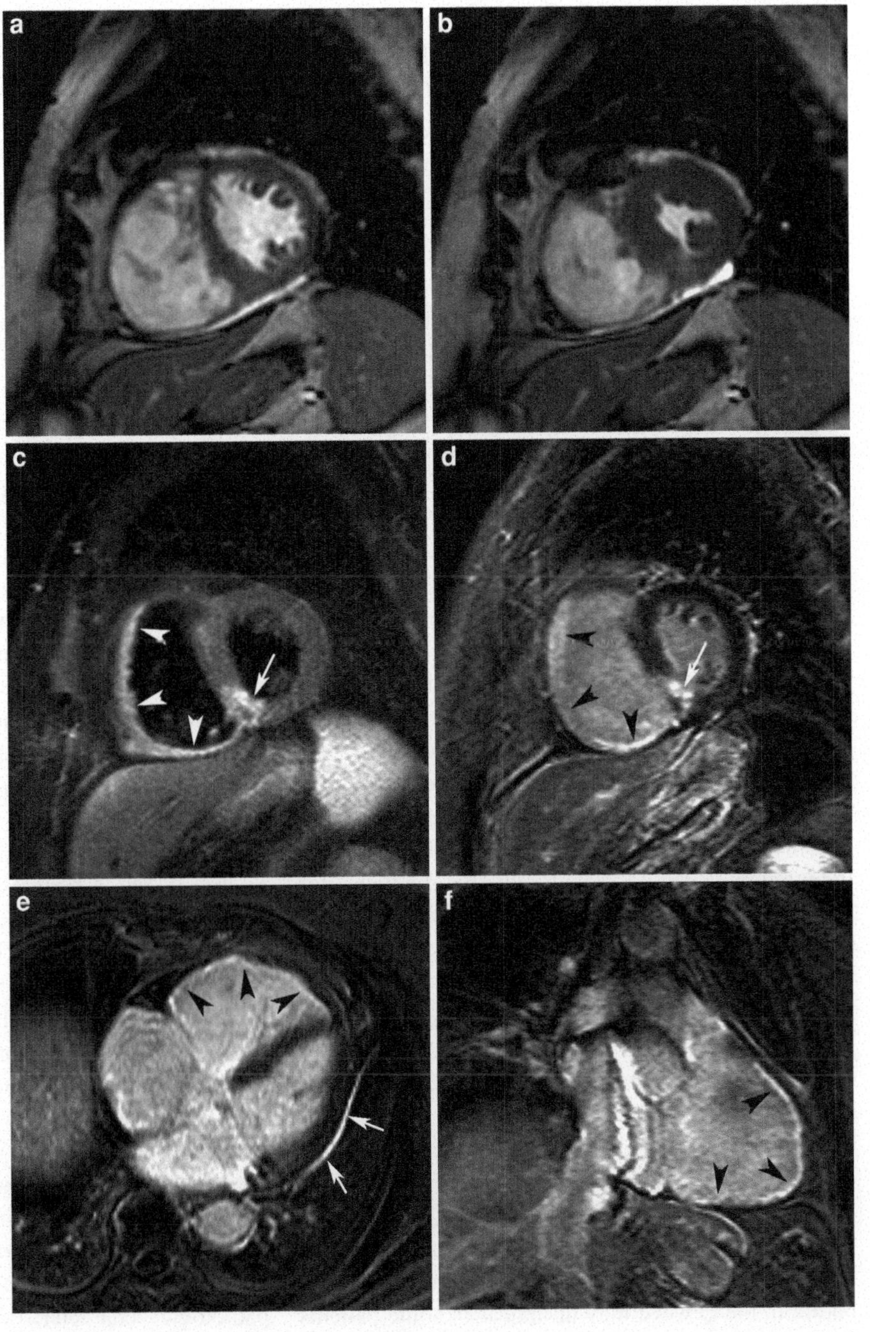

Fig. 31 Nearly isolated RV infarction in an 82-year-old woman. Short-axis cine at end diastole (**a**) and end systole (**b**), short-axis T2w-imaging (**c**). Late Gd imaging in short-axis (**d**), horizontal long-axis (**e**) and RV vertical long-axis (**f**). Moderately dilated and dysfunctional RV (EDV: 197 ml, EF: 39%) and nearly normal LV volumes and function (EDV: 109 ml, EF: 63%). Diffuse RV myocardial edema (*arrowheads*, **c**) with limited edema in inferoseptal LV wall (*arrow*, **c**). Late Gd imaging shows diffuse RV myocardial enhancement (*arrowheads*, **d**, **e**, **f**). Focal transmural enhancement in inferoseptal LV wall (*arrow*, **d**). Note the presence of some pericardial enhancement along the lateral LV border (*arrows*, **e**)

(Fig. 31). Animal and clinical studies have shown that RV is more resistant to prolonged ischemia than the LV with faster and better functional recovery despite similar initial dysfunction (Kinch and Ryan 1994; Laster et al. 1993, 1994). This can be attributed to a more favorable oxygen demand/supply profile for RV. Lack of RV recovery however, is associated with persistent hemodynamic compromise and high mortality rate (Zornoff et al. 2002; Larose et al. 2007). MRI is increasingly being used to study RV ischemic injury in MI patients. Assessment of reversible and irreversible ischemic injury in a thin and trabeculated RV wall is definitely more challenging, necessitating optimized approaches such as thinner slices, fat-saturation pre-pulses and optimized inversion times for late Gd MRI. Despite some limitations, MRI has definitely contributed not only by a better depiction but also by a better understanding of RV ischemic injury. It has become clear that the current established techniques for RV infarct detection, such as clinical investigation, ECG with right precordial leads, and echocardiography underestimate the true incidence of RV ischemic injury in acute inferior LV infarcts, with RV inferior wall enhancement in approximately 50% of patients (Kumar et al. 2006) (Fig. 26). Moreover, RV ischemic injury is not limited to inferior infarcts but is often found in anterior LV infarcts as well (Jenssen et al. 2010; Masci et al. 2010b) (Fig. 7). Taking into account that up to 30% of the RV free wall is perfused by the LAD coronary artery, a considerable portion of the RV myocardium is at risk in LAD infarcts. Fortunately, the RV myocardial salvage post-reperfusion is large and the resultant RV infarct size small (Bodi et al. 2010; Masci et al. 2010b) (Fig. 26). Acute RV dysfunction is related to the presence of RV ischemic injury, and the extent of RV myocardial edema is an independent predictor of global functional recovery. Remarkably, in a recent study we found at 4-month follow-up post-infarction besides resolvement of RV myocardial edema, a significant decrease in the extent and frequency of RV myocardial enhancement (Masci et al. 2010b). Potential explanations include volume shrinkage due to infarct healing but other mechanisms such as acute, temporary enhancement of the reversible injured, edematous portion of the jeopardized myocardium should be equally considered.

5.2.7 Unrecognized or Silent Myocardial Infarction

The diagnosis of healed MI is usually based on standard electrocardiography, in particular the presence of pathologic Q waves (Sheifer et al. 2001). The prevalence of unrecognized MI is therefore underestimated since non-Q-wave MIs are not taken into account. In addition, the Q wave may disappear in some patients late after MI. (Cox 1967). In the last couple of years several studies have shown, using late Gd MRI as morphologic in vivo validation technique, that ECG significantly underestimates the true prevalence of myocardial scarring due to prior MI (Kwong et al. 2006, 2008; Barbier et al. 2006; Meijs et al. 2009). In a recent study by Krittayaphong et al. involving 1,366 patients, using the 2007 criteria established by the universal definition of MI proposed by the joint ESC/ACC Foundation/American Heart Association/World Heart Foundation, ECG yielded a sensitivity, specificity, positive and negative predictive value, and accuracy of 46, 93, 79, 75, 75%, respectively (Thygesen et al. 2007; Krittayaphong et al. 2009). ECG-positive MIs had typically a greater size of MI, lower LV ejection fraction and poorer wall motion score compared with those without ECG evidence of MI. Barbier et al. found in 49 of 259 randomly selected 70-year-old subjects (19.8%) an unrecognized MI (Barbier et al. 2006). Since the presence of myocardial scar, even in small quantities, portends a strong and independent predictor of MACE, use of late Gd imaging may be indicated especially in elderly patients, or those with increased risk factors such as diabetic patients (Fig. 32) (Barbier et al. 2006; Kwong et al. 2008; Meijs et al. 2009; Cheong et al. 2009; Steel et al. 2009) (see also Sect. 5.2.1).

5.2.8 In Vivo Morphologic Validation of ECG using Contrast Enhanced MRI

Assessment of the electrical cardiac activity using 12-lead electrocardiography is the front-line technique in the diagnosis of acute MI as well to detect prior myocardial infarction (healed infarction) (Thygesen et al. 2007). In patients presenting with acute coronary syndrome, the patient's triage and treatment is to a large extent based on ECG changes indicative of new ischemia (new ST-T changes or new left bundle branch block), and development of pathological Q waves. The ECG allows the clinician to suggest the infarct-related artery, and to estimate the amount of myocardium at risk, and in ST-segment elevation infarcts, the degree of ST-resolution post-reperfusion reflects the success of reperfusion (Thygesen et al. 2007). Whereas a great deal of our knowledge of ECG-changes in IHD is based on pathologic correlations in animal work and autopsy studies described in the mid of the last century, contrast enhanced MRI allowing to in vivo study the pathologic characteristics of MI has prompted towards a reassessment and reinterpretation of our common understanding of the ECG (Myers et al. 1948a, b, c; Wu et al. 2001). First, it is a misnomer to consider a Q-wave infarction as transmural (Spodick 1980; Phibbs 1984; Sievers et al. 2004). Several MRI studies have shown that the primary determinant of the presence of a Q-wave is the total size of the underlying territorial infarction rather than its transmural extent (Moon et al. 2004; Kaandorp et al.

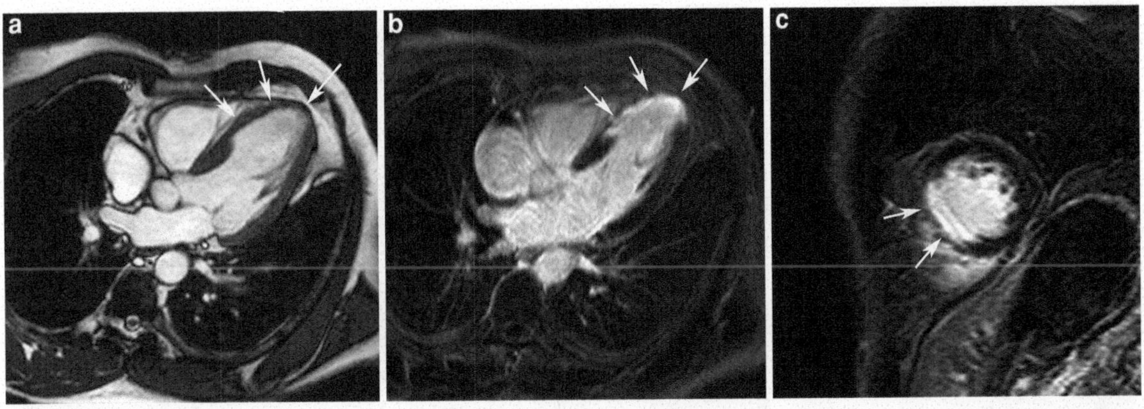

Fig. 32 Unrecognized myocardial infarction in a 53-year-old man referred for cardiac MRI to exclude hypertrophic cardiomyopathy and/or cardiac amyloidosis. Cine imaging in horizontal long-axis shows thinning of the apical half of the ventricular septum (*arrows*, **a**) with severe hypokinesia. Late Gd imaging in horizontal long-axis (**b**) and short-axis (**c**) plane show nearly complete transmural enhancement in apical half of ventricular septum and LV apex. Subsequent coronary angiography showed total occlusion of the mid LAD coronary angiography (not shown). The only patient complaint was that running (before 3 times per week) had become more difficult. At ECG a pathologic Q-wave was found in lead III

2005a; Engblom et al. 2005; Bodi et al. 2006; Plein et al. 2008b). The larger the endocardial extent of MI, the more likely there will be Q-wave on the ECG (Engblom et al. 2007). Second, ECG-derived estimates of infarct size correlate at best, only modestly with late Gd MRI, overestimating small infarcts and underestimating large infarcts (Geerse et al. 2009; Weir et al. 2010a, b). Importantly, the lateral LV territories are electrically silent and therefore may present with little ECG alteration (Rovai et al. 2007). Lateral infarcts can be very similar in magnitude to anterior infarcts and should not be considered low risk (Smalling 2009). Martin et al. proposed, using late Gd imaging as gold standard, the term ST-segment deviation MI including ST-segment depression MI besides ST-segment elevation MI for an improved detection of acute myocardial infarction, especially for those caused by occlusion of the left circumflex coronary artery (Martin et al. 2007). Recently, a multi-specialist team has defined a new terminology of the LV walls and proposed a new classification of Q-wave myocardial infarction based on cardiac MRI correlations (Cerqueira 2002; Bayés de Luna et al. 2006a). The new classification defining the most commonly occurring patterns of Q waves and Q-wave equivalents matched well with late Gd MRI necrotic areas (Bayés de Luna et al. 2006a, b; Cino et al. 2006). Importantly, 17% of MIs detected by late Gd imaging presented normal ECGs (Cino et al. 2006).

5.2.9 Serum Markers of Myocardial Necrosis Versus Contrast Enhanced MRI

Myocardial cell death is typically characterized by a release of different proteins into the circulation from the damaged myocytes. At present, the preferred biomarker is cardiac troponin (I or T), which has a nearly absolute myocardial tissue specificity as well as high clinical sensitivity (Thygesen et al. 2007). If troponin assays are not available, the best alternative is CK-MB. Since the release characteristics are complex, one of the crucial questions is what approach provides the best estimate of myocardial infarct size. Till date, several studies have used late Gd MRI as in vivo validation technique, but the results are not straightforward. Although all studies showed a significant correlation between rise in biomarkers and imaging findings, some of them used peak values (Haase et al. 2004; Ingkanisorn et al. 2004), while others proposed use of a single point measurement either early (i.e. 24–48 h) (Hallén et al. 2009) or late (i.e., 72–96 h) (Steen et al. 2006; Younger et al. 2007) post-infarction.

5.3 Patterns of Enhancement Depending on Infarct Location

As already discussed above, the tissue enhancement in MI, although acute or healed, is non-specific and merely reflects a disturbance in local alterations of

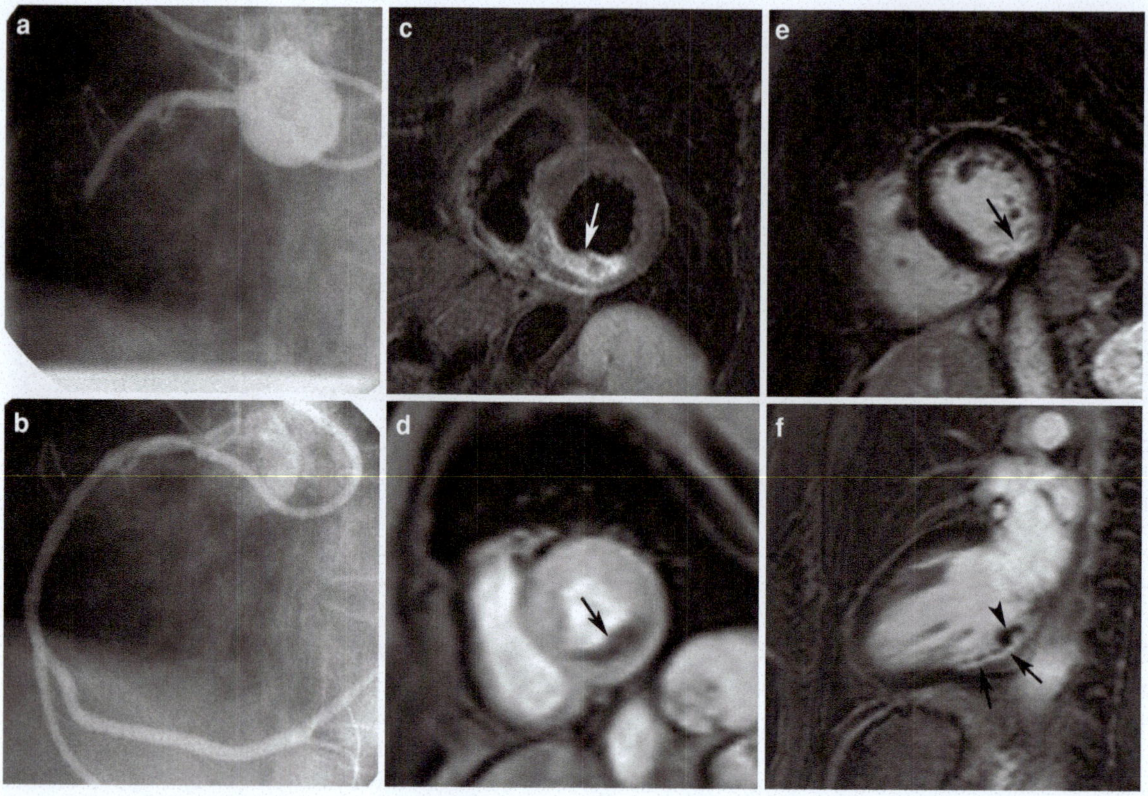

Fig. 33 Example of an acute inferior LV infarction in a 79-year-old patient due to occlusion of the RCA. Coronary angiography before (**a**) and after (**b**) PCI shows occlusion of the RCA at the middle segment with restoration of the patency post-PCI and stent placement. Comprehensive MR study after PCI shows edema in the inferior wall on T2w-imaging (*arrow*, **c**). First pass perfusion shows extensive mainly subendocardial perfusion defect in the inferior wall (*arrow*, **d**) while late Gd imaging in short-axis (**e**) and vertical long-axis (**f**) show focal late enhancement (*arrows*, **e**, f) with microvascular obstruction (*arrowhead*, **f**)

perfusion, tissue metabolism and loss of normal myocardial matrix. Differential diagnosis in clinical circumstances may therefore be less obvious, especially in cases with atypical presentations. There are, however, a few markers by which to attribute a certain pattern of myocardial enhancement with a higher degree of certainty in the IHD category. First, regardless of the MI location, the pattern of enhancement always presents as spreading outward from the endocardium. Whether the infarction itself is subendocardial or transmural, the subendocardium is always involved. Furthermore, the infarct location can always be traced back to a certain 'culprit' artery, which is to say, although the supply territories of the three major coronary arteries are variable depending on coronary artery anatomy, the infarction is always located within the anatomical territory supplied by one coronary artery (or one of its side branches), and the intensity of abnormalities increases toward the distal perfusion territory of that coronary artery. The use of these two criteria may already allow the physician to differentiate between myocardial enhancement due to MI and that seen in other diseases such as in myocarditis, which is known to present a more diffused multifocal enhancement pattern, often subepicardially located and not infrequently accompanied by pericardial enhancement (Mahrholdt et al. 2004) (see "Heart Muscle Diseases").

In inferior infarctions, the enhancement is usually located in the basal (segments 3–4) and midventricular (segments 9–10) inferior LV wall (Fig. 33) and may extend towards the lateral LV wall (segments 5–11) (Fig. 25c) as well as towards the RV inferior wall (Fig. 26). Lateral MIs typical-involve the lateral LV wall and sometimes may be extensive involving the entirety of the lateral wall (segments 5–6–11–12–16)

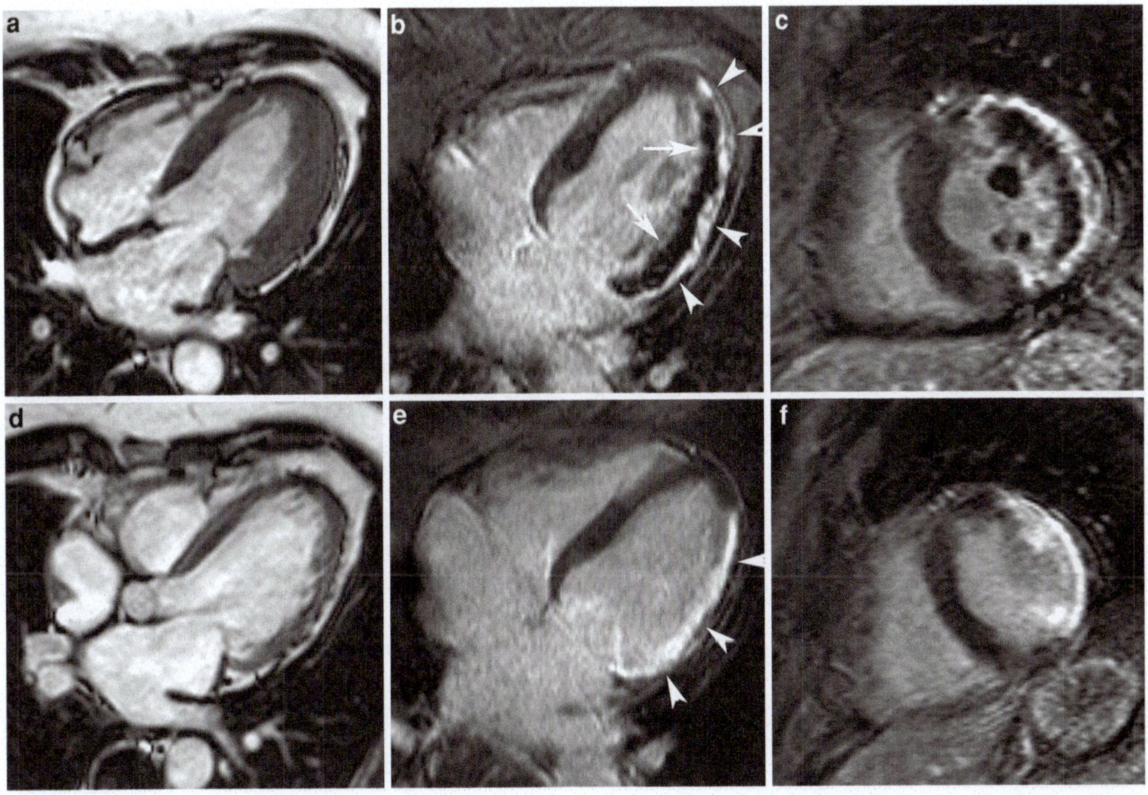

Fig. 34 Example of an extensive lateral LV infarction early post-infarction (i.e. day 4) (**a–c**), and at 4-month follow-up (**d–f**). Cine imaging in horizontal long-axis (**a**, **d**), late Gd imaging in horizontal long-axis (**b**, **e**) and short-axis (**c**, **f**). Early post-infarction, important wall thickening is noticed involving the entire lateral LV wall, while at follow-up important wall thinning has occurred. Late Gd imaging at day 4 shows extensive transmural infarction (*arrowheads*, **b**) with large microvascular obstruction (*arrows*, **b**). At follow-up a thin strongly enhancing scar remains (*arrows*, **e**)

(Fig. 34). Anterior infarcts that are variable in size, typically involve the anterior or anteroseptal wall showing a variable extend to the septum and antero-lateral wall. Longitudinally, they usually involve the mid—and apical LV portion and LV apex but may extend toward the basal LV portion (segments 1–2–6–7–8–12–13–14–17) (Fig. 35). Smaller sized infarctions, often at atypical locations (e.g., mid-septum), can be seen when coronary artery side branches are involved (Fig. 32), and micro-infarctions can be seen after PCI or stent placements (see Sect. 5.6).

5.4 Infarct-Related Complications

Complications related to MI, such as aneurysm formation, thrombus formation, valve leakage, associated pericardial effusion or post-infarction pericarditis, are best visualized by cardiac MRI using a comprehensive approach. MRI is useful to depict and differentiate true from false ventricular aneurysms (Figs. 36 and 37). The latter, defined as rupture of the myocardium contained by pericardial adhesions, typically present a smaller orifice compared to the maximal internal diameter, whereas in true aneurysms, still containing some myocardial elements in its wall, dimensions are similar. Moreover, pericardial enhancement was invariably found in false aneurysms but only in 3/18 patients with true aneurysm (Konen et al. 2005).

Ventricular thrombus formation is a frequent complication of MI occurring in 12% of anterior MIs, and is more common in cases of aneurysm formation (Chiarella et al. 1998). Thrombus detection is of paramount importance, since the presence is an indication for strict anticoagulation therapy to avoid

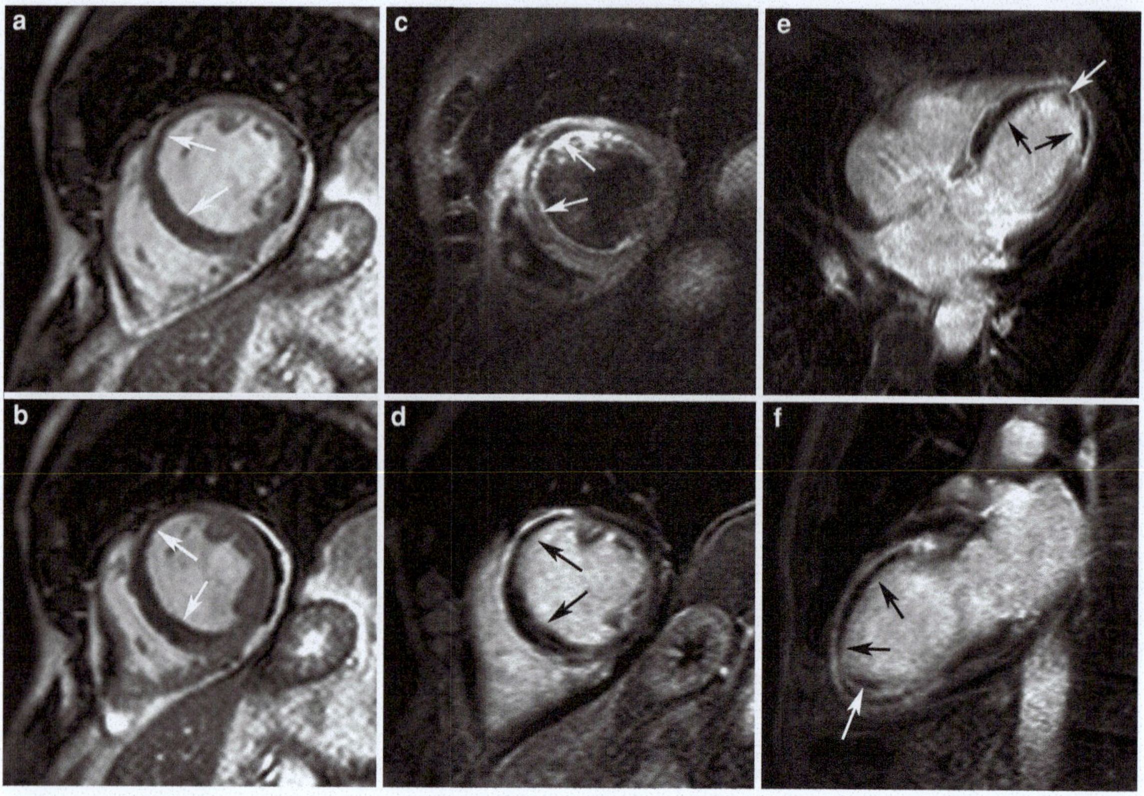

Fig. 35 Example of a severe antero-septo-apical LV infarction. Short-axis cine imaging at end diastole (**a**) and end systole (**b**) (following contrast administration). Short-axis T2w-imaging (**c**) and late Gd imaging in short-axis (**d**), horizontal long-axis (**e**) and vertical long-axis (**f**). Post-contrast cine imaging shows extensive hypointense zone (corresponding to microvascular obstruction) in the anteroseptal LV wall exploiting a-to dyskinetic wall motion pattern (*arrows*, **a**, **b**). Evidence of myocardial hemorrhage in the jeopardized myocardium with edema extending toward the adjacent RV wall (*arrows*, **c**). Late Gd imaging shows extensive enhancement in the antero-septo-apical region with large microvascular obstruction (*black arrows*, **d**, **e**, **f**). Note the presence of a small apical thrombus (*white arrow*, **e**, **f**)

potential neurological and peripheral embolic events. Thrombi are easily missed on transthoracic echocardiography especially when located in the LV apex or when trapped within the endocardial trabeculations. Using a combination of late Gd imaging and cine imaging, ventricular thrombi are well demonstrated and differentiated from stagnant or slow flow (Keeley and Hillis 1996; Mollet et al. 2002; Weinsaft et al. 2008). Thrombi are best visualized early after contrast administration, taking advantage of the high contrast of the blood pool (Figs. 15–38). They typically appear as hypo-intense filling-defects, whereas thrombus enhancement on late imaging can be found in organized clots (Barkhausen et al. 2002; Donato et al. 2009). Differentiation with no-reflow zones is usually straightforward because the hypo-intense zone is located in the myocardium. Use of a longer inversion time (e.g., 500 ms) may facilitate depiction of thrombi especially when adjacent to normal myocardium (Fig. 38).

Pericardial inflammation can occur early post-infarction and is typically found in transmural infarctions. This condition should be differentiated from late post-infarction pericarditis (Dressler's syndrome). Imaging, in particular MRI, is helpful in depicting associated pericardial pathology (Fig. 39) (Bogaert and Francone 2009) (see "Pericardial Disease").

Mitral valve leakage post-infarction is related to valve ring dilatation due to adverse LV remodeling and/or

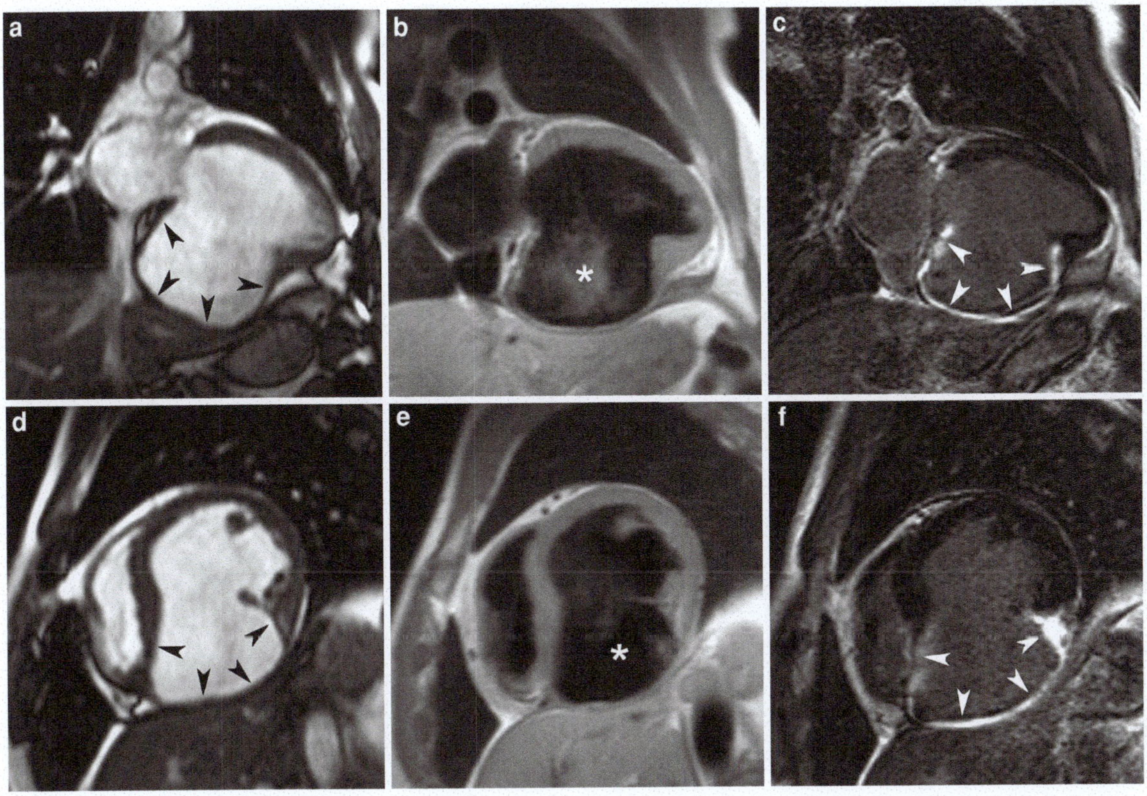

Fig. 36 Post-infarction aneurysm formation in a 63-year-old patient with previous inferior wall infarction. Cine imaging, T1w-imaging and late Gd imaging in vertical long-axis (**a**, **b**, **c**, respectively) and in short-axis plane (**d**, **e**, **f**, respectively). Presence of a broad-based aneurysm with extensive wall thinning (10 × 4 cm) originating from the inferior LV wall (*arrowheads*, *). Note the strong enhancement of the aneurysmatic wall at late Gd imaging (*arrowheads*, **c**, **f**). Histology of the aneurysm showed a thin, completely fibrotic scar without remaining myocardial tissue

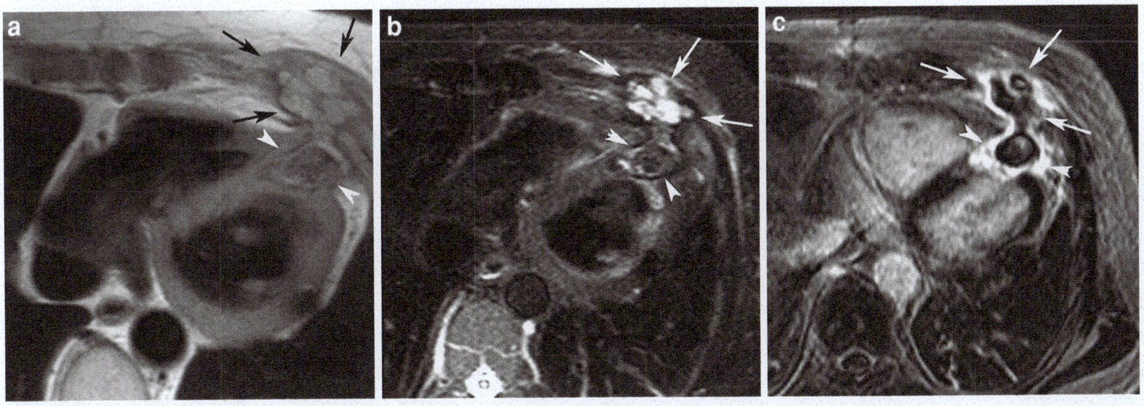

Fig. 37 False aneurysm in a 70-year-old man presenting with pulsatile mass in left hemithorax. History of previous anteroseptal LV infarction with aneurysmectomy in 1982. Presence of an irregular defined, inhomogeneous mass in left hemithorax (*arrows*, **a**, **b**, **c**) extending to the LV apex (*arrowheads*, **a**, **b**, **c**). Strong peripheral enhancement is shown at late Gd imaging (**c**). The false aneurysm was surgically resected

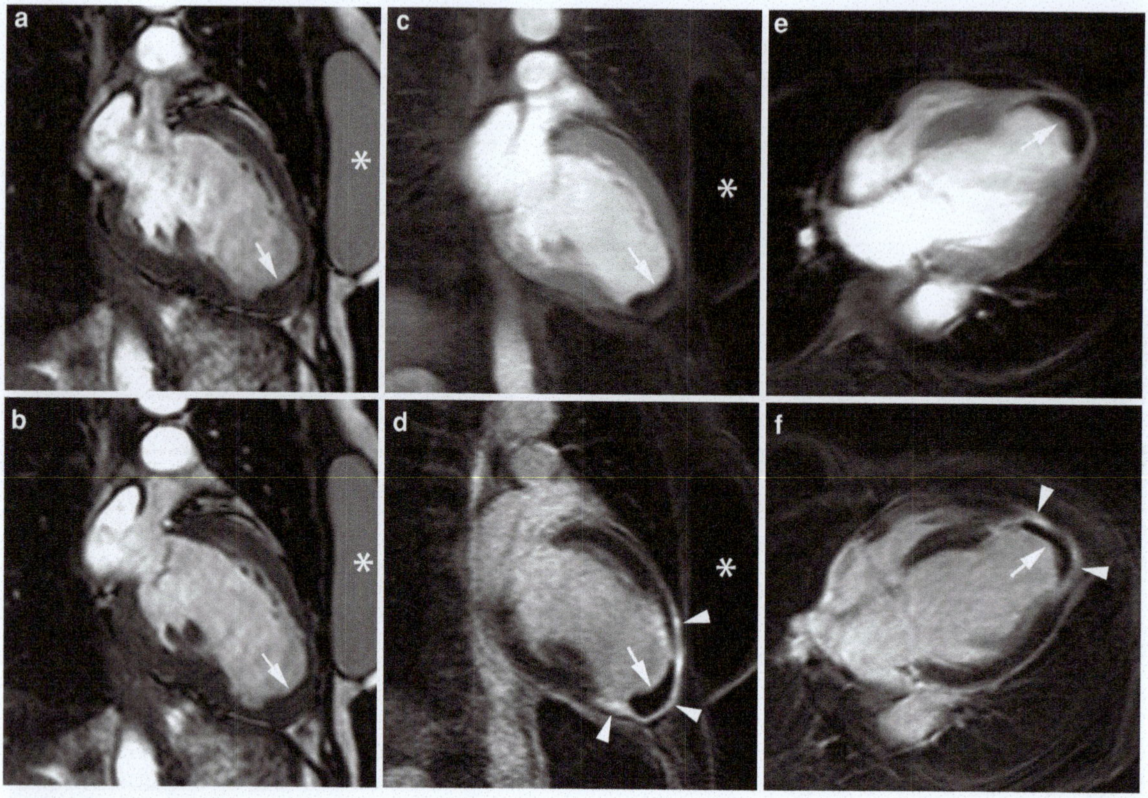

Fig. 38 Thrombus formation in a female patient with an acute apical myocardial infarction. Vertical long-axis cine imaging at end diastole (**a**) en end systole (**b**). Contrast-enhanced MRI in vertical long-axis (**c**, **d**) and horizontal long-axis plane (**e**, **f**) obtained early post-contrast administration using long inversion time (**c**, **e**) and using the late Gd imaging technique (**d**, **f**). At cine imaging the LV apex appears thick (*arrow*, **a**, **b**) but is akinetic. The true nature of the thick LV apex becomes evident at contrast-enhanced MRI. Presence of a dark structure molded over the LV apex in clear contrast with the enhancing myocardium and bright LV cavity (*arrow*, **c**, **e**). In particular, early Gd imaging with long inversion time allows good discrimination between thrombus and myocardium. At late imaging the infarcted myocardium is strongly enhanced (*arrowheads*, **d**, **f**) while the thrombus is dark (*arrow*, **d**, **f**). Although microvascular obstruction can present in a similar way, the thrombus is clearly located on the inside of the thin myocardial wall. Presence of a silicone breast prosthesis (*)

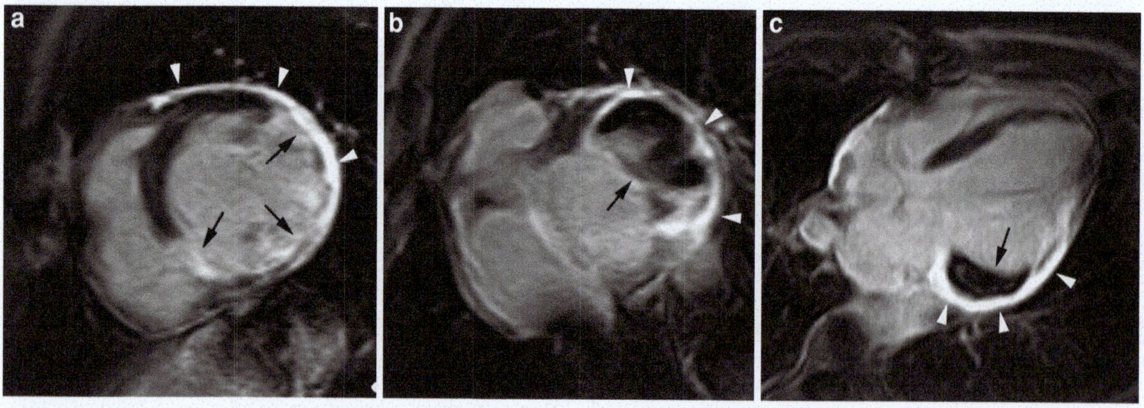

Fig. 39 Post-infarction aneurysm, thrombus and pericarditis. Late Gd imaging in short-axis (**a**, **b**) and in horizontal long-axis (**c**). Transmural enhancement of the inferolateral basal segment, as well as enhancement of the overlying pericardium (*arrowheads*, **a**–**c**) and aneurysmal dilation of the expanded infarction (*arrows*, **a**). Presence of large thrombus in the ventricular aneurysm (*arrows*, **b**–**c**)

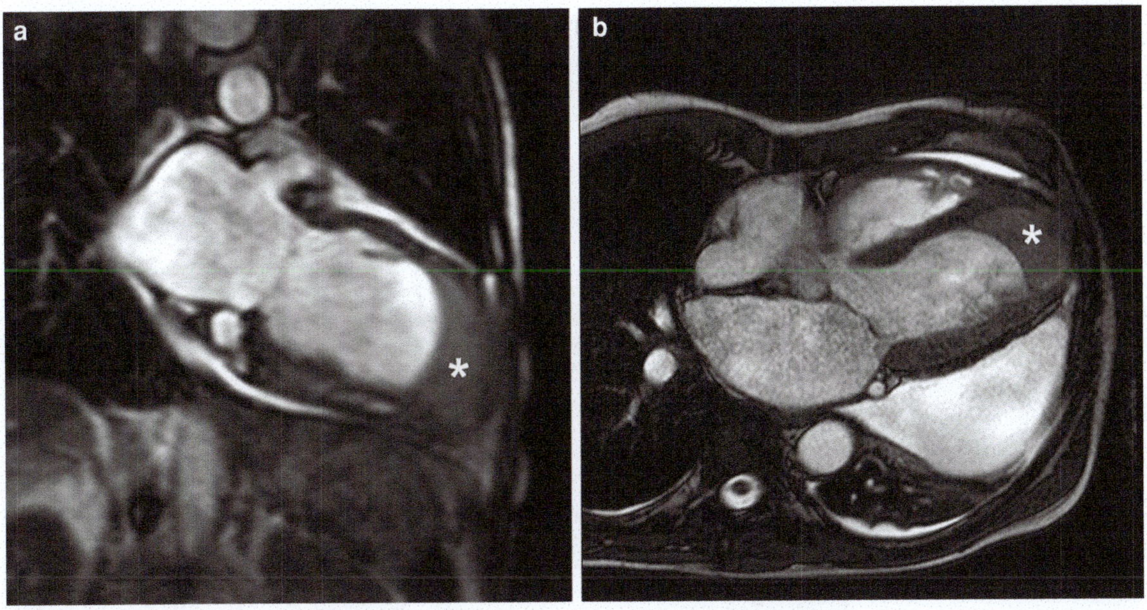

Fig. 40 Subendocardial dissecting myocardial hematoma in a patient with a recent apical myocardial infarction admitted with cardiogenic shock. Cine imaging in vertical (**a**) and horizontal (**b**) long-axis. Presence of a sharply defined, slightly hyperintense structure in LV apex clearly discernable from the LV blood pool and adjacent myocardium. Dynamic imaging showed deformation of the structure during cardiac contraction. Presence of an important pericardial effusion, mainly along the left lateral cardiac border

concomitant papillary muscle infarction. High-spatial resolution 3D contrast enhanced MRI techniques improve detection of papillary infarction (Peters et al. 2009). In a recent study by Tanimoto et al. the posterior papillary muscle was more frequently involved than the anterior papillary muscle (77 vs. 26%, $p<0.001$), but papillary muscle infarction was not necessarily associated with mitral regurgitation, and did not influence post-infarct LV remodeling (Tanimoto et al. 2010). In another study, in particular the presence of bilateral papillary muscle necrosis was related to mitral regurgitation (Okayama et al. 2011). MRI may be occasionally helpful in detecting rare complications such as ventricular septal defects or intramural dissecting myocardial hematoma (Fig. 40) (Jahnke et al. 2007a; Jun et al. 2007).

5.5 Infarct Healing and Ventricular Remodeling

Infarct healing, scar formation and adaptive ventricular remodeling are intricate processes that have been extensively studied in animal models and patients with an acute MI over the previous decades (Pfeffer and Braunwald 1989; Holmes et al. 2005). The magnitude and direction of changes are determined by several parameters such as infarct size, location and transmurality, extent of myocardial stunning, patency of the infarct-related artery, collateral circulation and presence of MVO, post-reperfusion myocardial hemorrhage (Fig. 41). In recent years, MRI has shown to be very helpful in better understanding the processes of infarct healing and ventricular remodeling (Kramer et al. 1993, 1996a, b, 1997; Bogaert et al. 1999, 2000; Moustakidis et al. 2002; Rademakers et al. 2003; Ganame et al. 2011) (Fig. 42). In particular, the comprehensive approach combining in vivo tissue characterization with functional data obtained with cine or tagging sequences is a major strength of MRI compared with other techniques, allowing to study evolution at long-term (Kramer et al. 2000; Schroeder et al. 2001; Garot et al. 2004; Engblom et al. 2009; Ibrahim et al. 2010; Ganame et al. 2011) (Fig. 3). In addition, diffusion-tensor cardiac MRI has been used to in vivo evaluate the structural correlates of functional remodeling after infarction (Walker et al. 2005; Wu et al. 2006, 2009).

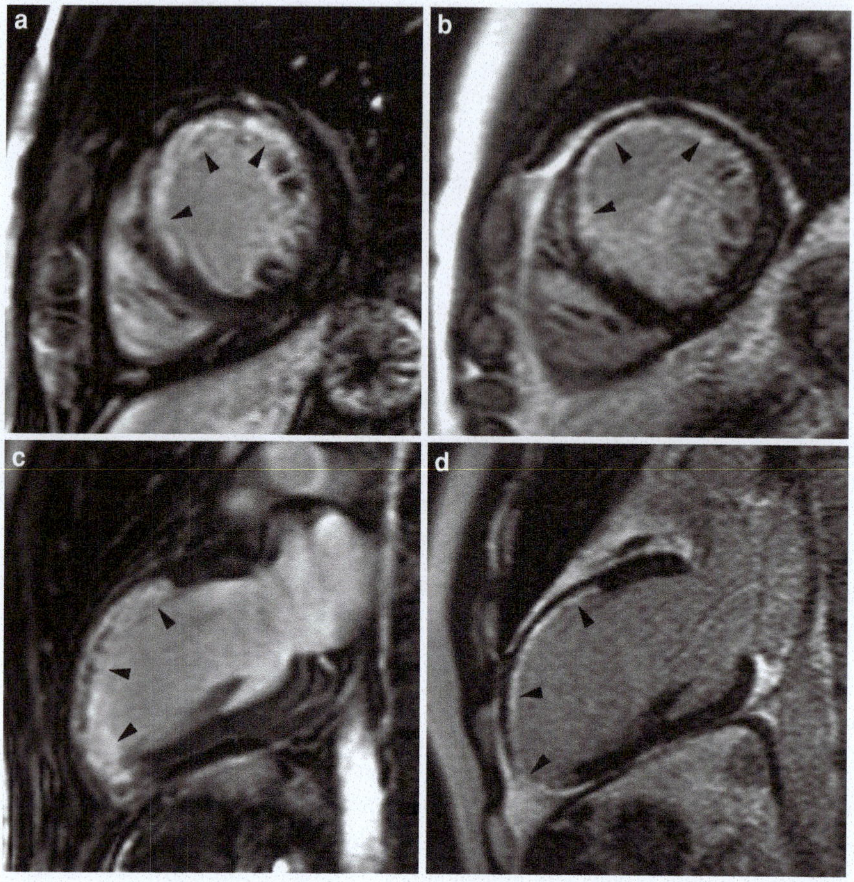

Fig. 41 Infarct healing and remodeling in a 54-year old patient after LAD occlusion. Late Gd imaging in short-axis (**a**, **b**) and vertical long-axis (**c**, **d**) in the acute phase (**a**, **c**) and at 4 months post-infarction (**b**, **d**). Early post-infarction (day 5), extensive, nearly complete transmural enhancement in anteroseptoapical LV wall (*arrowheads*, **a–c**) with small no-reflow areas at the endocardial border. Note the significant thinning of the infarcted myocardium (due to processes of infarct healing) at follow-up (*arrowheads*, **b**, **d**). Note the mild increase in thickness of the unenhanced rim in the infarct territory

5.6 Peri-Procedural Necrosis

Mild elevations in cardiac biomarkers are common after successful PCI and coronary bypass surgery, and are associated with future adverse events (Prasad et al. 2006; Larose 2006). The Universal Definition states that troponin is the preferred biomarker and an elevation of more than 3× the 99th percentile URL is defined as a *PCI-related MI* (*MI type 4a*) (Thygesen et al. 2007). The potential of late Gd MRI to depict myocardial necrosis as small as 1–2 g has enabled to better understand the underlying mechanisms of PCI-related myocardial necrosis (Ricciardi et al. 2001; Selvanayagam et al. 2004a, b, 2005a, b; Porto et al. 2006). Two types of myonecrosis-related types of enhancement have been described, i.e. "adjacent" myonecrosis in the neighborhood of the stent related to side branch occlusion (Fig. 43), and "distal" myonecrosis due to distal embolization of plaque material. The latter may lead to a reduction in MPR index at 24 h after PCI, and are confined to the segments with injury but do not affect the entire supply territory of the culprit vessel (Selvanayagam et al. 2007). Thrombus aspiration during primary PCI improves myocardial reperfusion and reduces the extent of periprocedural necrosis (Sardella et al. 2009). Other efforts to minimize peri-procedural necrosis include careful analysis of side branch anatomy (Porto et al. 2006). It was recently shown by late Gd imaging that subtle peri-procedural myocardial necrosis (less than 1g) frequently occurs, being undetected using the new universal definition of myocardial infarction (Locca et al. 2010). Lim et al. 2011 showed using late Gd imaging as reference technique that measurement of CK-MB is more clinically relevant than troponin for diagnosing MI type 4a. In addition, also other procedures such as chest compression and external defibrillation may result in release of cardiac biomarkers (Müllner et al. 1998). Here too, MRI yields promise to accurately depict subtle myocardial damage (Masci et al. 2007).

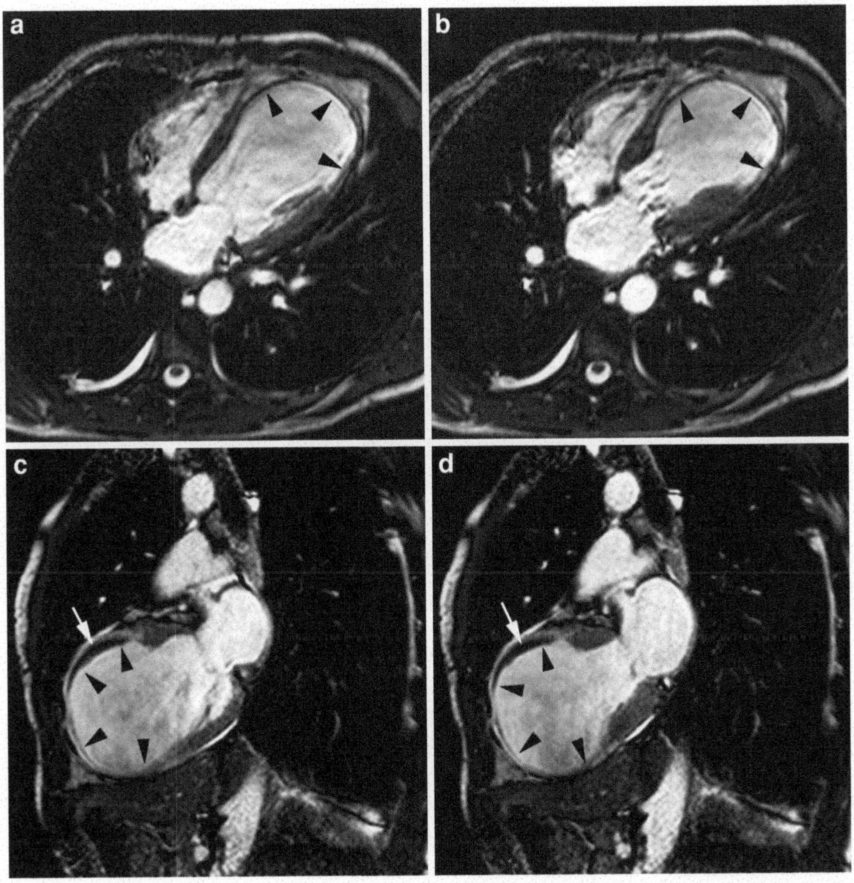

Fig. 42 Adverse LV remodeling with apical aneurysm formation in a 52-year-old patient with a late presentation of myocardial infarction. Cine imaging (post-contrast administration) in the horizontal (**a**, **b**) and vertical (**c**, **d**) at end diastole (**a**, **c**) and end systole (**b**, **d**). Extreme thinning of the entire LV apex with important aneurysmal bulging (*arrowheads*, **a–d**). The aneurysmal LV apex is dyskinetic. Presence of a mural thrombus along the infarcted anterior LV wall (*arrow*, **c**, **d**)

5.7 Role of MRI in Patients with Acute Chest Pain

Growing evidence has been fostering the role of cardiac MRI in the evaluation of patients with acute chest pain (Assomull et al. 2007; Arai 2007). In these patients, ACCF/AHA guidelines recommend a non invasive approach in those with low likelihood for MI or with severe co-morbidities. Similarly, ESC guidelines recommend non-invasive imaging in patients with acute chest pain but repetitive negative troponins and normal or undetermined electrocardiogram (ECG). Although the diagnosis of ST-segment elevation MI is straightforward, the majority of patients with acute chest pain admitted in the emergency department do not have ACS. This scenario is further complicated by the universal definition of MI based on ACC/ESC consensus document, which indicates cardiac troponin and ECG as the cornerstone tests for diagnosing acute MI. As a matter of fact, cardiac troponin is a highly sensitive but poorly specific marker of ischemic myocardial damage, since any condition provoking myocyte necrosis will result in a rise in cardiac troponin (Steg et al. 2009). Additionally, the increase in cardiac tropinin is limited to a narrow time window reducing their sensitivity to depict subacute MI. Similarly, ECG changes overlap between ischemic and non-ischemic heart disease, and a small acute MI may not induce typical ECG abnormalities. In these circumstances, a comprehensive cardiac MRI exam is of great value in diagnosing and eventually, differentiating acute MI from other entities clinically presenting similarly such as peri-myocarditis, tako-tsubo (or stress) cardiomyopathy or acute aortic disease (Assomull et al. 2007; Arai 2007; Eitel et al. 2008). In the latter condition, however, it should be kept in mind that cardiac computed tomography is the preferential imaging technique for diagnosing acute aortic syndrome (e.g., aortic dissection, intramural hemorrhage). In patients presenting with acute chest pain, troponin rise but normal coronary angiograms, cardiac MRI may yield findings

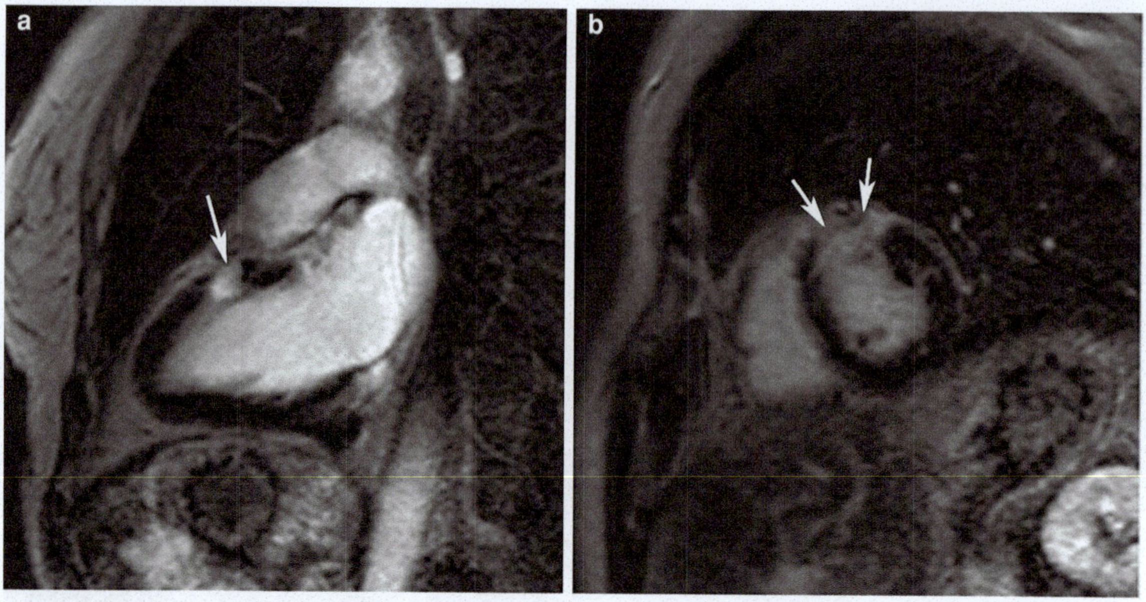

Fig. 43 Peri-procedural necrosis ('adjacent type') in a 55-year-old woman during PCI. Late Gd imaging in vertical long-axis (**a**) and midventricular short-axis (**b**). Patient experienced chest pain during PCI with parde curves on ECG and rise in troponins. MRI shows focal transmural enhancement in the anterior LV wall (*arrows*, **a**, **b**) at the level of coronary artery stent. Cine imaging shows focal severe hypokinesia of the mid-anterior wall

typical of acute myocarditis in as many as 30–50% of the cases (see "Heart Muscle Diseases"). Occassionally, MRI may reveal findings of an acute MI. Retrospective analysis of the 'normal' coronary angiograms usually reveals occlusion of one of the CA side branches (Fig. 44). In tako-tsubo cardiomyopathy, which is characterized by typical angina chest pain, ECG changes and normal coronary angiography, cardiac MRI may reveal akinesia or dyskinesia of the LV apex and edema on T2w-imaging, whereas the pattern of myocardial enhancement on late Gd imaging, when present, is typically different from that of acute myocarditis or acute MI (Fig. 45). However, it has to be kept in mind that only few clinical trials tested the value of cardiac MRI in patients with acute chest pain admitted to emergency department. Of note, Kwong et al. 2003 reported that late Gd MRI (T2w-imaging was not performed) had a sensitivity of 84% and specificity of 85% in diagnosing ACS in patients with chest pain and absent ST-segment elevation. Other authors, by adding T2w-imaging to the study protocol improved the overall accuracy of cardiac MRI in detecting acute MI yielding a sensitivity of 85% and specificity of 96% (Curry et al. 2008). According to data by Kwong et al., cardiac MRI was feasible in emergency department setting, and only 11% of patients were excluded from analysis (5% because of claustrophobia). However, in the routine clinical practice there are several constraints limiting the application of cardiac MRI in patients presenting to medical attention because of acute chest pain, such as the current limited capability to accommodate MRI studies in emergency.

6 Chronic Ischemic Cardiomyopathy

6.1 Ischemic Heart Disease and Heart Failure

Ischemic heart disease is the principal cause of heart failure, and its prevalence continues to increase (Mann and Bristow 2005; Gheorghiade et al. 2006) (see "Heart Failure and Heart Transplantation"). Heart failure poses an enormous medical and financial burden on our society. Patients in whom CAD is the underlying cause have significantly worse prognosis than patients with nonischemic heart failure. The onset of heart failure in CAD patients may be abrupt (e.g., following acute MI) or insidious. Patients have single or multi-vessel CAD

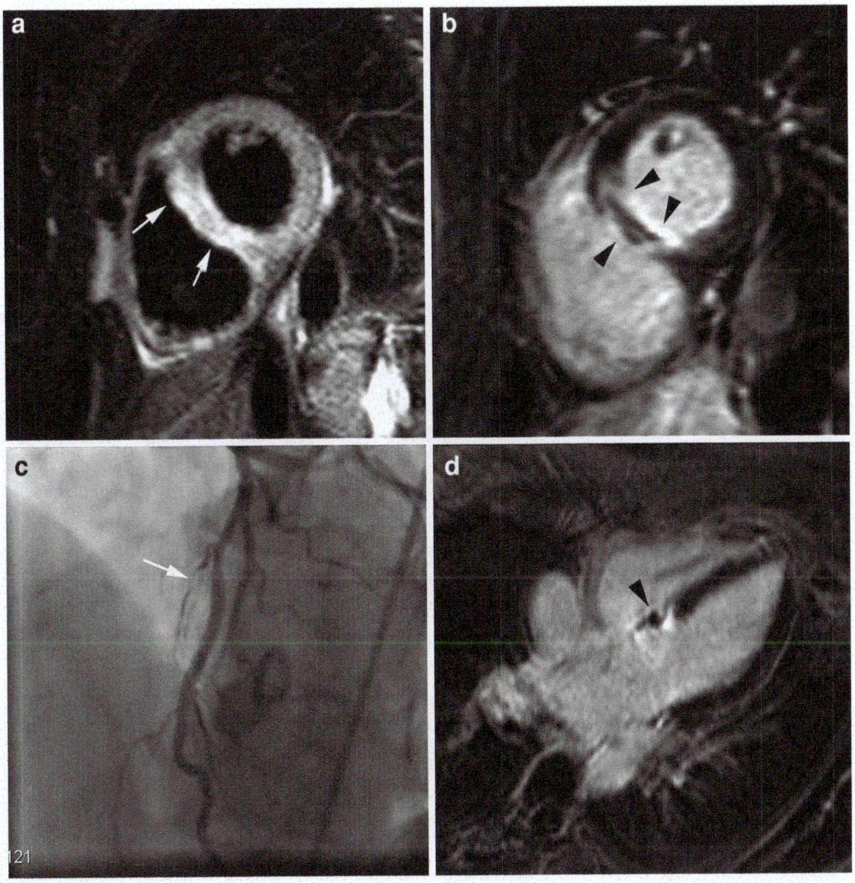

Fig. 44 Non ST-segment elevation MI (NSTEMI) in a 50-year-old woman. Short-axis T2w-imaging (**a**) and late Gd imaging (**b**). Coronary angiography (**c**) and late Gd imaging in horizontal long-axis plane (**d**). Patient admitted with NSTEMI but no critical stenoses on main coronary arteries, except 95% stenosis on first septal perforator (*arrow*, **c**). Subsequent MRI shows focal myocardial in basal part of ventricular septum (*arrows*, **a**) exhibiting dyskinetic wall motion pattern on cine imaging (not shown). Late Gd imaging shows transmural enhancement with central zone of micro-vascular obstruction in the jeopardized basal ventricular septum (*arrowheads*, **b**, **d**)

disease and typically present with dilated ventricles showing regional or more generalized ventricular dysfunction. Even if results of prospectively controlled studies of revascularization in these patient groups are still lacking, there is substantial evidence that patients with reversible LV dysfunction may benefit from a revascularization procedure, and thereby improve regional and global ventricular functions, reverse the maladaptive remodeling process, improve exercise capacity and decrease symptoms of heart failure and increase long-term prognosis (Bax et al. 2001; Schinkel et al. 2007). However, since the dysfunctional ventricle or myocardium in CAD often contains a mixture of different ischemic substrates (i.e. stunned, ischemic, hibernating, necrotic, scarred myocardium) within the same perfusion territory or within the ventricle, characterization of these ischemic substrates, in particular assessment of the viability, is of utmost importance to determine whether a patient may benefit from a revascularization procedure (see also Sect. 2) (Underwood et al. 2004; Wu et al. 2011) (Figs. 46 and 47). At present, different strategies for viability assessment using a variety of techniques are available. MRI has emerged as one of the preferential techniques to characterize the ischemic substrate and to determine myocardial viability. This technique can be used to assess the different aspects of the myocardium related to viability. On the one hand, MRI has emulated approaches used by other techniques, such as assessment of wall thickness or myocardial contractility reserve used by echocardiography (Baer et al. 1992, 2000). On the other hand, MRI has the unique capability to noninvasively visualize even subtle amounts of myocardial scar formation, or to measure metabolic spectra using MR spectroscopy (Wagner et al. 2003; Bottomley et al. 2009) (Fig. 48).

6.2 Myocardial Viability Assessment

A first approach to assess myocardial viability is measurement of segmental end-diastolic wall thickness (EDWT). In case of a history of previous MI,

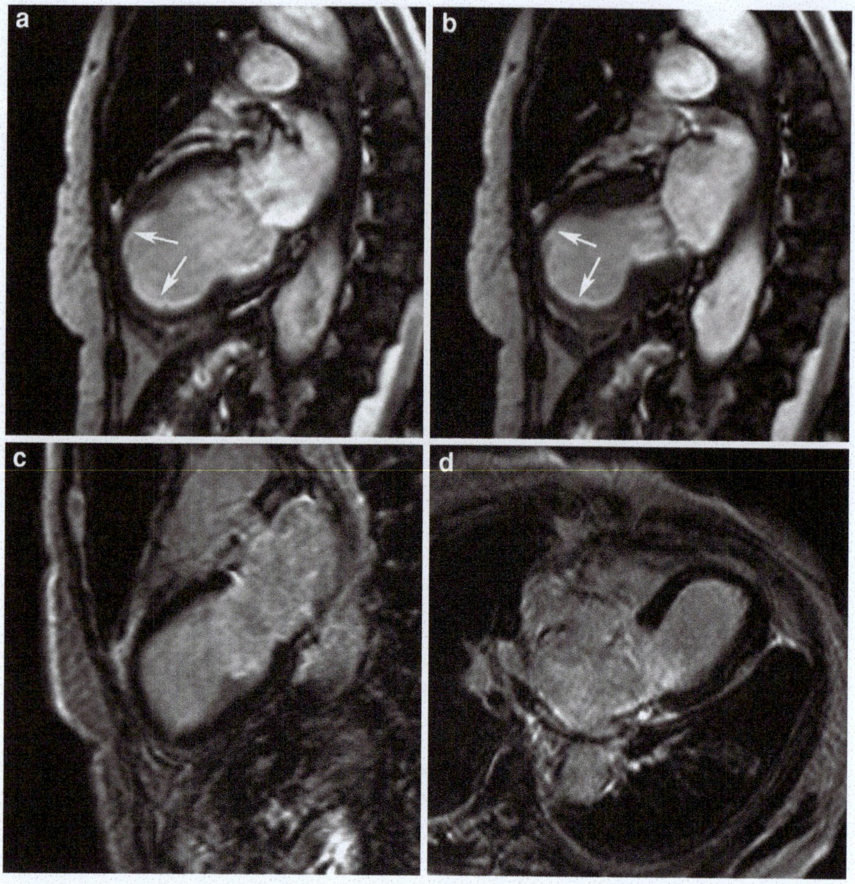

Fig. 45 Tako-Tsubo cardiomyopathy in an 81-year-old woman. Vertical long-axis cine imaging at end diastole (**a**) and end systole (**b**). Late Gd imaging in vertical long-axis (**c**) and horizontal long-axis image plane (**d**). Cine imaging shows severe contraction abnormalities with akinesia of the entire LV apex (*arrows*, **a**, **b**). Late Gd imaging, however, shows no abnormal myocardial enhancement

infarct healing with scar formation leads to a wall thinning of the infarcted region, and the amount of wall thinning is related to the degree of infarct transmurality (Baer et al. 1992, 1995) (Fig. 48). This approach appears very sensitive (95%, range 94–100%), but not specific (41%, range 19–53%) for prediction of functional recovery, indicating that thinned myocardium (<6 mm) has a low likelihood to improve function after revascularization and accurately reflects scar tissue (Kaandorp et al. 2005b; Schinkel et al. 2007). A substantial percentage of segments with preserved wall thickness, however, does not improve in function following revascularization. The most likely explanation is the presence of subendocardial infarction with preserved wall thickness. Kühl et al. found that the use of non-enhanced rim thickness by late Gd imaging (cut-off value: 3.0 mm) is superior to EDWT (cut-off: 5.4 mm) for viability assessment (Kühl et al. 2006). Moreover, thinned myocardial segments may undergo a process of "reverse remodeling" after successful myocardial revascularization with recovery of function and regain in regional wall thickness (John et al. 2005).

A second approach is the contractile reserve assessment during low dose dobutamine stress (Fig. 48) (see Sect. 4.2). In patients with chronic LV dysfunction, dysfunctional but viable (hibernating) segments improve contractility during low-dose (5–10 μg/kg body weight) dobutamine infusion (i.e. increased systolic wall thickening >2 mm), whereas contractility in non-viable scarred segments remain unchanged or worsen during stress imaging (Baer et al. 1995; Dendale et al. 1995, 1997). Since the contractility reserve is limited, the increase in contractility is typically followed by a worsening of function ("biphasic response") (Senior and Lahiri 1995). Dobutamine stress MRI has a good specificity (83%, range 70–95%) but moderate sensitivity (74%, range 50–89%), values that are in line with those of dobutamine echocardiography (Kaandorp et al. 2005b; Schinkel et al. 2007).

Contrast enhanced MRI using late Gd imaging, the third approach, detects scar tissue but not viability

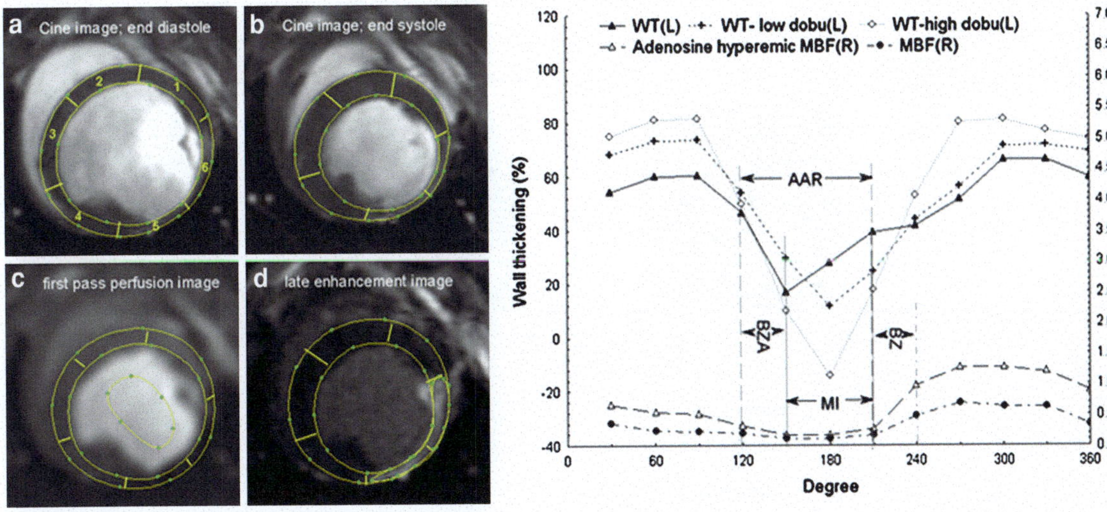

Fig. 46 Assessment of the different ischemic substrates in an animal model with chronic myocardial hypoperfusion using comprehensive MRI, including cine imaging at rest (**a**, **b**) and during low and high-dose dobutamine stress, first pass perfusion imaging at rest (**c**) and during adenosine stress, and late Gd imaging (**d**). Copper-coated stent-induced CA stenosis in LCx induces chronic hypoperfusion in lateral LV wall, defined as area at risk (*AAR*). The AAR contains a mixture of irreversibly (infarcted '*MI*') and reversibly (border zone area at risk '*BZA*') damaged myocardium. Stress-induced changes in wall thickening (*WT*) and myocardial blood flow (*MBF*) are heavily determined by the ischemic substrate as shown in the figure. In the x-axis is shown the regional values in circumferential direction (360°). Abbreviations, *BZ* border zone outside the area-at-risk. Courtesy PhD thesis, Ming Wu, Leuven

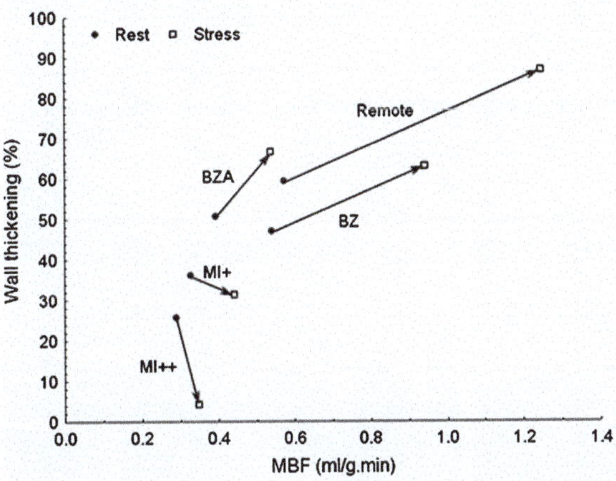

Fig. 47 Changes in regional myocardial blood flow (MBF) and function (wall thickening) in regions with different ischemic substrates from rest to stress. Abbreviations, *BZ* border zone, *BZA* border zone area-at-risk; MI+, infarct with <50% transmurality; MI++, infarct with >50% transmurality. Courtesy PhD thesis, Ming Wu, Leuven

(see also Sect. 3.4.3) (Fig. 49). Ramani et al. noted that hyperenhancement frequently occurs in dysfunctional myocardium in patients with stable CAD, and is associated with nonviability obtained by SPECT imaging and dobutamine echocardiography, whereas absence of hyperenhancement correlates with measures of viability, regardless of resting contractile function (Ramani et al. 1998). In particular, the likelihood of improvement in regional contractility after revascularization decreases progressively as the transmural extent of hyperenhancement before revascularization increases (Kim et al. 2000) (Figs. 49 and 50). In dysfunctional segments without hyperenhancement 78% improved contractility post-revascularization, compared to 2% of segments with scar tissue extending >75% of the LV wall. This technique has an excellent sensitivity (95%, range 91–99) but a low specificity (45%, range 37–54) (Kaandorp et al. 2005b). The relative low specificity can be ascribed to several factors: (1) short-term follow-up between revascularization and assessment of left ventricular function (time course of hibernating myocardium functional recovery can protract up to 14 months), (2) false positive results including those due to procedural injury, (3) incomplete revascularization, (4) tethering of the adjacent scarring segments.

Because none of the above approaches is perfect in predicting or excluding functional recovery after

Fig. 48 Overview of MRI strategies currently used to assess myocardial viability in patients presenting symptoms of chronic myocardial ischemia and LV dysfunction

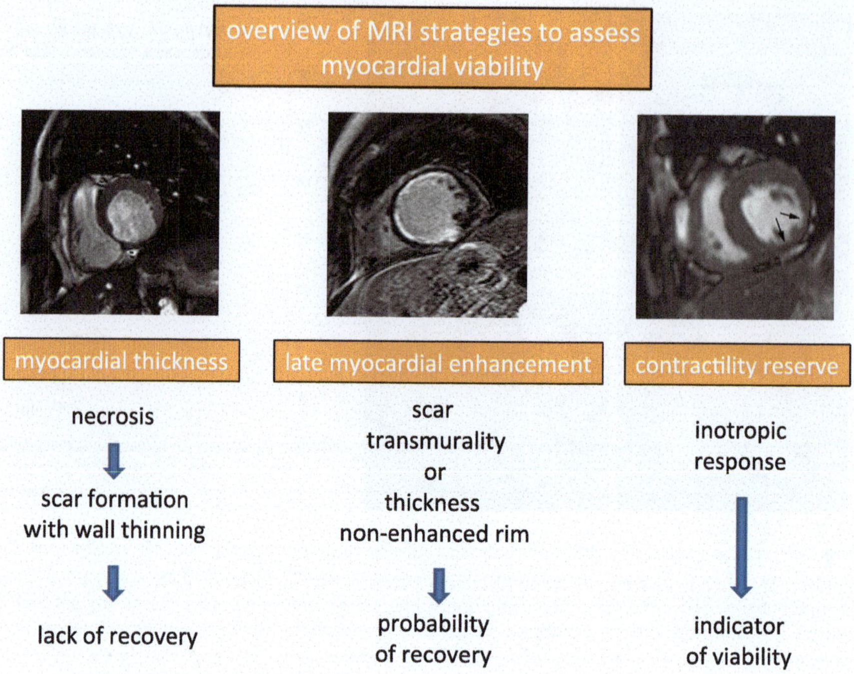

Fig. 49 Late Gd imaging (*short-axis plane*) in a 57-year-old patient with severe, long-standing three-vessel disease and chronic myocardial ischemia. Images show a dilated LV with absence of myocardial enhancement suggesting viable but dysfunctional myocardium

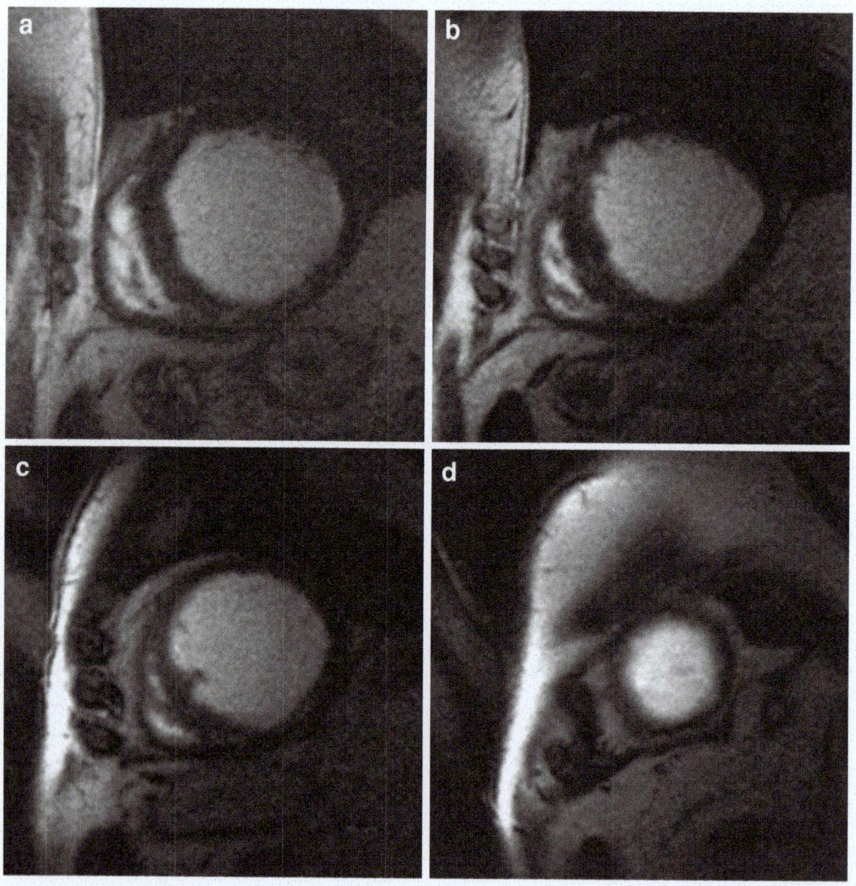

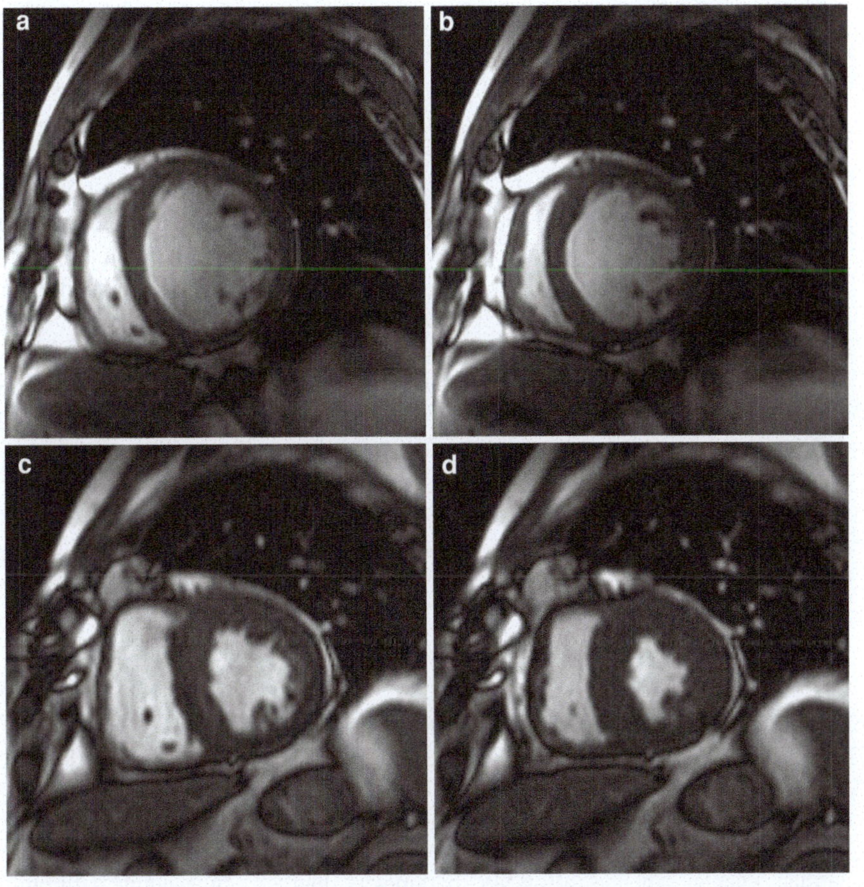

Fig. 50 Cine imaging (short-axis plane) in the same patient as in Fig. 49 before (**a**, **b**) and 4 months after (**c**, **d**) CABG surgery. End-diastolic (**a**, **c**) and end-systolic (**b**, **d**) time frames. Significant improvement in decrease in LV end-diastolic volume (EDV) and increase in ejection fraction (EF) with improved systolic wall thickening after CABG. Before surgery EDV: 450 ml, EF: 17%; and after surgery EDV: 200 ml, EF: 47.5%

revascularization, an integrated use of MRI techniques may improve diagnostic accuracy. Kaandorp et al. proposed to start with late Gd imaging to depict myocardial scarring and determine the transmural extent. Especially in dysfunctional segments with an intermediate extent of scar tissue (transmurality 25–50%), the likelihood of recovery is uncertain and in a second step dobutamine stress MRI may be valuable to differentiate between those with versus those without contractility reserve (Kaandorp et al. 2004). As mentioned earlier the thickness of the non-enhanced epicardial rim may provide additional value regarding viability (Kühl et al. 2006).

Finally, it should be emphasized that viability imaging with MRI is part of a more comprehensive approach providing accurate data on ventricular volumes and global function, enabling visualization and quantification of associated valvular heart disease (e.g., mitral regurgitation) and depiction of complications such as ventricular aneurysms or thrombus formation (Mollet et al. 2002).

6.3 Cardiac Resynchronization Therapy

Cardiac resynchronization therapy (CRT) has emerged as a highly effective therapy for heart failure (Aggarwal et al. 2009). Imaging, and in particular MRI, offers great promise to accurately depict patients who will benefit from this treatment (see "Heart Failure and Heart Transplantation"). Although MRI can be used for coronary venous depiction, its role is predominantly in myocardial scar imaging using late Gd imaging and in assessing cardiac dyssynchrony using cine techniques such as myocardial tagging, DENSE and tissue velocity mapping (see "Cardiac Function").

7 Prognosis Assessment

Prediction of clinical outcome and prognosis assessment are important in patients with suspected or known CAD. There is growing evidence that cardiac MRI is an increasingly important tool in the management of cardiovascular disease (Flett et al. 2009; Bingham and Hachamovitch 2011).

In patients with suspected CAD, a negative stress perfusion MRI study yields a high negative predictive value for future MACE, whereas stress perfusion defects predict subsequent MACE (Bodi et al. 2007; Jahnke et al. 2007b; Pilz et al. 2008; Steel et al. 2009; Korosoglou et al. 2010a). Similarly, dobutamine-stress induced WMAs are associated with future cardiac events (Hundley et al. 2002; Rerkpattanapipat et al. 2002; Kuijpers et al. 2004b; Jahnke et al. 2007b; Korosoglou et al. 2010a). In particular, this technique exhibits high prognostic utility for identifying women who may be at risk (Wallace et al. 2009; Coelho-Filho et al. 2011). Whereas an LV ejection fraction <40% is associated with future MACE independent of risk factors for CAD, a positive stress test in patients with mild to moderate reduction in LV ejection fraction (40–55%) forecasts future hard events (Dall'Armellina et al. 2008). In the study by Bingham and Hachamovitch (2011), 908 consecutive patients who underwent combined MRI (including stress perfusion, LV volumes and function, myocardial enhancement, aortic flow) for suspicion of CAD and myocardial ischemia, were followed for 2.6 ± 1.2 years. A normal CMR study yielded a low risk of cardiac events, whereas all CMR parameters had incremental value for prediction of adverse events over pre-MRI data. Two studies have shown that concomitant LV hypertrophy, defined as LV wall thickness $\geq$12 mm or LV mass > 96 g/m^2 in men and >77 g/m^2 is an independent predictor of MACE and should be reported in those referred for stress MRI, particularly in those without inducible ischemia (Walsh et al. 2009; Charoenpanichkit et al. 2010). LV hypertrophy bears a similar risk for future events as those patients presenting stress-induced WMA. Moreover, in patients without a history of MI but a clinical suspicion of CAD, presence of myocardial enhancement even in small amounts, reflecting ischemia-related myocardial scarring, carries an increased risk for future MACE (Kwong et al. 2006, 2008; Steel et al. 2009).

In patients with ACS in whom MI is excluded by cardiac biomarkers and non-diagnostic electrocardiograms, adenosine stress perfusion MRI is a more accurate predictor of future cardiac events than traditional cardiac risk factors (Ingkanisorn et al. 2006).

In acute MI, MRI has not only become the reference technique for infarct sizing but also because of its unique capability for characterization of the infarct and jeopardized myocardium, MRI is rapidly emerging as the technique to evaluate which infarct characteristics bear poor prognosis (Dall'Armellina et al. 2010). Although the extent of myocardial necrosis is a major determinant in predicting adverse remodeling and patient outcome (Wu et al. 2008; Larose et al. 2010; Ganame et al. 2011), it has become obvious that parameters other than purely infarct size should be taken into account (Bodi et al. 2009). These include MVO (Wu et al. 1998a; Hombach et al. 2005; Bruder et al. 2008; Cochet et al. 2009), post-reperfusion myocardial hemorrhage (Ganame et al. 2009), the peri-infarct area (Saeed et al. 2001; Yan et al. 2006; Schmidt et al. 2007) and myocardial salvage (Eitel et al. 2010; Masci et al. 2010a). Also in patients with non ST-segment elevation MI, persistent MVO is an independent predictor of MACE (Cochet et al. 2010). Since some phenomena such as MVO and myocardial hemorrhage seem to be related to infarct size, further research in large patient trials is needed to elucidate whether these parameters are truly independent, or should be considered as markers of infarct severity expression.

In ischemic cardiomyopathy patients with severely reduced LVEF, the extent of myocardial enhancement is associated with increased mortality or the need for cardiac transplantation (Kwon et al. 2009). In another study involving 857 consecutive patients with and without LV dysfunction and a median follow-up of 4.4 years, myocardial enhancement using a myocardial scar index (i.e, sum of transmurality scores of all 17 segments divided by 17) was a strong and independent predictor of all cause mortality/cardiac transplantation, even in the presence of traditional well-known prognosticators such as ejection fraction, congestive heart failure and age (Cheong et al. 2009).

8 Clinical Imaging Strategies: Practical Recipes

An important issue is the integration of the above MRI techniques into clinical routine. A major constraint in scanning cardiac patients is definitely the length of the scan procedure. Depending on the

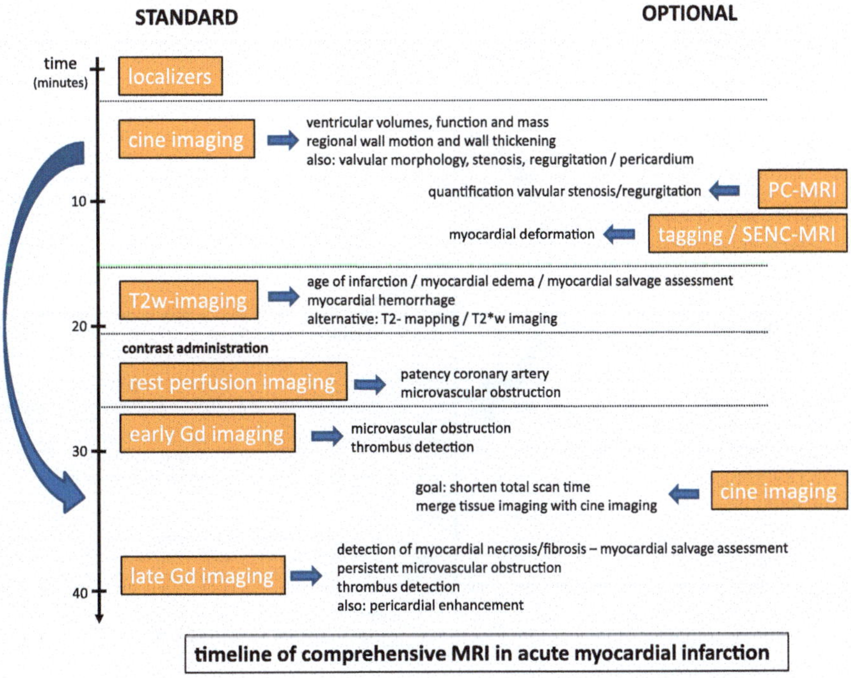

Fig. 51 Timeline of comprehensive MRI exam in a patient with acute myocardial infarction. The standard sequences are shown on the *left*, the optional sequences on the *right*. To shorten total imaging time cine imaging can be performed following contrast administration Abbreviations: *PC-MRI* phase-contrast, *MRI*; *SENC-MRI* strain-encoding MRI

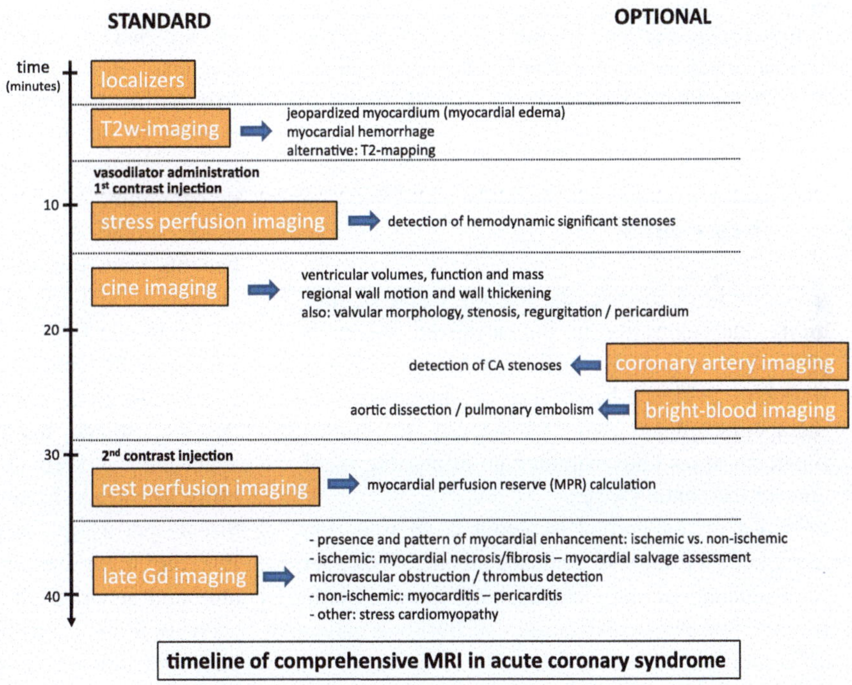

Fig. 52 Timeline of comprehensive MRI exam in a patient with acute coronary syndrome. The standard sequences are shown on the *left*, the optional sequences on the *right*

patient's general condition the MRI study should be finished preferably in less than 45 min. Besides sufficient training and experience in the field of cardiac MRI, use of standardized imaging protocols has shown to be very helpful in improving the success rate of cardiac MRI studies. Several optimized, comprehensive approaches for studying the different subgroups of IHD patients are nowadays available (Karamitsos et al. 2009; Lockie et al. 2009; Kim et al. 2010; Hundley et al. 2010; Dall'Armellina et al. 2010). In Figs. 51–53 we have provided a scheme of how different MRI techniques can be integrated into a

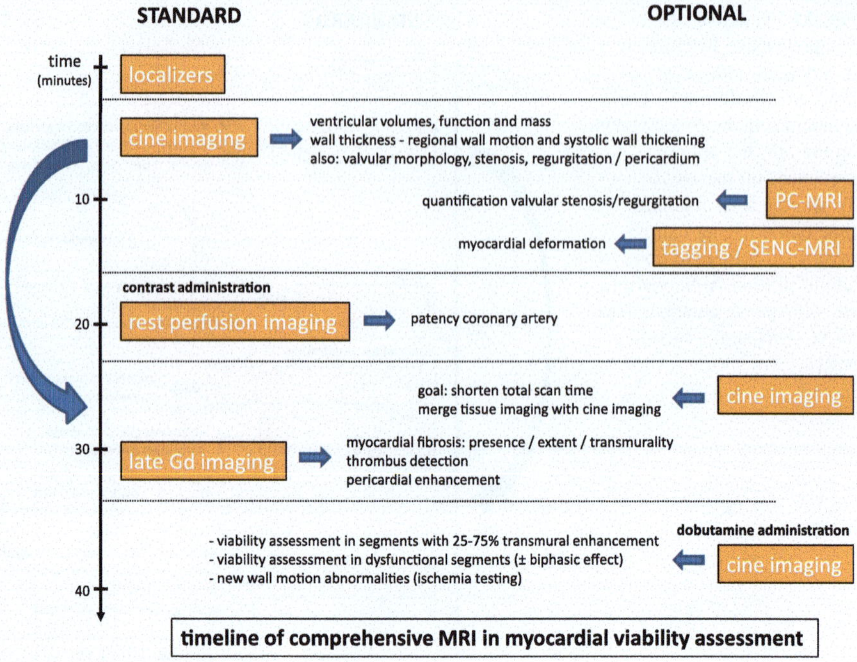

Fig. 53 Timeline of comprehensive MRI exam in myocardial viability assessment. The standard sequences are shown on the *left*, the optional sequences on the *right*. To shorten total imaging time cine imaging can be performed following contrast administration. Abbreviations: *PC-MRI* phase-contrast MRI, *SENC-MRI*, sensitivity-encoding MRI

comprehensive approach to study different types of IHD patients. As shown in these figures, the choice and sequence of MRI techniques can and should be adapted to each individual situation.

9 Key Points

- Ischemic heart disease, the leading cause of morbidity and mortality in industrialized countries, poses an enormous financial burden on our society. Rational, evidence-based use of diagnostic and therapeutic means will be needed to prevent financial lapses and guarantee an affordable medicine in the coming years.
- Presence of myocardial ischemia is an important risk factor for adverse clinical outcome. However, only stenotic coronary lesions that induce ischemia benefit from revascularization and improve patient outcome.
- The myocardium has a limited regenerative capacity, and loss of myocardial tissue results in altered loading conditions on the remaining myocardium.
- Sustained coronary artery occlusion ensues a cascade of events in the downstream myocardium, resulting in irreversible myocardial damage soon (i.e., 30 min), progressing in a transmural wave front of necrosis towards the subepicardium over the next 3–6 h.
- Irreversible myocardial damage initiates a complex process of inflammation and infarct healing ultimately resulting in fibrotic scarring of the damaged myocardium.
- Since chronic, dysfunctional but viable myocardium benefits from revascularization, improving patient symptoms, viability assessment is an important pillar in chronic IHD and CAD-related heart failure.
- Current MRI techniques allow to accurately assess stress-induced myocardial ischemia, to characterize the jeopardized myocardium in acute coronary syndrome, as well as determine myocardial viability in chronic ischemia.
- Stress perfusion imaging and stress function imaging in patients with suspected CAD are valuable and accurate alternatives to other techniques such as SPECT imaging or stress echocardiography, and moreover, can be integrated in a more comprehensive MRI approach, such as myocardial scar imaging yielding prognostic information.
- Although infarct sizing remains important in determining infarct severity and patient prognosis, it has become obvious, thanks to a major contribution of MRI that tissue characterization of the reversible and irreversible damaged myocardium of

the jeopardized region yields additional important diagnostic and prognostic information.

- Functional recovery post-revascularization in chronic ischemic myocardium is determined by the presence and transmural extent of infarct-related myocardial scarring. Late Gd MRI is an accurate quantitative tool for scar imaging. Diagnostic accuracy for predicting recovery can be improved adding low-dose functional stress imaging to study the contractility reserve of the non-enhanced subepicardial rim.

Acknowledgments The authors express their gratitude to Dr. P.G. Masci, MD, Pisa, Italy for his critical input in the preparation of this chapter.

References

Abdel–Aty H, Zagrosek A, Schulz–Menger J et al (2004) Delayed enhanced and T2-weighted cardiovascular magnetic resonance imaging differentiate acute from chronic myocardial infarction. Circulation 109:2411–2416

Abdel–Aty H, Cocker M, Meek C, Tyberg JV, Friedrich MG (2009) Edema as a very early marker for acute myocardial ischemia: a cardiovascular magnetic resonance study. J Am Coll Cardiol 53:1194–1201

Achenbach S, Raggi P (2010) Imaging of coronary atherosclerosis by computed tomography. Eur Heart J 31: 1442–1448

Adzamli IK, Blau M, Pfeffer MA et al (1993) Phosphonate-modified Gd-DTPA complexes. III. The detection of myocardial infarction by MRI. Magn Reson Med 29: 505–511

Aggarwal NR, Martinez MW, Gersh BJ, Careonthaitawee P (2009) Role of cardiac MRI and nuclear imaging in cardiac resynchronization therapy. Nat Rev Cardiol 6:759–770

Alderman EL, Stadius M (1992) The angiographic definitions of the bypass angioplasty revascularization investigation. Cor Art Dis 3:1189–1207

Aletras AH, Tilak GS, Natanzon A et al (2006) Retrospective determination of the area at risk for reperfused acute myocardial infarction with T2-weighted cardiac magnetic resonance imaging. Histopathological and displacement encoding with stimulated echoes (DENSE) functional validations. Circulation 113:1865–1870

Aletras AH, Kellman P, Derbyshire A, Arai AE (2008) Acut$_2$E TSE-SSFP: a hybrid method for T2-weighted imaging of edema in the Heart. Magn Reson Med 59:229–235

Al-Saadi N, Nagel E, Gross M et al (2000a) Noninvasive detection of myocardial ischemia from perfusion reserve based on cardiovascular magnetic resonance. Circulation 101:824–834

Al-Saadi N, Nagel E, Gross M et al (2000b) Improvement of myocardial perfusion reserve early after coronary intervention: assessment with cardiac magnetic resonance imaging. J Am Coll Cardiol 36:1557–1564

Amado LC, Gerber BL, Gupta SN et al (2004) Accurate and objective infarct sizing by contrast-enhanced magnetic resonance imaging in a canine myocardial infarction model. J Am Coll Cardiol 44:2383–2389

Andersen HR, Falk E, Nielsen D (1987) Right ventricular infarction: frequency, size and topography in coronary heart disease: a prospective study comprising 107 consecutive autopsies from a coronary care unit. J Am Coll Cardiol 10:1223–1232

Arai AE (2007) False positive or true positive Troponin in patients presenting with chest pain but 'normal' coronary arteries: lessons from cardiac MRI. Eur Heart J 28:1175–1177

Arheden H, Saeed M, Higgins CB et al (1999) Measurement of the distribution volume of gadopentetate dimeglumine at echo-planar MR imaging to quantify myocardial infarction: comparison with 99mTC-DTPA autoradiography in rats. Radiology 211:698–708

Asanuma T, Tanabe K, Ochiai K et al (1997) Relationship between progressive microvascular damage and intramyocardial hemorrhage in patients with reperfused anterior myocardial infarction. myocardial contrast echocardiographic study. Circulation 96:448–453

Assomull RG, Lyne JC, Keean N et al (2007) The role of cardiovascular magnetic resonance in patients presenting with chest pain, raised Troponin, and unobstructed coronary arteries. Eur Heart J 28:1242–1249

Baer FM, Smolarz K, Jungehulsing M et al (1992) Chronic myocardial infarction: assessment of morphology, function, and perfusion by gradient echo magnetic resonance imaging and 99mTc-methoxyisobutyl-isonitrile SPECT. Am Heart J 123:636–645

Baer FM, Voth E, Theissen P et al (1994) Gradient-echo magnetic resonance imaging during incremental dobutamine infusion for the localization of coronary artery stenoses. Eur Heart J 15:218–225

Baer FM, Voth E, Schneider C, Theissen P, Schicha H, Sechtem U (1995) Comparison of low-dose dobutamine-gradient-echo magnetic resonance imaging and positron emission tomography with [18F] Fluorodeoxyglucose in patients with chronic coronary artery disease. A functional and morphological approach to the detection of residual myocardial viability. Circulation 91:1006–1015

Baer FM, Theissen P, Crnac J et al (2000) Head to head comparison of dobutamine-transesophageal echocardiocardiography and dobutamine-magnetic resonance imaging for the detection of left ventricular functional recovery in patients with chronic coronary artery disease. Eur Heart J 21:981–991

Baks T, van Geuns R-J, Biagini E et al (2006) Effects of primary angioplasty for acute mycardial infarction on early and late infarct and left ventricular wall characteristics. J Am Coll Cardiol 47:40–44

Barbier CE, Bjerner T, Johansson L, Lind L, Ahlström H (2006) Myocardial scars more frequent than expected. Magnetic resonance imaging detects potential risk group. J Am Coll Cardiol 48:765–771

Barkhausen J, Hunold P, Eggebrecht H et al (2002) Detection and characterization of intracardiac thrombi on MR imaging. AJR 179:1539–1544

Baroldi G, Silver MD, De Maria R, Parodi O, Pellegrini A (1997) Lipomatous metaplasia in the left ventricular scar. Can J Cardiol 13:65–71

Bashour TT, Mason D (1990) Myocardial hibernation and embalment. Am Heart J 119:706–708

Basso C, Corbetti F, Silva C et al (2007) Morphologic validation of reperfused hemorrhagic myocardial infarction by cardiovascular magnetic resonance. Am J Cardiol 100: 1322–1327

Bauner KU, Muehling O, Wintersperger BJ, Winnik E, Reiser MF, Huber A (2007) Inversion recovery single-shot TurboFLASH for assessment of myocardial infarction at 3 Tesla. Invest Radiol 42:361–371

Bax JJ, Visser FC, Poldermans D et al (2001) Time course of functional recovery of stunned and hibernating segments after surgical revascularization. Circulation 104:I314–I318

Bayés de Luna A, Wagner G, Birnbaum Y et al (2006a) A new terminology for left ventricular walls and location of myocardial infarcts that present Q wave based on the standard of cardiac magnetic resonance imaging. A statement for healthcare professionals from a committee appointed by the International Society for Holter and Noninvasive electrocardiography. Circulation 114:1755–1760

Bayés de Luna A, Cino JM, Pujadas S et al (2006b) Concordance of electrographic patterns and healed myocardial infarction location detected by cardiovascular magnetic resonance. Am J Cardiol 97:443–451

Becker LC, Jeremy RW, Schaper J et al (1999) Ultrastructural assessment of myocardial necrosis occuring during ischemia and 3-h reperfusion in the dog. Am J Physiol 46: H243–H252

Beek AM, Kühl HP, Bondarenko O et al (2003) Delayed contrast-enhanced magnetic resonance imaging for the prediction of regional functional improvement after acute myocardial infarction. J Am Coll Cardiol 42:895–901

Beek AM, Bondarenko O, Afsharzada F, van Rossum AC (2009) Quantification of late gadolinium enhanced CMR in viability assessment in chronic ischemic heart disease: a comparison to functional outcome. J Cardiovasc Magn Reson 11:6

Bekkers SCAM, Backes WH, Kim RJ et al (2009) Detection and characteristics of microvascular obstruction in reperfused acute myocardial infarction using an optimized protocol for contrast-enhanced cardiovascular magnetic resonance imaging. Eur Radiol 19:2904–2912

Bekkers SCAM, Yazdani SK, Virmani R, Waltenberger J (2010) Microvascular obstruction. Underlying pathophysiology and clinical diagnosis. J Am Coll Cardiol 55:1649–1660

Beller GA (2000) Noninvasive assessment of myocardial viability. N Engl J Med 343:1488–1490

Beller GA (2001) Coronary heart disease in the first 30 years of the 21st century: challenges and opportunities. Circulation 103:2428–2435

Berbari R, Kachenoura N, Frouin F, Herment A, Mousseaux E, Bloch I (2009) An automated quantification of the transmural myocardial infarct extent using cardiac DE-MR images. Conf Proc IEEE Eng Med Biol Soc 4403–4406

Bernhardt P, Spiess J, Levenson B et al (2009) Combined assessment of myocardial perfusion and late gadolinium enhancement in patients after percutaneous coronary intervention or bypass grafts. A multicenter study of an integrated cardiovascular magnetic resonance protocol. J Am Coll Cardiol Img 2000:1292–1300

Berry C, Kellman P, Mancini C et al (2010) Magnetic resonance imaging delineates the ischemic aera at risk and myocardial salvage in patients with acute myocardial infarction. Circ Cardiovasc Imaging 3:527–535

Bingham SE, Hachamovitch R (2011) Incremental prognostic significance of combined cardiac magnetic resonance imaging, adenosine stress perfusion, delayed enhancement, and left ventricular function over preimaging information for the prediction of adverse events. Circulation 123: 1509–1518

Blume U, Lockie T, Stehning C et al (2009) Interleaved T1 and T2 relaxation time mapping for cardiac applications. J Magn Reson Imaging 29:480–487

Bodi V, Sanchis J, Lopez-Lereu MP et al (2005) Usefulness of a comprehensive cardiovascular magnetic resonance imaging assessment for predicting recovery of left ventricular wall motion in the setting of myocardial stunning. J Am Coll Cardiol 46:1747–1752

Bodi V, Sanchis J, Guillem MS et al (2006) Analysis of Q-waves after infarction with body surface map: relationship with infarct size. Int J Cardiol 111:399–404

Bodi V, Sanchis J, Lopez-Lereu MP et al (2007) Prognostic value of dipyridamole stress cardiovascular magnetic resonance imaging in patients with known or suspected coronary artery disease. J Am Coll Cardiol 50:1174–1179

Bodi V, Sanchis J, Nunez J et al (2009) Prognostic value of a comprehensive cardiac magnetic resonance assessment soon after a first ST-segment elevation myocardial infarction. J Am Coll Cardiol Img 2:835–842

Bodi V, Sanchis J, Mainar L et al (2010) Right ventricular involvement in anterior myocardial infarction: a translational approach. Cardiovasc Res 87:601–608

Bogaert J, Francone M (2009) Cardiovascular magnetic resonance in pericardial diseases. J Cardiovasc Magn Reson 11:14

Bogaert J, Rademakers F (2001) Regional nonuniformity of the human left ventricle. A 3D MR myocardial tagging study. Am J Physiol 280:H610–H620

Bogaert J, Maes A, Van de Werf F et al (1999) Functional recovery of subepicardial myocardial tissue in transmural myocardial infarction after successful reperfusion. An important contribution to the improvement of regional and global left ventricular function. Circulation 99:36–43

Bogaert J, Bosmans H, Maes A et al (2000) Remote myocardial dysfunction after acute anterior myocardial infarction: impact of left ventricular shape on regional function. A magnetic resonance myocardial tagging study. J Am Coll Cardiol 35:1525–1534

Bogaert J, Kalantzi M, Rademakers FE, Dymarkowski S, Janssens S (2007) Determinants and impact of microvascular obstruction in successfully reperfused ST-segment elevation myocardial infarction. Assessment by magnetic resonance imaging. Eur Radiol 17:2572–2580

Bondarenko O, Beek AM, Twisk JW, Visser CA, van Rossum AC (2008) Time course of functional recovery after revascularization of hibernating myocardium: a contrast-enhanced cardiovascular magnetic resonance study. Eur Heart J 29: 2000–2005

Bottomley PA, Wu KC, Gerstenblith G, Schulman SP, Steinberg A, Weiss RG (2009) Reduced myocardial creatine kinase flux in human myocardial infarction. An in vivo

phosphorus magnetic spectroscopy study. Circulation 119:1918–1924
Brady TJ, Goldman MR, Pykett IL et al (1982) Proton nuclear magnetic resonance imaging of regionally ischemic canine hearts: effect of paramagnetic proton signal enhancement. Radiology 144:343–347
Braunwald E, Kloner RA (1982) The stunned myocardium: prolonged, postischemic ventricular dysfunction. Circulation 66:1146–1149
Bremerich J, Saeed M, Arheden H et al (2000) Normal and infarcted myocardium: differentiation with cellular uptake of manganese at MR imaging in a rat model. Radiology 216:524–530
Bresnahan GF, Roberts R, Shell WE, JJr Ross, Sobel BE (1974) Deleterious effects due to hemorrhage after myocardial infarction. Am J Cardiol 33:82–86
Bruder O, Breuckmann F, Jensen C et al (2008) Prognostic impact of contrast-enhanced CMR early after acute ST segment elevation myocardial infarction (STEMI) in a regional STEMI network: results of the "Herzinfarktverbund Essen". Herz 33:136–142
Buda AJ, Zotz RJ, Gallagher KP (1987) The effect of inotropic stimulation on normal and ischemic myocardium after coronary occlusion. Circulation 76:163–172
Camici PG (2007) Is the chest pain in cardiac syndrome X due to subendocardial ischemia? Eur Heart J 28:1539–1540
Camici PG, Crea F (2007) Coronary microvascular dysfunction (2007). N Engl J Med 356:830–840
Canby RC, Reeves RC, Evanochko WT et al (1987) Proton nuclear magnetic resonance relaxation times in severe myocardial ischemia. J Am Coll Cardiol 10:412–420
Carlson M, Ubachs JFA, Hedström E, Heiberg E, Jovinge S, Arheden H (2009) Myocardium at risk after acute infarction in humans on cardiac magnetic resonance. Quantitative assessment during follow-up and validation with single-photon emission computed tomography. J Am Coll Cardiol Img 2:569–576
Cerqueira M (2002) Standardized myocardial segmentation and nomenclature for tomographic imaging of the heart: a statement for healthcare professionals from the Cardiac Imaging Committee of the Council on Clinical Cardiology of the American Heart Association. Circulation 105:539–542
Charoenpanichkit C, Morgan TM, Hamilton CA et al (2010) Left ventricular hypertrophy influences cardiac prognosis in patients undergoing dobutamine cardiac stress testing. Circ Cardiovasc Imaging 3:392–397
Cheng ASH, Pegg TJ, Karamitsos TD et al (2007) Cardiovascular magnetic resonance perfusion imaging at 3-Tesla for the detection of coronary artery disease. A comparison with 1.5-tesla. J Am Coll Cardiol 49:2440–2449
Cheong BYC, Muthupillai R, Wilson JM et al (2009) Prognostic significance of delayed-enhancement magnetic resonance imaging. Survival of 857 patients with and without left ventricular dysfunction. Circulation 120:2069–2076
Chiarella F, Santoro E, Domenicucci S et al (1998) Predischarge two-dimensional echocardiographic evaluation of left ventricular thrombosis after acute myocardial infarction in the GISSI-3 study. Am J Cardiol 81:822–827
Choi SI, Choi SH, Kim ST et al (2000) Irreversibly damaged myocardium at MR imaging with a necrotic tissue-specific contrast agent in a cat model. Radiology 215:863–868
Choi KM, Kim RJ, Gubernikoff G, Vargas JD, Parker M, Judd RM (2001) Transmural extent of acute myocardial infarction predicts long-term improvement in contractile function. Circulation 104:1101–1107
Cigarroa CG, de Filippi C, Brickner ME et al (1993) Dobutamine stress echocardiography identifies hibernating myocardium and predicts recovery of left ventricular function after coronary revascularization. Circulation 88: 430–436
Cino JM, Carreras F, Cygankiewicz I et al (2006) Utility of contrast-enhanced cardiovascular magnetic resonance (CE-CMR) to assess how likely is an infarct to produce a typical ECG pattern. J Cardiovasc Magn Reson 8:335–344
Cochet AA, Lorgis L, Lalande A et al (2009) Major prognostic impact of persistent microvascular obstruction as assessed by contrast-enhanced cardiac magnetic resonance in reperfused acute myocardial infarction. Eur Radiol 19: 2117–2126
Cochet A, Lalande A, Lorgis L et al (2010) Prognostic value of microvascular damage determined by cardiac magnetic resonance in non ST-segment elevation myocardial infarction: comparison between first-pass and late gadolinium-enhanced images. Invest Radiol 45:725–732
Coelho-Filho OR, Seabra LF, Mongeon F et al (2011) Stress myocardial perfusion imaging by CMR provides strong prognostic value to cardiac events regardless of patient's sex. J Am Coll Cardiol Img 4:850–861
Cook SC, Ferketich AK, Raman SV (2009) Myocardial ischemia in asymptomatic adults with repaired aortic coarctation. Int J Cardiol 133:95–101
Costa MA, Shoemaker S, Futamatsu H et al (2007) Quantitative magnetic resonance perfusion imaging detects anatomic and physiologic coronary artery disease as measured by coronary angiography and fractional flow reserve. J Am Coll Cardiol 50:514–522
Cox CJ (1967) Return to normal of the electrocardiogram after myocardial infarction. Lancet 1:1194–1197
Croisille P, Moore CC, Judd RM et al (1999) Differentiation of viable and nonviable myocardium by the use of three-dimensional tagged MRI in 2-day-old reperfused canine infarcts. Circulation 99:284–291
Cullen JH, Horsfield MA, Reek CR et al (1999) A myocardial perfusion reserve index in humans using first-pass contrast-enhanced magnetic resonance imaging. J Am Coll Cardiol 33:1386–1394
Curry RC, Shash K, Nagurney JT et al (2008) Cardiac magnetic resonance with T2-weighted imaging improves detection of patients with acute coronary syndrome in the emergency department. Circulation 118:837–844
Cury RC, Cattani CAM, Gabure LAG et al (2006) Diagnostic performance of stress perfusion and delayed-enhancement MR imaging in patients with coronary artery disease. Radiology 240:39–45
Dall'Armellina E, Morgan TM, Mandapaka S et al (2008) Prediction of cardiac events in patients with reduced left ventricular ejection fraction with dobutamine cardiovascular magnetic resonance assessment of wall motion score index. J Am Coll Cardiol 52:279–286
Dall'Armellina E, Karamitsos TD, Neubauer S, Choudbury RP (2010) CMR for characterization of the myocardium in acute coronary syndromes. Nat Rev Cardiol 7:624–636

de Roos A, Doornbos J, van der Wall EE, van Voorthuisen AE (1988) MR imaging of acute myocardial infarction: value of Gd-DTPA. AJR 150:531–534

de Roos A, Van Rossum AC, Van Der Wall E et al (1989) Reperfused and nonreperfused myocardial infarction: Diagnostic potential of Gd-DTPA-enhanced MR imaging. Radiology 172:717–720

de Waha S, Desch S, Eitel I et al (2010) Impact of early vs. late microvascular obstruction assessed by magnetic resonance imaging on long-term outcome after ST-elevation myocardial infarction: a comparison with traditional prognostic markers. Eur Heart J 31:2660–2668

Dendale PAC, Franken RP, Waldmann GJ et al (1995) Low-dosage dobutamine magnetic resonance imaging as an alternative to echocardiography in the detection of viable myocardium after acute infarction. Am Heart J 130: 134–140

Dendale P, Franken PR, van der Wall EE, de Roos A (1997) Wall thickening at rest and contractile reserve early after myocardial infarction: correlation with myocardial perfusion and metabolism. Cor Art Dis 8:259–264

Desmet W, Bogaert J, Dubois C et al (2011) High-dose intracoronary adenosine for myocardial salvage in patients with acute ST-segment elevation myocardial infarction. Eur Heart J 32(7):867

Detsky JS, Paul G, Dick AJ, Wright GA (2009) Reproducible classification of infarct heterogeneity using fuzzy clustering on multi-contrast delayed enhancement magnetic resonance imaging. IEEE Trans Med Imaging 28:1606–1614

Di Bella G, Masci PG, Ganame J, Dymarkowski S, Bogaert J (2008) Images in cardiovascular medicine. Liquefaction necrosis of mitral annulus calcification: detection and characterization with cardiac magnetic resonance imaging. Circulation 117:e292–e294

Donato R, Ganame J, Bogaert J (2009) Contrast-enhancing left ventricular apical thrombus. Eur Heart J 30:1977

Dulce MC, Duerinckx AJ, Hartiala J et al (1993) MR imaging of the myocardium using nonionic contrast medium: signal-intensity changes in patients with subacute myocardial infarction. AJR Am J Roentgenol 160:963–970

Dymarkowski S, Ni Y, Miao Y et al (2002) Value of T2-weighted MRI early after myocardial infarction in dogs: comparison with bis-gadolinium-mesoporphyrin enhanced T1-weighted MRI and functional data from cine MRI. Invest Radiol 37(2):77–85

Edelman RR, Wallner B, Singer A et al (1990) Segmented turboFLASH: method for breath-hold MR imaging of the liver with flexible contrast. Radiology 177:515–521

Eichstaedt HW, Felix R, Dougherty FC et al (1986) Langer M, Rutsch W, Schmutzler H. Magnetic resonance imaging (MRI) in different stages of myocardial infarction using the contrast agent gadolinium-DTPA. Clin Cardiol 9:527–535

Eichstaedt HW, Felix R, Danne O et al (1989) Imaging of acute myocardial infarction by magnetic resonance tomography (MRT) using the paramagnetic relaxation substance gadolinium-DTPA. Cardiovasc Drugs Ther 3:779–788

Eitel I, Behrendt F, Schindler K et al (2008) Differential diagnosis of suspected apical ballooning syndrome using contrast-enhanced magnetic resonance imaging. Eur Heart J 29:2651–2659

Eitel I, Desch S, Fuernau G et al (2010) Prognostic significance and determinants of myocardial salvage assessed by cardiovascular magnetic resonance in acute reperfused myocardial infarction. J Am Coll Cardiol 55:2470–2479

Eitel I, Kubusch K, Strohm O et al (2011) Prognostic value and determinants of a hypointense infarct core in T2-weighted cardiac magnetic resonance in acute reperfused ST-elevation myocardial infarction. Circ Cardiovasc Imaging, 4:354–362

Engblom H, Hedström E, Heiberg E, Wagner GS, Pahlm O, Arheden H (2005) Size and transmural extent of first-time reperfused myocardial infarction assessed by cardiac magnetic resonance can be estimated by 12-lead electrocardiogram. Am Heart J 150:920e1–920e9

Engblom H, Carlsson MB, Hedström E et al (2007) The endocardial extent of reperfused first-time myocardial infarction is more predictive of pathologic Q waves than is infarct transmurality: a magnetic resonance imaging study. Clin Physiol Funct Imaging 27:101–108

Engblom H, Hedström E, Heiberg E, Wagner GS, Pahlm O, Arheden H (2009) Rapid initial reduction of hyperenhanced myocardium after reperfused first myocardial infarction suggests recovery of the peri-infarction zone. One-year follow-up by MRI. Circ Cardiovasc Imaging 2:47–55

Escolano J (2010) Long-term trends in public finances. Fiscal Affairs Department. International Monetary Fund. September 24, 2010, Tokyo Japan (www.imf.org/external/oap/pdf/julio.pdf)

Fedele F, Montesano T, Ferro-Luzzi M et al (1994) Identification of viable myocardium in patients with chronic coronary artery disease and left ventricular dysfunction: role of magnetic resonance imaging. Am Heart J 128: 484–489

Feiring AJ, Johnson MR, Kioschos JM, Kirchner PT, Marcus ML, White CW (1987) The importance of the determination of the myocardial area at risk in the evaluation of the outcome of acute myocardial infarction in patients. Circulation 75:980–987

Fenchel M, Franow A, Stauder NI et al (2005) Myocardial perfusion after angioplasty in patients suspected of having single-vessel coronary artery disease: improvement detected at rest-stress first-pass perfusion MR imaging–initial experience. Radiology 237:67–74

Fieno DS, Kim RJ, Chen E-L, Lomasney JW, Klocke FJ, Judd RM (2000) Contrast-enhanced magnetic resonance imaging of myocardium at risk. Distinction between reversible and irreversible injury throughout infarct healing. J Am Coll Cardiol 36:1985–1991

Fishbein MC, Y-Rit J, Lando U, Kanmatsuse K, Mercier JC, Ganz W (1980) The relationship of vascular injury and myocardial hemorrhage to necrosis after reperfusion. Circulation 62:1274–1279

Flacke SJ, Fischer SE, Lorenz CH (2001) Measurement of the gadopentetate dimeglumine partition coefficient in human myocardium in vivo: normal distribution and elevation in acute and chronic infarction. Radiology 218:703–710

Flacke S, Allen JS, Chia JM et al (2003) Characterization of viable and nonviable myocardium at MR imaging: comparison of gadolinium-based extracellular and blood pool contrast materials versus manganese-based contrast materials in a rat myocardial infarction model. Radiology 226:731–738

Flett AS, Westwood MA, Davies LC, Mathur A, Moon JC (2009) The prognostic implications of cardiovascular magnetic resonance. Circ Cardiovasc Imaging 2:243–250

Foltz WD, Yang Y, Graham JJ, Detsky JS, Wright GA, Dick AJ (2006) MRI relaxation fluctuations in acute reperfused hemorrhagic infarction. Magn Reson Med 53:1311–1319

Foo TKF, Ho VB, Saranathan M et al (2005) Feasibility of integrating high-spatial-resolution 3D breath-hold coronary MR angiography with myocardial perfusion and viability examinations. Radiology 235:1025–1030

Francone M, Bucciarelli-Ducci C, Carbone I et al (2009) Impact of primary coronary angioplasty delay on myocardial salvage, infarct size, and microvascular damage in patients with ST-segment elevation myocardial infarction. Insight from cardiovascular magnetic resonance. J Am Coll Cardiol 54:2145–2153

Friedrich MG (2010) Myocardial edema–a new clinical entity? Nat Rev Cardiol 7:292–296

Friedrich MG, Abdel-Aty H, Taylor A et al (2008) The salvaged area at risk in reperfused acute myocardial infarction as visualized by cardiovascular magnetic resonance. J Am Coll Cardiol 51:1581–1587

Funaro S, La Torre G, Madonna M et al (2009) Incidence, determinants, and prognostic value of reverse left ventricular remodelling after primary percutaneous coronary intervention: results of the Acute Myocardial Infarction Contrast Imaging (AMICI) multicenter study. Eur Heart J 30:566–575

Fuster V (1999) Epidemic of cardiovascular disease and stroke: the three main challenges. Circulation 99:1132–1137

Fuster V, Sanz J, Viles-Gonzalez JF, Rajagopalan S (2006) The utility of magnetic resonance imaging in cardiac tissue regeneration trials. Nat Clin Pract Cardiovasc Med 3(1):S2–S7

Galiuto L, Lombardo A, Maseri A et al (2003) Temporal evolution and functional outcome of no-reflow: sustained and spontaneously reversible patterns following successful coronary recanalization. Heart 89:731–737

Ganame J, Messalli G, Dymarkowski S et al (2009) Impact of myocardial hemorrhage on left ventricular function and remodelling in patients with reperfused acute myocardial infarction. Eur Heart J 30:662–670

Ganame J, Messalli G, Masci PG et al (2011) Time course of infarct healing and left ventricular remodelling in patients with reperfused ST-segment elevation myocardial infarction using comprehensive magnetic resonance imaging. Eur Radiol 21:693–701

Garcia-Dorado D, Théroux P, Solares J et al (1990) Determinants of hemorrhagic infarcts. Histologic observations from experiments involving coronary occlusion, coronary reperfusion, and reocclusion. AJP 137:301–311

Garot J, Pascal O, Diéhold B et al (2002) Alterations of systolic left ventricular twist after acute myocardial infarction. Am J Physiol 282:H357–H362

Garot J, Lima JAC, Gerber BL et al (2004) Spatially resolved imaging of myocardial function with strain-encoded MR: comparison with delayed contrast-enhanced MR imaging after myocardial infarction. Radiology 233:596–602

Gebker R, Jahnke C, Manka R et al (2008) Additional value of myocardial perfusion imaging during dobutamine stress magnetic resonance for the assessment of coronary artery disease. Circ Cardiovasc Imaging 1:122–130

Gebker R, Jahnke C, Hucko T et al (2010a) Dobutamine stress magnetic resonance imaging for the detection of coronary artery disease in women. Heart 96:616–620

Gebker R, Mirelis JG, Jahnke C et al (2010b) Influence of left ventricular hypertrophy and geometry on diagnostic accuracy of wall motion and perfusion magnetic resonance imaging during dobutamine stress. Circ Cardiovasc Imaging 3:507–514

Geerse DA, Wu KC, Gorgels AP, Zimmet J, Wagner GS, Miller JM (2009) Comparison between contrast-enhanced magnetic resonance imaging and Selvester QRS scoring system in estimating changes in infarct size between the acute and chronic phases of myocardial infarction. Ann Noninvasive Electrocardiol 14:360–365

Gerber BL, Rochitte CE, Melin JA et al (2000) Microvascular obstruction and left ventricular remodeling early after acute myocardial infarction. Circulation 101:2734–2741

Gerber BL, Rochitte CE, Bluemke DA et al (2001) Relation between Gd-DTPA contrast enhancement and regional inotropic response in the periphery and center of myocardial infarction. Circulation 104:998–1004

Gerber BL, Raman SV, Nayak K et al (2008) Myocardial first-pass perfusion cardiovascular magnetic resonance: history, theory, and current state of the art. J Cardiovasc Magn Reson 10:18

Gheorghiade M, Sopko G, De Luca L et al (2006) Navigating the crossroads of coronary artery disease and heart failure. Circulation 114:1202–1213

Gibbons RJ, Valeti US, Araoz PA, Jaffe AS (2004) The quantification of infarct size. J Am Coll Cardiol 44: 1533–1542

Giri S, Chung Y-C, Merchant A et al (2009) T2 quantification for improved detection of myocardial edema. J Cardiovasc Magn Reson 11:56–68

Goldfarb JW, Roth M, Han J (2009) Myocardial fat deposition after left ventricular myocardial infarction: assessment by using MR water-fat separation imaging. Radiology 253:65–73

Gould K (1978) Noninvasive assessment of coronary stenosis by myocardial perfusion imaging during pharmacologic coronary vasodilatation: I. Physiologic basis and experimental validation. Am J Cardiol 41:267–278

Gould KL (2009) Does coronary flow trump coronary anatomy? J Am Coll Cardiol Img 2:1009–1023

Gropler RJ, Siegel BA, Sampathkumaran K et al (1992) Dependence of recovery of contractile function on maintenance of oxidative metabolism after myocardial infarction. J Am Coll Cardiol 19:989–997

Haase J, Bayar R, Hackenbroch M (2004) Relationship between size of myocardial infarctions assessed by delayed contrast-enhanced MRI after primary PCI, biochemical markers, and time to intervention. J Interven Cardiol 17:367–373

Hallén J, Buser P, Schwitter J et al (2009) Relation of cardiac troponin I measurements at 24 and 48 hours to magnetic resonance-determined infarct size in patients with ST-elevation myocardial infarction. Am J Cardiol 104: 1472–1477

Hayat SA, Janardhanan R, Moon JC, Pennell DJ, Senior R (2006) Comparison between myocardial contrast echocardiography and single-photon emission computed tomography for predicting transmurality of acute myocardial infarction. Am J Cardiol 97:1718–1721

Heidary S, Patel H, Chung J et al (2010) Quantitative tissue characterization of infarct core and border zone in patients with ischemic cardiomyopathy by magnetic resonance is associated with future cardiovascular events. J Am Coll Cardiol 55:2762–2768

Hendel RC, Patel MR, Kramer CR et al (2006) ACCF/ACR/SCCT/SCMR/ASNC/NASCI/SCAI/SIR 2006 Appropriateness criteria for cardiac computed tomography and cardiac magnetic resonance imaging. J Am Coll Cardiol 48: 1475–1497

Herijgers P, Laycock SK, Ni Y et al (1997) Localization and determination of infarct size by Gd-mesoporphyrin enhanced MRI in dogs. Int J Cardiac Imaging 13:499–507

Higgins CB, Herfkens R, Lipton MJ et al (1983) Nuclear magnetic resonance imaging of acute myocardial infarction in dogs: alterations in magnetic relaxation times. Am J Cardiol 52:184–188

Higginson LAJ, White F, Heggtveit HA, Sanders TM, Bloor CM, Covell JW (1982) Determinants of myocardial hemorrhage after coronary reperfusion in the anesthetized dog. Circulation 65:62–69

Hillenbrand HB, Kim RJ, Parker MA et al (2000) Early assessment of myocardial salvage by contrast-enhanced magnetic resonance imaging. Circulation 102:1678–1683

Hochman JS, Choo H (1987) Limitation of myocardial infarct expansion by reperfusion independent of myocardial salvage. Circulation 75:299–306

Holman ER, van Jonbergen HP, van Dijkman PR et al (1993) Comparison of magnetic resonance imaging studies with enzymatic indexes of myocardial necrosis for quantification of myocardial infarct size. Am J Cardiol 71:1036–1040

Holmes JW, Borg TK, Covell JW (2005) Structure and mechanics of healing myocardial infarcts. Annu Rev Biomed Eng 7:223–253

Hombach V, Grebe O, Merkle N et al (2005) Sequelae of acute myocardial infarction regarding cardiac structure and function and their prognostic significance as assessed by magnetic resonance imaging. Eur Heart J 26:549–557

Hsu LY, Natanzon A, Kellman P, Hirsch GA, Aletras AH, Arai AE (2006a) Quantitative myocardial infarction on delayed enhancement MRI. Part I: animal validation of an automated feature analysis and combined thresholding infarct sizing algorithm. J Magn Reson Imaging 23:298–308

Hsu LY, Rhoads KL, Holly JE, Kellman P, Aletras AH, Arai AE (2006b) Quantitative myocardial perfusion analysis with a dual-bolus contrast-enhanced first-pass MRI technique in humans. J Magn Reson Imaging 23:315–322

Hsu LY, Ingkanisorn WP, Kellman P, Aletras AH, Arai AE (2006c) Quantitative myocardial infarction on delayed enhancement MRI. Part II: clinical application of an automated feature analysis and combined thresholding infarct sizing algorithm. J Magn Reson Imaging 23:309–314

Huang T-Y, Liu Y-J, Stemmer A, Poncelet BP (2007) T2 Measurement of the human myocardium using a T2-prepared transient-state trueFISP sequence. Magn Reson Med 57:960–966

Huber AM, Schoenberg SO, Hayes C, Spannagl B, Engelmann MG, Franz WM, Reiser MF (2005) Phase-sensitive inversion-recovery MR imaging in the detection of myocardial infarction. Radiology 237:854–860

Huber A, Bauner K, Wintersperger BJ et al (2006) Phase-sensitive inversion recovery (PSIR) single-shot TrueFISP for assessment of myocardial infarction at 3 tesla. Invest Radiol 41:148–153

Huber A, Hayes C, Spannagl B et al (2007) Phase-contrast inversion recovery single-shot balanced steady-state free precession for detection of myocardial infarction during a single breathhold. Acad Radiology 14:1500–1508

Hundley WG, Hamilton CA, Clarke GD et al (1999) Visualization and functional assessment of proximal and middle left anterior descending coronary stenoses in humans with magnetic resonance imaging. Circulation 99:3248–3254

Hundley WG, Morgan TM, Neagle CM, Hamilton CA, Rerkpattanapipat P, Link KM (2002) Magnetic resonance imaging determination of cardiac prognosis. Circulation 106:2328–2333

Hundley WD, Bluemke DA, Finn JP et al (2010) ACCF/ACR/AHA/NASCI/SCMR 2010 Expert consensus document on cardiovascular magnetic resonance. A report of the American College of Cardiology Foundation Task Force on Expert Consensus Documents. Circulation 121:2462–2508

Ibanez B, Prat-González S, Speidl WS et al (2007) Early metoprolol administration before coronary reperfusion results in increased myocardial salvage. Analysis of ischemic myocardium at risk using cardiac magnetic resonance. Circulation 115:2909–2916

Ibrahim T, Nekolla SG, Hörnke M et al (2005) Quantitative measurement of infarct size by contrast-enhanced magnetic resonance imaging early after acute myocardial infarction. Comparison with single-photon emission tomography using Tc99m-sestamibi. J Am Coll Cardiol 45:544–552

Ibrahim T, Bülow HP, Hackl T et al (2007) Diagnostic value of contrast-enhanced magnetic resonance imaging and single-photon emission computed tomography for detection of myocardial necrosis early after acute myocardial infarction. J Am Coll Cardiol 49:208–216

Ibrahim T, Hackl T, Nekolla SG et al (2010) Acute myocardial infarction: serial cardiac MR imaging shows a decrease in delayed enhancement of the myocardium during the 1st week after reperfusion. Radiology 254:88–97

Ingkanisorn WP, Rhoads KL, Aletras AH, Kellman P, Arai AE (2004) Gadolinium delayed enhancement cardiovascular magnetic resonance correlates with clinical measures of myocardial infarction. J Am Coll Cardiol 43:2253–2259

Ingkanisorn WP, Kwong RY, Bohme NS et al (2006) Prognosis of negative adenosine stress magnetic resonance in patients presenting to an emergency department with chest pain. J Am Coll Cardiol 47:1427–1432

Ito H, Tomooka T, Sakai N, Yu H et al (1992) Lack of myocardial perfusion immediately after successful thrombolysis. A predictor of poor recovery of left ventricular function in anterior myocardial infarction. Circulation 85: 1699–1705

Ito H, Maruyama A, Iwakura K et al (1996) Clinical implications of the 'no-reflow' phenomenon. A predictor of complications and left ventricular remodeling in reperfused anterior wall myocardial infarction. Circulation 93 :223–228

Jahnke C, Paetsch I, Gebker R, Bornstedt A, Fleck E, Nagel E (2006) Accelerated 4D dobutamine stress MR imaging with k-t BLAST: feasibility and diagnostic performance. Radiology 241:718–728

Jahnke C, Hetzer R, Komoda T, Fleck E, Paetsch I (2007a) Images in cardiovascular medicine. Intramural dissecting hemorrhage of the myocardium. Circulation 115:e457–e459

Jahnke C, Nagel E, Gebker R (2007b) Prognostic value of cardiac magnetic resonance stress tests: adenosine stress perfusion and dobutamine stress wall motion imaging. Circulation 115:1769–1776

Jahnke C, Gebker R, Manka R, Schnackenburg B, Fleck E, Paetsch I (2010) Navigator-gated 3D blood oxygen level dependent CMR at 3.0T for detection of stress-induced myocardial ischemic reactions. J Am Coll Cardiol Img 3:375–384

Janssens S, Dubois C, Bogaert J et al (2006) Autologous bone marrow-derived stem-cell transfer in patients with ST-segment elevation myocardial infarction: double-blind, randomised controlled trial. Lancet 367:113–121

Jennings RB, Hawkins HK, Lowe JE et al (1978) Relation between high-energy phosphate and lethal injury in myocardial ischemia in the dog. Am J Pathol 92:187–214

Jenssen CJ, Jochims M, Hunold P et al (2010) Right ventricular involvement in acute left ventricular myocardial infarction: prognostic implications of MRI findings. AJR 194:592–598

John AS, Dreyfus GD, Pennell DJ (2005) Images in cardiovascular medicine. Reversible wall thinning in hibernation predicted by cardiovascular magnetic resonance. Circulation 111:e24–e25

Johnston DL, Brady TJ, Ratner AV et al (1985) Assessment of myocardial ischemia with proton magnetic resonance: effects of a three hour coronary occlusion with and without reperfusion. Circulation 71:595–601

Judd RM, Lugo-Olivieri CH, Arai M et al (1995a) Physiological basis of myocardial contrast enhancement in fast magnetic resonance images of 2-day-old reperfused canine infarcts. Circulation 92:1902–1910

Judd RM, Atalay MK, Rottman GA et al (1995b) Effects of myocardial water exchange on T1 enhancement during bolus administration of MR contrast agents. Magn Reson Med 33:215–223

Jugdutt BI, Khan MI (1992) Impact of increased infarct transmurality on remodeling and function during healing after anterior myocardial infarction in the dog. Can J Physiol Pharmacol 70:949–958

Jun SL, Chanani NK, Moore P, Higgins CB (2007) Images in cardiovascular medicine. Magnetic resonance imaging of a posttraumatic myocardial infarction and ventricular septal defect with a closure device in place. Circulation 115:e13–e15

Kaandorp TA, Bax JJ, Schuijf JD et al (2004) Head-to-head comparison between contrast-enhanced magnetic resonance imaging and dobutamine magnetic resonance imaging in men with ischemic cardiomyopathy. Am J Cardiol 93: 1461–1464

Kaandorp TAM, Bax JJ, Lamb HJ et al (2005a) Which parameters on magnetic resonance imaging determine Q waves on the electrocardiogram. Am J Cardiol 95:925–929

Kaandorp TAM, Lamb HJ, van der Wall EE, de Roos A, Bax JJ (2005b) Cardiovascular MR to assess myocardial viability in chronic ischaemic LV dysfunction. Heart 91:1359–1365

Karamitsos T, Francis JM, Myerson S, Selvanayagam JB, Neubauer S (2009) The role of cardiovascular magnetic resonance imaging in heart failure. J Am Coll Cardiol 54:1407–1424

Keeley EC, Hillis LD (1996) Left ventricular mural thrombus after acute myocardial infarction. Clin Cardiol 19:83–86

Kelle S, Hamdan A, Schnackenburg B et al (2008) Dobutamine stress cardiovascular magnetic resonance at 3 Tesla. J Cardiovasc Magn Reson 10:44

Kelle S, Roes SD, Klein C, Kokocinski T, de Roos A, Fleck E, Bax JJ, Nagel E (2009) Prognostic value of myocardial infarct size and contractile reserve using magnetic resonance imaging. J Am Coll Cardiol 54:1770–1777

Kellman P, Arai AE, McVeigh ER et al (2002) Phase-sensitive inversion recovery for detecting myocardial infarction using gadolinium-delayed hyperenhancement. Magn Reson Med 47(2):372–383

Kellman P, Dyke CK, Aletras AH et al (2004) Artifact suppression in imaging of myocardial infarction using B1-weighted phased-array combined phase-sensitive inversion recovery dagger. Magn Reson Med 51(2):408–412

Kellman P, Aletras AH, Mancini C, McVeigh ER, Arai AE (2007) T2-Prepared SSFP improves diagnostic confidence in edema imaging in acute myocardial infarction compared to turbo spin echo. Magn Reson Med 57:891–897

Kellman P, Hernando D, Shah S et al (2009) Multi-echo Dixon fat and water separation method for detecting fibro-fatty infiltration in the myocardium. Magn Reson Med 61: 215–221

Kim RJ, Chen EL, Lima JA et al (1996) Myocardial Gd-DTPA kinetics determine MRI contrast enhancement and reflect the extent and severity of myocardial injury after acute reperfused infarction. Circulation 94:3318–3326

Kim RJ, Fieno DS, Parrish TB et al (1999) Relationship of MRI delayed contrast enhancement to irreversible injury, infarct age, and contractile function. Circulation 100: 1992–2002

Kim RJ, Wu E, Rafael A et al (2000) The use of contrast-enhanced magnetic resonance imaging to identify reversible myocardial dysfunction. N Engl J Med 343:1445–1453

Kim RJ, Shah DJ, Judd RM (2003) How we perform delayed enhancement imaging. J Cardiovasc Magn Reson 5: 505–514

Kim RJ, Albert TSE, Wible JH et al (2008) Performance of delayed-enhancement magnetic resonance imaging with Gadoversetamide contrast for the detection and assessment of myocardial infarction. An international, multicenter, double-blinded, randomized trial. Circulation 117: 629–637

Kim HW, Farzaneh A, Kim RJ (2010) Cardiovascular magnetic resonance in patients with myocardial infarction. Current and emerging applications. J Am Coll Cardiol 55:1–16

Kinch J, Ryan T (1994) Right ventricular Infarction. N Engl J Med 330:1211–1217

Kino A, Zuehlsdorff S, Sheehan JJ, Weale PJ, Carroll TJ, Jerecic R, Carr JC (2009) Three-dimensional phase-sensitive inversion-recovery turbo FLASH sequence for the evaluation of left ventricular myocardial scar. AJR 193:W381–W388

Klein C, Nekolla SG, Bengel FM et al (2002) Assessment of myocardial viability with contrast-enhanced magnetic resonance imaging. Comparison with positron emission tomography. Circulation 105:162–167

Klein C, Schmal TR, Nekolla SG, Schnackenburg B, Fleck E, Nagel E (2007) Mechanism of late gadolinium enhancement in patients with acute myocardial infarction. J Cardiovasc Magn Reson 9:653–658

Klem I, Heitner JF, Shah DJ et al (2006) Improved detection of coronary artery disease by stress perfusion cardiovascular magnetic resonance with the use of delayed enhancement infarction imaging. J Am Coll Cardiol 47:1630–1638

Kloner RA, Jennings RB (2001) Consequences of brief ischemia: stunning, preconditioning and their clinical implications. Circulation 104:2981–2989

Kloner RA, Ganote CE, Jennings RB (1974) The 'no-reflow' phenomenon after temporary coronary occlusion in the dog. J Clin Invest 54:1496–1508

Klumpp B, Fenchel M, Hoevelborn T, Helber U, Scheule A, Claussen C, Miller S (2006) Assessment of myocardial viability using delayed enhancement magnetic resonance imaging 3.0 Tesla. Invest Radiol 41:661–667

Knuesel PR, Nanz D, Wyss C et al (2003) Characterization of dysfunctional myocardium by positron emission tomography and magnetic resonance: relation to functional outcome after revascularization. Circulation 108(9):1095–1100

Konen E, Merchant N, Gutierrez C et al (2005) True versus false left ventricular aneurysm: differentiation with MR imaging–initial experience. Radiology 236:65–70

Korosoglou G, Futterer S, Humpert PM et al (2009a) Strain-encoded cardiac MR during high-dose dobutamine stress testing: comparison to cine imaging and to myocardial tagging. J Magn Reson Imaging 29:1053–1061

Korosoglou G, Lossnitzer D, Schellberg D et al (2009b) Strain-encoded cardiac magnetic resonance imaging as an adjunct for dobutamine stress testing. Incremental value to conventional wall motion analysis. Circ Cardiovasc Imaging 2:132–140

Korosoglou G, Elhmidi Y, Steen H et al (2010a) Prognostic value of high-dose dobutamine stress magnetic resonance imaging in 1, 493 consecutive patients. Assessment of myocardial wall motion and perfusion. J Am Coll Cardiol 56:1225–1234

Korosoglou G, Lehrke S, Wochele A et al (2010b) Strain-encoded CMR for the detection of inducible ischemia during intermediate stress. J Am Coll Cardiol Img 3:361–371

Kraitchman DL, Sampath S, Castillo E et al (2003) Quantitative ischemia detection during cardiac magnetic resonance stress testing by use of FastHARP. Circulation 107:2025–2030

Kramer CM, Hundley WG (2010) Steadily straining toward clinical utility. Real-time quantitative CMR of myocardial deformation during stress. J Am Coll Cardiol Img 3: 372–374

Kramer CM, Lima JA, Reichek N et al (1993) Regional differences in function within noninfarcted myocardium during left ventricular remodeling. Circulation 88:1279–1288

Kramer CM, Rogers WJ, Theobald TM et al (1996a) Remote noninfarcted regional dysfunction soon after first anterior myocardial infarction. A magnetic resonance tagging study. Circulation 94:660–666

Kramer CM, Ferrari VA, Rogers WJ et al (1996b) Angiotensin-converting enzyme inhibition limits dysfunction in adjacent noninfarcted regions during left ventricular remodeling. J Am Coll Cardiol 27:211–217

Kramer CM, Rogers WJ, Theobald TM et al (1997) Dissociation between changes in intramyocardial function and left ventricular volumes in the eight weeks after first anterior myocardial infarction. J Am Coll Cardiol 30:1625–1632

Kramer CP, Rogers WJ, Mankad S, Theobald TM, Pakstis DL, Hu Y-L (2000) Contractile reserve and contrast uptake pattern by magnetic resonance imaging and functional recovery after reperfused myocardial infarction. J Am Coll Cardiol 36:1835–1840

Krittayaphong R, Maneesai A, Chaithiraphan V, Saiviroonporn P, Chaipet O, Udompunturak S (2009) Comparison of diagnostic and prognostic value of different electrocardiographic criteria to delayed-enhancement magnetic resonance imaging for healed myocardial infarction. Am J Cardiol 103:464–470

Kühl HP, Beek AM, van der Weerdt AP et al (2003) Myocardial viability in chronic ischemic heart disease: comparison of contrast-enhanced magnetic resonance imaging with (18)F-fluorodeoxyglucose positron emission tomography. J Am Coll Cardiol 41:1341–1348

Kühl HP, Papavasilliu TS, Beek AM et al (2004) Myocardial viability: rapid assessment with delayed contrast-enhanced MR imaging with three-dimensional inversion-recovery prepared pulse sequence. Radiology 230:576–582

Kühl HP, van der Weerdt A, Beek A, Visser F, Hanrath P, van Rossum A (2006) Relation of end-diastolic wall thickness and the residual rim of viable myocardium by magnetic resonance imaging to myocardial viability assessed by fluorine-18 deoxyglucose positron emission tomography. Am J Cardiol 97:452–457

Kuijpers D, Janssen CHC, van Dijkman PRM, Oudkerk M (2004a) Dobutamine stress MRI. Part I. Safety and feasibility of dobutamine cardiovascular magnetic resonance in patients suspected of myocardial ischemia. Eur Radiol 14:1823–1828

Kuijpers D, van Dijkman PRM, Janssen CHC, Vliegenthart R, Zijlstra F, Oudkerk M (2004b) Dobutamine stress MRI. Part II. Risk stratification with dobutamine cardiovascular magnetic resonance in patients suspected of myocardial ischemia. Eur Radiol 14:2046–2052

Kuijpers D, Yiu K, van Dijkman PRM et al (2003) Dobutamine cardiovascular magnetic resonance for the detection of myocardial ischemia with the use of myocardial tagging. Circulation 107:1592–1597

Kumar A, Abdel-Aty H, Kriedemann I et al (2006) Contrast-enhanced cardiovascular magnetic resonance imaging of right ventricular infarction. J Am Coll Cardiol 48: 1969–1976

Kurita T, Sakuma H, Onishi K et al (2009) Regional myocardial perfusion reserve determined using myocardial perfusion magnetic resonance imaging showed a direct correlation with coronary flow velocity reserve by Doppler flow wire. Eur Heart J 30:444–452

Kwon DH, Halley CM, Carrigan TP et al (2009) Extent of left ventricular scar predicts outcomes in ischemic cardiomyopathy patients with significantly reduced systolic function. A delayed hyperenhancement cardiac magnetic resonance study. J Am Coll Cardiol Img 2:34–44

Kwong RY, Schussheim AE, Rekhraj S et al (2003) Detecting acute coronary syndrome in the emergency department with cardiac magnetic resonance imaging. Circulation 107:531–537

Kwong RY, Chan AK, Brown KA et al (2006) Impact of unrecognized myocardial scar detected by cardiac magnetic resonance imaging on event-free survival in patients presenting with signs or symptoms or coronary artery disease. Circulation 113:2733–2743

Kwong RY, Sattar H, Wu H et al (2008) Incidence and prognositic implication of unrecognized myocardial scar characterized by cardiac magnetic resonance in diabetic patients without clinical evidence of myocardial infarction. Circulation 118:1011–1020

Lamfers EJP, Hooghoudt TEH, Hertzberger DP, Schut A, Stolwijk PWJ, Verheugt FWA (2003) Abortion of acute ST-segment elevatuion myocardial infarction after reperfusion: incidence, patients' characteristics, and prognosis. Heart 89:496–501

Lanza GA, Buffon A, Sestito A et al (2008) Relation between stress-induced myocardial perfusion defects on cardiovascular magnetic resonance and coronary microvascular dysfunction in patients with cardiac syndrome X. J Am Coll Cardiol 51:466–472

Larose E (2006) Below radar. Contributions of cardiac magnetic resonance to the understanding of myonecrosis after percutaneous coronary intervention. Circulation 114: 620–622

Larose E, Ganz P, Reynolds G, Dorbala S, Di Carli MR, Brown KA, Kwong RY (2007) Right ventricular dysfunction assessed by cardiovascular magnetic resonance imaging predicts poor prognosis late after myocardial infarction. J Am Coll Cardiol 49:855–862

Larose E, Rodés-Cabau J, Pibarot P et al (2010) Predicting late myocardial recovery and outcomes in the early hours of ST-segment elevation myocardial infarction. J Am Coll Cardiol 55:2459–2469

Laster SB, Shelton TJ, Barzilai B, Goldstein JA (1993) Determinants of the recovery of right ventricular performance following experimental chronic right coronary artery occlusion. Circulation 88:696–708

Laster SB, Ohnishi Y, Saffitz JE, Goldstein JA (1994) Effects of reperfusion on ischemic right ventricular dysfunction. Disparate mechanisms of benefit related to duration of ischemia. Circulation 90:1398–1409

Lauterbur PC, Dias MM, Rudin AM (1978) Augmentation of tissue water proton spin-lattice relaxation rates by in vivo addition of paramagnetic ions. In: Dutton PL, Leigh JS, Scarpa A (eds) International symposium on frontiers of biological energetics of electrons to tissues. Academic, New York, pp 752–759

Lee JT, Ideker RE, Reimer KA (1981) Myocardial infarct size and location in relation to the coronary vascular bed at risk in man. Circulation 64:526–534

Lee DC, Simonetti OP, Harris KR et al (2004) Magnetic resonance versus radionuclide pharmacological stress perfusion imaging for flow-limiting stenoses of varying severity. Circulation 110:58–65

Lim CCS, van Gaal WJ, Testa L et al (2011) With the "Universal Definition", measurement of creatine kinase-myocardial band rather than troponin allows more accurate diagnosis of periprocedural necrosis and infarction after coronary intervention. J Am Coll Cardiol 57:653–661

Lima JA, Judd RM, Bazille A, Schulman SP, Atalar E, Zerhouni EA (1995) Regional heterogeneity of human myocardial infarcts demonstrated by contrast-enhanced MRI. Potential mechanisms. Circulation 92:1117–1125

Liu X, Huang Y, Pokreisz P et al (2007) Nitric oxide inhalation improves microvascular flow and decreases infarction size after myocardial ischemia and reperfusion. J Am Coll Cardiol 50:808–817

Lloyd-Jones D, Adams RJ, Brown TM et al (2010) Heart disease and stroke statistics–2010 update: a report from the American Heart Association. Circulation 121: e46–e215

Locca D, Bucciarelli-Ducci C, Ferrante G et al (2010) New universal definition of myocardial infarction. Applicable after complex percutaneous coronary interventions? J Am Cardiol Intv 3:950–958

Lockie T, Nagel E, Redwood S, Plein S (2009) The use of cardiovascular magnetic resonance imaging in acute coronary syndromes. Circulation 119:1671–1681

Look DC, Locker DR (1970) Time saving in measurement of NMR and EPR relaxation times. Rev Sci Instrum 41: 250–251

Lotan CS, Miller SK, Bouchard A et al (1990) Detection of intramyocardial hemorrhage using high-field proton (1H) nuclear magnetic resonance imaging. Cathet Cardiovasc Diagn 20:205–211

Lotan CS, Bouchard A, Cranney CB, Bishop SP, Pohost GM (1992) Assessment of postreperfusion myocardial hemorrhage using proton NMR imaging at 1.5T. Circulation 86:1018–1025

Lubbers DD, Janssen CHC, Kuijpers D et al (2008) The addtional value of first pass myocardial perfusion imaging during peak dose of dobutamine stress cardiac MRI for the detection of myocardial ischemia. Int J Cardiovasc Imaging 24:69–76

Lücke C, Schindler K, Lehmkuhl L et al (2010) Prevalence and functional impact of lipomatous metaplasia in scar tissue following myocardial infarction evaluated by MRI. Eur Radiol 20:2074–2083

Maes A, Flameng W, Nuyts J et al (1994) Histological alterations in chronically hypoperfused myocardium: correlation with PET findings. Circulation 90:735–745

Mahrholdt H, Wagner A, Holly TA et al (2002) Reproducibility of chronic infarct size measurement by contrast-enhanced magnetic resonance imaging. Circulation 106:2322–2327

Mahrholdt H, Goedecke C, Wagner A et al (2004) Cardiovascular magnetic resonance assessment of human myocarditis. A comparison to histology and molecular biology. Circulation 109:1250–1258

Mahrholdt H, Wagner A, Judd RM, Sechtem U, Kim RJ (2005) Delayed enhancement cardiovascular magnetic resonance assessment of non-ischaemic cardiomyopathies. Eur Heart J 26:1461–1474

Manka R, Vitanis V, Boesiger P, Flammer AJ, Plein S, Kozerke S (2010) Clinical feasibility of accelerated, high signal resolution myocardial perfusion imaging. J Am Coll Cardiol Img 3:710–717

Mann DL, Bristow MR (2005) Mechanisms and models in heart failure: the biomechanical model and beyond. Circulation 111:2837–2849

Marie PY, Angioï M, Carteaux JP et al (2001) Detection and prediction of acute heart transplant rejection with the myocardial T2 determination provided by a black-blood magnetic resonance imaging sequence. J Am Coll Cardiol 37:825–831

Martin TN, Groenning BA, Murray HM et al (2007) ST-segment deviation analysis of the admission 12-lead electrocardiogram as an aid to early diagnosis of acute myocardial infarction with a cardiac magnetic imaging gold standard. J Am Coll Cardiol 50:1021–1028

Masci PG, Dymarkowski S, Bogaert J (2007) Images in cardiovascular medicine. Papillary muscle infarction after cardiopulmonary resuscitation. Circulation 116:e308–e309

Masci PG, Dymarkowski S, Rademakers FE, Bogaert J (2009) Determination of regional ejection fraction in patients with myocardial infarction by using late gadolinium enhancement and cine MR: feasibility study. Radiology 250:50–60

Masci PG, Ganame J, Strata E et al (2010a) Myocardial salvage by CMR correlates with LV remodeling and early ST-segment resolution in acute myocardial infarction. J Am Coll Cardiol Img 3:45–51

Masci PG, Francone M, Desmet W et al (2010b) Right ventricular ischemic injury in patients with acute ST-segment elevation myocardial infarction. Characterization with cardiovascular magnetic resonance. Circulation 122:1405–1412

Matheijssen NA, de Roos A, van der Wall EE et al (1991) Acute myocardial infarction: comparison of T2-weighted and T1-weighted gadolinium-DTPA enhanced MR imaging. Magn Reson Med 17:460–469

Mather AN, Lockie T, Nagel E et al (2009) Appearance of microvascular obstruction on high resolution first-pass perfusion, early and late gadolinium enhancement CMR in patients with acute myocardial infarction. J Cardiovasc Magn Reson 11:33–41

Mather AN, Fairbairn TA, Ball SG, Greenwood JP, Plein S (2010) Reperfusion haemorrhage as determined by cardiovascular MRI is a predictor of adverse left ventricular remodelling and markers of late arrhythmic risk. Heart 97:463–1459

Matsumura K, Jeremy RW, Schaper J et al (1998) Progression of myocardial necrosis during reperfusion of ischemic myocardium. Circulation 97:795–804

McCrohon JA, Moon JCC, Prasad SK et al (2003) Differentiation of heart failure related to dilated cardiomyopathy and coronary artery disease using gadolinium-enhanced cardiovascular magnetic resonance. Circulation 108:54–59

McNamara MT, Wesbey GE, Brasch RC et al (1985) Magnetic resonance imaging of acute myocardial infarction using a nitroxyl spin label (PCA). Invest Radiol 20:591–595

McNamara MT, Tscholakoff D, Revel D et al (1986) Differentiation of reversible and irreversible myocardial injury by MR imaging with and without gadolinium-DTPA. Radiology 158:765–769

Meijs MFL, Bots ML, Cramer MJM et al (2009) Unrecognised myocardial infarction in subjects at high vascular risk: prevalence and determinants. Heart 95:728–732

Mewton N, Bonnefoy E, Revel D, Ovize M, Kirkorian G, Croisille P (2009) Presence and extent of cardiac magnetic resonance microvascular obstruction in reperfused non-ST-elevated myocardial infarction and correlation with infarct size and myocardial enzyme release. Cardiology 113:50–58

Meyer C, Strach K, Thomas D et al (2008) High-resolution myocardial stress perfusion at 3T in patients with suspected coronary artery disease. Eur Radiol 18:226–233

Mikami Y, Sakuma H, Nagata M et al (2009) Relationship between signal intensity on T2-weighted MR images and presence of microvascular obstruction in patients with acute myocardial infarction. AJR 193:W321–W326

Mollet NR, Dymarkowski S, Volders W et al (2002) Visualization of ventricular thrombi with contrast-enhanced magnetic resonance imaging in patients with ischemic heart disease. Circulation 106:2873–2876

Moon JCC, Perez De Arenaza D et al (2004) The pathologic basis of Q-wave and non-Q-wave myocardial infarction. A cardiovascular magnetic resonance study. J Am Coll Cardiol 44:554–560

Morton G, Plein S, Nagel E (2010a) Noninvasive coronary angiography using computed tomography versus magnetic resonance imaging. Ann Intern Med 152:827–828

Morton G, Schuster A, Perera D, Nagel E (2010b) Cardiac magnetic resonance imaging to guide complex revascularization in stable coronary artery disease. Eur Heart J 31:2209–2216

Moustakidis P, Maniar HS, Cupps BP et al (2002) Altered left ventricular geometry changes the border zone temporal distribution of stress in an experimental model of left ventricular aneurysm: a finite element model study. Circulation 106(I):I-168–I-175

Müllner M, Oschatz E, Sterz F et al (1998) The influence of chest compressions and external defibrillation on the release of creatine kinase-MB and cardiac troponin T in patients resuscitated from out-of-hospital cardiac arrest. Resuscitation 38:99–105

Murry CE, Reinecke H, Pabon LM (2006) Regeneration gaps: observations on stem cells and cardiac repair. J Am Coll Cardiol 47:1777–1785

Myers GB, Howard A, Klein M, Stofer BE (1948a) Correlation of the electrocardiographic and pathologic findings in anteroseptal infarction. Am Heart J 36:535–575

Myers GB, Howard A, Stofer BE (1948b) Correlation of the electrocardiographic and pathologic findings in lateral infarction. Am Heart J 37:374–417

Myers GB, Howard A, Stofer BE (1948c) Correlation of the electrocardiographic and pathologic findings in posterior infarction. Am Heart J 38:547–582

Nagel E, Lehmkuhl HB, Bocksch W et al (1999) Noninvasive diagnosis of ischemia-induced wall motion abnormalities with the use of high-dose dobutamine stress MRI: comparison with dobutamine stress echocardiography. Circulation 99:763–770

Nagel E, Klein C, Paetsch I et al (2003) Magnetic resonance perfusion measurement for the noninvasive detection of coronary artery disease. Circulation 108:432–437

Nandalur KR, Dwamena BA, Choudhri AF, Nandalur MR, Carlos RC (2007) Diagnostic performance of stress cardiac magnetic resonance imaging in the detection of coronary artery disease. A meta-analysis. J Am Coll Cardiol 50: 1343–1353

Natanzon A, Aletras AH, Hsu L-Y, Arai AE (2005) Determining canine myocardial area at risk with manganese-enhanced MR imaging. Radiology 236:589–866

Neill W, Ingwall J, Andrews E et al (1986) Stabilization of the derangement in adenosine triphosphate metabolism during sustained, partial ischemia in the dog heart. J Am Coll Cardiol 8:894–900

Neubauer S (2007) The failing heart–an engine running out of fuel. N Engl J Med 356:1140–1151

Ni Y, Marchal G, Yu J et al (1995) Localization of metalloporphyrin induced "specific" enhancement in experimental liver tumors: comparison of magnetic resonance imaging, microangiographic and histologic findings. Acad Radiol 2:687–699

Ni Y, Petré C, Miao Y et al (1997) Magnetic resonance imaging–histomorphologic correlation studies on paramagnetic metalloporphyrins in rat models of necrosis. Invest Radiol 32:770–779

Ni Y, Pislaru C, Bosmans H et al (1998) Validation of intracoronary delivery of metalloporphyrin as an in vivo histochemical staining for myocardial infarction with MR imaging. Acad Radiol 5(1):537–541

Niccoli G, Burzotta F, Galiuto L, Crea F (2009) Myocardial no-reflow in humans. J Am Coll Cardiol 54:281–292

Nienaber CA, Brunken RC, Sherman CT (1991) Metabolic and functional recovery of ischemic human myocardium after coronary angioplasty. J Am Coll Cardiol 18:966–978

Nijveldt R, Beek AM, Hirsch A et al (2008) Functional recovery after acute myocardial infarction. Comparison between angiography, electrocardiography, and cardiovascular magnetic resonance measures of microvascular injury. J Am Coll Cardiol 52:181–189

Nijveldt R, Hofman MBM, Hirsch A, Beek AM, Umans VAWM, Algra PR, Piek JJ, van Rossum AC (2009) Assessment of microvascular obstruction and prediction of short-term remodeling after acute myocardial infarction: cardiac MR imaging study. Radiology 250:363–370

Nishimura T, Kobayashi H, Ohara Y et al (1989) Serial assessment of myocardial infarction by using gated MR imaging and Gd-DTPA. AJR Am J Roentgenol 153(4):715–720

O'Regan DP, Ahmed R, Karunanithy N et al (2009) Reperfusion hemorrhage following acute myocardial infarction: Assessment with T2* mapping and effect on measuring the area at risk. Radiology 250:916–922

Ochiai K, Shimada T, Murakami Y et al (1999) Hemorrhagic myocardial infarction after coronary reperfusion detected in vivo by magnetic resonance imaging in humans: prevalence and clinical implications. J Cardiovasc Magn Reson 1:247–256

Okayama S, Uemara S, Soeda T et al (2011) Clinical significance of papillary muscle late enhancement detected via cardiac magnetic resonance imaging in patients with single old myocardial infarction. Int J Cardiol 146: 73–79

Orn S, Manhenke C, Anand IS, Squire I, Nagel E, Edvardsen T, Dickstein K (2007) Effect of left ventricular scar size, location, and transmurality on left ventricular remodeling with healed myocardial infarction. Am J Cardiol 99: 1109–1114

Orn S, Manhenke C, Greve OJ, Larsen AI, Bonarjee VVS, Edvardsen T, Dickstein K (2009) Microvascular obstruction is a major determinant of infarct healing and subsequent left ventricular remodelling following primary percutaneous coronary intervention. Eur Heart J 30:1978–1985

Ortiz-Pérez JT, Meyers SN, Lee DC et al (2007) Angiographic estimates of myocardium at risk during acute myocardial infarction: validation study using cardiac magnetic resonance Imaging. Eur Heart J 28:1750–1758

Ortiz-Pérez JT, Rodriguez J, Sheridan NM et al (2008) Correspondence between the 17-segment model and coronary arterial anatomy using contrast-enhanced cardiac magnetic resonance imaging. JACC Cardiovasc Imaging 1:282–293

Ortiz-Pérez JT, Lee DC, Meyers SN, Davidson CJ, Bonow RO, Wu E (2010) Determinants of myocardial salvage during acute myocardial infarction. Evaluation of a combined angiographic and CMR myocardial salvage index. J Am Coll Cardiol Img 3:491–500

Oshinski JN, Yang Z, Jones JR et al (2001) Imaging time after Gd-DTPA injection is critical in using delayed enhancement to determine infarct size accurately with magnetic resonance imaging. Circulation 104:2838–2842

Paetsch I, Föll D, Kaluza A et al (2005) Magnetic resonance stress tagging in ischemic heart disease. Am J Physiol Heart Circ Physiol 288:H2708–H2714

Paetsch I, Jahnke C, Ferrari VA et al (2006) Determination of interobserver variability for identifying inducible left ventricular wall motion abnormalities during dobutamine stress magnetic resonance imaging. Eur Heart J 27:1459–1464

Panting JR, Gatehouse PD, Yang GZ et al (2002) Abnormal subendocardial perfusion in cardiac syndrome x detected by cardiovascular magnetic resonance imaging. N Engl J Med 346:1948–1953

Patterson RE, Jones-Collins BA, Aamodt R et al. (1993) Differences in collateral myocardial blood flow following gradual vs abrupt coronary occlusion. Cardiovasc Res 17:207–213

Peters DC, Appelbaum EA, Nezafat R et al (2009) Left ventricular infarct size, peri-infarct zone, and papillary scar measurements: a comparison of high-resolution 3D and conventional 2D late gadolinium enhancement cardiac MRI. J Magn Reson Imaging 30:794–800

Pfeffer MA, Braunwald E (1989) Ventricular remodeling after myocardial infarction. Experimental observations and clinical implications. Circulation 81:1161–1172

Pfisterer ME, Zellweger MJ, Gersh BJ (2010) Management of stable coronary artery disease. Lancet 375:763–772

Phibbs B (1984) Transmural versus Q wave infarction. J Am Coll Cardiol 4:1332

Pilz G, Jeske A, Klos M et al (2008) Prognostic value of normal adenosine-stress cardiac magnetic resonance imaging. Am J Cardiol 101:1408–1412

Pislaru SV, Ni Y, Pislaru C et al (1999) Noninvasive measurements of infarct size after thrombolysis with a necrosis-avid MRI contrast agent. Circulation 99:690–696

Plein S, Ridgway JP, Jones TR et al (2002) Coronary artery disease: assessment with a comprehensive MR imaging protocol–initial results. Radiology 225:300–307

Plein S, Greenwood JP, Ridgway JP, Cranny G, Ball SG, Sivananthan MU (2004) Assessment of non-ST segment elevation acute coronary syndromes with cardiac magnetic resonance imaging. J Am Coll Cardiol 44:2173–2181

Plein S, Kozerke S, Suerder D et al (2008a) High spatial resolution myocardial perfusion cardiac magnetic resonance for the detection of coronary artery disease. Eur Heart J 29:2148–2155

Plein S, Younger JF, Sparrow P, Ridgway JP, Ball SG, Greenwood JP (2008b) Cardiovascular magnetic resonance of scar and ischemia burden early after acute ST elevation and non-ST elevation myocardial infarction. J Cardiovasc Magn Reson 10:47–55

Pomeroy OH, Wendland M, Wagner S et al (1989) Magnetic resonance imaging of acute myocardial ischemia using a manganese chelate, Mn-DPDP. Invest Radiol 24:531–536

Porto I, Selvanayagam JB, Van Gaal WJ et al (2006) Plaque volume and occurrence and location of periprocedural myocardial necrosis after percutaneous coronary intervention. Insights from delayed-enhancement magnetic resonance imaging, thrombolysis in myocardial infarction myocardial perfusion grade analysis, and intravascular ultrasound. Circulation 114:662–669

Prasad A, Singh M, Lerman A et al (2006) Isolated elevation in Troponin T after percutaneous coronary intervention is associated with higher long-term mortality. J Am Coll Cardiol 48:1765–1770

Rademakers FE, Marchal G, Mortelmans L, Marchal G, Bogaert J (2003) Evolution of regional performance after an acute myocardial infarction in humans using magnetic resonance tagging. J Physiol 546:777–787

Rahimtoola SH (1989) The hibernating myocardium. Am Heart J 117:211–220

Raman SV, Simonetti OP, Winner MW III et al (2010) Cardiac magnetic resonance with edema imaging identifies myocardium at risk and predicts worse outcome in patients with non-ST-segment elevation acute coronary syndrome. J Am Coll Cardiol 55:2480–2488

Ramani K, Judd RM, Holly TA et al (1998) Contrast magnetic resonance imaging in the assessment of myocardial viability in patients with stable coronary artery disease and left ventricular dysfunction. Circulation 98:2687–2694

Rehr RB, Peshock RM, Malloy CR (1986) Improved in vivo magnetic resonance imaging of acute myocardial infarction after intravenous paramagnetic contrast agent administration. Am J Cardiol 57:864–868

Rehwald WG, Fieno DS, Chen EL et al (2002) Myocardial magnetic resonance imaging contrast agent concentrations after reversible and irreversible ischemic injury. Circulation 105:224–229

Reimer KA, Jennings RB (1970) The wavefront progression of myocardial ischemic cell death. II. Transmural progression of necrosis within the framework of ischemic bed size (myocardium at risk) and collateral flow. Lab Invest 40:633–644

Reimer KA, Jennings RB (1979) The changing anatomic reference base of evolving myocardial infarction. Circulation 60:866–876

Reimer KA, Jennings RB, Cobb FR et al (1985) Animal models for protecting ischemic myocardium: results of the NHLBI Cooperative Study. Comparison of unconscious and conscious dog models. Circ Res 56:651–665

Rerkpattanapipat P, Morgan TM, Neagle CM et al (2002) Assessment of preoperative cardiac risk with magnetic resonance imaging. Am J Cardiol 90:416–419

Ricciardi MJ, Wu E, Davidson CJ et al (2001) Visualization of discrete microinfarction after percutaneous coronary intervention associated with mild creatine kinase-MB elevation. Circulation 103:2780–2783

Rieber J, Huber A, Erhard I et al (2006) Cardiac magnetic resonance perfusion imaging for the functional assessment of coronary artery disease: a comparison with coronary angiography and fractional flow reserve. Eur Heart J 27:1465–1471

Rivas F, Cobb FR, Bache RJ, Greenfield JC (1976) Relationship between blood flow to ischemic regions and extent of myocardial infarction. Circ Res 38:439–447

Rochitte CE, Lima JA, Bluemke DA et al (1998) Magnitude and time course of microvascular obstruction and tissue injury after acute myocardial infarction. Circulation 98:1006–1014

Roes SD, Kelle S, Kaandorp TA et al (2007) Comparison of myocardial infarct size assessed with contrast-enhanced magnetic resonance imaging and left ventricular function and volumes to predict mortality in patients with healed myocardial infarction. Am J Cardiol 100:930–936

Roes SD, Borleffs JW, van der Geest RJ et al (2009) Infarct tissue heterogeneity assessed with contrast-enhanced MRI predicts spontaneous ventricular arrhythmia in patients with ischemic cardiomyopathy and implantable cardioverter-defibrillator. Circ Cardiovasc Imaging 2:183–190

Rogers WJ, Kramer CM, Geskin G et al (1999) Early contrast-enhanced MRI predicts late functional recovery after reperfused myocardial infarction. Circulation 99:744–750

Rokey R, Verani MS, Bolli R et al (1986) Myocardial infarct size quantification by MR imaging early after coronary artery occlusion in dogs. Radiology 158:771–774

Rovai D, Di Bella G, Rossi G et al (2007) Q wave prediction of myocardial infarction location, size and transmural extent at magnetic resonance imaging. Cor Art Dis 18:381–389

Ruffolo RR Jr (1987) The pharmacology of dobutamine. Am J Med Sci 294:244–248

Saeed M, Wagner S, Wendland MF et al (1989) Occlusive and reperfused myocardial infarcts: differentiation with Mn-DPDP–enhanced MR imaging. Radiology 172:59–64

Saeed M, Bremerich J, Wendland MF et al (1999) Reperfused myocardial infarction as seen with use of necrosis-specific versus standard extracellular MR contrast media in rats. Radiology 213:247–257

Saeed M, Lund G, Wendland MF et al (2001) Magnetic resonance characterization of the peri-infarction zone of reperfused myocardial infarction with necrosis-specific and extracellular nonspecific contrast media. Circulation 10:871–876

Sardella G, Mancone M, Bucciarelli-Ducci C et al (2009) Thrombus aspiration during primary percutaneous coronary intervention improves myocardial reperfusion and reduces infarct size: the EXPIRA (thrombectomy with export catheter in infarct-related artery during primary percutaneous coronary intervention) prospective, randomized trial. J Am Coll Cardiol 53:309–315

Schaefer S, Malloy CR, Katz J et al (1988) Gadolinium-DTPA-enhanced nuclear magnetic resonance imaging of reperfused myocardium: identification of the myocardial bed at risk. J Am Coll Cardiol 12:1064–1072

Scheffler K, Hennig JT (2001) Quantification with inversion recovery TrueFISP. Magn Reson Med 45:720–723

Schinkel AF, Bax JJ, Poldermans D, Elhendy A, Ferrari R, Rahimtoola SH (2007) Hibernating myocardium: diagnosis and patient outcomes. Curr Probl Cardiol 32:375–410

Schmidt A, Azevedo CF, Cheng A et al (2007) Infarct tissue heterogeneity by magnetic resonance imaging identifies enhanced cardiac arrhythmia susceptibility in patients with left ventricular dysfunction. Circulation 115:2006–2014

Schroeder AP, Houlind K, Pedersen EM, Nielsen TT, Egeblad H (2001) Serial magnetic resonance imaging of global and regional left ventricular remodeling during 1 year after acute myocardial infarction. Cardiology 96:106–114

Schuijf JD, Kaandorp TA, Lamb HJ et al (2004) Quantification of myocardial infarct size and transmurality by contrast-enhanced magnetic resonance imaging in men. Am J Cardiol 94:284–288

Schulz-Menger J, Gross M, Messroghli D et al (2003) Cardiovascular magnetic resonance of acute myocardial infarction at a very early stage. J Am Coll Cardiol 42:513–518

Schwitter J, Nanz D, Kneifel S et al (2001) Assessment of myocardial perfusion in coronary artery disease by magnetic resonance. A comparison with positron emission tomography and coronary angiography. Circulation 103:2230–2235

Schwitter J, Wacker CM, Van Rossum AC et al (2008) MR-Impact: comparison of perfusion-cardiac magnetic resonance with single-photon emission computed tomography for the detection of coronary artery disease in a multicentre, multivendor, randomized trial. Eur Heart J 29:480–489

Selvanayagam JB, Kardos A, Francis JM et al (2004a) Value of delayed-enhancement cardiovascular magnetic resonance imaging in predicting myocardial viability after surgical revascularization. Circulation 110:1535–1541

Selvanayagam JB, Petersen SE, Francis JM et al (2004b) Effects of off-pump versus on-pump coronary surgery on reversible and irreversible myocardial injury. A randomized trial using cardiovascular magnetic resonance imaging and biochemical markers. Circulation 109:345–350

Selvanayagam JB, Jerosch-Herold M, Porto I et al (2005a) Resting myocardial blood flow is impaired in hibernating myocardium. A magnetic resonance study of quantitative perfusion assessment. Circulation 112:3289–3296

Selvanayagam JB, Porto I, Channon K et al (2005b) Troponin elevation after percutaneous coronary intervention directly represents the extent of irreversible myocardial injury. Insights from cardiovascular magnetic resonance imaging. Circulation 111:1027–1032

Selvanayagam JB, Cheng ASH, Jerosch-Herold MJ et al (2007) Effect of distal embolization on myocardial perfusion reserve after percutaneous coronary intervention. A quantitative magnetic resonance perfusion study. Circulation 116:1458–1464

Senior R, Lahiri A (1995) Enhanced detection of myocardial ischemia by stress dobutamine echocardiography utilizing the "biphasic" response of wall thickening during low and high dose dobutamine infusion. J Am Coll Cardiol 26:26–32

Sensky PR, Jivan A, Hudson NM et al (2000) Coronary artery disease: combined stress MR imaging protocol–one stop evaluation of myocardial perfusion and function. Radiology 215:608–614

Setser RM, Chung YC, Weaver JA, Stillman AE, Simonetti OP, White RD (2005) Effect of inversion time on delayed-enhancement magnetic resonance imaging with and without phase-sensitive reconstruction. J Magn Reson Imaging 21:650–655

Sheifer SE, Manolio TA, Gersh BJ (2001) Unrecognized myocardial infarction. Ann Intern Med 135:801–811

Sievers B, John B, Brandts B, Franken U, van Bracht M, Trappe H-J (2004) How reliable is electrocardiography in differentiating transmural from non-transmural myocardial infarction? A study with contrast magnetic resonance as gold standard. Int J Cardiol 97:417–423

Simonetti OP, Finn JP, White RV, Laub G, Henry DA (1996) "Black blood" T2-weighted inversion-recovery MR imaging of the heart. Radiology 199:49–57

Simonetti OP, Kim RJ, Fieno DS et al (2001) An improved MR imaging technique for the visualization of myocardial infarction. Radiology 218(1):215–223

Singh S, Kalra MK, Gilman MD et al (2011) Adaptive statistical iterative reconstruction technique for radiation dose reduction in chest CT: a pilot study. Radiology 259:565–573

Sinusas AJ, Trautman KA, Bergin JD et al (1990) Quantification of area at risk during coronary occlusion and degree of myocardial salvage after reperfusion with technetium-99m methoxyisobutyl isonitrile. Circulation 82:1424–1437

Smalling RW (2009) Ischemic time. The new gold standard for ST-segment elevation myocardial infarction care. J Am Coll Cardiol 54:2154–2156

Sobel BE, Bresnahan GF, Shell WE, Yoder RD (1972) Estimation of infarct size and its relation to prognosis. Circulation 46:640–648

Spodick DH (1980) Transmural versus nontransmural infarction. Circulation 62:447–448

Steel K, Broderick R, Gandla V et al (2009) Complementary prognostic values of stress myocardial perfusion and late gadolinium enhancement imaging by cardiac magnetic resonance in patients with known or suspected coronary artery disease. Circulation 120:1390–1400

Steen H, Giannitsis E, Futterer S, Merten C, Juenger C, Katus HA (2006) Cardiac troponin T at 96 hours after acute myocardial infarction correlates with infarct size and cardiac function. J Am Coll Cardiol 48:2192–2194

Steg PG, FitzGerald G, Fox KAA (2009) Risk stratification in non-ST-segment elevation acute coronary syndromes: troponin alone is not enough. Am J Med 122:107–108

Strach K, Meyer C, Schild H, Sommer T (2006) Cardiac stress MR imaging with dobutamine. Eur Radiol 16:2728–2738

Stuber AM, Schoenberg SO, Hayes C, Spannagl B, Engelmann MG, Franz WM, Reiser MF (2005) Phase-sensitive inversion-recovery MR imaging in the detection of myocardial infarction. Radiology 237:854–860

Sutton MGSJ, Sharpe N (2000) Left ventricular remodeling after myocardial infarction. Pathophysiology and therapy. Circulation 101:2981–2988

Tanimoto T, Imanishi T, Kitabata H et al (2010) Prevalence and clinical detection of papillary muscle infarction detected by late gadolinium-enhanced magnetic resonance imaging in patients with ST-segment elevation myocardial infarction. Circulation 122:2281–2287

Tarantini G, Cacciavillani L, Corbetti F et al (2006a) Duration of ischemia is a major determinant of transmurality and severe microvascular obstruction after primary angioplasty. A study performed with contrast-enhanced magnetic resonance. J Am Coll Cardiol 46:1229–1235

Tarantini G, Razzolini R, Cacciavillani L et al (2006b) Influence of transmurality, infarct size, and severe microvascular obstruction on left ventricular remodeling and function after primary coronary angioplasty. Am J Cardiol 98:1033–1040

Taylor AJ, Al-Saadi N, Abdel-Aty H, Schulz-Menger J, Messroghli DR, Friedrich MG (2004) Detection of acutely impaired microvascular reperfusion after infarct angioplasty with magnetic resonance imaging. Circulation 109:2080–2085

Taylor AM, Dymarkowski S, Verbeken E, Bogaert J (2006) Dection of pericardial inflammation with late-enhancement cardiac magnetic resonance imaging: initial results. Eur Radiol 16:569–574

Thiele H, Nagel E, Paetsch I et al (2001) Functional cardiac MR imaging with steady-state free precession (SSFP) significantly improves endocardial border delineation without contrast agents. J Magn Reson Imaging 14:362–367

Thiele H, Kappl MJE, Conradi S, Niebauer J, Hambrecht R, Schuler G (2006) Reproducibility of chronic and acute infarct size measurement by delayed enhancement-magnetic resonance imaging. J Am Coll Cardiol 47:1641–1645

Thiele H, Kappl MJ, Linke A et al (2007) Influence of time-to-treatment, TIMI-flow grades, and ST-segment resolution on infarct size and infarct transmurality as assessed by delayed enhancement magnetic resonance imaging. Eur Heart J 28:1433–1439

Thygesen K, Alpert JS, White HD (2007) on behalf of the Joint ESC/ACCF/AHA/WHF Task Force for the Redefinition of Myocardial Infarction (2007) Universal definition of myocardial infarction. Circulation 116:2634–2653

Tilak GS, Hsu LY, Hoyt RF Jr, Arai AE, Aletras AH (2008) In vivo T2-weighted magnetic resonance imaging can accurately determine the ischemic area at risk for 2-day-old nonreperfused myocardial infarction. Invest Radiol 43:7–15

Tonino PA, De Bruyne B, Pijls NH et al (2009) Fractional flow reserve versus angiography for guiding percutaneous coronary intervention. N Engl J Med 360:213–224

Tops LF, Roest AA, Lamb HJ et al (2005) Intraatrial repair of transposition of the great arteries: use of MR imaging after exercise to evaluate regional systemic right ventricular function. Radiology 237:861–867

Tscholakoff D, Higgins CB, Sechtem U et al (1986) Occlusive and reperfused myocardial infarcts: effect of Gd-DTPA on ECG-gated MR imaging. Radiology 160:515–519

Tumkosit M, Puntawangkoon C, Morgan TM et al (2009) Left ventricular infarct size assessed with 0.1 mmol/kg of gadobenate dimeglumine correlates with that assessed with 0.2 mmol/kg of gadopentate dimeglumine. J Comput Assist Tomogr 33:328–333

Underwood SR, Bax JJ, vom Dahl J et al (2004) Imaging techniques for the assessment of myocardial hibernation. Report of a Study Group of the European Society of Cardiology. Eur Heart J 25:815–836

van Dijkman PR, van der Wall EE, de Roos A et al (1991) Acute, subacute, and chronic myocardial infarction: quantitative analysis of gadolinium-enhanced MR images. Radiology 180(1):147–151

van Rugge FP, Holman ER, van der Wall EE et al (1993) Quantitation of global and regional left ventricular function by cine magnetic resonance imaging during dobutamine stress in normal human subjects. Eur Heart J 14:456–463

van Rugge FP, van der Wall EE, Spanjersberg SJ et al (1994) Magnetic resonance imaging during dobutamine stress for detection and localization of coronary artery disease. Quantitative wall motion analysis using a modification of the centerline method. Circulation 90:127–138

Vermeltfoort IA, Bondarenko O, Raijmakers PG et al (2007) Is subendocardial ischemia present in patients with chest pain and normal coronary angiograms? A cardiovascular MR study. Eur Heart J 28:1554–1558

Wagner A, Mahrholdt H, Holly TA et al (2003) Contrast-enhanced MRI and routine single photon emission computed tomography (SPECT) perfusion imaging for detection of subendocardial myocardial infarcts: an imaging study. Lancet 361:374–379

Wahl A, Gollesch A, Paetsch I et al (2003) Safety and feasibility of high-dose dobutamine-atropine stress MRI for diagnosis of myocardial ischemia: experience in 1000 consecutive cases. J Cardiovasc Magn Reson 5:51 (abstract)

Walker JC, Ratcliffe MB, Zhang P et al (2005) MRI-based finite-element analysis of left ventricular aneurysm. Am J Physiol Heart Circ Physiol 289:H692–H700

Wallace EL, Morgan TM, Walsh TF et al (2009) Dobutamine cardiac magnetic resonance result predict cardiac prognosis in women with known or suspected ischemic heart disease. J Am Coll Cardiol Img 2:299–307

Walsh TF, Dall'Armellina E, Chughtai H et al (2009) Adverse effect of increased left ventricular wall thickness on five year outcomes of patients with negative dobutamine stress. J Cardiovasc Magn Reson 11:25

Watkins S, McGeoch R, Lyne J et al (2009) Validation of magnetic resonance myocardial perfusion imaging with fractional flow reserve for the detecton of significant coronary heart disease. Circulation 120:2207–2213

Weinsaft JW, Kim HW, Shah HW et al (2008) Detection of left ventricular thrombus by delayed-enhancement cardiovascular magnetic resonance. Prevalence and markers in patients with systolic dysfunction. J Am Coll Cardiol 52:148–157

Weir RAP, Murphy CA, Petrie CJ et al (2010a) Microvascular obstruction remains a portent of adverse remodeling in optimally treated patients with left ventricular systolic dysfunction after acute myocardial infarction. Circ Cardiovasc Imaging 3:360–367

Weir RAP, Martin TN, Murphy CA et al (2010b) Comparison of serial measurements of infarct size and left ventricular ejection fraction by contrast-enhanced cardiac magnetic resonance imaging and electrocardiographic QRS scoring in reperfused anterior ST-elevation myocardial infarction. J Electrocardiol 43:230–236

Weissleder R, Lee A, Khaw B et al (1992) Antimyosin-labeled monocrystalline iron oxide allows detection of myocardial infarct: MR antibody imaging. Radiology 182:381–385

Wesbey GE, Higgins CB, McNamara MT et al (1984) Effect of gadolinium-DTPA on the magnetic relaxation times of normal and infarcted myocardium. Radiology 153:165–169

Wilke N, Jerosch-Herold M, Wang Y et al (1997) Myocardial perfusion reserve: assessment with multisection, quantitative, first-pass MR imaging. Radiology 204:373–384

Williams ES, Kaplan JI, Thatcher F et al (1980) Prolongation of proton spin lattice relaxation times in regionally ischemic tissue from dog hearts. J Nucl Med 21:449–453

Wisenberg G, Prato FS, Carroll SE et al (1988) Serial nuclear magnetic resonance imaging of acute myocardial infarction with and without reperfusion. Am Heart J 115:510–518

Wolf GL, Baum L (1983) Cardiovascular toxicity and tissue proton T1 response to manganese injection in the dog and rabbit. AJR Am J Roentgenol 141:193–197

Wright J, Adriaenssens T, Dymarkowski S, Desmet W, Bogaert J (2009) Quantification of myocardial area at risk with T2-weighted CMR. Comparison with contrast-enhanced CMR and coronary angiography. J Am Coll Cardiol Img 2:825–831

Wu KC, Zerhouni EA, Judd RM et al (1998a) Prognostic significance of microvascular obstruction by magnetic resonance imaging in patients with acute myocardial infarction. Circulation 97:765–772

Wu KC, Kim RK, Bluemke DA et al (1998b) Quantification and time course of microvascular obstruction by contrast-enhanced echocardiography and magnetic resonance imaging following acute myocardial infarction and reperfusion. J Am Coll Cardiol 32:1756–1764

Wu E, Judd RM, Vargas JD (2001) Visualisation of presence, location, and transmural extent of healed Q-wave and non–Q-wave myocardial infarction. Lancet 357:21–28

Wu M-T, Tseng W-Y, Su M-Y et al (2006) Diffusion tensor magnetic resonance imaging mapping the fiber architecture remodeling in human myocardium after infarction. Correlation with viability and wall motion. Circulation 114:1036–1045

Wu E, Ortiz JT, Tejedor P, Lee DC et al (2008) Infarct size by contrast enhanced cardiac magnetic resonance is a stronger predictor of outcomes than left ventricular ejection fraction or end-systolic volume index: prospective cohort study. Heart 94:730–736

Wu M-T, Su M-Y, Huang Y-L et al (2009) Sequential changes of myocardial microstructure in patients with postmyocardial infarction by diffusion-tensor cardiac MR. Correlation with left ventricular structure and function. Circ Cardiovasc Imaging 2:32–40

Wu M, D'Hooge J, Ganame J et al (2011) Non-invasive characterization of the area-at-risk using magnetic resonance imaging in chronic ischemia. Cardiovasc Research 89:166–174

Yan AT, Shayne AJ, Brown KA et al (2006) Characterization of the peri-infarct zone by contrast-enhanced cardiac magnetic resonance imaging is a powerful predictor of post-myocardial infarction mortality. Circulation 114:32–39

Yeh RW, Sidney S, Chandra M, Sorel M, Selby JV, Go AS (2010) Population trends in the incidence and outcomes of acute myocardial infarction. N Engl J Med 362:2155–2165

Yelgec NS, Dymarkowski S, Ganame J, Bogaert J (2007) Value of MRI in patients with a clinical suspicion of acute myocarditis. Eur Radiol 17:2211–2217

Yellon DM, Hausenloy DJ (2007) Myocardial reperfusion injury. N Engl J Med 357:1121–1135

Younger JF, Plein S, Barth J, Ridgway JP, Ball SG, Greenwood JP (2007) Troponin-I concentration 72 hours after myocardial infarction correlates with infarct size and presence of microvascular obstruction. Heart 93:1547–1551

Zornoff LAM, Skali H, Pfeffer MA et al (2002) Right ventricular dysfunction and risk of heart failure and mortality after myocardial infarction. J Am Coll Cardiol 39:1450–1455

Heart Muscle Diseases

J. Bogaert and A. M. Taylor

Contents

1	**Introduction**	275
2	**MRI Strategies to Study Heart Muscle Diseases**	276
3	**Cardiac or Ventricular Hypertrophy**	279
4	**Primary Cardiomyopathies**	284
4.1	Hypertrophic Cardiomyopathy	284
4.2	Dilated Cardiomyopathy	297
4.3	Restrictive Cardiomyopathy	302
4.4	Arrhythmogenic Right Ventricular Cardiomyopathy/Dysplasia	304
4.5	Left Ventricular Non-Compaction Cardiomyopathy	309
4.6	Inflammatory Cardiomyopathy or Myocarditis	312
4.7	Stress Cardiomyopathy or Tako-Tsubo Cardiomyopathy	320
4.8	Peripartum Cardiomyopathy	321
4.9	Tachycardia-Induced Cardiomyopathy	321
5	**Secondary Cardiomyopathies**	323
5.1	Infiltrative and Storage Disease	323
5.2	Endomyocardial Disease	328
5.3	Toxicity (Substance Abuse, Recreational Drugs, Heavy Metals)	330
5.4	Cancer Treatment-Induced Cardiac Toxicity	331
5.5	Inflammatory, Autoimmune and Vasculitic Disease	333
5.6	Endocrine Disorders	337
5.7	Neuromuscular/Neurological Disorders—Myopathies	338
5.8	Uremic Cardiomyopathy	338
6	**Congenital Myocardial Disorders in the Adult Population**	339
7	**Key Points**	341
References		341

Abstract

Heart muscle diseases or cardiomyopathies represent an important and heterogeneous group of cardiac diseases. Imaging is an essential pillar in assessment of the phenotypic expression of this group of diseases, indispensable for disease classification, obligatory to evaluate the degree of dysfunction, and appealing for risk stratification. This chapter focuses on the emerging role of MRI to assess this complex group of diseases. Since MRI provides unique information on myocardial tissue characteristics and functional properties, the focus is not only on the diagnosis, differential diagnosis, follow-up of disease progression, and evaluation of response to treatment of cardiomyopathies but this technique is increasingly being used for risk stratification of potential harmful complications, such as cardiac arrhythmias, heart failure, and sudden cardiac death.

1 Introduction

Heart muscle diseases or cardiomyopathies represent an important and heterogeneous group of cardiac diseases. The identification of several new disease

J. Bogaert (✉)
Department of Radiology,
University Hospitals Casthuisberg,
Catholic University of Leuven,
Herestraat 49, 3000 Leuven, Belgium
e-mail: jan.bogaert@uz.kuleuven.ac.be

A. M. Taylor
Centre for Cardiovascular Imaging,
UCL Institute of Cardiovascular Science
and Great Ormond Street Hospital for Children,
London, UK

J. Bogaert et al. (eds.), *Clinical Cardiac MRI*, Medical Radiology. Diagnostic Imaging,
DOI: 10.1007/174_2011_358, © Springer-Verlag Berlin Heidelberg 2012

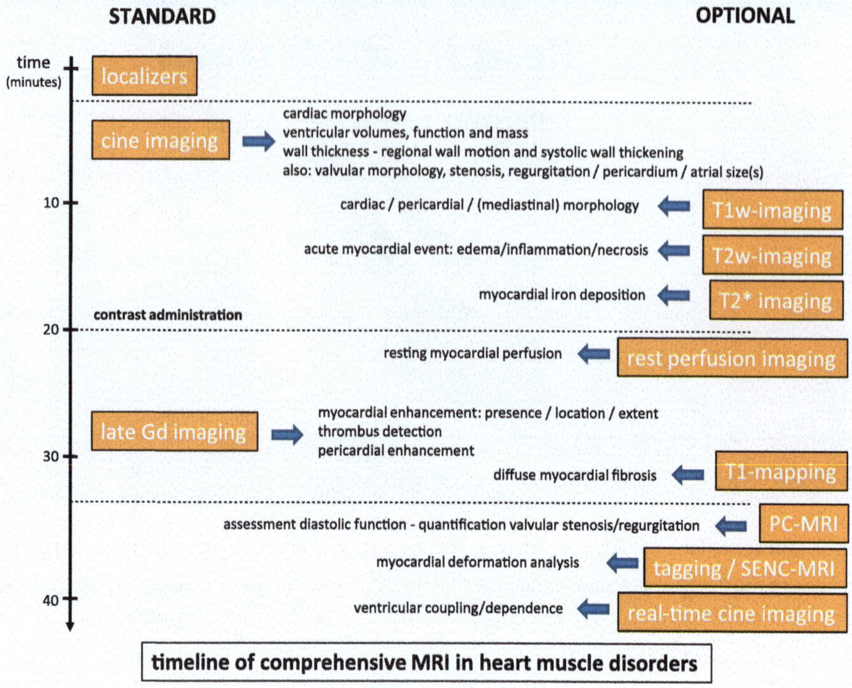

Fig. 1 Timeline for studying patients with heart muscle disorders. On the *left*, the standard MRI sequences that are used in the majority of patients, and the information that can be obtained with each sequence are shown. On the *right* the optional sequences that can be chosen depending on the clinical question, or on the information that need to be obtained are shown. Abbreviations: *PC* phase contrast; *SENC* strain encoding

entities affecting the myocardium, dramatic advances in diagnosis especially in the field of molecular genetics, and precise knowledge of causation over the past decade have led to the development of a new, contemporary classification, affording more clarity in this complex group of diseases and their basic disease mechanisms (Maron et al. 2006a; Watkins et al. 2011). Today, cardiomyopathies can be most effectively classified as those solely or predominantly confined to the heart muscle ("primary cardiomyopathies") and those who show pathological myocardial involvement as part of a generalized systemic (multi-organ) disorder ("secondary cardiomyopathies"). The considerable overlap, clinically, morphologically, functionally, and genetically between heart muscle diseases, hampers and renders any attempt toward classification arbitrary (Watkins et al. 2011). Moreover, several cardiovascular diseases not included as cardiomyopathies may affect the myocardium, cause systolic or diastolic dysfunction and impede differentiation with heart muscle diseases. Cardiac imaging is an essential pillar in assessment of the phenotypic expression of genetic heart muscle diseases, indispensable for disease classification, and obligatory to evaluate the degree of dysfunction. This chapter focuses on the emerging role of MRI to assess this complex group of diseases. Since MRI provides unique information on myocardial tissue characteristics and functional properties, the focus is not only on the diagnosis, differential diagnosis, follow-up of disease progression and evaluation of response to treatment of cardiomyopathies but this technique is increasingly being used for risk stratification of potential harmful complications, such as cardiac arrhythmias, heart failure, and sudden cardiac death.

2 MRI Strategies to Study Heart Muscle Diseases

Today, cardiac MRI sequences have been tailored toward comprehensive evaluation of heart muscle diseases (Fig. 1). Within a scan period of 30–45 min, cardiac and pericardial morphology, systolic and diastolic functional indices, myocardial perfusion and tissue properties, and valvular function can be assessed. To achieve the highest achievable output of an MRI study, it is mandatory to possess proper clinical information before study onset, enabling the MRI examination to be fine-tuned using appropriate sequences and imaging planes. For instance, it is obvious that the approach is different in arrhythmogenic right ventricular cardiomyopathy/dysplasia (ARVC/D) than in patients with suspected cardiac amyloidosis or hemochromatosis.

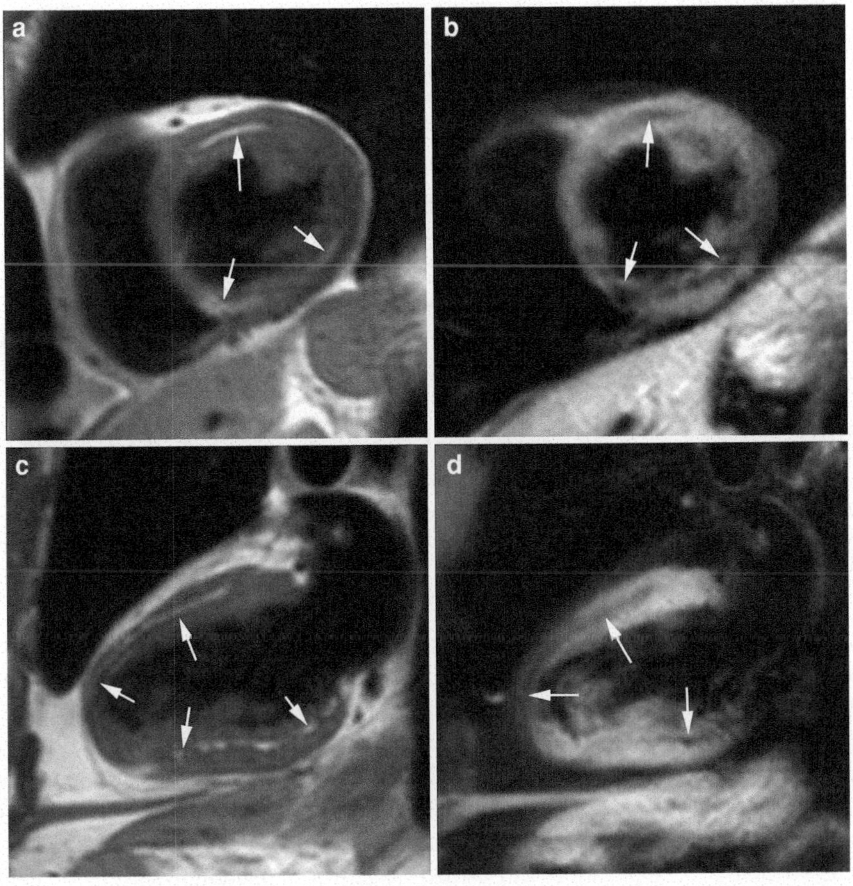

Fig. 2 Comprehensive use of MRI for myocardial tissue characterization. T1w-imaging in short-axis (**a**, **b**) and vertical long-axis (**c**, **d**), without (**a**, **c**) and with (**b**, **d**) fat-suppression techniques. While normal myocardium has a homogeneous intensity, the midwall is diffusely hyperintense on T1w-imaging (*arrows*, **a**, **c**), similar to the signal intensity of the surrounding epicardial and mediastinal fat. Using fat-suppression, the midwall hyperintense signal is nulled (*arrows*, **b**, **d**) proving the fatty nature. Findings consistent of lipomatous metaplasia

Dark-blood imaging, using fast spin-echo (SE) sequences, provides detailed morphological images of the heart, pericardium, and great vessels. The myocardium has a gray appearance, similar to that of skeletal muscle, and is clearly distinguishable from the adjacent bright epicardial fat and dark intracavitary blood. Myocardial T1- and T2-relaxation times, for a 1.5 T scanner, are 800 and 33 ms, respectively. Myocardial disorders may manifest themselves by changes in relaxation times. This phenomenon can be used, at least to a certain degree, for tissue characterization. Fatty myocardial replacement, for instance, is visible as bright foci within the myocardium on T1-weighted SE MRI (*'T1w-imaging'*) (Fig. 2). Depending on its location and association with other findings, this may fit in lipomatous metaplasia commonly found post-infarction. Also in ARVC/D, lipomatous replacement is a common finding though differentiation with benign conditions of fatty replacement such as benign senile dystrophy may be challenging. Bright myocardium on T2-weighted imaging (*'T2w-imaging'*) is suggestive of acute myocardial injury, representing myocardial edema with or without necrosis, and may be found for instance in patients with recent myocardial infarction as well as in acute myocarditis patients.

Bright-blood imaging, using balanced steady-state free precession (b-SSFP) sequences, has become the reference sequence for dynamic functional imaging (*'cine imaging'*) of the heart (see "Cardiac MR Physics" and "Cardiac Function"). Moreover, because of its high spatial and contrast resolution, image quality of cine images is often superior to dark-blood images, allowing detailed cardiac morphologic assessment (Fig. 3). Using multi-slice 2 or 3D imaging, complex anatomical variations can be appropriately unraveled, while dynamic imaging allows evaluation of intracardiac or transvalvular flow patterns, for example in patients with obstructive hypertrophic cardiomyopathy (HCM) depiction of flow acceleration in the LV outflow tract and mitral valve regurgitation (Fig. 4). Cine imaging, using real-

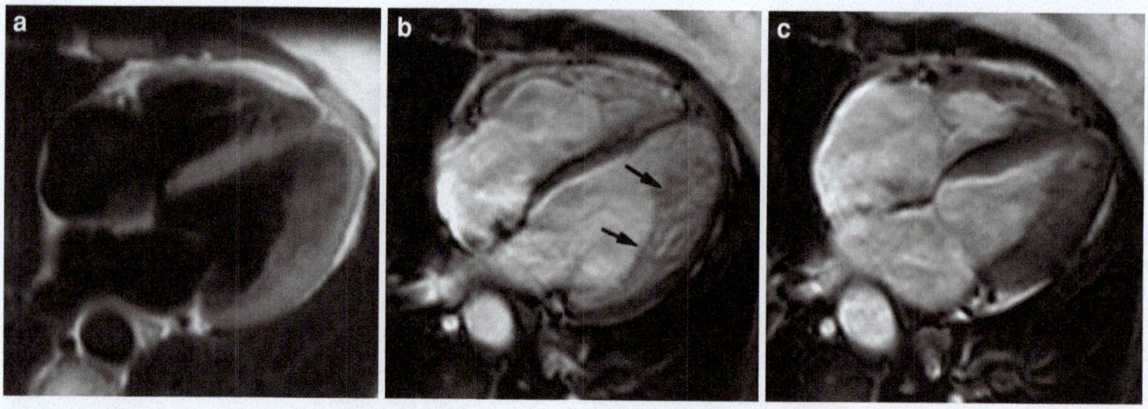

Fig. 3 Dark-blood versus bright-blood imaging in a 56-year-old woman with LV non-compaction cardiomyopathy (LVNC). The patient was referred for MRI because of thickened LV lateral wall on transthoracic echocardiography. T1w-imaging (**a**), cine imaging at end diastole (**b**), and end systole (**c**) in horizontal long-axis. While the LV lateral wall appears thickened on T1w-imaging and end-systolic cine imaging, the prominent trabecular network (*arrows*, **b**) is well visible on end-diastolic cine imaging in the lateral and apical part of the LV, confirming the diagnosis of LVNC. Likely stagnant blood between these prominent trabeculations causes a pseudo-thickening of the lateral wall on dark-blood imaging

time sequences during free breathing, can be exploited for instance to assess the physiological interaction between ventricles (i.e., ventricular coupling), thereby providing valuable information to differentiate between restrictive cardiomyopathy (RCM) and constrictive pericarditis. Phase-contrast MRI (PC-MRI) allows for accurate quantification of flow velocities and volumes. The applications of PC-MRI range from assessment of valvular pathology (quantification) stenosis and/or regurgitation), evaluation of diastolic indices, to quantification of myocardial velocities. Other dynamic MRI techniques, such as myocardial tagging, have shown helpful to analyze wall deformation and to quantify myocardial strain patterns helping in better understanding pathophysiology of heart muscle disorders. Contrast-enhanced three-dimensional MR angiography (ceMRA) can be applied in selected cases, for instance to exclude aortic coarctation in patients with unexplained LV myocardial hypertrophy.

Paramagnetic, gadolinium-based contrast agents are nowadays routinely used in the assessment of patients with heart muscle diseases (Matsuoka et al. 1993). Their administration enables an improved discrimination between normal and pathological myocardium, which is not only helpful in diagnosing myocardial diseases, but may yield prognostic information as well (Mahrholdt et al. 2005; Moon et al. 2003a). Increased early global myocardial contrast uptake, compared to the uptake in skeletal muscle, may be useful to depict myocarditis (Friedrich et al. 1998), while focal myocardial enhancement patterns may provide valuable information directing toward specific heart muscle disorders (Mahrholdt et al. 2005). In particular, the introduction of contrast-enhanced inversion-recovery MRI with late or delayed imaging by Simonetti et al. in 2001 (‘*late Gd imaging*’), has undoubtedly led to a paradigm shift in the field of non-invasive myocardial imaging. For a variety of myocardial diseases, this technique has become a valuable alternative to endomyocardial biopsy (EMB) (Cooper 2009). Briefly, (see “Cardiac MR Physics” for a detailed explanation), normal myocardium on late Gd imaging normally appears dark, while pathological (e.g., fibrotic or necrotic) myocardium appears bright. Although the myocardial enhancement itself is non-specific, the pattern, location, and extent of enhancement not only enables differentiation between ischemic (i.e., related to underlying coronary artery disease) and non-ischemic origins, but also differentiation between groups with non-ischemic-related disorders (Mahrholdt et al. 2005) (Fig. 5). However, since the late Gd imaging technique is designed for depicting of focal myocardial diseases, diseases diffusely or microscopically (beyond the spatial resolution of MRI) affecting the myocardium, such as diffuse myocardial fibrosis, can yield falsely negative findings on late Gd imaging, explaining some discrepancies between MRI and histology (Mahrholdt et al. 2004). Diffuse myocardial fibrosis occurs as part of normal aging but this process of

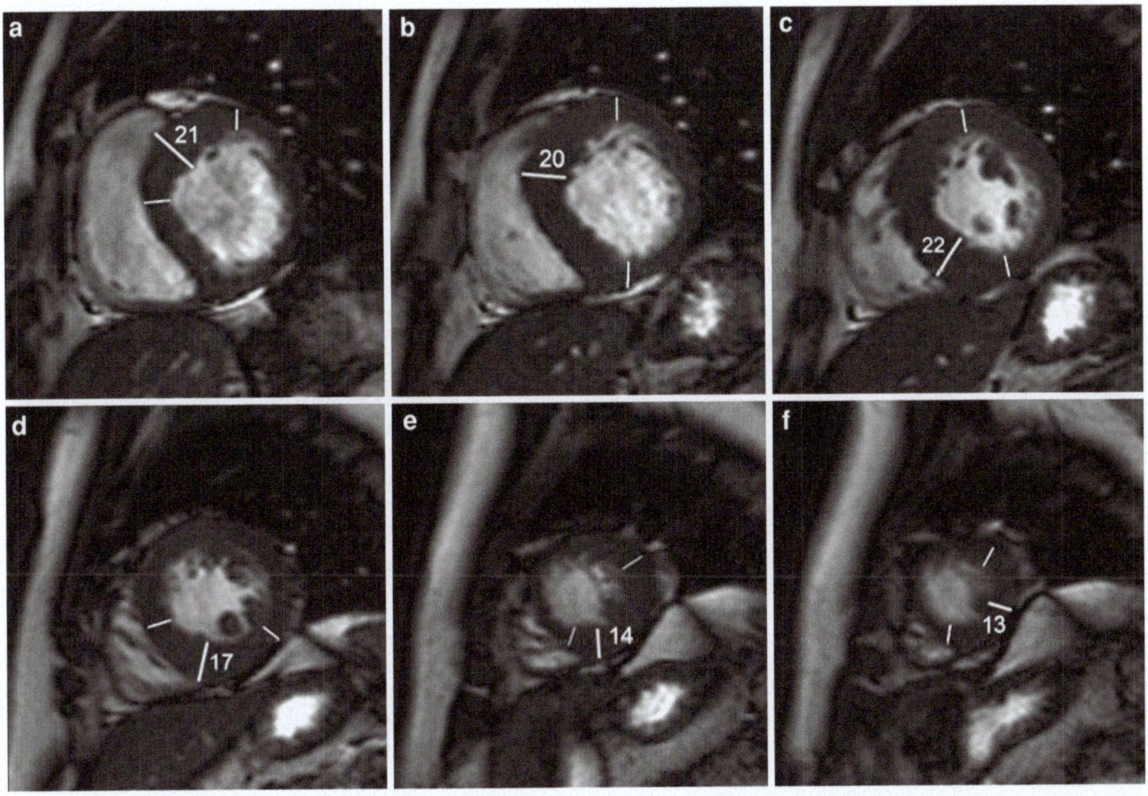

Fig. 4 Use of bright-blood (cine) imaging for morphologic cardiac assessment in asymmetric septal HCM. Selection of six short-axis cine images at end diastole from LV base (**a**) toward LV apex (**f**). For each slice, the thickest part is measured (mm) as well as the extent of hypertrophy indicated using a cut-off of 12 mm. The spiraling pattern of hypertrophy can be well appreciated on these images, following a counter-clockwise spiral when looking from LV apex

collagen deposition is accelerated in diseases as hypertension, aortic stenosis, cardiomyopathy hereby decreasing myocardial compliance and leading to dyspnea, diastolic dysfunction, heart failure, arrhythmia, and is associated with poor clinical outcomes (Moreo et al. 2009; Jellis et al. 2010). Similar to regional myocardial scarring, diffuse myocardial fibrosis alters gadolinium contrast kinetics causing shortening of myocardial T1 relaxation time. The latter is correlated with the myocardial collagen content. T1-mapping techniques to calculate post-contrast myocardial T1 have been recently proposed, and preliminary results have shown appealing results to depict diffuse myocardial fibrosis (Iles et al. 2008; Flett et al. 2010; Jellis et al. 2010). Basically, this is achieved using fast gradient-echo sequences with multiple increasing inversion times (50–1000 ms) performed at a fixed time point (e.g., 15 min) after contrast administration. Flett et al. (2010) proposed the use of a gadolinium infusion to achieve equilibrium contrast. These images are then processed with a curve fitting technique to generate T1 maps. The clinical value of these T1-mapping techniques needs further assessment. Finally, a free bonus of the late Gd imaging technique is that concomitant cardiac pathology, such as pericardial pathology or intracavitary thrombus formation, can be accurately depicted (Mollet et al. 2002; Bogaert et al. 2004; Bogaert and Francone 2009).

3 Cardiac or Ventricular Hypertrophy

The heart is capable of remodeling in response to environmental demands, a phenomenon called *cardiac plasticity*, and a variety of physiological and pathological stimuli can induce it to grow (*hypertrophy*) or to shrink (*atrophy*) (Hill and Olson 2007). Adaptive hypertrophy is usually associated with alternations in cardiac geometry (size and shape), myocardial mass, and function (Frey et al. 2004; Maron and Pelluccia

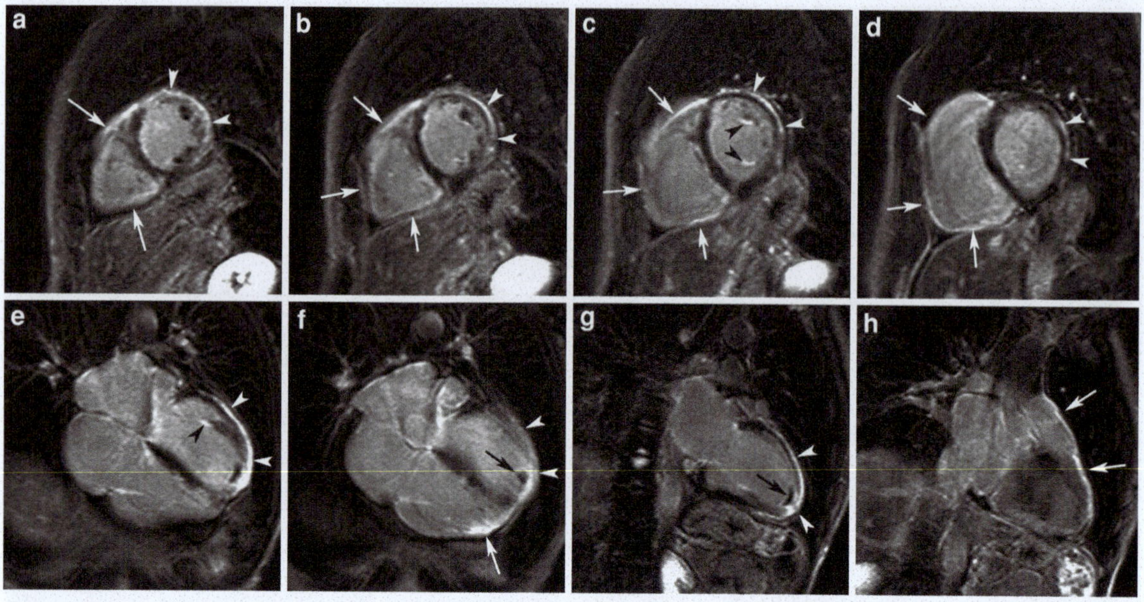

Fig. 5 Late Gd imaging in a 52-year-old man with dilated cardiomyopathy. Short-axis imaging (**a–d**), horizontal (**e–f**), and vertical (**g–h**) long-axis imaging. Diffuse and strong enhancement is found in the left (*arrowheads*, **a–g**) and right ventricle (*white arrows*, **a–d**, **f**, **h**). While the myocardial enhancement, representing myocardial fibrosis, in RV wall is transmural, in the LV the subepicardial part of the lateral wall and apex are involved. Note the presence of a small mural thrombus in LV apex (*black arrow*, **f–g**). The pattern of enhancement is typically non-ischemic

2006; Dorn 2007; Bluemke et al. 2008). It is characterized by an increase in the volume of myocytes ("intracellular remodeling") and concomitant changes in the extracellular matrix (i.e., the amount and physical properties of collagen). While tissue properties remain normal in physiological hypertrophy, they are altered in pathological hypertrophy leading to increased myocardial stiffness and diastolic dysfunction, and represent an important and independent risk factor for major cardiovascular complications, including heart failure and sudden cardiac death (SCD) (Maron 2003). Differentiation between cardiac hypertrophy and cardiomyopathies is often challenging. Ventricular hypertrophy is expressed by changes in total myocardial mass, and relative wall thickness (RWT) (wall thickness to chamber radius ratio). Because of its high accuracy and reproducibility for assessing ventricular size and shape three-dimensionally, MRI is increasingly used to study cardiac hypertrophy and to evaluate cardiac remodeling in large epidemiologic studies (Gatzka 2002; Heckbert et al. 2006; Meijs et al. 2007; Bluemke et al. 2008).

Regular and intensive physical training leads to physiological cardiac hypertrophy, the so-called "*athlete's heart*". In 1975, Morganroth et al. (1975) postulated that the type of cardiac morphological adaptation observed in athletes corresponded with the type of hemodynamic stimulus imposed on the ventricles during repeated exercise. Endurance training (e.g., long-distance running or cycling), as a consequence of prolonged repetitive volume overload, leads to an eccentric form of hypertrophy, principally characterized by increased ventricular chamber size with a proportional increase in wall thickness (increased wall mass, but unchanged RWT) (Pluim et al. 1999). The cardiac adaptation is typically "balanced", i.e., similar changes are found in left and right ventricles (Scharlag et al. 2002; Vogelsang et al. 2008) (Fig. 6). In contrast, strength (or resistance) training (e.g., weightlifting), as a consequence of pressure overload during strenuous resistive exercise predominantly develops a concentric form of hypertrophy with increased ventricular wall thickness, but unchanged cavity size (increased wall mass and increased ventricular RWT), underpinning the elevated ventricular mass. In a meta-analysis of cardiac structure and function in athlete's hearts, Pluim et al. found a geometric pattern more complicated than postulated by Morganroth et al. (Pluim et al. 1999).

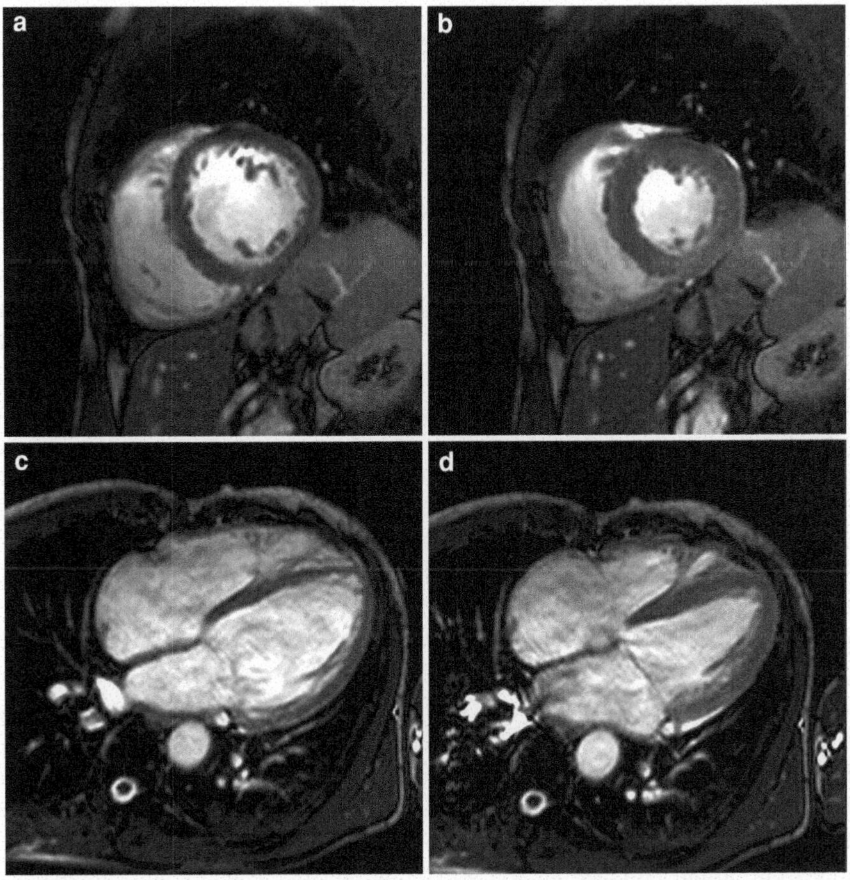

Fig. 6 Physiological cardiac hypertrophy in a triathlete. Cine imaging in short-axis (**a**, **b**) and horizontal long-axis (**c**, **d**), end-diastolic (**a**, **c**) and end-systolic (**b**, **d**) time frame. The ventricular remodeling is balanced, i.e., left ventricle: EDV_I: 129 ml/m^2, ESV_I: 70 ml/m^2, LV mass index 77 g/m^2, LV EF: 46%; right ventricle: EDV_I 142 ml/m^2, $RVESV_I$ 85 ml/m^2, RV EF: 40%. LV end-diastolic diameter: 62 mm, end-systolic diameter: 44 mm. LV septal wall thickness: 10 mm, lateral wall: 9 mm. The resting EF's are lower than to those obtained in untrained healthy volunteers. During exercise, the cardiac output is primarily increased by increase in stroke volume (and thus ejection fraction), less by increase in heart rate

In endurance-trained athletes, a significant increase in RWT was found, while strength-trained athletes showed an increase in LV diameter in addition to an increase in LV wall thickness. The combined endurance- and strength-trained athletes showed a significant increase in RWT and the highest increase in LV internal diameter. Although broadly adopted in scientific and medical literature, the "Morganroth hypothesis" is based on cross-sectional rather than longitudinal studies using relatively insensitive echocardiographic measurements to estimate ventricular remodeling. Longitudinal exercise training studies using appropriate techniques such as MRI are warranted to more accurately explore the relation between the type and intensity of training and cardiac adaptation (Naylor et al. 2008). Also, the process of normalizing (or scaling) cardiac size for between-subject differences in body size and composition is critical to correctly interpret cardiac hypertrophy and remodeling (Dewey et al. 2008). It might be that the increased LV mass observed in some athletes merely reflect a 'larger than normal' body size. An allometric (exponential) rather than a ratiometric (linear) may better indicate the normalcy of cardiovascular size and function for a given patient size (Bluemke et al. 2008; Dewey et al. 2008). Despite all these arguments, it is beyond doubt that training leads to enlargement of ventricular cavity size, and increase in wall thickness or LV mass (Naylor et al. 2008; Vogelsang et al. 2008). Physiological increases in wall thickness are mild, even in elite athletes. End-diastolic wall thicknesses usually do not exceed 13 mm in male, and 11 mm in female athletes. Values above 16 mm should be regarded as definitely abnormal (Belenkov et al. 1992; Maron et al. 1995). Diastolic indices in athletes are normal or slightly enhanced (i.e., increased E/A ratio). With the associated bradycardia, early diastolic filling is prolonged and the contribution of atrial contraction to ventricular filling reduced. Not only gender, but also race has a significant impact on cardiac adaptation to sport activities. Black athletes develop a greater magnitude of physiological hypertrophy (11.3 ± 1.6 mm; range 8–16 mm) than white athletes (10 ± 1.5 mm; range 7–14 mm), but the wall changes are matched with concomitant increase in LV volumes and they present normal diastolic indices (Basavarajaiah et al. 2008a).

Correct decision-making is crucial in trained athletes presenting with borderline increased LV wall thickness (>12 to <16 mm), as it may prevent SCD due to (unrecognized) HCM, which is the most common cause of exercise-related SCD in young athletes in the United States, or conversely reassure the athlete, enabling them to continue safely as competitors (Lauschke and Maisch 2008; Basavarajaiah et al. 2008b). Recent work has shown that the prevalence of HCM is extremely rare in highly trained athletes (none in 3,500 athletes) (Basavarajaiah et al. 2008b). In subjects presenting a "gray zone" LV wall thickness detraining for 12 weeks or alternatively genetic testing for HCM can be recommended. Since in athlete's heart the increase in wall thicknesses is balanced with an increase in LV cavity size, Petersen et al. proposed an MRI-derived end-diastolic wall thickness to LV volume ratio (mm × m^2 × ml) to differentiate between athlete's heart and pathological LV hypertrophy (i.e., HCM, aortic stenosis, hypertensive heart disease) (Petersen et al. 2005a). Using a receiver operating curve-determined cut-off value for diastolic wall-to-volume ratio of <0.15 mm/m^2/ml, athlete's hearts could be differentiated from all forms of pathological cardiac hypertrophy with 99% specificity and 80% sensitivity.

Pathological cardiac hypertrophy is found in a variety of cardiac diseases including cardiomyopathies, increased afterload (e.g., aortic or pulmonary stenosis, systemic or pulmonary arterial hypertension), increased preload (e.g., volume overload due to valvular regurgitation), and may occur as a compensatory mechanism following myocardial infarction. Similar to physiological hypertrophy, two basic patterns have been described, i.e., concentric hypertrophy with increased wall thickness and unchanged cavity dimensions, stroke volume and ejection fraction due to pressure overload (e.g., aortic stenosis or systemic arterial hypertension), and eccentric hypertrophy with no or minimal increase in wall thickness, increased LV chamber volume, stroke volume and reduced ejection fraction due to volume overload (e.g., aortic valve insufficiency) (Rudin et al. 1991) (Fig. 7). In clinical practice; however, the spectrum of geometric adaptations is more complex, and is most likely matched to systemic hemodynamics and ventricular load (Ganau et al. 1992). The majority of untreated patients with systemic arterial hypertension, for instance, have a normal LV mass and wall thickness, whilst the "typical" hypertensive concentric hypertrophy occurs in a minority of patients. Hypertensive patients may also present with asymmetric LV hypertrophy, characterized by a septal/posterior wall thickness ratio >1.5 at end-diastole (Cuspidi et al. 1997). The beneficial effects of this compensatory hypertrophic response to increased cardiac afterload, i.e., to reduce LV wall stress, are counteracted by several unwanted side-effects of the increase in LV mass, i.e., increase in myocardial oxygen consumption, reduced coronary reserve, increased cardiac fibrosis, propensity for cardiac failure due to systolic and diastolic dysfunction, and arrhythmogenesis, all contributing to an increased mortality (Frey et al. 2004). In the Multiethnic Study of Atherosclerosis (MESA), 5,098 participants underwent cardiac MRI and were followed up for a median of 4 years, body size-adjusted LV mass alone predicted incident heart failure, while concentric ventricular remodeling predicted incident stroke and coronary heart disease (Bluemke et al. 2008).

Cardiac MRI combined with MR angiography of the thoraco-abdominal aorta and renal arteries provides a comprehensive evaluation to study hypertensive patients, allowing to detect secondary causes of hypertension (e.g., aortic coarctation and renal artery stenosis) and to assess the impact on the heart (Maceira et al. 2008b). Late Gd imaging enables detection of areas of focal myocardial fibrosis, to visualize myocardial damage caused by microvascular abnormalities and concomitant coronary heart disease, while T1-mapping techniques are appealing to depict diffuse myocardial fibrosis (Fig. 7). In a small number of hypertensive patients, myocardial enhancement was reported in the septal and lateral LV wall, typically located in the midwall layers (Maceira et al. 2008a; Meijs et al. 2007). Moreover, MR spectroscopy showed an association between impairment in high-energy phosphate metabolism and diastolic dysfunction in hypertensive patients (Lamb et al. 1999). Ventricular torsion, measured by MRI tagging, was different in athletes (preserved torsion) and aortic stenosis patients with pathological cardiac hypertrophy (increased torsion, and prolonged apical untwisting) (Stuber et al. 1999). These observations contribute to a better understanding of pathophysiology of cardiac hypertrophy, such as diastolic dysfunction in pressure-overloaded hearts.

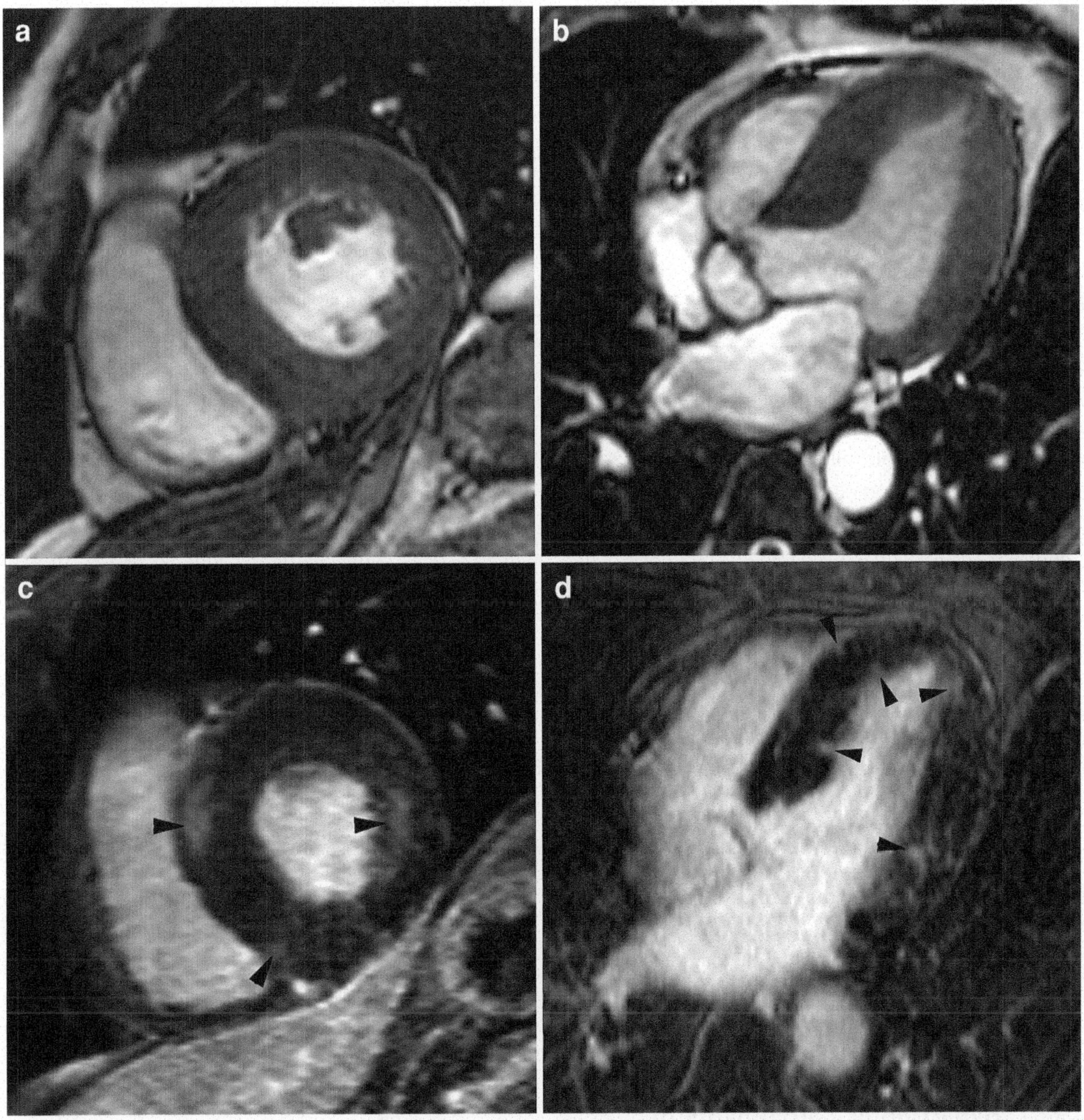

Fig. 7 Severe pathological concentric LV hypertrophy in a 56-year-old male with a long-standing calcified aortic stenosis, and a gradient over the stenotic valve of 125 mm Hg (measured by PC-MRI). Cine imaging in short-axis (**a**) and horizontal long-axis (**b**) (end-diastolic time frame). Late Gd imaging in short-axis (**c**), and horizontal long-axis (**d**). Although the hypertrophy is concentric and severe (LV wall mass: 270 gram), the hypertrophy is most pronounced in the ventricular septum (end-diastolic wall thickness of 25 mm). On late Gd imaging multiple areas of focal myocardial enhancement are shown throughout the myocardium (*arrowheads*, **c**, **d**). Although the precise nature of this focal enhancement is unknown, it may represent small micro-infarctions (ischemia-related or emboligenic) and/or areas of macroscopic replacement fibrosis

In summary, cardiac MRI should be considered a key imaging modality to study the patterns of geometric and tissue remodeling in physiological and pathological cardiac hypertrophy. Right and LV ventricular volumes, mass, and function can be assessed with a higher accuracy and reproducibility than with echocardiography, enabling sample size to be reduced in studies that need to assess ventricular volumes, mass, and function (Bellenger et al. 2000). Moreover, the degree of adverse myocardial tissue remodeling can be depicted using contrast-enhanced MRI techniques.

4 Primary Cardiomyopathies

Cardiomyopathies, a term introduced by Harvey and Brigden more than half a century ago, represent a heterogeneous group of heart diseases characterized by direct involvement of the myocardium in conjunction with cardiac dysfunction (Brigden et al. 1957; Harvey et al. 1964). The identification of novel entities, the improvement of molecular genetics and the recent emerging of channelopathies have led to the development of a new classification (Maron et al. 2006a; Charron et al. 2010; Watkins et al. 2011). *Primary cardiomyopathies*, which are exclusively or predominantly confined to the heart muscle, are categorized as genetic, acquired, or mixed, whereas *secondary cardiomyopathies* are characterized in the context of systemic disorders. Despite the increasing awareness of these pathologies and the efforts of cardiovascular research towards a better depiction, the correct diagnosis may be challenging and sometimes elusive. This difficulty may have critical consequences on patient management and treatment. The development of cardiac imaging has facilitated the diagnosis and classification of cardiomyopathies. Although transthoracic echocardiography still represents the imaging modality of choice, MRI has emerged as an important technique in the diagnosis and characterization of cardiomyopathies.

4.1 Hypertrophic Cardiomyopathy

The characteristic finding of HCM is an inappropriate myocardial hypertrophy in the absence of an obvious cause for the hypertrophy, such as systemic hypertension or aortic stenosis (Maron et al. 2006a). HCM is the most common inherited cardiomyopathy with an estimated prevalence of 0.2%, and is caused by mutations in one of the genes encoding sarcomeric proteins (Charron et al. 2010; Watkins et al. 2011). Familial clustering is often observed, and the disease is genetically transmitted in about 60% of individuals with HCM (Crilley et al. 2003; Keren et al. 2008). The natural history and clinical presentation of HCM are highly variable. Symptoms are caused by intraventricular obstruction usually of the left ventricular outflow tract (LVOT), myocardial ischemia, diastolic dysfunction, heart failure, and ventricular arrhythmias. Although patients might be completely asymptomatic, HCM is the most commonly identified cause of premature SCD due to ventricular arrhythmias in young individuals and apparently healthy athletes (Maron et al. 2003b; Keren et al. 2008). Histologically, HCM is characterized by a disorganization and malalignment of the myofibrils, i.e., *myofibrillar disarray*, and various patterns of myocardial fibrosis. Though myofibrillar disarray is not unique to HCM, it is clearly more extensive in HCM than in secondary myocardial hypertrophy from pressure overload or congenital heart disorders (Bulkley et al. 1977; Maron et al. 1981). Besides, accumulating data supports that abnormalities in HCM are not limited to the myocardium but structurally may involve other parts of the heart such as the mitral valve apparatus (Maron et al. 2011). MRI has emerged as a prime player not only in assessing HCM patients but moreover yields promise in the preclinical diagnosis as well as in screening the relatives of known HCM patients (Crilley et al. 2003; Nagueh and Mahmarian 2006).

With the current arsenal of MRI sequences, a comprehensive assessment is achievable, including assessment of the phenotypic expression, cardiac systolic and diastolic function, hemodynamic obstruction and mitral regurgitation, myocardial perfusion, myocardial tissue characterization, and post-treatment evaluation: this technique has shown of great value in the differential diagnosis with other forms of benign and malignant myocardial hypertrophy (Fig. 8).

4.1.1 Phenotypic Expression

Mutations in the genes encoding sarcomeric proteins may lead to a wide spectrum of phenotypic expressions including not only HCM but also dilated, restrictive, and non-compaction cardiomyopathy, emphasizing the crucial role of cardiac imaging in the assessment of the phenotypic expression in inherited heart muscle disorders (Hoedemakers et al. 2007; Watkins et al. 2011). MRI provides routinely high-resolution morphologic images with excellent delineation of endo- and epicardial myocardial borders encompassing the entire heart enabling detailed 3D assessment of the phenotypic expression, to measure

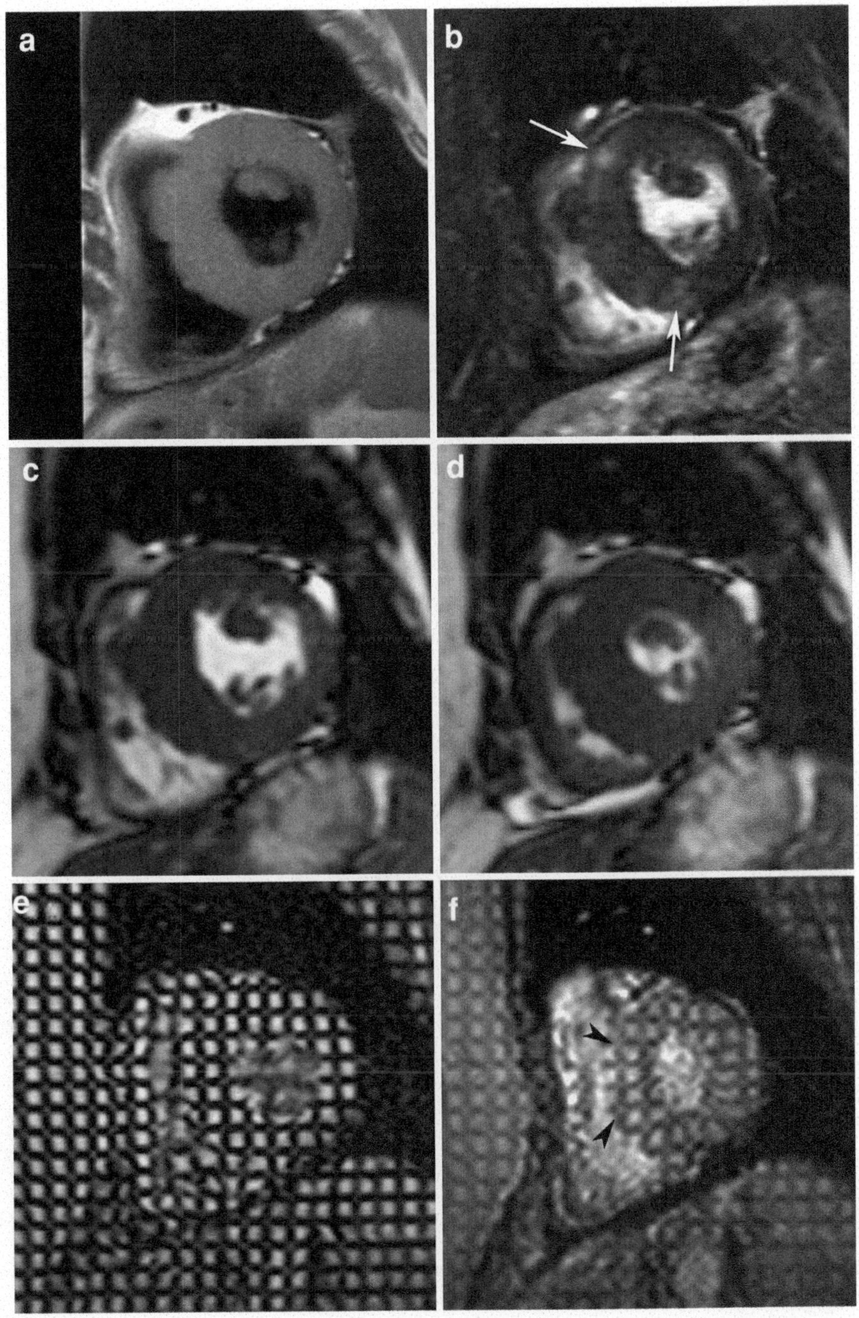

Fig. 8 Comprehensive MRI in a 57-year-old woman with severe form of obstructive hypertrophic cardiomyopathy. T1w-imaging (**a**), late Gd imaging (**b**), cine imaging at end diastole (**c**) and end systole (**d**), and SPAMM myocardial tagging at end diastole (**e**) and end systole (**f**). This approach allows for evaluation of the presence, location and extent of hypertrophy, and for assessment of myocardial wall motion and deformation pattern. Late Gd imaging enables depiction of the areas of increased signal intensity in the thickened regions, reflecting myocardial fibrosis (*arrows*, **b**). Decreased systolic deformation in the thickened regions visible by SPAMM imaging (*arrowheads*, **f**)

myocardial mass and to quantify segmental wall thickness; also in areas that are difficult to assess by echocardiography, such as the anterolateral free wall, apex, and RV free wall (Rickers et al. 2005; Maron et al. 2007; Maron et al. 2009) (Figs. 3 and 9).

The typical phenotypic expression is that of a hypertrophied, non-dilated left ventricle. The distribution of the hypertrophy is often asymmetrical, segmental, or confined to relatively small regions of the LV chamber (Klues et al. 1995) (Fig. 10). In 70% of patients, the anterior portion of the ventricular septum and the anterior LV wall are involved (Fig. 11). Abnormalities are usually most prominent in the basal segments (Maron et al. 2009). Less frequent locations

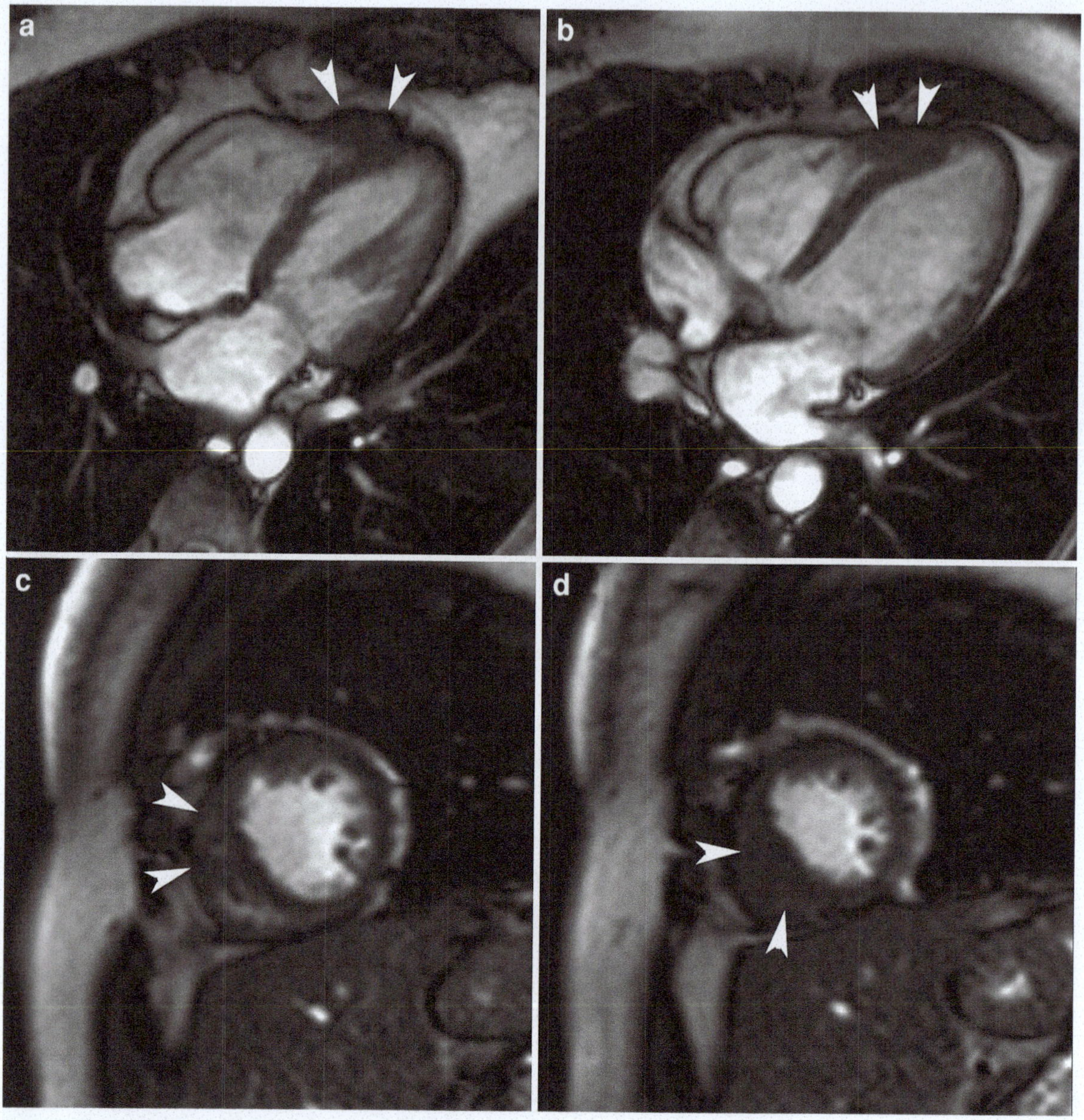

Fig. 9 Focal form of hypertrophic cardiomyopathy in a 47-year-old woman with familial history of hypertrophic cardiomyopathy. Cine imaging in horizontal long-axis (**a**, **b**) and short-axis (**c**, **d**), showing end-diastolic (**a**, **c**) and end-systolic (**b**, **d**) time frames. The focal thickening of the apical RV free wall extending to the apical part of the ventricular septum can be well appreciated on MRI (*arrowheads*)

of myocardial hypertrophy include: the mid- and lower portion of the ventricular septum often extending to the inferior wall, the anterolateral wall, and the apex (Fig. 12). HCM may present in about 5% of patients as severe concentric LV hypertrophy. In a recent analysis of the spatial 3D spread of hypertrophy, we found that the majority of patients with so-called asymmetrical septal HCM follows a spiral pattern of hypertrophy in longitudinal direction following a counter-clockwise spiral, when viewed from LV apex (unpublished data) (Fig. 13). The magnitude of spiraling; however, was largely variable.

Concomitant abnormalities in morphology and function of the papillary muscles are often present.

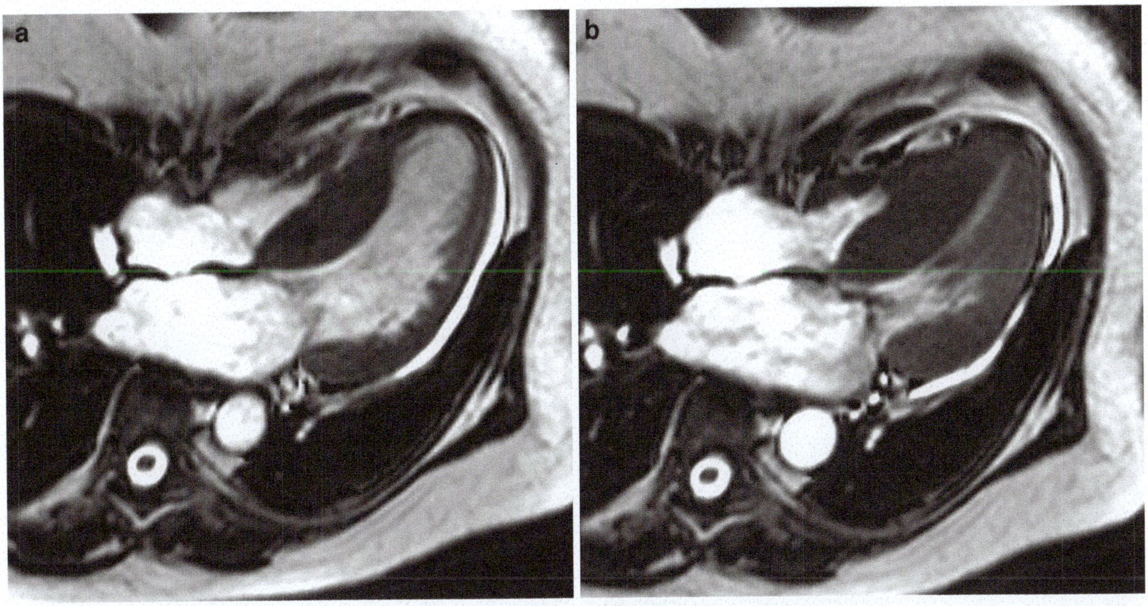

Fig. 10 Asymmetrical septal HCM in a 57-year-old patient (same patient as in Fig 8). Cine imaging at end diastole (**a**) and end systole (**b**) in horizontal long-axis plane. The thickened appearance of the basal and mid-portion of the ventricular septum can be well appreciated on this horizontal long-axis view

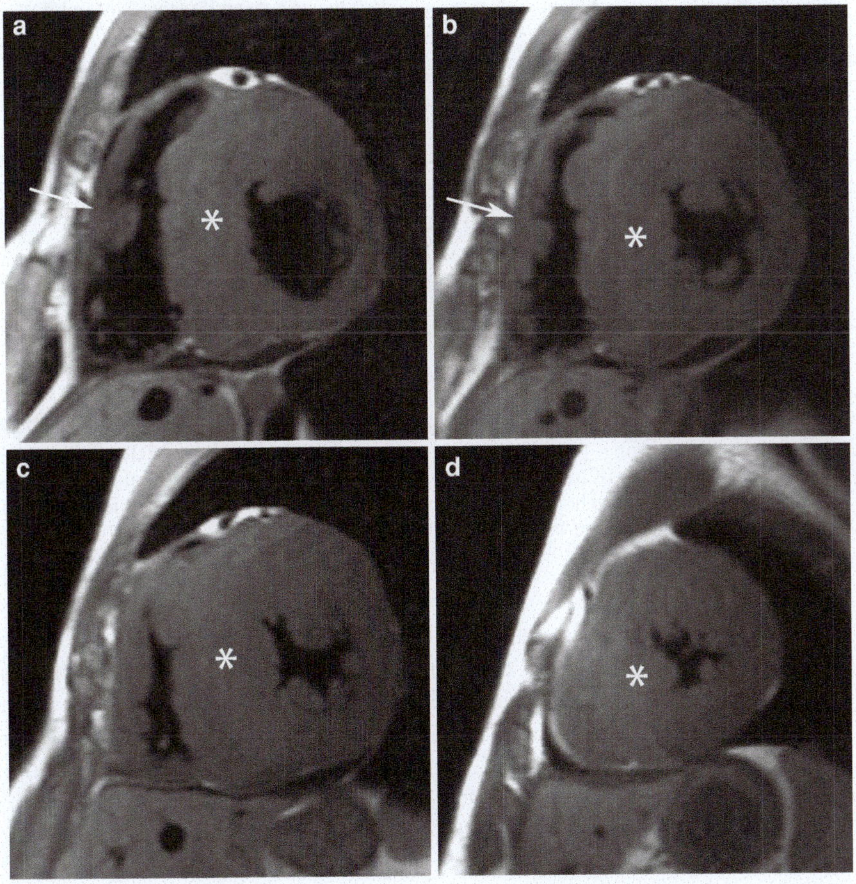

Fig. 11 Extreme form of hypertrophic, obstructive cardiomyopathy in a young male teenager. T1w-imaging in cardiac short-axis (**a–d**). The spread of the myocardial hypertrophy (*) can be well appreciated. The ventricular septum, and adjacent anterior and inferior wall are extensively thickened with end-diastolic wall thicknesses exceeding 50 mm ("asymmetrical septal" form). The total LV mass exceeds 500 g. Note the concomitant hypertrophy of the RV free wall (*arrow*), and the presence of a small pericardial effusion

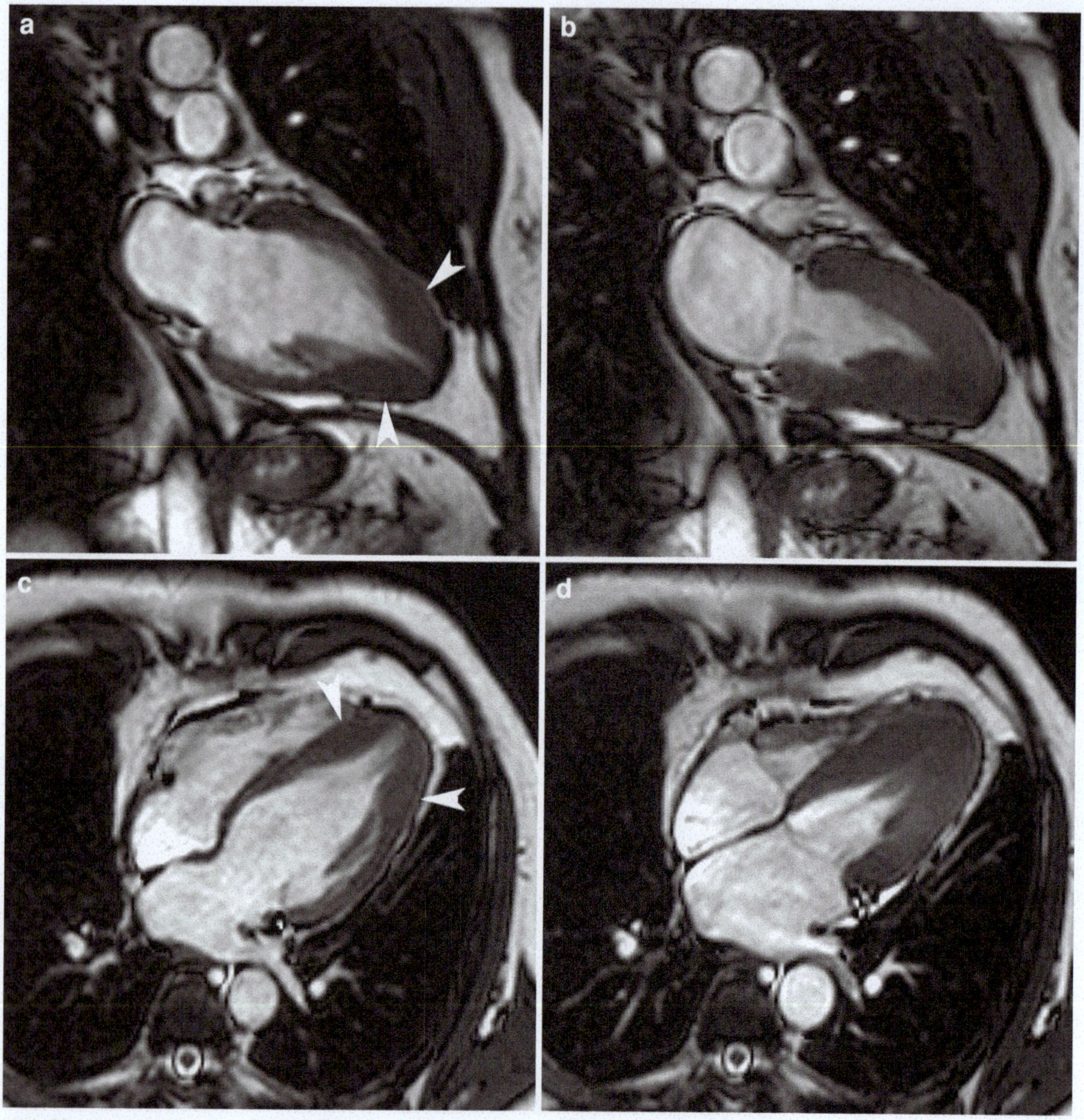

Fig. 12 Apical form of HCM in a 54-year-old man. Cine imaging in vertical (**a**, **b**) and horizontal long-axis plane (**c**, **d**), end-diastolic (**a**, **c**), and end-systolic (**b**, **d**) time frames. Circumferential thickening of the LV apex with maximal end-diastolic wall thickness of 21 mm

Morphologic abnormalities include hypertrophy, variation in appearance (e.g., bifid papillary muscle) and number of papillary muscles, and abnormal enhancement on late Gd MRI. Increased anteroapical displacement of the anterolateral papillary muscle may contribute to the severity of LVOT obstruction (Harrigan et al. 2008; Kwon et al. 2008). Of note is that the RV is also frequently involved, supporting the hypothesis that HCM represents a myocardial affliction potentially affecting both ventricles (Maron et al. 2007) (Figs. 8 and 9). A minority of patients (5–10%) with HCM show progressive adverse ventricular remodeling that eventually may lead to an 'end-stage' dilated HCM (Thaman et al. 2004; Harris et al. 2006; Keren et al. 2008).

Though the pattern of remodeling is heterogeneous including impaired LV contractility, cavitary dilatation, and wall thinning of the thickened segments,

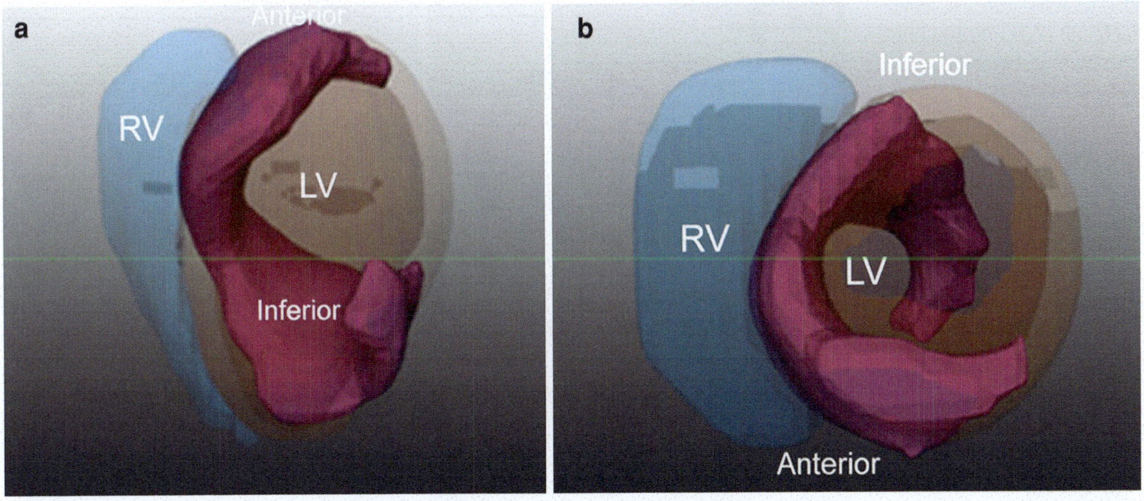

Fig. 13 Spiral nature of HCM. Virtually-rendered 3D data, viewed from the side (**a**), and from a longitudinal perspective (**b**). The hypertrophied myocardium is shown in pink, starting anterobasally and moving in a counter clock-wise spiral toward the LV apex (viewed from the LV apex)

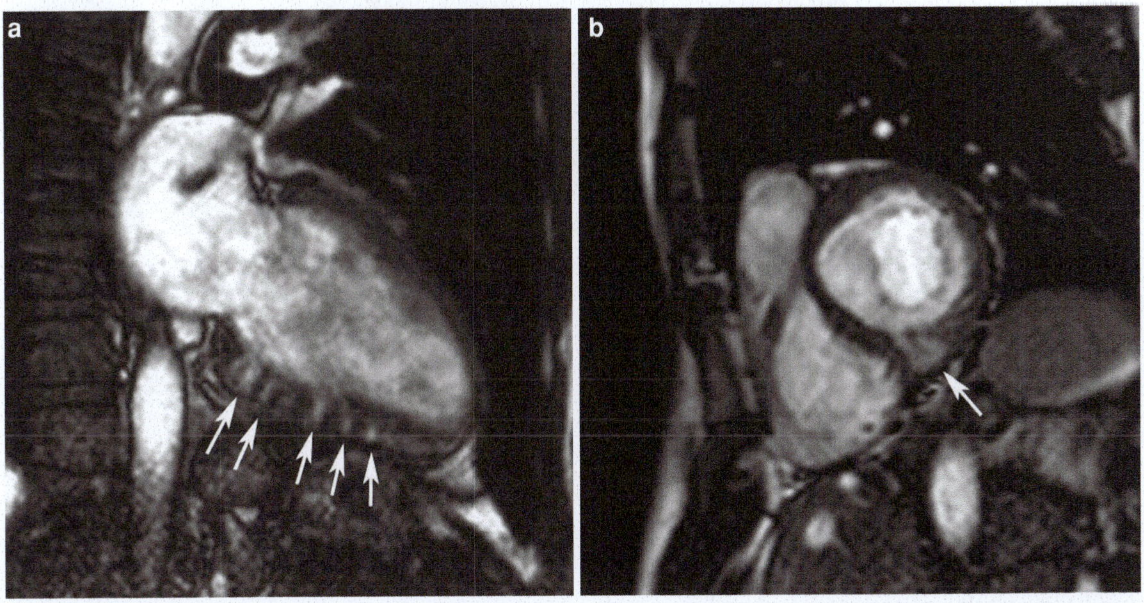

Fig. 14 Deep muscular clefts in inferoseptal LV wall in a 47-year-old man presenting with severe sensorimotoric polyneuropathy and histologic evidence of skeletal myopathy. Cine imaging in vertical (**a**) and horizontal long-axis (**b**) show multiple deep muscular cleft in the inferoseptal LV wall (*arrows*)

timely recognition is important to prevent heart failure and SCD. Deep muscular clefts in the basal LV inferoseptal wall have been reported in HCM mutation carriers who have not yet developed myocardial hypertrophy, but because this type of cleft may be found in normal volunteers and other cardiac diseases, it is currently unclear whether this belongs to the phenotypic expression of HCM (Fig. 14) (Germans et al. 2006; Johansson et al. 2007).

HCM is considered when the wall thickness exceeds 15 mm. In some cases the increase in wall thickness may be extreme. Borderline increases in

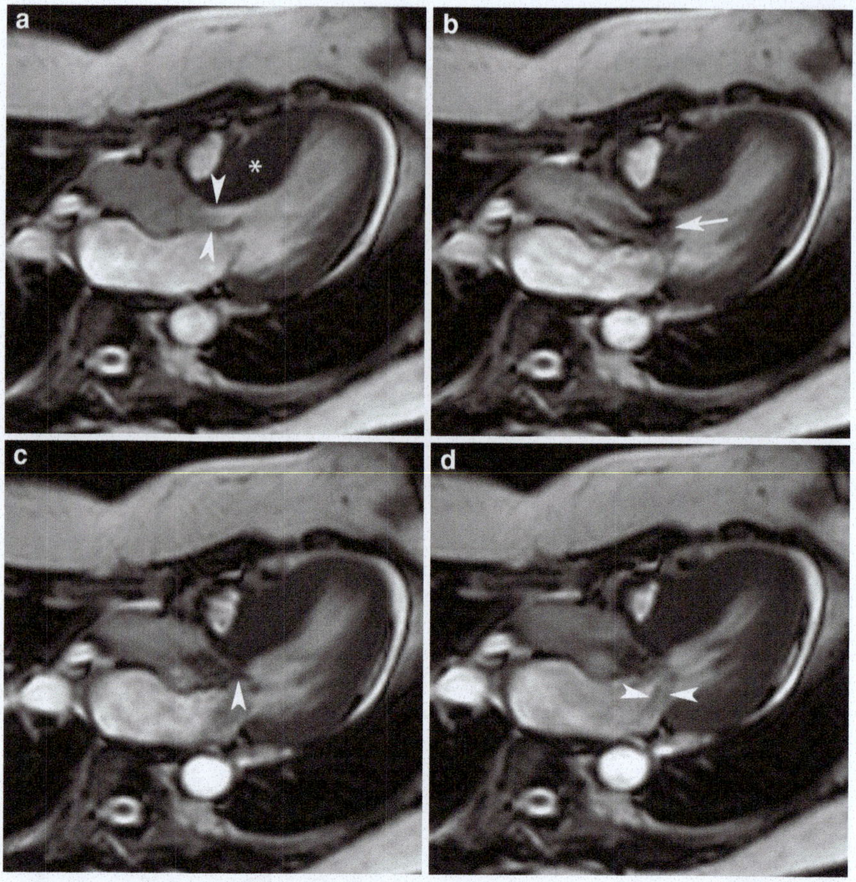

Fig. 15 Asymmetrical septal HCM with LVOT obstruction. Thickening of the basal ventricular septum (24 mm)(*, **a**) with narrowing of the LVOT (*arrowheads*, **b**). Flow acceleration during onset of cardiac systole visible of signal void jet (*arrow*, **b**). Subsequent systolic anterior motion (SAM) of the anterior mitral valve leaflet (*arrowhead*, **c**) that comes in contact with the thickened septum. As a consequence, mitral regurgitation occurs because of non-closure of the leaflets

wall thickness (i.e., 12–15 mm) are more difficult to interpret, especially in athletes who may present with physiological hypertrophy, in patients with concomitant diseases such as arterial hypertension, or in parts of the left ventricle that in normal conditions have a thinner wall such as the LV apex. Whereas the diagnosis of HCM is usually straightforward in asymmetrical septal forms, concentric forms of HCM are more difficult to diagnose because a variety of other heart muscle diseases and myocardial remodeling related to no heart muscle disorders may present in a similar way.

The less common apical form of HCM, a non-obstructive variant, typically presents with T wave inversion in the anterolateral leads on electrocardiogram, and has a high prevalence in Japan (Abelmann and Lorell 1989) (Fig. 12). Because of near-field problems of the echo probe, apical HCM is often difficult to assess by echocardiography, and MRI should be considered the preferred imaging technique (Casolo et al. 1989; Moon et al. 2004a). Three different types have been described: (a) true apical form with a spadelike configuration, (b) involvement of the apex and symmetric hypertrophy of the four ventricular wall segments, and (c) involvement of the apex with asymmetric involvement of the wall segments, i.e., non-spade apical form (Suzuki et al. 1993; Soler et al. 1997).

Another form of HCM is mid-ventricular hypertrophy. These patients may present with a gradient between the LV apical region and the remainder of the chamber. This may progress to a non-contractile apical aneurysm (about 2% of HCM patients) eventually with apical thrombus formation (Abelmann and Lorell 1989; Maron et al. 2008a). Typically the aneurysms show a strong enhancement on late Gd imaging, suggestive of extensive myocardial scarring. For correct appraisal of myocardial wall thicknesses, measurements should be performed perpendicular through the myocardial wall using the end-diastolic cine MR images. We recommend a set of short-axis cine MR images completely encompassing the

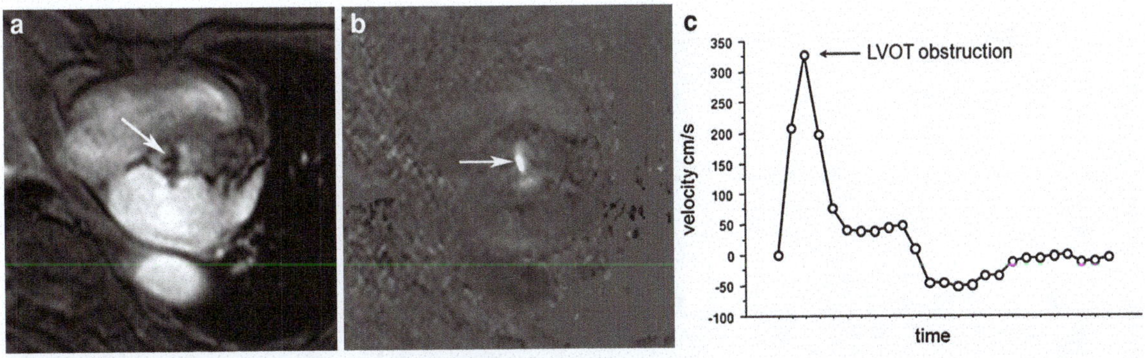

Fig. 16 Assessment of hemodynamic compromise in LVOT by PC-MRI (same patient as Fig. 15). Magnitude (**a**) and phase (**b**) image of PC-MRI, and corresponding flow curve (**c**). Severe flow acceleration in LVOT starting in early systole visible as a small high-signal intensity zone (*arrow*, **b**). Complete obstruction of the LVOT occurring 125 ms after onset of systole with cessation of the forward flow during the remainder of the cardiac cycle. The peak velocity at the moment of obstruction was 3.25 m/s corresponding to a gradient of 42 mm Hg

ventricles, in combination with vertical and horizontal long-axis views. The latter need to be perfectly positioned for correct judgment of wall dimensions particular in apical HCM. Additional views are needed to study the LVOT (see below). It is important to emphasize that it is a misconception to take LV mass index as requirement for establishing the clinical diagnosis of HCM (Olivotto et al. 2008), as about 20% of patients with a definite HCM phenotype present with a normal LV mass index by MRI, correlating only weakly with maximal wall thickness.

In a recent paper by Maron et al. (2011), it was nicely shown using MRI that the mitral valve apparatus is frequently phenotypically involved, even in gene carriers without phenotypic expression of HCM. Abnormalities typically consist in elongation of the anterior (26 ± 5 mm vs. 19 ± 5 mm in control subjects, $P < 0.001$), the posterior (14 ± 4 mm vs. 10 ± 3 mm in control subjects, $P < 0.01$), or both mitral valve leaflets. Moreover, elongated mitral valve leaflets are important determinants of LVOT obstruction (see below), in particular in patients in whom anterior mitral leaflet length exceeds twofold the transverse dimension of the outflow tract.

4.1.2 Hemodynamic Compromise

A crucial step in the diagnosis of HCM patients is the evaluation of hemodynamic compromise, which is confined in about 25% of patients to the level of the LVOT, less commonly to the mid-ventricular level. Myocardial hypertrophy causing focal narrowing of the ventricular lumen may lead to altered flow dynamics with flow acceleration, concomitant pressure drop, and the presence of an intraventricular gradient between the distal and proximal chamber (Fig. 15). This typically occurs during systole and ranges from mild degrees of flow impairment to complete flow obstruction (Fig. 16). A gradient $\geq$50 mm Hg is considered obstructive. The obstruction may be present at rest ('resting obstructive HCM') or may be provoked by exercise, the Valsalva maneuver, or administration of amyl nitrite ('latent obstructive HCM'). LVOT obstruction is related with dyspnea and syncope, predisposes to atrial enlargement due to concomitant mitral regurgitation and the development of atrial arrhythmias, and is associated with increased risk of death, while mid-ventricular forms are associated with apical aneurysm formation. Recently, Maron et al. mentioned that HCM is predominantly a disease of LVOT obstruction, reporting the need to study the heart during exercise in patients with no or small subaortic gradient at rest (Maron et al. 2006b). Of the 63% of patients belonging to the latter group, more than half of them developed a gradient >50 mm Hg during exercise, and the exercise-induced obstruction could largely account for the symptoms of heart failure. As mentioned above, elongated anterior mitral leaflets contribute to the severity of hemodynamic compromise (Maron et al. 2011). In HCM patients with mid-ventricular obstruction (>30 mm Hg), the latter is an independent predictor of adverse outcome (i.e., SCD and potentially lethal arrhythmic events), and is frequently related with the formation of an apical LV aneurysm (Minami et al. 2011).

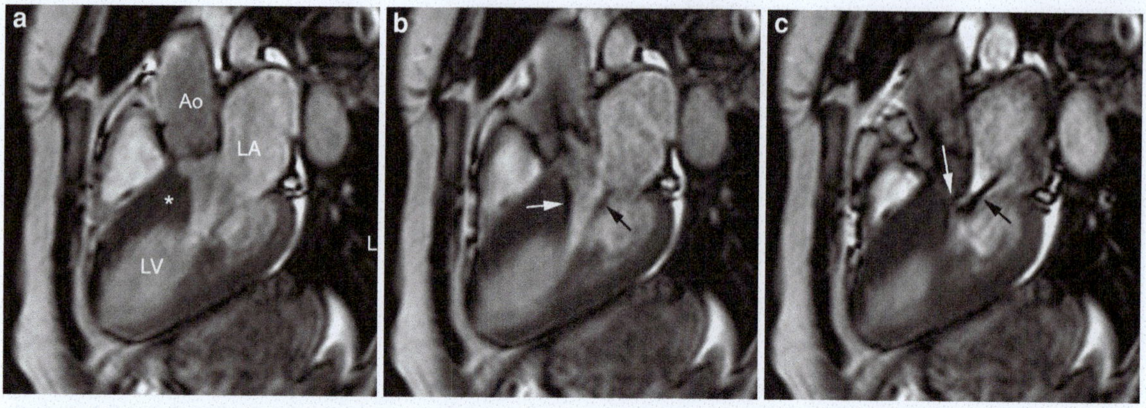

Fig. 17 "Venturi"-effect in hypertrophic (obstructive) cardiomyopathy. Cine imaging at end diastole (**a**), early systole (**b**), and mid systole (**c**). Important thickening of the basal ventricular septum (*), causing LVOT narrowing. LV contraction leads to flow acceleration in the narrowed LVOT, visible as an area of signal void (*arrow*, **b**). The subsequent pressure drops cause SAM, leading to mitral regurgitation (*black arrow*, **c**) and left atrial enlargement

Use of MRI in depicting LVOT (sub)-obstruction is targeted on: (a) depiction and quantification of flow acceleration with measurement of peak velocities, (b) measurement of LVOT area, and (c) visualization and quantification of the presence and severity of mitral regurgitation. The LVOT in HCM patients can be best studied starting with a series of parallel cine MR images along the LV inflow-outflow tract view ('three-chamber view') (see "Cardiovascular MR Imaging Planes and Segmentation"). Flow acceleration and turbulence cause signal void during systole (Park et al. 1992), which is usually most pronounced over the thickened part of the basal ventricular septum. Moreover, the LV inflow-outflow tract view enables evaluation of the presence and severity of associated systolic anterior motion (SAM) of the anterior mitral valve leaflet. This is caused by the pressure drop in the narrowed LVOT causing an anterior suction of the leaflet with eventual apposition to the thickened septum causing a partial or complete outflow obstruction (the so-called "Venturi effect") (Fig. 17). A direct consequence of SAM is the presence of a moderate to severe mitral regurgitation, usually occurring during mid to late systole with secondary left atrial enlargement, which is usually well depicted in the LV inflow-outflow tract view. SAM produces greater mitral regurgitation if the posterior leaflet is limited in its ability to move anteriorly, participate in SAM, and coapt effectively. To quantify the peak velocity and thus to calculate the gradient between the LV cavity and remainder of the LVOT, PC-MRI is used with the image plane positioned perpendicular through the LVOT where the signal void is best visible. To avoid aliasing the VENC should be adjusted to the expected peak velocities (see "valvular heart disease"). The same sequence can be used to measure the severity of mitral regurgitation. Because the regurgitant jet is often excentrically located, one should be careful to correctly position the slice of interest. A combination of vertical and horizontal long-axis views enables to evaluate the degree of left atrial enlargement. Finally, the LVOT area and area changes during the cardiac cycle can be quantified using planemetry from a series of cine MRI sequences obtained perpendicular through the LVOT. An outflow tract area smaller than 2.7 cm^2 in systole by MRI yielded a 100% sensitivity and specificity by MRI to differentiate obstructive (including latent forms) from non-obstructive HCM (Schulz-Menger et al. 2006).

4.1.3 Cardiac Function

Diastolic and systolic dysfunction is common in patients with HCM. Abnormalities in diastolic function characterized by restrictive filling are related to increased chamber stiffness and impaired ventricular relaxation (Steward et al. 1968). At present, diastolic dysfunction is thought to be one of the major pathophysiological mechanisms in HCM, frequently leading to diastolic heart failure and adverse prognosis. Diastolic dysfunction can occur either without important hypertrophy, the so-called '*restrictive phenotype*' of HCM, or earlier than systolic dysfunction in the course of the typical HCM phenotype.

This restrictive phenotype is an uncommon presentation, but is associated with poor prognosis (Kubo et al. 2007). Although echocardiography with Doppler flow and tissue imaging is still the preferred imaging modality to assess diastolic function and to depict subtle changes in LV relaxation, PC-MRI can be used to assess mitral inflow patterns as well as pulmonary venous flow patterns for evaluating presence of a restrictive physiology (see "Cardiac Function"). Myocardial tagging techniques can be applied to assess ventricular untwisting during isovolemic relaxation as parameter of ventricular relaxation, but the time-consuming post-processing hampers integration in routine clinical imaging.

The impact of myocardial hypertrophy on global and regional systolic function can be precisely assessed with cine MRI. HCM patients typically present with normal or decreased ventricular cavities, usually presenting with high-ejection fractions and low end-systolic values. In patients with severe HCM, especially at mid-ventricular and apical level, near-complete compression of the ventricular cavity may occur during cardiac contraction. Remarkably, this increased global functionality is achieved with a markedly reduced contractility within the thickened myocardial segments, which is due to muscle disorganization (Maron et al. 1987; Arrivé et al. 1994; Bogaert et al. 2003; Aletras et al. 2011).

MRI strain imaging techniques, such as myocardial tagging and displacement encoding with stimulated echoes (DENSE), have been useful in providing insight into the myocardial strain characteristics in HCM patients (Maier et al. 1992; Young et al. 1994; Kramer et al. 1994; Dong et al. 1994; Aletras et al. 2011). Systolic strains, i.e., circumferential and longitudinal shortening as well as wall thickening, are invariably reduced in the hypertrophied myocardium and the severity is inversely related to the magnitude of hypertrophy (Figs. 8, 9 and 10). On the other hand, ventricular torsion is significantly increased in HCM patients, partially explaining why ventricular ejection performance may be normal while segmental myocardial function is distinctly abnormal.

4.1.4 Myocardial Ischemia

While ventricular fibrillation is the principal cause of SCD in HCM patients (Spirito et al. 1997), the final mechanism triggering cardiac arrest is, as yet, incompletely clarified. However, our knowledge by which LV hypertrophy relates to higher risk for malignant ventricular arrhythmias and SCD has definitely benefited from novel imaging modalities, in particular cardiac MRI. The risk of SCD is related to the magnitude, rather than the distribution of LV hypertrophy (Maron et al. 2003a, b). Myocardial ischemia seems an important player in the pathogenesis of ventricular arrhythmias. Autopsy findings have shown presence of myocardial ischemic damage, either acute or subacute or in the form of fibrotic scars in young HCM patients with SCD (Basso et al. 2000). This can be attributed to a reduced capillary density caused by hypertrophy and to dysplasia of the small intramural coronary arterioles caused by pressure necrosis due to extravascular compression contributing to a phenomenon of microvascular dysfunction (Knaapen et al. 2008; Kwon et al. 2009). This causes a blunted vasodilator response in HCM patients, indicative of microvascular dysfunction, particularly in the endocardium, and in proportion to the magnitude of hypertrophy (Kawada et al. 1999; Varnava et al. 2000; Petersen et al. 2007; Sotgia et al. 2008). Microvascular dysfunction and subsequent myocardial ischemia are considered a potentially important pathway toward myocardial replacement fibrosis.

4.1.5 Myocardial Fibrosis

Myocardial fibrosis is a hallmark of HCM and a proposed substrate for arrhythmias and heart failure. It is usually interpreted as a secondary response to long-standing disease, including ischemia, microvascular dysfunction, and obstruction. However, recent observations have challenged this interpretation showing that the stimulus for myocardial fibrosis is an early manifestation of sarcomere-gene mutations that may be present before occurrence of cardiac morphological features of HCM (Ho et al. 2010). Myocardial fibrosis is present in the majority of patients with overt HCM, and corresponds with impairment in myocardial energy metabolism, and correlates with the severity of ventricular remodeling and dysfunction (Bogaert et al. 2003; Debl et al. 2006; Esposito et al. 2008; Rudolf et al. 2009). Use of late Gd imaging has become a well-accepted technique to depict focal myocardial fibrosis correlating well with the autopsy findings (Choudbury et al. 2002; Moon et al. 2004b).

Myocardial fibrosis typically occurs only in hypertrophied regions, with multiple patchy foci

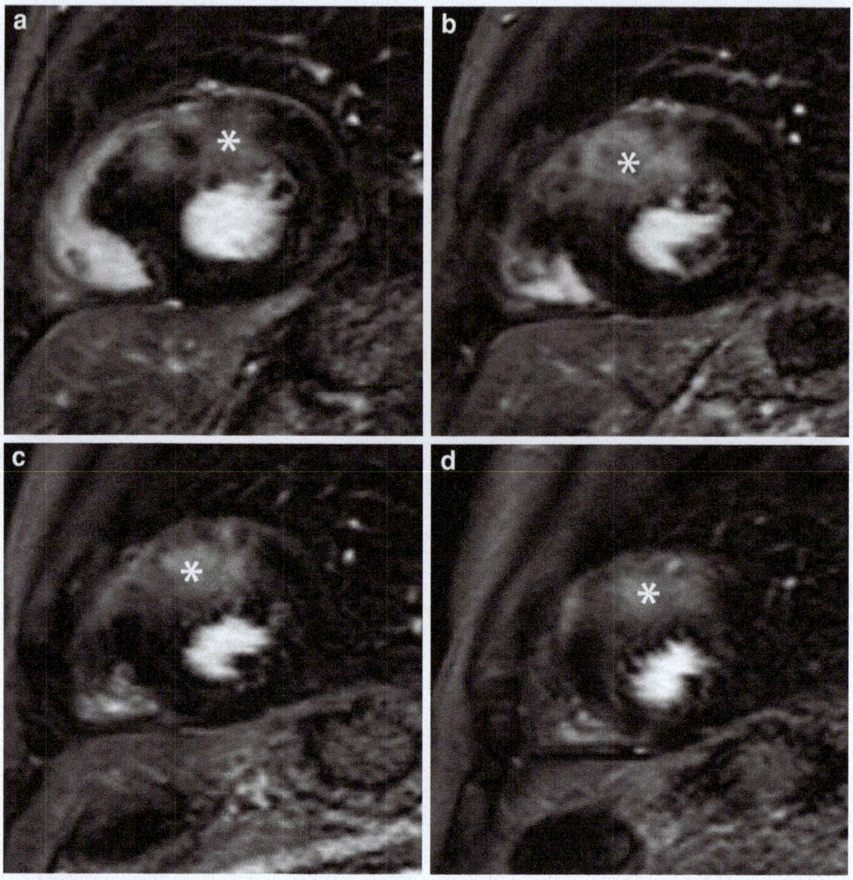

Fig. 18 Typical enhancement pattern in HCM. Late Gd imaging in four short-axis levels. Irregularly defined inhomogeneous 'cloudy' enhancement (*) in the thickened myocardium

predominantly involved in the mid-ventricular wall, junctions of the interventricular septum and the right ventricular free wall (Choudbury et al. 2002) (Fig. 18). The location of scarring is related (but not exclusively) to decreased regional systolic wall thickening (Aletras et al. 2011) (Fig. 19), which does not correspond to the perfusion territories of the epicardial coronary arteries (Fig. 20). There is an increasing body of evidence that the presence and extent of myocardial fibrosis, visualized by late Gd imaging, in patients with HCM, is an independent predictor of adverse outcome, i.e., SCD, sustained ventricular tachycardia or fibrillation, and heart failure (Fig. 21) (Varnava et al. 2001; Moon et al. 2003a; Suk et al. 2008; Leonardi et al. 2009; Rubinshtein et al. 2010; O'Hanlon et al. 2010). Also in patients with no, or minimal symptoms, late Gd imaging adds prognostic value to conventional criteria for risk stratification (Miller et al. 2007; Adabag et al. 2008). Moreover, myocardial enhancement is related not only to an increased risk for SCD, but also to the presence of progressive disease and prediction of systolic and diastolic dysfunction (Maron et al. 2008b; Motoyasu et al. 2008; Moreo et al. 2009; Olivotto et al. 2010; Bruder et al. 2010).

Extensive myocardial scarring is invariably associated with end-stage dilated HCM (Harris et al. 2006; Melacini et al. 2010), and is more extensive than in patients with dilated cardiomyopathy (DCM) (Matoh et al. 2007). To achieve a reliable estimate of the extent of myocardial enhancement, Harrigan et al. proposed a semi-automated tresholding of six (or more) SDs above the mean signal intensity of visual normal remote myocardium to define myocardial enhancement in HCM patients (Harrigan et al. 2011).

4.1.6 Evaluation of Post Treatment

The effects of medical treatment (either β-blocker or Verapamil) on symptomatic LVOT obstruction can be accurately accessed by MRI, which can identify patients with refractory LVOT increased gradient that need addition of other drugs like disopyr-

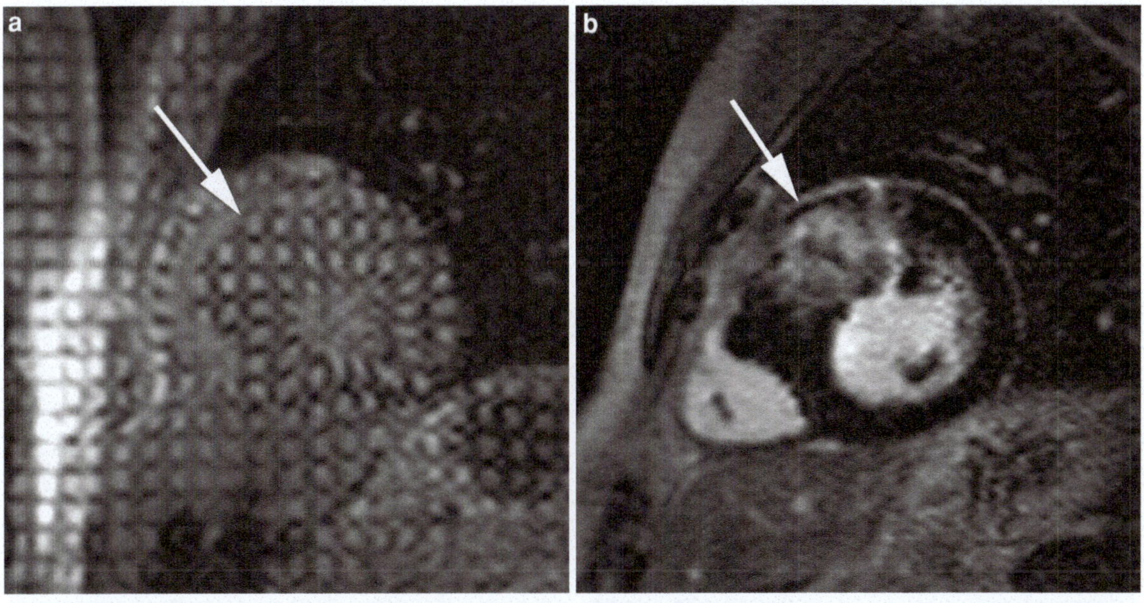

Fig. 19 Relation between myocardial deformation and myocardial scarring in HCM. Short-axis SPAMM myocardial tagging (mid-systolic time frame) (**a**) and late Gd imaging (**b**). Diffuse inhomogeneous enhancement in the thickened myocardium (*arrow*, **b**) with impaired myocardial deformation (*arrow*, **a**). From Bogaert et al. (2004). Reprinted with permission from American Roentgen Ray Society

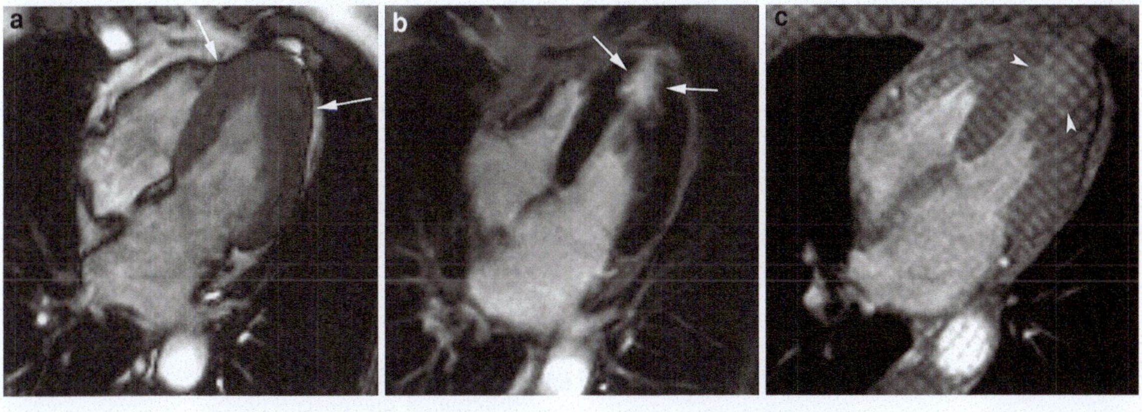

Fig. 20 Myocardial enhancement in apical HCM. Vertical long-axis cine imaging (**a**), late Gd imaging (**b**), and SPAMM myocardial tagging (mid-systolic time frame) (**c**). Important hypertrophy of the apical half of the LV (*arrows*, **a**) with strong enhancement on late Gd imaging mainly subendocardially located in the thickened apex (*arrows*, **b**). SPAMM tagging performed following contrast administration nicely shows the lack of deformation being most pronounced in the enhancing myocardium (*arrowheads*, **c**)

amide. Additionally the success of drug-refractory mechanical treatment on LVOT obstruction, like surgical septal myomectomy or catheter-based septal alcohol ablation or septal coiling, can be accurately assessed with the same technique (Sigwart 1995; Mazur et al. 2001; Valeti et al. 2007). Using a combination of cine imaging, PC-MRI, and late Gd imaging, one can locate the site of septal reduction, evaluate the extent of myocardial necrosis, quantify the LVOT orifice, and measure LVOT flow velocities (Schulz-Menger et al. 2000a; Wu et al. 2001; van Dockum et al. 2004; Valeti et al. 2007; Durand et al.

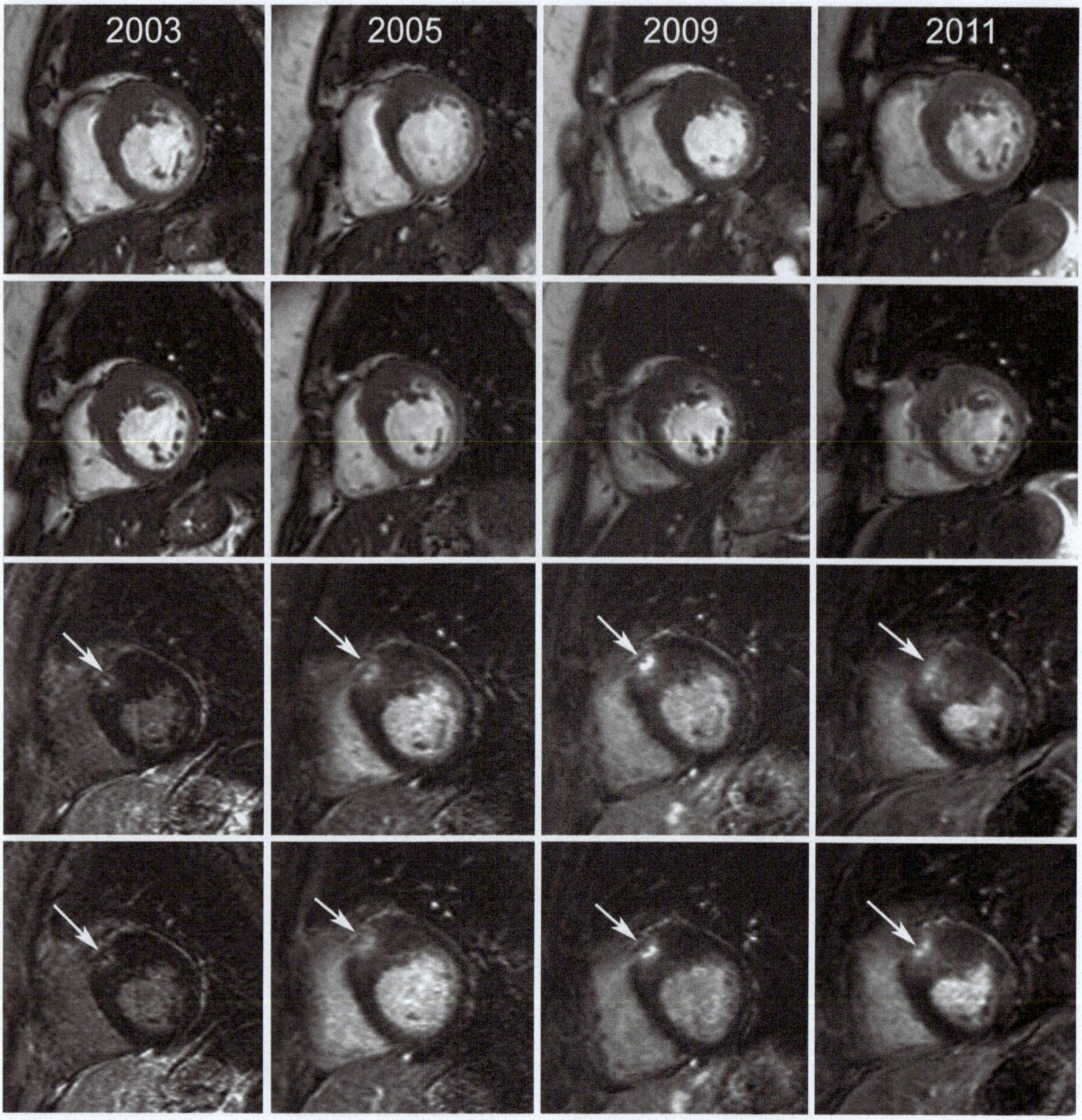

Fig. 21 Spontaneous evolution of asymmetric septal HCM with four MRI studies over a period of 8 years (2003–2011) in a 57-year-old woman with familial history of HCM. The *two upper rows* show end-diastolic short-axis cine images at two levels, while the *two lower rows* show late Gd imaging using the same slice positions. While there is no progression in terms of hypertrophy (i.e., maximal wall thickness nor LV mass) over time (*two upper columns*), we notice a progressive increase in size and signal intensity over time of the subepicardial zone of late Gd enhancement in the anteroseptal LV wall, suggesting progressive myocardial fibrosis formation

2008) (Fig. 22). Occlusion of one or more septal branches by selective coiling or infusion of ethanol of the LAD coronary artery creates an occlusive septal infarction. Subsequent infarct healing with scar formation and associated thinning of the basal interventricular septum results in LVOT dilatation, decrease in pressure gradient and symptomatic improvement (Schulz-Menger et al. 2000a). Late Gd imaging is a valuable tool to detect and measure the infarcted area, detecting in which patients this area is too small or located outside the target area, and therefore may not achieve a substantial reduction of

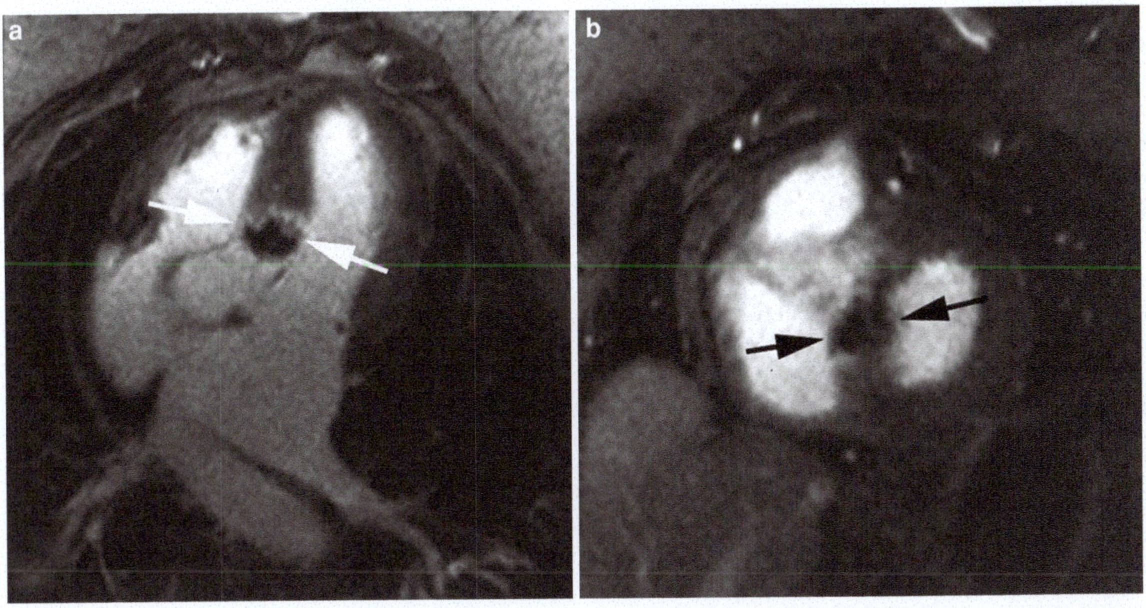

Fig. 22 Asymmetric septal obstructive HCM in a 54-year-old woman treated with alcoholization of first septal perforator coronary artery to reduce LVOT obstruction. Late Gd imaging in LVOT view (**a**) and basal short-axis view (**b**). Presence of a large hypo-intense zone surrounded by thin hyperintense rim in thickened septum (*arrows*), corresponding to occlusive infarct caused by alcoholization. From Bogaert et al. (2004). Reprinted with permission from American Roentgen Ray Society

the LVOT obstruction. Not infrequently the induced infarcts are located on the right side of the interventricular septum, have smaller sizes and less reduction in the LVOT gradient. Large infarcts may cause potentially hazardous conduction abnormalities or ventricular arrhythmias (van Dockum et al. 2004; McCann et al. 2004). Reduction of LVOT obstruction in symptomatic patients is associated with reverse LV remodeling with a significant reduction in myocardial mass and improvement in contractile function in the remote myocardium (van Dockum et al. 2005; van Dockum et al. 2006). The above findings indicate that LVOT obstruction is at least in part afterload-dependent and reversible.

4.2 Dilated Cardiomyopathy

DCM is the most common cardiomyopathy worldwide and is characterized by dilation and impaired contraction of the left, right or both ventricles in the absence of abnormal loading conditions (e.g., hypertension and valve disease) or coronary artery disease (CAD) sufficient to cause global systolic impairment (Elliott et al. 2008; Jefferies and Towbin 2010). Though most often secondary to abnormal loading or ischemic damage, DCM can also be described as primary (genetic, mixed, or acquired) or secondary to other causes (e.g., infiltrative or autoimmune), and thus DCM can be considered to represent a final common pathway that is the end result of myocardial damage. Although the cause of DCM is often not definable (idiopathic DCM), genetic inheritance is found in about 20–35% of patients, and a variety of cytotoxic agents (e.g., alcohol, chemotherapeutic agents and illicit drugs), metabolic abnormalities, inflammatory and infectious causes, neuromuscular causes can also results in DCM (Dec and Fuster 1994; Jefferies and Towbin 2010; Charron et al. 2010). Although many patients are asymptomatic, patients usually present with symptoms of left heart failure. Right heart failure may be present, and is an aggravating factor (Sun et al. 1997; Hombach et al. 2009), but is not necessary for the diagnosis of DCM. Other, potentially life-treatening symptoms of DCM are ventricular arrhythmias, conduction abnormalities, syncope, SCD, and increased risk of thromboembolic events. A certain number of patients present with advanced heart failure and severe LV systolic dysfunction, but show normal or mildly dilated ventricles

(<10–15% above normal range)—i.e., mildly dilated DCM (Elliott et al. 2008).

Histologically, DCM is characterized by myocyte apoptosis and hypertrophy, with myocyte elongation that explains the increase in chamber size in combination with normal or thinned myocardial walls (Beltrami et al. 1995). This causes a typical eccentric ventricular hypertrophy with a typically decreased wall thickness to chamber diameter ratio, thereby increasing the sphericity of the ventricle. The net result is a significant increase in wall stress, which has a negative impact on systolic ventricular performance (Fujita et al. 1993). A second, important histological feature is an excessive deposition of collagen and decreased capillary density. Both reactive (interstitial and perivascular) and reparative (replacement) patterns of fibrosis are seen in DCM (Proclemer et al. 1997; Hughes and McKenna 2005). The fibrosis is thought to reflect inflammation as well as microvascular ischemia.

The role of cardiac imaging in general, and MRI in particular, in studying DCM patients is to assess the severity of ventricular dilatation, dysfunction, and contraction abnormalities, to diagnose diastolic dysfunction, to visualize and quantify concomitant valve regurgitation, and to depict thrombus formation (Fig. 23). Though the above information can be obtained with echocardiography, the added value of performing MRI in DCM patients is undoubted. Cardiac MRI can characterize myocardial tissue using T2w-imaging and T2 mapping techniques, T2* quantification, and late Gd imaging, providing data about myocardial edema and inflammation, iron deposition (see iron deposition cardiomyopathy), and myocardial necrosis/fibrosis (Raman et al. 2010), thus being a valuable non-invasive substitute for endomyocardial biopsy (EMB). Moreover, imaging is becoming increasingly important in risk assessment, therapy planning, and determination of prognosis.

Imaging should include assessment of extracardiac abnormalities such as pleural effusion or azygos vein and superior vena cava dilatation that may be indicative of left and right heart failure, respectively. *Firstly*, cine MRI is the reference technique to quantify cardiac chamber size, ventricular function and mass, to assess myocardial wall thicknesses and segmental function, and to calculate wall thickness to chamber radius ratio in DCM patients (Semelka et al. 1990; Buser et al. 1990; Gaudio et al. 1991; Strohm et al. 2001). In addition, myocardial tagging techniques can be of interest to unravel the impact on myocardial deformation (MacGowan et al. 1997; Rademakers et al. 2003). Typically, the left (and right) ventricle shows a moderate to severe degree of ventricular dilatation with moderate to very low ejection fraction (e.g., lower than 20%) (Fig. 24). Atria may be enlarged, but usually less extensive than the ventricles. Ventricular stroke volumes are often within normal limits or only modestly impaired because of the dilatation. However, these should be corrected for the presence of concomitant valve regurgitation (Fig. 25). Segmental wall motion is usually severely hypokinetic to dyskinetic with a variable degree of dyssynchrony, the latter often in association with bundle branch block (Masci et al. 2010a), and related to the presence of myocardial fibrosis (see below) (Tigen et al. 2010). The degree of segmental dysfunction is related not only to an increase in wall stress, as a consequence of the (non-compensated) eccentric hypertrophy, but also due to an intrinsic impairment in myocardial contractility (Fujita et al. 1993; Rademakers et al. 2003). At least in some DCM patients the myocardial trabeculations along the LV free wall may be more prominent than in normals (Imai et al. 1992) (Fig. 26). Though some groups have used an approach to express and quantify the degree of (hyper)-trabeculation, differentiation with other pathologies such as non-compaction cardiomyopathy (see Sect. 4.1.5) may be challenging (Fernandez-Golfin et al. 2009; Jacquier et al. 2010; Dawson et al. 2011). Diastolic abnormalities are not uncommon in DCM patients, and may be present in the right ventricle showing normal volumes and systolic function (Suzuki et al. 1991).

Secondly, there is an accumulating body of evidence that MRI may be useful in depicting fibrosis in DCM patients. Late Gd imaging has shown to be of great help in differentiating between CAD and non-CAD-related causes of LV dilatation and dysfunction, which is important in further therapy planning (Koito et al. 1996; Wu et al. 2001; McCrohon et al. 2003) (Figs. 5 and 27). Ischemically dilated cardiomyopathies typically show subendocardial or transmural enhancement, representing myocardial scarring, in coronary artery perfusion territories (see "Ischemic Heart Disease"), whereas DCM patients most often show no myocardial enhancement, less commonly linear or patchy midwall enhancement not respecting

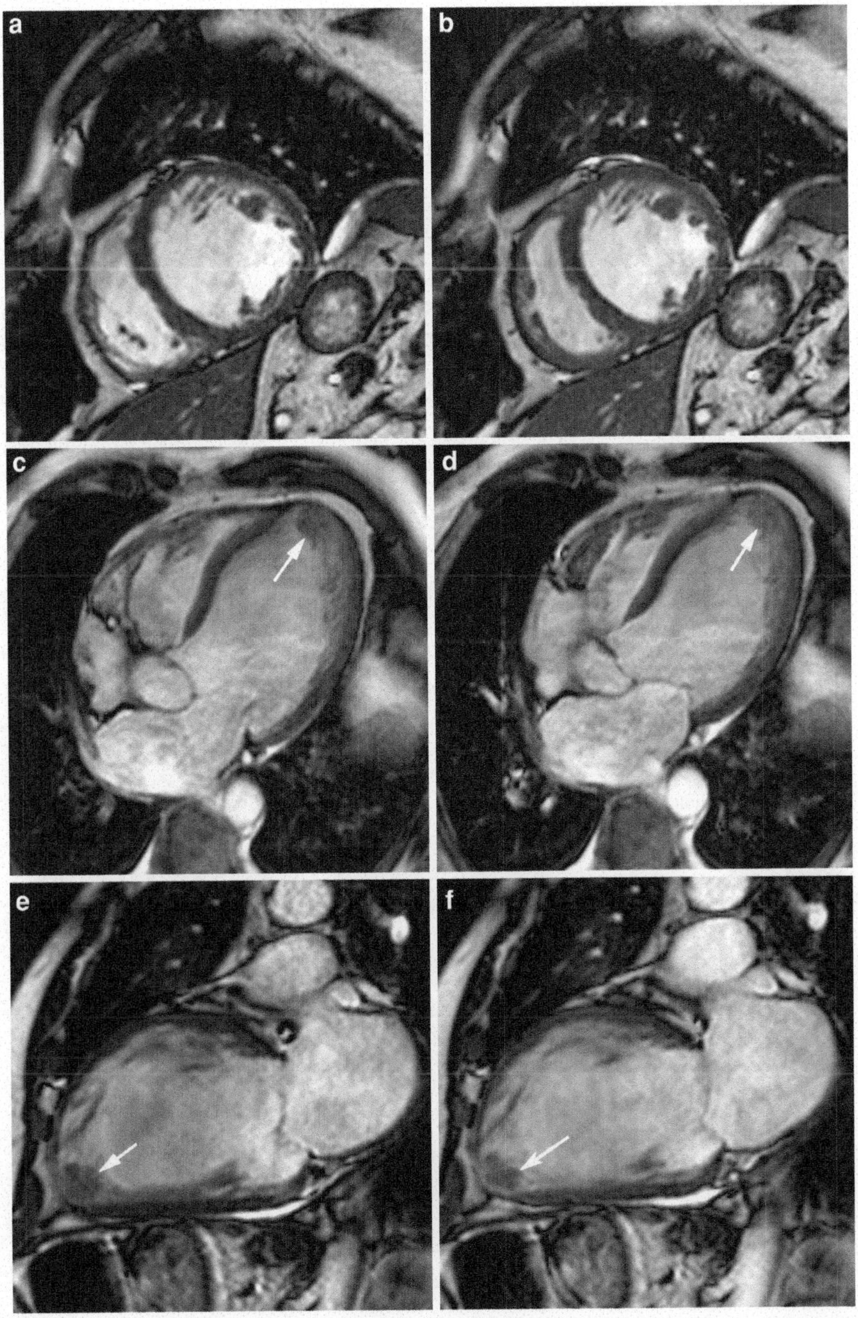

Fig. 23 Idiopathic DCM in a 53-year-old man. Cine imaging in short-axis (**a**, **b**), horizontal long-axis (**c**, **d**), and vertical long-axis (**e**, **f**), at end diastole (*left column*) and end systole (*right column*). Important LV dilation with severely diminished global and regional function (end-diastolic volume: 463 ml, end-systolic volume: 417 ml, stroke volume: 46 ml, ejection fraction: 10%). Mural thrombus in LV apex (*arrow*, **c–d**). Note the moderate hypertrophy of the trabeculations along the LV lateral wall, and the left atrial enlargement due to mitral regurgitation secondary to the LV enlargement. No myocardial abnormalities on late Gd imaging (not shown). Normal luminal appearance of coronary arteries on coronary artery catheterization

coronary artery perfusion territories and not necessarily limited to the LV, but also involving the RV may be seen (Fig. 27) (Wu et al. 2001; McCrohon et al. 2003; Soriano et al. 2005). This midwall enhancement likely reflects segmental fibrosis. Finally, a small number of DCM patients show a typical ischemic pattern of enhancement, corresponding with healed infarcts. Coronary angiography in these patients not infrequently reveals normal coronary arteries, questioning whether recanalization of the occlusive coronary artery occurred or whether the infarct was due to embolization from minimally stenotic, but unstable plaques. This group of patients should be considered to most likely have LV dysfunction related to CAD, although CAD can coexist with DCM. The latter combination should be

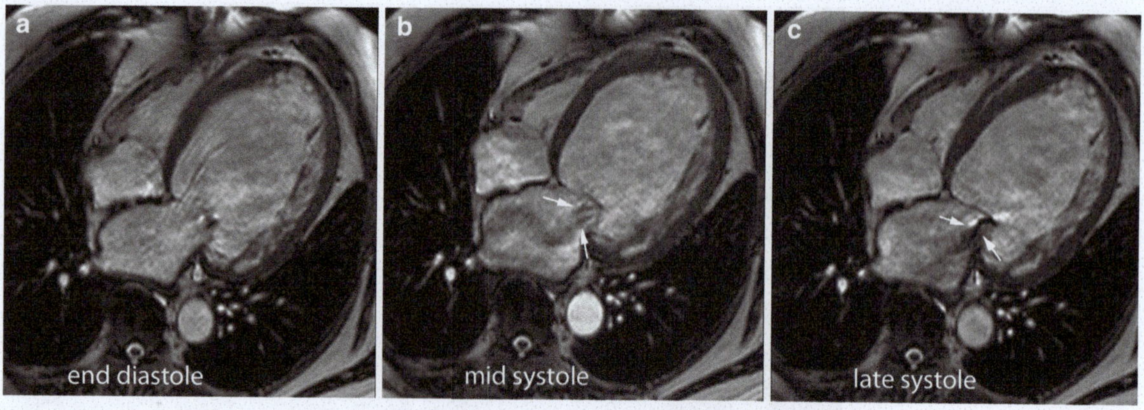

Fig. 24 Extreme form of DCM in a 63-year-old man. Cine imaging in horizontal long-axis at end diastole (**a**), mid systole (**b**), and late systole (**c**). Extreme LV dilatation (EDV: 877 ml, EF: 12%) and moderate RV dilatation (EDV: 248 ml, EF: 42%). Important mitral regurgitation (*arrows*, **b**, **c**) due to mitral valve ring dilatation. Regurgitant volume of 45 ml measured by PC-MRI

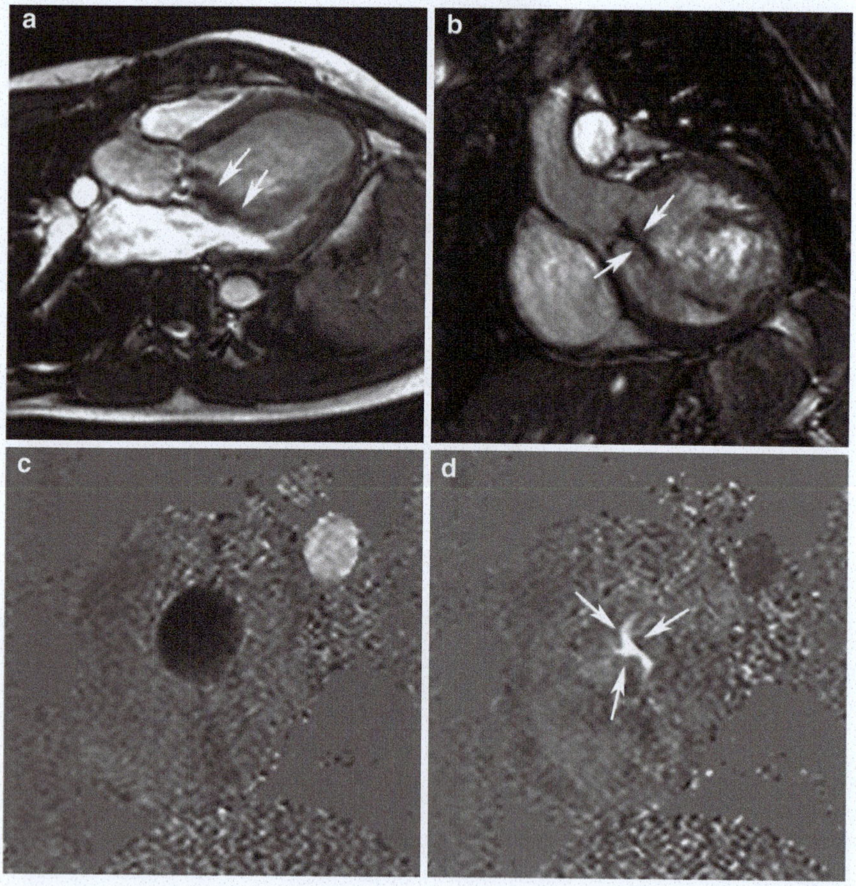

Fig. 25 Non-DCM-related cause of LV dilatation in a 21-year-old man with Marfan disease and severe aortic regurgitation. Cine imaging in LVOT view (**a**) and short-axis view (**b**), diastolic time frames. PC-MRI of the aorta valve (level just beneath the valve) at systole (**c**) and diastole (**d**). Severe dilation of LV EDV (500 ml) with EF of 51%. The regurgitant aortic jet is well visible on cine imaging as a black jet (*arrows*, **a**, **b**), as well on PC-MRI (*arrows*, **d**)

considered in particular in patients with non-extensive infarctions.

Besides depiction of the underlying cause of ventricular dilation and dysfunction, late Gd imaging is appealing for risk stratifying DCM patients. Several groups have found in non-ischemic cardiomyopathy patients that the presence of midwall myocardial enhancement (>25% of wall thickness) is predictive

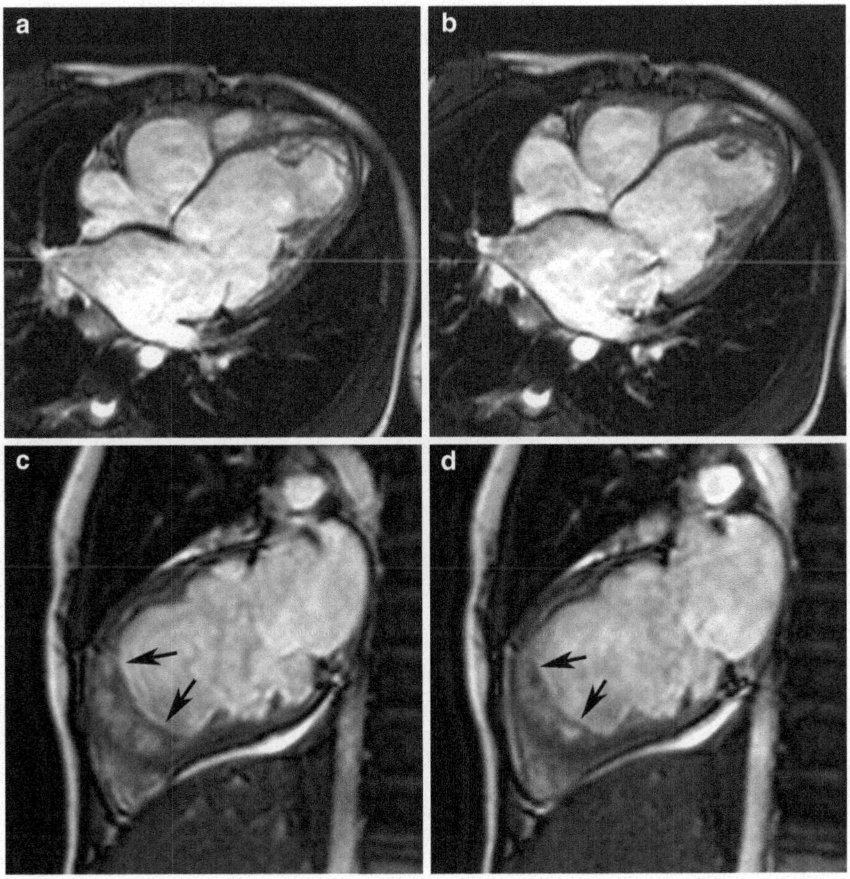

Fig. 26 Dilated dysfunctional left ventricle in a 19-year-old woman. Cine imaging in horizontal long-axis (**a**, **b**) and vertical long-axis (**c**, **d**) at end diastole (*left*) and end systole (*right*). Extremely thin-walled ventricles in particular of the ventricular septum, with pronounced appearance of the trabeculations in LV apex (*arrows*, **c**, **d**). The left ventricle has an EDV of 260 ml and EF of 11%. Differentiation between DCM with compensatory trabecular hypertrophy and Left ventricular non-compaction cardiomyopathy (LVNC) is challenging is this case

of inducible ventricular tachycardia, thus allowing for the identification of high-risk patients, and the need for device therapy (Nazarian et al. 2005; Assomull et al. 2006; Wu et al. 2008; Shimizu et al. 2010). Especially in DCM patients with mildly to moderately decreased ejection fraction, late Gd imaging adds predictive value. Patients with abnormal myocardial enhancement might benefit from prophylatic ICD placement (Lakdawala and Givertz 2010). In a recent study by Hombach et al. (2009) including 141 DCM patients; however, midwall myocardial enhancement was not associated with an independent prognostic impact, stressing the need for large prospective studies in this field.

Bogun et al. (2009) used late Gd imaging to plan appropriate mapping and ablation strategy in a small group of DCM patients. The location of the scar (endo vs. epicardial) was important to determine the optimal approach for ablation. Moreover, catheter ablation appeared to be unsuccessful in patients with a predominantly intramural scar. Heart failure patients with no evidence of myocardial scarring by late Gd imaging respond more favorably to β-blockade therapy with functional improvement and reverse ventricular remodeling than those with myocardial scar (Bello et al. 2003).

As mentioned above, a major limitation of the late Gd imaging technique is that diffusely spread pathology such as diffuse myocardial fibrosis is missed because the sequence is optimized to depict focal myocardial pathology. This probably explains the normal findings on late Gd imaging in the majority of DCM patients (McCrohon et al. 2003). Alternative approaches (e.g., T1-mapping) are currently under investigation for depicting diffuse myocardial fibrosis. Deposition of collagen increases the extracellular space, which results in an increased interstitial accumulation of gadolinium contrast at steady state, an increased myocardial partition coefficient, and a shortening of T1-relaxation times (Jerosch-Herold et al. 2008; Iles et al. 2008; Han et al. 2009; Sueyoshi et al. 2010). The expansion of the extracellular space

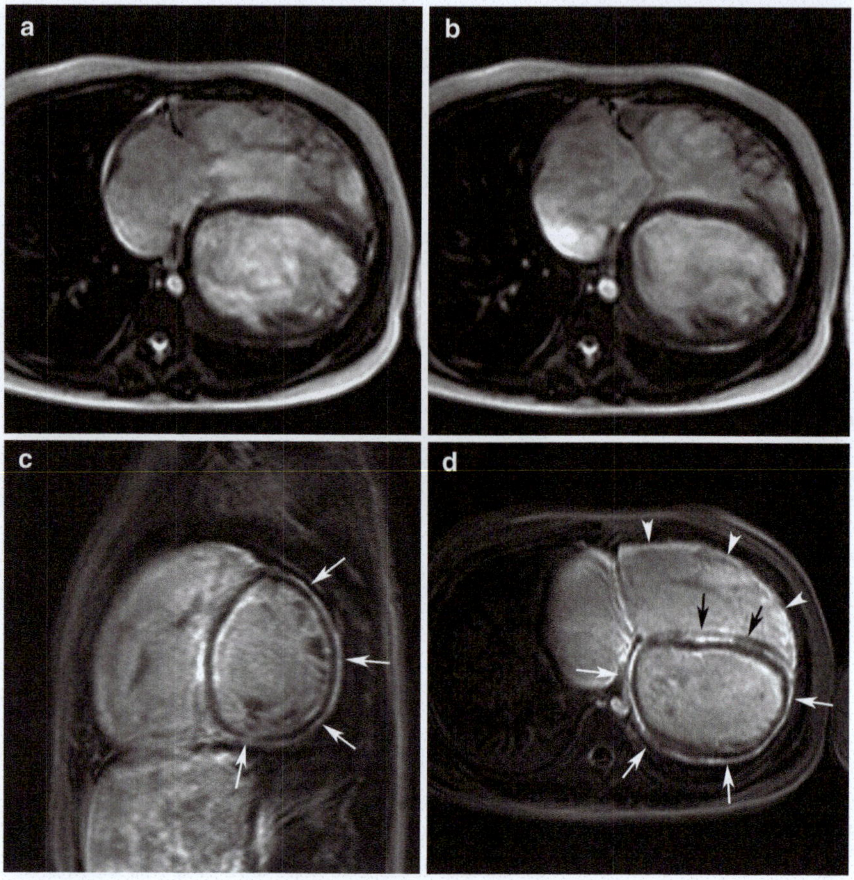

Fig. 27 Extreme form of DCM in an 11-year-old girl involving both ventricles, presenting with heart failure NYHA IV. Cine imaging in horizontal long-axis at end diastole (**a**) and end systole (**b**). Late Gd imaging in short-axis (**c**) and horizontal long-axis (**d**). Important dilatation and dysfunction of both ventricles, i.e., LV EDV: 324 ml, LV EF: 9%, RV EDV: 520 ml, EF: 7%. Late Gd imaging shows diffuse strong enhancement of the subepicardial LV enhancement (*white arrows*, **c**, **d**), midwall septal enhancement (*black arrows*, **d**) and diffuse RV enhancement (*arrowheads*, **d**)

and thus the increase in myocardial fibrosis are correlated with the impairment in myocardial blood flow, the degree of ventricular dilation and contractile dysfunction as well as diastolic dysfunction in DCM patients (Knaapen et al. 2006; Jerosch-Herold et al. 2008; Moreo et al. 2008; Sueyoshi et al. 2010).

Thirdly, DCM can occur at a late stage following acute myocarditis characterized by chronic inflammation, ventricular dilatation and dysfunction, and persistence of the viral proteins in the myocardium (Elliott et al. 2008). Because this subgroup of DCM patients may favorably respond to immunomodulatory therapy, depiction of chronic inflammation is important. Whereas the role of MRI in assessing acute myocarditis patients is well established and diagnostic criteria have been defined (Lake Louise Criteria) (Friedrich et al. 2009) (see Sect. 4.1.6), its role in assessing chronic myocarditis patients is less clear. Mahrholdt et al. (2004) reported a significant decrease in extent of midwall/subepicardial focal myocardial enhancement at 3-month follow-up in patients with acute myocarditis. This is most likely to represent residual inflammation or fibrotic sequela of prior, possibly subclinical myocarditis. In patients with chronic myocarditis, De Cobelli et al. (2006) found a similar pattern of focal myocardial enhancement as in acute myocarditis patients, corresponding with chronic inflammation at EMB in up to 70% of patients. More recently, two studies showed that chronic myocardial inflammation is associated with generalized myocardial edema and an increase of global myocardial enhancement whereas the above-described focal myocardial enhancement pattern using the late Gd imaging technique had low sensitivity and specificity (Gutberlet et al. 2008; Voigt et al. 2011).

4.3 Restrictive Cardiomyopathy

RCM is the least common form of cardiomyopathy. The hallmark of this cardiomyopathy is an increased stiffness of the myocardium leading to impairment of

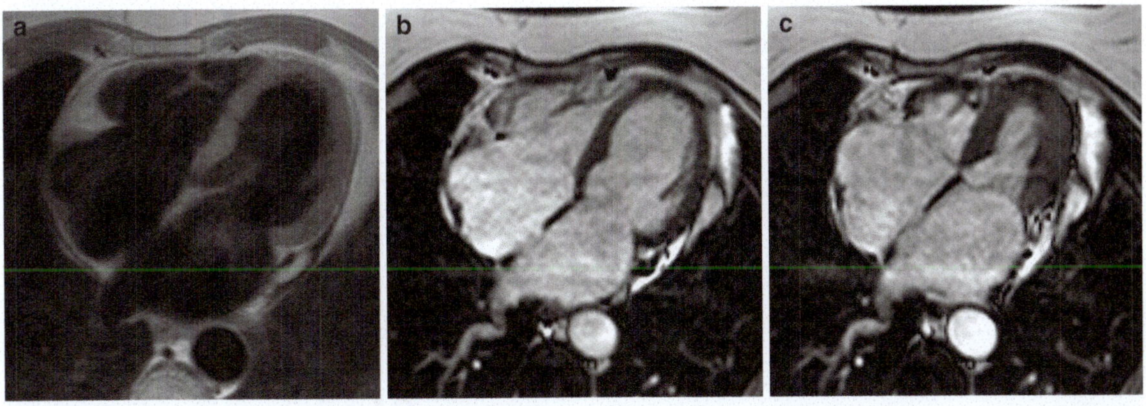

Fig. 28 Idiopathic RCM in 73-year-old woman presenting with increased filling pressures. T1w-imaging (**a**), cine imaging at end diastole (**b**), and end systole (**c**) in horizontal long-axis. The ventricles have a normal configuration and normal systolic function. The main hallmark of RCM is increased myocardial stiffness leading to increased filling pressures, and diastolic dysfunction. As a consequence the atria are markedly enlarged. Note the presence of a small pericardial effusion laterally to the left atrioventricular groove

ventricular filling, diastolic dysfunction and ultimately heart failure (Nihoyannopoulos and Dawson 2009). RCM has always been difficult to define because a wide range of different pathologies involving the myocardium and/or endocardium may present with a restrictive physiology (Kushwaha et al. 1997). Besides idiopathic (or primary) forms, RCM may result from myocardial fibrosis, myocardial infiltrative (e.g., amyloidosis, sarcoidosis) and storage diseases (e.g., hemochromatosis and Fabry's disease), and from a variety of endomyocardial diseases (e.g., endomyocardial fibrosis, hypereosinophilic syndrome and radition—see secondary cardiomyopathies). In addition, restrictive inflow physiology may be found in other myocardial disorders such as HCM, or in hypertensive heart disease.

Primary RCM presents with normal or reduced ventricular volumes, and myocardial wall thicknesses within normal limits. In contrast, there is a disproportionate enlargement of the atria due to increased ventricular filling pressures, often worsened by a concomitant presence of mitral and tricuspid regurgitation (Fig. 28). Though systolic function in RCM is traditionally considered to be normal—RCM is considered to exclusively affect diastolic function—there is a vast amount of evidence that systolic dysfunction is part of RCM, but the dysfunction is not shown on the routinely used functional systolic parameters (e.g., ejection fraction) (Zile et al. 2004). During systole, energy is generated and stored into the myocardium, which is released during isovolemic relaxation causing active suction of blood during the first part of diastole. The mechanism of energy storage/release is the twisting/untwisting process of the ventricle, which can be studied accurately with myocardial tagging techniques (Rademakers et al. 1992; Tan et al. 2009; Prasad et al. 2010). Abnormalities typically increase during exercise (Westermann et al. 2008; Tan et al. 2009). It is estimated that at least one-half of patients presenting with symptoms and signs of heart failure will have a normal LV ejection fraction, having a survival similar to that of patients with reduced ejection fraction (Bhatia et al. 2006; Owan et al. 2006; Rademakers and Bogaert 2006).

Impaired ventricular filling with diastolic dysfunction is not only the hallmark in RCM, but is also seen in constrictive pericarditis. Differentiation between both entities can be difficult on clinical grounds, but is critical for decision-making regarding the therapeutic approach, since constrictive pericarditis requires surgical resection or stripping of the pericardium, whereas medical treatment is indicated for RCM (Schwefer et al. 2009) (see also "Pericardial Disease").

Similar to other cardiomyopathies, the role of MRI in assessing RCM is comprehensive, ranging from morphologic assessment of the heart and pericardium, assessment of systolic and diastolic functional parameters (Fig. 29), evaluation of ventricular coupling (Fig. 30), quantifying valve regurgitation, to myocardial tissue characterization. Though in many

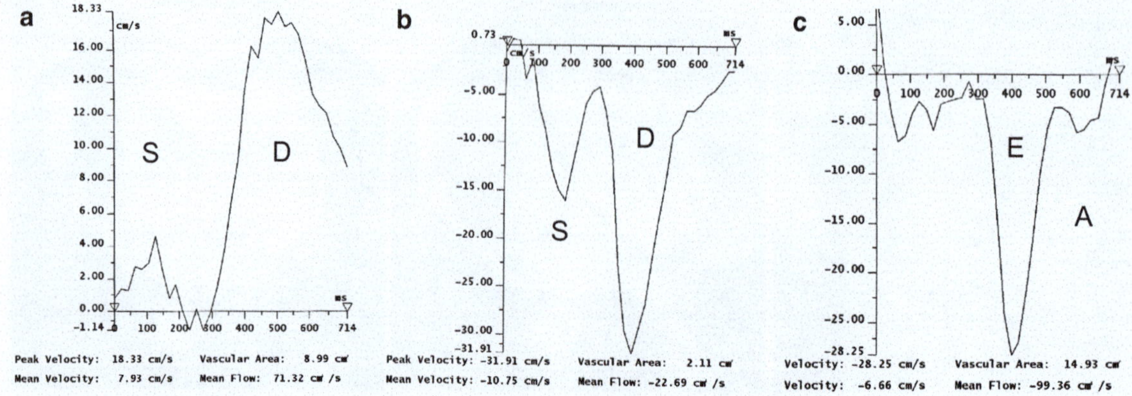

Fig. 29 Typical flow curves in RCM, using PC-MRI. Flow pattern in the inferior vena cava (**a**), pulmonary vein (**b**), and mitral valve (**c**). The *x*-axis represents time during the cardiac cycle (0 ms corresponds with R-wave of QRS complex). The *y*-axis is flow velocity (cm/sec). Systolic forward venous flow (*S*) is diminished due to increased atrial pressures (**a**, **b**). The latter are necessary to compensate for the decreased myocardial compliance. As a consequence, early ventricular filling (*E*) is typically enhanced (**c**), while the contribution of atrial contraction (*A*) to ventricular filling is minimal. At the venous level, forward flow is maximal during early diastolic ventricular filling (*D*), while later during the cardiac cycle, forward flow may be abolished or even reversed. Without assessment of the respiratory variation of these flow curves, differentiation between RCM and constrictive pericarditis is often not possible

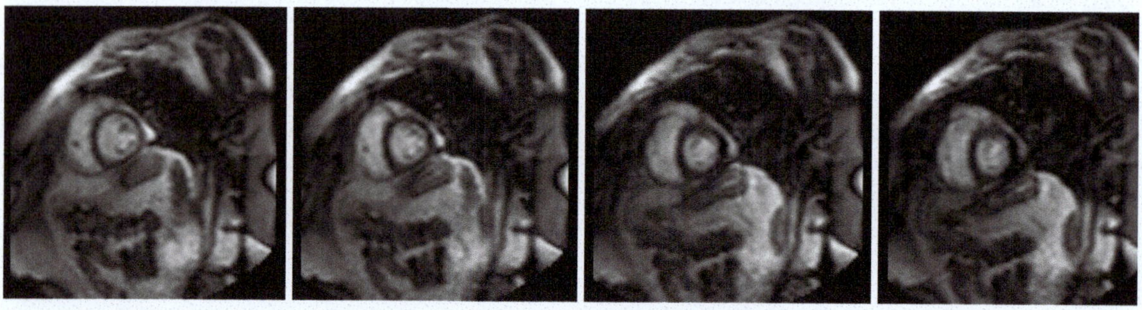

Fig. 30 Ventricular septal motion in a patient with RCM. Real-time MRI in cardiac short-axis, using real-time cine imaging (acquisition time per image 60 ms) during deep inspiration and expiration. Four consecutive heart beats after onset of inspiration at the moment of early ventricular filling. In contrast to patients with constrictive pericarditis (see Fig. 27 in "Pericardial Disease"), the position and motion of the ventricular septum during early ventricular filling is minimally influenced by respiration. In some patients, due to the increased myocardial stiffness, the respiratory variation in septal motion is even diminished compared with healthy persons

cases, the etiology of RCM is possible only by EMB and histological analysis, several secondary cardiomyopathies causing RCM can nowadays be accurately depicted with MRI (Cooper et al. 2007).

4.4 Arrhythmogenic Right Ventricular Cardiomyopathy/Dysplasia

Arrhythmogenic right ventricular cardiomyopathy/dyplasia (ARVC/D), first described in 1736, is a rare inherited heart muscle disease that may be the cause of SCD particularly in young people and athletes (Basso et al. 2009). The estimated prevalence in the general population ranges from 1 in 1.000 to 1 in 5,000. ARVC/D is mainly a disease of the cardiomyocyte junction, caused by mutations in genes encoding desmosomal proteins, with both autosomal dominant and autosomal recessive (e.g., Naxos diseas and Carvajal syndrome) inheritance patterns (Fontaine et al. 1998; Basso et al. 2009; Watkins et al. 2011). These mutations compromise the intercellular adhesion causing a "wear and tear" with myocyte loss and inflammatory myocarditis and repair with fibrofatty tissue (Sen-Chowdhry et al. 2008). Though initially regarded as a pathological entity exclusively involving the RV, the LV may be structurally and functionally involved, suggesting that the broader term arrhythmogenic cardiomyopathy may be more appropriate to (re)-define this disease entity (Pinamonti et al. 2011).

The myocardial areas structurally more vulnerable to mechanical stress such as the inferior, apical, and infundibular part of the thin-walled right ventricle ("the so-called *triangle of dysplasia*") and the inferolateral wall of the LV are prone to involvement in ARVC/D. The replacement by fibrofatty tissue starts from the epicardium and may become transmural, leading to wall thinning and aneurysm formation, associated with dysfunction (systolic bulging) and in later stages ventricular dilatation and dysfunction. The electrical impulse conduction may be impaired due to the fibrofatty replacement causing the typical epsilon waves and electrical instability that precipitates ventricular arrhythmias and SCD (Fontaine et al. 1998; Corrado et al. 2000; Basso et al. 2009). Recently, it has been reported that myocarditis may selectively affect the RV causing structural abnormalities, including microaneurysms, and arrhythmic manifestations typical of ARVC/D (Pieroni et al. 2009).

The clinical presentation of ARVC/D is highly variable. It is generally considered that this disorder is progressive. The natural history and presentation is a function of both cardiac electrical instability and progressive ventricular dysfunction. Four different clinicopathological phases of this disorder have been described (Basso et al. 2009):

(1) A subclinical phase with concealed RV structural abnormalities and no symptoms even though SCD may be the first manifestation of the disease, usually in young people during competitive sports or intense physical exercise,
(2) An overt RV electrical disorder with symptomatic RV arrhythmias (that may cause cardiac arrest) in association with overt RV structural and functional abnormalities,
(3) RV failure due to progressive loss of myocardium with severe dilatation and dysfunction in the presence of preserved LV function, and
(4) Biventricular failure due to significant LV involvement that can mimic DCM.

This traditional classification scheme has recently been challenged by novel imaging and genetic findings reporting a higher occurrence of LV involvement, mentioning three distinct patterns of ARVC/D, besides the traditional RV phenotype with LV involvement in a late stage of the disease, a left dominant phenotype with early and prominent LV manifestations, and a biventricular phenotype with simultaneous involvement of both ventricles (Norman et al. 2005; Sen-Chowdhry et al. 2008; Jain et al. 2010; Pinamonti et al. 2011). Though these findings support the adoption of the broader term arrhythmogenic cardiomyopathy, other groups do not share this opinion (Dalal et al. 2009) emphasizing that ARVC/D remains an *enigmatic disease* and the diagnosis of this disorder is often challenging, especially in its early stages (Sen-Chowdhry et al. 2010).

Nowadays, the diagnosis is targeted toward early detection of concealed forms of ARVC/D and risk stratification to prevent SCD, such as restriction of physical exercise, anti-arrhythmic drugs, and AICD insertion (Basso et al. 2009). In 1994, the Task Force of the working group on cardiomyopathies proposed minor and major diagnostic criteria for AVRC/D (Table 1), that recently have been modified to improve the diagnosis and management of this condition (McKenna et al. 1994; Marcus et al. 2010). Although the initial criteria were highly specific they lacked sensitivity for early and familial disease. Therefore, the diagnostic criteria encompassing structural, histological, electrocardiographic, arrhythmic, and genetic features of the disease have been modified incorporating knowledge obtained with emerging diagnostic modalities (e.g., MRI) and advances in the genetics of ARVC/D (Marcus et al. 2010). The diagnosis of ARVC/D is made if two major criteria are present, or one major plus two minor criteria are present, or four minor criteria, from different groups, are present.

The revised task force criteria to assess global and regional dysfunction and structural alternations (i.e., criterium I) in ARVC/D by MRI are based on: (a) assessment of regional wall motion of the RV free wall, and (b) quantification of RV volume or RV ejection fraction. This criterium is considered as *major* if regional RV akinesia or dyskinesia or dyssynchronous RV contraction is found in combination with a ratio of RV end-diastolic volume to BSA $\geq$110 ml/m^2 (male) or $\geq$100 ml/m^2 (female) *or* an RV ejection fraction $\leq$40%, and as minor if regional RV akinesia or dyskinesia or dyssynchronous RV contraction is found in combination with a ratio of RV

Table 1 Original criteria for ARVC/D

1. Family history
major: familial history confirmed at necropsy/surgery
minor: familial history of sudden death (<35 years of age) due to suspected ARVD/C
familial history (clinical diagnosis based on present criteria)
2. ECG depolarization/conduction abnormalities
major: epsilon waves or localized prolongation (>110 ms) of QRS complex right precordial leads (V1–V3)
minor: late potentials on signal averaged ECG
3. ECG repolarization abnormalities
minor: inverted T-waves in right precordial leads (V2 and V3) in people >12 years of age in absence of right bundle branch block
4. Arrhythmias (minor)
sustained or nonstained left bundle branch block-type ventricular tachycardia documented on ECG or Holter monitoring or during exercise
frequent ventricular extrasystoles (>1,000/24 h on Holter monitoring)
5. Global or regional dysfunction and structural alterations
major: severe dilatation and reduction of RV ejection fraction with no or minor LV involvement
localized RV aneurysms
akinetic or dyskinetic areas with diastolic bulging
severe segmental dilatation of RV
minor: mild global RV dilatation or ejection fraction reduction with normal LV
mild segmental dilatation of RV
regional RV hypokinesia
6. Tissue characteristics of walls
major: fibrofatty replacement of myocardium on endomyocardial biopsy

Adapted from Corrado et al. 2000

end-diastolic volume to BSA $\geq$100 to <110 ml/m^2 (male) or $\geq$90 to <100 ml/m^2 (female) *or* an RV ejection fraction >40 to $\leq$45% (Marcus et al. 2010) (Fig. 31). In contrast to the original task force criteria, RV hypokinesia is not included in the revised task force criteria. The sensitivity and specificity for a major criterium is 76–68 and 90–98% for males and females, respectively, and for a minor criterium is 79–89 and 85–97% for males and females, respectively. However, in recent work by Vermes et al. (2011) assessing the impact of the revised criteria on the prevalence of ARVC/D in a retrospective study by MRI, it was shown that compared to the original Task Force criteria, the revised criteria significantly reduced the overall prevalence of major and minor criteria, and although the revised criteria yielded high specificity, sensitivity was not improved stressing questioning whether these novel criteria truly improve early diagnosis of ARVC/D.

To ensure a complete assessment of regional wall motion, not only of RV, but also the LV in ARVC/D patients, we recommend a combination of cine MRI in short- and long-axis directions (Fig. 32). Accurate interpretation of cardiac MRI in ARVC/D patients requires a great deal of expertise; otherwise there is a major risk of 'over-calling' ARVC/D, yielding an unacceptable high false-positive rate (Sen-Chowdhry et al. 2006). For instance, in normal subjects the RV free wall at the vicinity of the insertion of the moderator band may appear hypokinetic, or a thin RV apex does not necessarily stand for ARVC/D. Thus, knowledge of the complex shape and contraction patterns of RV is an absolute requirement for everyone dealing with assessment of this group of patients (Fritz et al. 2005).

Though the diagnosis of fibrofatty replacement is made by EMB, MRI is increasingly used as a surrogate for in vivo pathology. EMB is invasive and carries the risk of perforation and tamponade. Moreover, the sensitivity of this test is low because, for reasons of safety, samples are usually taken from the interventricular septum, a region uncommonly involved by ARVC/D. As a non-invasive technique, MRI can be performed, if necessary, repetitively and also in mutation carriers. Moreover, the entire heart can be completely evaluated and importantly the functional impact of structural abnormalities can be immediately assessed.

Already in the 1980s the value of MRI to detect intramyocardial adipose deposits was reported by Casolo et al. (1987). Adipose tissue has high-signal intensity on T1w-imaging and stands in clear contrast to the intermediate signal intensity of the myocardium, thus providing a non-invasive means of depicting fatty replacement. However, when applied to the thin RV free wall, depiction of intramyocardial fat and differentiation form epicardial fat remains, in our experience, challenging, explaining why different approaches have been proposed in order to optimize image quality and improve the depiction of myocardial fat (Berkowitz et al. 2009; Kellman et al. 2009).

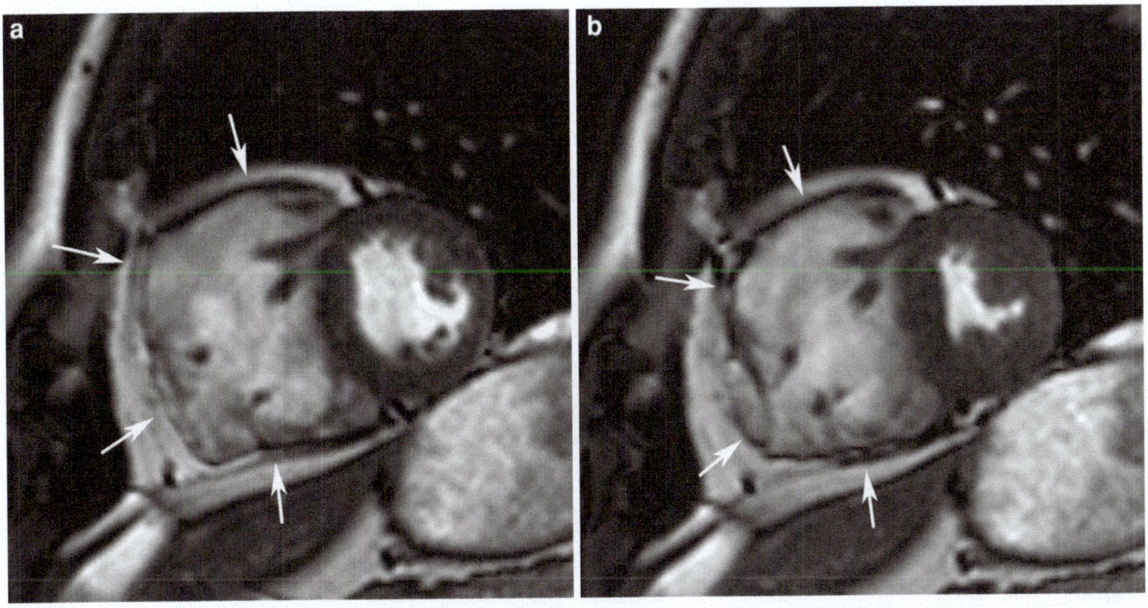

Fig. 31 Severe RV dilatation and dysfunction in a patient with ARVC/D. Short-axis cine imaging at end diastole (**a**) and end systole (**b**). Important RV dilatation (EDV: 304 ml) and systolic dysfunction (EF: 22%). Focal RV wall thinning showing a- to dyskinetic wall motion (*arrows*, **a**, **b**). Normal size and function of left ventricle

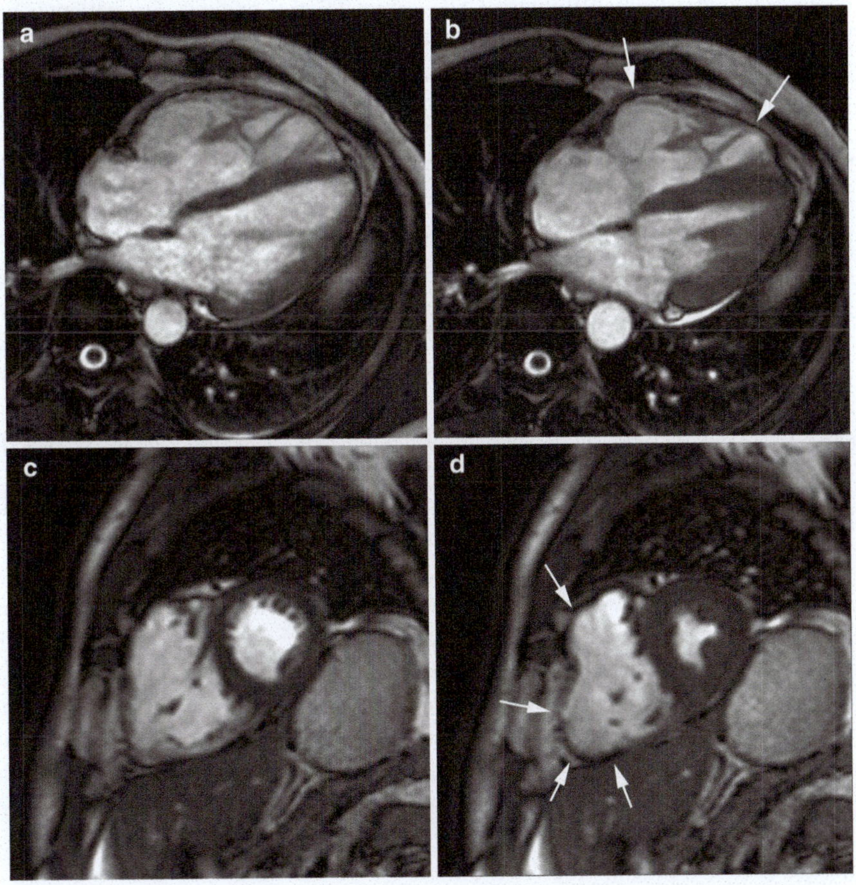

Fig. 32 Cine imaging in a 51-year-old patient with ARVC/D, i.e., horizontal long-axis (**a**, **b**) and short-axis (**c**, **d**), end-diastolic (*left*) and end-systolic (*right*) image frames. Moderate RV dilatation (EDV: 221 ml) and dysfunction (EF: 35%). Several regions show severely diminished contractility (*arrows*, **b**, **d**), the spread of abnormalities can be best appreciated using a combination of short and long-axis image planes

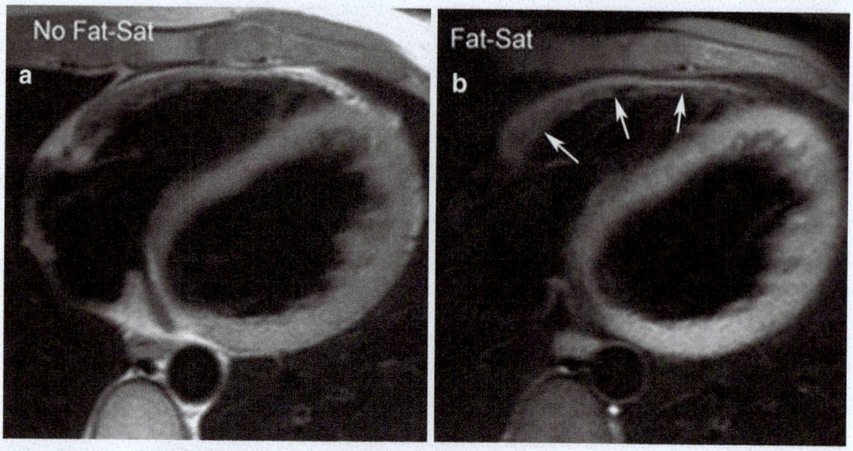

Fig. 33 Combined non-fat suppressed (**a**) and fat suppressed (**b**) T1w-imaging to assess the RV free wall (*arrows*, **b**) in ARVC/D

Furthermore, in ARVC/D patients presenting with ventricular arrhythmias and irregular contraction patterns image quality is often degraded hampering adequate interpretation. Castillo et al. (2004) recommended use of 5 mm thin slices with a 5 mm slice spacing, use of a relatively small field of view (240–280 mm) and a double inversion-recovery fast SE sequence, with a double RR interval TR, a short TE of 30 ms, and an echo train length of 24–32 or less according to the breath-hold capability of the patient. To avoid wrap-around aliasing artifact, the posterior elements of the cardiac phased-array coil were switched off. Additional use of spectrally selective fat-suppression improving the contrast-to-noise ratio was recommended (Fig. 33) (Abarra et al. 2004; Castillo et al. 2004). Tandri et al. (2006) using a similar MRI protocol as described above found a sensitivity and specificity for depicting fat infiltration of 84 and 79%, respectively, with an interobserver agreement of 0.74 (kappa-value). Intramyocardial fat, however, was not only observed in 84% of patients meeting the task force criteria for ARVC/D but also in 34% of patients with idiopathic RV outflow tract tachycardia and in 4% of normal subjects, emphasizing that fat is not necessarily synomyonous for ARVC/D. These findings confirm previous studies demonstrating that presence of intramyocardial fat is not an infrequent feature in normal hearts, especially in the anterolateral and apical RV wall and is considered as a part of the aging process (Burke et al. 1998; Kimura et al. 2010) (Fig. 34).

Several other groups have reported morphological and functional abnormalities similar to ARVC/D in patients with idiopathic RV outflow tract tachycardia, including fixed wall thinning, fatty myocardial infiltration and local bulging (Carlson et al. 1994; Globits et al. 1997; Proclemer et al. 1997; White et al. 1998). In contrast to ARVC/D patients, these patients have normal RV volumes and functions. The findings by Tandri et al. (2004), however, contradicted the above observations showing similar structural and functional findings in patients with idiopathic RV outflow tachycardia and controls.

Since myocardial inflammation and fibrotic replacement are two key features of ARVC/D, contrast-enhanced imaging improves the diagnostic accuracy of MRI. Several small studies have shown a good agreement between the presence of replacement fibrosis in the RV on biopsy and myocardial enhancement on late Gd MRI in ARVC/D patients (Hunold et al. 2005; Tandri et al. 2005; Pfluger et al. 2008) (Figs. 35, 36 and 37). Although larger registry data are needed, late Gd MRI defined RV fibrosis diagnosis yields promise to be used as minor criteria for the diagnosis of ARVC/D, especially in those patients in whom EMB is not performed. However, other entities such as patients with prior myocardial infarction, myocarditis, sarcoidosis or DCM may present RV myocardial enhancement as well (Soriano et al. 2005; Pieroni et al. 2009; Masci et al. 2010b; Raman et al. 2010) (Fig. 5). The late Gd imaging technique faces similar challenges regarding the depiction of abnormal myocardial enhancement in the thin RV free wall. Use of late Gd imaging may be furthermore of interest to evaluate concomitant (or predominant) LV involvement in ARVC/D patients (Sen-Chowdhry et al. 2007, 2008; Dalal et al. 2009).

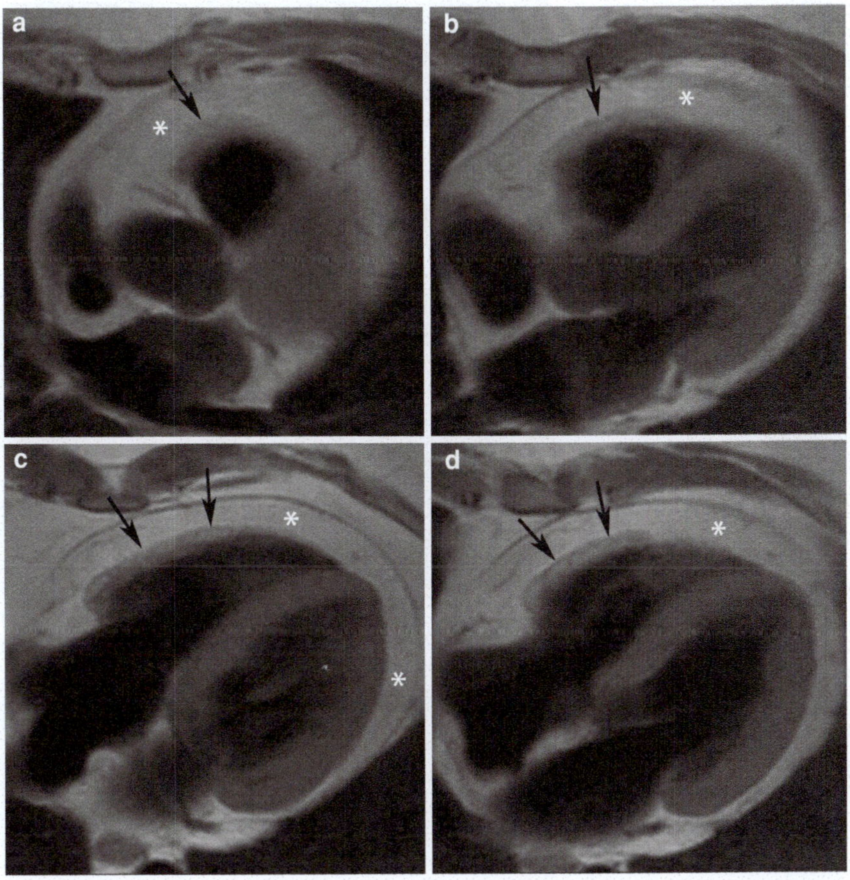

Fig. 34 Benign fatty replacement of RV free wall in a 62-year-old woman. Cardiac MRI was performed because of suspected pericardial fluid on echocardiography. Axial T1w-imaging at 4 levels (**a–d**). Note the presence of an abundant amount of epicardial fat (*), probably mistaken for pericardial fluid on echocardiography. Moreover, the RV free wall has a thickened appearance with speckled appearance due to diffuse fatty infiltration (*arrows*). There is also a lipomatous hyperplasia of the atrial septum

Finally, fibrofatty replacement induces a series of abnormalities that may be of use in the diagnosis of ARVC/D. Initially heavy fatty infiltration may lead to wall hypertrophy (>8 mm) with trabecular disarray and hypertrophy of the moderator band (Tandri et al. 2003) (Fig. 33). Later stages, with segmental loss of myocytes and fibrosis, lead to extreme wall thinning (<2 mm) with single or multiple aneurysm formation or outpouching of the RV wall.

Uhl's anomaly of the right ventricle is an unusual, congenital cardiac disorder with almost complete absence of RV myocardium, normal tricuspid valve, and preserved septal and LV myocardium (Uhl 1952). Since this disease bears some similarities with ARVC/D and idiopathic RV outflow tract tachycardia, it is unclear whether these are different expressions of the same condition, or whether they should be considered as separate entities (Pamuru et al. 2010). The role of MRI in this entity is limited to case studies, confirming extreme thinning of RV wall with RV dilatation, showing akinetic wall motion (Otmani et al. 2007).

4.5 Left Ventricular Non-Compaction Cardiomyopathy

Left ventricular non-compaction (LVNC), also called non-compaction cardiomyopathy or isolated ventricular non-compaction, is considered a distinct cardiomyopathy, which has been categorized as unclassified cardiomyopathy by the WHO—International Society and Federation of Cardiology task force in 1995 (Richardson et al. 1996) and recently been listed among the group of genetic cardiomyopathies (Maron et al. 2006a, b; Watkins et al. 2011). This entity is also called LV hypertrabeculation because of presence of prominent trabeculations (Finsterer et al. 2002) (Fig. 38), or as spongy myocardium because of the spongy appearance of the non-compacted

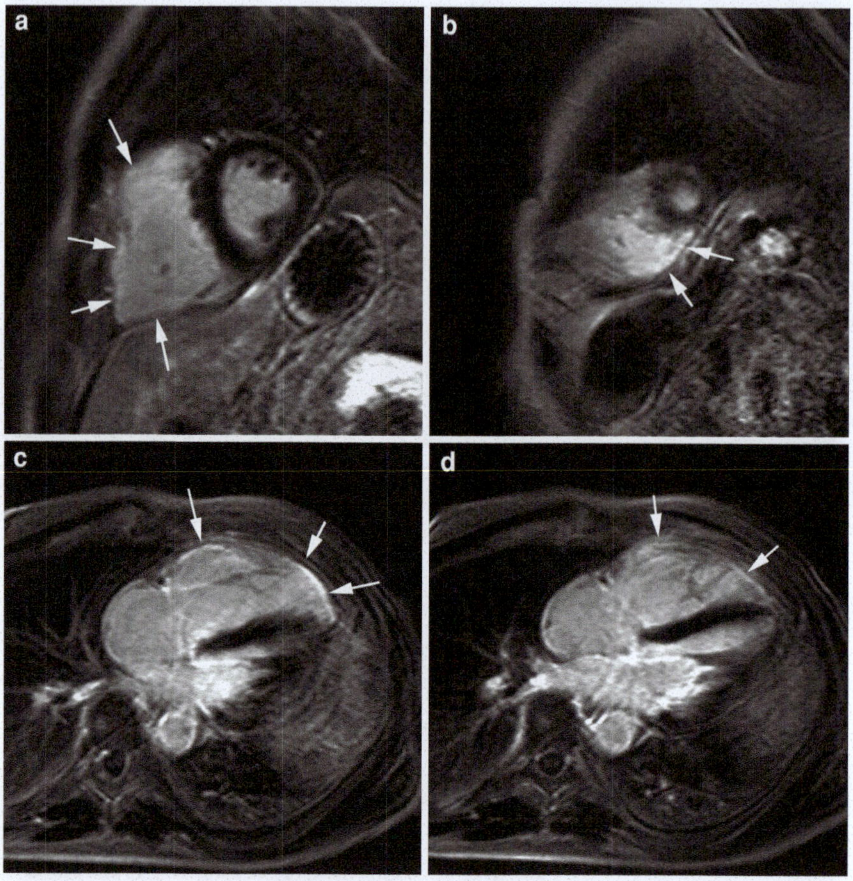

Fig. 35 Late Gd imaging in ARVC/D imaging (same patient as in Fig. 32). Short-axis (**a**, **b**) and axial plane (**c**, **d**). Focal strong enhancement is found in RV free wall (*arrows*, **a–d**). The areas of enhancement correspond to the dysfunctional areas on cine imaging (see Fig. 31)

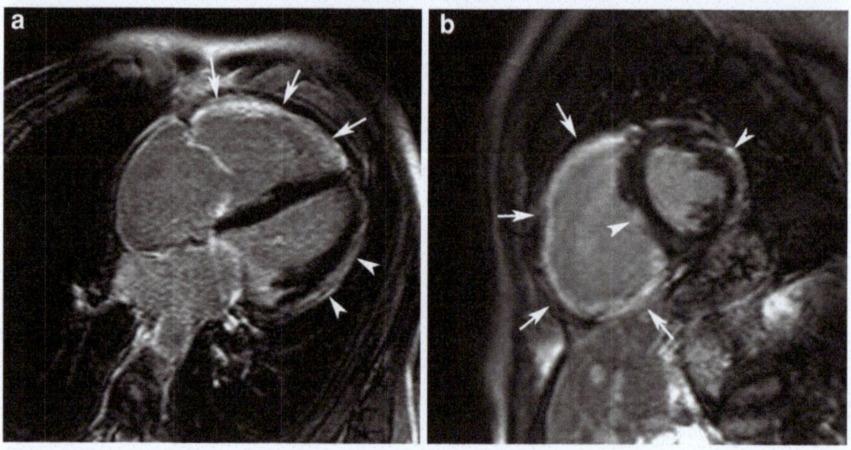

Fig. 36 Late Gd imaging in a 60-year-old patient with ARVC/D. Horizontal long-axis (**a**) and short-axis (**b**) plane. Diffuse, strong enhancement is found in the entire RV wall (*arrows*) as well as focal subepicardial enhancement along the LV lateral wall (*arrowheads*)

myocardium, referring to the myocardium found in non-mammalian vertebrates lacking epicardial coronary arteries, such as fish, amphibians, and reptiles (Angelini et al. 1999). LVNC can be associated with congenital heart abnormalities (non-isolated form) and is found in both pediatric and adult populations (Fig. 39). Though genetic defects are found in half of LVNC patients, some have suggested that LVNC may actually represent an acquired pathology, while other reports have shown regression of non-compaction. Moreover, the link between gene defect and phenotypic expression remains unclarified. One generally

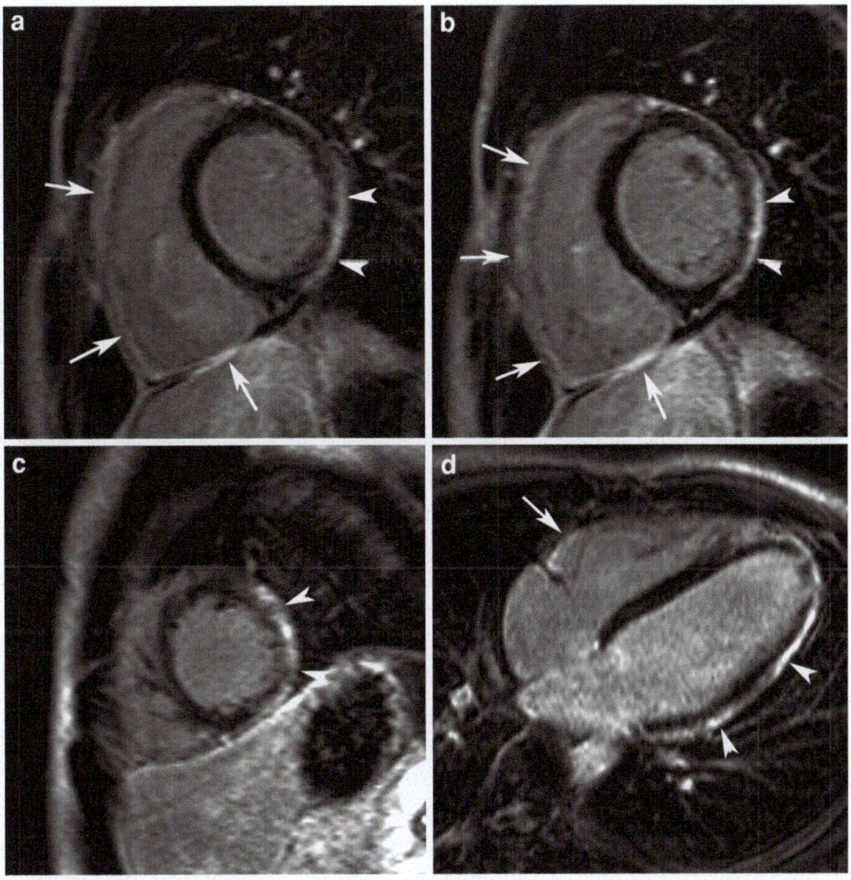

Fig. 37 Late Gd imaging in a 24-year-old man with familial history of ARVC/D who underwent screening with MRI. Short-axis imaging (**a–c**), horizontal long-axis (**d**). Besides enhancement in RV free wall (*arrows*), strong subepicardial enhancement is present in LV, mainly in the lateral wall (*arrowheads*). These findings in combination with a strong familial history are highly suspected of ARVC/D

accepted hypothesis is that LVNC is caused by an intrauterine arrest (between week 5 and 8) of the process of compaction of the loosely interwoven meshwork of myocardial fibers, which normally progresses from epi- to endo-cardium and from cardiac base to apex (Elshershari et al. 2001; Pignatelli et al. 2003). As a result, LVNC patients present with prominent trabeculations, deep intertrabecular recesses and a thin epicardial compacta.

A second hypothesis suggests that the prominent trabeculations represent an adaptive mechanism to compensate for abnormally contracting myocardium. Evidence is given by the observation of myocardial fibrosis, suggesting that myocarditis may be responsible for some cases (Captur and Nihoyannopoulos 2010). In a recent paper by Nucifora et al. (2011), myocardial enhancement by late Gd imaging was found in 55% of patients with LVNC, and the presence was related to clinical severity and LV systolic dysfunction (Fig. 40).

Most commonly, the apical and mid-ventricular part of the inferior and lateral LV wall are affected, whereas involvement of the anterior wall and septum and the basal segments is much less common (Oechslin et al. 2000). Occasionally, the RV may be involved as well (Fig. 38). LVNC patients may be asymptomatic or present clinically with heart failure, systemic embolism, and ventricular arrhythmias (Pignatelli et al. 2003). This disorder is not infrequently associated with neuromuscular disorders (Stöllberger et al. 2011). The natural history and prognosis are probably better than previously thought (Lofiego et al. 2007).

Attempts to define diagnostic morphologic criteria have been challenging, mainly because of the lack of an easy-to-use criterium enabling differentiation of LVNC patients from normal subjects and other disease entities. As a consequence, currently four different echocardiography-based classification schemes have been proposed (Chin et al., Jenni et al., Stollberger et al., Belanger et al.), potentially leading to confusion and

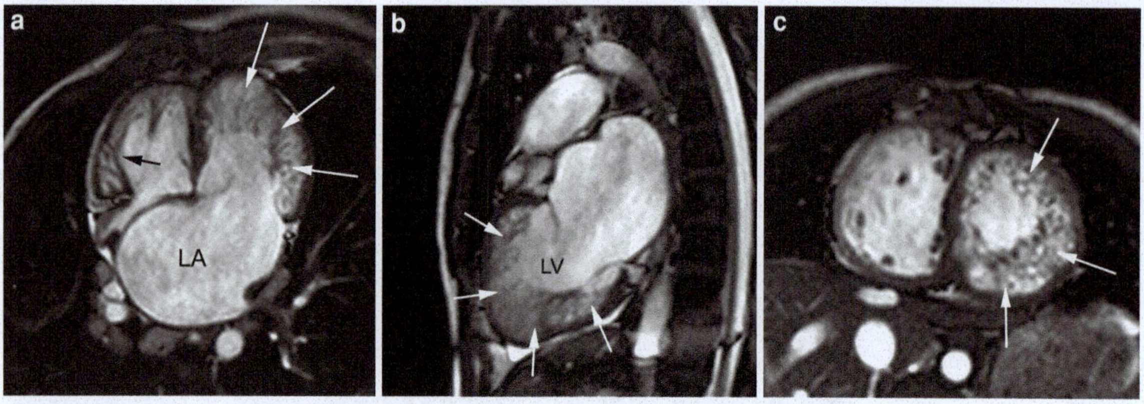

Fig. 38 LVNC in a 26-year-old man. Cine imaging in horizontal long-axis (**a**), vertical long-axis (**b**), and short-axis (**c**). Very prominent trabecular network (*white arrows*) along the entire LV lateral wall and LV apex. Thinning of the compacta of the LV lateral wall. Also in the RV, a prominent network is visible (*black arrow*). Note important dilation of the left atrium (LA)

disagreement (Belanger et al. 2008; Captur and Nihoyannopoulos 2010). In brief, these criteria take into account the two-layered appearance of the myocardial wall, the ratio of non-compacted to compacted myocardium (NC/C ratio), the number of visible trabeculations apically to the papillary muscles, and the presence of deep intertrabecular spaces visualized on color Doppler imaging. In a recent study by Kohli et al. it was shown that these diagnostic criteria are likely to be too sensitive, with up to one-fourth of heart failure patients and 8% of control sujects fulfilling one or more criteria for LVNC (Kohli et al. 2008; Anderson 2008). Other papers, including MRI findings, in contrast, suggest that the echocardiographic criteria might be too strict, and that techniques such as MRI may enhance detection of more subtle forms of LVNC (McCrohon et al. 2002; Borreguero et al. 2004; Pignatelli et al. 2003). The superior spatial and contrast resolution of MRI makes this technique intrinsically appealing for detection of LVNC. The location and extent of the trabecular network, and the thickness of the trabeculations and compacta can be well visualized using a combination of cine MRI in different cardiac imaging planes (Fig. 3). These sequences, moreover, allow the impact of morphologic abnormalities on regional and global function to be assessed.

Late Gd imaging may reveal underlying myocardial pathology such as replacement fibrosis (Dodd et al. 2008; Alsaileek et al. 2008; Nucifora et al. 2011) (Fig. 40). In 2005b, Petersen et al. established MRI criteria using an NC/C ratio similar to Jenni et al. and Chen et al. A ratio >2.3 in diastole distinguished LVNC from normals, athletes, and a series of cardiac diseases with a sensitivity and specificity of 86 and 99%, respectively (Petersen et al. 2005b). Jacquier et al. (2010) quantified the trabeculated LV mass. The percentage of trabeculated LV mass in controls was 12 $\pm$ 5 versus 32 $\pm$ 10% in LVNC patients. A trabeculated LV mass value >20% predicted the diagnosis of LVNC with a sensitivity and specificity of 94 and 94%, respectively. Though promising, the applicability of the above MRI criteria in daily clinical practice needs further confirmation, as reliable calculation of trabecular mass may be challenging and time-consuming. Finally, in recent work by Dawson et al. (2011), data were provided regarding normal age- and gender values for segmental thicknesses of the non-compacted ('trabecular') and compacted layer at end diastole and end systole. These data will be of great help in interpreting MRI studies performed patients with suspected LVNC.

In summary, our knowledge regarding this enigmatic disease is increasing, though there are many unanswered questions (Oechslin and Jenni 2011) (Fig. 41). The advent of novel techniques such as MRI will definitely help in better understanding the phenotypic expression and in determining accurate diagnostic and prognostic criteria.

4.6 Inflammatory Cardiomyopathy or Myocarditis

Myocarditis, or inflammatory cardiomyopathy, is defined as an inflammatory infiltrate of the

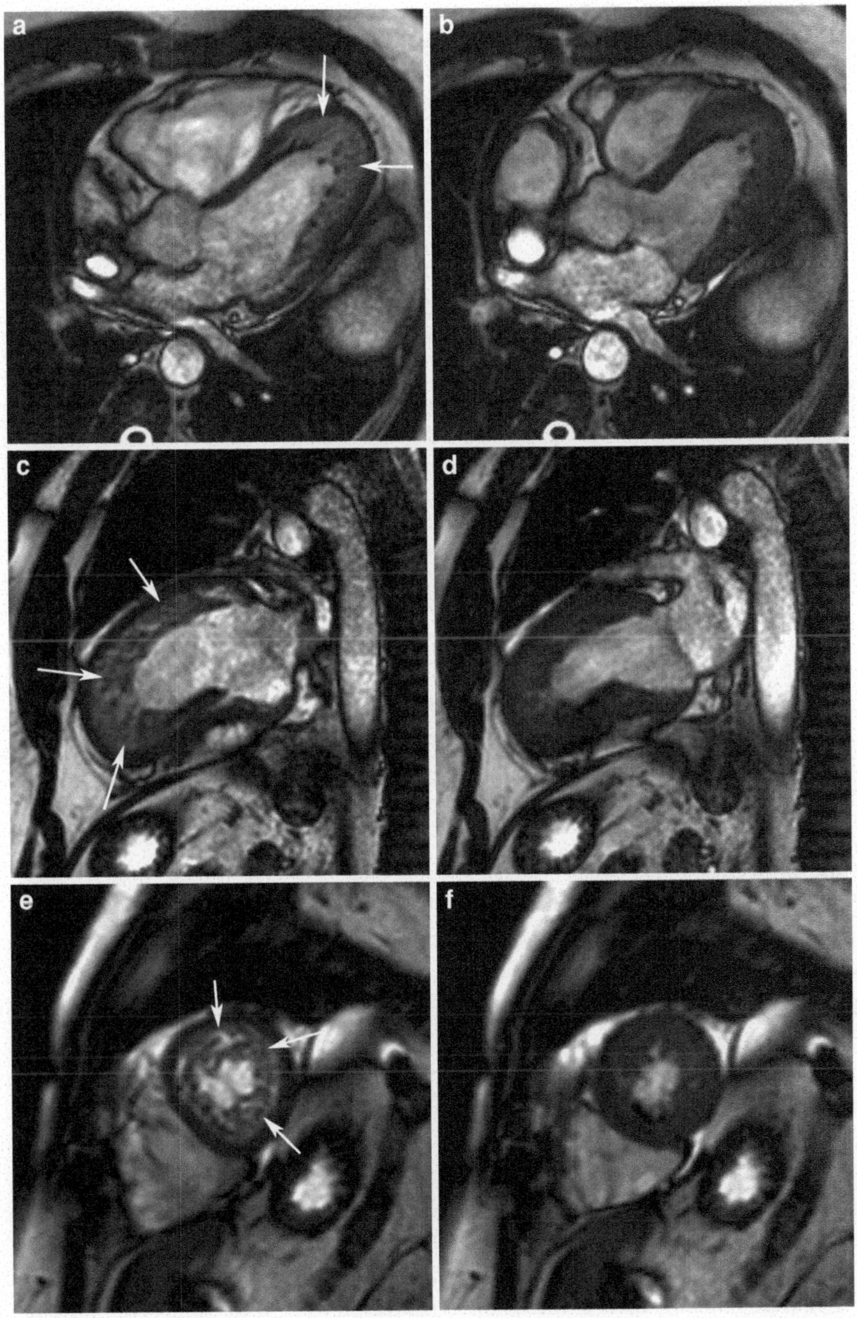

Fig. 39 LVNC in combination with Ebstein's disease in a 55-year-old man. Cine imaging in horizontal long-axis, (**a**, **b**), vertical long-axis (**c**, **d**), and short-axis (**e**, **f**), end-diastolic (*left*) and end-systolic (*right*) time frames. Note the prominent trabecular network mainly in LV apex (*arrows*). Presence of an obliquely oriented tricuspid valve with apically implanted septal papillary muscle (abnormalities well visible on dynamic viewing)

myocardium with necrosis or degeneration of adjacent myocytes, not typical of CAD-related ischemic damage (Aretz et al. 1986). Myocarditis may be isolated or part of a systemic disorder. Infectious disease is the major cause, but myocarditis may also be triggered by (auto)-immune reactions and pharmacological agents and transplant rejection. Though virtually any infectious agent may cause myocarditis, the majority of cases in recent years are linked to parvovirus B19 and human herpesvirus 6 infection, while coxsackie B and adenovirus associated myocarditis has become rare (Mahrholdt et al. 2006; Cooper 2009). It is important to note that myocarditis may occur concomitantly with other cardiomyopathies, in particular a

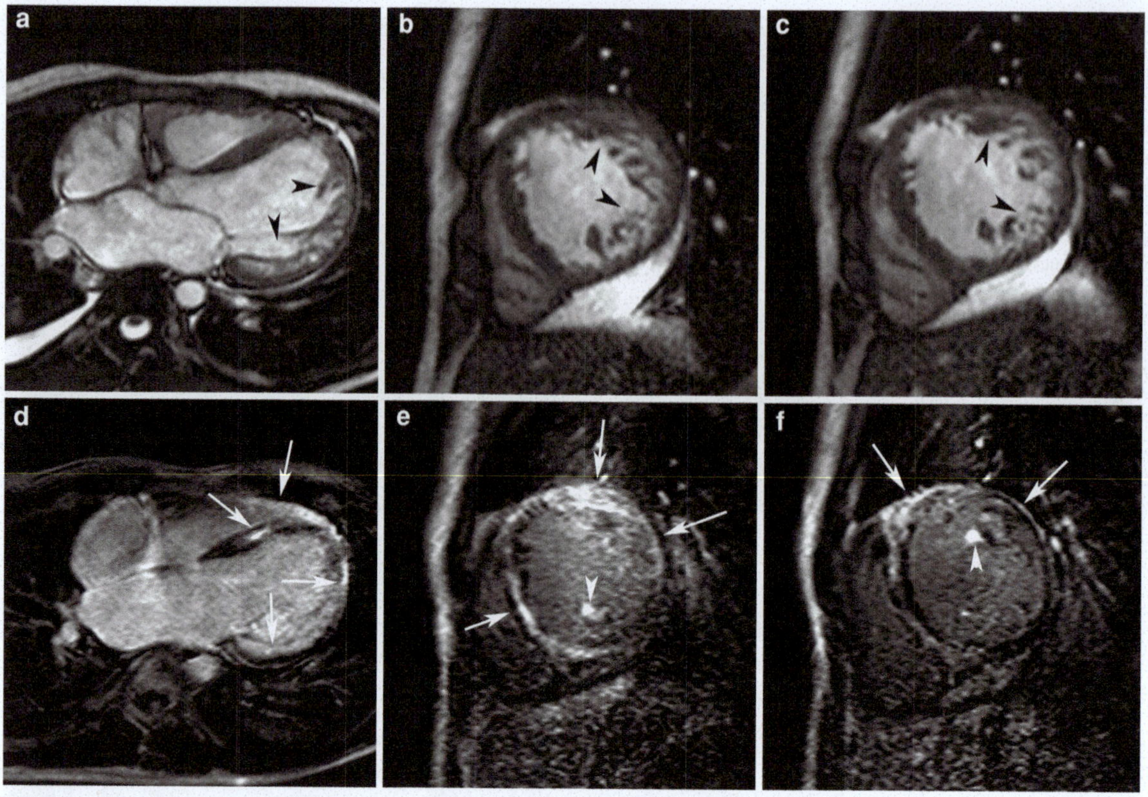

Fig. 40 Myocardial fibrosis in LVNC in a 24-year-old man. Cine imaging in horizontal long-axis (**a**), and short-axis (**b**, **c**). Late Gd imaging in horizontal long-axis (**d**) and short-axis (**e**, **f**). Presence of prominent trabeculations along the LV lateral wall (*arrowheads*, **a–c**). Following contrast administration multiple areas of enhancement are seen, in LV anterior wall, midwall of septum, papillary muscles, and RV free wall (*arrows*, **d–f**)

high percentage of ARVC/D patients show associated myocarditis (Cooper 2009).

Myocarditis is an insidious disease with a varied clinical presentation. Although the clinical course of myocarditis is usually benign with spontaneous recovery, approximately 5–10% of patients will progress toward DCM and ultimately may need a cardiac transplantation. Moreover, it is estimated that myocarditis is the underlying cause of SCD in adults <40 years of age in about 20% of cases (Feldman and McNamara 2000). Early recognition of myocarditis is often hampered by lack of specific symptoms at initial presentation (Lieberman et al. 1991). One should consider the possibility of myocarditis in patients showing an "acute coronary syndrome"-like presentation with normal coronary arteries, and increased serum cardiac biomarkers (Mahrholdt et al. 2006; Assomull et al. 2007; Yelgec et al. 2007). It was found that chest pain symptoms are caused by coronary spasm and are related to parvovirus B19 infection (Yilmaz et al. 2008a).

Patients usually follow a benign course, with normal or only mildly dilated ventricles, and often a normal LV function. A second distinct form of clinical presentation is that of subacute, new-onset congestive heart failure, which is associated with herpes 6 or combined parvovirus B19/herpes 6 virus infections (Mahrholdt et al. 2006). These patients usually show more severe LV dilatation and dysfunction, with only half of the patients improving during follow-up. A third presentation is malaise with signs of flu-like syndrome with fever and arthralgia. Patients with chronic persistent myocarditis usually show no ventricular dysfunction despite foci of myocyte necrosis.

The diagnosis of myocarditis is challenging, in particular due to the insensitivity of most traditional diagnostic tests (Cooper 2009). The ECG may show non-specific findings such as ventricular arrhythmias or heart block, ST elevation (mimicking acute myocardial infarction), or changes similar to pericarditis.

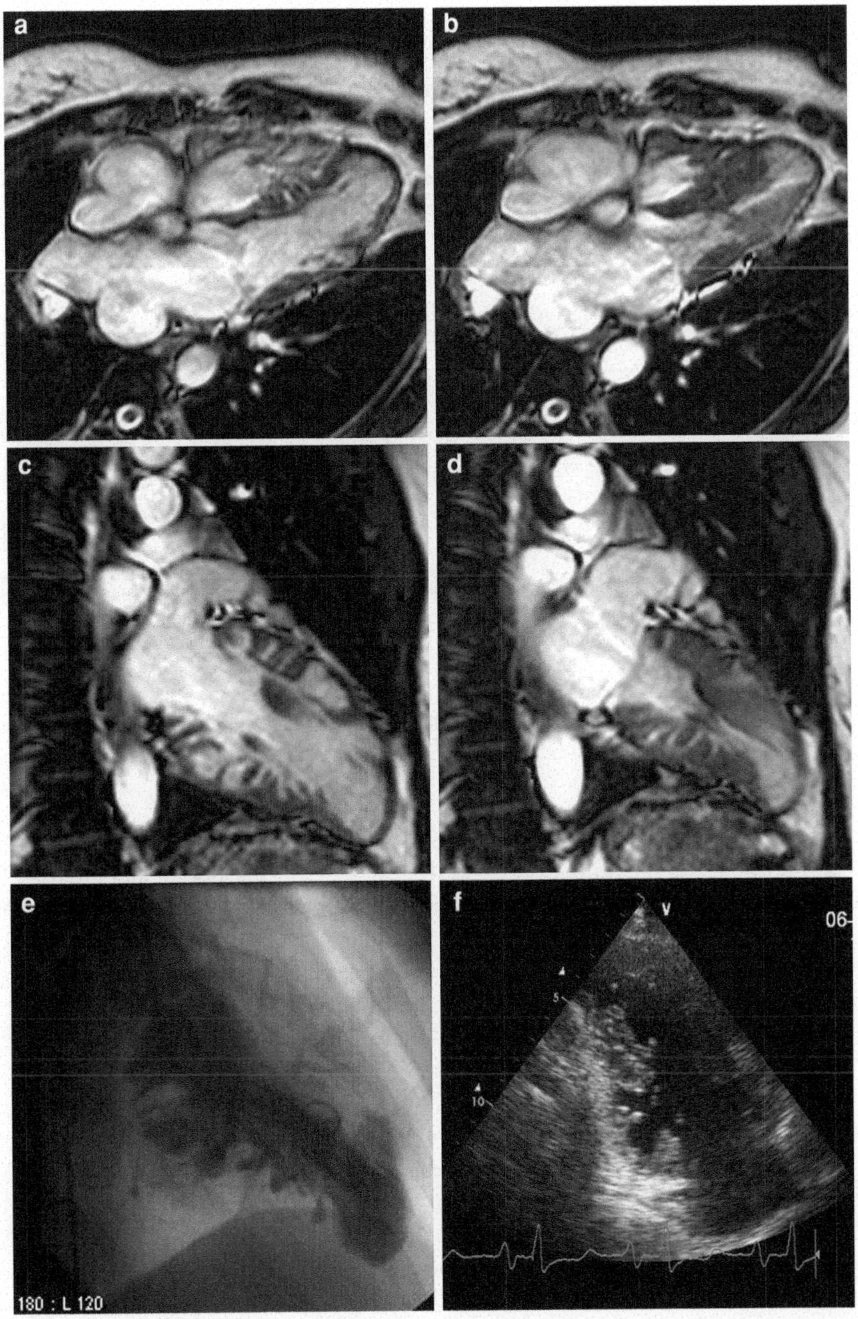

Fig. 41 Extreme form of LVNC, saw-tooth cardiomyopathy, or atypical presentation of HCM in a 49-year-old woman. Cine imaging in horizontal (**a**, **b**) and vertical long-axis (**c**, **d**), end-diastolic view (**a**, **c**), end-systolic view (**b**, **d**). Contrast ventriculography, vertical long-axis view (**e**), and echocardiography, long-axis view (**f**). Presence of diffuse saw-tooth like indentations in LV and RV with very thin compacta and thick compactions. Though this case was diagnosed as LVNC, the MRI questions whether it is actually an unclassified, novel form of cardiomyopathy, such as saw-tooth cardiomyopathy (Davlouros et al. 2009)

Echocardiography is of limited value in the diagnosis of myocarditis, and is primarily used to rule out other causes of heart failure. Laboratory tests may show leukocytosis, elevated sedimentation rate, eosinophilia, and elevated serum cardiac biomarkers (Smith et al. 1997). Endomyocardial biopsy, using the histopathological (Dallas) or immunohistological criteria, is used to depict myocardial inflammation, myocytolysis, and viral genome detection (Kindermann et al. 2008), and is indicated in patients with unexplained, new-onset heart failure, and in those who do not have response to usual treatment within 1 or 2 weeks to rule out fulminant or giant-cell myocarditis (Cooper et al. 2007). Though safe in experienced hands, EMB is prone to sampling error with a relatively low sensitivity and negative predictive

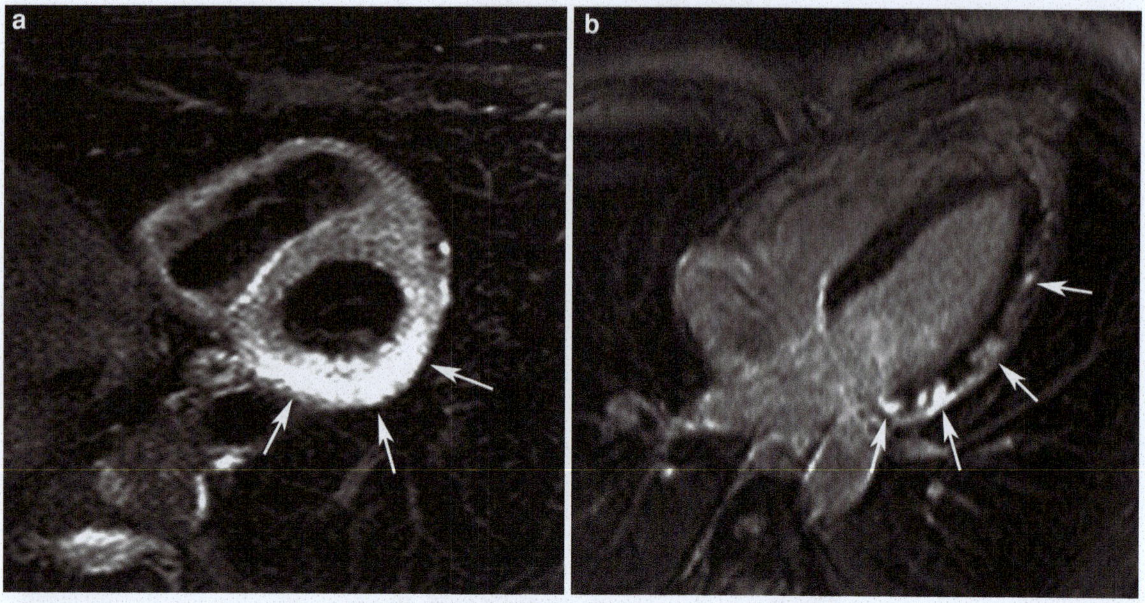

Fig. 42 Acute myocarditis in a 48-year-old man, presenting with acute dyspnea and chest pain, showing increased Troponin I levels (7.4 μg/L), ST-elevations in V4–V6, I, II, aVL, and normal coronary arteries on coronary angiography. Short-axis T2w-imaging (**a**) and horizontal long-axis late Gd imaging (**b**). T2w-imaging shows myocardial edema in infero- lateral wall of the LV (*arrows*, **a**), while late Gd maging shows several subepicardial foci of myocardial enhancement along the lateral wall (*arrows*, **b**) with some associated pericardial enhancement

value, but a high positive predictive value (Feldman and McNamara 2000; Yilmaz et al. 2010).

Since the first publications in the early 1990s, there is now substantial evidence that MRI is an important tool in the diagnosis of myocarditis, offering the clinician valuable information that cannot be achieved by EMB (Gagliardi et al. 1991; Friedrich et al. 1998; Mahrholdt et al. 2004, 2005, 2006; Abdel-Aty et al. 2005; Cooper 2009; Zagrosek et al. 2009; Yilmaz et al. 2010). In a German registry, involving 11,040 patients from 20 centers, myocarditis/cardiomyopathies was the most important indication (32%) for a cardiac MRI study (Bruder et al. 2009). An expert panel has recently established recommendations including indications for MRI in patients with suspected myocarditis, MRI protocol standards and diagnostic MRI criteria for myocarditis (i.e., "Lake Louise Criteria") (Friedrich et al. 2009). In brief, a comprehensive MRI examination should provide information on: (a) cardiac and pericardial morphology, (b) ventricular volumes, function and mass, and (c) myocardial tissue characterization (myocardial edema, hyperemia-capillary leakage, myocardial necrosis—fibrosis). To achieve these goals, a combination of cine MRI, T2w-imaging, T1w-imaging before and after contrast administration, and late Gd imaging is recommended. This approach provides a useful tool to monitor reversible and irreversible myocardial tissue injury over the course of myocarditis, to differentiate acute from healed myocarditis, to depict concomitant pericardial effusion and pericarditis, and to evaluate functional consequences of improvement/deterioration over time.

Myocardial edema, caused by lymphocyte infiltrate, is visible on T2w-imaging as bright myocardium, and represents reversibly/irreversibly damaged myocardium (Fig. 42). Whereas focal edema is generally depicted without difficulty, global edema is more challenging to diagnose. The proposed strategy is to compare myocardial signal intensity (SI) on T2w-imaging with SI of a skeletal muscle. A ratio SI-myocardium/SI-skeletal muscle ('edema ratio') >1.9 is suspecious of diffuse myocardial edema (Abdel-Aty et al. 2005) (Fig. 43). However, in systemic inflammation with involvement of skeletal muscle this approach is of limited value. Moreover, it is questionable whether T2w-imaging is sensitive enough to depict myocarditis with less severe

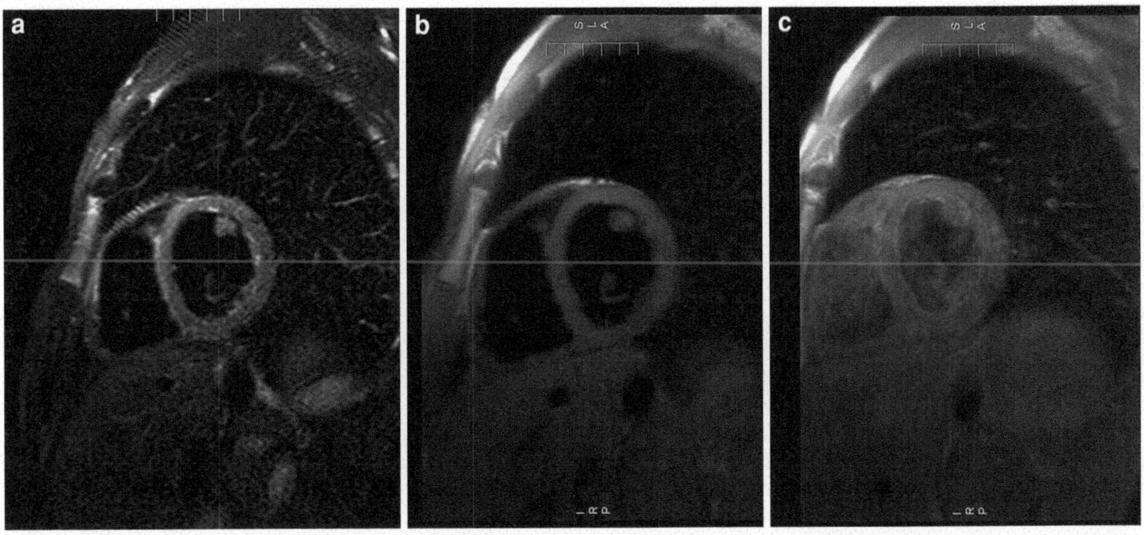

Fig. 43 MRI approach for depiction of global myocardial edema and myocardial hyperemia in acute myocarditis. Mid-ventricular short-axis T2w-imaging (**a**), T1w-imaging before (**b**), and early after (**c**) contrast administration. The difference in signal intensity between myocardial and skeletal muscle provides information regarding the presence of generalized myocardial edema (**a**), while the differences in contrast uptake between myocardial and skeletal muscle can be used to determine the degree of myocardial hyperemia (**b**, **c**)

inflammation (i.e., borderline myocarditis) (De Cobelli et al. 2006). To depict diffuse *myocardial hyperemia and capillary leakage* in the inflamed myocardium, the increased uptake of contrast agent during the early vascular phase is calculated using T1w-imaging, which is obtained by the ratio of the myocardial SI before and early (<3 min) post-contrast administration, and compared to that of skeletal muscle (global relative enhancement ratio). A ratio >4 (1.5T GE scanner) >5 (1.5T Siemens scanner) is concordant with myocardial hyperemia and increased capillary leakage (Fig. 43) (Zagrosek et al. 2009). In patients with co-existent myositis, an absolute myocardial SI increase of 45% post-contrast can be used as threshold (Laissy et al. 2002). *Myocardial necrosis* (acute phase) *and fibrosis* (chronic phase) are shown on late Gd imaging. The enhancement pattern is typically non-ischemic, enabling rule out of acute myocardial infarction in patients presenting with "acute-coronary-syndrome"-like symptoms. Most frequently, the subepicardial part of the lateral free LV wall is involved, a pattern found in the majority of patients with parvovirus B19 (Mahrholdt et al. 2006) (Fig. 42). Not infrequently, the enhancement may extend to the adjacent pericardium ± a small pericardial effusion (Yelgec et al. 2007; Ong et al. 2011). The second most frequent pattern is midwall enhancement of the interventricular septum (Fig. 44), and seems to be frequently associated with human herpes 6 virus genome. Other locations are the inferolateral and anteroseptal LV walls. The enhancement may be multifocal or diffuse in distribution. Functionally, wall motion is usually mildly to moderate impaired in the regions showing myocardial edema/enhancement.

A combined use of all three tissue-based MRI parameters for tissue characterization increases the diagnostic accuracy in acute and chronic myocarditis (Abdel-Aty et al. 2005; Gutberlet et al. 2008). Moreover, a diagnostic synergy can be achieved using a combined MRI and EMB approach, thereby overcoming some limitations when these techniques are individually applied (Baccouche et al. 2009). Though initially stated that EMB directed toward the areas of myocardial enhancement increased diagnostic accuracy (Mahrholdt et al. 2004), this was not confirmed in a recent large patient study, most likely because the enhanced areas do not necessarily reflect active/chronic inflammation (Yilmaz et al. 2010). Follow-up studies in acute myocarditis patients show a reversal of the myocardial edema ratio and global relative enhancement ratio that is paralleled by a significant

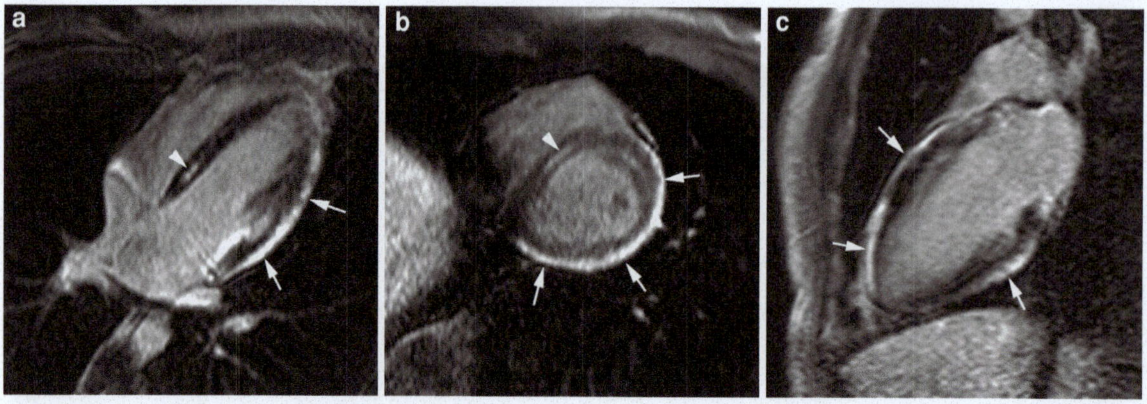

Fig. 44 Myocarditis in a 22-year-old man presenting with arrhythmias. Late Gd imaging in horizontal long-axis (**a**), short-axis (**b**), and vertical long-axis (**c**). Besides strong subepicardial myocardial enhancement in the anterior-lateral and inferior LV wall (*arrows*), focal midwall enhancement is shown in the basal part of the ventricular septum (*arrowhead*, **a**, **b**)

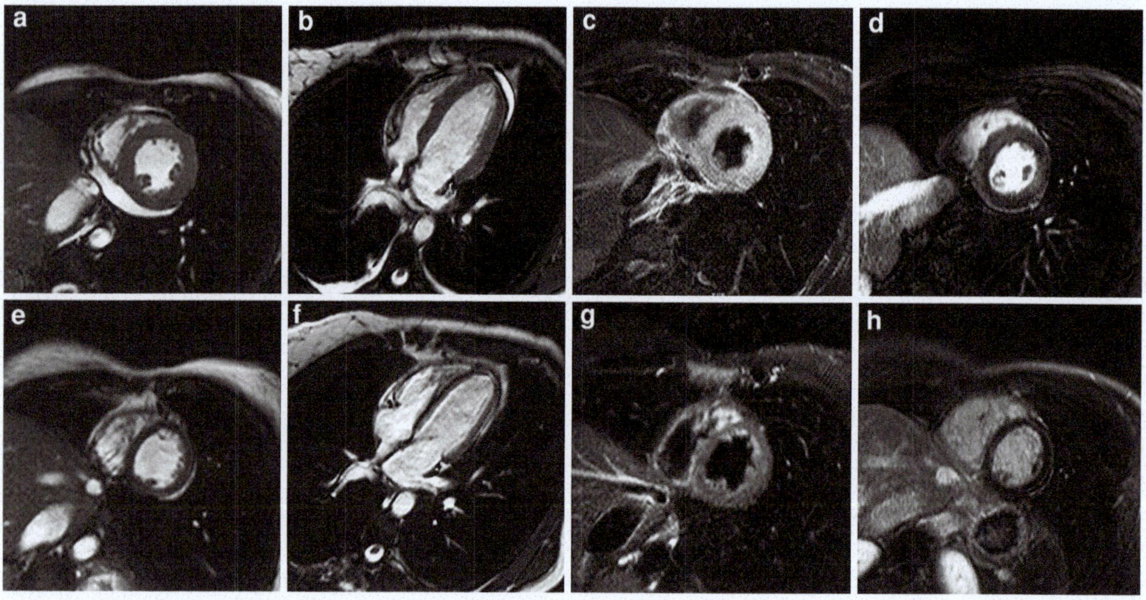

Fig. 45 Severe, acute myocarditis in a 41-year-old woman with follow-up MRI study 10 months later. Cine imaging in cardiac short-axis (**a**, **e**) and horizontal long-axis (**b**, **f**). T2w-imaging (**c**, **g**) and late Gd imaging (**d**, **h**) in cardiac short-axis. *Upper row*, MRI during acute phase; *lower row*, follow-up MRI. The most prominent finding in the acute phase is the edematously thickened myocardial wall (wall thickness 13 mm), showing high signal intensity on T2w-imaging (**c**), some inhomogeneous enhancement (**d**), and the presence of a mild pericardial effusion. Decreased LV function (EF: 42%). At follow-up, the myocardial edema has completely resolved (**g**), wall thicknesses have normalized (wall thickness 8 mm), LV function normalized (EF: 67%), and the pericardial effusion has disappeared. Late Gd imaging shows some mild enhancement subepicardially in LV lateral wall, and in midwall of the ventricular septum

decrease in LV mass and improvement in LV ejection fraction (Zagrosek et al. 2008, 2009) (Fig. 45). In most patients, the abnormal myocardial enhancement persists at follow-up, reflecting irreversible damage, though the spatial extent significantly decreases (Fig. 46) (Mahrholdt et al. 2004; Zagrosek et al. 2009). In patients with suspected chronic myocarditis, increased edema ratio and global relative enhancement ratio reflects myocardial inflammation whereas abnormal myocardial enhancement yields

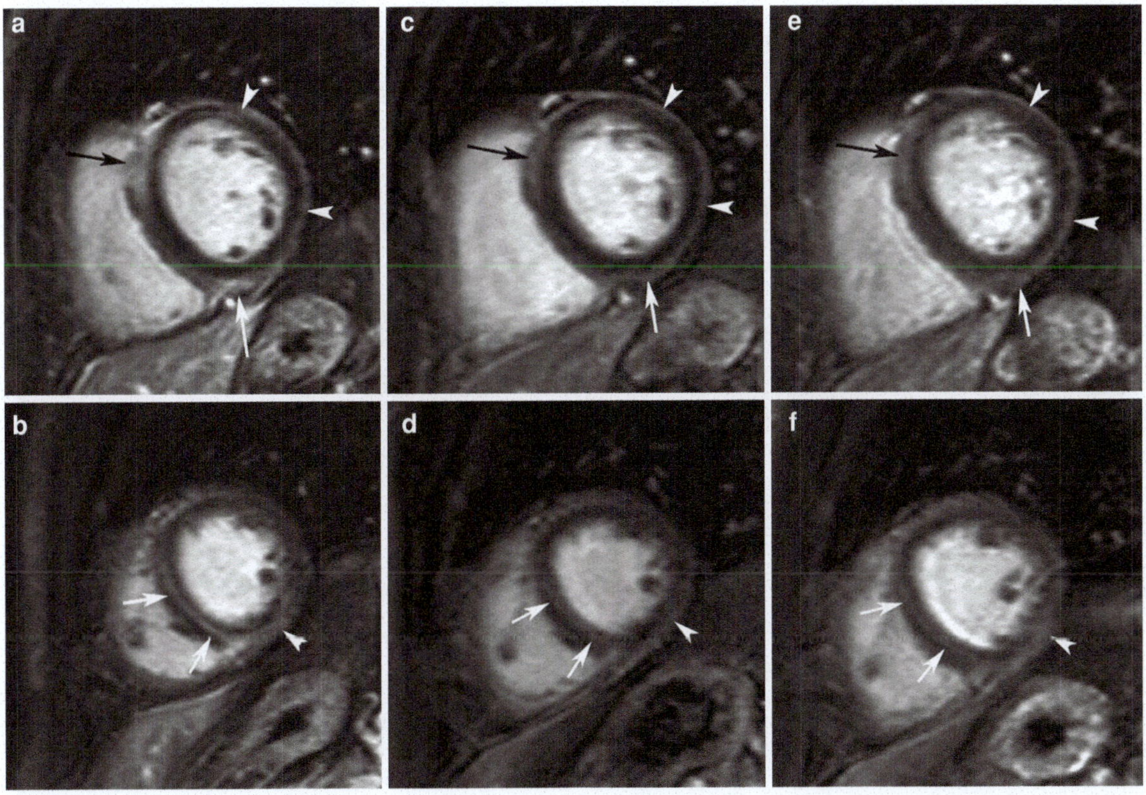

Fig. 46 Acute myocarditis in a 45-year-old man. Short-axis late Gd imaging at admission (**a**, **b**), at 1 month (**c**, **d**) and at 9 months (**e**, **f**). The evolution of time of the areas of late enhancement can be well appreciated. While LV function completely normalized over time (improvement EF from 40 to 67%), the areas of myocardial enhancement persist, though the extent and intensity of enhancement decreases

low sensitivity and accuracy (Gutberlet et al. 2008). Improved techniques for tissue characterization such as T1 and T2 mapping are needed to further improve diagnostic accuracy.

Lyme disease is caused by the spirochete *Borrelia burgdorferi*, and is characterized by a multisystem disorder primarily affecting the skin, joints, heart, and central nervous system (Nathwani et al. 1990). The most common cardiac manifestation of Lyme disease is transient atrioventricular block due to direct affects on the conduction system. Other manifestations such as rhythm disturbances, myopericarditis, and heart failure are less common (van der Linde 1991). The cardiac manifestations are usually self-limiting, though it has been suggested that *B. burgdorferi* may be associated with, or even play an etiological role in, the development of DCM (Stanek et al. 2004). MRI abnormalities of Lyme carditis include myopericarditis with myocardial wall thickening and myocardial enhancement, the presence of mild to moderate pericardial effusion, and regional and/or global ventricular dysfunction (Bergler et al. 1993; Globits et al. 1994; Munk et al. 2007; Naik et al. 2008).

Chagas' Disease (American trypanosomiasis) caused by Trypanosoma cruzi is endemic in Latin America, where it is one of the leading causes of death (WHO Expert Committee 1984). Cardiac involvement is crucial in the patient's prognosis, presenting as lymphocytic myocarditis with several degrees of myocardial fibrosis. Patients present with severely impaired LV function and refractory heart failure, or have episodes of sustained ventricular tachycardia without severe LV dysfunction (Bellotti et al. 1996). Contrast-enhanced MRI is helpful in depicting areas of myocardial inflammation and fibrosis (Kalil-Filho and de Albuquerque 1995; Bellotti et al. 1996). The pattern of enhancement is non-ischemic involving the mid-wall and subepicardial part of the apical and basal inferolateral LV wall segments (Rochitte et al. 2007). The patient's

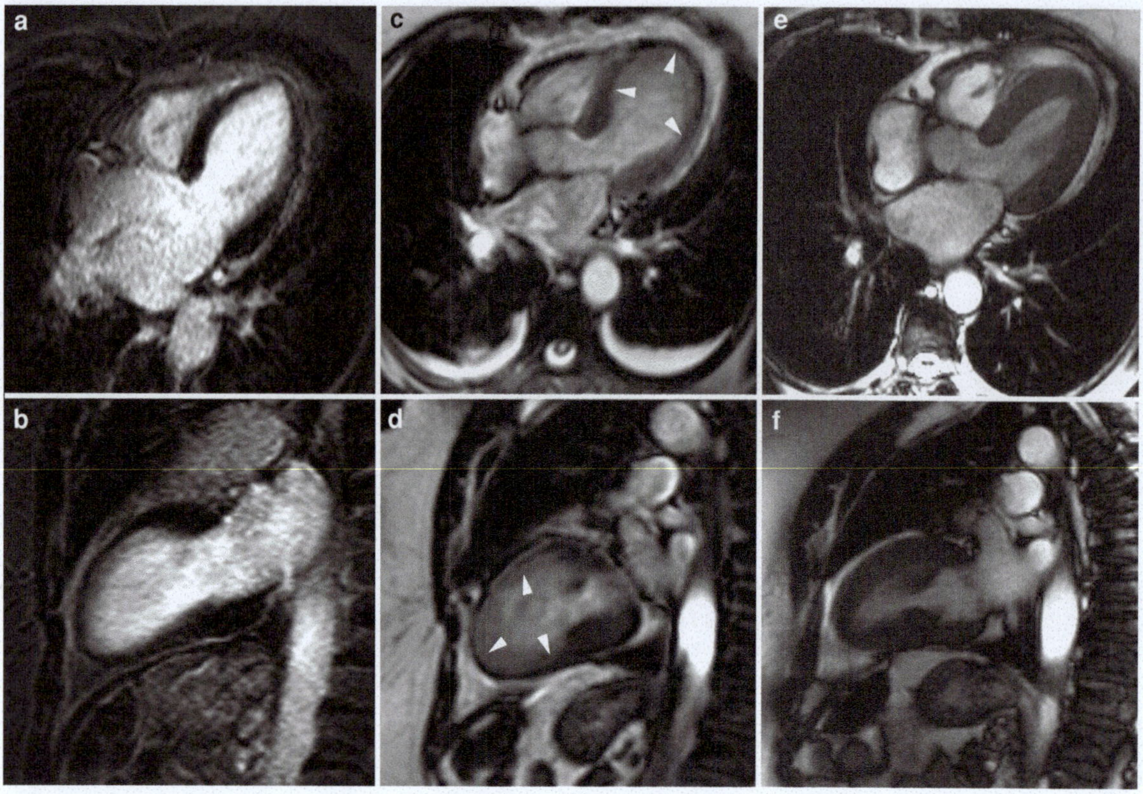

Fig. 47 Apical ballooning in a 60-year-old woman after a (non-traumatic) car accident. The patient complained of interscapular chest pain, and soon developed pulmonary edema and severe LV dysfunction. On cardiac catheterization normal coronary arteries were found. Late Gd imaging in vertical long-axis (**a**) and horizontal long-axis plane (**b**). Cine imaging (end-systolic frame) at admission (**c**, **d**) and 3 weeks later (**e**, **f**). No evidence of myocardial infarction on late Gd imaging (nor at follow-up MRI). Bulging and akinesia of the apical half of the LV (*arrowheads*, **c**, **d**), with profound reduction in LV function (EF: 32%). Note also the presence of bilateral pleural effusion (**c**). Three weeks later, the LV has regained its normal configuration, and regional and global function are completely normalized. The pleural effusion has disappeared

"geographic" history may be of importance in the diagnosis of this condition (Marcu et al. 2007).

4.7 Stress Cardiomyopathy or Tako-Tsubo Cardiomyopathy

Tako-Tsubo cardiomyopathy, also called *stress cardiomyopathy*, *transient LV apical ballooning*, or *apical ballooning syndrome* represents a reversible LV dysfunction with acute myocardial infarction-like ST-segment elevation without coronary artery lesions and with minimal myocardial enzymatic release (Tsukihashi et al. 2001; Abe and Kondo 2002; Abe et al. 2003; Desmet et al. 2003). The typical presentation is apical LV akinesia causing "apical ballooning" with preserved function (or even hypercontractility) in the basal segments. Supportive treatment leads to spontaneous recovery in nearly all patients, and the prognosis is excellent (Prasad et al. 2008) (Fig. 47). The finding of left ventriculography in the acute phase corresponds to a "*tako-tsubo*", which in Japanese means an octopus fishing pot with a round bottom and a narrow neck. Another descriptive name for this entity is "*ampulla cardiomyopathy*". Recently, several variants of stress cardiomyopathy, such as transient mid-ventricular ballooning syndrome—"inverted Tako-Tsubo", transient apical-sparing cardiomyopathy and RV Tako-Tsubo cardiomyopathy, have been described suggesting that this stress-related cardiac dysfunction does not exclusively affect the LV apex, but may involve other parts of the LV as well as the RV (Haghi et al. 2006;

Hurst et al. 2006; Syed et al. 2008; Bulut et al. 2009; Eitel et al. 2011).

The clinical course may closely resemble acute myocardial infarction, acute coronary syndrome, or acute myocarditis. Emotional and physical stresses are the most frequent precipitating factors; and this disorder preferentially affects elderly woman (Desmet et al. 2003; Abe et al. 2003; Sharkey et al. 2005). At present, the causal relation between stress and this syndrome has not been clarified. Several hypotheses have been presented, ranging from spasms of the epicardial coronary arteries, over stress-related impairment of the coronary microcirculation, to catecholamine-related cardiotoxicity with activation of cardiac adrenoreceptors (Ako et al. 2002; Akashi et al. 2002; Tsukihashi et al. 2001; Ueyama et al. 2002; Galiuto et al. 2010). In some patients catecholamine-producing neuroendocrine tumors (pheochromocytoma) may cause a stress-like cardiomyopathy (de Souza et al. 2008). This reversible LV dysfunction in stress cardiomyopathy can be considered as an atypical presentation of myocardial stunning. Although myocardial stunning is usually observed in ischemic heart disease (Braunwald and Kloner 1982), and is accompanied by a coronary event with segmental dysfunction, the reversible dysfunction in "tako-tsubo" cardiomyopathy is not limited to a specific coronary artery territory, but involves the apical part of the LV and not infrequently also the RV apex (Syed et al. 2008).

Although most cases of "tako-tsubo" cardiomyopathy are described on the left ventriculography during cardiac catheterization, MRI is appealing in the diagnosis and follow-up of this infrequent myocardial disorder. The apical ballooning and dysfunction, as well as the functional recovery, can be well demonstrated on long-axis, cine MRI (Figs. 45 and 47). MRI is of particular interest to differentiate this entity from acute myocarditis or acute myocardial infarction (Eitel et al. 2008). Typically, these patients show no evidence of myocardial damage on late Gd imaging, but often show signs of myocardial edema on T2w-imaging, and increased global myocardial enhancement in the dysfunctional apical region indicative of inflammation (Eitel et al. 2010, 2011; Stensaeth et al. 2010). Finally, MRI can be used to depict the presence of an extra-adrenal pheochromocytoma as cause of stress cardiomyopathy.

4.8 Peripartum Cardiomyopathy

Peripartum cardiomyopathy is defined as LV dysfunction and symptoms of heart failure that develop between 1-month antepartum and 5-months postpartum, and is characterized by myocardial inflammation with or without concomitant pericarditis. The precise etiology of this myocardial disorder is unknown, but possible mechanisms include: myocarditis, an abnormal immune response to pregnancy, a maladaptive process to the hemodynamics of pregnancy, and prolonged tocolysis (Sliwa et al. 2006). Presentation is similar to that of patients with DCM, and is mainly one of exclusion of other causes. The patients have a high risk for venous, arterial, and cardiac thrombus formation. About half of the patients with peripartum cardiomyopathy recover without complications. The prognosis is poor in patients with persistent cardiomyopathy (>6 months). A similar entity occurring early in pregnancy has recently been described, probably representing a continuum of a spectrum of the same disease (Elkayam et al. 2005). Pregnancy-associated cardiomyopathy might be, therefore, a more appropriate term. MRI has a role in the assessment of ventricular function and functional recovery, to detect thrombus formation, and to rule out myocardial damage (Fig. 48). Since different pathophysiological mechanisms may be involved in peripartum cardiomyopathy, edema imaging and late Gd imaging may reveal patterns of both inflammatory and non-inflammatory cardiomyopathy (Baruteau et al. 2010). Since only a limited number of studies are available, larger scale studies are needed to better determine the contribution of MRI for diagnosis and prognosis.

4.9 Tachycardia-Induced Cardiomyopathy

Prolonged cardiac tachyarrhythmias of atrial or ventricular origin can cause reversible cardiomyopathy characterized by LV dilatation and reduced ejection fraction. In contrast to patients with idiopathic DCM, tachycardia treatment by control of rhythm or rate leads to a complete or partial improvement of cardiac function and reversed ventricular remodeling (Fig. 49) (Huffman et al. 2010). An MRI examination can provide valuable information regarding

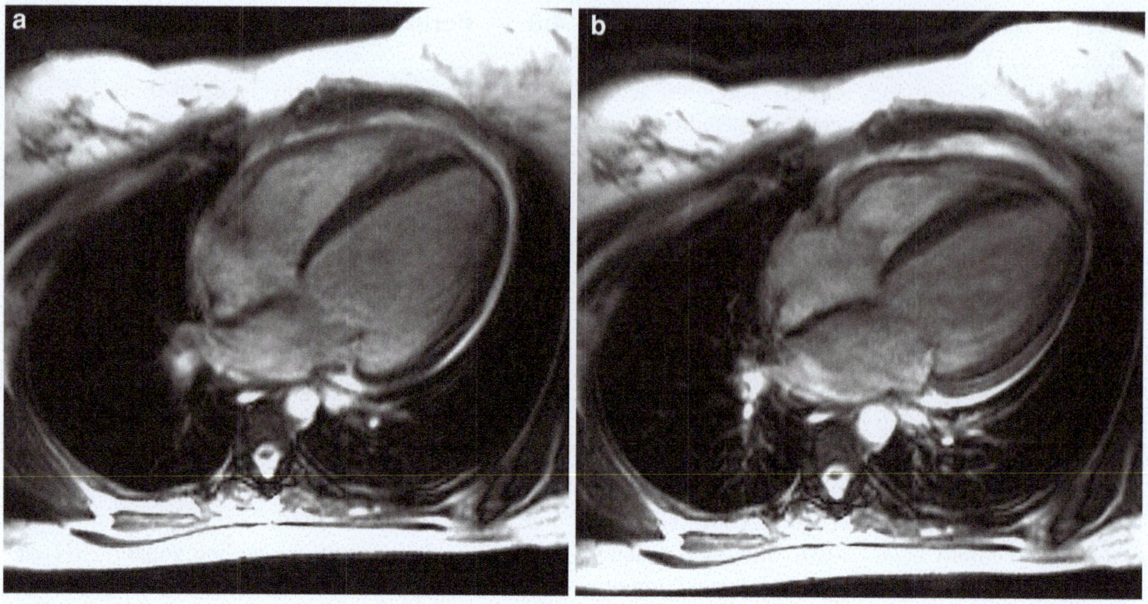

Fig. 48 Peripartum cardiomyopathy in a 29-year-old woman, one month post childbirth presenting with cardiac failure. Horizontal long-axis cine imaging, at end diastole (**a**) and end systole (**b**). Dilated left ventricle with severely compromised LV function (EF: 19%). No evidence of myocardial damage on late Gd imaging (not shown)

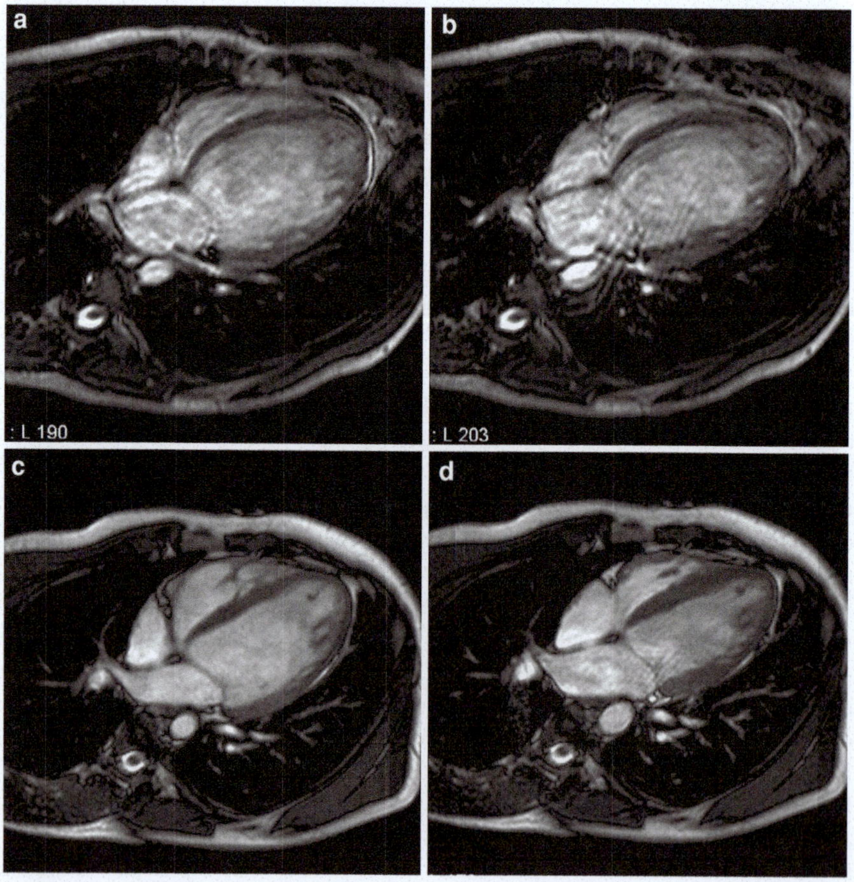

Fig. 49 Tachycardia-induced cardiomyopathy in a 25-year-old man with continuous runs of atrial tachycardia (160/min). Cine imaging before (**a**, **b**), and 9 months following successful ablation (**c**, **d**). End-diastolic (**a**, **c**) and end-systolic (**b**, **d**) time frames. Severe LV dilation (EDV: 504 ml) and systolic dysfunction (EF: 9%) before ablation, with severe motion artifacts due to arrhythmias. Reversed LV remodeling post-ablation with decrease in LV EDV (236 ml) and significant improvement in LV EF (49%)

ventricular volumes and function, depict (ir)reversible myocardial damage, and visualize associated findings such as atrial appendage thrombus formation in patients with atrial arrhythmias.

5 Secondary Cardiomyopathies

5.1 Infiltrative and Storage Disease

5.1.1 Amyloid Heart Disease

Amyloidosis is an uncommon systemic disorder characterized by the extracellular deposition of amyloid in one or more organs. Cardiac deposition, leading to infiltrative cardiomyopathy/RCM ('amyloidotic cardiomyopathy'), is a common feature of amyloidosis, and it is the presence and severity of cardiac involvement that drives the prognosis (Rahman et al. 2004; Falk and Dubrey 2010). Cardiac involvement may be the presenting feature of the disease, or may be discovered while investigating a patient presenting with non-cardiac amyloidosis. The predominant manifestation is diastolic heart failure due to myocardial infiltration, but in patients with involvement of intramyocardial vessels symptoms of chronic myocardial ischemia may be the presenting complaint. Congo red staining is the recognized technique to histologically depict amyloid. New biochemical staining techniques enable further differentiation among the various types of amyloid, such as the AL (light chain), the hereditary transthyretin-related form (ATTRm), and wild-type (non-mutant) transthyretin-related amyloidosis (ATTRwt) systemic "senile" type, and secondary forms of systemic amyloidosis. Rarely, the amyloid deposition may exclusively affect the atria (isolated atrial amyloid type). Although the therapeutic means are still limited and the treatment is generally unsatisfactory, the diagnosis is important to exclude potentially curable conditions that it may mimic.

Nowadays, diagnosis and treatment are targeted toward an earlier depiction of cardiac amyloid deposition with determination of the type of amyloid, aiming to improve patient prognosis. In recent work by Rapezzi et al. (2009), it was shown that amyloidotic cardiomyopathies should be considered as separate entities depending on the type of amyloidosis. For instance, AL cardiac amyloidosis was associated with only mild increases in wall thickness, but these patients had a high frequency of hemodynamic derangement, while the ATTRwt and ATTRm types had markedly increased wall thickness, but less frequently hemodynamic alternations.

Though a high index of suspicion is still required, the diagnosis of cardiac amyloid disease has definitely benefited from the availability of non-invasive cardiac imaging techniques, in particular MRI, which is generally recognized as a very promising diagnostic modality. Deposition of amyloid fibrils in myocardial tissue and valve leaflets typically causes a thickening of ventricular and atrial walls and valve leaflets. The ventricular cavities have a normal or reduced size, while the atria are usually enlarged due to the diastolic dysfunction and/or valvular dysfunction due to amyloid deposition. Pleural and pericardial effusions are not infrequently seen. A severe concentric hypertrophy of both normal-sized ventricles in the absence of arterial hypertension or valvular heart disease is suspicious for amyloidosis (Fig. 50). Cardiac amyloidosis may present as asymmetric septal hypertrophy hereby mimicking HCM.

Functionally, cardiac amyloid disease predominantly causes diastolic dysfunction characterized by abnormal relaxation and restrictive inflow physiology, while measures of global systolic function (i.e., ejection fraction) are only decreased late in the disease. However, measures of strain and strain rate have shown an early impairment of longitudinal contraction, reflecting subendocardial systolic dysfunction, hence stressing that it is likely a misnomer to consider cardiac amyloidosis as purely affecting diastolic function (Koyama et al. 2003; Falk and Dubrey 2010).

Cardiac MRI offers the clinician an excellent tool to get a detailed view on the above-described morphological and functional abnormalities in cardiac amyloidosis, to differentiate cardiac amyloidosis from other disease entities having a similar clinical presentation, to depict concomitant findings such as thrombus formation, pericardial and pleural effusion, and to depict patients with increased risk of death (Melacini et al. 2010). In analogy with other ischemic and non-ischemic myocardial diseases, late Gd imaging is highly appealing for improved tissue characterization in amyloid heart disease. The pattern of myocardial enhancement seems primarily determined by the distribution and severity of amyloid deposition (Fig. 51) (Maceira et al. 2005; Vogelsberg

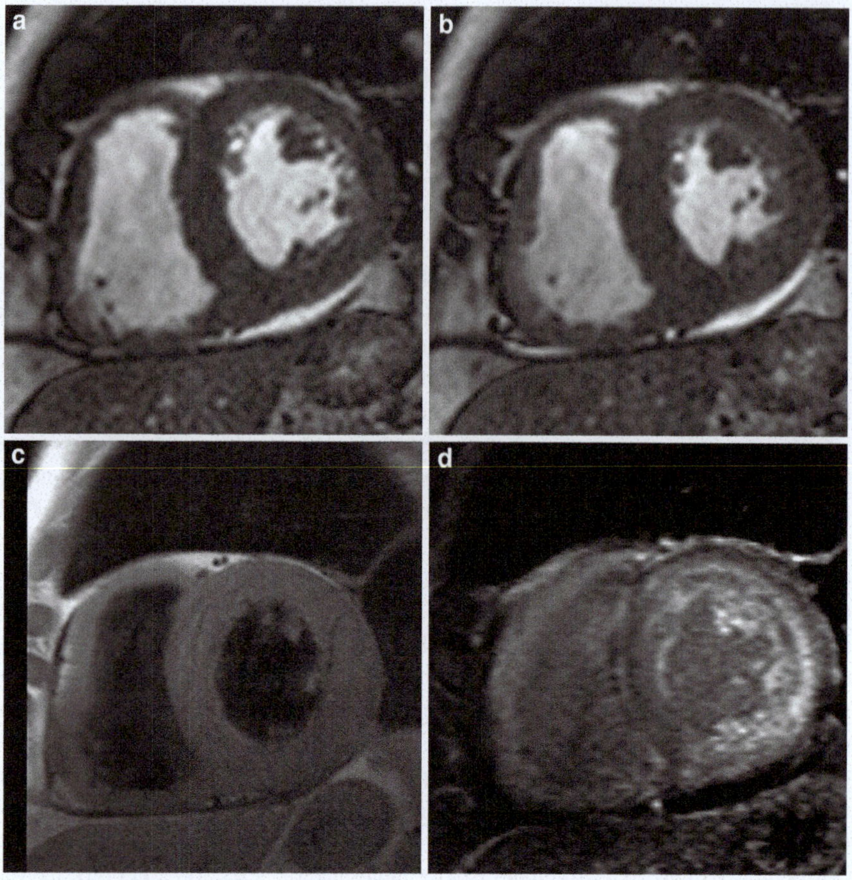

Fig. 50 Cardiac amyloidosis in a 67-year-old man. Cine imaging at end diastole (**a**) and end systole (**b**). T1w-imaging (**c**) and late Gd imaging (**d**). All images acquired in mid-ventricular short-axis. Important biventricular hypertrophy with severely reduced function (LV EF: 25%, RV EF: 26%). While the myocardial signal is homogeneous on T1w-imaging, strong inhomogeneous enhancement is seen on late Gd imaging mainly involving the anterior, lateral and inferior segments

et al. 2008; Syed et al. 2010). The latter causes an increase of the extracellular space altering the myocardial contrast kinetics. Though the initial studies showed an enhancement pattern extensively involving the myocardium, preferential involvement of the subendocardium of both ventricles hereby creates a zebra enhancement pattern (Maceira et al. 2005; Van Geluwe et al. 2006; Vogelsberg et al. 2008), involvement of the midwall and subepicardium, creating a diffuse homogeneous or heterogeneous myocardial enhancement not limited to the LV but enhancement of right ventricle and atria is increasingly reported (Fig. 52) (Syed et al. 2010). The latter enhancement pattern is typically found in ATTRm patients (Di Bella et al. 2010). Patchy focal enhancement is infrequently found, but may be related to less advanced stages presenting normal wall thicknesses. Furthermore, it should be noted that in some patients on late Gd imaging the ventricular cavities may appear relatively dark with a myocardium that remains bright using the normal range of inversion times (suboptimal myocardial nulling) (Syed et al. 2010). If the administration as well as the dosage of gadolinium is correctly performed, this pattern should immediately raise the suspicion of cardiac amyloidosis, especially in the presence of other signs of cardiac amyloidosis such as myocardial hypertrophy. The pattern can be explained by altered gadolinium kinetics in the blood and myocardium, i.e., diffuse myocardial enhancement in combination with increased clearance of gadolinium from the blood pool, providing small differences in T1-relaxation time between blood and myocardium (Maceira et al. 2005). Although late Gd imaging findings are strongly associated with clinical, morphological, functional, and biochemical markers of prognosis, it is currently unclear whether myocardial enhancement on late Gd imaging is an independent predictor of patient prognosis, emphasizing the need for larger patient studies including patients with less extensive cardiac involvement as well (Maceira et al. 2008b; Austin et al. 2009; Ruberg et al. 2009; Migrino et al.

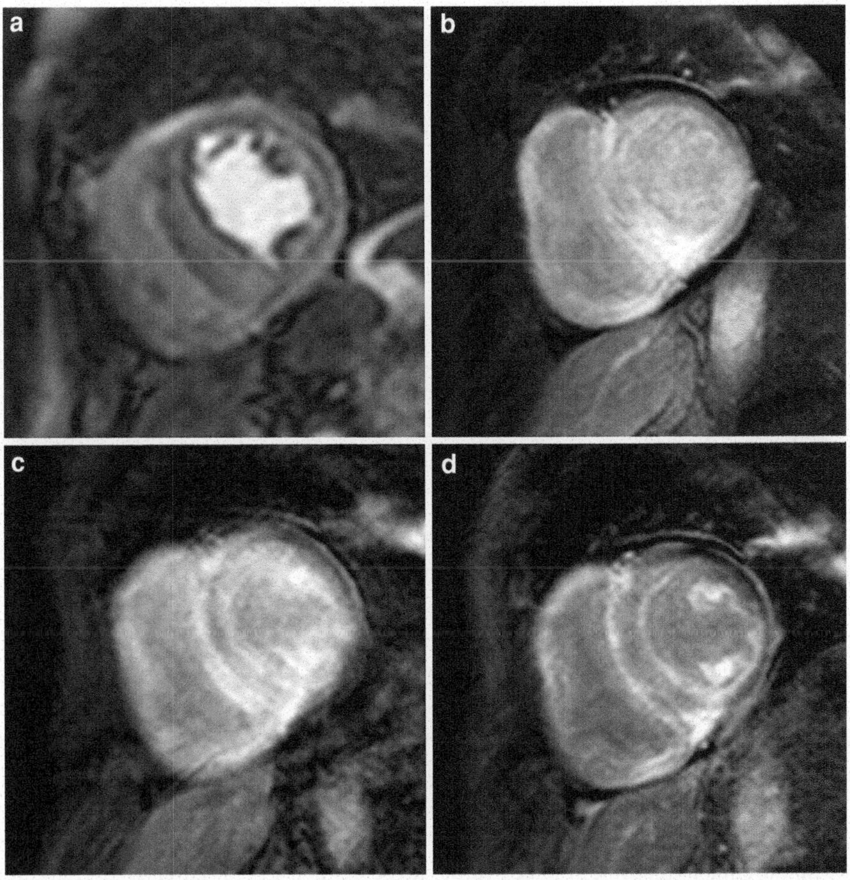

Fig. 51 Cardiac amyloidosis in a 70-year-old man. Time-related changes in myocardial enhancement. Perfusion imaging (**a**), late Gd imaging at 5,10, and 15 min following contrast administration (images **b**, **c**, and **d**, respectively). Strong inhomogeneous myocardial enhancement is present becoming preferentially subendocardially and subepicardially located in the LV and RV as well as in both papillary muscles at later imaging (**d**). Courtesy of Ilse Crevits, MD, Roeselare, Belgium

2009; Mekinian et al. 2010; Syed et al. 2010). Although some patterns have been associated with early stages of cardiac amyloidosis (see above), the precise role of late Gd imaging in depicting mild forms of amyloid heart is not yet defined. Moreover, it is of interest to further explore the relation between the type of enhancement and type of amyloidosis (Di Bella et al. 2010). Finally, since a considerable number of amyloidosis patients have renal impairment, gadolinium administration may be contraindicated because of the risk of nephrogenic systemic sclerosis. Alternative approaches such as the use of T2w-imaging have shown not be useful in depicting myocardial amyloid deposition (Sparrow et al. 2009).

5.1.2 Iron Overload Cardiomyopathy

Iron overload cardiomyopathy or myocardial siderosis is defined as the presence of systolic or diastolic cardiac dysfunction secondary to increased deposition of iron in the heart independent from other concomitant processes (Liu and Olivieri 1994). Iron is an essential element needed for many metabolic and biological processes, but given that the body cannot actively excrete this metal, iron overload will result in accumulation in parenchymal organs causing damage (Gujja et al. 2010). It can result from primary or secondary hemochromatosis. Primary hemochromatosis is caused by specific gene mutations involved in iron metabolism leading to increased gastrointestinal absorption, and usually presents late in life. Secondary hemochromatosis usually occurs in patients requiring chronic blood transfusion, such as thalassemia, sickle cell anemia, with red cell transfusion starting at a young age. Myocardial iron load is positively correlated with the number of blood units given (Lesnefsky et al. 1992; Jensen et al. 2001). Other conditions in which iron overload may occur in body organs include chronic alcoholic disease and chronic hemodialysis.

Recognition and intervention in an early stage of the disease is important, but very challenging because most patients are initially asymptomatic while patients presenting with heart failure complaints may be refractory

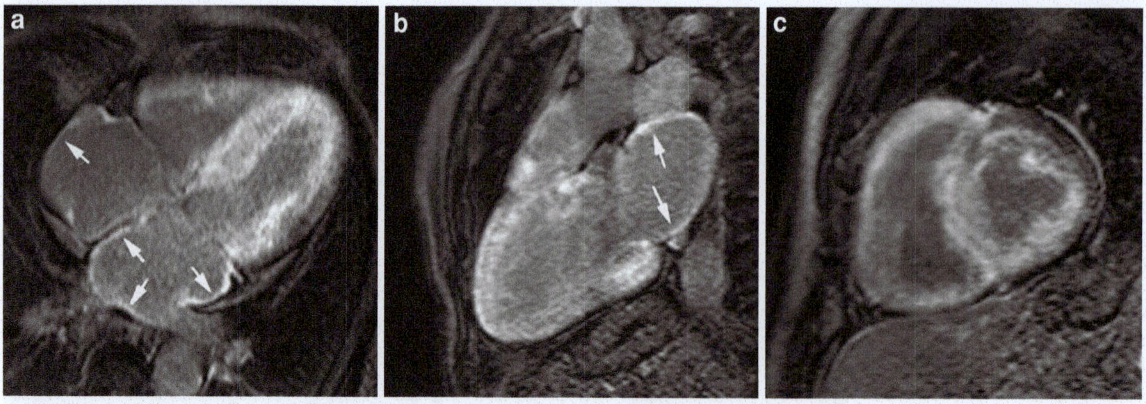

Fig. 52 Cardiac amyloidosis (senile type) in a 75-year-old man. Late Gd imaging in horizontal (**a**), vertical (**b**) long-axis, and cardiac short-axis (**c**). Strong myocardial enhancement is seen in both ventricles mainly subendocardially, as well in both atria (*arrows*, **a**, **b**). Courtesy of Ilse Crevits, MD, Roeselare, Belgium

to treatment. Timely chelation therapy may delay or prevent the occurrence of toxic DCM. Though EMB enables deciption and quantification of the amount of myocardial iron deposition, the iron deposition tends to be patchy and thus biopsies may miss the areas of deposition providing a false negative result. Also, it is invasive procedure, and as a consequence, not useful as tool for screening asymptomatic patients (Gujja et al. 2010). Non-invasive cardiac imaging, such as echocardiography, has a limited value in screening patients for myocardial iron deposition. Myocardial wall thickness and end-diastolic chamber diameter may be mildly increased. Diastolic dysfunction showing a restrictive physiology usually precedes systolic dysfunction (Benson et al. 1989). Ventricular dilatation and dysfunction usually do not appear until the iron concentration reaches a critical level, but then there is often a rapid deterioration in cardiac function. Abnormal wall motion, such as reduced longitudinal shortening, detectable with tissue Doppler echocardiography, precedes global ventricular dysfunction, enabling depiction of iron deposition at an earlier stage, but the abnormalities are not specific for this disorder (Vogel et al. 2003).

MRI is currently the only available non-invasive method with the potential to identify the presence of iron in the heart, to quantify the myocardial iron load, and to monitor iron chelation therapy (Chan et al. 1992; Jensen et al. 2003; Tanner et al. 2007). Moreover, because myocardial iron deposition is not related to deposition in other organs, organ-specific measurements are indispensable (Anderson et al. 2001).

The presence of iron disturbs the magnetic field homogeneity and thereby shortens tissue T2 relaxation time (Stark et al. 1985; Hardy and Henkelman 1989): the higher the iron content, the shorter the T2 relaxation time. Where earlier studies used SE sequences for quantitative evaluation of the iron content, nowadays breath-hold multi-echo gradient-echo sequences are used to calculate the T2* (T2star) of the myocardium (Anderson et al. 2001; Westwood et al. 2003a, b). The number of echoes used may vary, but the principle remains the same. The idea is to image the myocardium with echo times with a different length, and measure the change in signal intensity across the echoes, a phenomenon called T2* decay. To derive T2*, an exponential trendline is fitted with an equation in the form $y = \text{Ke}^{-\text{TE/T2*}}$ where K represents a constant (Westwood et al. 2003a). Typically, a mid-ventricular short-axis slice is used for determining myocardial iron deposition, whereby myocardial T2* is calculated in a large region of the interventricular septum, excluding regions in the proximity of the coronary veins and lungs because of the risk of susceptibility artifacts (Carpenter et al. 2011). In addition, liver T2* can be measured as well to determine liver iron load (Kirk et al. 2009). The technique is currently well validated showing a good reproducibility (also between different MRI vendors) (Westwood et al. 2003a, b; He et al. 2008). Normal values for myocardial T2* at 1.5 T field strength are 33.3 ± 7.8 ms, with a lower limits of 17.7 ms (mean—2SD). Similar normal values are reported for myocardial T2* at 3T, i.e., 33.3 ± 8.3 ms (Storey et al. 2007).

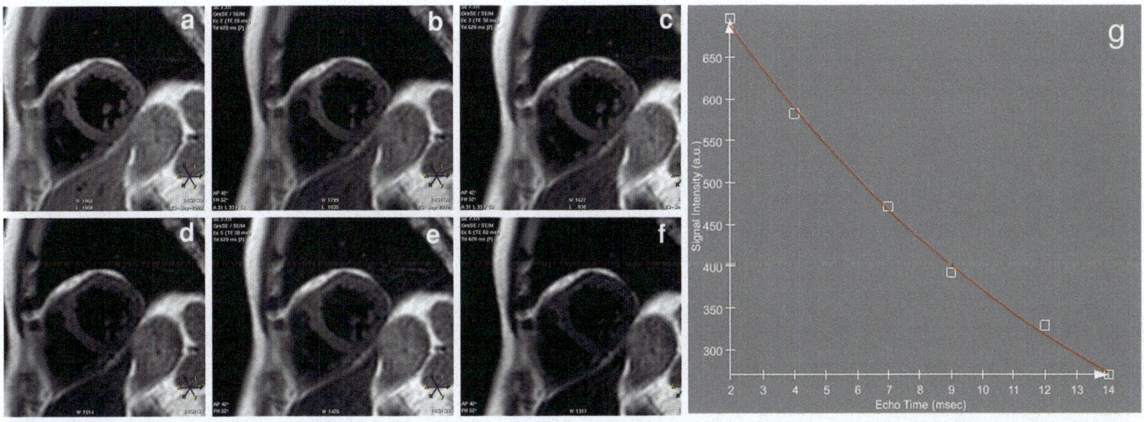

Fig. 53 Hereditary hemochromatosis in a 56-year-old man. T2* imaging using GRASE MRI with 6 echoes (**a–f**), and corresponding T2* map (**g**). The myocardial T2* was 13 ms (normal value at 1.5 Tesla: 33.3 ± 7.8 ms). The patient had no evidence of systolic nor diastolic dysfunction

In patients with myocardial iron overload, T2* values are typically <20 ms (range of clinical interest: 5–20 ms) (Fig. 53). Myocardial iron load measurements are usually combined with functional and volumetric MRI measures, to obtain information about ventricular volumes and mass as well as systolic and diastolic functional indices. The decline in T2* is inversely related with LV ejection fraction (Mavrogeni et al. 2009). Kirk et al. (2009) showed in a recent multicenter prospective study involving 652 thalassemia major patients that myocardial T2* identifies patients at high risk of heart failure and arrhythmia from myocardial siderosis, and this measurement is superior to other measures such as serum ferritin and liver iron. A myocardial T2* < 10 ms increases the risk of heart failure within the first year significantly, and the risk rises steeply with further reduction in T2* (i.e., <6 ms). Arrhythmias, mainly of atrial origin, occurred predominantly in patients with myocardial T2* < 20 ms. In summary, T2* MRI has marked potential to significantly reduce heart-failure-related death in transfusion dependent anemias using effective cardiac chelation therapy (Tanner et al. 2007; Kirk et al. 2009).

5.1.3 Glycogen and Other Metabolic Storage Diseases

Cardiac involvement in metabolic storage diseases such as type I or II glycogenosis, Anderson-Fabry, Gaucher and Neimann-Pick diseases, galactosialidosis, and mucopolysaccharidosis is common and represents an important cause of morbidity and mortality in these patients. The accumulation in cardiac structures leads to a variety of cardiac signs and symptoms, including LV hypertrophy, diastolic dysfunction, arrhythmias, ischemia due to small-vessel disease, and heart failure. The ventricular wall thickening may mimic other cardiac diseases such as HCM (Fig. 54). Though in clinical practice, echocardiography is the prime imaging modality, there is accumulating evidence that MRI is of interest in the diagnosis, differential diagnosis and evaluation of disease progression and enzyme-replacement therapy in storage diseases. Approximately 50% of Fabry patients show myocardial enhancement on late Gd imaging in the basal inferolateral LV wall, usually involving the mid and subepicardial part of the myocardial wall (Fig. 55) (non-ischemic pattern) (Moon et al. 2003b, c). Focal myocardial scarring causes the enhancement, which may be the substrate for arrhythmias and SCD (Moon et al. 2006). In terminal stage patients the basal inferolateral LV wall may show extensive thinning (Takenaka et al. 2008) and severely reduced regional function. Moreover, there is evidence that early disease recognization and initiation of enzyme-replacement therapy is associated with significant reduction in myocardial mass and improvement in myocardial function and exercise capacity, whereas mild to severe forms of myocardial fibrosis show no improvement (Beer et al. 2006; Weidemann et al. 2009).

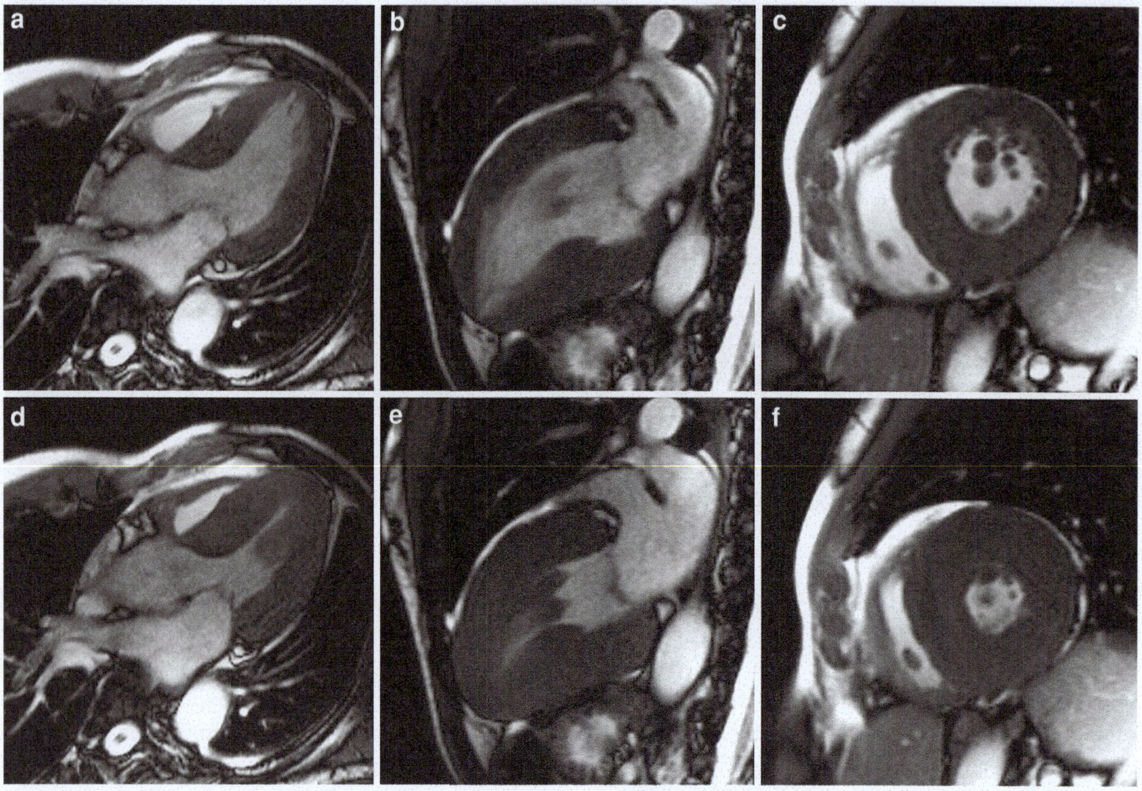

Fig. 54 Anderson-Fabry's disease in 46-year-old man. Cine imaging in horizontal long-axis (**a**, **d**), vertical long-axis (**b**, **e**), and short-axis (**c**, **f**). End-diastolic images *upper row*, end-systolic *lower row*. Severe concentric LV hypertrophy (LV mass: 315 g). Although global LV function is preserved, the regional function (wall thickening) is significantly impaired

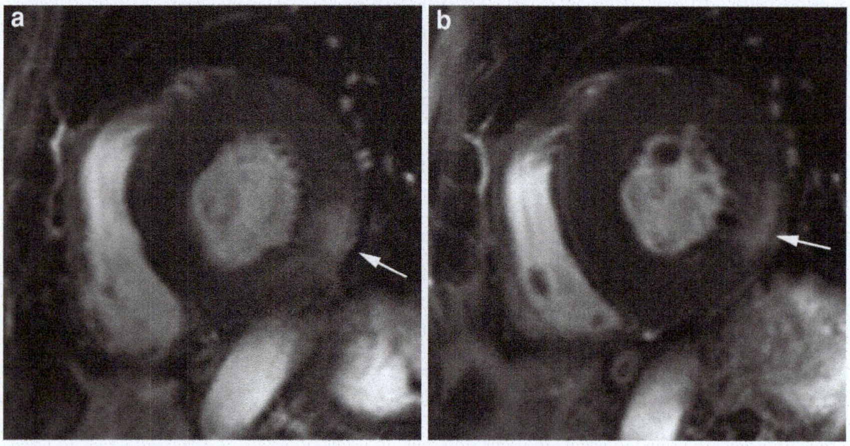

Fig. 55 Late Gd imaging in Anderson-Fabry's disease (same patient as 9.54). Two short-axis levels (**a**, **b**). Concentric LV hypertrophy with focal zone of late enhancement subepicardially in infero LV lateral wall (*arrow*)

5.2 Endomyocardial Disease

Endomyocardial disease is a common form of secondary restrictive cardiomyopathy, and includes Löffler endocarditis and endomyocardial fibrosis (Parrillo 1990). Although they were previously thought to be two variants of a single disease, these entities have not only a different geographical distribution, but also a different clinical presentation. *Löffler endocarditis* occurs in temperate countries, has

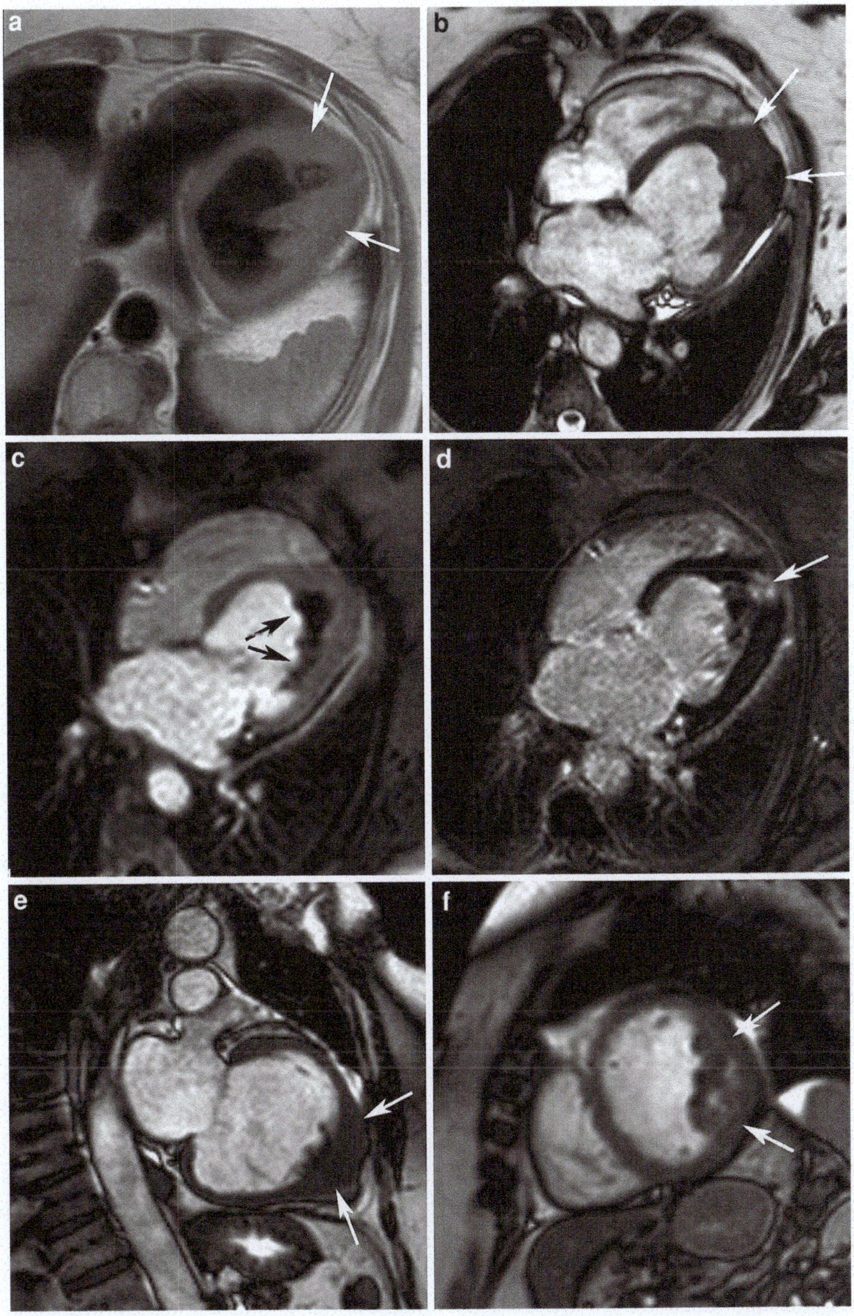

Fig. 56 Endomyocardial disease in 78-year-old woman. Horizontal long-axis T1w-imaging (**a**), cine imaging (**b**), first-pass perfusion imaging (**c**), late Gd imaging (**d**). Vertical long-axis cine imaging (**e**) and short-axis imaging (**f**). Important thickening of the LV apex obliterating the cavity (*arrows*, **a**, **b**, **e**). Large area of non-perfusion during first-pass imaging most likely representing thrombus formation (*arrows*, **c**), while on late Gd imaging area of enhancement visible in LV apex representing myocardial fibrosis (*arrow*, **d**). The papillary muscles seem to be involved in the inflammatory-fibrotic process (*arrows*, **f**). Courtesy of Ilse Crevits, MD, Roeselare, Belgium

a more aggressive and rapidly progressive course, and is related to hypereosinophilia, while *endomyocardial fibrosis* occurs most commonly in equatorial Africa and is not related to hypereosinophilia (Mocumbi et al. 2008). The restrictive pattern is caused by an intensive endocardial fibrotic wall thickening of the apex and subvalvular regions of one or both ventricles, which may cause an inflow obstruction to blood (Fig. 56). The underlying pathogenesis of Löffler endocarditis is complex and probably related to hypereosinophilia, with a toxic effect of eosinophils on the heart causing necrosis, endomyocarditis, and intramyocardial thrombus formation (Fig. 57) (Weller and Bubley 1994). In the later phase, localized or

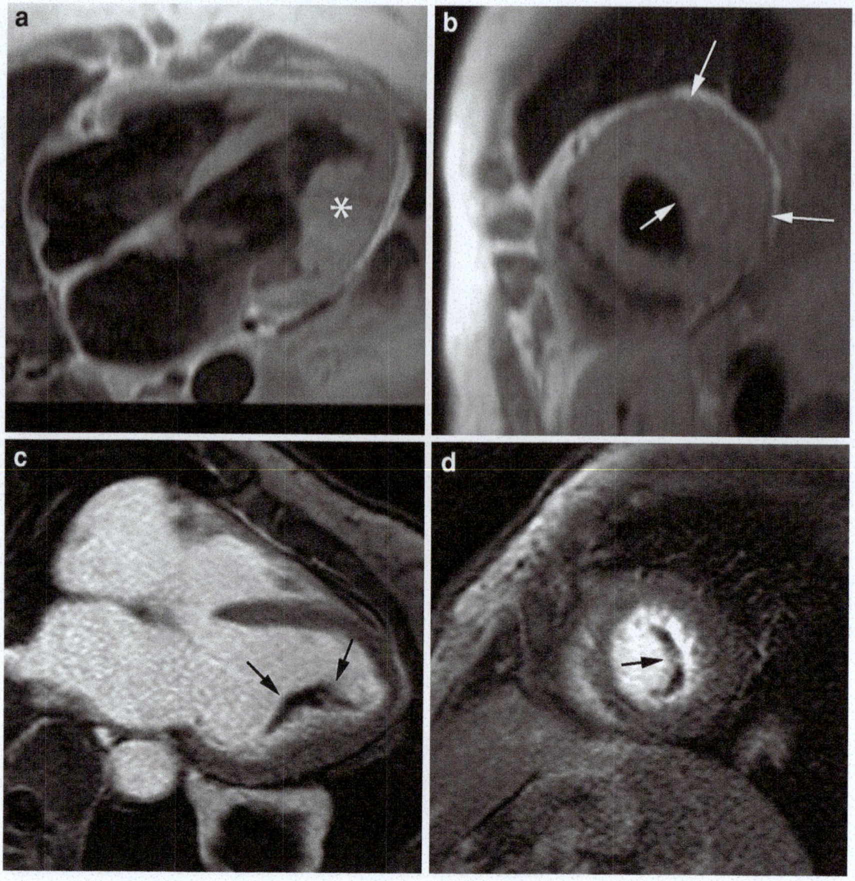

Fig. 57 Endomyocardial disease in 72-year-old woman with hypereosinophilia and restrictive filling pattern. T1w-imaging in horizontal long-axis and short-axis (**a**, **b**), late Gd imaging in horizontal long-axis and short-axis (**c**, **d**). T1w-imaging shows important thickening of the LV lateral wall (*, **a**)(*arrows*, **b**). Late Gd imaging nicely show the presence of a mural thrombus (*arrows*, **c**, **d**) adjacent to a mildly thickened lateral wall. Adapted from Bogaert et al. (2004)

extensive replacement fibrosis causes thickening and deformation of the ventricular wall. Atrioventricular valve regurgitation, as a result of progressive scarring of the chordae tendinae, may occur, with enlargement of the atria. The increased stiffness of the ventricles and the reduction of the ventricular cavity by organized thrombus cause a restrictive filling pattern. Recently, major and minor diagnostic (echocardiographic) criteria have been defined for endomyocardial fibrosis (Mocumbi et al. 2008). A comprehensive MRI approach enables depiction of the fibrous endocardial thickening, myocardial inflammation, apical or subvalvular obliteration, chordal deformation with valvular regurgitation, thrombus formation, and the restrictive physiology. Importantly, such an assessment is of high value for excluding entities such as apical hypertrophic cardiomyopathy, LV non-compaction cardiomyopathy, and liquefaction necrosis of the mitral valve (see Figs. 43 and 44) (D'Silva et al. 1992; Lombardi et al. 1995; Chandra et al. 1996b; Pitt et al. 1996; Huong et al. 1997; Di Bella et al. 2008; Coelho-Filho et al. 2010; Francone et al. 2010).

5.3 Toxicity (Substance Abuse, Recreational Drugs, Heavy Metals)

Cardiovascular complications of excessive use of ethanol, cocaine, and other recreational drugs, often in combination with cigarette smoking, have become an important cause of cardiovascular-related morbidity and mortality in young adults. Although an extensive discussion of these substances and their effects on the heart is beyond the scope of this chapter, in this section a brief description is provided about the cardiac side-effects of the most frequently-used recreational drugs.

Substance abuse should be considered in young patients presenting with chest pain. The role of cardiac imaging, including cardiovascular MRI, is to evaluate the impact of substance abuse on cardiac

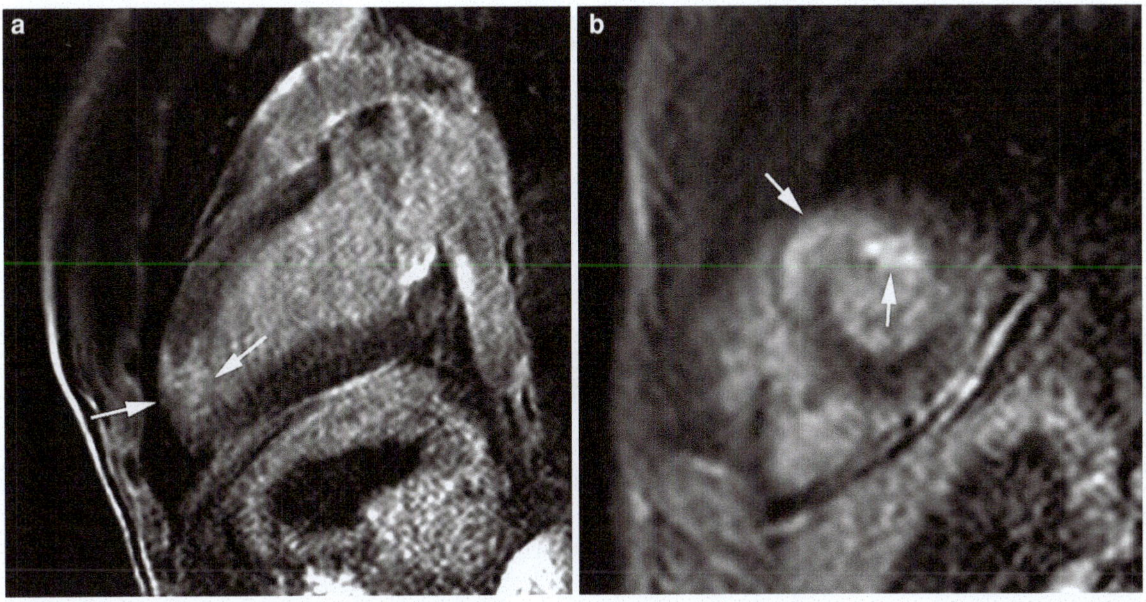

Fig. 58 Cocaine-induced or related myocardial damage (ischemia?, necrosis?, myocarditis?) in a 20-year-old man, who was admitted with ventricular tachycardia and fibrillation. The patient showed ST-segment abnormalities on ECG and elevated cardiac troponins. Late Gd imaging in the vertical long-axis (**a**) and short-axis (**b**) shows well-delineated, focal zone with abnormal transmural enhancement in LV apex (*arrows*)

morphology, ventricular and valvular function, to rule out structural myocardial damage (e.g., myocardial infarction and myocarditis), and to detect other complications such as endocarditis with abscess or pseudoaneurysm formation, and aortic dissection. The abuse of alcohol is associated with chronic cardiomyopathy, hypertension, and arrhythmia. Abstinence or using alcohol in moderation can reverse these cardiovascular problems (Awtry and Philippides 2010). Alcohol is also distinguished among the substances of abuse by having possible protective effects against CAD and stroke when used in moderate amounts.

Substance abuse with cocaine is associated with multiple cardiovascular conditions, including myocardial infarction, myocarditis, endocarditis, aortic dissection, LV hypertrophy, arrhythmias, sudden death, and cardiomyopathy (Kloner and Rezkalla 2003) (Fig. 45). Cocaine can potentiate the physiological actions of catecholamines and has direct effects on voltage-dependent sodium ion channels related to local anesthetic properties. The effects of cocaine can be augmented with concomitant alcohol consumption and cigarette smoking. Acute myocardial ischemia caused by cocaine may be related to in situ thrombosis and/or coronary vasospasm (Fig. 58).

Amphetamines (e.g., speed, ice and ecstasy) have many of the cardiovascular toxicities seen with cocaine, including acute and chronic cardiovascular diseases. Heroin and other opiates can cause arrhythmias and non-cardiac pulmonary edema, and may reduce cardiac output. Cardiovascular problems are less common with cannabis (marijuana) than with opiates, but major cognitive disorders may be seen with its chronic use. It is still controversial whether caffeine can cause hypertension and coronary artery disease, and questions have been raised about its safety in patients with heart failure and arrhythmia (Frishman et al. 2003a, b). Toxic metals, such as cadmium, arsenic, and lead may pose serious risks to human health and cause damage to the vascular system and be cardiotoxic (Kang 2003).

5.4 Cancer Treatment-Induced Cardiac Toxicity

With new anticancer therapies, many patients have an increased life expectancy. Treatment-related co-morbidities, in particular cardiac toxicity, have therefore become an issue for cancer survivors (Jurcut et al. 2008). Anthracyclines are highly potent cytotoxic

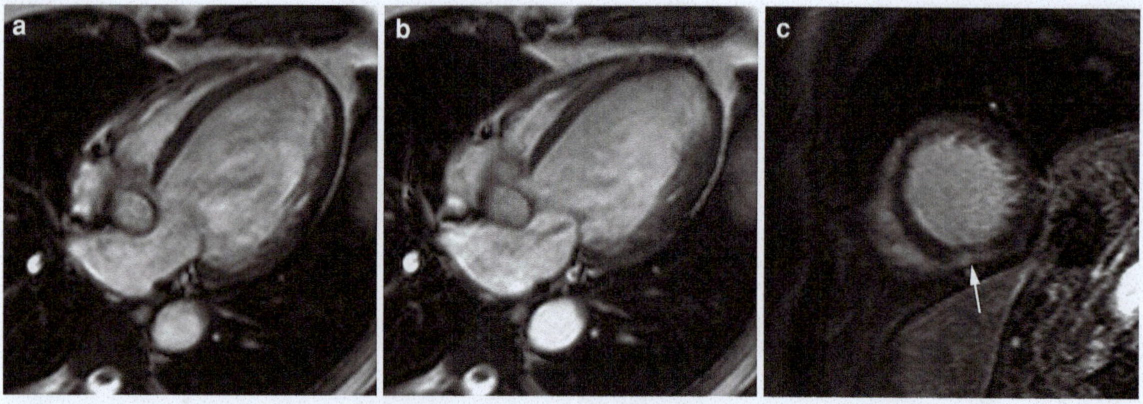

Fig. 59 Anthracycline cardiotoxicity in a 60-year-old man with previous chemotherapy for osteosarcoma, presenting with cardiac failure. Horizontal long-axis cine imaging at end diastole (**a**) and end systole (**b**), short-axis late Gd imaging (**c**). Important LV dilation and dysfunction (EDV: 269 ml, EF: 23%). Presence of a moderately severe mitral regurgitation. Late Gd imaging shows area of enhancement in LV inferior wall (*arrow*, **c**) (midwall to subepicardium). The enhancement pattern is non-ischemic (the patient presented with normal coronary arteries). Though non-specific, the enhancement is likely to represent myocardial damage (scarring) caused by anthracycline toxicity

drugs that are included in polychemotherapeutic regimens for treatment of a variety of solid tumors and hematologic malignancies. Because of increased survival due to these treatments, there is an increased number of patients who has been exposed to anthracycline chemotherapy (Bleyer 1990; Singal and Iliskovic 1998). These patients are at risk of premature cardiac disease, related to a dose-dependent cardiotoxic effect of anthracycline resulting in congestive heart failure, sometimes years after completion of chemotherapy (Von Hoff et al. 1979; Lipshultz et al. 1991) (Fig. 59). Other cardiac abnormalities include dilated and restrictive cardiomyopathy, and subtler changes in cardiac function. As there is no safe threshold dose—anthracyclines are burdened by their cardiotoxicity.

Detection of anthracycline-induced cardiotoxity is usually performed by echocardiography, looking for impairment in LV ejection fraction (Yoon et al. 2010). Since changes may be subtle, especially in early phases, there is a need for other functional parameters that more reliably depict early anthracycline cardiotoxicity (Eidem 2008; Jurcut et al. 2008). Though of potential great value, the role of MRI is currently rather marginally investigated. It was shown using MRI that LV ejection fraction significantly decreased between 3 and 28 days post-treatment in patients having a normal ejection fraction before the start of treatment (Wassmuth et al. 2001). Interestingly, pronounced increase in myocardial enhancement early post-treatment predicted significant loss of ejection fraction at follow-up. These findings were recently confirmed in an animal model showing that increased myocardial enhancement post-treatment forecasted a subsequent drop in LV ejection fraction and corresponded with intracellular vacuolization consistent with doxorubicin cardiotoxicity, whereas lack of myocardial enhancement predicted no drop in LV ejection fraction or unanticipated death (Lightfoot et al. 2010).

Other chemotherapeutic agents such as high-dose cyclophosphamide are potentially cardiotoxic as well but the role of MRI is less well explored than for anthracyclince-induced toxicity. Radiotherapy, with or without chemotherapy, is often used as treatment for breast cancer, lung cancer, and mediastinal lymphoma. Radiation-induced cardiac damage may occur when the heart is in the irradiation field, and is related to total irradiation dose, extent of involvement and duration of follow-up post-radiotherapy. Virtually all parts of the heart can suffer radiation damage causing constrictive pericarditis, myocardial ischemia and myocardial fibrosis, valve thickening, and regurgitation and diastolic dysfunction (Zinzani et al. 1996; Lund et al. 1996; Heidenreich et al. 2005). The risk of cardiac events, such as myocardial infarction or SCD, is increased in patients with known cardiovascular risk factors and in those receiving combined chemoradiotherapy (Glanzmann et al. 1998; Myrehaug et al. 2010). The possible incidence of radiation-induced cardiovascular disease and its putative mechanisms of action were recently reviewed in a UK health Protection Agency document (Circulatory Disease Risk—Report of the independent Advisory Group on Ionising Radiation Health Protection Agency 2010. ISBN 978-0-85951-676-1).

5.5 Inflammatory, Autoimmune and Vasculitic Disease

5.5.1 Sarcoidosis

Sarcoidosis is a chronic multisystem granulomatous disorder of unknown etiology. Cardiac involvement is clinically evident in only 5% of patients with sarcoidosis, while at autopsy myocardial lesions are found in 20–60% (Silverman et al. 1978; Virmani et al. 1980). Cardiac involvement can cause fatal ventricular tachyarrhythmias, conduction abnormalities, and congestive heart failure (Sharma 2003). Though most patients with cardiac sarcoidosis have a subclinical, asymptomatic course, the risk of SCD due to ventricular arrhythmias or conduction block is substantial accounting for 30–65% of fatalities. Consensus criteria for the diagnosis of cardiac sarcoidosis have been established by the Japanese Ministry of Health and Welfare (Table 2) (Smedema et al. 2005; Patel et al. 2009). These results of various diagnostic tests, including tissue biopsy, electrocardiography, echocardiography, and myocardial scintigraphy are used to diagnose or exclude cardiac sarcoidosis.

However, most criteria including EMB suffer from low sensitivity, low specificity, or both (Smedema et al. 2005). Endomyocardial biopsy yields, because of the focal myocardial involvement of sarcoidosis, sensitivity values as low as 20%, questioning whether it can be considered as the 'gold standard'. Moreover, with the proposed imaging modalities a large amount of myocardial damage may be required before abnormalities become evident (Patel et al. 2009), making the diagnosis of cardiac sarcoidosis challenging, and emphasizing the need for more accurate techniques. If cardiac manifestation occurs in a patient with multisystem sarcoidosis, especially when presenting with typical symptoms of cardiac sarcoidosis the diagnosis is relatively clear. However, in patients where cardiac dysfunction is the first or sole manifestation of sarcoidosis, the diagnosis may be challenging (White et al. 2010). Early diagnosis and effective treatment (e.g., aggressive use of corticosteroids, immunosuppressive, and immune modulator therapy, AICD in patients at risk) are absolutely necessary to improve the long-term prognosis.

Table 2 Modified guidelines for the diagnosis of cardiac sarcoidosis based on the study report on diffuse pulmonary diseases from the Japanese Ministry of Health and Welfare, 1993

1. Histologic diagnosis group: EMB demonstrates epitheloid granulomata without caseating granulomata
2. Clincial diagnosis group: in patients with histologic diagnosis of extracardiac sarcoidosis, cardiac sarcoidosis is suspected when "a" and at least one of criteria "b" to "d" is present, and other etiologies such as hypertension and coronary artery disease have been excluded:
a. Complete RBBB, left-axis deviation, AV block, VT, PVC, or pathological Q or ST-T change on resting or ambulatory ECG
b. Abnormal wall motion, regional wall thinning, or dilation of the left ventricle on echocardiographic studies
c. Perfusion defect by ^{201}thallium-myocardial scintigraphy or abnormal accumulation on ^{67}Ga-citrate or ^{99}m TCPYP myocardial scintigraphy
d. Abnormal intracardiac pressure, low cardiac output, or abnormal wall motion or depressed ejection fraction of the left ventricle on cardiac catheterization

AV atrioventricular, *EMB* endomyocardial biopsy, *PVC* premature ventricular contraction, *RBBB* right bundle branch block, *VT* ventricular tachycardia

There is a steadily growing body of evidence that MRI is of significant value in the diagnosis of cardiac sarcoidosis (Chandra et al. 1996a; Matsuki and Matsuo 2000; Shimada et al. 2001; Vignaux et al. 2002a, b; Smedema et al. 2005; Matoh et al. 2008; Ichinose et al. 2008; Patel et al. 2009; Cheong et al. 2009; Manins et al. 2009; Schulz-Menger et al. 2000b). Moreover, this technique may be of help in guiding EMB toward pathological areas (Niida et al. 2008), and in monitoring disease response to treatment (Patel et al. 2009). If we take the three successive histogical stages of sarcoidosis into consideration, i.e., edema, non-caseating epitheloid granulomatous infiltration, and replacement fibrosis with myocardial scarring, a comprehensive MRI examination including edema imaging, late Gd imaging, and cine imaging should be recommended (Figs. 60 and 61). Though non-specific, myocardial edema is indicative of increased free myocardial water content, representing reversible or irreversible myocardial damage, and usually points in the direction of an acute or active inflammatory

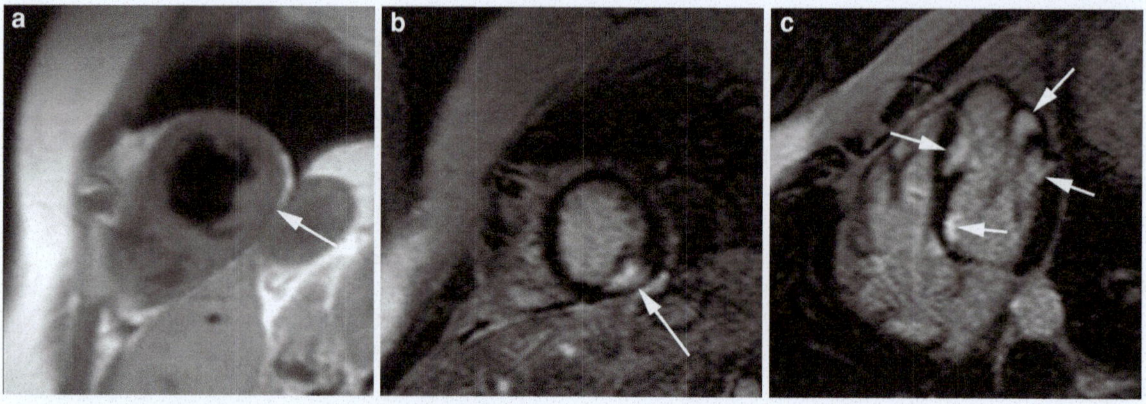

Fig. 60 Cardiac sarcoidosis in a 41-year-old woman presenting with asymptomatic atrioventricular block. Short-axis T1w-imaging (**a**), late Gd imaging in short-axis (**b**) and horizontal long-axis (**c**). T1w-imaging shows mild thickening of the infero-lateral LV wall (*arrow*, **a**). On late Gd imaging this area shows strong enhancement (*arrows*, **b**), while on horizontal long-axis imaging several areas of strong enhancement are found throughout the LV wall (*arrows*, **c**), likely to represent several non-caseating granulomas. Splenic biopsy in this patient revealed non-caseating granulomas. Adapted from Bogaert et al. (2004)

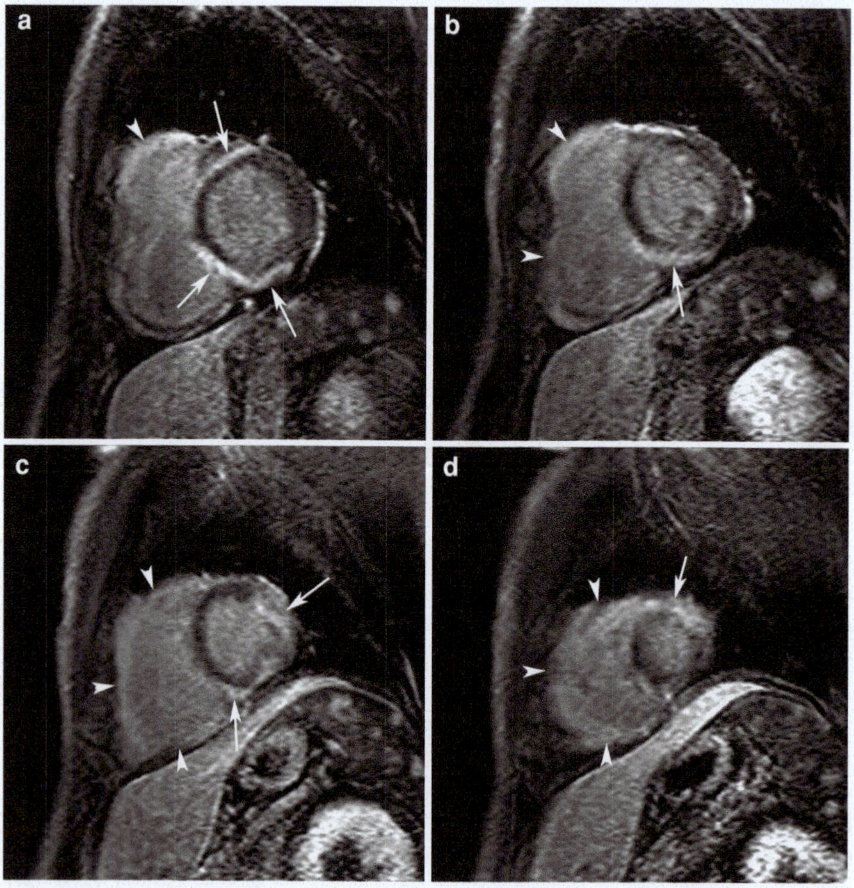

Fig. 61 Cardiac sarcoidosis in a 47-year-old man presenting with decreased biventricular function, enlarged mediastinal and hilar lymph nodes. Late Gd imaging in short-axis shows multiple preferentially subepicardial areas of LV enhancement extending to the ventricular septum (*arrows*), and important RV enhancement (*arrowheads*). The pattern of enhancement is clearly non-ischemic, and in combination with enlarged lymph nodes suggests the possibility of cardiac sarcoidosis. Cardiac and skin biopsy showed granulomatous inflammation

component. Myocardial enhancement by late Gd imaging in cardiac sarcoidosis does occur in a variety of patterns potentially involving every part of RV and LV. Current data suggest that in about 20–25% of patients with extracardiac sarcoidosis, but without evidence of cardiac sarcoidosis, abnormal myocardial enhancement is found (Smedema et al. 2005; Patel et al. 2009). Both CAD patterns with subendocardial to transmural involvement and non-CAD types of enhancement (midwall/subepicardial) have been reported (Ichinose et al. 2008; Ohira et al. 2008; Patel et al. 2009; Cheong et al. 2009; Manins et al. 2009). In a recent study by Patel et al. the RV subendocardial part of the interventricular septum was relatively commonly involved as well as the RV free wall (Patel et al. 2009). Other groups have reported relatively frequent involvement of the inferobasal and inferolateral LV wall (Smedema et al. 2005; Cheong et al. 2009). Abnormal myocardial enhancement in a patient with extracardiac sarcoidosis is strongly suspicious for myocardial involvement. In patients with a CAD pattern of enhancement, previous myocardial infarction or CAD disease should be ruled out. In patients without evidence of extracardiac sarcoidosis, the diagnosis of cardiac sarcoidosis is less evident because other diseases (e.g., ARVC/D, myocarditis, or DCM) may present in a similar way (Yared et al. 2008; White et al. 2010). A clue toward the possibility of cardiac sarcoidosis is given by the often, patchy nature of myocardial enhancement, though some case reports have mentioned a diffuse subepicardial enhancement. One should always look for extracardiac signs of sarcoidosis, e.g., mediastinal and hilar adenopathy, on the MR images, which is of great help in the differential diagnosis. Cine MRI enables measurement of ventricular volumes and function, to assess wall thicknesses, and the impact of structural abnormalities on regional function. Several studies have shown that the global extent of myocardial enhancement is significantly correlated to ventricular dilatation and dysfunction (Ichinose et al. 2008; Matoh et al. 2008). Two studies have shown that late Gd imaging is significantly more sensitive for determining cardiac involvement than the consensus criteria established by the Japanese Ministry of Health (Table 2), supporting the integration of novel imaging techniques such as MRI into the diagnostic assessment of cardiac sarcoid (Smedema et al. 2005; Patel et al. 2009). Furthermore, there may be a role of MRI in determining patient outcome and in monitoring response to treatment. Patel et al. (2009) reported a higher rate of adverse events and cardiac death in patients with abnormal myocardial enhancement, compared to those without damage. The same group reported the persistence of myocardial enhancement by late Gd imaging without evidence of new areas of enhancement, in a small group of patients ($n = 6$) with 6-month follow-up data. Since this group did not include edema imaging, it may be of interest to investigate if changes in myocardial edema can be exploited to evaluate treatment response.

In summary, the role of MRI in depicting cardiac involvement in sarcoidosis patients is emerging, holding promise that MRI criteria will be integrated into future revised consensus criteria. Further investigation, however, is needed to better understand the presentation of cardiac sarcoidosis by MRI, in particular how this entity can be differentiated from other myocardial disorders, to enhance our knowledge regarding the specificity and negative predictive value of MRI, and to define in larger, preferably multicenter studies its role in patient management and risk stratification. Finally, it is of note that use of MRI in patient follow-up will always be limited because a considerable number of patients will receive an AICD.

5.5.2 Granulomatosis with Polyangiitis

Granulomatosis with polyangiitis, formerly called '*Wegener's granulomatosis*', is a systemic inflammatory disorder of unknown etiology. Cardiac involvement occurs in 6–44% of patients (Grant et al. 1994). Pericarditis and pericardial effusion are found in 50% of patients with cardiac involvement (Forstot et al. 1980) (Fig. 62). Coronary arteritis involving the proximal aorta with dilation and wall thickening is found in another 50% of patients. Myocarditis with granuloma, which may produce acute cardiac failure and progress to cardiomyopathy, is seen in 25%. Wegener's granulomatosis may also present as mass lesions within the ventricles and may result in obstruction (Kosovsky et al. 1991). Non-invasive cardiac imaging modalities, such as transthoracic and transesophageal echocardiography, and MRI, may be helpful in identifying and delineating cardiac and proximal aortic involvement in Wegener's granulomatosis and in following the response to treatment (Kosovsky et al. 1991; Goodfield et al. 1995). Myocardial involvement is characterized on late Gd imaging as patchy focal subendocardial or midwall enhancement involving both ventricles (To et al. 2007).

5.5.3 Vasculitis

Churg-Strauss syndrome is a rare form of systemic vasculitis. Involvement of the heart is a major

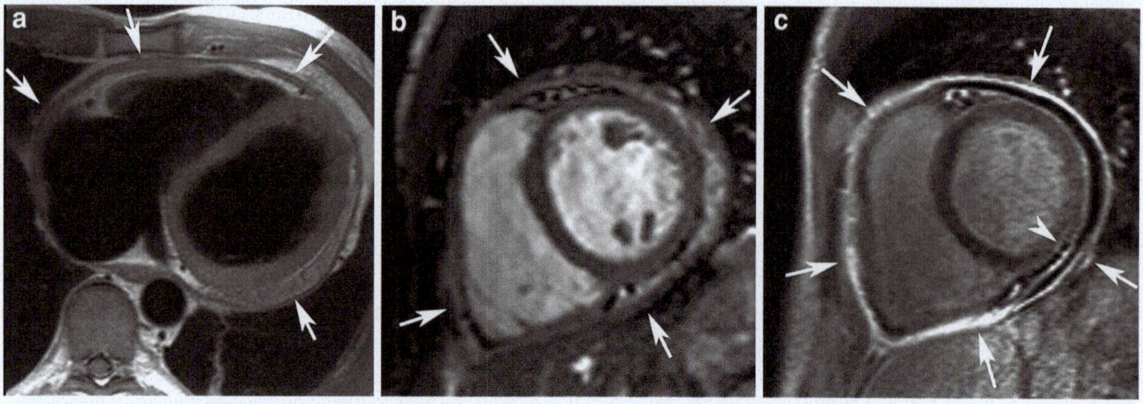

Fig. 62 Cardiac involvement in a 38-year-old man with granulomatosis with polyangiitis. Axial T1w-imaging (**a**), short-axis cine imaging (**b**), and late Gd imaging (**c**). Presence of a mild pericardial effusion showing high-signal intensity on T1w-imaging (probably high-protein content), thickened pericardial layers (*arrows*, **a**, **b**). Strong pericardial enhancement is seen following contrast administration (*arrows*, **c**), with subtle zone of subepicardial myocardial enhancement in LV inferior wall (*arrowhead*, **c**)

contributor to disease-related death. Cardiac manifestations include impaired LV function, valvular insufficiency, pericardial effusion, endomyocarditis, thrombus formation, and heart failure with abnormalities on MRI in up to 62% of patients (Neumann et al. 2009; Dennert et al. 2010). The most severe cardiac manifestion is endomyocarditis ± thrombus formation, eventually causing fatal outcome. Similar to other forms of myocarditis, MRI enables depiction of myocardial edema, increased early myocardial contrast uptake and abnormal late myocardial enhancement reflecting inflammation/necrosis—fibrosis. The functional consequences, and concomitant findings such as pericardial effusion, valve regurgitation and thrombus formation can be evaluated with a single non-invasive examination (Wassmuth et al. 2008). Myocardial enhancement is found most frequently in the anteroseptal and lateral involving all myocardial layers (Marmursztejn et al. 2009). Hansch et al. (2009) reported frequent subendocardial first-pass perfusion defects corresponding to the areas of myocardial edema in these patients. In patients treated with immunosuppressive therapy, MRI shows normalization or regression of myocardial enhancement (Marmursztejn et al. 2010). Also for other small and medium vessel vasculitides, MRI is of great value for evaluating cardiac involvement (Kane and Keogh 2009).

5.5.4 Autoimmune Disease

Systemic lupus erythematosus (SLE) is a multi-organ inflammatory disorder mainly affecting women and associated with high cardiovascular morbidity and mortality. The most common cardiac manifestations are non-bacterial "verrucous" endocarditis (Libman-Sacks endocarditis), pericardial effusion, pericardial thickening, and myocarditis. Although the latter is clinically evident in 10% of patients, the incidence at autopsy approaches 40%. Although the experience of MRI in SLE is still limited, there may be role to depict disease activity using a similar approach as in patients with myocarditis, i.e., myocardial edema ratio, global myocardial enhancement, and late Gd imaging in combination with functional imaging (Singh et al. 2005; Abdel-Aty et al. 2008; O'Neill et al. 2009). Myocardial enhancement in SLE seems to predominantly involve the midwall (Edwards et al. 2007).

Systemic sclerosis is a connective tissue disease clinically characterized by widespread vascular lesions and fibrosis of the skin and major organs including lungs, kidneys, and heart. Cardiac involvement, including primary myocardial involvement, is very common and recognized as a poor prognostic factor. The myocardial damage, subsequently causing myocardial fibrosis, is most likely to be related to repeated ischemic injury. The role of MRI is focused on depiction of microvascular impairment or ischemia using stress perfusion MRI, and visualization of myocardial necrosis and fibrosis using late Gd imaging with late imaging either with an ischemic pattern (subendocardial) or non-ischemic pattern (mid-myocardial layer) (Kahan and Allanore

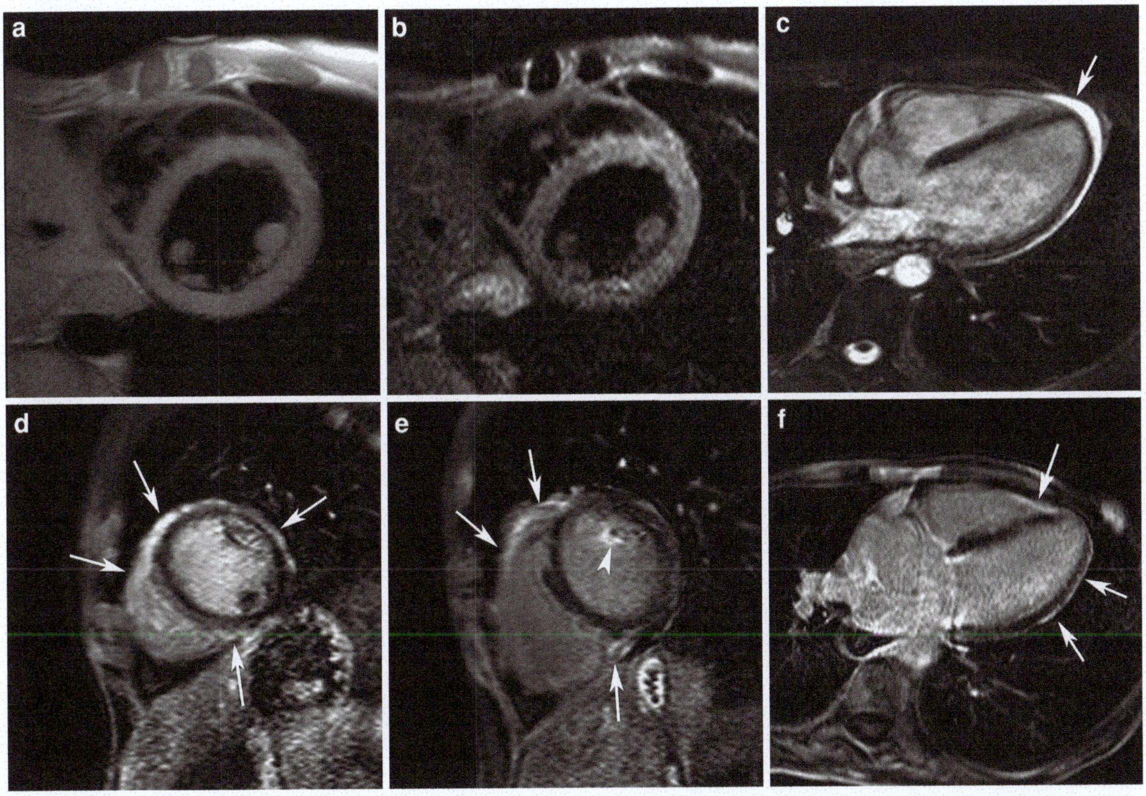

Fig. 63 Severe systemic sclerosis in a 36-year-old man with cardiac, muscle, skin, and pulmonary involvement. T1w (**a**) and T2w-imaging (**b**) in cardiac short-axis. Horizontal long-axis cine imaging (**c**). Late Gd imaging in short-axis (**d**, **e**) and horizontal long-axis (**f**). Moderate LV dilatation and dysfunction (EDV: 243 ml, EF: 45%). Mild amount of pericardial fluid (*arrow*, **c**). Myocardial enhancement is found subepicardially in LV (*arrows*, **d**, **e**, **f**), transmurally in RV (*arrows*, **d**, **f**) and focally in papillary muscles (*arrowhead*, **e**)

2006; Nassenstein et al. 2008; Hachulla et al. 2009; Kobayashi et al. 2008) (Fig. 63). *Dermatomyositis* and *polymyositis* infrequently involve the heart, but are associated with poor prognosis. MRI may be of help in depicting myocardial fibrosis and evaluate the effects of treatment (Allenore et al. 2006).

5.6 Endocrine Disorders

Diabetic cardiomyopathy describes the diabetes-associated changes in structure and function of the myocardium not directly attributable to confounding factors such as CAD or hypertension. In many patients, in particular those with type 2 diabetes, the simultaneous presence of these co-morbidities may augment the development of LV hypertrophy, thereby increasing susceptibility to ischemic injury, and increasing the overall likelihood of developing heart failure (Boudina and Abel 2010). The natural history is characterized by a latent subclinical period, during which there is evidence of diastolic dysfunction and LV hypertrophy, before clinical deterioration and systolic heart failure ensue (Khavandi et al. 2009). There is a growing body of evidence that diabetes inflicts a direct insult on the myocardium, with cellular, structural, and functional changes manifest as the diabetic myocardial phenotype. Several mechanisms are implicated in the pathogenesis of diabetic cardiomyopathy. For an extensive explanation we would like to refer to following review papers (Khavandi et al. 2009; Gropler et al. 2010; Boudina and Abel 2010).

Use of MRI in this patient population is of interest for several reasons. This technique is the gold standard to evaluate morphological and geometrical ventricular remodeling and to measure systolic function, and provides reliable data regarding diastolic function. As extensively discussed within this chapter, late Gd imaging MRI has become the preferred technique for depicting and to categorizing the pattern of myocardial fibrosis, while T1 mapping yields promise for the depiction of diffuse myocardial fibrosis (Maya and Villarreal 2010). Moreover, ^{1}H and ^{31}P MR spectroscopy have been shown to be good diagnostic tools in recognizing subtle changes in myocardial metabolism in diabetic cardiomyopathy patients, such as myocardial steatosis and changes in phosphocreatine/ATP ratio (Rijzewijk et al. 2008; Maya and Villarreal 2010; Ng et al. 2010).

The cardiovascular system is a principal target of thyroid hormones. Alterations in thyroid hormone metabolism may alter cardiac function, which is reversible after normalization of thyroid function. It has been shown using MRI that in patients with mild (subclinical) *hypothyroidism* cardiac preload is decreased and afterload increased leading to a reduction in stroke volume and cardiac output (Ripoli et al. 2005). In contrast, *hyperthyroidism* causes tachycardia, hyperdynamic circulation with increased preload and stroke volume, and decreased exercise capacity (Biondi and Kahaly 2010). Cardiac complications of untreated hyperthyroidism (i.e., toxic multinodular goiter, toxic adenoma, Graves disease) include atrial enlargement, atrial fibrillation with increased risk of stroke, congestive heart failure, autoimmune myocarditis, cardiac valve involvement, specific cardiomyopathies, and pulmonary hypertension (Biondi and Kahaly 2010).

5.7 Neuromuscular/Neurological Disorders—Myopathies

Friedreich's ataxia is a neurodegenerative disease characterized by progressive limb and gait ataxia, areflexia, pyramidal signs in the legs. This automosal recessive disorder is often associated with HCM (concentric or asymmetric) that may progress toward a DCM (Fig. 64). The underlying mechanism that triggers HCM, is the production of frataxin. It is suggested that this protein of unknown function causes oxidative stress or respiratory chain dysfunction. It has been shown that Idebenone, a potent free radical scavanger, may protect the myocardium against this oxidative stress, and thus be effective at controlling cardiac hypertrophy in Friedreich's ataxia. A reduction in LV mass has been reported in Friedreich's ataxia patients after 6 months of Idebenone treatment (Hausse et al. 2002). Though LV mass calculations in this study were performed with echocardiography, MRI has the advantage to be a more accurate and highly reproducible technique for wall mass calculations and should be recommended to perform these kinds of repeated follow-up studies (Meyer et al. 2007).

Duchenne mucular dystrophy is an X-linked, recessive disease caused by mutation in the dystrophin gene. This disorder is clinically associated with skeletal myopathy and DCM, leading to heart failure and causing death in 30% of patients. Patients with the less common *mucular dystrophy type Becker-Kiener* often show myocardial damage, with late Gd MRI subepicardially in the (infero)-lateral wall, which is associated with decreased LV ejection fraction (Silva et al. 2007; Yilmaz et al. 2008b). In *myopathies* the heart is frequently affected in addition to the skeletal muscle. Since cardiac abnormalities are highly heterogeneous resembling almost all different entities described in this chapter, MRI may have a role in evaluating the morphologic substrate and the functional consequences (Finsterer and Stöllberger 2008).

5.8 Uremic Cardiomyopathy

Patients with end-stage renal failure have an increased risk of premature cardiovascular disease, in particular of SCD, accounting for almost 40% of deaths in this population. Uremic cardiomyopathy is defined on echocardiography as LV hypertrophy, dilation and systolic dysfunction. Two contrast-enhanced MRI studies, performed prior to the concerns of nephrogenic systemic fibrosis (NSF) have substantially contributed to our understanding of uremic cardiomyopathy (Mark et al. 2006; Schietinger et al. 2008). LV hypertrophy is a common finding in end-stage renal failure and chronic hemodialysis patients. Increased myocardial enhancement is prevalent, with the extent related to LV hypertrophy. Three patterns of myocardial enhancement have been found: (1) infarct-related, (2) diffuse ("amyloid-like"), and (3) focal non-infarct related-pattern. The latter pattern is more prevalent in hypertrophied, dysfunctional LV segments, most likely representing myocardial fibrosis and/or infiltrative process. Though this may represent a marker for SCD, because of risk of NSF with the use of gadolinium chelates, late Gd imaging is currently not possible in this population.

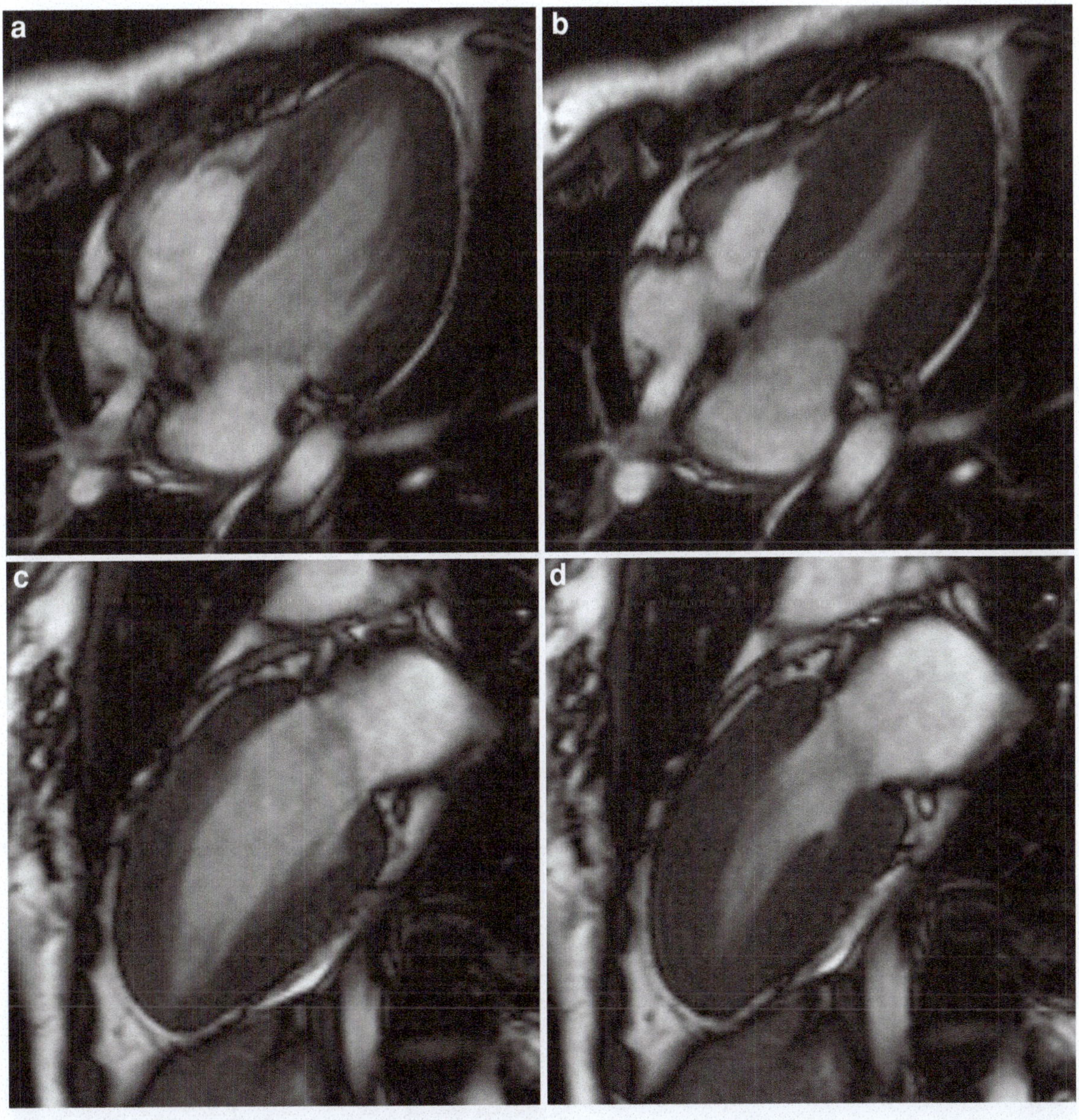

Fig. 64 Concentric LV hypertrophy in a 22-year-old woman with Friedreich's ataxia. Cine imaging in horizontal long-axis (**a**, **b**) and vertical long-axis (**c**, **d**), end diastole (*left*)–end systole (*right*). Homogeneously thickened myocardial wall (maximal wall thickness at end diastole: 17 mm)

6 Congenital Myocardial Disorders in the Adult Population

When performing cardiac MRI studies on a regular basis, a series of myocardial disorders may be encountered usually in adults, who do not fit with one of the above discussed non-ischemic myocardial abnormalities nor with ischemic heart disease. Knowledge of cardiac anatomy (see "Cardiac Anatomy") and congenital heart disorders (see "Congenital Heart Disease") may be helpful to recognize these entities that often can be considered as congenital. For instance, congenitally corrected transposition of the great arteries may be asymptomatic until adult life. Ventricular diverticula, congenital aneurysms or spontaneously closed

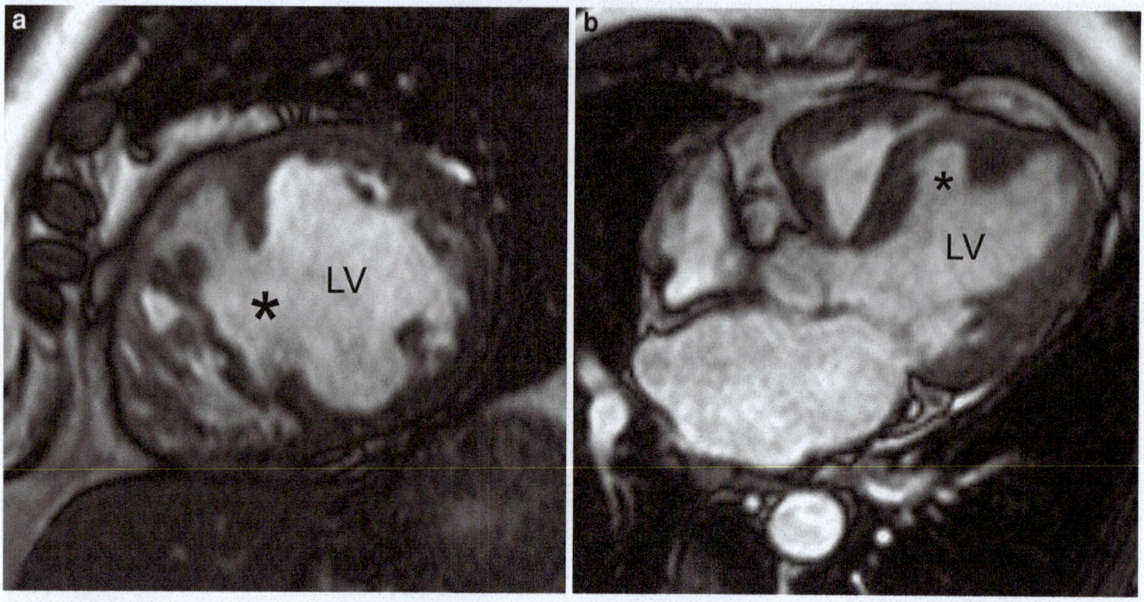

Fig. 65 Spontaneously closed muscular ventricular septal defect in a 65-year-old male suspected of ischemic myocardial disease. Cine imaging in short-axis (**a**) and horizontal long-axis (**b**). A large defect (*) is visible in the middle third of the ventricular septum. However, the patient had no symptoms of interventricular shunt and flow measurements through the great vessels revealed similar flow volumes. Hypertrophy of the RV muscular trabeculations has spontaneously sealed the defect. This phenomenon is not infrequent in muscular, even large, ventricular septal defects

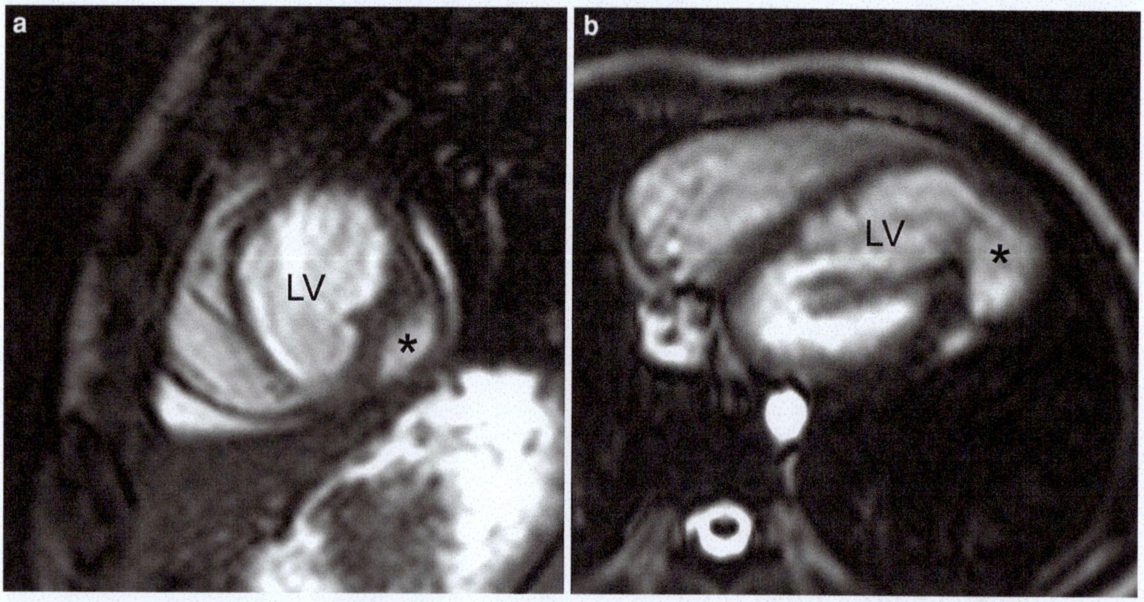

Fig. 66 Congenital LV diverticulum in a 8-year-old girl. Cine imaging in short-axis (**a**) and horizontal long-axis (**b**). Presence of a well-delineated outpouching (*) in apicolateral part of LV in communication with the ventricular cavity by a rather small neck. In contrast to an LV aneurysm, usually the result of an infarction, this diverticulum shows contraction during systole, because it contains a muscular wall

ventricular septal defects are rare entities, but can be well recognized using a comprehensive MRI approach (Figs. 65 and 66).

7 Key Points

- MRI provides essential, often unique, information regarding heart muscle diseases, and therefore should be part of the diagnostic investigation in patients with this group of cardiac diseases.
- Using a comprehensive MRI approach, adapted to the specific clinical question, valuable information can be provided regarding morphology, tissue characterization, and the impact on cardiac function.
- Not only the presence of abnormalities, but also the relation of abnormalities with regard to the rest of the heart, and the presence and type of adaptive cardiac remodeling can be accurately assessed using a combination of bright-blood and black-blood imaging in different imaging planes.
- T2w-imaging is of interest for depicting myocardial edema in acute myocardial events, such as myocarditis, stress cardiomyopathy, and/or acute myocardial information.
- T2* imaging is the preferred technique to non-invasively measure the presence of myocardial iron deposition and to monitor chelation therapy.
- Contrast-enhanced MRI, using late Gd imaging, provides accurate information regarding the presence of fibrotic myocardial replacement.
- Though the enhancement as such is aspecific, the pattern/location of enhancement is helpful to discriminate between ischemic and non-ischemic origin. Moreover, the presence of enhancement suggests cardiac involvement in many secondary cardiomyopathies (e.g., sarcoidosis).
- There is growing evidence that depiction of myocardial fibrosis in HCM patients using late Gd imaging is a marker of increased risk for malignant arrhythmias and adverse remodeling.
- T1-mapping techniques yield promising results to depict the presence of diffuse myocardial fibrosis.
- Fibrous or fibrofatty replacement and not fatty replacement is the pathological substrate of ARVC/D. Pure fatty replacement can occur as a normal aging process.

References

Abarra S, Migrino RQ, Sosnovik D, Leichter JA, Brady TJ, Holmvang G (2004) Value of fat suppression in the MRI evaluation of suspected arrhythmogenic right ventricular dysplasia. AJR 182:587–591

Abdel-Aty H, Boyé P, Zagrosek A et al (2005) Diagnostic performance of cardiovascular magnetic resonance in patients with suspected acute myocarditis. Comparison of different approaches. J Am Coll Cardiol 45:1815–1822

Abdel-Aty H, Siegle N, Natusch A et al (2008) Myocardial tissue characterization in systemic lupus erythematosus: value of a comprehensive cardiovascular magnetic resonance approach. Lupus 17:561–567

Abe Y, Kondo M (2002) Apical ballooning of the left ventricle: a distinct entity? Heart 89:974–976

Abe Y, Kondo M, Matsuoka R, Araki M, Dohyama K, Tanio H (2003) Assessment of clinical features in transient left ventricular apical ballooning. J Am Coll Cardiol 41: 737–742

Abelmann WH, Lorell BH (1989) The challenge of cardiomyopathy. J Am Coll Cardiol 13:1219–1239

Adabag AS, Maron BJ, Appelbaum E et al (2008) Occurrence and frequency of arrhythmias in hypertrophic cardiomyopathy in relation to delayed enhancement on cardiovascular magnetic resonance. J Am Coll Cardiol 51:1369–1374

Akashi Y, Nakazawa K, Sakakibara M, Miyake F, Sasaka (2002) Reversible left ventricular dysfunction "Takotsubo" cardiomyopathy related to catecholamine cardiotoxicity. J Electrocardiol 35:351–356

Ako J, Kozaki K, Yoshizumi M, Ouchi Y (2002) Transient left ventricular apical ballooning without coronary artery stenosis: a form of stunning-like phenomenon? J Am Coll Cardiol 39:741–742

Aletras AH, Tilak GS, Hsu LY, Arai AE (2011) Heterogeneity of intramural function in hypertrophic cardiomyopathy: mechanistic insights from late gadolinium enhancement and high-resolution DENSE strain maps. Circ Cardiovasc Imaging 4:425–434

Allenore Y, Vignaux O, Arnaud L et al (2006) Effects of corticosteroids and immunosuppressors on idiopathic inflammatory myopathy related myocarditis evaluated by magnetic resonance imaging. Ann Rheum Dis 65:249–252

Alsaileek AA, Syed I, Seward JB, Julsrud P (2008) Myocardial fibrosis of left ventricle: magnetic resonance imaging in noncompaction. J Magn Reson Imaging 27:621–624

Anderson RH (2008) Ventricular non-compaction—a frequently ignored finding? Eur Heart J 29:10–11

Anderson LJ, Holden S, Davis B et al (2001) Cardiovascular T2-star (T2*) magnetic resonance for the early diagnosis of myocardial iron overload. Eur Heart J 22:2171–2179

Angelini A, Melacini P, Barbero F, Thiene G (1999) Evolutionary persistence of spongy myocardium in humans. Circulation 99:2475

Aretz HT, Billingham ME, Edwards WD et al (1986) Myocarditis: a histopathologic definition and classification. Am J Cardiovasc Pathol 1:3–14

Arrivé L, Assayag P, Russ G, Najmark D, Brochet E, Nahum H (1994) MRI and cine MRI of asymmetric septal hypertrophic cardiomyopathy. J Comput Assist Tomogr 18:376–382

Assomull RG, Prasad SK, Lyne J et al (2006) Cardiovascular magnetic resonance, fibrosis, and prognosis in dilated cardiomyopathy. J Am Coll Cardiol 48:1977–1985

Assomull RG, Lyne JC, Keenan N et al (2007) The role of cardiovascular magnetic resonance in patients presenting with chest pain, raised Troponin, and unobstructed coronary arteries. Eur Heart J 28:1242–1249

Austin BA, Tang WH, Rodriguez ER et al (2009) Delayed hyper-enhancement magnetic resonance imaging provides incremental diagnostic and prognostic utility in suspected cardiac amyloidosis. J Am Coll Cardiol Img 2:1369–1377

Awtry EH, Philippides GJ (2010) Alcohol and cocaine-associated cardiomyopathies. Prog Cardiovasc Dis 52: 289–299

Baccouche H, Mahrholdt H, Meinhardt G et al (2009) Diagnostic synergy of non-invasive cardiovascular magnetic resonance and invasive endomyocardial biopsy in troponin-positive patients without coronary artery disease. Eur Heart J 30:2869–2879

Baruteau AE, Leurent G, Martins RP et al (2010) Peripartum cardiomyopathy in the era of cardiac magnetic resonance imaging: first results and perspectives. Int J Cardiol 144:143–145

Basavarajaiah S, Boraita A, Whyte G, Wilson M, Carby L, Shah A, Sharma S (2008a) Ethnic differences in left ventricular remodeling in highly-trained athletes. J Am Coll Cardiol 51:2256–2262

Basavarajaiah S, Wilson M, Whyte G, Shah A, McKenna W, Sharma S (2008b) Prevalence of hypertrophic cardiomyopathy in highly trained athletes. J Am Coll Cardiol 51: 1033–1039

Basso C, Thiene G, Corrado D, Buja G, Melacini P, Nava A (2000) Hypertrophic cardiomyopathy and sudden cardiac death in the young: pathologic evidence of myocardial ischemia. Hum Pathol 31:988–998

Basso C, Corrado D, Marcus FI, Nava A, Thiene G (2009) Arrhythmogenic right ventricular dysplasia. Lancet 373: 1289–1300

Beer M, Weidemann F, Breunig F, Knoll A et al (2006) Impact of enzyme replacement therapy on cardiac morphology and function and late enhancement in Fabry's cardiomyopathy. Am J Cardiol 97:1515–1518

Belanger AR, Miller MA, Donthireddi UR, Najovits AJ, Goldman ME (2008) New classification scheme of left ventricular noncompaction and correlation with ventricular performance. Am J Cardiol 102:92–96

Belenkov Y, Vikhert OA, Belichenko OI, Arabidze GG (1992) Magnetic resonance imaging of cardiac hypertrophy in malignant arterial hypertension. Am J Hypertens 5: 195S–199S

Bellenger NG, Davies LC, Francis JM, Coats AJS, Pennell DJ (2000) Reduction in sample size for studies of remodeling in heart failure by the use of cardiovascular magnetic resonance. J Cardiovasc Magn Reson 2:271–278

Bello D, Shah DJ, Farah GM (2003) Gadolinium cardiovascular magnetic resonance predicts reversible myocardial dysfunction and remodeling in patients with heart failure undergoing β-blocker therapy. Circulation 108:1945–1953

Bellotti G, Bocchi EA, de Moreas A et al (1996) In vivo detection of *Trypanosoma cruzi* antigens in hearts of patients with chronic Chagas' heart disease. Am Heart J 131:301–317

Beltrami CA, Finato N, Rocco M et al (1995) The cellular basis of dilated cardiomyopathy in humans. J Mol Cell Cardiol 27:291–305

Benson L, Liu P, Olivieri N, Rose V, Freedom R (1989) Left ventricular function in young adults with thalassemia. Circulation 80:274

Bergler KJ, Sochor H, Stanek G, Globits S, Ullrich R, Glogar D (1993) Indium 111-monoclonal antimyosin antibody and magnetic resonance imaging in the diagnosis of acute Lyme myopericarditis. Arch Intern Med 153:2696–2700

Berkowitz SJ, Macedo R, Malayeri AA et al (2009) Axial black blood turbo spin echo imaging of the right ventricle. Magn Reson Med 61:307–314

Bhatia SR, Tu JV, Lee DS et al (2006) Outcome of heart failure with preserved ejection fraction in a population-based study. N Engl J Med 355:260–269

Biondi B, Kahaly GJ (2010) Cardiovascular involvement in patients with different causes of hyperthyroidism. Nat Rev Endocrinol 6:431–443

Bleyer WA (1990) The impact of childhood cancer on the United States and the world. CA Cancer J Clin 40:355–367

Bluemke DA, Kronmal RA, Lima JAC, Liu K, Olson J, Burke GL, Folsom AR (2008) The relationship of left ventricular mass and geometry to incident cardiovascular events. J Am Coll Cardiol 52:2148–2155

Bogaert J, Francone M (2009) Cardiovascular magnetic resonance in pericardial diseases. J Cardiovasc Magn Reson 11:14

Bogaert J, Goldstein M, Tannouri F, Golzarian J, Dymarkowski S (2003) Late myocardial enhancement in hypertrophic cardiomyopathy using contrast-enhanced magnetic resonance imaging. Am J Roentgenol AJR 180:981–985

Bogaert J, Taylor AM, Van Kerckhove F, Dymarkowski S (2004) Use of inversion-recovery contrast-enhanced MRI technique for cardiac imaging: spectrum of diseases. Am J Roentgenol AJR 182:609–615

Bogun FM, Desjardins B, Good E et al (2009) Delayed-enhanced magnetic resonance imaging in nonischemic cardiomyopathy. Utility for identifying the ventricular arrhythmia substrate. J Am Coll Cardiol 53:1138–1145

Borreguero LJJ, Corti R, de Soria RF, Osende JI, Fuster V, Badimon JJ (2004) Diagnosis of isolated noncompaction of the myocardium by magnetic resonance imaging. Circulation 105:e177–e178

Boudina S, Abel ED (2010) Diabetic cardiomyopathy, causes and effects. Rev Endocr Metab Disord 11:31–39

Braunwald E, Kloner RA (1982) The stunned myocardium: prolonged, postischemic ventricular dysfunction. Circulation 66:1146–1156

Brigden W (1957) The noncoronary cardiomyopathies. Lancet II:1179–1243

Bruder O, Schneider S, Nothnagel D et al (2009) EuroCMR (European Cardiovascular Magnetic Resonance) registry: result of the German pilot phase. J Am Coll Cardiol 54: 147–1466

Bruder O, Wagner A, Jensen CJ et al (2010) Myocardial scar visualized by cardiovascular magnetic resonance imaging

predicts major adverse events in patients with hypertrophic cardiomyopathy. J Am Coll Cardiol 56:875–887
Bulkley BH, Weisfeldt ML, Hutchins GM (1977) Asymmetric septal hypertrophy and myocardial fiber disarray. Features of normal, developing and malformed hearts. Circulation 56:292–298
Bulut A, Rav-Acha M, Aydin O et al (2009) "Inverted Tako-Tsubo": transient apical-sparing cardiomyopathy. Int J Cardiol 134:e35–e38
Burke AP, Farb A, Tashko G, Virmani R (1998) Arrhythmogenic right ventricular cardiomyopathy and fatty replacement of the right ventricular myocardium. Are they different diseases? Circulation 97:1571–1580
Buser PT, Wagner S, Auffermann W et al (1990) Three-dimensional analysis of the regional contractility of the normal and the cardiomyopathic left ventricle using cine-magnetic resonance imaging (in German). Z Kardiol 79:573–579
Captur G, Nihoyannopoulos P (2010) Left ventricular non-compaction: genetic heterogeneity, diagnosis and clinical course. Int J Cardiol 140:145–153
Carlson MD, White RD, Trohman RG et al (1994) Right ventricular outflow tract ventricular tachycardia: detection of previously unrecognized anatomic abnormalities using cine magnetic resonance imaging. J Am Coll Cardiol 24: 720–727
Carpenter JP, He T, Kirk P et al (2011) On T2* magnetic resonance and cardiac iron. Circulation 123:1519–1528
Casolo GC, Poggesi L, Boddi M et al (1987) ECG-gated magnetic resonance imaging in right ventricular dysplasia. Am Heart J 113:1245–1248
Casolo GC, Trotta F, Rostagno C et al (1989) Detection of apical hypertrophic cardiomyopathy by magnetic resonance imaging. Am Heart J 117:468–472
Castillo E, Tandri H, Rodriguez R et al (2004) Arrhythmogenic right ventricular dysplasia: ex vivo and in vivo fat detection with black-blood MR imaging. Radiology 232:38–48
Chan PCK, Liu P, Cronin C, Heathcote J, Uldall R (1992) The use of nuclear magnetic resonance imaging in monitoring total body iron in hemodialysis patients with hemosiderosis treated with erythropoietin and phlebotomy. Am J Kidney Dis 19:484–489
Chandra M, Silverman ME, Oshinski J, Pettigrew R (1996a) Diagnosis of cardiac sarcoidosis aided by MRI. Chest 110:562–565
Chandra M, Pettigrew RI, Eley JW, Oshinski JN, Guyton RA (1996b) Cine-MRI-aided endomyocardectomy in idiopathic hypereosinophilic syndrome. Ann Thorac Surg 62: 1856–1858
Charron P, Arad M, Arbustini E et al (2010) Genetic counseling and testing in cardiomyopathies: a position statement of the European Society of Cardiology Working Group on Myocardial and Pericardial Diseases. Eur Heart J 31:2715–2726
Cheong BYC, Muthupillai R, Nemeth M et al (2009) The utility of delayed-enhancement magnetic resonance imaging for identifying nonischemic myocardial fibrosis in asymptomatic patients with biopsy-proven systemic sarcoidosis. Sarcoidosis Vasc Diffuse Lung Dis 26:39–46
Choudbury L, Mahrholdt H, Wagner A et al (2002) Myocardial scarring in asymptomatic or mildly symptomatic patients with hypertrophic cardiomyopathy. J Am Coll Cardiol 40:2156–2164
Coelho-Filho OR, Mongeon F-P, Mitchell RN et al (2010) Löffler endocarditis presenting with recurrent polymorphic ventricular tachycardia diagnosed by cardiac magnetic resonanc imaging. Circulation 122:96–99
Cooper LT (2009) Myocarditis. N Engl J Med 360:1526–1538
Cooper LT, Baughman KL, Feldman AM et al (2007) The role of endomyocardial biopsy in the management of cardiovascular disease. A scientific statement from the American Heart Association, the American College of Cardiology, and the European Society of Cardiology. Circulation 116: 2216–2233
Corrado D, Fontaine G, Marcus FI et al (2000) Arrhythmogenic right ventricular dysplasia/cardiomyopathy. Need for an international registry. Circulation 101:e101–e106
Crilley JG, Boehm EA, Blair E et al (2003) Hypertrophic cardiomyopathy due to sarcomeric gene mutations is characterized by impaired energy metabolism irrespective of the degree of hypertrophy. J Am Coll Cardiol 41:1776–1782
Cuspidi C, Lonati L, Sampieri L, Leonetti G, Zanchetti A (1997) Physiological versus pathological hypertrophy. The athlete and the hypertensive. In: Zanchetti A et al (eds) Hypertension and the heart. Plenum Press, New York, pp 145–158
D'Silva SA, Kohli A, Dalvi BV, Kale PA (1992) MRI in right ventricular endomyocardial fibrosis. Am Heart J 123: 1390–1392
Dalal D, Tandri H, Judge DP et al (2009) Morphologic variants of familial arrhythmogenic right ventricular dysplasia/cardiomyopathy. A genetics-magnetic resonance imaging correlation study. J Am Coll Cardiol 53:1289–1299
Davlouros PA, Danias PG, Karatza AA, Kiaffas MG, Alexopoulos D (2009) Saw-tooth cardiomyopathy. J Cardiovasc Magn Reson 16:54
Dawson DK, Maceira AM, Raj VJ, Graham C, Pennell DJ, Kilner PJ (2011) Regional thicknesses and thickening of compacted and trabeculated myocardial layers of the normal left ventricle studied by cardiovascular magnetic resonance. Circ Cardiovasc Imaging 4:139–146
De Cobelli F, Pieroni M, Esposito A et al (2006) Delayed gadolinium-enhanced cardiac magnetic resonance in patients with chronic myocarditis presenting with heart failure or recurrent arrhythmias. J Am Coll Cardiol 47: 1649–1654
de Souza F, Altenburg R, Curi Gismondi O, Cunha Neto SH, de Mattos MA (2008) Tako-tsubo-like cardiomyopathy and extra-adrenal pheochromocytoma: case report and literature review. Clin Res Cardiol 97:397–401
Debl K, Djavidani B, Buchner S et al (2006) Delayed hyperenhancement in magnetic resonance imaging of left ventricular hypertrophy caused by aortic stenosis and hypertrophic cardiomyopathy: visualization of focal fibrosis. Heart 92:1447–1451
Dec GW, Fuster V (1994) Idiopathic dilated cardiomyopathy. N Engl J Med 331:1564–1574
Dennert RM, van Paassen P, Schalla S et al (2010) Cardiac involvement in Churg-Strauss syndrome. Arthritis Rheum 62:627–634

Desmet WJR, Adriaenssens BFM, Dens JAY (2003) Apical ballooning of the left ventricle: first series in white patients. Eur Heart J 89:1027–1031

Dewey FE, Rosenthal D, Murphy DJ, Froelicher VF, Ashley EA (2008) Does size matter. Clinical applications of scaling cardiac size and function for body size. Circulation 117: 2279–2287

Di Bella G, Masci PG, Ganame J, Dymarkowski S, Bogaert J (2008) Liquefaction necrosis of the mitral annulus calcification: detection and characterization with cardiac magnetic resonance imaging. Circulation 117:e292–e294

Di Bella G, Minutoli F, Mazzeo A et al (2010) MRI of cardiac involvement in transthyretin familial amyloid polyneuropathy. AJR 195:W394–W399

Dodd JD, Holmvang G, Hoffmann U et al (2008) Quantification of left ventricular noncompaction and trabecular delayed hyperenhancement with cardiac MRI: correlation with clinical severity. AJR 189:974–980

Dong SJ, MacGregor JH, Crawley AP et al (1994) Left ventricular wall thickness and regional systolic function in patients with hypertrophic cardiomyopathy. Circulation 90:1200–1209

Dorn GWII (2007) The fuzzy logic of physiological cardiac hypertrophy. Hypertension 49:962–970

Durand E, Mousseaux E, Coste P et al (2008) Non-surgical septal myocardial reduction by coil embolization for hypertrophic obstructive cardiomyopathy: early and 6 months follow-up. Eur Heart J 29:348–355

Edwards NC, Ferro CJ, Townend JN, Steeds RP (2007) Myocardial disease in systemic vasculitis and autoimmune disease detected by cardiovascular magnetic resonance. Rheumatology 46:1208–1209

Eidem BW (2008) Identification of anthracycline cardiotoxicity: left ventricular ejection fraction is not enough. J Am Soc Echocardiogr 21:1290–1292

Eitel I, Behrendt F, Schindler K et al (2008) Differential diagnosis of suspected apical ballooning syndrome using contrast-enhanced magnetic resonance imaging. Eur Heart J 29:2651–2659

Eitel I, Lücke C, Grothoff M et al (2010) Inflammation in takotsubo cardiomyopathy: insights form cardiovascular magnetic resonance imaging. Eur Radiol 20:422–431

Eitel I, von Knobelsdorff-Brenkenhoff F, Bernhardt P et al (2011) Clinical characteristics and cardiovascular magnetic resonance findings in stress (Takotsubo) cardiomyopathy. JAMA 306:277–286

Elkayam U, Akhter MW, Singh H et al (2005) Pregnancy-associated cardiomyopathy. Clinical characteristics and a comparison between early and late presentation. Circulation 111:2050–2055

Elliott P, Andersson B, Arbustini E et al (2008) Classification of the cardiomyopathies: a position statement from the European Society of Cardiology working group on myocardial and pericardial diseases. Eur Heart J 29:270–276

Elshershari H, Okutan V, Celiker A (2001) Isolated noncompaction of the ventricular myocardium. Cardiol Young 11:472–475

Esposito A, De Cobelli F, Perseghin G et al (2008) Impaired left ventricular energy metabolism in patients with hypertrophic cardiomyopathy is related to the extension of fibrosis at delayed gadolinium-enhanced magnetic resonance imaging. Heart 95:228–233

Falk RH, Dubrey SW (2010) Amyloid heart disease. Prog Cardiovasc Dis 52:347–361

Feldman AM, McNamara D (2000) Myocarditis. N Engl J Med 343:1388–1398

Fernandez-Golfin C, Pachon M, Corros C et al (2009) Left ventricular trabeculae: quantification in different cardiac diseases and impact on left ventricular morphological and functional parameters assessed with cardiac magnetic resonance. J Cardiovasc Med 10:827–833

Finsterer J, Stöllberger C (2008) Primary myopathies and the heart. Scand Cardiovasc J 42:9–24

Finsterer J, Stöllberger C, Feichtinger H (2002) Histological appearance of left ventricular hypertrabeculation/noncompaction. Cardiology 98:162–164

Flett AS, Hayward MP, Ashworth MT et al (2010) Equilibrium contrast cardiovascular magnetic resonance for the measurement of diffuse myocardial fibrosis. Preliminary validation in humans. Circulation 122:138–144

Fontaine G, Fontaliran F, Frank R (1998) Arrhythmogenic right ventricular cardiomyopathies. Clinical forms and main differential diagnoses. Circulation 97:1532–1535

Forstot JZ, Overlie PA, Neufeld GK, Harmon CE, Forstot SL (1980) Cardiac complications of Wegener's granulomatosis: a case report of complete heart block and review of the literature. Semin Arthritis Rheum 10:148–154

Francone M, Iacucci I, Mangia M, Carbone I (2010) Endomyocardial disease related to idiopathic hypereosinophilic syndrome: a cardiac magnetic resonance evaluation. Pediatr Cardiol 31:921–922

Frey N, Katus HA, Olson EN, Hill JA (2004) Hypertrophy of the heart. A new therapeutic target? Circulation 109: 1580–1589

Friedrich MG, Strohm O, Schulz-Menger J, Marciniak H, Luft FC, Dietz R (1998) Contrast-enhanced magnetic resonance imaging visualizes changes in the course of viral myocarditis. Circulation 97:1802–1809

Friedrich MG, Sechtem I, Schulz-Menger J et al (2009) Cardiovascular magnetic resonance in myocarditis: a JACC white paper. J Am Coll Cardiol 53:1475–1487

Frishman WH, Del Vecchio A, Sanal S, Ismail A (2003a) Cardiovascular manifestations of substance abuse part 1: cocaine. Heart 5:187–201

Frishman WH, Del Vecchio A, Sanal S, Ismail A (2003b) Cardiovascular manifestations of substance abuse part 2: alcohol, amphetamines, heroin, cannibs, and caffeine. Heart 5:253–271

Fritz J, Solaiyappan M, Tandri H et al (2005) Right ventricle shape and contraction patterns and relation to magnetic resonance imaging findings. J Comput Assist Tomogr 29:725–733

Fujita N, Duerinckx AJ, Higgins CB (1993) Variation in left ventricular regional wall stress with cine magnetic resonance imaging: normal subjects versus dilated cardiomyopathy. Am Heart J 125:1337–1345

Gagliardi MG, Bevilacqua M, Di Renzi P, Picardo S, Passariello R, Marcelletti C (1991) Usefulness of magnetic resonance imaging for diagnosis of acute myocarditis in infants and children, and comparison with endomyocardial biopsy. Am J Cardiol 68:1089–1091

Galiuto L, Ranieri De Caterina A, Porfidia A et al (2010) Reversible coronary microvascular dysfunction: a common

pathogenetic mechanism in apical ballooning or Tako-Tsubo syndrome. Eur Heart J 31:1319–1327
Ganau A, Devereux RB, Roman MJ (1992) Patterns of left ventricular hypertrophy and geometric remodeling in essential hypertension. J Am Coll Cardiol 19:1550–1558
Gatzka CD (2002) Left ventricular hypertrophy, cardiac imaging and cardiac electric activity. J Hypertens 20: 2153–2156
Gaudio C, Tanzilli G, Mazzarotto P et al (1991) Comparison of left ventricular ejection fraction by magnetic resonance imaging and radionuclide ventriculography in idiopathic dilated cardiomyopathy. Am J Cardiol 67:411–415
Gaudio C, Pelliccia F, Tanzilli G, Mazzarotto P, Cianfrocca C, Marino B (1992) Magnetic resonance imaging for assessment of apical hypertrophy in hypertrophic cardiomyopathy. Clin Cardiol 15:164–168
Germans T, Wilde AAM, Dijkmans PA et al (2006) Structural abnormalities of the inferoseptal left ventricular wall detected by cardiac magnetic resonance imaging in carriers of hypertrophic cardiomyopathy mutations. J Am Coll Cardiol 48:2518–2523
Glanzmann C, Kaufmann P, Jenni R et al (1998) Cardiac risk after mediastinal irradiation for Hodgkin's disease. Radiother Oncol 46:51–62
Globits S, Bergler KJ, Stanek G, Ullrich R, Glogar D (1994) Magnetic resonance imaging in the diagnosis of acute Lyme carditis. Cardiology 85:415–417
Globits S, Kreiner G, Frank H et al (1997) Significance of morphological abnormalities detected by MRI in patients undergoing successful ablation of right ventricular outflow tract tachycardia. Circulation 96:2633–2640
Goodfield NER, Bhandari S, Plant WD, Morley-Davies A, Sutherland GR (1995) Cardiac involvement in Wegener's granulomatosis. Br Heart J 73:110–115
Grant SCD, Levy RD, Venning MC, Ward C, Brooks NH (1994) Wegener's granulomatosis and the heart. Br Heart J 71:82–86
Gropler RJ, Beanlands RSB, Dilsizian V et al (2010) Imaging myocardial metabolic remodeling. J Nucl Med 51:88S–101S
Gujja P, Rosing DR, Tripodi DJ, Shizukuda Y (2010) Iron overload cardiomyopathy. Better understanding of an increasing disorder. J Am Coll Cardiol 56:1001–1012
Gutberlet M, Spors B, Thoma T et al (2008) Suspected chronic myocarditis at cardiac MR: diagnostic accuracy and association with immunohistologically detected inflammation and viral persistence. Radiology 246:401–409
Hachulla AL, Launay D, Gaxotte V et al (2009) Cardiac magnetic imaging in systemic sclerosis: a cross-sectional observational study of 52 patients. Ann Rheum Dis 68: 1878–1884
Haghi D, Athanasiadis A, Papavassiliu T et al (2006) Right ventricular involvement in Takotsubo cardiomyopathy. Eur Heart J 27:2433–2439
Han Y, Peters DC, Dokhan B, Manning WJ (2009) Shorter difference between myocardium and blood optimal inversion time suggests diffuse fibrosis in dilated cardiomyopathy. J Magn Reson Imaging 30:967–972
Hansch A, Pfeil A, Rzanny R, Neumann T, Kaiser WA (2009) First-pass myocardial perfusion abnormalities in Churg-Strauss syndrome with cardiac involvement. Int J Cardiovasc Imaging 25:501–510
Hardy P, Henkelman RM (1989) Transverse relaxation rate enhancement caused by magnetic particles. Magn Reson Imaging 7:265–275
Harrigan CJ, Appelbaum E, Maron BJ et al (2008) Significance of papillary muscle abnormalities identified by cardiovascular magnetic resonance in hypertrophic cardiomyopathy. Am J Cardiol 101:668–673
Harrigan CJ, Peters DC, Gibson CM et al (2011) Hypertrophic cardiomyopathy: quantification of late gadolinium enhancement with contrast-enhanced cardiovascular MR imaging. Radiology 258:128–133
Harris KM, Spirito P, Maron MS et al (2006) Prevalence, clinical profile, and significance of left ventricular remodeling in the end-stage of hypertrophic cardiomyopathy. Circulation 114:216–225
Harvey WP, Segal JP, Gurel T (1964) The spectrum of primary myocardial disease. Prog Cardiovasc Dis 7:17–42
Hausse AO, Aggoun Y, Bonnet D et al (2002) Idebenone and reduced cardiac hypertrophy in Friedreich's ataxia. Heart 87:346–349
He T, Kirk P, Firmin DN et al (2008) Multi-center transferability of a breath-hold T2 technqiue for myocardial iron assessment. J Cardiovasc Magn Reson 10:11
Heckbert SR, Post W, Pearson GDN et al (2006) Traditional cardiovascular risk factors in relation to left ventricular mass, volume, and systolic function by cardiac magnetic resonance imaging. J Am Coll Cardiol 48:2285–2292
Heidenreich PA, Hancock SL, Vagelos RH, Lee BK, Schnittger I (2005) Diastolic dysfunction after mediastinal irradiation. Am Heart J 150:977–982
Hill JA, Olson EN (2007) Cardiac plasticity. Mechanisms of disease. N Engl J Med 358:1370–1380
Ho CY, López B, Coelho-Filho OR (2010) Myocardial fibrosis as an early manifestation of hypertrophic cardiomyopathy. N Engl J Med 363:552–563
Hoedemaekers YM, Caliskan K, Majoor-Krakauer D et al (2007) Cardiac B-myosin heavy chain defects in two families with non-compaction cardiomyopathy: linking non-compaction to hypertrophic, restrictive, and dilated cardiomyopathies. Eur Heart J 28:2732–2737
HombachV MerkleN, Torzewski J et al (2009) Electrocardiographic and cardiac magnetic resonance imaging parameters as predictors of a worse outcome in patients with idiopathic dilated cardiomyopathy. Eur Heart J 30:2011–2018
Huffman C, Wagman G, Fudim M et al (2010) Reversible cardiomyopathies—a review. Transplant Proc 42:3673–3678
Hughes SE, McKenna WJ (2005) New insights into the pathology of inherited cardiomyopathy. Heart 91:257–264
Hunold P, Wieneke H, Bruder O et al (2005) Late enhancement: a new feature in MRI of arrhythmogenic right ventricular cardiomyopathy. J Cardiovasc Magn Reson 7:649–655
Huong DL, Wechsler B, Papo T et al (1997) Endomyocardial fibrosis in Behçet's disease. Ann Rheum Dis 56:205–208
Hurst RT, Askew JW, Reuss CS et al (2006) Transient midventricular ballooning syndrome. A new variant. J Am Coll Cardiol 48:579–583

Ichinose A, Otani H, Oikawa M et al (2008) MRI of cardiac sarcoidosis: basal and subepicardial localization of myocardial lesions and their effect on left ventricular function. AJR Am J Roentgenol 191:862–869
Iles L, Pfluger H, Phrommintikul A et al (2008) Evaluation of diffuse myocardial fibrosis in heart failure with cardiac magnetic resonance contrast-enhanced T1 mapping. J Am Coll Cardiol 52:1574–1580
Imai H, Kumai T, Sekiya M et al (1992) Left ventricular trabeculae evaluated with MRI in dilated cardiomyopathy and old myocardial infarction. J Cardiol 22:83–90
Jacquier A, Thuny F, Jop B et al (2010) Measurement of trabeculated left ventricular mass using cardiac magnetic resonance imaging in the diagnosis of left ventricular non-compaction. Eur Heart J 31:1098–1104
Jain A, Shehata ML, Stuber M et al (2010) Prevalence of left ventricular regional dysfunction in arrhythmogenic right ventricular dysplasia. A tagged MRI study. Circ Cardiovasc Imaging 3:290–297
Jefferies JL, Towbin JA (2010) Dilated cardiomyopathy. Lancet 375:752–762
Jellis C, Martin J, Narula J, Marwick TH (2010) Assessment of nonischemic myocardial fibrosis. J Am Coll Cardiol 56:89–97
Jensen PD, Jensen FT, Christensen T, Heickendorff L, Jensen LG, Ellegaard J (2001) Indirect evidence for the potential ability of magnetic resonance imaging to evaluate the myocardial iron content in patients with transfusional iron overload. MAGMA 12:153–166
Jensen PD, Jensen FT, Christensen T, Eiskjaer H, Baandrup U, Nielsen JL (2003) Evaluation of myocardial iron by magnetic resonance imaging during iron chelation therapy with deferrioxamine: indication of close relation between myocardial iron content and chelatable iron pool. Blood 101:4632–4639
Jerosch-Herold M, Sheridan DC, Kushner JD et al (2008) Cardiac magnetic resonance imaging of myocardial contrast uptake and blood flow in patients affected with idiopathic or familial dilated cardiomyopathy. Am J Physiol Heart Circ Physiol 295:H1234–H1242
Johansson B, Maceira AM, Babu-Narayan SV, Moon JC, Pennell DJ, Kilner PJ (2007) Clefts can be seen in the basal inferior wall of the left ventricle and the interventricular septum in healthy volunteers as well as patients by cardiovascular magnetic resonance. J Am Coll Cardiol 50:1294–1297
Jurcut R, Wildiers H, Ganame J, D'hooge J, Paridaens R, Voigt JU (2008) Detection and monitoring of cardiotoxicity-what does modern cardiology offer? Support Care Cancer 16: 437–445
Kahan A, Allanore Y (2006) Primary myocardial involvement in systemic sclerosis. Rheumatology 45:iv14–iv17
Kalil-Filho R, de Albuquerque CP (1995) Magnetic resonance imaging in Chagas' heart disease. Rev Paul Med 113:880–883
Kane GC, Keogh KA (2009) Involvement of the heart by small and medium vessel vasculitis. Curr Opin Rheumatol 21:29–34
Kang YJ (2003) New understanding in cardiotoxicity. Curr Opin Drug Discov Devel 6:110–116
Kawada N, Sakuma H, Yamakado T et al (1999) Hypertrophic cardiomyopathy: MR measurement of coronary blood flow and vasodilator flow reserve in patients and healthy subjects. Radiology 21:129–135
Kellman P, Hernando D, Shah S et al (2009) Multiecho Dixon fat and water separation method for detecting fibrofatty infiltration in the myocardium. Magn Reson Med 61:215–221
Keren A, Syrris P, McKenna WJ (2008) Hypertrophic cardiomyopathy: the genetic determinants of clinical disease expression. Nat Clin Pract Cardiovasc Med 5:158–168
Khavandi K, Khavandi A, Asghar O et al (2009) Diabetic cardiomyopathy—a distinct disease? Best Pract Res Clin Endocrinol Metab 23:347–360
Kimura F, Matsuo Y, Nakajima T et al (2010) Myocardial fat at cardiac imaging: how can we differentiate pathologic form physiologic fatty infiltration. Radiographics 30:1587–1602
Kindermann I, Kindermann M, Kandolf R et al (2008) Predictors of outcome in patients with suspected myocarditis. Circulation 118:639–648
Kirk P, Roughton M, Porter JB et al (2009) Cardiac T2* magnetic resonance for prediction of cardiac complications in thalassemia major. Circulation 120:1961–1968
Kloner RA, Rezkalla SH (2003) Cocaine and the heart. N Engl J Med 348:487–488
Klues HG, Schiffers A, Maron BJ (1995) Phenotypic spectrum and patterns of left ventricular hypertrophy in hypertophic cardiomyopathy: morphologic observations and significance as assessed by two-dimensional echocardiography in 600 patients. J Am Coll Cardiol 26:1699–1708
Knaapen P, Götte MJW, Paulus WJ et al (2006) Does myocardial fibrosis hinder contractile function and perfusion in idiopathic dilated cardiomyopathy? PET and MR imaging study. Radiology 240:380–388
Knaapen P, Germans T, Camici PG et al (2008) Determinants of coronary microvascular dysfunction in symptomatic hypertrophic cardiomyopathy. Am J Physiol Heart Circ Physiol 294:H986–H993
Kobayashi H, Yokoe I, Hirano M et al (2008) Cardiac magnetic resonance imaging with pharmacological stress perfusion and delayed enhancement in asymptomatic patients with systemic sclerosis. J Rheumatol 36:106–112
Kohli SK, Pantazis AA, Shah JS et al (2008) Diagnosis of left-ventricular non-compaction in patients with left-ventricular systolic dysfunction: time for a reappraisal of diagnostic criteria. Eur Heart J 29:89–95
Koito H, Suzuki J, Ohkubo N, Ishiguro Y, Iwasaka T, Inada M (1996) Gadolinium-diethylenetriamine pentaacetic acid enhanced magnetic resonance imaging of dilated cardiomyopathy: clinical significance of abnormally high signal intensity of left ventricular myocardium. J Cardiol 28:41–49
Kosovsky PA, Ehlers KH, Rafal RB, Williams WM, O'Loughlin JE, Markisz JA (1991) MR imaging of cardiac mass in Wegener granulomatosis. J Comput Assist Tomogr 15: 1028–1030
Koyama J, Ray-Sequin PA, Falk RH et al (2003) Longitudinal myocardial function assessed by tissue velocity, strain, and strain rate tissue Doppler echocardiography in patients with AL (primary) cardiac amyloidosis. Circulation 107: 2446–2452
Kramer CM, Reichek N, Ferrari VA, Theobald T, Dawson J, Axel L (1994) Regional heterogeneity of function in hypertrophic cardiomyopathy. Circulation 90:186–194
Kubo T, Gimeno JR, Bahl A et al (2007) Prevalence, clinical significance, and genetic basis of hypertrophic cardiomyopathy with restrictive phenotype. J Am Coll Cardiol 49:2419–2426

Kushwaha SS, Fallon JT, Fuster V (1997) Restrictive cardiomyopathy. N Engl J Med 336:267–276

Kwon DH, Setser RM, Thamilarasan M et al (2008) Abnormal papillary muscle morphology is independently associated with increased left ventricular outflow tract obstruction in hypertrophy cardiomyopathy. Heart 94:1295–1301

Kwon DH, Smedira NG, Rodriguez ER et al (2009) Cardiac magnetic resonance detection of myocardial scarring in hypertrophic cardiomyopathy. Correlation with histopathology and prevalence of ventricular tachycardia. J Am Coll Cardiol 54:242–249

Laissy JP, Messin B, Varenne O et al (2002) MRI of acute myocarditis: a comprehensive approach based on various imaging sequences. Chest 122:1638–1648

Lakdawala NK, Givertz MM (2010) Dilated cardiomyopathy with conduction disease and arrhythmia. Circulation 122:527–534

Lamb HJ, Beyerbacht HP, van der Laarse A et al (1999) Diastolic dysfunction in hypertensive heart disease is associated with altered myocardial metabolism. Circulation 99:2261–2267

Lauschke J, Maisch B (2008) Athlete's heart of hypertrophic cardiomyopathy? Clin Res Cardiol 98:80–88

Leonardi S, Raineri C, De Ferrari GM et al (2009) Usefulness of cardiac magnetic resonance in assessing the risk of ventricular arrhythmias and sudden death in patients with hypertrophic cardiomyopathy. Eur Heart J 30:2003–2010

Lesnefsky EJ, Allen KG, Carrea FP, Horwitz LD (1992) Ironcjatalyzed reactions cause lipid peroxidation in the intact heart. J Mol Cell Cardiol 24:1031–1038

Lieberman EB, Hutchins GM, Herskowitz A, Rose NR, Baughman KL (1991) Clinicopathologic description of myocarditis. J Am Coll Cardiol 18:1616–1626

Lightfoot JC, D'Agostino RB, Hamilton CA et al (2010) Novel approach to early detection of doxorubicin cardiotoxicity by gadolinium-enhanced cardiovascular magnetic resonance imaging in an experimental model. Circ Cardiovasc Imaging 3:550–558

Lipshultz SE, Colan SD, Gelber RD et al (1991) Late cardiac effects of doxorubicin therapy for acute lymphoblastic leukemia in childhood. N Engl J Med 324:808–815

Liu P, Olivieri N (1994) Iron overload cardiomyopathies: new insights into an old disease. Cardiovasc Drugs Ther 8:101–110

Lofiego C, Biagini E, Pasquale F et al (2007) Wide spectrum of presentation and variable outcomes of isolated left ventricular non-compaction. Heart 93:65–71

Lombardi C, Rusconi C, Faggiano P, Lanzani G, Campana C, Arbustini E (1995) Successful reduction of endomyocardial fibrosis in a patient with idiopathic hypereosinophilic syndrome. A case report. Angiology 46:345–351

Lund MB, Ihlen H, Voss BM et al (1996) Increased risk of heart valve regurgitation after mediastinal radiation for Hodgkin's disease: an echocardiographic study. Heart 75:591–595

Maceira AM, Joshi J, Prasad SK et al (2005) Cardiovascular magnetic resonance in cardiac amyloidosis. Circulation 111:186–193

Maceira AM, Prasad SK, Pennell DJ, Mohiaddin RH (2008a) Integrated evaluation of the hypertensive patient with cardiovascular magnetic resonance. Int J Cardiol 125:383–390

Maceira AM, Prasad SK, Hawkins PN, Roughton M, Pennell DJ (2008b) Cardiovascular magnetic resonance and prognosis in cardiac amyloidosis. J Cardiovasc Magn Reson 10:54–64

MacGowan GA, Shapiro EP, Azhari H et al (1997) Shortening in the fiber and cross-fiber directions in the normal human left ventricle and in idiopathic dilated cardiomyopathy. Circulation 96:535–541

Mahrholdt H, Goedecke C, Wagner A et al (2004) Cardiovascular magnetic resonance assessment of human myocarditis. A comparison to histology and molecular biology. Circulation 109:1250–1258

Mahrholdt H, Wagner A, Judd RM, Sechtem U, Kim RJ (2005) Delayed enhancement cardiovascular magnetic resonance assessment of non-ischaemic cardiomyopathies. Eur Heart J 26:1461–1474

Mahrholdt H, Wagner A, Deluigi C et al (2006) Presentation, patterns of myocardial damage, and clinical course of viral myocarditis. Circulation 114:1581–1590

Maier SE, Fischer SE, McKinnon GC, Hess OM, Kraeyenbuehl HP, Boesiger P (1992) Evaluation of left ventricular segmental wall motion in hypertrophic cardiomyopathy with myocardial tagging. Circulation 86:1919–1928

Manins V, Habersberger J, Pfluger H, Taylor AJ (2009) Cardiac magnetic resonance imaging in the evaluation of cardiac sarcoidosis: an Australian single-center experience. Int J Med 39:77–82

Marcu CB, beek AM, van Rossum AC (2007) Chagas' heart disease diagnosed on MRI: the importance of patient "geographic" history. Int J Cardiol 1147:e58–e60

Marcus FI, McKenna WJ, Sherrill D et al (2010) Diagnosis of arrhythmogenic right ventricular cardiomyopathy/dyplasia. Proposed modification of the task force criteria. Circulation 121:1533–1541

Mark PB, Johnston N, Groenning BA et al (2006) Redefinition of uremic cardiomyopathy by contrast-enhanced cardiac magnetic resonance imaging. Kidney Int 69:1839–1845

Marmursztejn J, Vignaux O, Cohen P et al (2009) Impact of cardiac magnetic resonance imaging for assessment of Churg-Strauss syndrome: a cross-sectional study in 20 patients. Clin Exp Rheumatol 27:S70–S76

Marmursztejn J, Cohen P, Duboc D et al (2010) Cardiac magnetic resonance imaging in Churg-Strauss-syndrome. Impact of immunosuppressants on outcome assessed in a prospective study on 8 patients. Clin Exp Rheumatol 28(1 Suppl 57):8–13

Maron BJ (2003) Sudden death in young athletes. N Engl J Med 349:1064–1075

Maron BJ, Pelliccia A (2006) The heart of trained athletes. Cardiac remodeling and the risk of sports, including sudden death. Circulation 114:1633–1644

Maron BJ, Anan TJ, Roberts WC (1981) Quantitative analysis of the distribution of cardiac muscle cell disorganization in the left ventricular wall of patients with hypertrophic cardiomyopathy. Circulation 63:882–894

Maron BJ, Bonow RO, Cannon ROI, Leon MB (1987) Hypertrophic cardiomyopathy: interrelations of clinical manifestations, pathophysiology, and therapy. N Engl J Med 316:780–789

Maron BJ, Pelliccia A, Spirito P (1995) Cardiac disease in young trained athletes. Insight into methods for

distinguishing athlete's heart from structural heart disease, with particular emphasis on hypertrophic cardiomyopathy. Circulation 91:1596–1602
Maron BJ, McKenna WJ, Danielson GK et al (2003a) American College of Cardiology/European Society of Cardiology clinical expert consensus document on hypertrophic cardiomyopathy. J Am Coll Cardiol 42:1687–1713
Maron MS, Olivotto I, Betocchi S et al (2003b) Effect of left ventricular outflow tract obstruction on clinical outcome in hypertrophy cardiomyopathy. N Engl J Med 348:295–303
Maron BJ, Towbin JA, Thiene G et al (2006a) Contemporary definitions and classification of the cardiomyopathies: an American Heart Association Scientific Statement from the Council on Clinical Cardiology, Heart Failure and Transplantation Committee; Quality of Care and Outcomes Research and Functional Genomics and Translational Biology Interdisciplinary Working Groups; and Council on Epidemiology and Prevention. Circulation 113: 1807–1816
Maron MS, Olvitoo I, Zenovich AG et al (2006b) Hypertrophic cardiomyopathy is predominantly a disease of left ventricular outflow tract obstruction. Circulation 114:2232–2239
Maron MS, Hauser TH, Dubrow E et al (2007) Right ventricular involvement in hypertrophic cardiomyopathy. Am J Cardiol 100:1293–1298
Maron MS, Finley JJ, Bos M et al (2008a) Prevalence, clinical significance, and natural history of left ventricular apical aneurysms in hypertrophic cardiomyopathy. Circulation 118:1541–1549
Maron MS, Appelbaum E, Harrigan CJ et al (2008b) Clinical profile and significance of delayed enhancement in hypertrophic cardiomyopathy. Circ Heart Fail 1:184–191
Maron MS, Maron BJ, Harrigan C et al (2009) Hypertrophic cardiomyopathy phenotype revisited after 50 years with cardiovascular magnetic resonance. J Am Coll Cardiol 54:220–228
Maron MS, Olivotto I, Harrigan C et al (2011) Mitral valve abnormalities identified by cardiovascular magnetic resonance represent a primary phenotypic expression of hypertrophic cardiomyopathy. Circulation 124:40–47
Masci PG, Marinelli M, Piacenti M et al (2010a) Myocardial structural, perfusion, and metabolic correlates of left bundle branch block mechanical derangement in patients with dilated cardiomyopathy. A tagged cardiac magnetic resonance and positron emission tomography study. Circ Cardiovasc Imaging 3:482–490
Masci PG, Francone M, Desmet W et al (2010b) Right ventricular ischemic injury in patients with acute ST-segment elevation myocardial infarction. Characterization with cardiovascular magnetic resonance. Circulation 122:1405–1412
Matoh F, Satoh H, Shiraki K et al (2007) Usefulness of delayed enhancement magnetic resonance imaging to differentiate dilated phase of hypertrophic cardiomyopathy and dilated cardiomyopathy. J Cardiac Fail 13:372–379
Matoh F, Satoh H, Shiraki K et al (2008) The usefulness of delayed enhancement magnetic resonance imaging for diagnosis and evaluation of cardiac function in patients with cardiac sarcoidosis. J Cardiol 51:179–188
Matsuki M, Matsuo M (2000) MR findings of myocardial sarcoidosis. Clin Radiol 55:323–325
Matsuoka H, Hamada M, Honda T et al (1993) Precise assessment of myocardial damage associated with secondary cardiomyopathies by use of Gd-DTPA-enhanced magnetic resonance imaging. Angiology 44:945–950
Mavrogeni S, Gotsis E, Verganelakis D et al (2009) Effect of iron overload on exercise capacity in thalassemic patients with heart failure. Int J Cardiovasc Imaging 25:777–783
Maya L, Villarreal FJ (2010) Diagnostic approaches for diabetic cardiomyopathy and myocardial fibrosis. J Moll Cell Cardiology 48:524–529
Mazur W, Nagueh SF, Lakkis NM et al (2001) Regression of left ventricular hypertrophy after nonsurgical septal reduction therapy for hypertrophic obstructive cardiomyopathy. Circulation 103:1492–1496
McCann GP, Van Dockum WG, Beek AM et al (2007) Extent of myocardial infarction and reverse remodeling assessed by cardiac magnetic resonance in patients with and without right bundle branch block following alcohol septal ablation for obstructive hypertrophic cardiomyopathy. Am J Cardiol 99:563–567
McCrohon JA, Richmond DR, Pennell DJ, Mohiaddin RH (2002) Isolated noncompaction of the myocardium. A rarity or missed diagnosis? Circulation 106:e22–e23
McCrohon JA, Moon JCC, Prasad SK et al (2003) Differentiation of heart failure related to dilated cardiomyopathy and coronary artery disease using gadolinium-enhanced cardiovascular magnetic resonance. Circulation 108:54–59
McKenna WJ, Thiene G, Nava A et al (1994) Diagnosis of arrhythmogenic right ventricular dysplasia/cardiomyopathy. Br Heart J 71:215–218
Meijs MFL, Bots ML, Vonken E-JA et al (2007) Rationale and design of the SMART Heart study. A prediction model for left ventricular hypertrophy in hypertension. Neth Heart J 15:295–298
Mekinian A, Lions C, Leleu X et al (2010) Prognosis assessment of cardiac involvement in systemic AL amyloidosis by magnetic resonance imaging. Am J Med 123:864–868
Melacini P, Basso C, Angelini A et al (2010) Clinicopathological profiles of progressive heart failure in hypertrophic cardiomyopathy. Eur Heart J 31:2111–2123
Meyer C, Schmid G, Görlitz S et al (2007) Cardiomyopathy in Friedreich's ataxia—assessment by cardiac MRI. Mov Disord 22:1615–1622
Migrino RQ, Christenson R, Szabo A, Bright M, Truran S, Hari P (2009) Prognostic implication of late gadolinium enhancement on cardiac MRI in light chain (AL) amyloidosis on long term follow-up. BMC Med Phys 9:5–11
Miller MA, Gomes JA, Fuster V (2007) Risk stratification of sudden cardiac death in hypertrophic cardiomyopathy. Nat Clin Pract Cardiovasc Med 4:667–676
Minami Y, Kajimoto K, Terajima Y et al (2011) Clinical implications of midventricular obstruction in patients with hypertrophic cardiomyopathy. J Am Coll Cardiol 57:2346–2355
Mocumbi AO, Ferreira MB, Sidi D, Yacoub MH (2008) A population study of endomyocardial fibrosis in a rural area of Mozambique. N Engl J Med 359:43–49
Mollet NR, Dymarkowski S, Volders W et al (2002) Visualization of ventricular thrombi with contrast-enhanced MRI in patients with ischemic heart disease. Circulation 106:2873–2876

Moon JCC, McKenna WJ, McCrohon JA, Elliot PM, Smith GC, Pennell DJ (2003a) Toward clinical risk assessment in hypertrophic cardiomyopathy with gadolinium cardiovascular magnetic resonance. J Am Coll Cardiol 41:1561–1567

Moon JCC, Mundy HR, Lee PJ, Mohiaddin RH, Pennell DJ (2003b) Myocardial fibrosis in glycogen storage disease type III. Circulation 107:e47

Moon JCC, Sachdev B, Elkington AG et al (2003c) Gadolinium enhanced cardiovascular magnetic resonance in Anderson-Fabry disease. Evidence for a disease specific abnormality of the myocardial interstitium. Eur Heart J 24:2151–2155

Moon JC, Fisher NG, McKenna WJ, Pennell DJ (2004a) Detection of apical hypertrophic cardiomyopathy by cardiovascular magnetic resonance in patients with non-diagnostic echocardiography. Heart 90:645–649

Moon JC, Reed E, Sheppard MN et al (2004b) The histologic basis of late gadolinium enhancement cardiovascular magnetic resonance in hypertrophic cardiomyopathy. J Am Coll Cardiol 43:2260–2264

Moon JC, Sheppard M, Reed E et al (2006) The histological basis of late gadolinium enhancement cardiovascular magnetic resonance in a patient with Anderson-Fabry disease. J Cardiovasc Magn Reson 8:479–482

Moreo A, Ambrosio G, De Chiara B et al (2009) Influence of myocardial fibrosis on left ventricular diastolic function. Noninvasive assessment by cardiac magnetic resonance and echo. Circ Cardiovasc Imaging 2:437–443

Morganroth J, Maron BJ, Henry WL, Epstein SE (1975) Comparative left ventricular dimensions in trained athletes. Ann Intern Med 82:521–524

Motoyasu M, Kurita T, Onishi K et al (2008) Correlation between late gadolinium enhancement and diastolic function in hypertrophic cardiomyopathy assessed by magnetic resonance imaging. Circ J 72:378–383

Munk PS, Ørn S, Larsen AI (2007) Lyme carditis: persistent local delayed enhancement by cardiac magnetic resonance imaging. Int J Cardiol 115:e108–e110

Myrehaug S, Pintelie M, Yun L et al (2010) A population-based study of cardiac morbidity among Hodgkin lymphoma patients with preexisting heart disease. Blood 116:2237–2240

Nagueh SF, Mahmarian JJ (2006) Noninvasive cardiac imaging in patients with hypertrophic cardiomyopathy. J Am Coll Cardiol 48:2410–2422

Naik M, Kim D, O'Brien F, Axel L, Srichai MB (2008) Images in cardiovascular medicine. Lyme carditis. Circulation 118:1881–1884

Nassenstein K, Breuckmann F, Huger M et al (2008) Detection of myocardial fibrosis in systemic sclerosis by contrast-enhanced magnetic resonance imaging. Rofo 180:1054–1060

Nathwani D, Hamlet N, Walker E (1990) Lyme disease: a review. Br J Gen Pract 40:72–74 (see comments)

Naylor LH, George K, O'Driscoll G, Green DJ (2008) The athlete's heart: a contemporary appraisal of the 'Morganroth hypothesis'. Sports Med 38:69–90

Nazarian S, Bluemke DA, Lardo AC et al (2005) Magnetic resonance assessment of the substrate for inducible ventricular tachycardia in nonischemic cardiomyopathy. Circulation 112:2821–2825

Neumann T, Manger B, Schmid M et al (2009) Cardiac involvement in Churg-Strauss syndrome: impact of endomyocarditis. Medicine (Baltimore) 88:236–243

Ng AC, Delgado V, Bertini M et al (2010) Myocardial steatosis and biventricular strain and strain rate imaging in patients with type 2 diabetes mellitus. Circulation 122:2538–2544

Nihoyannopoulos P, Dawson D (2009) Restrictive cardiomyopathies. Eur J Echocardio 10:iii23–iii33

Niida T, Isoda K, Sasaki M et al (2008) Late gadolinium enhanced high resolution magnetic resonance imaging reveals pathophysiological condition of cardiac sarcoidosis. Int Heart J 50:263–266

Norman M, Simpson M, Mogensen J et al (2005) Novel mutation in desmoplakin causes arrhythmogenic left ventricular cardiomyopathy. Circulation 112:636–642

Nucifora G, Aquaro GD, Pingitore A, Masci PG, Lombardi M (2011) Myocardial fibrosis in isolated left ventricular non-compaction and its relation to disease severity. Eur J Heart Failure 13:170–176

O'Hanlon R, Grasso A, Roughton M et al (2010) Prognostic significance of myocardial fibrosis in hypertrophic cardiomyopathy. J Am Coll Cardiol 56:867–874

O'Neill SG, Woldman S, Bailliard F et al (2009) Cardiac magnetic resonance imaging in patients with systemic lupus erythematosus. Ann Rheum Dis 68(9):1478–1481

Oechslin E, Jenni R (2011) Left ventricular non-compaction revisited: a distinct phenotype with genetic heterogeneity? Eur Heart J 32:1446–1456

Oechslin EN, Attenhofer Jost CH, Rojas JR et al (2000) Long-term follow-up of 34 adults with isolated left ventricular noncompaction: a distinct cardiomyopathy with poor prognosis. J Am Coll Cardiol 36:493–500

Ohira H, Tsujino I, Ishimaru S (2008) Myocardial imaging with 18F-fluoro-2-deoxyglucose positron emission tomography and magnetic resonance imaging in sarcoidosis. Eur J Nucl Med Mol Imaging 35:933–941

Olivotto I, Maron MS, Autore C et al (2008) Assessment and significance of left ventricular mass by magnetic resonance in hypertrophic cardiomyopathy. J Am Coll Cardiol 52:559–566

Olivotto I, Maron BJ, Appelbaum E et al (2010) Spectrum and clinical significance of systolic function and myocardial fibrosis assessed by cardiovascular magnetic resonance in hypertrophic cardiomyopathy. Am J Cardiol 106:261–267

Ong P, Athansiadis A, Hill S et al (2011) Usefulness of pericardial effusion as new diagnostic criterion for noninvasive detection of myocarditis. Am J Cardiol 108:445–452

Otmani A, Leborgne L, Renard C et al (2007) Electrocardiogram, electrocardiography, and magnetic resonance imaging characteristics in Uhl's disease. Circulation 115:e11–e12

Owan TE, Hodge DO, Herges RM et al (2006) Trends in prevalence and outcome of heart failure with preserved ejection fraction. N Engl J Med 355:251–259

Pamuru PR, Dokuparthi MVN, Remersu S, Calambur N, Nallari P (2010) Comparison of Uhl's anomaly, right ventricular outflow tract ventricular tachycardia (RVOT VT) and arrhythmogenic right ventricular dysplasia/cardiomyopathy (ARVD/C) with an insight into genetics of ARVD/C. Indian J Med Res 131:35–45

Park JH, Kim YM, Chung JW, Park YB, Han JH, Han MC (1992) MR imaging of hypertrophic cardiomyopathy. Radiology 185:441–446

Parrillo JE (1990) Heart disease and the eosinophil. N Engl J Med 323:1560–1561

Patel MR, Cawley PJ, Heitner JF et al (2009) Detection of myocardial sarcoidosis in patients with sarcoidosis. Circulation 120:1969–1977

Petersen SE, Selvanayagam JB, Francis JM et al (2005a) Differentiation of athlete's heart from pathological forms of cardiac hypertrophy by means of geometric indices derived from cardiovascular magnetic resonance. J Cardiovasc Magn Reson 7:551–558

Petersen SE, Selvanayagam JB, Wiesmann F et al (2005b) Left ventricular non-compaction. Insight from cardiovascular magnetic resonance imaging. J Am Coll Cardiol 46: 101–105

Petersen SE, Jerosch-Herold M, Hudsmith LE (2007) Evidence for microvascular dysfunction in hypertrophic cardiomyopathy. New insights from multiparametric magnetic resonance imaging. Circulation 115:2418–2425

Pfluger HB, Phrommintikul A, Mariani JA, Cherayath JG, Taylor AJ (2008) Utility of myocardial fibrosis and fatty infiltration detected by cardiac magnetic resonance imaging in the diagnosis of arrhythmogenic right ventricular dysplasia–a single centre experience. Heart Lung Circ 17:478–483

Pieroni M, Dello Russo A, Marzo F et al (2009) High prevalence of myocarditis mimicking arrhythmogenic right ventricular cardiomyopathy. Differential diagnosis by electroanatomic mapping-guided endomyocardial biopsy. J Am Coll Cardiol 53:681–689

Pignatelli RH, McMahon CJ, Dreyer WJ et al (2003) Clinical characterization of left ventricular noncompaction in children. A relatively common form of cardiomyopathy. Circulation 108:2672–2678

Pinamonti B, Dragos AM, Pyxaras SA et al (2011) Prognostic predictors in arrhythmogenic right ventricular cardiomyopathy: results from a 10-year registry. Eur Heart J 32: 1105–1113

Pitt M, Davies MK, Brady AJ (1996) Hypereosinophilic syndrome: endomyocardial fibrosis. Heart 76:377–378

Pluim BM, Zwinderman AH, van der Laarse A, van der Wall EE (1999) The athlete's heart. A meta-analysis of cardiac structure and function. Circulation 100:336–344

Prasad A, Lerman A, Rihal CS (2008) Apical ballooning syndrome (Tako-Tsubo or stress cardiomyopathy): a mimic of acute myocardial infarction. Am Heart J 155:408–417

Prasad A, Hastings JL, Shibata S et al (2010) Characterization of static and dynamic left ventricular function in patients with heart failure with a preserved ejection fraction. Circ Heart Fail 3:617–626

Proclemer A, Basadonna PT, Slavich GA, Miani D, Fresco C, Fioretti PM (1997) Cardiac magnetic resonance imaging findings in patients with right ventricular outflow tract premature contractions. Eur Heart J 18:2002–2010

Rademakers FE, Bogaert J (2006) Cardiac dysfunction in heart failure with normal ejection fraction: MRI measurements. Prog Cardiovasc Dis 49:215–227

Rademakers FE, Buchalter MB, Rogers WJ et al (1992) Dissociation between left ventricular untwisting and filling. Accentuation by catecholamines. Circulation 85:1572–1581

Rademakers FE, Marchal G, Mortelmans L, Van de Werf F, Bogaert J (2003) Evolution of regional performance after an acute anterior myocardial infarction in humans using magnetic resonance tagging. J Physiol 546:777–787

Rahman JE, Helou EF, Gelzer-Bell R (2004) Noninvasive diagnosis of biopsy-proven cardiac amyloidosis. J Am Coll Cardiol 43:410–415

Raman SV, Basso C, Tandri H, Taylor MRG (2010) Imaging phenotype vs genotype in nonhypertrophic heritable cardiomyopathies. Dilated cardiomyopathy and arrhythmogenic right ventricular cardiomyopathy. Circ Cardiovasc Imaging 3:753–765

Rapezzi C, Merline G, Quarta C et al (2009) Systemic cardiac amyloidosis. Disease profiles and clinical courses of the 3 main types. Circulation 120:1203–1212

Richardson P, McKenna W, Bristow M et al (1996) Report of the 1995 World Health Organization/International Society and Federation of Cardiology Task Force on the definition and classification of cardiomyopathies. Circulation 93:841–842

Rickers C, Wilke N, Jerosch-Herold M et al (2005) Utility of cardiac magnetic resonance imaging in the diagnosis of hypertrophic cardiomyopathy. Circulation 112:855–861

Rijzewijk LJ, van der Meer RW, Smit JW et al (2008) Myocardial steatosis is an independenet predictor of diastolic dysfunction in type 2 diabetes mellitus. J Am Coll Cardiol 52:1793–1799

Ripoli A, Pingitore A, Favilli B et al (2005) Does subclinical hypothyroidism affect cardiac pump performance? Evidence from a magnetic resonance imaging study. J Am Coll Cardiol 45:439–445

Rochitte CE, Nacif MD, de Oliveira Junior AC et al (2007) Cardiac magnetic resonance in Chagas' disease. Artif Organs 31:259–267

Ruberg FL, Appelbaum E, Davidoff R et al (2009) Diagnostic and prognostic utility of cardiovascular magnetic resonance imaging in light-chain cardiac amyloidosis. Am J Cardiol 103:544–549

Rubinshtein R, Glockner JF, Ommen SR et al (2010) Characteristics and clinical significance of late gadolinium enhancement by contrast-enhanced magnetic resonance imaging in patients with hypertrophic cardiomyopathy. Circ Heart Fail 3:51–58

Rudin M, Pedersen B, Umemura K, Zierhut W (1991) Determination of rat heart morphology and function in vivo in two models of cardiac hypertrophy by means of magnetic resonance imaging. Basic Res Cardiol 86:165–174

Rudolf A, Abdel-Aty H, Bohl S et al (2009) Noninvasive detection of fibrosis applying contrast-enhanced cardiac magnetic resonance in different forms of left ventricular hypertrophy. Relation to remodeling. J Am Coll Cardiol 53:284–291

Scharlag J, Schneider G, Urhausen A, Rochette V, Kramann B, Kindermann W (2002) Athete's heart. Right and left ventricular mass and function in male endurance athletes and untrained individuals determined by magnetic resonance imaging. J Am Coll Cardiol 40:1856–1863

Schietinger BJ, Brammer GM, Wang H et al (2008) Patterns of late gadolinium enhancement in chronic hemodialysis patients. J Am Coll Cardiol Img 1:450–456

Schulz-Menger J, Strohm O, Waigand J, Uhlich F, Dietz R, Friedrich MG (2000a) The value of magnetic resonance imaging of the left ventricular outflow tract in patients with

hypertrophic obstructive cardiomyopathy after septal artery embolization. Circulation 101:1764–1766
Schulz-Menger J, Strohm O, Dietz R, Friedrich MG (2000b) Visualization of cardiac involvement in patients with systemic sarcoidosis applying contrast-enhanced magnetic resonance imaging. MAGMA 11:82–83
Schulz-Menger J, Abdel-Aty H, Busjahn A et al (2006) Left ventricular outflow tract planimetry by cardiovascular magnetic resonance differentiates obstructive from non-obstructive hypertrophic cardiomyopathy. J Cardiovasc Magn Reson 8:741–746
Schwefer M, Aschenbach R, Heidemann J, Mey C, Lapp H (2009) Constrictive pericarditis, still a diagnostic challenge: comprehensive review of clinical management. Eur J Cardiohoracic Surg 36:502–510
Semelka RC, Tomei E, Wagner S et al (1990) Interstudy reproducibility of dimensional and functional measurements between cine magnetic resonance studies in the morphologically abnormal left ventricle. Am Heart J 119: 1367–1373
Sen-Chowdhry S, Prasad SK, Syrris P et al (2006) Cardiovascular magnetic resonance in arrhythmogenic right ventricular cardiomyopathy revisited. Comparison with task force criteria and genotype. J Am Coll Cardiol 48:2132–2140
Sen-Chowdhry S, Syrris P, Ward D, Asimaki A, Sevdalis E, McKenna WJ (2007) Clinical and genetic characterization of families with arrhythmogenic right ventricular dysplasia/cardiomyopathy provides novel insights into patterns of disease expression. Circulation 115:1710–1720
Sen-Chowdhry S, Syrris P, Prasad SK et al (2008) Left dominant arrhythmogenic cardiomyopathy. An underrecognized clinical entity. J Am Coll Cardiol 52:2175–2187
Sen-Chowdhry S, Syrris P, Pantazis A et al (2010) Mutational heterogeneity, modifier genes, and environmental influence to phenotypic diversity of arrhythmogenic cardiomyopathy. Circ Cardiovasc Genet 3:323–330
Sharkey SW, Lesser JR, Zenovich AG et al (2005) Acute and reversible cardiomyopathy provoked by stress in women form the United States. Circulation 111:472–479
Sharma OP (2003) Diagnosis of cardiac sarcoidosis. An imperfect science, a hesitant art. Chest 123:18–19
Shimada T, Shimada K, Sakane T et al (2001) Diagnosis of cardiac sarcoidosis and evaluation of the effects of steroid therapy by gadolinium-DTPA-enhanced magnetic resonance imaging. Am J Med 110:520–527
Shimizu I, Iguchi N, Watanabe H et al (2010) Delayed cardiovascular magnetic resonance as a novel technique to predict cardiac events in dilated cardiomyopathy patients. Int J Cardiol 142:224–229
Sigwart U (1995) Non-surgical reduction for hypertrophic obstructive cardiomyopathy. Lancet 346:211–214
Silva MC, Meira ZM, Giannetti G et al (2007) Myocardial delayed enhancement by magnetic resonance imaging in patients with muscular dystrophy. J Am Coll Cardiol 49:1874–1879
Silverman KJ, Hutchins GM, Bulkley BH (1978) Cardiac sarcoid: a clinicopathologic study of 84 unselected patients with systemic sarcoidosis. Circulation 58:1204–1211
Simonetti OP, Kim RJ, Fieno DS et al (2001) An improved MR imaging technique for the visualization of myocardial infarction. Radiology 218:215–223
Singal PK, Iliskovic N (1998) Doxorubicin-induced cardiomyopathy. N Engl J Med 339:900–905
Singh JA, Woodard PK, Davilla-Roman VG et al (2005) Cardiac magnetic resonance imaging abnormalities in systemic lupus erythematosus: a preliminary report. Lupus 14:137–144
Sliwa K, Flett J, Elkayam Y (2006) Peripartum cardiomyopathy. Lancet 368:687–693
Smedema JP, Snoep G, van Kroonenburgh MPG et al (2005) Evaluation of the accuracy of gadolinium-enhanced magnetic resonance in the diagnosis of cardiac sarcoidosis. J Am Coll Cardiol 45:1683–1690
Smith SC, Ladenson JH, Mason JW, Jaffe AS (1997) Elevations of cardiac troponin I associated with myocarditis. Experimental and clinical correlates. Circulation 95:163–168
Soler R, Rodriguez E, Rodriguez JA, Perez ML, Penas M (1997) Magnetic resonance imaging of apical hypertrophic cardiomyopathy. J Thorac Imaging 12:221–225
Soriano CJ, Ridocci F, Estornell J, Jimenez J, Martinez V, De Velasco JA (2005) Noninvasive diagnosis of coronary artery disease in patients with heart failure and systolic dysfunction of uncertain etiology, using late gadolinium-enhanced cardiovascular magnetic resonance. J Am Coll Cardiol 45:743–748
Sotgia B, Sciagrà R, Olivotto I et al (2008) Spatial resolution between coronary microvascular dysfunction and delayed contrast enhancement in patients with hypertrophic cardiomyopathy. J Nucl Med 49:1090–1096
Sparrow P, Amirabadi A, Sussman MS, Paul N, Merchant N (2009) Quantitative assessment of myocardial T2 relaxation times in cardiac amyloidosis. J Magn Reson Imaging 30:942–946
Spirito P, Seidman CE, MCKenna WJ, Maron BK (1997) The management of hypertrophic cardiomyopathy. N Engl J Med 336:775–785
Stanek G, Gray J, Strie F, Wormser G (2004) Lyme borreliosis. Lancet Infect Dis 4:197–198
Stark DD, Mosely ME, Bacon BR et al (1985) Magnetic resonance imaging and spectroscopy of hepatic iron overload. Radiology 154:137–142
Stensaeth KH, Fossum E, Hoffmann P et al (2010) Takotsubo cardiomyopathy in acute coronary syndrome; clinical features and contribution of cardiac magnetic resonance during the acute and convalescent phase. Scand Cardiovasc J 45:77–85
Steward S, Mason D, Braunwald E (1968) Impaired rate of left ventricular filling in idiopathic hypertrophic subaortic stenosis and valvular aortic stenosis. Circulation 37:8–14
Stöllberger C, Blazek G, Wegner C, Winkler-Dworak M, Finsterer J (2011) Neuromuscular and cardiac comorbidity determines survival in 140 patients with left ventricular hypertrabeculation/noncompaction. Int J Cardiol 148:120–123
Storey P, Thompson AA, Carqueville CL et al (2007) R2* imaging at 3T and comparison with 1.5. J Magn Reson Imaging 25:540–547
Strohm O, Schulz-Menger J, Pilz B, Osterziel KJ, Dietz R, Friedrich MG (2001) Measurement of left ventricular dimensions and function in patients with dilated cardiomyopathy. J Magn Reson Imaging 13:367–371
Stuber M, Scheidegger MB, Fischer SE et al (1999) Alterations in the local myocardial motion pattern in patients suffering

from pressure overload due to aortic stenosis. Circulation 100:361–368

Sueyoshi E, Sakamoto I, Uetani M (2010) Contrast-enhanced myocardial inversion time at the null point for detection of left ventricular myocardial fibrosis in patients with dilated and hypertrophic cardiomyopathy: a pilot study. AJR Am J Roentgenol 294:W293–W298

Suk T, Edwards C, Hart H, Christiansen JP (2008) Myocardial scar detected by contrast-enhanced cardiac magnetic resonance imaging is associated with ventricular tachycardia in hypertrophic cardiomyopathy patients. Heart Lung Circ 17:370–374

Sun JP, James KB, Yang XS et al (1997) Comparison of mortality rates and progression of left ventricular dysfunction in patients with idiopathic dilated cardiomyopathy and dilated versus nondilated right ventricular cavities. Am J Cardiol 80:1583–1587

Suzuki J, Caputo GR, Masui T, Chang JM, O'Sullivan M, Higgins CB (1991) Assessment of right ventricular diastolic and systolic function in patients with dilated cardiomyopathy using cine magnetic resonance imaging. Am Heart J 122:1035–1040

Suzuki J, Watanabe F, Takenaka K et al (1993) New subtype of apical hypertrophic cardiomyopathy identified with nuclear magnetic resonance imaging as an underlying cause of markedly inverted T waves. J Am Coll Cardiol 22:1175–1181

Syed IS, Prasad A, Oh JK (2008) Apical ballooning syndrome or aborted acute myocardial infarction? Insights from cardiovascular magnetic resonance imaging. Int J Cardiovasc Imaging 24:875–882

Syed IS, Glockner JF, Feng DL et al (2010) Role of cardiac magnetic resonance imaging in the detection of cardiac amyloidosis. J Am Coll Cardiol Img 3:155–164

Takenaka T, Teraguchi H, Yoshida A et al (2008) Terminal stage cardiac findings in patient with cardiac Fabry disease: an electrocardiographic, echocardiographic, and autopsy study. J Cardiol 51:50–59

Tan YT, Wenzelburger F, Lee E et al (2009) The pathophysiology of heart failure with normal ejection fraction. Exercise echocardiography reveals complex abnormalities of both systolic and diastolic function involving torsion, untwist, and longitudinal motion. J Am Coll Cardiol 54:36–46

Tandri H, Calkins H, Nasir K et al (2003) Magnetic resonance imaging findings in patients meeting task force criteria for arrhythmogenic right ventricular dysplasia. J Cardiovasc Electrophysiol 14:476–482

Tandri H, Bluemke DA, Ferrari VA et al (2004) Findings on magnetic resonance imaging of idiopathic right ventricular outflow tachycardia. Am J Cardiol 94:1441–1445

Tandri H, Saranathan M, Rodriguez ER et al (2005) Noninvasive detection of myocardial fibrosis in arrhythmogenic right ventricular cardiomyopathy using delayed-enhancement magnetic resonance imaging. J Am Coll Cardiol 45:98–103

Tandri H, Castillo E, Ferrari VA et al (2006) Magnetic resonance imaging of arrhythmogenic right ventricular dysplasia. Sensitivity, specificity, and observer variability of fat detection versus functional analysis of the right ventricle. J Am Coll Cardiol 48:2277–2284

Tanner MA, Galanello R, Dessi C et al (2007) A randomized, placebo-controlled, double-blind trial of the effect of combined therapy with deferoxamine and deferiprone on myocardial iron in thalassemia major using cardiovascular magnetic resonance. Circulation 115:1876–1884

Thaman R, Gimeno JR, Reith S et al (2004) Progressive left ventricular remodeling in patients with hypertrophic cardiomyopathy and severe left ventricular hypertrophy. J Am Coll Cardiol 44:398–405

Tigen K, Karaahmet T, Kirma C et al (2010) Diffuse late gadolinium enhancement by cardiovascular magnetic resonance predicts significant intraventricular systolic dyssynchrony in patients with non-ischemic dilated cardiomyopathy. J Am Soc Echocardiogr 23:416–422

To A, De Zoysa J, Christiansen JP (2007) Cardiomyopathy associated with Wegener's granulomatosis. Heart 93:984

Tsukihashi K, Ueshima K, Uchida T et al (2001) Transient left ventricular apical ballooning without coronary artery stenosis: a novel heart syndrome mimicking acute myocardial infarction. J Am Coll Cardiol 38:11–18

Ueyama T, Kasamatsu K, Hano T, Yamamoto K, Tsuruo Y, Nishio I (2002) Emotional stress induces transient left ventricular hypocontraction in the rat via activation of cardiac adrenoceptors. A possible animal of Tako-Tsubo cardiomyopathy. Circ J 66:712–713

Uhl HSM (1952) A previously undescribed congenital malformation of the heart: almost total absence of the myocardium of the right ventricle. Bull Johns Hopkins Hosp 91:197–205

Valeti US, Nishimura RA, Holmes DR et al (2007) Comparison of surgical septal myectomy and alcohol septal ablation with cardiac magnetic resonance imaging in patients with hypertrophic obstructive cardiomyopathy. J Am Coll Cardiol 49:350–357

van der Linde MR (1991) Lyme carditis: clinical characteristics of 105 cases. Scand J Infect Dis Suppl 77:81–84

van Dockum WG, ten Gate FJ, ten Berg JM et al (2004) Myocardial infarction after percutaneous transluminal septal myocardial ablation in hypertrophic obstructive cardiomyopathy: evaluation by contrast-enhanced magnetic resonance imaging. J Am Coll Cardiol 43:27–34

van Dockum WG, Beek AM, ten Gate FJ et al (2005) Early onset and progression of left ventricular remodeling after alcohol septal ablation in hypertrophic obstructive cardiomyopathy. Circulation 111:2503–2508

van Dockum WG, Kuijer JPA, Götte MJW et al (2006) Septal ablation in hypertrophic cardiomyopathy improves systolic myocardial function in the lateral (free) wall: a follow-up study using CMR tissue tagging and 3D strain analysis. Eur Heart J 27:2833–2839

Van Geluwe F, Dymarkowski S, Crevits I, De Wever W, Bogaert J (2006) Amyloidosis of the heart and respiratory system. Eur Radiol 16:2358–2365

Varnava AM, Elliot PM, Sharma S, McKenna WJ, Davies MJ (2000) Hypertrophic cardiomyopathy: the interrelation of disarray, fibrosis, and small vessel disease. Heart 84:476–482

Varnava AM, Elliot PM, Mahon N, Davies MJ, McKenna WJ (2001) Relation between myocyte disarray and outcome in hypertrophic cardiomyopathy. Am J Cardiol 88:275–279

Vermes E, Strohm O, Otmani A et al (2011) Impact of the revision of arrhythmogenic right ventricular cardiomyopathy/dysplasia task force criteria on its prevalence by CMR criteria. J Am Coll Cardiol Img 4:282–287

Vignaux O, Dhote R, Duboc D et al (2002a) Detection of myocardial involvement in patients with sarcoidosis applying T2-weighted, contrast-enhanced, and cine magnetic resonance imaging: initial results of a prospective study. J Comput Assist Tomogr 26:762–767
Vignaux O, Dhote R, Duboc D et al (2002b) Clinical significance of myocardial magnetic resonance abnormalities in patients with sarcoidosis. A 1-year follow-up study. Chest 122:1895–1901
Virmani R, Burcs JC, Robcrts WC (1980) Cardiac sarcoidosis: a major cause of sudden death in young individuals. Chest 77:423–428
Vogel M, Anderson LJ, Holden S, Deanfield JE, Pennell DJ, Walker JM (2003) Tissue Doppler echocardiography in patients with thalassaemia detects early myocardial dysfunction related to myocardial iron overload. Eur Heart J 24:113–119
Vogelsang TW, Hanel B, Kristoffersen US et al (2008) Effect of eight weeks of endurance training on right and left ventricular volume and mass in untrained obese subjects: a longitudinal study. Scand J Med Sci Sports 18:354–359
Vogelsberg H, Mahrholdt H, Deluigi C et al (2008) Cardiovascular magnetic resonance in clinically suspected cardiac amyloidosis. J Am Coll Cardiol 51:1022–1030
Voigt A, Elgeti T, Durmus T et al (2011) Cardiac magnetic resonance imaging in dilated cardiomyopathy in adults—towards identification of myocardial inflammation. Eur Radiol 21:925–935
Von Hoff D, Layard M, Basa P (1979) Risk factors for doxorubicin-induced congestive heart failure. Ann Intern Med 91:710–717
Wassmuth R, Lentzsch S, Erbruegger U et al (2001) Subclinical cardiotoxic effects of anthracyclines as assessed by magnetic resonance imaging–a pilot study. Am Heart J 141:1007–1013
Wassmuth R, Göbel U, Natusch A et al (2008) Cardiovascular magnetic resonance imaging detects cardiac involvement in Churg-Strauss syndrome. J Card Fail 14:856–860
Watkins H, Ashrafian H, Redwood C (2011) Inherited cardiomyopathies. N Engl J Med 364:1643–1656
Weidemann F, Niemann M, Breunig F et al (2009) Long-term effects of enzyme replacement therapy on Fabry cardiomyopathy. Evidence for a better outcome with early treatment. Circulation 119:524–529
Weller PF, Bubley GJ (1994) The idiopathic hypereosinophilic syndrome. Blood 83:2759–2779
Westermann D, Kasner M, Steendijk P et al (2008) Role of left ventricular stiffness in heart failure with normal ejection fraction. Circulation 117:2051–2060
Westwood M, Anderson LJ, Firmin DN et al (2003a) A single breath-hold multi-echo T2* cardiovascular magnetic resonance technique for diagnosis of myocardial iron overload. J Magn Reson Imag 18:33–39
Westwood M, Anderson LJ, Firmin DN et al (2003b) Interscanner reproducibility of cardiovascular magnetic resonance T2* measurements of tissue iron in thalassemia. J Magn Reson Imag 18:616–620
White RD, Trohman RG, Flamm SD et al (1998) Right ventricular arrhythmia in the absence of arrhythmogenic dysplasia: MR imaging of myocardial abnormalities. Radiology 207:743–751
White J, Sutton T, Kerr A (2010) Isolated primary cardiac sarcoidosis. MRI diagnosis and monitoring of treatment response with cardiac enzymes. Circ Heart Fail 3:e28–e29
World Health Organization Expert Committee (1984) Chagas disease. In: World Health Organization technical report series 697. WHO, Geneva, pp 50–55
Wu E, Judd RM, Vargas JD et al (2001) Visualisation of the presence, location and transmural extent of healed Q-wave and non-Q-wave myocardial infarction. Lancet 357:21–28
Wu KC, Weiss RG, Thiemann DR et al (2008) Late gadolinium enhancement by cardiovascular magnetic resonance heralds an adverse prognosis in nonischemic cardiomyopathy. J Am Coll Cardiol 51:2414–2421
Yared K, Johri AM, Soni AV et al (2008) Cardiac sarcoidosis imitating arrhythmogenic right ventricular dysplasia. Images in cardiovascular medicine. Circulation 118: e113–e115
Yelgec NS, Dymarkowski S, Ganame J, Bogaert J (2007) Value of MRI in patients with a clinical suspicion of acute myocarditis. Eur Rad 17:2211–2217
Yilmaz A, Mahrholdt H, Athanasiadis A et al (2008a) Coronary spasm as the underlying cause for chest pain in patients with PVB19 myocarditis. Heart 94:1456–1463
Yilmaz A, Gdynia H-J, Baccouche H et al (2008b) Cardiac involvement in patients with Becker muscular dystrophy: new diagnostic and pathophysiological insights by a CMR approach. J Cardiovasc Magn Reson 10:50
Yilmaz A, Kindermann I, Kindermann M et al (2010) Comparative evaluation of left and right ventricular endomyocardial biopsy. Differences in complication rate and diagnostic performance. Circulation 122:900–909
Yoon GJ, Telli ML, Kao DP et al (2010) Left ventricular dysfunction in patients receiving cardiotoxic cancer therapies are clinicians responding optimally? J Am Coll Cardiol 56:1644–1650
Young AA, Kramer CM, Ferrari VA, Axel L, Reichek N (1994) Three-dimensional left ventricular deformation in hypertrophic cardiomyopathy. Circulation 90:854–867
Zagrosek A, Wassmuth R, Abdel-Aty H et al (2008) Relation between myocardial edema and myocardial mass during the acute and convalescent phase of myocarditis–a CMR study. J Cardiovasc Magn Reson 10:19
Zagrosek A, Abdel-Aty H, Boyé P et al (2009) Cardiac magnetic resonance monitors reversible and irreversible myocardial injury in myocarditis. J Am Coll Cardiol Img 2:131–138
Zile MR, Baicu CF, Gaasch WH (2004) Diastolic heart failure—abnormalities in active relaxation and passive stiffness of the left ventricle. N Engl J Med 350:1953–1959
Zinzani PL, Gherlinzoni F, Piovaccari G et al (1996) Cardiac injury as late toxicity of mediastinal radiation therapy for Hodgkin's disease patients. Haematologica 81:132–137

Pulmonary Hypertension

Shahin Moledina and Vivek Muthurangu

Contents

1 **Introduction** 355
1.1 Clinical Pulmonary Hypertension 356
1.2 Epidemiology 356
1.3 Symptoms 356
1.4 Treatment Strategies 356
1.5 Role of Imaging in Pulmonary Hypertension 356

2 **Cine Imaging** 357
2.1 Volumetry and Mass 357
2.2 Interventricular Septal Configuration 358
2.3 Vascular Distension 359

3 **Flow Assessment** 359
3.1 Great Vessel Flow 360
3.2 Atrioventricular Flow 361

4 **MR Angiography** 361
4.1 Thromboembolic Pulmonary Hypertension 361
4.2 Non-Embolic Disease 362

5 **Late Gadolinium Imaging** 362

6 **Whole-Heart 3D SSFP** 362

7 **Computed Tomography** 363

8 **Conclusion** 363

9 **Key Points** 364

References 364

S. Moledina
UCL Centre for Cardiovascular Imaging
and Great Ormond Street Hospital for Children,
London, WC1N 3JH, UK

V. Muthurangu (✉)
Cardio-respiratory Unit,
Great Ormond Street Hospital for Children,
London, WC1N 3JH, UK
e-mail: v.muthurangu@ucl.ac.uk

Abstract

In this chapter the basics of MRI physics will be addressed. It will start with an overview of MR signal generation and relaxation. Then the concept of magnetization preparation will be explored in the context of cardiac imaging. The next sections will address the physics behind spatial encoding and motion compensation. Finally specific cardiac MRI sequences will be discussed including a discussion of optimization. By the end of the chapter the reader should have a better understanding of basic MRI physics and a greater ability to optimise sequences.

1 Introduction

Pulmonary hypertension (PH) encompasses a collection of conditions all characterized by elevated blood pressure in the pulmonary arteries. Although they have differing etiologies, they share similarities in their symptoms and prognosis. Disease severity is largely driven by the extent pulmonary arterial involvement, (traditionally expressed in terms of pressure or vascular resistance) and the effect this has on right ventricular (RV) function. Thus, assessment of the pulmonary vasculature and the RV are key in the management of PH. However, the RV and pulmonary circulation have complex geometries, and due to their position in the thorax are difficult to access by traditional imaging modalities. Both MRI and CT are unencumbered by considerations of acoustic windows and can acquire data in three dimensions. This renders them potentially useful in the assessment of patients with PH and correspondingly there has been an explosion in PH studies

J. Bogaert et al. (eds.), *Clinical Cardiac MRI*, Medical Radiology. Diagnostic Imaging,
DOI: 10.1007/174_2011_413, © Springer-Verlag Berlin Heidelberg 2012

utilizing MRI and CT. The aim of this chapter is to provide an overview of how MRI and to a lesser extent CT, can be used to assess PH.

1.1 Clinical Pulmonary Hypertension

PH is defined hemodynamically as a mean resting pulmonary artery pressure exceeding 25 mm Hg, the normal being 14 mm Hg (Badesch et al. 2009). Pathologically it is characterized by progressive luminal narrowing of the distal small pulmonary arteries leading to an increased pulmonary vascular resistance. At the same time, the central pulmonary arteries become stiff and dilated. These vascular changes result in increased afterload to the RV, which initially undergoes adaptive hypertrophy, but later experiences maladaptive dilatation, fibrosis and valve regurgitation resulting in RV failure. PH can occur in isolation (idiopathic pulmonary arterial hypertension), or in association with a broad range of conditions. It is therefore classified clinically into five broad groups sharing similarities in pathophysiology, clinical presentation and therapeutic response (Simonneau et al. 2009). These groups are: (1) pulmonary arterial hypertension (PAH), (2) PH due to left heart disease, (3) PH associated with lung disease, (4) chronic thromboembolic PH, and (5) PH with multifactorial mechanisms.

1.2 Epidemiology

Overall PH is a rare condition. The incidence of idiopathic PAH in adults is approximately 1–2 per million and in children is approximately 0.5 per million (Moledina et al. 2010). However, the prevalence of PH in the presence of other conditions is much higher. For instance, between 5.8 and 28 percent of adults with congenital heart disease have PH (Lowe et al. 2011), while the prevalence in patients with connective tissue disease is estimated at 7–12% (Simonneau et al. 2009). In patients with chronic obstructive pulmonary disease, the prevalence maybe as high as 60% (Minai et al. 2010).

1.3 Symptoms

The symptoms of PH are non-specific and include dyspnoea and exercise intolerance. As a result PH is often diagnosed late with patients having consulted a number of healthcare professionals before final diagnosis. Regardless of the etiology, the presence of PH is associated with significantly reduced quality-of-life and survival. The median survival in adults with IPAH before the availability of treatment was 2.8 years (D'Alonzo et al. 1991) and for children was less than 1 year (Houde et al. 1993). In connective tissue disease PAH is associated with a 45% 1 year survival if untreated (Condliffe et al. 2009). Thankfully, new treatments are becoming available that have significantly improved prognosis.

1.4 Treatment Strategies

Since the 1980s a number of therapies have become available for the treatment of pulmonary arterial hypertension and there are still more in late phase clinical trials. These drugs have been shown to improve clinical status and exercise capacity and a meta-analysis of randomized clinical trials has demonstrated improved survival (Galie et al. 2009). Indications are that earlier treatment results in improved clinical status (Galie et al. 2008). It is imperative therefore that PH is detected at the earliest opportunity.

Drug treatments remain expensive and have potential side effects. Most treatment guidelines advocate sequential combination therapy. This requires reliably identifying patients who either deteriorate or fail to improve on first line treatment prior to escalating therapy. Since current drug treatments do not represent a cure, the final treatment available is lung transplantation. This further requires an objective means by which to identify patients most likely to succumb to the disease. Hemodynamic studies have repeatedly demonstrated that RV function is the major determinant of outcome in this patient group (D'Alonzo et al. 1991).

1.5 Role of Imaging in Pulmonary Hypertension

The thorough assessment of patients with PH necessitates a sequential approach. This includes screening and diagnosis, identification of etiology, monitoring of treatment response and finally risk stratification and prognostication.

Screening and diagnosis of patient groups at risk of developing PH requires identification of abnormalities consistent with PH. This can be done invasively with measurement of pulmonary artery pressure, or non-invasively by assessing tricuspid regurgitate jet velocity or right heart function.

Once the diagnosis of PH is made, attention should shift to identifying potential causes or associated conditions. In conjunction with history, examination and laboratory tests, imaging is focused at identifying thromboembolic disease, lung parenchymal disease, veno-occlusive disease, left heart disease and congenital heart disease.

Following initial diagnosis and initiation of treatment close follow-up with regular assessment of treatment response is required to identify those who would benefit from escalation of therapy or listing for lung transplantation. An important aspect of this is that it enables management based on prognosis as well as treatment response.

Imaging obviously has a major role to play in all of these areas. Traditionally, echocardiography has been the mainstay of non-invasive assessment. However, MRI (and CT) has many advantages that have made them increasingly important in the management of PH. In the rest of this chapter, different MR techniques will be discussed in terms of optimization for PH and clinical utility. Finally the role of CT will be discussed.

2 Cine Imaging

Gradient echo imaging with its short repetition times permits the acquisition of cine MR images and allows assessment of the dynamic nature of the cardiovascular system. These sequences can be used for the volumetric quantification of ventricular function, assessing ventricular interactions and measuring vascular distension through the cardiac cycle.

Due to its superior blood pool contrast b-SSFP imaging has become the most widely accepted cine imaging technique. However, since dyspnea is the most common symptom encountered in PH, breath holds may be poorly tolerated. This is problematic, as most cardiac gated cine imaging requires breath holds and breathing artifact can significantly reduce image quality. Scanning protocols must therefore utilize maneuvers to minimize the duration of breath holds.

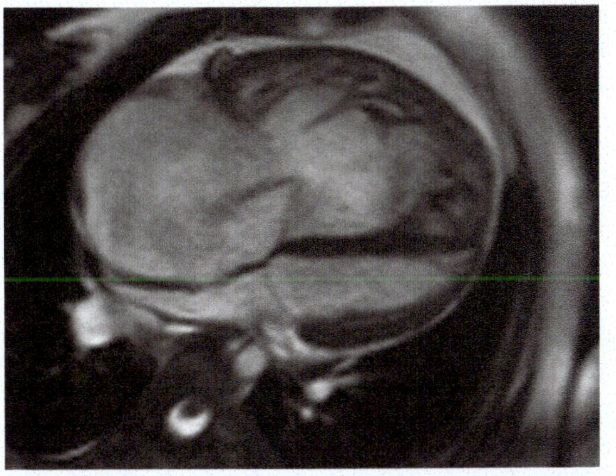

Fig. 1 Four chamber balanced SSFP image from a patient with idiopathic pulmonary hypertension. The RV is dilated and hypertrophied. Tricuspid regurgitation is present and results in loss of signal

These include application of rectangular field of view, partial Fourier encoding, parallel imaging techniques or the reduction in spatial resolution (by reducing matrix size). Alternatively, cine imaging can be achieved by utilizing real-time sequences such as radial *k*–*t* SENSE (Muthurangu et al. 2008) obviating the need for breath holding altogether. These relatively new real-time imaging techniques have been validated for the assessment of RV volumes. Once optimized cine sequences can be used a several different ways to help in the assessment of PH.

2.1 Volumetry and Mass

RV dilatation, hypertrophy and reduced contractility correlate with hemodynamics and prognosis. It is therefore vital that these parameters are assessed accurately. This requires careful optimization to suit the physiology and symptoms of patients with PH.

2.1.1 Scan Planning

The RV has a complex geometry, which effects the assessment of its volume and function. Furthermore in the presence of PH, the RV undergoes dilatation and hypertrophy; further increasing it is complex 3D morphology (Fig. 1). Due to this complexity, no single imaging plane is likely to be ideally suited for RV volumetric and mass analysis. In the normal RV, longitudinal shortening of the RV is thought to be the major determinant of global RV systolic function. This results in through plane motion of the tricuspid annulus with relation to imaging planes orientated in the short axis resulting in potential errors in volumetric analysis. A study comparing imaging in the RV short axis plane with trans-axial imaging in healthy volunteers found that acquisition in the trans-axial plane resulted in more reproducible measures of RV volume (Jauhiainen et al. 2002). The RV remodeling, which accompanies PH results in reduction in longitudinal function and recent work suggests that transverse shortening is an important determinant of global RV function in these patients (Kind et al. 2010). Therefore the optimal scanning plane for multi-slice volumetric assessment of the RV in PH is yet to be defined and may depend on the degree of RV dilation. Irrespective of the plane chosen, what is important is cross-referencing segmentation to cine images in another plane (i.e. using the four-chamber to aid segmentation of the short axis).

It should be noted that RV stroke volume calculated from flow measurements in the pulmonary artery and those derived from volumetric analysis correlate well in the absence of valvar regurgitation. However, both tricuspid and pulmonary regurgitation are common in patients with PH thus volumetric analysis overestimates 'true' or 'effective' stoke volume.

2.1.2 Clinical Studies

Significant RV dilatation occurs in the presence of PH with both RV end systolic and end diastolic dimensions increased as compared to controls (Hoeper et al. 2001). Importantly, several studies have shown that RV parameters are associated with survival. In one study of adults with IPAH, an RVEDVi $\geq$ 84 ml/m^2 was associated with poorer survival (van Wolferen et al. 2007). In the same study reduced left ventricular (LV)EDVi ($\leq$40 ml/m^2) and reduced RV stoke volume index ($\leq$25 ml/m^2) were also strong predictors of poor survival. Similar results have been replicated in children with mixed etiologies of PH, where effective RV ejection fraction was a powerful predictor of survival.

Assessment of disease progression and response to therapy has also been performed using MRI. Progressive RV dilatation, reduced LVEDVi and reduced RVSV after 1-year follow-up have been shown to correlate with worse survival (van Wolferen et al. 2007). Conversely, treatment with prostacyclin is associated with improvement in RVSV, which correlates with improvements in six-minute-walk distance (Roeleveld et al. 2004). While in chronic thromboembolic PH, improvement in RV ejection fraction following pulmonary endarterectomy correlates with the decrease in mean pulmonary artery pressure (Kreitner et al. 2004).

Assessment of the ventricle does not stop with quantification of volumes and function. It is also important in diseases like PH to assess the myocardium. RV mass index (RV mass divided by LV mass) of greater than 0.6 had a sensitivity of 84% and specificity of 71% for detecting PH in one study of a mixed PH population (Saba et al. 2002). The diagnostic accuracy was better than Doppler echocardiography in that patient group. Furthermore RV mass index correlated with invasively measured mean pulmonary artery pressure ($r = 0.8$), again better than Doppler echocardiography in the same study. Similar results have been obtained for patients with systemic sclerosis (Hagger et al. 2009) and IPAH (Katz et al. 1993). Furthermore RV mass index has been shown to correlate with survival both in IPAH (van Wolferen et al. 2007) and in systemic sclerosis (Hagger et al. 2009).

Quantification of RV mass can also provide insights into direct effects of the disease and its treatment on the myocardium. In one randomized control trial of treatment with sildenafil verses bosentan (Wilkins et al. 2005), sildenafil therapy was associated reduction in RV mass. There is also evidence that chronic reduction in LV preload such as is seen in chronic thromboembolic PH is associated with reduced LV mass which recovers when pulmonary arterial obstruction is relieved (Hardziyenka et al. 2011).

2.2 Interventricular Septal Configuration

The right and left ventricular cavity are separated by the interventricular septum and its movement can therefore provide insight into the relative pressure difference between the two chambers at any point in the cardiac cycle. Under normal circumstances LV pressure exceeds RV pressure at every point through the cardiac cycle. The LV short axis is therefore circular with the inter-ventricular septum concave

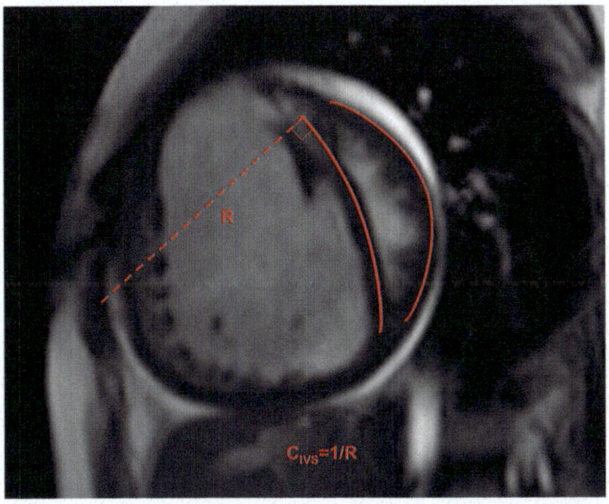

Fig. 2 Mid-ventricular short axis view from a patient with pulmonary hypertension. The interventricular septum bows leftwards. Septal curvature is defined by deriving, R, the radius of a circle whos arc is the interventricular septum. Septal curvature, C_{IVS}, is equal to $1/R$. In order to normalise for patient size curvature is calculated for the LV free wall and the curvature ratio is calculated. Ratio $= C_{IVS}/C_{LV}$. A ratio of 1 implies no bowing, negative values indicate leftward bowing

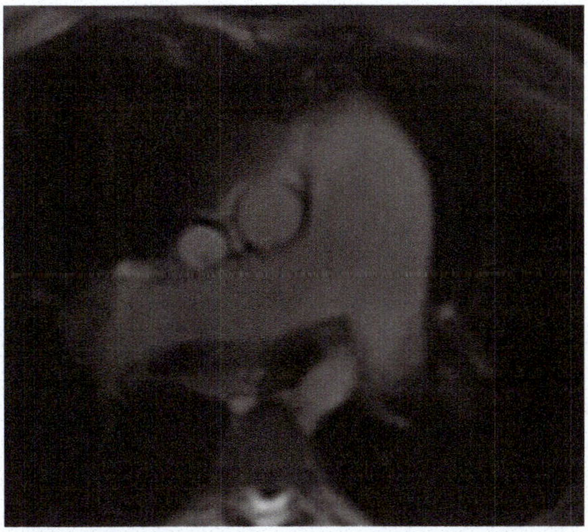

Fig. 3 Dilated central pulmonary arteries in a patient with pulmonary hypertension

towards the LV cavity. Under conditions of increased RV systolic pressure the inter-ventricular septum bows leftwards. The curvature of the inter-ventricular can be measured as demonstrated in Fig. 2. Increased RV afterload also results in an increased duration of RV free wall contraction such that RV systole continues even after LV diastole has begun (Marcus et al. 2008). The intraventricular septum can therefore bow toward the LV in early LV diastole even when the peak RV systolic pressure is sub-systemic.

In one study, the curvature of the inter-ventricular septum expressed as a ratio of the curvature of the LV free wall was found to correlate with RV systolic pressure (Roeleveld et al. 2005b). Another study derived cut off values for curvature ratio of 0.67, which had an 87% sensitivity and 100% specificity for detecting PH (Dellegrottaglie et al. 2007).

2.3 Vascular Distension

Since PH is associated with proximal vessel dilatation and stiffening, measurement of the size and the distensability of the main pulmonary artery provide insight into haemodynamics (Fig. 3). A cine acquisition placed perpendicular to the pulmonary trunk permits measurement of the minimum (minA) and maximum (maxA) cross sectional areas. This provides information about the degree of vessel dilatation and distensability and a number of studies have assessed the utility of these measures. In one such study with same day MRI and cardiac catheterization, a PA pulsatility (maxA−minA/minA × 100%) of <40% detected the presence of resting PH with a sensitivity of 93% and a specificity of 63%. Interestingly, PA pulsatility was also reduced in patients with exercise induced PH, often considered an early phenotype, compared to healthy controls suggesting that this may be a useful measure for the early detection of PH. In addition, there was a modest correlation with PA pressure and resistance (Sanz et al. 2009). In a separate pilot study (Jardim et al. 2007), a pulmonary artery distensibility (maxA−minA/maxA × 100%) of >10% was able to detect acute vasodilator responders with a sensitivity of 100%, but a specificity of only 56%. Finally, in a large study with 48 months follow-up PA pulsatility, also referred to as relative area change, was strongly predictive of survival (Gan et al. 2007).

3 Flow Assessment

Quantification of blood flow velocity and volume are important in the assessment of PH. Absolute flow volume, i.e. cardiac output is reduced in PH, and flow characteristics are altered as the result of altered mechanical properties of the pulmonary vascular bed.

The most commonly applied method for the quantification of flow in the great vessels is velocity encoded phase contrast MRI acquired during free breathing. The accuracy of velocity encoded phase contrast MRI has been repeatedly demonstrated both in phantom experiments and in vivo. However, severe PH is associated with a change in flow from a laminar or plug flow pattern to a helical flow pattern (Mauritz et al. 2008; Reiter et al. 2008). Such swirling flow patterns have been shown to result in inaccuracies in the quantification of through plain flow. The exact mechanism for these inaccuracies is unknown, but they may result through the accrual of phase by virtue of the component of flow in the inplane direction. It is therefore imperative to acquire additional flow data for the accurate assessment of pulmonary artery flow. This may be done by acquiring through plane flow in the proximal branch pulmonary arteries or alternatively summing pulmonary venous flow. In the absence of intracardiac shunts LV stroke volume may be used.

In the case of high velocity eccentric flow jets, such as are seen with tricuspid regurgitation in PH, velocity encoded phase-contrast MR has potential limitations in assessing peak flow velocity and can underestimate peak velocity. Nevertheless, one small study has demonstrated good correlation between PA systolic pressure measured by right heart catheter and that derived by applying the modified Bernoulli equation to PC-MRI derived peak TR velocity (Nogami et al. 2009).

Peak flow velocity is reduced and there is a shorter time to peak velocity (acceleration time) in the main pulmonary artery. A 'notch', mid-systolic decrease in PA flow velocity, is present representing early wave reflection as a result of both pulmonary artery stiffening and a more proximal site of wave reflection (Fig. 4). Pulmonary regurgitation is detected in approximately one third of patients.

Discrepancies between aortic and pulmonary artery net flow may indicate the presence of shunt lesions and should prompt close assessment of cardiovascular anatomy to identify the responsible lesion. In particular, assessment should focus on the atrial and ventricular septums, the pulmonary venous connections and the presence or absence of significant systemic to pulmonary artery connections, such as persistent arterial ducts or aorto-pulmonary windows.

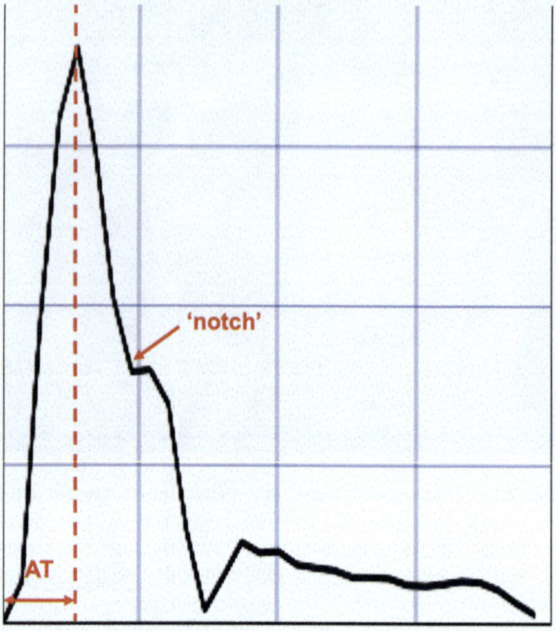

Fig. 4 A typical volumetric flow curve from a phase contrast sequence in the pulmonary artery of a patient with PH. Note the short acceleration time (*AT*) and the mid systolic deceleration '*notch*'

3.1 Great Vessel Flow

Pulmonary artery dilatation and reduced stroke volume are necessarily accompanied by a reduction in average flow velocity. A study investigating pulmonary artery flow characteristics measured with phase contrast magnetic resonance imaging (Sanz et al. 2007) found that average velocity within the main pulmonary artery correlated with pulmonary artery pressure and resistance ($r = 0.73$–0.86). The threshold value for average flow velocity of 11.7 cm/s revealed PAH with a sensitivity of 92.9% and a specificity of 82.4%.

Pulmonary valve regurgitation is prevalent in patients with PH and its severity (regurgitation fraction) correlates with functional status of patients. Transcatheter re-valvation has been associated with improved functional status and reduction in RV volume (Lurz et al. 2009).

Acceleration time (AT), the time from the onset of flow to the peak velocity, is shorter in PH compared with healthy controls, and may be used as an additional marker for the presence of disease. In some studies, AT was found to correlate negatively with mean PA pressure (Tardivon et al. 1994); however, this has not been a consistent finding (Roeleveld et al. 2005a; Ley et al. 2007), and AT cannot be used to predict PA pressure.

Doppler echocardiographic studies have examined mid-systolic deceleration, notching and demonstrated its correlation with hemodynamics and outcome (Hardziyenka et al. 2007; Urboniene et al. 2010). Such flow profiles are readily demonstrated by MRI (Alunni et al. 2010) and hemodynamic correlates are bound to follow.

3.2 Atrioventricular Flow

A phase contrast MR sequence applied perpendicular to the flow across the tricuspid and mitral valves permits simultaneous analysis of the filling patterns of both left and right ventricles. PH is associated with a restrictive filling pattern (ration of early to late filling $E/A < 1$) across the tricuspid valve. There is also delayed onset of tricuspid inflow compared to mitral inflow. The magnitude of the interventricular delay correlates with systolic PA pressure (Alunni et al. 2010). However, tricuspid regurgitation is not easily assessed using velocity encoded MR alone. In fact it requires both MR volumetry and velocity encoded PCMR.

3.2.1 Tricuspid Regurgitation

The tricuspid valve is designed to operate at low pressures. In the presence of PH, tricuspid valve regurgitation is common. This leads to volume loading of the ventricle and pump inefficiency and is therefore an important determinant of overall ventricular function. Calculation of tricuspid valve regurgitation fraction combines data from volumetry and flow. In brief, tricuspid regurgitation fraction equals RV stroke volume minus pulmonary artery forward volume (measured by velocity encoded phase contrast MR) divided by RV stroke volume multiplied by 100% (Kon et al. 2004). One small study of patients with mainly IPAH found similar RV volumes in patients with 'normal' cardiac output as those with poor cardiac output the major difference between groups being the severity of TR (Hoeper et al. 2001). The severity of TR has also been shown to be of significance in prognosis of children with PH.

4 MR Angiography

Spatial resolution of contrast enhanced magnetic resonance angiography (ce-MRA) continues to improve. However, even with the application of parallel imaging techniques acquisition of coronal high resolution datasets, at 1.5 T, ce-MRA requires breath holds estimated at approximately 20–25 s. In a patient population where dyspnea is the most prevalent symptom such sequences are likely to result in technically inadequate studies in a large proportion. An alternative strategy of acquiring two sagittal data sets, one for each lung, has been tried with some success (Kreitner et al. 2007). Using this method, isotropic data with voxel sizes ranging from 1 to 1.2 mm^3 have been achieved in patients with PH performing breathholds of between 12 and 14 s.

4.1 Thromboembolic Pulmonary Hypertension

Thromboembolic disease is an important cause of PH and its identification is essential since pulmonary endarterectomy can be curative in selected patients. Contrast enhanced MRA of the pulmonary arteries using gadolinium has been assessed for its diagnostic accuracy in this regard. A meta-analysis of studies using ce-MRA for diagnosing acute pulmonary embolus (with pulmonary angiography as the gold standard) found that the sensitivity of this approach ranged from 77 to 100% and the specificity from 95 to 98% (Stein et al. 2003). However, the included studies were relatively small, having between 30 and 118 patients. A more recent multi-centre prospective study (Stein et al. 2010) including 371 adults shed further light on the diagnostic accuracy of this modality. An important finding was that a quarter of studies were deemed technically inadequate. Of those studies deemed technically adequate ce-MRA had a sensitivity of 78% and specificity of 99% for detecting pulmonary embolus. The sensitivity was further increased by inclusion of magnetic resonance venography of the lower limb; however, this technique was technically difficult and less than 50% of patients had technically adequate results.

In a study comparing ce-MRA with digital subtraction angiography in chronic thromboembolic PH, MR vessel detection was as good as digital subtraction angiography down to the level of segmental arteries. For sub segmental vessels ce-MRA detected 93% of the vessels detected on DSA (Kreitner et al. 2007).

Due to these limitations ce-MRA is not recommended as a sole screening tests for chronic thromboembolic PH, and most international guideline

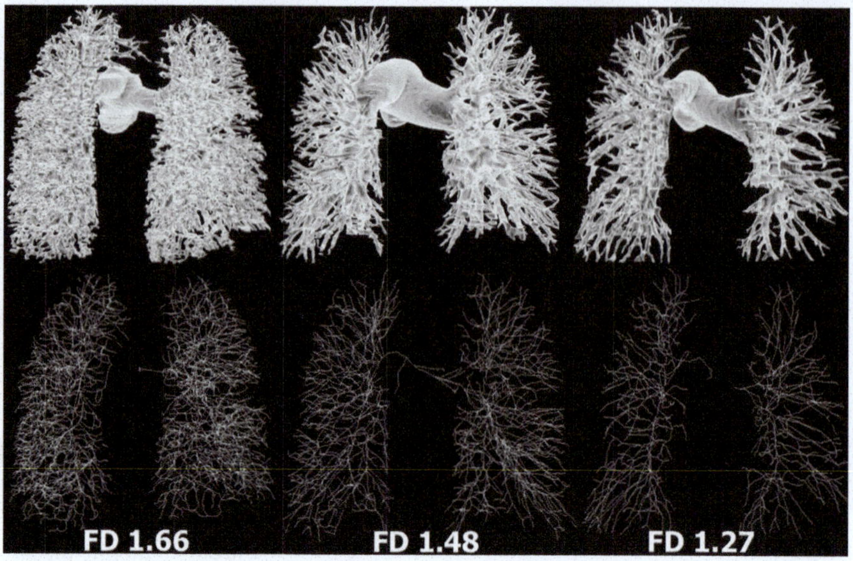

Fig. 5 CT angiographs showing increased pruning with increasing disease severity (quantified by fractal dimension—FD)

groups continue to recommend ventilation perfusion scintigraphy followed by pulmonary angiography or CT pulmonary angiography instead.

4.2 Non-Embolic Disease

As the obliterative pathological process proceeds the pulmonary vascular tree becomes pruned distally and tortuous more proximally. These changes can be appreciated on pulmonary angiography and also result in increased heterogeneity of flow, which is detectable on time resolved angiography. The clinical significance of these changes is yet to be established with MRI, but has been demonstrated for CT pulmonary angiography (Fig. 5).

5 Late Gadolinium Imaging

In addition to ventricular remodeling described above, increased RV afterload is associated with myocyte apoptosis, inflammation and fibrosis. Thus, quantification of myocardial fibrosis may be a useful indicator of RV wall stress. Areas of delayed contrast enhancement are typically found at the insertion points of the RV into the interventricular septum (Fig. 6). These zones correspond with areas of increased mechanical stress. Delayed contrast enhancement has also been noted extending into the interventricular septum, particularly in patients with leftward bowing off the interventricular septum. A case report of a pathological MRI correlate has raised the possibility that delayed contrast enhancement results from an accentuation of normal insertion point myocardial architecture as opposed to pathological fibrosis. Either way the extent of delayed contrast enhancement is inversely related to measures of RV systolic function (Blyth et al. 2005; Shehata et al. 2011).

6 Whole-Heart 3D SSFP

Identification of previously undiagnosed congenital heart lesions, and in particular shunt lesions, should actively be addressed when assessing patients with PH. Cardiac MRI is now considered the gold standard for assessment of anatomy in adult patients with congenital heart disease. 3D b-SSFP imaging is particularly well suited to assessment intracardiac and proximal great vessel anatomy. Since whole-heart 3D b-SSFP is respiratory navigated and ECG triggered there is no necessity for breath holding. Mild resting tachypnea may theoretically narrow the acquisition window; however, in practice this is rarely a problem. Furthermore, patients have a relative resting tachycardia often resulting in more rapid data acquisition. Valve regurgitation, particularly tricuspid and pulmonary, can result in signal dropout.

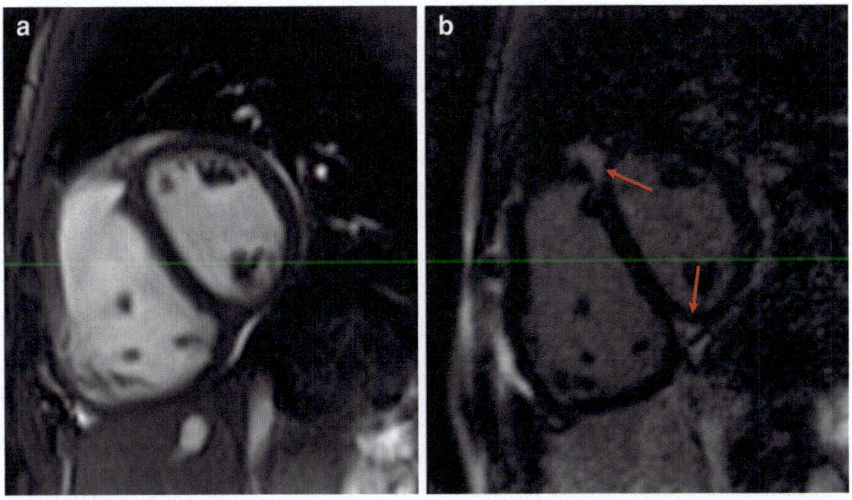

Fig. 6 A mid-ventricular short axis frame from a cine sequence (*left*) with a corresponding image balanced SSFP inversion recovery sequence (*right*). Areas of late enhancement are seen at the insertion points of the RV into the interventricular septum (*arrows*)

7 Computed Tomography

The principal role of CT in assessment of PH is to demonstrate features of secondary forms of PH. The development of multi-slice CT has made it possible to image the complete lung parenchyma at high resolution in less than 10 s, producing isotropic data at sub millimeter resolution. This duration of breath holding is achievable for the majority of patients in question. An additional benefit of the increased image acquisition speed is the ability to perform CT pulmonary angiography of sufficient resolution to depict sub-segmental arteries.

Parenchymal lung disease such as chronic obstructive airways disease (COPD) or lung fibrosis can be detected and differentiated. Furthermore, the rarer pulmonary veno-occlusive disease is evident and has characteristic features of thickened into lobular septa, poorly defined nodular opacities and lymph adenopathy. This is an important differential diagnosis since its clinical manifestation can mirror that of IPAH; however, pulmonary vasodilators may result in pulmonary oedema and worsening of the patient. Emphysema appears as a decrease in mean lung density whereas fibrotic lung disease is associated with an increase in density and changes including honeycombing, reticular opacities and the groundglass attenuation. These diseases result in progressive alveolar hypoxaemia leading to hypoxic vasoconstriction.

CT pulmonary angiography is often considered the first line cross-sectional imaging modality for evaluation of acute pulmonary embolism. Furthermore, in chronic thromboembolic PH, CT angiography can distinguish more surgically amenable central disease from distal disease, which appears as mosaic attenuation.

Finally, a number of studies have reported on the use of ECG gated CT in PH. Since this produces isotropic 4D volumes which can be reconstructed in any imaging plane it theoretically permits analysis of parameters which have been described in the section on cine MRI e.g. vessel distension, septal bowing and global indices of ventricular function. Blood tissue contrast however, is mainly determined by local concentration of contrast agent and therefore highly dependent on timing of acquisition. Furthermore, temporal resolution is lower than that for cine MRI. Finally, the dose of ionising radiation is increased compared with ECG triggered acquisition. These are likely to remain limitations to routine use of gated CT in the serial assessment patients with PH.

8 Conclusion

Numerous studies have now confirmed the clinical utility of cardiac MRI (and CT) in patients with PH. MRI can be considered the gold standard for the assessment of ventricular volumes and function as well as for the non-invasive quantification of blood flow. However, whilst these are extremely important in determining clinical outcome, the disease resides in the distal pulmonary vessels. To understand the disease fully one must either visualize the vasculature or measure its effects on the pulmonary haemodynamics. This reveals two of the limitation of MRI; its resolution and its inability to measure pressure. Exciting work is underway to mitigate these. By combining MRI with direct pressure measurement by cardiac catheterization it is now possible to accurately quantify pulmonary vascular resistance and compliance (see "MR Guided Cardiac Catheterisation"). Experimental work using this methodology will soon produce even more complete assessments of afterload such as impedance spectra and wave intensity analysis. Load independent measures of ventricular function can also be derived from pressure volume loops of the RV. Thus cross sectional imaging is likely to play an increasingly important role in the field of PH.

9 Key Points

- Signs of PH should be sought on imaging studies of patients with unexplained dysnea.
- Cardiac MRI derived parameters of cardiac function and blood flow correlate with haemodynamics, functional status and prognosis in patients with PH and offer a non-invasive means for assessment.
- Scanning protocols should be adjusted to take account of dyspnoea and altered physiology in order to maximise yield from studies in this patient group.

References

Alunni JP, Degano B, Arnaud C, Tetu L, Blot-Souletie N, Didier A, Otal P, Rousseau H, Chabbert V (2010) Cardiac MRI in pulmonary artery hypertension: correlations between morphological and functional parameters and invasive measurements. Eur Radiol 20:1149–1159

Badesch DB, Champion HC, Sanchez MA, Hoeper MM, Loyd JE, Manes A, Mcgoon M, Naeije R, Olschewski H, Oudiz RJ, Torbicki A (2009) Diagnosis and assessment of pulmonary arterial hypertension. J Am Coll Cardiol 54:S55–S66

Blyth KG, Groenning BA, Martin TN, Foster JE, Mark PB, Dargie HJ, Peacock AJ (2005) Contrast enhanced-cardiovascular magnetic resonance imaging in patients with pulmonary hypertension. Eur Heart J 26:1993–1999

Condliffe R, Kiely DG, Peacock AJ, Corris PA, Gibbs JS, Vrapi F, Das C, Elliot CA, Johnson M, Desoyza J, Torpy C, Goldsmith K, Hodgkins D, Hughes RJ, Pepke-Zaba J, Coghlan JG (2009) Connective tissue disease-associated pulmonary arterial hypertension in the modern treatment era. Am J Respir Crit Care Med 179:151–157

D'alonzo GE, Barst RJ, Ayres SM, Bergofsky EH, Brundage BH, Detre KM, Fishman AP, Goldring RM, Groves BM et al (1991) Survival in patients with primary pulmonary hypertension. Results from a national prospective registry. Ann Intern Med 115:343–349

Dellegrottaglie S, Sanz J, Poon M, Viles-Gonzalez JF, Sulica R, Goyenechea M, Macaluso F, Fuster V, Rajagopalan S (2007) Pulmonary hypertension: accuracy of detection with left ventricular septal-to-free wall curvature ratio measured at cardiac MR. Radiology 243:63–69

Galie N, Manes A, Negro L, Palazzini M, Bacchi-Reggiani ML, Branzi A (2009) A meta-analysis of randomized controlled trials in pulmonary arterial hypertension. Eur Heart J 30:394–403

Galie N, Rubin L, Hoeper M, Jansa P, Al-Hiti H, Meyer G, Chiossi E, Kusic-Pajic A, Simonneau G (2008) Treatment of patients with mildly symptomatic pulmonary arterial hypertension with bosentan (EARLY study): a double-blind, randomised controlled trial. Lancet 371:2093–2100

Gan CT, Lankhaar JW, Westerhof N, Marcus JT, Becker A, Twisk JW, Boonstra A, Postmus PE, Vonk-Noordegraaf A (2007) Noninvasively assessed pulmonary artery stiffness predicts mortality in pulmonary arterial hypertension. Chest 132:1906–1912

Hagger D, Condliffe R, Woodhouse N, Elliot CA, Armstrong IJ, Davies C, Hill C, Akil M, Wild JM, Kiely DG (2009) Ventricular mass index correlates with pulmonary artery pressure and predicts survival in suspected systemic sclerosis-associated pulmonary arterial hypertension. Rheumatology (Oxford) 48:1137–1142

Hardziyenka M, Campian ME, Reesink HJ, Surie S, Bouma BJ, Groenink M, Klemens CA, Beekman L, Remme CA, Bresser P, Tan HL (2011) Right ventricular failure following chronic pressure overload is associated with reduction in left ventricular mass evidence for atrophic remodeling. J Am Coll Cardiol 57:921–928

Hardziyenka M, Reesink HJ, Bouma BJ, de Bruin-bon HA, Campian ME, Tanck MW, van den Brink RB, Kloek JJ, Tan HL, Bresser P (2007) A novel echocardiographic predictor of in-hospital mortality and mid-term haemodynamic improvement after pulmonary endarterectomy for chronic thrombo-embolic pulmonary hypertension. Eur Heart J 28:842–849

Hoeper MM, Tongers J, Leppert A, Baus S, Maier R, Lotz J (2001) Evaluation of right ventricular performance with a right ventricular ejection fraction thermodilution catheter and MRI in patients with pulmonary hypertension. Chest 120:502–507

Houde C, Bohn DJ, Freedom RM, Rabinovitch M (1993) Profile of paediatric patients with pulmonary hypertension judged by responsiveness to vasodilators. Br Heart J 70:461–468

Jardim C, Rochitte CE, Humbert M, Rubenfeld G, Jasinowodolinski D, Carvalho CR, Souza R (2007) Pulmonary artery distensibility in pulmonary arterial hypertension: an MRI pilot study. Eur Respir J 29:476–481

Jauhiainen T, Jarvinen VM, Hekali PE (2002) Evaluation of methods for MR imaging of human right ventricular heart volumes and mass. Acta Radiol 43:587–592

Katz J, Whang J, Boxt LM, Barst RJ (1993) Estimation of right ventricular mass in normal subjects and in patients with primary pulmonary hypertension by nuclear magnetic resonance imaging. J Am Coll Cardiol 21:1475–1481

Kind T, Mauritz GJ, Marcus JT, van de Veerdonk M, Westerhof N, Vonk-Noordegraaf A (2010) Right ventricular ejection fraction is better reflected by transverse rather than longitudinal wall motion in pulmonary hypertension. J Cardiovasc Magn Reson 12:35

Kon MW, Myerson SG, Moat NE, Pennell DJ (2004) Quantification of regurgitant fraction in mitral regurgitation by cardiovascular magnetic resonance: comparison of techniques. J Heart Valve Dis 13:600–607

Kreitner KF, Kunz RP, Ley S, Oberholzer K, Neeb D, Gast KK, Heussel CP, Eberle B, Mayer E, Kauczor HU, Duber C (2007) Chronic thromboembolic pulmonary hypertension—assessment by magnetic resonance imaging. Eur Radiol 17:11–21

Kreitner KF, Ley S, Kauczor HU, Mayer E, Kramm T, Pitton MB, Krummenauer F, Thelen M (2004) Chronic thromboembolic pulmonary hypertension: pre- and postoperative assessment with breath-hold MR imaging techniques. Radiology 232:535–543

Ley S, Mereles D, Puderbach M, Gruenig E, Schock H, Eichinger M, Ley Zaporozhan J, Fink C, Kauczor HU (2007) Value of MR phase-contrast flow measurements for functional assessment of pulmonary arterial hypertension. Eur Radiol 17:1892–1897

Lowe BS, Therrien J, Ionescu-Ittu R, Pilote L, Martucci G, Marelli AJ (2011) Diagnosis of pulmonary hypertension in the congenital heart disease adult population impact on outcomes. J Am Coll Cardiol 58:538–546

Lurz P, Nordmeyer J, Coats L, Taylor AM, Bonhoeffer P, Schulze-Neick I (2009) Immediate clinical and haemodynamic benefits of restoration of pulmonary valvar competence in patients with pulmonary hypertension. Heart 95:646–650

Marcus JT, Gan CT, Zwanenburg JJ, Boonstra A, Allaart CP, Gotte MJ, Vonk-Noordegraaf A (2008) Interventricular mechanical asynchrony in pulmonary arterial hypertension: left-to-right delay in peak shortening is related to right ventricular overload and left ventricular underfilling. J Am Coll Cardiol 51:750–757

Mauritz GJ, Marcus JT, Boonstra A, Postmus PE, Westerhof N, Vonk-Noordegraaf A (2008) Non-invasive stroke volume assessment in patients with pulmonary arterial hypertension: left-sided data mandatory. J Cardiovasc Magn Reson 10:51

Minai OA, Chaouat A, Adnot S (2010) Pulmonary hypertension in COPD: epidemiology, significance, and management: pulmonary vascular disease: the global perspective. Chest 137:39S–51S

Moledina S, Hislop AA, Foster H, Schulze-Neick I, Haworth SG (2010) Childhood idiopathic pulmonary arterial hypertension: a national cohort study. Heart 96:1401–1406

Muthurangu V, Lurz P, Critchely JD, Deanfield JE, Taylor AM, Hansen MS (2008) Real-time assessment of right and left ventricular volumes and function in patients with congenital heart disease by using high spatiotemporal resolution radial k-t SENSE. Radiology 248:782–791

Nogami M, Ohno Y, Koyama H, Kono A, Takenaka D, Kataoka T, Kawai H, Kawamitsu H, Onishi Y, Matsumoto K, Matsumoto S, Sugimura K (2009) Utility of phase contrast MR imaging for assessment of pulmonary flow and pressure estimation in patients with pulmonary hypertension: comparison with right heart catheterization and echocardiography. J Magn Reson Imaging 30:973–980

Reiter G, Reiter U, Kovacs G, Kainz B, Schmidt K, Maier R, Olschewski H, Rienmueller R (2008) Magnetic resonance-derived 3-dimensional blood flow patterns in the main pulmonary artery as a marker of pulmonary hypertension and a measure of elevated mean pulmonary arterial pressure. Circ Cardiovasc Imaging 1:23–30

Roeleveld RJ, Marcus JT, Boonstra A, Postmus PE, Marques KM, Bronzwaer JG, Vonk-Noordegraaf A (2005a) A comparison of noninvasive MRI-based methods of estimating pulmonary artery pressure in pulmonary hypertension. J Magn Reson Imaging 22:67–72

Roeleveld RJ, Marcus JT, Faes TJ, Gan TJ, Boonstra A, Postmus PE, Vonk-Noordegraaf A (2005b) Interventricular septal configuration at mr imaging and pulmonary arterial pressure in pulmonary hypertension. Radiology 234:710–717

Roeleveld RJ, Vonk-Noordegraaf A, Marcus JT, Bronzwaer JG, Marques KM, Postmus PE, Boonstra A (2004) Effects of epoprostenol on right ventricular hypertrophy and dilatation in pulmonary hypertension. Chest 125:572–579

Saba TS, Foster J, Cockburn M, Cowan M, Peacock AJ (2002) Ventricular mass index using magnetic resonance imaging accurately estimates pulmonary artery pressure. Eur Respir J 20:1519–1524

Sanz J, Kariisa M, Dellegrottaglie S, Prat-Gonzalez S, Garcia MJ, Fuster V, Rajagopalan S (2009) Evaluation of pulmonary artery stiffness in pulmonary hypertension with cardiac magnetic resonance. JACC Cardiovasc Imaging 2:286–295

Sanz J, Kuschnir P, Rius T, Salguero R, Sulica R, Einstein AJ, Dellegrottaglie S, Fuster V, Rajagopalan S, Poon M (2007) Pulmonary arterial hypertension: noninvasive detection with phase-contrast MR imaging. Radiology 243:70–79

Shehata ML, Lossnitzer D, Skrok J, Boyce D, Lechtzin N, Mathai SC, Girgis RE, Osman N, Lima JA, Bluemke DA, Hassoun PM, Vogel-Claussen J (2011) Myocardial delayed enhancement in pulmonary hypertension: pulmonary hemodynamics, right ventricular function, and remodeling. Am J Roentgenol 196:87–94

Simonneau G, Robbins IM, Beghetti M, Channick RN, Delcroix M, Denton CP, Elliott CG, Gaine SP, Gladwin MT, Jing ZC, Krowka MJ, Langleben D, Nakanishi N, Souza R (2009) Updated clinical classification of pulmonary hypertension. J Am Coll Cardiol 54:S43–S54

Stein PD, Chenevert TL, Fowler SE, Goodman LR, Gottschalk A, Hales CA, Hull RD, Jablonski KA, Leeper KV Jr, Naidich DP, Sak DJ, Sostman HD, Tapson VF, Weg JG, Woodard PK (2010) Gadolinium-enhanced magnetic resonance angiography for pulmonary embolism: a multicenter prospective study (PIOPED III). Ann Intern Med 152:434–443 W142-3

Stein PD, Woodard PK, Hull RD, Kayali F, Weg JG, Olson RE, Fowler SE (2003) Gadolinium-enhanced magnetic resonance angiography for detection of acute pulmonary embolism: an in-depth review. Chest 124: 2324–2328

Tardivon AA, Mousseaux E, Brenot F, Bittoun J, Jolivet O, Bourroul E, Duroux P (1994) Quantification of hemodynamics in primary pulmonary hypertension with magnetic resonance imaging. Am J Respir Crit Care Med 150:1075–1080

Urboniene D, Haber I, Fang YH, Thenappan T, Archer SL (2010) Validation of high-resolution echocardiography and magnetic resonance imaging vs. high-fidelity catheterization in experimental pulmonary hypertension. Am J Physiol Lung Cell Mol Physiol 299:L401–L412

van Wolferen SA, Marcus JT, Boonstra A, Marques KM, Bronzwaer JG, Spreeuwenberg MD, Postmus PE, Vonk-Noordegraaf A (2007) Prognostic value of right ventricular mass, volume, and function in idiopathic pulmonary arterial hypertension. Eur Heart J 28:1250–1257

Wilkins MR, Paul GA, Strange JW, Tunariu N, Gin-Sing W, Banya WA, Westwood MA, Stefanidis A, Ng LL, Pennell DJ, Mohiaddin RH, Nihoyannopoulos P, Gibbs JS (2005) Sildenafil versus endothelin receptor antagonist for pulmonary hypertension (SERAPH) study. Am J Respir Crit Care Med 171:1292–1297

Heart Failure and Heart Transplantation

S. Dymarkowski and J. Bogaert

Contents

1 **Key Points** 367

2 **Introduction** 368

3 **MR Imaging Biomarkers in Heart Failure** 369
3.1 Ventricular Function 369
3.2 Tissue Characterization 370

4 **Imaging in Cardiac Resynchronization Therapy** 373
4.1 MR Imaging of Dyssynchrony 373
4.2 MR Imaging of Myocardial Scar and Site of LV Pacing 374

5 **Heart Transplantation** 376
5.1 Detection of Allograft Rejection 376
5.2 Long-Term Allograft Surveillance 377
5.3 Detection of Complications 380

References 381

Abstract

Heart failure (HF) may be the result of all forms of cardiac disease. Therefore, the development of accurate diagnostic tools for proper selection of therapeutic options is necessary to achieve good response rates in revascularization or resynchronization therapies. The same statement is true for implantation of cardioverter/defibrillators (ICD). Quantification of LV and RV function by MR imaging in patients with HF is quite routinely performed as a surrogate biomarker of baseline status or as a treatment follow-up tool, and can be considered as the standard of reference for quantification of LV and RV volumes and function. Further in this chapter, the role of cardiac MR imaging in resynchronization therapy (CRT) will be discussed, related to imaging of and quantification of the amount of scar tissue and the spatial relation of the myocardial scar to the site of LV pacing, since these are considered important parameters for CRT response. Finally, we will show that a comprehensive MRI exam may be used to noninvasively detect transplant vasculopathy and transplant-related complications.

1 Key Points

Non-invasive serial MRI assessment of LV remodeling provides important information regarding outcome and therapy response in patients with LV dysfunction and heart failure (HF). The limited measurement variability and reproducibility maximizes the value of the data obtained.

S. Dymarkowski (✉) · J. Bogaert
Department of Radiology, University Hospitals, Catholic University of Leuven, Herestraat 49, 3000 Leuven, Belgium
e-mail: steven.dymarkowski@uz.kuleuven.ac.be

J. Bogaert et al. (eds.), *Clinical Cardiac MRI*, Medical Radiology. Diagnostic Imaging,
DOI: 10.1007/174_2011_356, © Springer-Verlag Berlin Heidelberg 2012

More evidence is arising that MRI can provide useful information in pre-CRT imaging, not only in visualizing dyssynchrony itself, but also in adequate mapping of myocardial scar tissue and detailed anatomical information of the cardiac veins and coronary sinus.

Results of MRI studies in acute allograft rejection remain unequivocal and are subject to a large standard deviation over different study populations. MRI after cardiac transplantation is especially well suited to monitor long-term effects of cardiac denervation and the corresponding cardiovascular adaptation. MRI offers a comprehensive evaluation of complications following transplantation surgery.

2 Introduction

Heart failure (HF) is a clinical syndrome that is most commonly described by symptoms such as fatigue and dyspnea upon exercise related to cardiac dysfunction. Clinical symptoms of congestion such as pulmonary edema and peripheral extremity swelling are usually present. It has various diagnostic criteria, and the term HF is often incorrectly used to describe other cardiac-related illnesses.

Heart failure is a common, debilitating and potentially lethal condition with gradually increasing prevalence. The incidence of HF augments with age, affecting those over the age of 65 by more than 10% (McMurray and Pfeffer 2005). This age-dependent increase is most likely multifactorial and might be influenced by the aging of the myocardium and the vasculature itself as well as the increased incidence of myocardial ischemia due to coronary heart disease.

Furthermore, improved management and treatment of both acute coronary syndromes and chronic ischemic heart disease has led to a dramatic decrease in case fatality rate of acute infarctions (AMI) and has improved survival rates in chronic disease states. Progress in treatment has nevertheless led to large cohorts of patients responsible for an enormous augmentation in health expenditure. Costs have been estimated to be as high as 2% of the total budget of the National Health Service in the United Kingdom, and more than $35 billion in the United States (Stewart et al. 2002; Rosamond et al. 2008). In its progressive nature, HF is known to have an annual mortality rate of 10%.

Table 1 Underlying causes of heart failure

Primary myocardial diseases
Ischemic heart disease
Acute myocardial infarction (AMI)
Chronic ischemia (hibernating myocardium)
Cardiomyopathies (CMP)
Idiopathic CMP
Metabolic CMP
Toxic CMP
Infiltrative CMP
Myocarditis
Disease states with increased ventricular load
Pressure overload
Aortic stenosis
Hypertension
Volume overload
Valvular disease
Hyperdynamic circulation (AV fistulas, uncorrected septal defects).
Restrictive heart disease
Constrictive pericarditis
Decreased myocardial compliance—Infiltrative CMP
Endocardial fibro-elastosis
Electrophysiologic disturbances
Tachycardias

The symptoms mentioned above are fairly non-specific, and it may be said that the attribution of these signs to cardiac disease in this population may be confounded by aging itself of by deconditioning. Furthermore, there might also be comorbid conditions that could mask the cardiac origin of the patient's complaints.

If we consider that HF may be the result of all forms of cardiac disease (ischemic, valvular, inflammatory, idiopathic,…; Table 1), the development of accurate diagnostic tools for proper selection of therapeutic options is necessary to achieve good response rates in revascularization or resynchronization therapies. The same statement is true for implantation of cardioverter/defibrillators (ICD). Since several clinical studies have described appropriate therapy in only about 20% of patients, the current cost-effectiveness of patient selection may be questioned (Birnie and Tang 2006; Sanders et al. 2010).

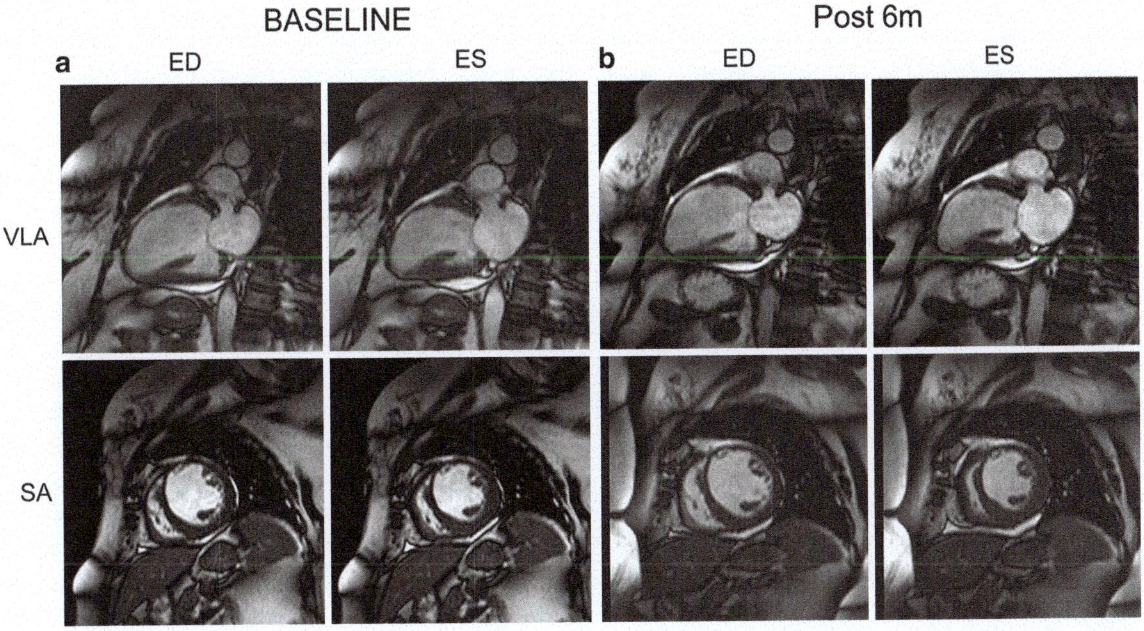

Fig. 1 **a** Inclusion stage b-SSFP cine MRI study in vertical long-axis (*top*) and short-axis (*bottom*) orientation of a 69-year-old heart failure patient included in a heart failure trial. Wall thinning in the anterior LV wall is observed. The ventricle appears dilated and globally hypokinetic. **b** Corresponding images of the follow-up study 6 months later show comparable morphologic and functional features. No additional negative remodeling effects can be observed. *ED* end-diastole, *ES* end-systole, *VLA* vertical long axis, *SA* short axis

Whether it concerns medical therapy, surgery or implantation of devices, patient treatment should seed a maximal clinical benefit with minimum adverse effects. In this strategy, imaging is often used to provide accurate functional biomarkers to provide measureable parameters in describing the patient's pathology and his/her response to therapy. In this setting, echocardiography remains the first-line modality for diagnosis, and several echocardiographic parameters have been defined to have clinical significance (Marwick 2010). Several researchers have expressed interest in using other imaging modalities to further refine the often difficult differential diagnosis and to aid in patient stratification. From the part of MR imaging, its largest virtue may be that it often provides several different relevant markers simultaneously in one single exam. Standardization in MR imaging strategies may in the future aid to promulgate this technique as a standard of reference in HF management. Currently, several trials are already underway to underline both the appropriateness and the importance of this new non-invasive imaging technique and to assess its importance of cost-management for the future (Taylor et al. 2010) (Fig. 1).

3 MR Imaging Biomarkers in Heart Failure

3.1 Ventricular Function

Under clinical circumstances, evaluation of ventricular volumes, mass and function already constitutes a large marker for decision-making since it is known that these parameters are major determinants of therapy response and prognosis and can serve as important surrogate markers. The majority of this information can be readily assessed in most patients with echocardiography or radionuclide ventriculography. Based on this information, patients will be guided to treatment regimens (surgery, cardiac resynchronization therapy (CRT), internal cardioverter defibrillator or drug trials). This fact stresses the accurate and reproducible quantification of LV and RV function for appropriate risk stratification and treatment allocation of patients (Remme and Swedberg 2001; Vardas et al. 2007).

Compared to echocardiography, quantification of LV and RV function by MR imaging is quite routinely performed using ECG-gated breath-hold cine MRI. The balanced steady-state free precession (SSFP) technique is preferred over the spoiled gradient-echo sequence for the acquisition of cine MRI, the latter being considered outdated due to less favorable blood-to-myocardium contrast. The image quality generated by these cine MRI sequences—together with systematic analysis—ensures highly reproducible measurements, independent of the field strength used (Hudsmith et al. 2006), and can be considered as the standard of reference for quantification of LV and RV volumes and function. The increased reliability of the endocardial border detection can be considered as an extra advantage in the presence of ventricular dilatation and slow flow, as is often seen in dilated cardiomyopathy of chronic myocardial hibernation.

A dilated ventricle can be generally covered in the short-axis direction by 12–16 slices of 6–8 mm thick. The nature of the diseases involved often mandate fast examination methods and more comfort for the patient. By using parallel imaging, the breath-hold period can usually be kept short. In case of significant artifacts during the acquisition of real-time (RT) ECG-triggered or ungated cine MRI can be used to achieve considerable shortening of examination time in high reproducibility. Similar to the breath-hold variants, interstudy and intraobserver variability of real-time cine shows a low variability and can be considered as an alternative and suitable tool for clinical routine and may be particularly relevant in patients with sub-optimal breath-holding ability and/or arrhythmia (Beer et al. 2010) (Fig. 2).

An important part of patients with clinical signs of cardiac failure will present with normal LV systolic function while the diastolic function is disturbed. Echocardiography is traditionally considered the most used clinical imaging modality for assessment of diastolic function, since the relationship between E/E′ (early mitral inflow velocity divided by the early diastolic longitudinal lengthening velocity) and end-diastolic pressure has been extensively studied and is a considered a good parameter for diastolic function (Sohn 2011; Paulus et al. 2007).

Inflow patterns can be easily assessed using phase contrast cine MRI (PC-MRI), and several studies have found an excellent correlation with echocardiography (Rathi et al. 2008). Nevertheless, from the practical side, venc MRI and the assessment of diastolic function is often underused in clinical practice.

3.2 Tissue Characterization

As shown in Table 1, HF can arise from a variety of pathologies, either ischemic or nonischemic. The treatment and outcome of these patients are very much relying on the exact cause of the disease state. Correct differential diagnosis is therefore of utmost importance for adequate treatment. Usually the presence of ischemic heart disease is confirmed or ruled out by conventional coronary angiography (Remme and Swedberg 2001). Performing an MR examination may further help to narrow down the diagnosis by identifying certain markers, either morphological, or depending on tissue relaxation parameters that are known to have altered in specific disease states (Mahrholdt et al. 2005). Especially if a genetic background is suspected, screening of an entire family can be considered as a non-invasive alternative for diagnosis. The specific changes that can be expected in ischemic and non-ischemic cardiomyopathies are discussed in detail in "Ischemic Heart Disease" and "Heart Muscle Diseases" and are only briefly summarized here.

In a first step, T2-weighted imaging, usually using triple-inversion recovery turbospin echo with fat saturation ''black-blood'' sequences, can be performed to detect edema of the myocardium.

This technique has been shown to increase the diagnostic accuracy of cardiac MR compared to late Gd MRI alone in patients with several potential causes of HF such as suspected acute myocarditis (Abdel-Aty et al. 2005), and has proven its role in acute coronary syndromes and in detecting myocardial edema related to cardiac transplant rejection (Marie et al. 2001).

In selected subgroups of patients, T2*-weighted measurements may be performed. This concerns mainly patients suspected of iron overload cardiomyopathy in thc sctting of hereditary hemochromatosis, post-transfusional hemosiderosis, or linked to myocardial iron overload secondary to liver or bone marrow pathology. By using T2*-weighted imaging, also called T2* relaxometry, the T2* relaxation value of myocardium is measured, using a black-blood sequence with several different echo times, usually six or more. While this process used to be quite time consuming, recently breath-hold versions of this sequence have become available and its use does not significantly lengthen a cardiac MR examination (He et al. 2007). The dephasing, or T2* decay of the

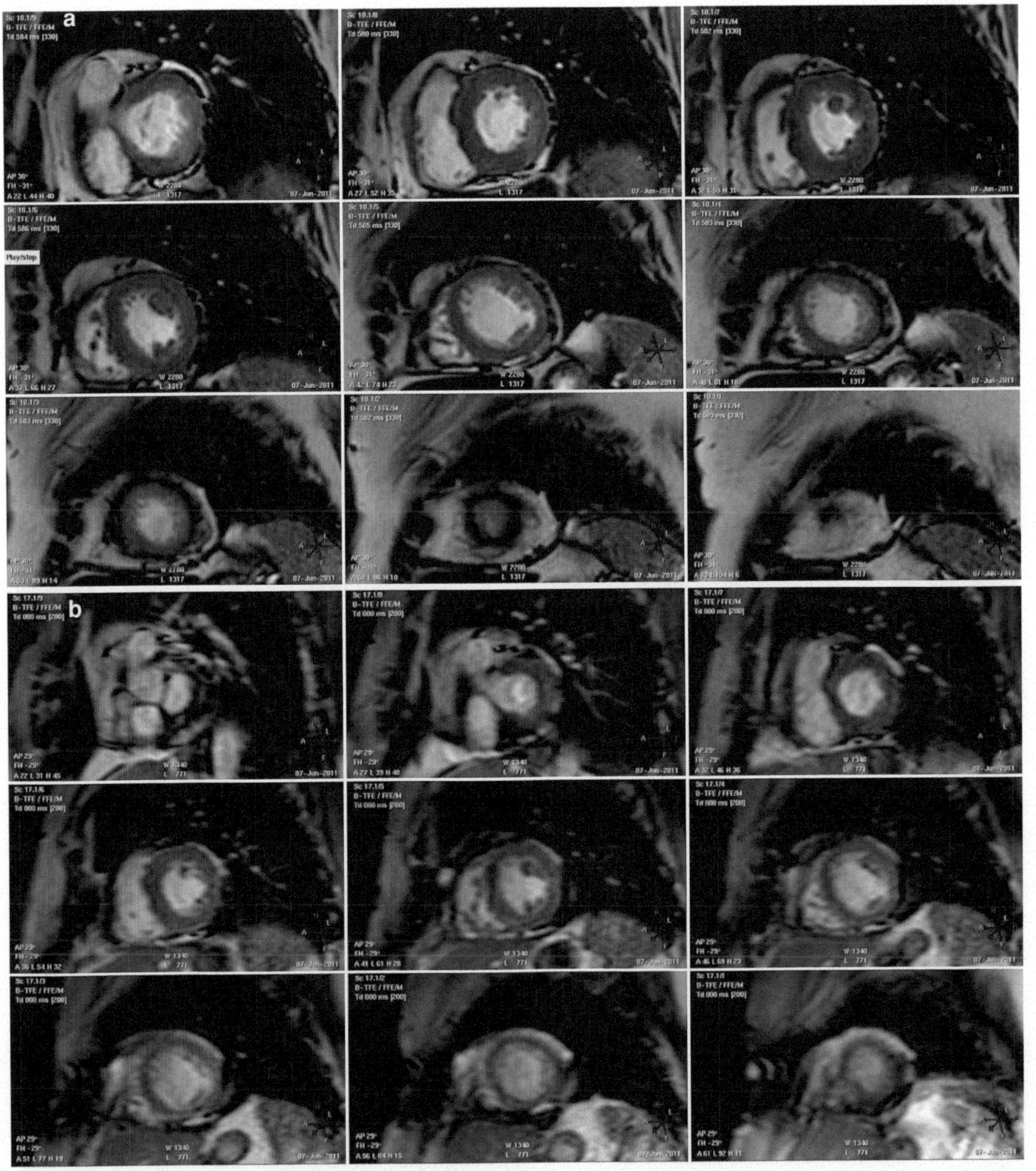

Fig. 2 Example of a breath-hold dataset (**a**) in a patient with a dilated cardiomyopathy compared to a free breathing short-axis cine MRI dataset (**b**), all end-diastolic images

myocardial signal is mapped in a graph or numerically expressed as a measure of myocardial iron content (Fig. 3). A T2* value of >30 ms is considered normal, between 10 and 20 ms moderately abnormal, and <10 ms severely abnormal (Kirk et al. 2009; Anderson et al. 2001).

Almost routine in any cardiac MR study, especially in HF patient is late Gd MRI, also known as delayed enhancement imaging. Imaging of the myocardial scar in patients with CAD will typically show either subendocardial or transmural contrast enhancement, with a distribution area corresponding

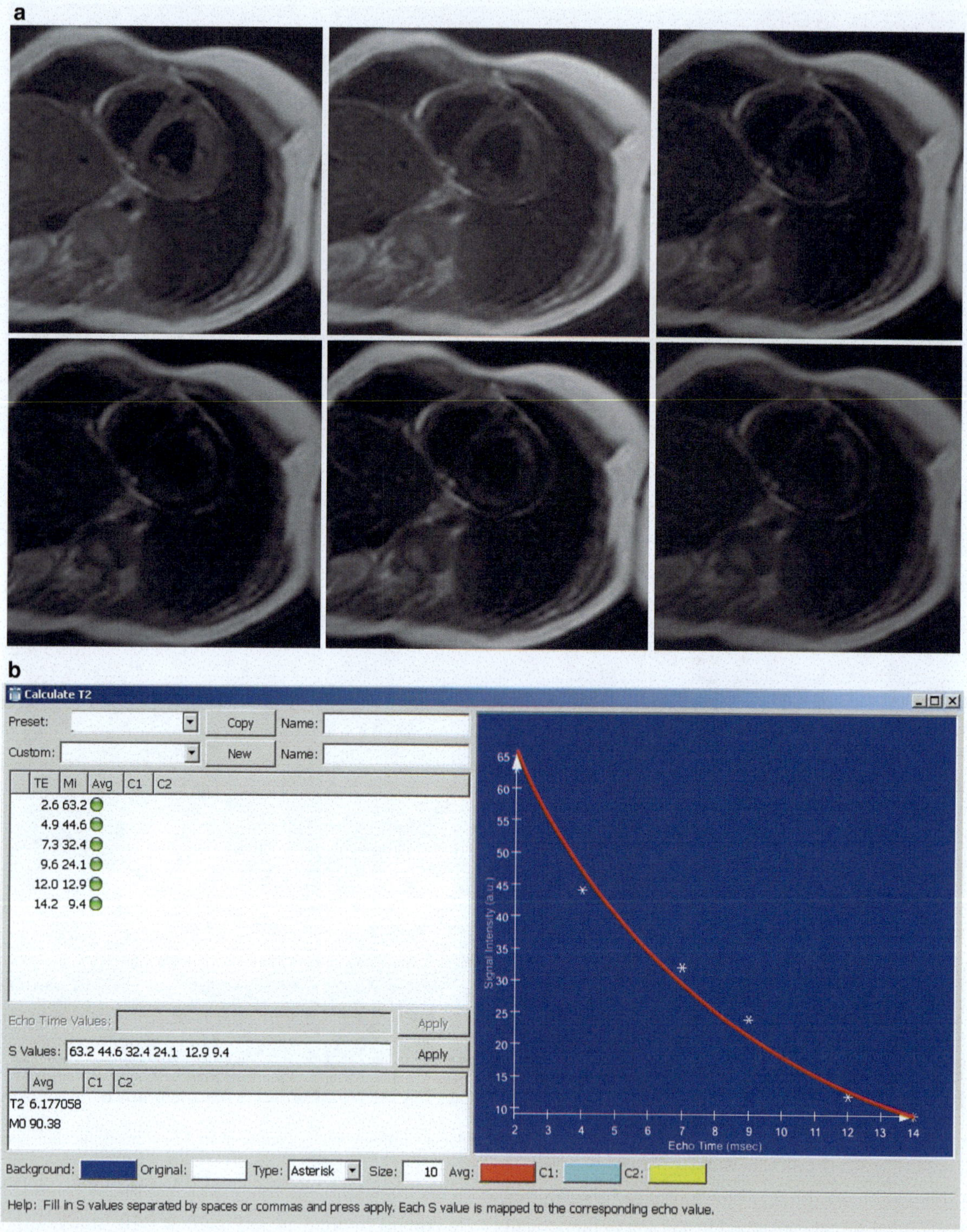

Fig. 3 T2* relaxometry in a patient with iron deposition disease. Input of measured signal intensities from a multi-echo gradient-echo sequence (**a**) into a self-developed software program provides both graphical and quantitative output (**b**)

to the vascular bed of an epicardial coronary artery. Conversely, patients with non-ischemic CMP may have either no detectable fibrosis at all or signs of myocardial fibrosis without mural or segmental localization characteristics for ischemic heart disease (i.e., midwall, subepicardial location, patchy distribution; Mahrholdt et al. 2005). Careful analysis of the pattern, intensity and localization of enhancing myocardial tissue may aid in the differential diagnosis of ischemic or non-ischemic CMP. Worldwide experience gained of the last 10 years has lead to the identification of specific enhancement patterns in myocarditis, both hypertrophic and dilated cardiomyopathy, Fabry disease, cardiac amyloid deposition disease, sarcoidosis, etc (Maceira et al. 2005, Moon et al. 2003a, 2003b). This is elaborated in more detail in "Heart Muscle Diseases".

4 Imaging in Cardiac Resynchronization Therapy

4.1 MR Imaging of Dyssynchrony

The implementation of Cardiac Resynchronixation Therapy- or CRT-has been shown to improve the general quality of life and survival rates in HF patients with reduced LV EF and wide QRS complex, generally with HF symptoms; a LV ejection fraction less than or equal to 35% and QRS duration on EKG of 120 ms or greater (Cleland et al. 2005). In CRT, a biventricular pacemaker is placed so that this may activate both the septal and lateral walls of the left ventricle. By pacing both sides of the left ventricle, the pacemaker can resynchronize a heart whose opposing walls do not contract in synchrony, which occurs in approximately 25–50% of HF patients. CRT devices have at least two leads, one in the right ventricle to stimulate the septum, and another inserted through the coronary sinus to pace the lateral wall of the left ventricle. Often, for patients in normal sinus rhythm, there is also a lead in the right atrium to facilitate synchrony with the atrial contraction. Thus, timing between the atrial and ventricular contractions, as well as between the septal and lateral walls of the left ventricle can be adjusted to achieve optimal cardiac function. Nevertheless, applying recent selection criteria for CRT, a significant number of HF patients do not respond to this therapy. For example, in the Multicenter InSync Randomized Clinical Evaluation (MIRACLE) and the Multicenter InSync Implantable Cardioverter Defibrillator (MIRACLE-ICD) trials, more than 30% of the patients did not show a favorable clinical response to CRT. The current triage of patients is mainly based on clinical symptoms and electrocardiographic data, while there is still little room for imaging studies. Several smaller trials have focused on the use of echocardiography to define parameters to more accurately select patients for CRT, but several larger multicenter trials could not confirm these results, questioning the role of mechanical dyssynchrony in patient selection for CRT, and sparking a worldwide controversy and vigorous debating on the topic if imaging should or should not be used as a selection tool for patients scheduled to undergo CRT (Delgado and Bax 2011; Sung and Foster 2011) (Fig. 4).

On this topic, several recent studies have called into question the reproducibility of echocardiography-based measurements of dyssynchrony (Gabriel et al. 2007). The international multicenter Predictors Of ResPonse to CrT (PROSPECT) study, which examined the role of echocardiography in identifying positive responders to CRT, did not find any TDI-based parameters that predicted a positive response to CRT (Chung et al. 2008).

MRI may provide alternate strategies to quantify this dyssynchrony. On cineMRI images, dyssynchrony can be qualitatively assessed or by analysis of the delineated images on a workstation, the amount of regional myocardial thickening and—wall motion and differences in end-systolic timing can be quantified and expressed graphically or in numbers (Fig. 5). Several differences in systolic time and maximal radial wall thickening between a control group and HF patients eligible for CRT have thus been quantified (Mischi et al. 2008; Ordas and Frangi 2005).

More complex methods to quantify myocardial strain include the use of MR tagging and strain encoded imaging (SENC), but several constrains limit the clinical applicability (Lardo et al. 2005; Osman et al. 2001). First of all, image analysis of tagged images can be very time consuming—several hours up to days per patient—and requires much user input. Secondly, MR tags usually appear quite faded in the second part of the cardiac cycle, due to inherent T1 relaxation recovery, so that all information regarding diastolic events is imaged in less than ideal

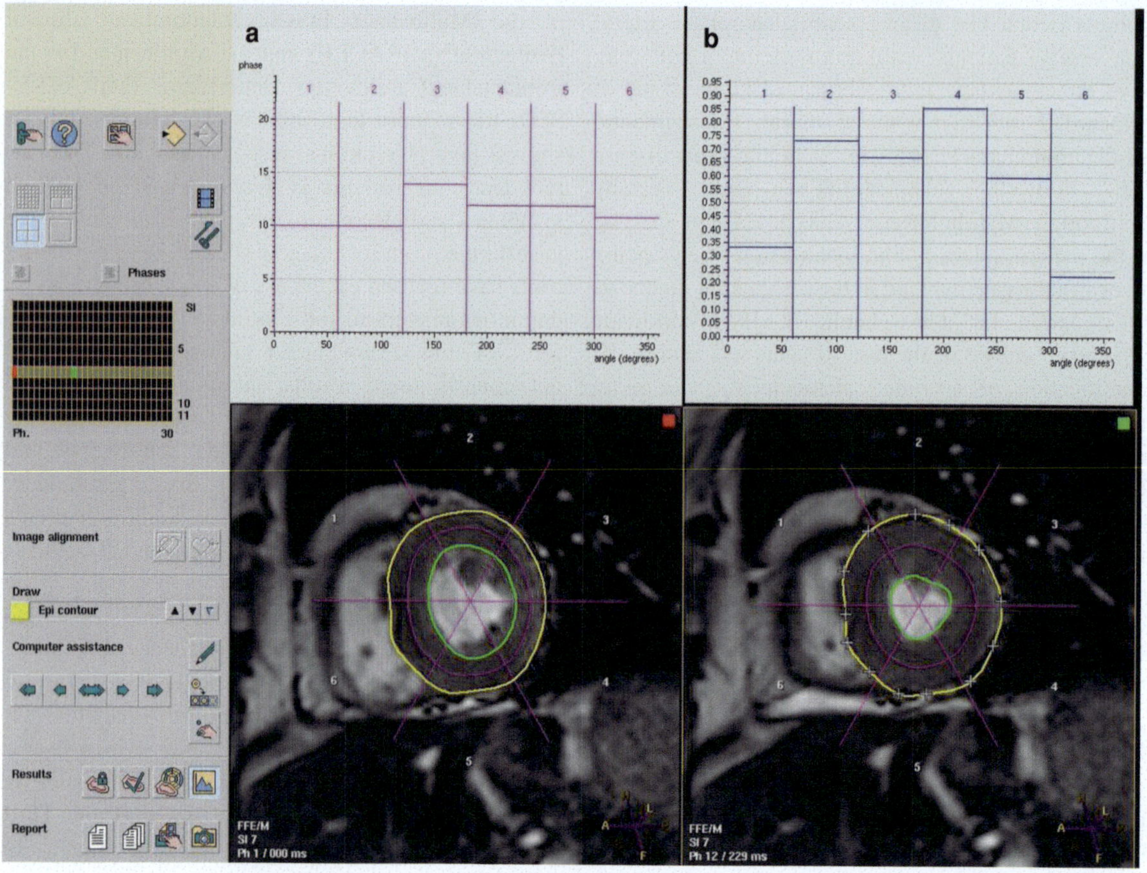

Fig. 4 Dyssynchrony measurements. After detailed delineation of endo-and epi-cardial contours and sectoring of the myocardium, both time to maximal wall thickening (graph **a**) as well as maximal wall thickening (**b**) are calculated

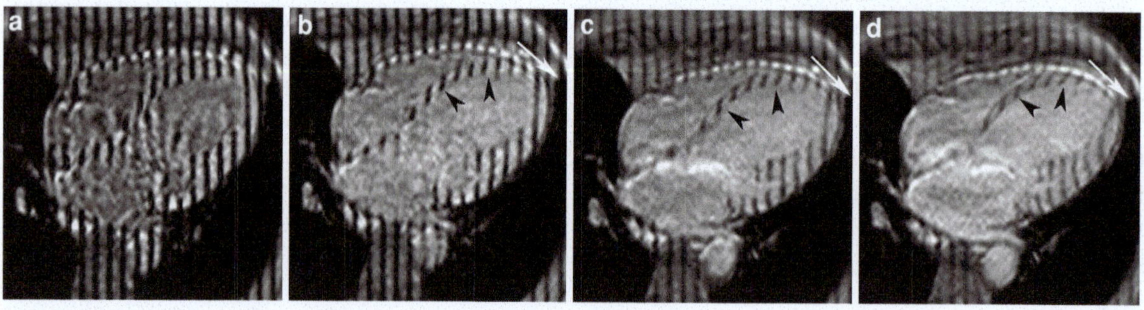

Fig. 5 Figure illustrating the use of MR tagging to demonstrate both systolic dyskinesia (*black arrowheads*) and 'rocking of the apex' (*white arrows*)

circumstances. Techniques such as C-SPAMM tagging overcome this last issue, but as it is true for most tagging technique, the analysis is mainly confined to research facilities and not yet part of a routine clinical cardiac MR exam. Therefore, the data on the clinical value in CRT is very limited.

4.2 MR Imaging of Myocardial Scar and Site of LV Pacing

As stated earlier, cardiac MR imaging in CRT does not limit itself to imaging of dyssynchrony, but also the quantification of the amount of scar tissue and the

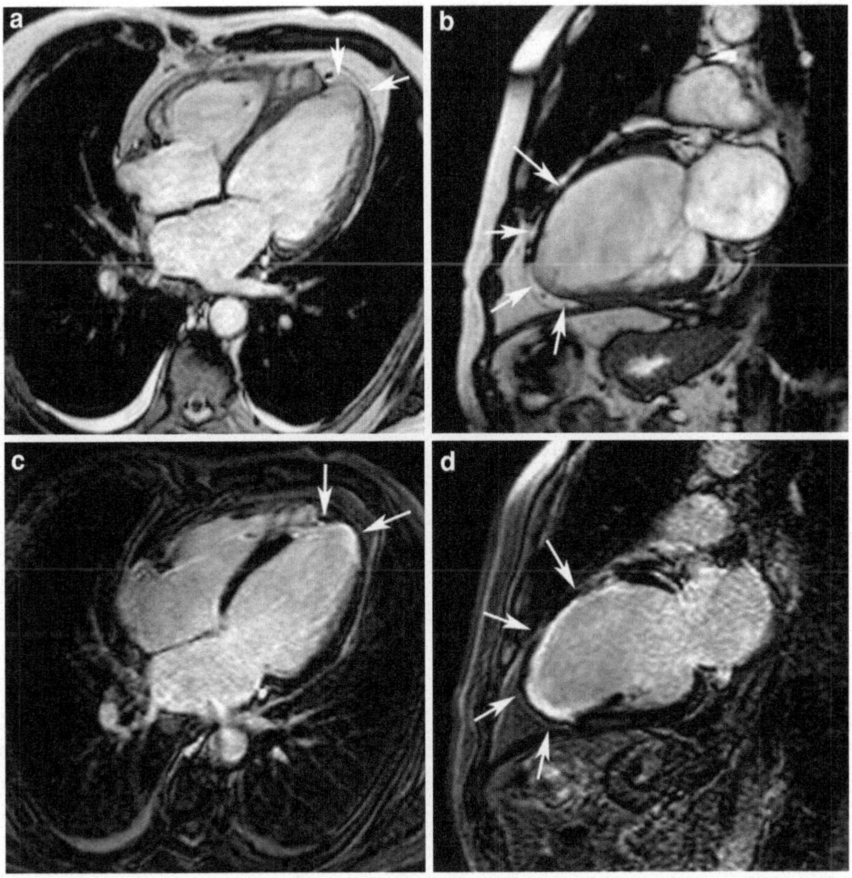

Fig. 6 Pre-CRT MRI study of a patient with extensive ischemic heart disease. Cine MRI shows negative remodeling (thinning of the apex and a considerable part of the anterior wall) due to an old LAD infarction (a, b; *arrows*) Late Gd MRI confirms the near-transmural aspect of this infarction (c, d; *arrows*)

spatial relation of the myocardial scar to the site of LV pacing are considered important parameters for CRT response.

Late Gd MRI is used to define the precise extent of infarcted myocardium, with excellent distinction between completely transmural and sub-endocardial extent of this scar (Adelstein and Saba 2007). This feature is quite unique in cardiac MRI. Many studies have found a significant direct relationship between scar burden and response to CRT and an inverse relationship between scar burden and the reduction LV end-diastolic volume post-CRT (Ypenburg et al. 2007). Currently, a cutoff value of 15% scar is found to be a positive marker for CRT response with 85% sensitivity and 90% specificity (White et al. 2006) (Fig. 6).

Also the site of scarring has been found to be an important parameter in CRT response. Studies have demonstrated an inversely proportional relationship between the extent of myocardial scarring and CRT response in cases of septal and inferolateral scar (Marsan et al. 2009; Bleeker et al. 2006). In this context, the ability of CMR to visualize the cardiac venous anatomy and myocardial scar tissue in a single examination becomes an interesting issue for optimal planning of the CRT implantation and identification of the ideal cardiac vein for the placement of the LV lead (Younger et al. 2009). The preferred sites for placement of a transvenous pacing are the lateral or posterior branches of the coronary. However, many variants of the anatomy of these veins exist with regard to vein diameter, course and angulations sinus (Gassis et al. 2006; Singh et al. 2005). Using a very simple adaptation of the routine 3D MRCA sequence, coronary venous anatomy can be acquired with good contrast between the blood vessels and the surrounding myocardial tissues. Since maximal benefit from CRT is likely achieved when the pacing leads are placed in the area with the greatest electrical and mechanical activation delay, analysis of both venous MR angiography images and the late Gd MRI images, the choice for either transvenous of epicardial lead placement may be motivated and the placement of a lead in an area of extensive scarring can be avoided, since this would very likely induce poor response to CRT.

5 Heart Transplantation

5.1 Detection of Allograft Rejection

Heart transplantation is an established treatment for selected patients with refractory HF. Long-term survival rates are superior to those resulting from other forms of therapy for that patient population. In addition, an improved quality of life has been reported by many patients. A vigilant eye remains necessary to detect acute allograft rejection, which remains one of the major causes of death during the first year post transplantation. Thus, a crucial factor in improving results is accurate evaluation of the severity and extent of cardiac rejection, with differentiation of rejection from other conditions such as infection (Walpoth et al. 1995).

In the early phase, myocardial rejection consists in interstitial edema and mononuclear cell infiltration, which progresses toward myocytolysis or myocyte necrosis (Sasaki et al. 1987). Therefore, early diagnosis and adequate treatment before the occurrence of myocardial necrosis are mandatory. However, the clinical presentation of acute cardiac rejection may be silent in patients receiving cyclosporine treatment. Right endomyocardial biopsy and histological grading is the gold standard for the detection of myocardial rejection (Caves et al. 1973; Billingham 1982). However, endomyocardial biopsy has several drawbacks: it is invasive and costly, 6–12 h is required before the diagnostic results become available, experienced pathologists are required for the histological diagnosis, and it is prone to sampling error (Nishimura et al. 1988; Smart et al. 1993).

Therefore, a non-invasive modality that would guide the timing of endomyocardial biopsy and assess the response to changes in immunosuppressive therapy would be advantageous. Several pathways to use MRI as a monitoring tool have been explored.

Since one of the early findings in cardiac rejection is an increase in the myocardial water content, principally due to myocardial edema, assessment of relaxation times theoretically provides a sensitive measure of rejection (Scott et al. 1983). Although animal studies have consistently shown increases in T2 relaxation times in cardiac transplants as early as 2 days after transplantation (Nishimura et al. 1987, 1988), studies in patients, however, have proved to be more contradictory. While some investigators have shown an increase in T2 relaxation times in patients with cardiac rejection (Smart et al. 1993; Marie et al. 2001), others could not confirm these results (Doornbos et al. 1990). A large degree of overlap between the T2 values of normal volunteers, patients without signs of cardiac rejection, and patients with such signs was observed. In other words, the absence of a demarcation value between normal or non-rejected and rejected myocardium precludes the clinical application of T2 relaxation times for assessment of cardiac rejection.

The contradictory results between these animal and patient studies can be explained in several ways. First, the signal intensity on T2-weighted images of supposedly abnormal myocardium may be influenced by presence of varying degrees of necrosis, edema and fibrosis, making measurement of T2 relaxation times difficult with present spatial resolution. Second, animal studies represent optimized conditions while the clinical situation is far more complex. Factors such as variable ischemia time of the donor heart or effects of cyclosporine therapy may contribute to changes in T2 relaxation time.

Several investigators have evaluated the role of contrast agents for the assessment of cardiac transplant rejection. Animal studies using extracellular Gd-DTPA have shown that in the absence of rejection, Gd-DTPA induced mild homogeneous myocardial enhancement (Nishimura et al. 1987; Kurland et al. 1989) while moderate and severe allograft rejection were characterized by one or more areas of intense myocardial enhancement. The extent and distribution of intense myocardial enhancement corresponded to the severity and extent of histological rejection. Studies using blood pool agents found statistically significant contrast enhancement differences between acutely rejecting heart transplants and non-rejecting ones at four minutes after injection of the contrast agent and increased with increasing time after injection, with relative contrast enhancement reflecting the histologically determined degree of rejection (Johansson et al. 2002).

In patients, these results have been under scrutiny for many years. Mousseux et al. reported myocardial

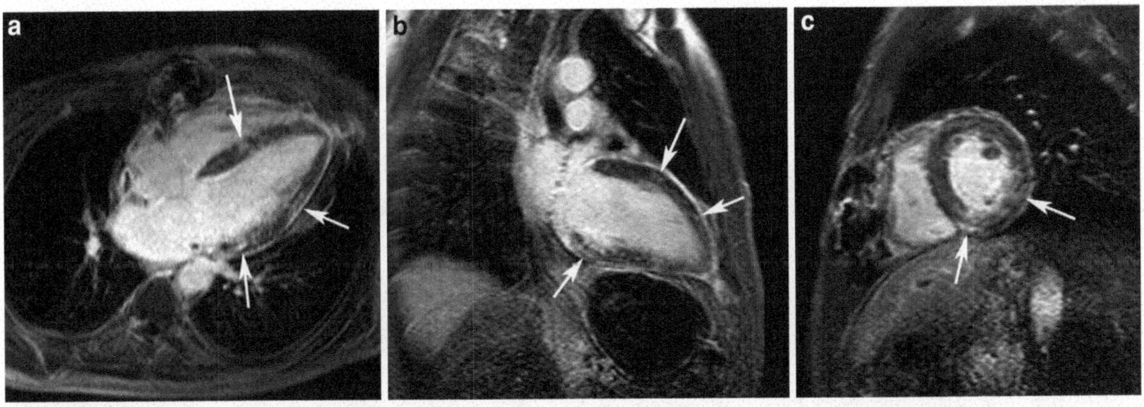

Fig. 7 Late Gd MRI images of a 41-year-old male cardiac transplant patient presenting with a slightly hypertrophic LV with good systolic function. EDV: 157 ml, ESV: 76 ml, EF: 52%, SV: 81 ml, CO: 7.1 l/min, mass: 172 g. Multifocal, low-intensity areas of enhancement (*arrows*) can be seen in multiple LV segments. Endomyocardial biopsies failed to reveal any signs of rejection

enhancement not to be significantly different in patients with mild histological rejection compared with those with moderate or severe rejection (Mousseaux et al. 1993) In a later paper using 3D CE-IR MRI techniques (Almenar et al. 2003), beside a trend toward increased myocardial uptake in patients with acute necrosis, analysis of myocardial perfusion and CE-IR MRI sequences did not reflect any significant changes. Later research reported typical chronic myocardial scar to be present in a significant number of patients with angiographically classified mild transplant coronary artery disease (Steen et al. 2008). In this study patients with only infarct-atypical late Gd MRI (diffuse spotted or intramural) were associated with significantly better left ventricular function compared to patients with infarct-typical or combined late Gd MRI patterns. It remains unclear however how many of these enhancing lesions are due to transplant coronary artery disease or to the rejection process itself (Fig. 7).

5.2 Long-Term Allograft Surveillance

It is important to realize that the transplanted heart does not provide the recipient with normal cardiac function. Cardiac physiology after heart transplantation is unique. When the native heart is removed, sympathetic and parasympathetic innervation is severed, causing resting hemodynamics to differ significantly, acutely and chronically, from those seen in healthy subjects. In addition, the renin-angiotensin-aldosterone regulation mechanism undergoes changes as a result of surgical denervation. Afferent control mechanisms and efferent responses are both altered, leading to important clinical abnormalities. The heart rate does not vary according to respiration and does not respond to Valsalva maneuvers or carotid massage. Other examples include altered cardiovascular responses to exercise, altered cardiac electrophysiology and altered responses to cardiac pharmacologic agents (Cotts and Oren 1997). Finally, most patients do not experience angina after cardiac transplant, because of denervation, although there are reports of angina during myocardial ischemia. Several authors have noted limited sympathetic reinnervation in some cardiac transplant recipients (Wilson et al. 1991; Bengel et al. 2001). This finding suggests that reinnervation may include a return of sympathetic neural mediation of heart rate, ventricular contractility and modulation of artery vasomotor tone. An improved understanding of the changes in cardiac physiology, which occur after heart transplant, may allow the care of these patients to be optimized.

It is known that patients develop high-ejection fractions and present with concentric hypertrophy in the later stages after transplantation. In a recent study by Wilhelmi et al. in a patient cohort 12.5 ± 1.4 years after heart transplantation, it was shown with Doppler echocardiography that ejection fraction increased to 71 ± 11.7%, left ventricular mass increased to 263.8 ± 111.4 g in males and 373.0 ± 181.1 g in females. Focused on right ventricular

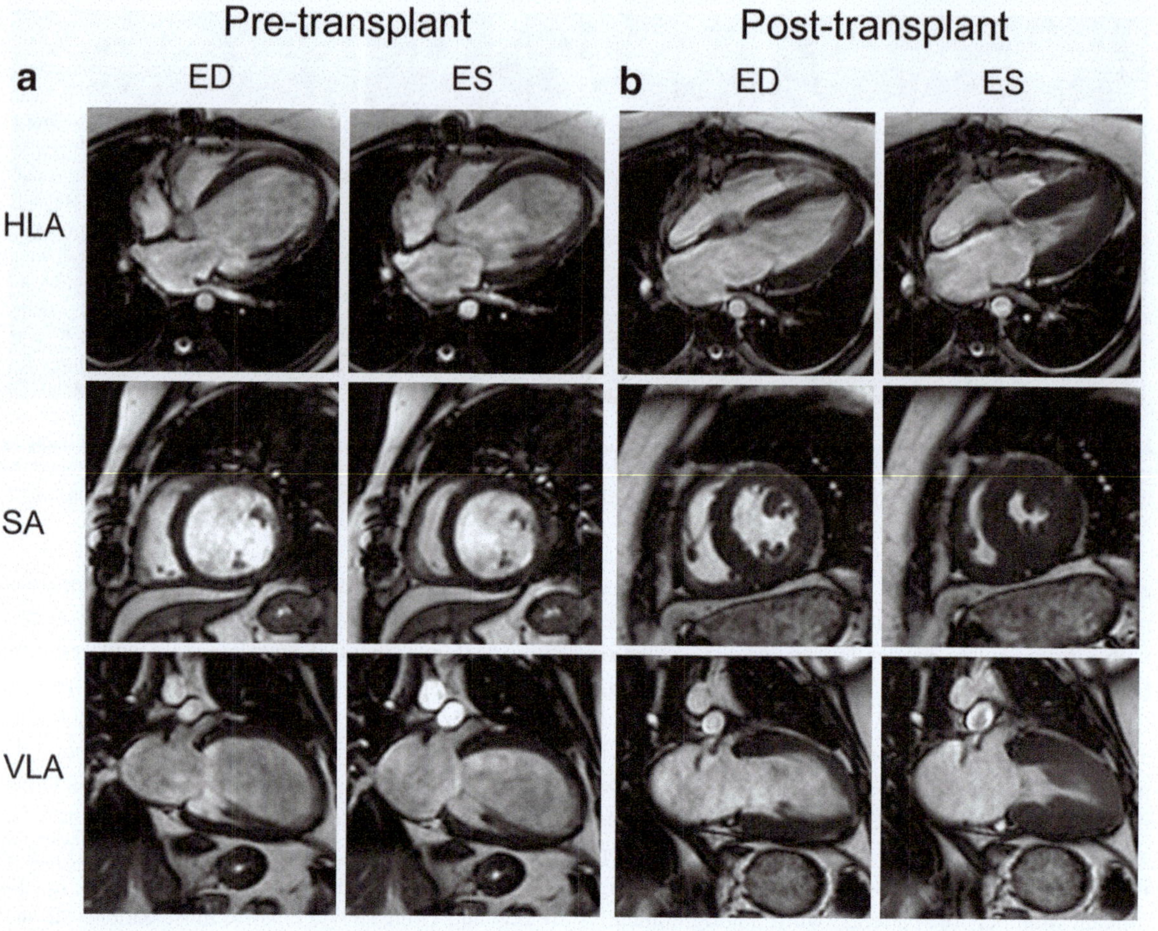

Fig. 8 Comparison of pre- and post-transplant MRI studies. **a** Cine MRI images for a 38-year-old patient with idiopathic dilated cardiomyopathy. The LV is dilated and severely hypokinetic (EDV 344 ml, ESV 290 ml, SV 54 ml, EF 23%). **b** Corresponding cine MRI series 3 years after transplantation. Note the surgically altered atrial anatomy (part donor and receptor atrium) and the good systolic function of the allograft (EDV 117 ml, ESV 44 ml, SV 73 ml, EF 62%). Measurement of the end-diastolic wall thickness (average 16 mm) and the total myocardial mass (235 g) indicates the patient has developed concentric hypertrophy

morphology, enlargement of both the right atrium and the right ventricle was observed in the majority of the patients (Wilhelmi et al. 2002).

MRI has a definite role in the long-term follow-up of patients after cardiac transplantation to assess cardiac morphology and function, since one of the major strengths of MRI in assessing cardiac diseases is the accurate assessment of ventricular function and mass. The excellent visualization of the myocardium on cine MRI and its endo- and epi-cardial surfaces allows to track changes in wall thickening and wall motion over time and has undisputed benefits in terms of accuracy over echocardiography (Bogaert et al. 1995). Cardiac MRI with b-SSFP cine studies can offer increased sensitivity of long-term follow-up studies and also allow to evaluate changes in time which otherwise would be missed (Barkhausen et al. 2001) (Fig. 8).

Furthermore, a comprehensive MRI exam may be used to non-invasively detect transplant vasculopathy. Due to the denervation of the allograft as mentioned above, transplant vasculopathy often lacks clinical symptoms and is the reason for frequent surveillance angiography in heart transplant recipients. By performing resting state and hyperemic MR perfusion measurements, myocardial perfusion reserve (MPR) and endomyocardial-to-epimyocardial perfusion ratio can be assessed. In a study by Mueling et al. transplant arteriopathy was detected, expressed as a decreased myocardial perfusion reserve with sensitivity and

Fig. 9 Images of 26-year-old male transplant patient, 5 years post transplant. The original pathology was non-compaction cardiomyopathy with cardiac failure. Current images show a hypertrophied and dilated LV with mildly reduced systolic function due to global hypokinesia. EDV: 252 ml, ESV: 140 ml, EF: 45%, SV: 113 ml, CO: 10.9 l/min, mass: 268 g. Both precontrast T1w and T2w MRI (a, b) show non-specific signal intensity alterations. C: Cine MRI. Late Gd MRI (**d–f**) reveals diffuse patchy enhancement of both LV and RV myocardium. Pathology showed signs of chronic humoral rejection

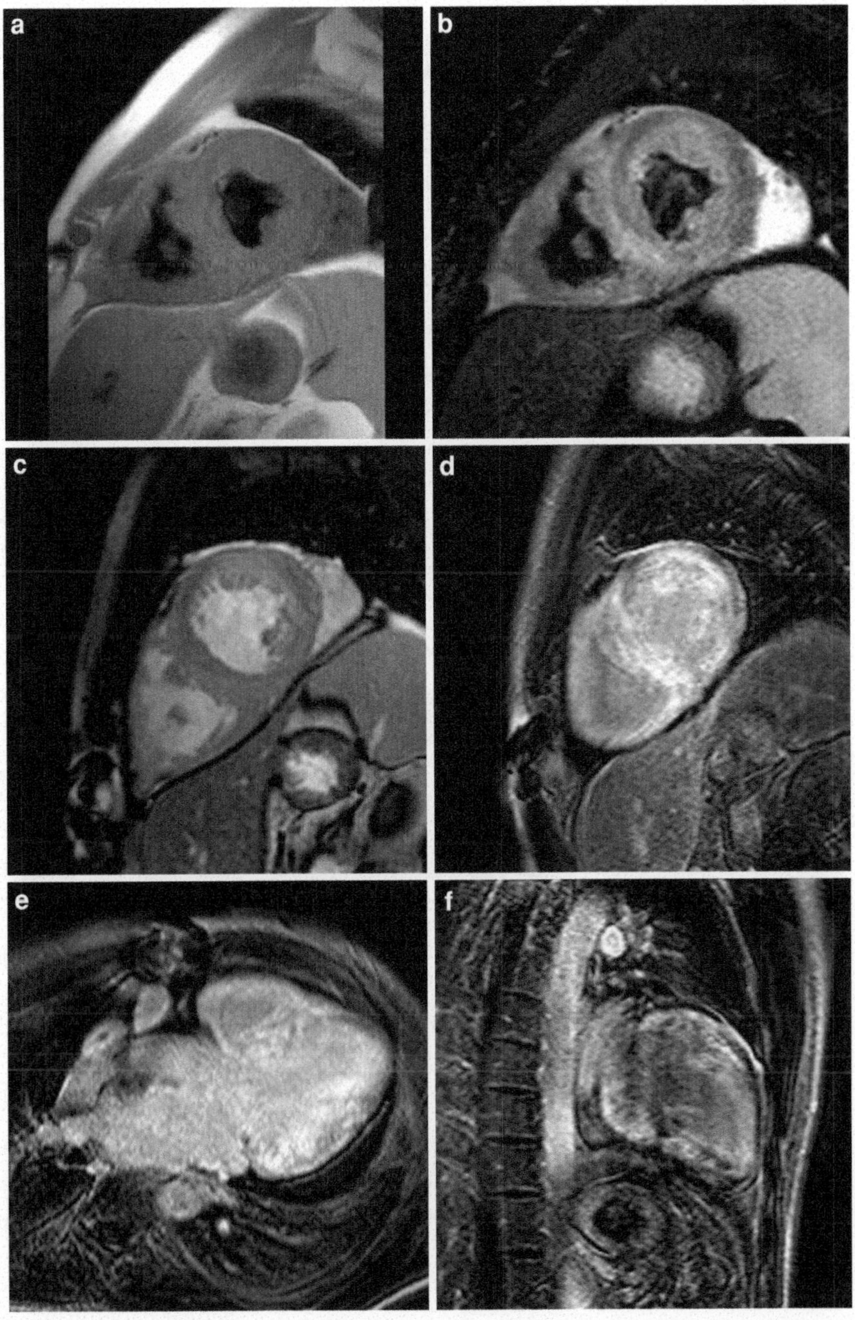

specificity of 100 and 85%, respectively (Muehling et al. 2003).

As already stated before, there is much speculation on the nature of late Gd MRI lesions in cardiac transplant patients. Currently, little is really known on the histological background of so-called 'typical' and 'atypical' enhancing myocardium post-transplantation (Steen et al. 2008), and further research with larger patient, potentially employing targeted biopsies in combination with immunohistological techniques is warranted to elucidate if these effects are due to transplant coronary artery disease or to the rejection process itself (Fig. 9).

The value of alternative approaches such as ^{31}P MR spectroscopy have been investigated by studying variations in cardiac high-energy phosphates in transplant

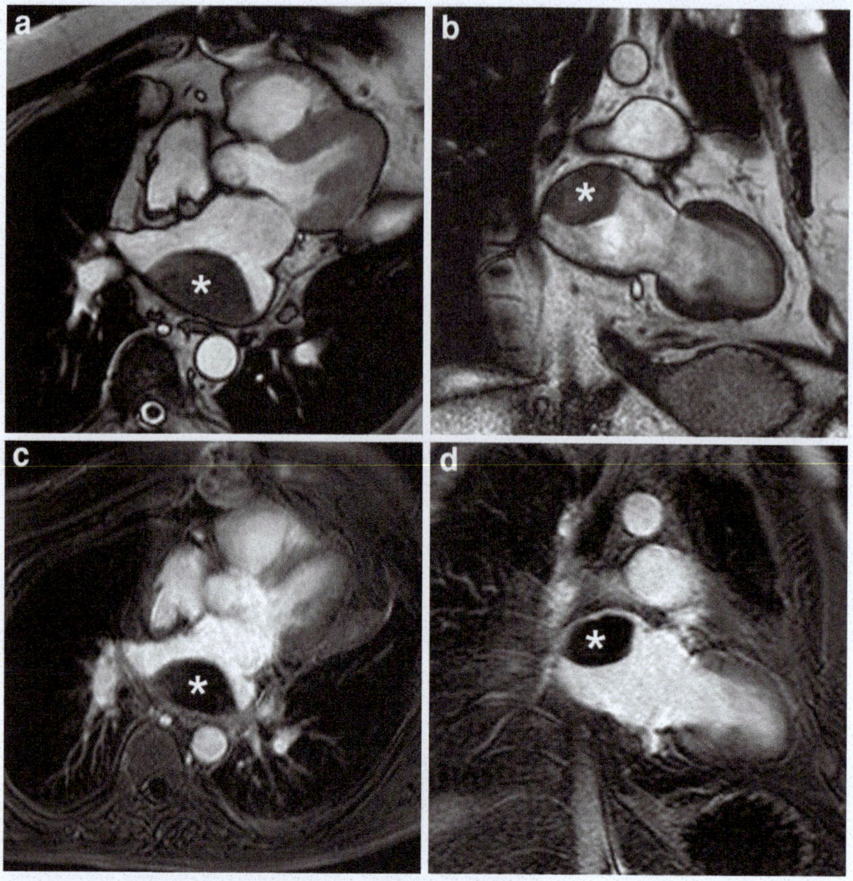

Fig. 10 Atrial thrombus formation. A large soft-tissue mass (asterisk) is located on the posterior wall of the left atrium in a 63-year-old male transplant patient. Top row: HLA (**a**) and VLA (**b**) cine MR images. The mass does not contain any internal flow on cine MR and does not enhance on late-Gd MRI (**c**, **d**). Findings consistent with thrombus formation. Note the enlarged size of the left atrium

patients (Caus et al. 2006). It was found that patients with transplant vasculopathy present with significantly lower phosphocreatine over adenosine triphosphate levels that compared to asymptomatic transplant patients and volunteers. Although promising as a non-invasive method to detect the potential early onset of transplant vasculopathy, lack of randomized multicenter trials and limited clinical distribution for the moment do not allow generalized conclusions for coronary angiograms. This may be relevant for coronary angiography follow-up and adjustments of immunotherapy regimen.

5.3 Detection of Complications

After transplantation both sections of the recipient and donor atria are intact but do not contract synergistically. The decreased atrial input results in a lower net stroke volume than that in a native heart. In the immediate post-operative period, a "stiff" heart develops causing a restrictive hemodynamic pattern that results in low-cardiac output. Low-cardiac output may be caused by one or more of the following: vasopressors used in the donor, ischemic injury at the time of donor procurement, denervation, high peripheral vascular resistance, edema and allograft rejection (Cotts and Oren 1997). Next to complications associated with restrictive heart disease and the difficult differential diagnosis with constrictive pericarditis, other complications such as pleural or pericardial effusion, hemorrhage and endocavitary processes, e.g., thrombus formation can be very well assessed with MRI.

Pericardial effusions may present as high intensity crescent-shaped structures within the myocardium and can contain linear densities, representing hemorrhagic content of fibrotic strands. Thrombus formation occurs most currently in the morphologically abnormal atria and is usually broad based on the atrial wall. Thrombi present on cine MRI as a heterogeneously intense soft-tissue mass, easily detectable if large, but smaller thrombi may be masqueraded on b-SSFP cine images, due to the intrinsic contrast mechanism of these sequences. Seen that the T2 and T1 values of the blood itself contribute more to the hyperintense signal than the intracardiac flow, a thrombus—or blood clot—can be nearly invisible in an abnormally shaped atrium with sluggish blood flow near the borders. Therefore it is recommended to acquire either T1- or T2-weighted TSE images, or to inject intravenous contrast and to acquire contrast-enhanced images series to improve visualization (Mollet et al. 2002). Thrombi will present as intermediate-to-high signal intensity on TSE images and as non-enhancing structures on CE-MRI images (Fig. 10).

References

Abdel-Aty H, Boye P, Zagrosek A et al (2005) Diagnostic performance of cardiovascular magnetic resonance in patients with suspected acute myocarditis: comparison of different approaches. J Am Coll Cardiol 45:1815–1822

Adelstein EC, Saba S (2007) Scar burden by myocardial perfusion imaging predicts echocardiographic response to cardiac resynchronization therapy in ischemic cardiomyopathy. Am Heart J 153:105–112

Almenar L, Iguala B, Martínez-Dolza L et al (2003) Utility of cardiac magnetic resonance imaging for the diagnosis of heart transplant rejection. Transpl Proc 35:1962–1964

Anderson LJ, Holden S, Davis B et al (2001) Cardiovascular T2-star (T2*) magnetic resonance for the early diagnosis of myocardial iron overload. Eur Heart J 22:2171–2179

Barkhausen J, Ruehm SG, Goyen M et al (2001) MR evaluation of ventricular function: true fast imaging with steady-state precession versus fast low-angle shot cine MR imaging: feasibility study. Radiology 219:264–269

Beer M, Stamm H, Machann W et al (2010) Free breathing cardiac real-time cine MR without ECG triggering. Int J Cardiol 145(2):380–382

Bengel FM, Ueberfuhr P, Schiepel N et al (2001) Effect of sympathetic reinnervation on cardiac performance after heart transplantation. N Engl J Med 345:731–738

Billingham ME (1982) Diagnosis of cardiac rejection by endomyocardial biopsy. Heart Transpl 1:25–30

Birnie DH, Tang AS (2006) The problem of nonresponse to cardiac resynchronization therapy. Curr Opin Cardiol 21:20–26

Bleeker GB, Kaandorp TA, Lamb HJ et al (2006) Effect of posterolateral scar tissue on clinical and echocardiographic improvement after cardiac resynchronization therapy. Circulation 113:969–976

Bogaert J, Bosmans H, Rademakers FE et al (1995) Left ventricular quantification with breath-hold MR imaging: comparison with echocardiography. MAGMA 3:5–12

Caus T, Kober F, Marin P et al (2006) Non-invasive diagnostic of cardiac allograft vasculopathy by 31P magnetic resonance chemical shift imaging. Eur J Cardiothorac Surg 29(1):45–49

Caves PK, Stinson EB, Graham AF et al (1973) Percutaneous transvenous endomyocardial biopsy. JAMA 225:288–291

Chung ES, Leon AR, Tavazzi L et al (2008) Results of the predictors of response to CRT (PROSPECT) trial. Circulation 117:2608–2616

Cleland JG, Daubert JC, Erdmann E et al (2005) The effect of cardiac resynchronization on morbidity and mortality in heart failure. N Engl J Med 352:1539–1549

Cotts WG, Oren RM (1997) Function of the transplanted heart: unique physiology and therapeutic implications. Am J Med Sci 314:164–172

Delgado V, Bax JJ (2011) Assessment of Systolic Dyssynchrony for Cardiac Resynchronization Therapy Is Clinically Useful. Circulation 123(6):640–655

Doornbos J, Verwey H, Essed CE, Balk AH, de Roos A (1990) MR imaging in assessment of cardiac transplant rejection in humans. J Comput Assist Tomogr 14(1):77–81

Gabriel RS, Bakshi TK, Scott AG et al (2007) Reliability of echocardiographic indices of dyssynchrony. Echocardiography 24:40–46

Gassis SA, Delurgio DB, Leon AR (2006) Progress in cardiovascular disease: Technical considerations in cardiac resynchronization therapy. Prog Cardiovasc Dis 48:239–255

He T, Gatehouse PD, Kirk P et al (2007) Black-blood T2* technique for myocardial iron measurement in thalassemia. J Magn Reson Imaging 25:1205–1209

Hudsmith LE, Petersen SE, Tyler DJ et al (2006) Determination of cardiac volumes and mass with FLASH and SSFP cine sequences at 1.5 vs. 3 Tesla: a validation study. J Magn Reson Imaging 24(2):312–318

Johansson L, Johnsson C, Penno E, Björnerud A, Ahlström H (2002) Acute cardiac transplant rejection: detection and grading with MR imaging with a blood pool contrast agent—experimental study in the rat. Radiology 225(1):97–103

Kirk P, Roughton M, Porter JB et al (2009) Cardiac T2* magnetic resonance for prediction of cardiac complications in thalassemia major. Circulation 120:1961–1968

Kurland RJ, West J, Kelley S et al (1989) Magnetic resonance imaging to detect heart transplant rejection: sensitivity and specificity. Transpl Proc 21:2537–2543

Lardo AC, Abraham TP, Kass DA (2005) Magnetic resonance imaging assessment of ventricular dyssynchrony: current and emerging concepts. J Am Coll Cardiol 46:2223–2228

Maceira AM, Joshi J, Prasad SK et al (2005) Cardiovascular magnetic resonance in cardiac amyloidosis. Circulation 111:186–193

Mahrholdt H, Wagner A, Judd RM et al (2005) Delayed enhancement cardiovascular magnetic resonance assessment of non-ischaemic cardiomyopathies. Eur Heart J 26:1461–1474

Marie PY, Angioi M, Carteaux JP et al (2001) Detection and prediction of acute heart transplant rejection with the myocardial T2 determination provided by a black-blood magnetic resonance imaging sequence. J Am Coll Cardiol 37:825–831

Marsan NA, Westenberg JJ, Ypenburg C et al (2009) Magnetic resonance imaging and response to cardiac resynchronization therapy: relative merits of left ventricular dyssynchrony and scar tissue. Eur Heart J 30:2360–2367

Marwick TH (2010) Echocardiography in the era of multimodality imaging. Heart Lung Circ 19(3):175–184

McMurray JJ, Pfeffer MA (2005) Heart failure. Lancet 365(9474):1877–1889

Mischi M, Van Den Bosch HM, Jansen AM et al (2008) Quantification of regional left ventricular dyssynchrony by magnetic resonance imaging. IEEE Trans Biomed Eng 55:985–995

Mollet NR, Dymarkowski S, Volders W et al (2002) Visualization of ventricular thrombi with contrast-enhanced magnetic resonance imaging in patients with ischemic heart disease. Circulation 106:2873–2876

Moon JC, Sachdev B, Elkington AG et al (2003a) Gadolinium enhanced cardiovascular magnetic resonance in Anderson-Fabry disease. Evidence for a disease specific abnormality of the myocardial interstitium. Eur Heart J 24:2151–2155

Moon JC, McKenna WJ, McCrohon JA et al (2003b) Toward clinical risk assessment in hypertrophic cardiomyopathy with gadolinium cardiovascular magnetic resonance. J Am Coll Cardiol 41:1561–1567

Mousseaux E, Farge D, Guillemain R et al (1993) Assessing human cardiac allograft rejection using MRI with Gd-DOTA. J Comput Assist Tomogr 17:237–244

Muehling OM, Wilke NM, Panse P et al (2003) Reduced myocardial perfusion reserve and transmural perfusion gradient in heart transplant arteriopathy assessed by magnetic resonance imaging. J Am Coll Cardiol 42:1054–1060

Nishimura T, Sada M, Sasaki H et al (1987) Cardiac transplantation in dogs: evaluation with gated MRI and Gd-DTPA contrast enhancement. Heart Vessels 3:141–145

Nishimura T, Sada M, Sasaki H et al (1988) Assessment of severity of cardiac rejection in heterotopic heart transplantation using indium-111 antimyosin and magnetic resonance imaging. Cardiovasc Res 22:108–112

Ordas S, Frangi A (2005) Automatic quantitative analysis of myocardial wall motion and thickening from long-and short-axis cine MRI studies. Conf Proc IEEE Eng Med Biol Soc 7:7028–7031

Osman NF, Sampath S, Atalar E (2001) Imaging longitudinal cardiac strain on short-axis images using strain-encoded MRI. Magn Reson Med 46:324–334

Paulus WJ, Tschope C, Sanderson JE et al (2007) How to diagnose diastolic heart failure: a consensus statement on the diagnosis of heart failure with normal left ventricular ejection fraction by the Heart Failure and Echocardiography Associations of the European Society of Cardiology. Eur Heart J 28:2539–2550

Rathi VK, Doyle M, Yamrozik J et al (2008) Routine evaluation of left ventricular diastolic function by cardiovascular magnetic resonance: a practical approach. J Cardiovasc Magn Reson 10:36

Remme WJ, Swedberg K (2001) Guidelines for the diagnosis and treatment of chronic heart failure. Eur Heart J 22:1527–1560

Rosamond W, Flegal K, Furie K et al (2008) Heart disease and stroke statistics–2008 update: a report from the American Heart Association Statistics Committee and Stroke Statistics Subcommittee. Circulation 117(4):e25–e146

Sanders GD, Kong MH, Al-Khatib SM et al (2010) Cost-effectiveness of implantable cardioverter defibrillators in patients over 65 years of age. Am Heart J 160:122–131

Sasaki H, Sada M, Nishimura T et al (1987) The expanded scope of effectiveness of nuclear magnetic resonance imaging to determine cardiac allograft rejection. Transpl Proc 19:1062–1064

Scott GE, Nath RL, Friedlich JA et al (1983) Usefulness of myocardial edema to assess heterotopic allograft rejection in dogs. Heart Transpl 2:232–237

Singh JP, Houser S, Heist EK et al (2005) The coronary venous anatomy: A segmental approach to aid cardiac resynchronization therapy. J Am Coll Cardiol 46:68–74

Smart FW, Young JB, Weilbaecher D et al (1993) Magnetic resonance imaging for assessment of tissue rejection after heterotopic heart transplantation. J Heart Lung Transpl 12:403–410

Sohn DW (2011) Heart failure due to abnormal filling of the heart. J Cardiol 57(2):148–159

Steen H, Merten C, Refle S et al (2008) HA. Prevalence of different gadolinium enhancement patterns in patients after heart transplantation. J Am. Coll Cardiol 52(14):1160–1167

Stewart S, Jenkins A, Buchan S et al (2002) The current cost of heart failure to the National Health Service in the UK. Eur J Heart Fail 4(3):361–371

Sung RK, Foster E (2011) Assessment of systolic dyssynchrony for cardiac resynchronization therapy is not clinically useful. Circulation 123(6):656–662

Taylor AJ, Cerqueira M, Hodgson JM et al (2010) ACCF/SCCT/ACR/AHA/ASE/ASNC/NASCI/SCAI/SCMR 2010 appropriate use criteria for cardiac computed tomography: a report of the American College of Cardiology Foundation Appropriate Use Criteria Task Force, the Society of Cardiovascular Computed Tomography, the American College of Radiology, the American Heart Association, the American Society of Echocardiography, the American Society of Nuclear Cardiology, the North American Society for Cardiovascular Imaging, the Society for Cardiovascular Angiography and Interventions, and the Society for Cardiovascular Magnetic Resonance. J Am Coll Cardiol 56(22):1864–1894

Vardas PE, Auricchio A, Blanc JJ et al (2007) Guidelines for cardiac pacing and cardiac resynchronization therapy: the task force for cardiac pacing and cardiac resynchronization therapy of the European society of cardiology. developed in collaboration with the European heart rhythm association. Eur Heart J 28:2256–2295

Walpoth BH, Lazeyras F, Tschopp A et al (1995) Assessment of cardiac rejection and immunosuppression by magnetic resonance imaging and spectroscopy. Transpl Proc 27:2088–2091

White JA, Yee R, Yuan X et al (2006) Delayed enhancement magnetic resonance imaging predicts response to cardiac resynchronization therapy in patients with intraventricular dyssynchrony. J Am Coll Cardiol 48:1953–1960

Wilhelmi M, Pethig K, Wilhelmi M et al (2002) Heart transplantation: echocardiographic assessment of morphology and function after more than 10 years of follow-up. Ann Thorac Surg 74:1075–1079

Wilson RF, Christensen BV, Olivari MT, Simon A, White CW, Laxson DD (1991) Evidence for structural sympathetic reinnervation after orthotopic cardiac transplantation in humans. Circulation 83(4):1210–1220

Younger JF, Plein S, Crean A et al (2009) Visualization of coronary venous anatomy by cardiovascular magnetic resonance. J Cardiovasc Magn Reson 11:26

Ypenburg C, Roes SD, Bleeker GB et al (2007) Effect of total scar burden on contrast-enhanced magnetic resonance imaging on response to cardiac resynchronization therapy. Am J Cardiol 99:657–660

Pericardial Disease

J. Bogaert and A. M. Taylor

Contents

1	**Introduction**	383
2	**Pericardial Anatomy and Physiology**	384
3	**MRI Techniques**	384
4	**Normal Pericardium**	386
5	**Congenital Pericardial Anomalies**	386
5.1	Pericardial Cyst	386
5.2	Pericardial Defect	387
5.3	Pericardial Diverticulum	390
6	**Acquired Pericardial Diseases**	390
6.1	Effuse Pericardial Disease	390
6.2	Pericardial Inflammation	393
6.3	Constrictive Pericarditis	393
6.4	Pericardial Masses	406
7	**Conclusions**	407
8	**Key Points**	407
References		407

J. Bogaert (✉)
Department of Radiology and Medical Imaging Research Center (MIRC), University Hospitals Gasthuisberg, Catholic University of Leuven, Herestraat 49, 3000 Leuven, Belgium
e-mail: jan.bogaert@uz.kuleuven.ac.be

A. M. Taylor
Cardiothoracic Unit, Institute of Child Health and Great Ormond Street Hospital for Children, London, UK

Abstract

The diagnosis of pericardial disease often remains challenging, even with modern cardiac imaging modalities. MRI has a lot to offer in the assessment of pericardial diseases, in the first place because it merges morphologic with functional imaging. A combined MRI approach including cine imaging, T1- and T2-weighted imaging and contrast-enhanced imaging allows tissue characterization of the pericardial abnormalities and assessment of the remainder of the heart, while phase-contrast MRI and real-time cine imaging can be used to assess the functional impact on cardiac filling. In this chapter the variety of congenital and acquired pericardial diseases is highlighted with particular emphasis on the value of MRI in the diagnosis and differential diagnosis.

1 Introduction

The pericardium, and pericardial diseases in particular, has received, in contrast to other parts of the heart, relatively limited interest. Today, despite improved knowledge of pathophysiology of pericardial diseases and the availability of a wide spectrum of diagnostic tools, the diagnostic challenge remains. The clinical presentation may be atypical, mimicking other cardiac, pulmonary or pleural diseases; in developed countries a shift in the epidemiology of constrictive pericarditis has been noted. Accurate decision-making is crucial considering the significant morbidity and mortality caused by complicated pericardial diseases, and the potential benefit of therapeutic interventions.

J. Bogaert et al. (eds.), *Clinical Cardiac MRI*, Medical Radiology. Diagnostic Imaging,
DOI: 10.1007/174_2011_337, © Springer-Verlag Berlin Heidelberg 2012

Imaging herein has an important role, and magnetic resonance imaging (MRI) is definitely one of the most versatile modalities to study the pericardium. It fuses excellent anatomic detail and tissue characterization with accurate evaluation of cardiac function and assessment of the hemodynamic consequences of pericardial constraint on cardiac filling. This chapter focuses on the current state of knowledge on how MRI can be used to study the most common pericardial diseases.

2 Pericardial Anatomy and Physiology

Although the normal pericardium is a thin, avascular, relatively inelastic, flask-shaped sac enveloping the heart, this structure is an important determinant of cardiac filling (Little and Freeman 2006; Troughton et al. 2004; Spodick et al. 1992). In most cases, evaluation of pericardial diseases extends beyond morphologic assessment, and the diagnostic challenge is to determine the impact of abnormal pericardium on cardiac filling. Anatomically, the pericardium is composed of two layers, an inner serous membrane and an outer fibrocollagenous layer (Spodick et al. 1992). The inner serosal layer, termed the visceral pericardium, is closely attached to the epicardial surface of the heart and covers a sub-epicardial layer of conjunctive tissue containing fat and coronary vessels. The serosal layer reflects back on itself to become the inner lining of the outer fibrous layer. Together, these layers form the parietal pericardium. The pericardium contains two major pericardial sinuses which are composed of different recesses (Groell et al. 1999). The transverse sinus is the connection between the two tubes of pericardium that envelops the great vessels. The aorta and pulmonary artery are enclosed in one anterosuperior tube, and the vena cava and pulmonary veins are enclosed in a more posterior tube. The oblique sinus lies behind the left atrium so that the posterior wall of the left atrium is actually separated from the pericardial space. This explains why a posterior pericardial effusion is seen behind the left atrium only when it is very large. The pericardial virtual cavity normally contains between 10 and 50 ml of an ultrafiltrate of plasma (Roberts and Spray 1976). The fluid is produced by the visceral pericardium and drainage of the cavity is toward both the thoracic duct and the right lymphatic duct.

The pericardium holds the heart within the anterior mediastinum, protecting it from adjacent organs. Its relative inelasticity provides constraint during diastolic filling, which limits chamber dilation, particularly of the thin-walled right atrium and ventricle (Troughton et al. 2004). While acute pericardial dilation is limited because of its exponential pressure–volume relation, chronic pericardial stress, e.g. slowly accumulating pericardial effusion or left ventricular remodeling, in contrast, may occur without pericardial constriction (Little and Freeman 2006; Freeman and LeWinter 1986; Freeman and Little 1986). As the pericardium slowly dilates, the pericardial pressure–volume relation shifts to the right, explaining why chronic pericardial effusion may become quite large without compressing the cardiac chambers (Taylor et al. 1967). The pericardium, moreover, equalizes compliance between right and thicker walled left ventricle, and produces interdependence of filling between ventricles, a phenomenon also called "ventricular coupling" (see constrictive pericarditis). Though, normally not physiologically important, ventricular coupling is exaggerated and a key diagnostic feature when intrapericardial pressure is increased (as in cardiac tamponade) or when the pericardial cavity is fixed (as in constrictive pericarditis) (Troughton et al. 2004; Freeman and LeWinter 1986; Freeman and Little 1986; Taylor et al. 1967; Janicki and Weber 1980; Freeman and LeWinter 1984). Finally, the pericardium also acts as a physiological intermediate between the pleural space and heart chambers, and the respiratory changes in intrathoracic pressure are directly transmitted to the sub-atmospheric pericardial cavity and subsequently to the cardiac chambers. Because of its thinner wall, this interaction is more pronounced on the right than on the left ventricle.

3 MRI Techniques

Today, comprehensive pericardial imaging should provide information on morphologic characteristics of the pericardium and cardiac structures, and assess the impact of pericardial diseases on cardiac function, in particular cardiac filling. Though MRI is traditionally considered, together with computed tomography (CT),

Table 1 MRI strategies to evaluate the pericardium

Pericardial morphology (*T1w imaging – cine imaging)*)
- pericardial width/localization/extent
- pericardial delineation
Pericardial layer/fluid characterization (*T1w- and T2w imaging /cine imaging/contrast-enhanced MRI using T1w imaging or late Gd imaging*)
Pericardial function
- motion pattern (*cine imaging*)
- fusion of pericardial layers (*MRI tagging*)
Cardiac morphology (*T1w-imaging, cine imaging*)
- size and shape of ventricles and atria
- myocardial morphology (restrictive cardiomyopathy)
Cardiac systolic function (*cine imaging*)
- regional and global systolic ventricular function
Cardiac filling (*PC-MRI*)
Ventricular coupling (*real-time cine imaging*)
- ventricular septal shape and septal motion patterns
- respiratory-related septal shift
Other findings (*T1w-imaging, cine imaging, late Gd imaging*)
- myocardial enhancement (associated myocarditis? myocardial infiltrative or storage disease?)
- caval vein size
- pleural fluid/ascites

as the preferred imaging modality to morphologically visualize the pericardium and pericardial space, MRI can substantially aid in clarifying the intricate relation between pericardial constraint and cardiac filling (Table 1). Black-blood T1-weighted spin-echo MRI ('T1w-imaging'), using fast, segmented sequences, is still the best approach to visualize, the heart, pericardium and mediastinum (Bogaert and Francone 2009; Misselt et al. 2008). Use of a small field of view and a saturation block positioned on the frontal chest wall may hereby improve pericardial visualization. Scanning in two perpendicular oriented planes through the heart guarantees optimal depiction of the entire pericardium, for instance, using a set of axial views combined with coronal or cardiac short-axis views. T2-weighted spin-echo MRI ('T2w imaging'), preferably using a short inversion-time inversion-recovery (STIR) sequence (also called "triple-inversion" spin-echo), is highly useful to depict myocardial edema (Aletras et al. 2006; Friedrich et al. 2008), and can also be applied to detect pericardial fluid and/or edema of the pericardial layers in patients with inflammatory pericarditis. Use of paramagnetic contrast agents can be recommended in case of pericardial masses, and inflammatory pericarditis to depict concomitant myocardial pathology (e.g. myocarditis) and may be useful to better differentiate between inflammatory and constrictive forms of pericarditis. Either T1-weighted spin-echo MRI or inversion-recovery gradient-echo MRI with delayed enhancement ('late Gd imaging') is used for post-contrast imaging (Klein et al. 2003; Bogaert et al. 2004; Taylor et al. 2006).

Cine imaging, using balanced steady-state free precession (SSFP) gradient-echo MRI sequences, is the reference technique used today to quantify global and regional cardiac systolic function. It is also used to rule out underlying RV or LV dysfunction, and moreover to measure atrial volumes/function in patients clinically suspected of constrictive pericarditis. Moreover, the high-spatial and temporal resolution of cine MRI can be applied to exploit new applications such as the assessment of pericardial mobility, which can help in depicting a rigid pericardium in patients with a non or minimally thickened constrictive pericarditis. The availability of new real-time cine imaging sequences enabled to study dynamic, fast-changing, physiologic events such as ventricular coupling (Francone et al. 2005). MRI tagging techniques may be used to detect fibrotic adhesion of pericardial layers or to diagnose myocardial involvement in constrictive pericarditis (Kojima et al. 1999). Assessment of diastolic heart function, though usually obtained with Doppler-echocardiography, can also be achieved with phase-contrast (PC) MRI technique (Bogaert and Francone 2009; Rademakers and Bogaert 2006; Paelinck et al. 2002). Analysis of pulmonary and/or systemic venous pattern in combination with cardiac inflow patterns through the atrioventricular valves can yield findings that are classic for restrictive cardiac filling. Similar to real-time cine imaging, real-time PC-MRI also provides information about the impact of respiration on venous flow and atrioventricular flow patterns enabling improved differentiation between constrictive pericarditis and restrictive cardiomyopathy.

To conclude, improvements in MRI technology have shifted the way this technique can be applied to study the pericardium from basically a static

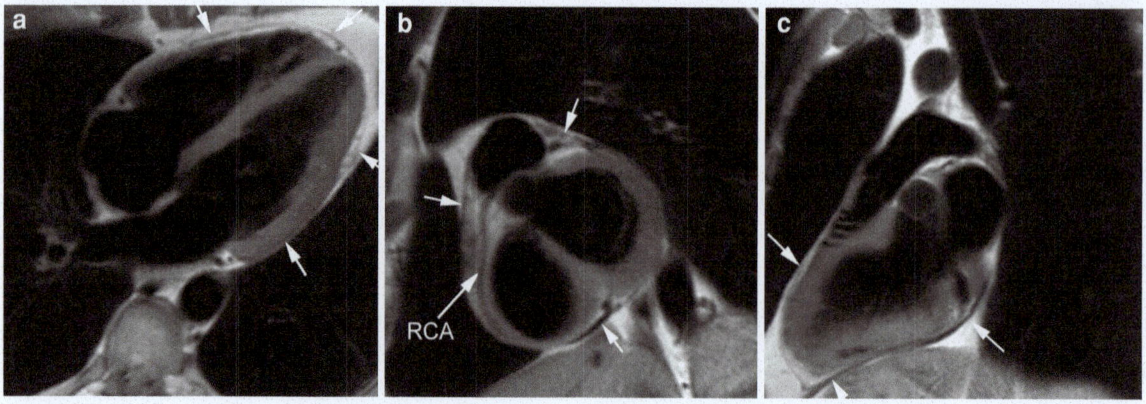

Fig. 1 Normal pericardium on T1w imaging in horizontal long-axis direction (**a**), short-axis (**b**), and vertical long-axis (**c**). The normal pericardium is visible as a thin curvilinear structure (*arrows*) with low-signal intensity surrounded by the bright epicardial and mediastinal fat (**a–c**). Pericardial visualization is often hampered along the free wall of the left ventricle (**a**, **b**)

morphologic assessment toward an integrated dynamic morphological functional approach, raising the hope to improve diagnostic testing of the often complex and intriguing group of pericardial disorders (Table 1).

4 Normal Pericardium

Normal pericardium is visible on T1w imaging as a thin, smooth, low-intensity curvilinear structure surrounded by high-intensity mediastinal and epicardial fat, or medium-intensity myocardium (Fig. 1) (Sechtem et al. 1986a; Stark et al. 1984). The low signal of adjacent lung parenchyma and paucity of surrounding fat, may hamper the pericardial visualization over the free wall of the left ventricle (Sechtem et al. 1986a). The transverse pericardial sinus, preaortic and retroaortic recesses can be identified in the majority of patients (Fig. 2) (Stark et al. 1984; Im et al. 1988). Especially the superior pericardial recessus should not be mistaken for a focal aortic dissection or enlarged lymph nodes (McMurdo et al. 1985; Solomon et al. 1990; Groell et al. 1999). The oblique sinus, which is actually separated from the remainder of the pericardial space, is well depicted only when it contains some pericardial fluid (Fig. 3). On cine imaging, the pericardial layers have low-signal intensity while pericardial fluid has a high-signal intensity (Fig. 4). Figure 5 shows the presentation of the normal pericardium on coronary MR angiography. Values of normal pericardial thickness on MRI, i.e., 1.2 mm in diastole to 1.7 mm in systole, exceed those found in anatomical studies of the heart, i.e., 0.4–1 mm (Sechtem et al. 1986b; Bogaert and Duerinckx 1995; Chako et al. 1995). The overestimation of pericardial thickness on MRI can be explained by motion of pericardial layers during image acquisition, lack of sufficient spatial resolution and chemical shift artifacts at the fat–fluid interface on cine imaging.

5 Congenital Pericardial Anomalies

5.1 Pericardial Cyst

Pericardial cysts are congenital encapsulated cysts implanted on the pericardium which are not connected with the pericardial cavity. They typically occur in the cardiophrenic sulcus (90%), most often right-sided (70%). On chest radiography, they present as a well-defined outpouching on the lateral heart border. On MRI, they appear as a well-defined homogeneous paracardiac structure, having the signal characteristics of water, implanted on the pericardium (Fig. 6) (Sechtem et al. 1986b). Pericardial cysts are usually asymptomatic, though rarely they may become symptomatic when compressing other cardiac structures (Fig. 7). Pericardial cysts should be differentiated from encapsulated pericardial effusions, and other cystic structures such as bronchogenic cysts and thymic cysts.

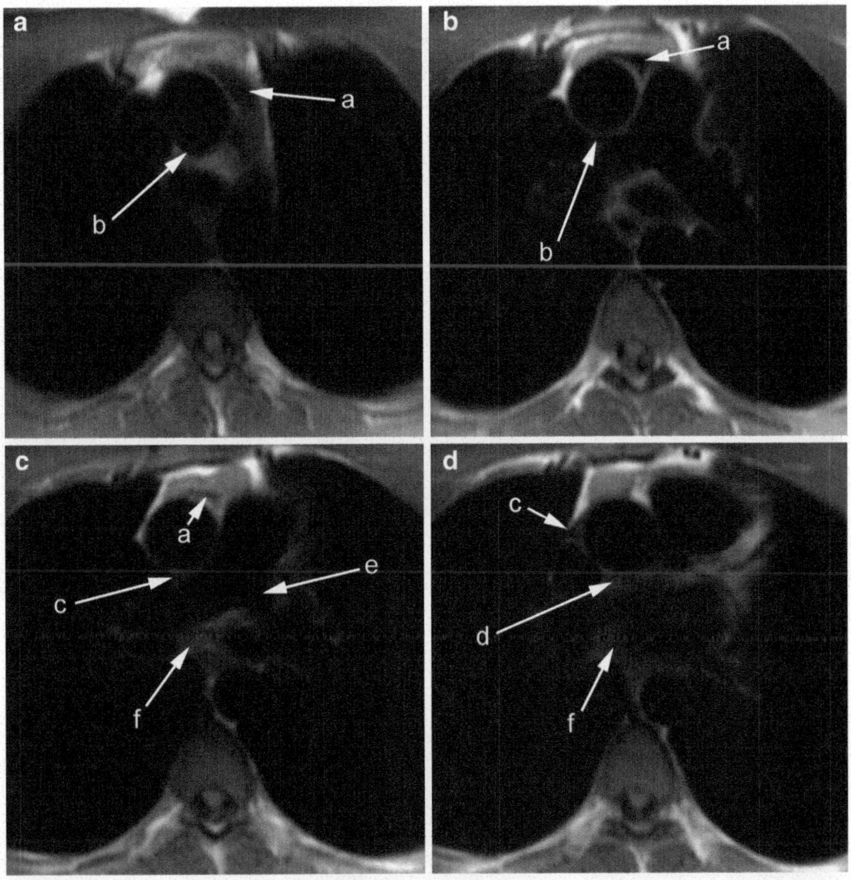

Fig. 2 Pericardial recesses. Axial T1w imaging at the level of the origin of the great vessels (**a–d**). Transverse sinus: superior aortic recess, anterior portion (**a**), posterior portion (**b**), right lateral portion (**c**); transverse sinus: inferior aortic recess (**d**) and the left pulmonic recess (**e**). The oblique sinus (**f**) lies behind the left atrium

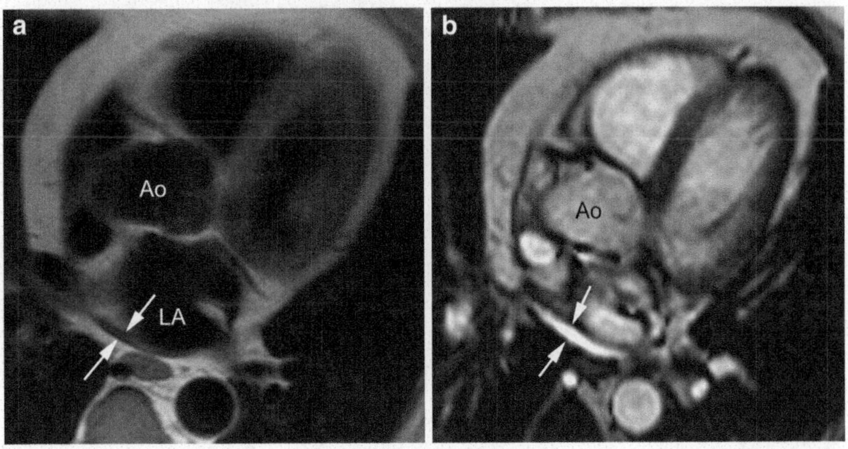

Fig. 3 Oblique pericardial sinus. T1w imaging (**a**) and cine imaging (**b**) in horizontal long-axis plane. The oblique sinus, containing a small amount of pericardial fluid, is visible as a curvilinear structure (*arrows*) behind the left atrium (*LA*). Abbrevations: Ao, aorta

5.2 Pericardial Defect

Congenital pericardial agenesis is an uncommon entity, and is considered to result from an abnormal embryonic development that may be secondary to abnormalities in the vascular supply of the pericardium. Pericardial defects occur in a spectrum ranging from a small defect to total absence of the pericardium. Partial defects (large more common than small partial defects) are far more common than total defects (Sechtem et al. 1986b; Amplatz and Moller 1993). It may be associated, in at least one-third of cases, with other malformations,

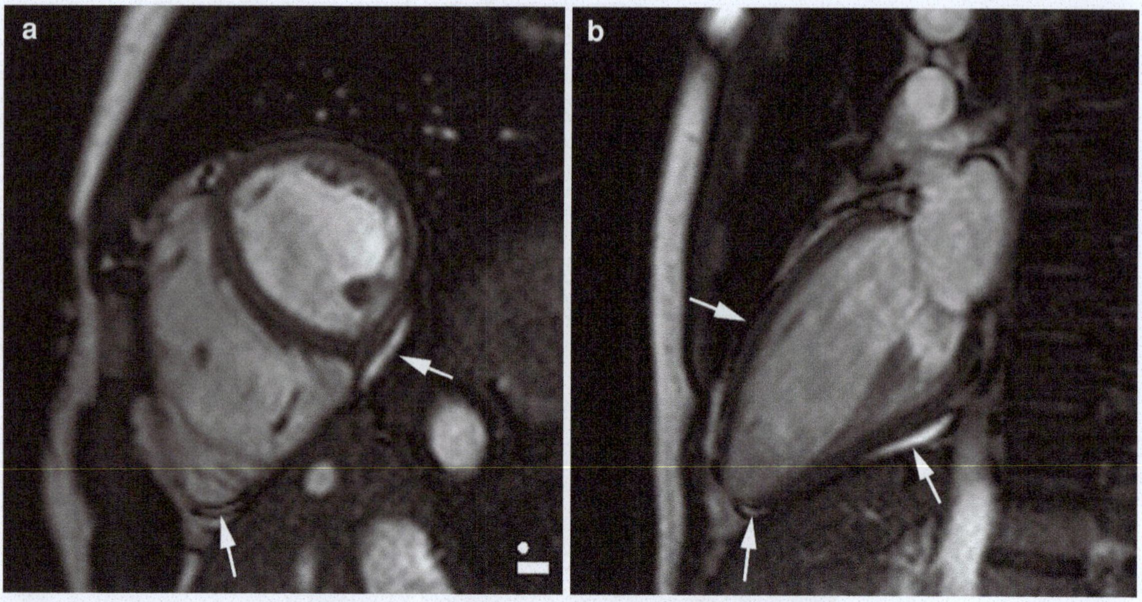

Fig. 4 Appearance of normal pericardium on cine imaging in cardiac short-axis (**a**) and vertical long-axis plane (**b**). The pericardial sac is visible as low-signal intensity line while pericardial fluid demonstrates a high-signal (*arrows*)

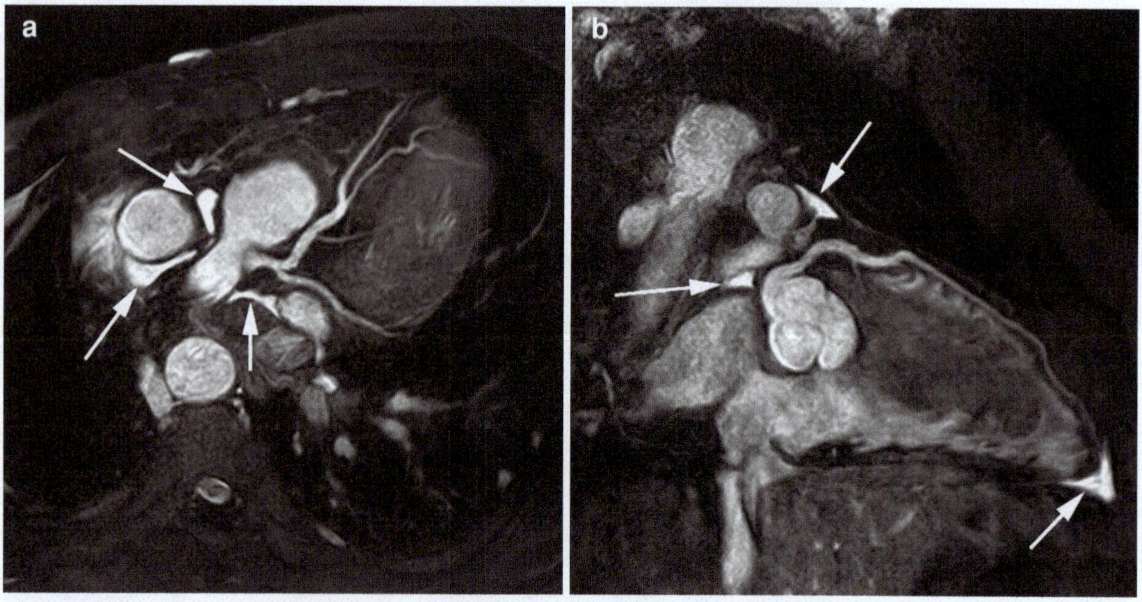

Fig. 5 Appearance of the pericardium and pericardial recesses on coronary MR angiography. Tangential view through left coronary artery tree (**a**) and perpendicular view through left main stem and left anterior descending coronary artery (**b**). Parts of the pericardium and pericardial recesses are visible as well-defined high-signal areas (*arrows*). The signal intensity of pericardial fluid is higher than the blood in the coronary arteries

particularly malformations of the heart (tetralogy of Fallot, atrial septal defect, patent ductus arteriosus) or other types of abnormalities (bronchogenic cyst or hiatus hernia) (Letanche et al. 1988; Lorell and Braunwald 1988). Cardiac structures or portions of the lung can herniate through the defect. The clinical presentation is variable. Patients are often asymptomatic, and the disease may be detected on routine chest

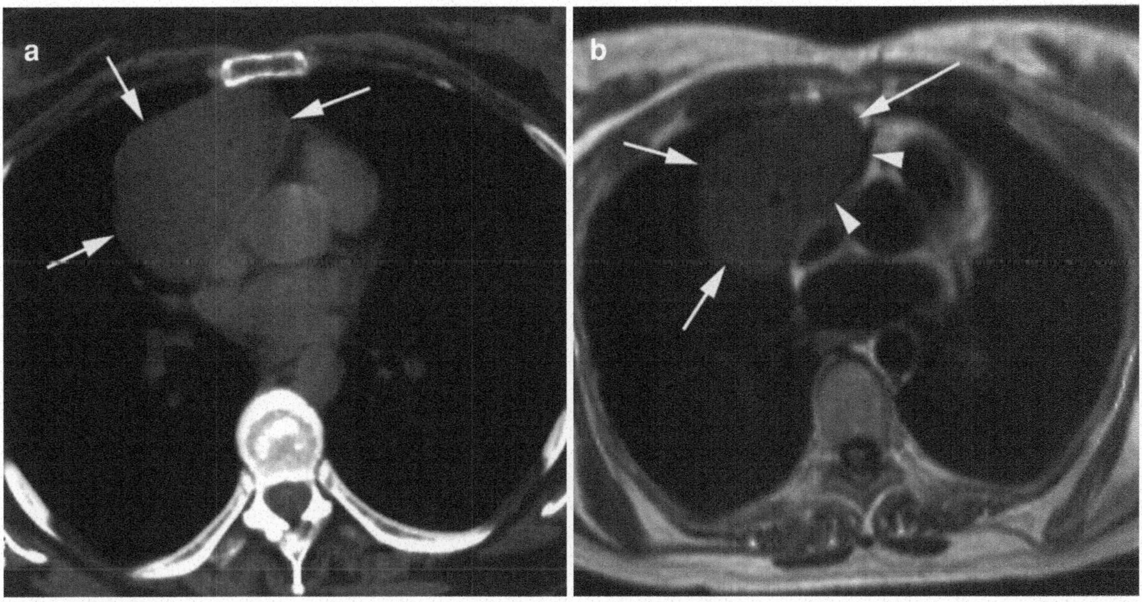

Fig. 6 Pericardial cyst. Axial non-enhanced CT (**a**) and T1w imaging (**b**). The pericardial cyst is visible as a well-delineated, homogeneous low-density (0 HU) and low-signal intensity soft-tissue structure visible along the right paracardiac border (*arrows*), implanted on a normal pericardium (*arrowheads*)

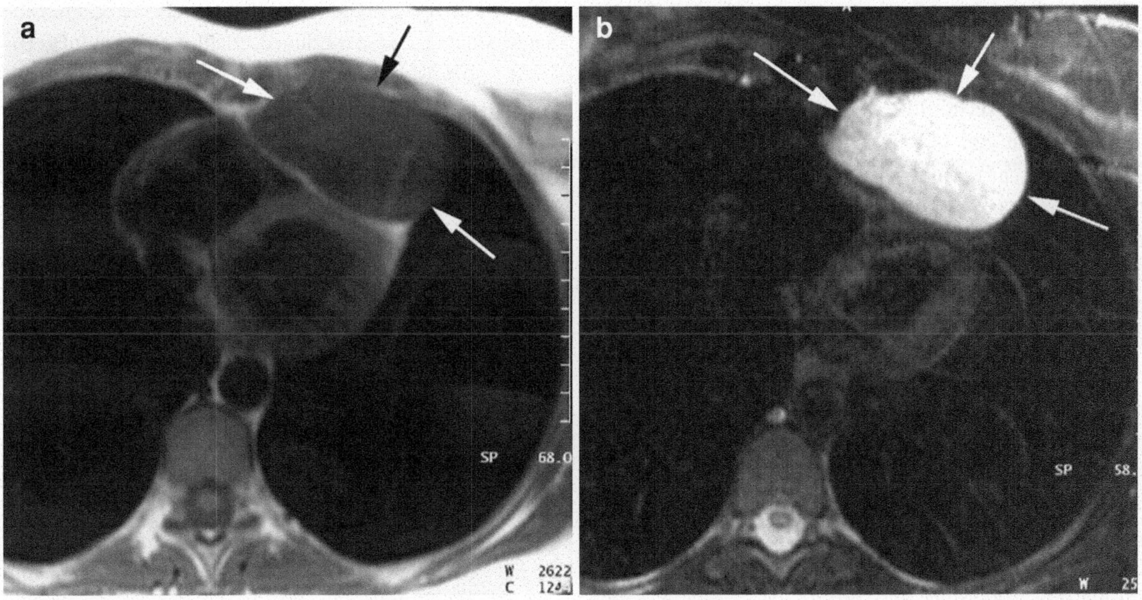

Fig. 7 Symptomatic pericardial cyst. Axial T1w imaging (**a**) and T2w imaging (**b**). Presence of a sharply delineated, well-defined, homogeneous soft-tissue structure with compression of the apex of right and left ventricle (*arrows*). The cyst has a low signal on T1w imaging and a very high signal on T2w imaging. The compression of the ventricles can be well appreciated on (dynamic) cine imaging

radiograph as an abnormal left cardiac contour (Glover et al. 1969). Symptoms occur when cardiac structures are transiently entrapped or incarcerated in the defect. Herniation of the left atrial appendage through a small defect may lead to infarction of the appendage or the left coronary artery might be compressed leading to ischaemia especially during exercise (Amplatz and Moller 1993).

The diagnosis of a pericardial defect is not straightforward, and may be challenging using MRI since in normal conditions the pericardium over the lateral side of the left ventricle, corresponding to the most frequent location of pericardial defects, is usually not well depicted because of a paucity of surrounding fat (Gutierrez et al. 1985). Thus, the diagnosis of a defect usually relies on other signs such as an abnormal location of cardiac structures with excessive levorotation or cardiac indentation at the location of the defect (Abbas et al. 2005; Scheuermann-Freestone et al. 2007). Since herniation is often intermittent in time, positional changes such as to positioning the patient in left lateral decubitus can be helpful in diagnosing pericardial defects. Functional examination may be helpful in establishing the diagnosis of congenital pericardial defect. While the normal cardiac apex is essentially stationary in the chest during the cardiac cycle, excessive mobility may be indicative of a pericardial defect (Psychidis-Papakyritsis et al. 2007).

5.3 Pericardial Diverticulum

Pericardial diverticulum is an exceedingly rare condition that can be congenital or acquired. It corresponds to a herniation through a defect in the parietal pericardium that communicates with the pericardial cavity (Sechtem et al. 1986b). Congenital diverticula results from a failure in the fusion of one of the mesenchymal lacunae that normally concurs to form the pericardial sac. They typically occur in the cardiophrenic angles and have the tendency to change in size over time. MRI is helpful in reaching a preoperative diagnosis. Although it resembles a pericardial cyst, the diagnosis of a diverticulum should be suspected when a complete wall cannot be identified in all parts of the lesion (Carretta et al. 2003).

6 Acquired Pericardial Diseases

6.1 Effuse Pericardial Disease

Abnormal fluid accumulation may be seen in heart failure, renal insufficiency, infection (bacterial, viral, tuberculous), neoplasm (carcinoma of lung, breast, lymphoma), trauma and myocardial infarction (Wang et al. 2003). Imaging is often required to confirm the presence, severity and extent of fluid; to characterize the nature of fluid; to rule out pericardial inflammation; to determine the hemodynamic impact on the heart; and to guide pericardiocentesis. For this purpose, echocardiography is the standard imaging modality. However, image quality and interpretation may be hampered by acoustic window, and in obese patients or in those with obstructive lung disease, necessitating additional imaging, such as CT or MRI. With exception of transesophageal echocardiography, this technique is generally unreliable for assessment of pericardial thickness, and may be of limited value in detecting loculated effusions (Troughton et al. 2004; Misselt et al. 2008; Bogaert and Francone 2009). Because the pericardial sac can be easily and completely visualized on MRI, this technique is superior to detect the distribution and amount of fluid accumulation than with echocardiography (Mulvagh et al. 1989). Although MRI can detect pericardial effusions as small as 30 ml (Fig. 8), a clear-cut relationship between the measured width of the pericardial space and total fluid volume cannot be established because pericardial fluid accumulation is often not homogeneously spread. Due to the gravitational dependency, focal fluid accumulation posterolateral to the left ventricle and along the inferolateral wall of the RV are not infrequent (Fig. 9) (Stark et al. 1984). Another common location is the superior pericardial recess. In general, a pericardial width greater than 4 mm should be regarded as abnormal. Moderate effusions (between 100 and 500 ml of fluid) are associated with a greater than 5 mm pericardial space anterior to the right ventricle (Sechtem et al. 1986a; Bogaert and Duerinckx 1995). Similar to ventricular volumetric quantification, multi-slice (cine) imaging can be used to quantify the precise amount of pericardial fluid.

Because the stretching capacity of the pericardial layers is limited, acute accumulation of pericardial contents (e.g. fluid, blood, air) can lead to cardiac chamber compression with decreased cardiac filling and subsequently impaired stroke volume, a phenomenon called "cardiac tamponade" (Mulvagh et al. 1989). The symptomatology can be dramatic, potentially lethal within minutes after onset. Symptoms are linked to the increase in pericardial pressure determined by the absolute volume of fluid, rate of fluid accumulation and the physical characteristics of the

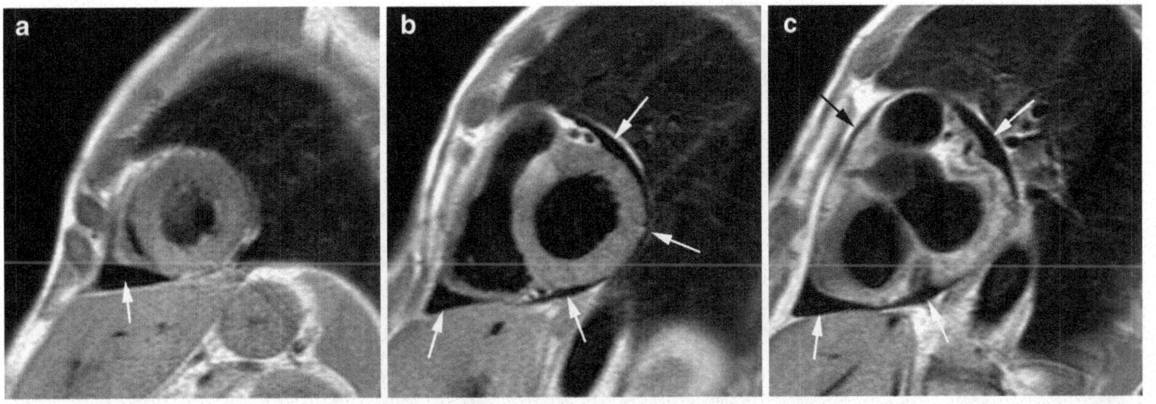

Fig. 8 Small pericardial effusion. Short-axis T1w imaging (**a–c**). MRI allows excellent appreciation of the spread of the fluid within the pericardial sac, which is predominantly located inferolateral to of the right ventricle and superolateral to the left ventricle located

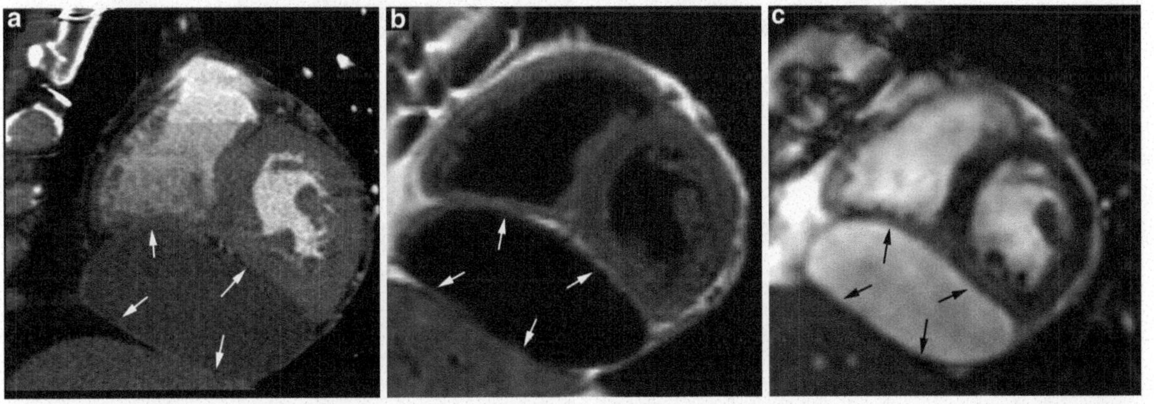

Fig. 9 Loculated pericardial effusion with cardiac compression. Short-axis computed tomography (**a**) T1w imaging (**b**) and cine imaging (**c**). Large oval-shaped pericardial effusion (*arrows*), inferiorly located to the heart. Note the compression on RV and LV. Courtesy: Marco Francone, MD, PhD, La Sapienza, Rome, Italy

pericardium (degree of stretching). The diagnosis of pericardial tamponade is a clinical one that is usually confirmed by echocardiography. Hallmarks of cardiac tamponade are the diastolic inversion or collapse of the RV free wall indicating intrapericardial pressure exceeding interventricular pressure; right atrial compression during early systole (Fig. 10); exaggerated respiratory variation in cardiac inflow; and abnormal flow patterns in the caval veins (Spodick 2003). Though, MRI has a limited role in the diagnosis of acute cardiac tamponade; chronic, less severe, forms can be encountered in patients with pericardial effusion on MRI (Fig. 10). Care should be taken to look for features of constriction, which can occur transiently in the resolution phase, after pericardiocentesis or with organized effusions (see effusive-constrictive pericarditis) (Troughton et al. 2004).

Analysis of MRI signals enables, at least to some extent, fluid characterization. Transudates typically have low-signal intensity on T1w imaging, and a high-signal intensity on T2w imaging . Exudates, having a high protein and cell content, increase T1-relaxation (higher signal intensity) and shorten T2-relaxation (lower signal intensity). However, because of motion artifacts, pericardial fluid characterization is not always feasible. In particular noninear motion of pericardial fluid during cardiac motion may falsely cause hyperintensities on T1w imaging within the effusion even in the presence of a simple transudate. Moreover characterization of small effusions may often be

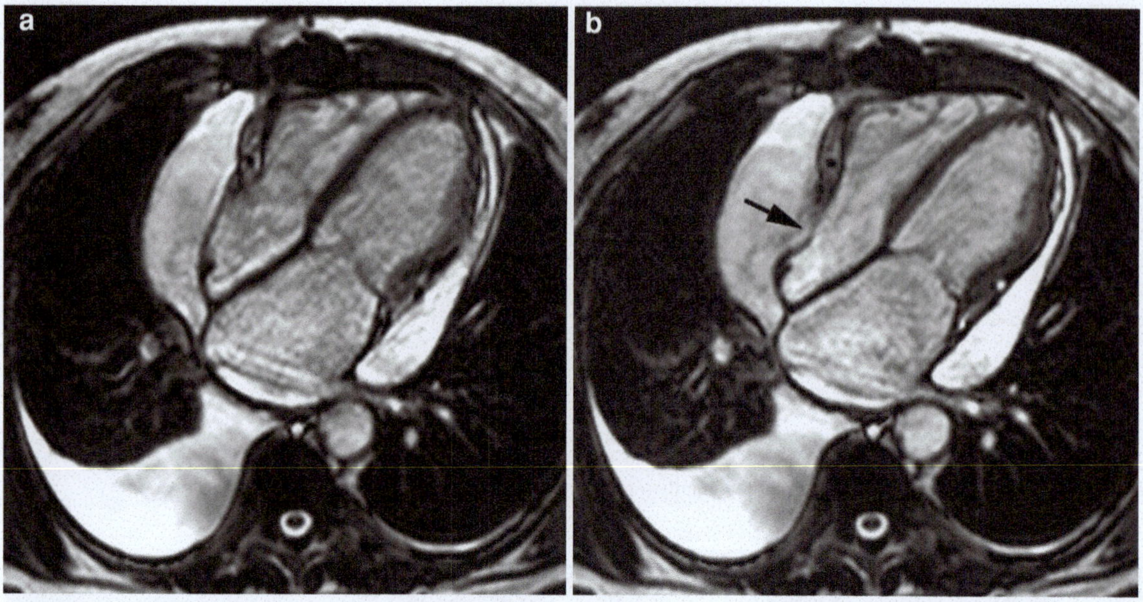

Fig. 10 Moderate pericardial effusion with signs of cardiac tamponade. Horizontal long-axis cine imaging at end-diastole (**a**) and mid-systole (**b**). A moderate pericardial effusion is present, most pronounced at the basal half of the heart. During systole collapse (*arrow*, **b**) of the right atrial wall occurs because the intrapericardial pressure exceeds the right atrial pressure. Note the presence of a moderate right-sided pleural effusion

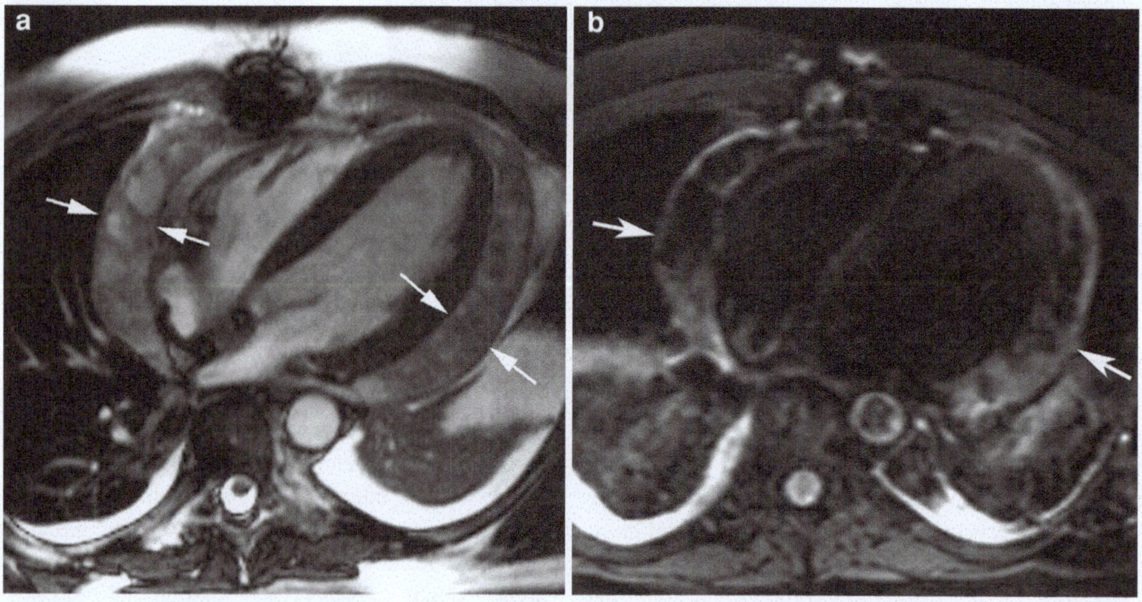

Fig. 11 Hemopericardium early post-aortic valve replacement. Axial cine imaging (**a**) and T2w imaging (**b**). In contrast with the high-signal of the bilateral pleural effusion, the signal of the pericardial fluid (*arrows*) on cine imaging and T2w imaging is highly inhomogeneous with presence of multiple fibrinous strands

difficult. The signal intensity of a hemorrhagic pericardial effusion is dependent on the duration of the disease (Fig. 11). With balanced SSFP-gradient-echo techniques, often a better characterization of the pericardial fluid content can be achieved such as the visualization of fibrinous strands or presence of coagulated blood. Other abnormalities helpful in the diagnosis are depiction of thickened pericardial blades with assessment of pericardial inflammation (Bogaert and Francone 2009; Taylor et al. 2006).

6.2 Pericardial Inflammation

Inflammation of the pericardium (*inflammatory pericarditis*) presents in many clinical settings and has a wide range of causes (Troughton et al. 2004). The acute presentation is an important differential in the assessment of acute chest pain, but pericarditis can also present in sub-acute or chronic forms. The symptoms are mainly related to the severity of pericardial inflammation. Although the true incidence and prevalence of pericarditis are difficult to measure, a prevalence of 1% in autopsy studies suggests that pericarditis may be subclinical (Troughton et al. 2004). In up to 30% of patients no cause of pericarditis can be defined (idiopathic). Infections (viral/bacterial/tuberculosis/fungal) are common causes of acute pericarditis. It can be noted that organisms responsible for myocarditis are commonly implicated. In developed countries, tuberculosis has become less common, but should still be considered in immunocompromised hosts (Little and Freeman 2006; Troughton et al. 2004; Restrepo et al. 2006). Radiation therapy for treatment of mediastinal tumors and breast cancer is an increasingly important cause of pericarditis and pericardial constriction. Pericarditis can be a manifestation of various systemic diseases (e.g. rheumatoid arthritis, systemic lupus erythematosus, and scleroderma); it can be secondary to primary or metastatic pericardial disease, and can be found in patients with uremia or following an acute myocardial infarction. The latter occurs early postinfarction and is typically found in transmural infarctions. This condition should be differentiated from late-post-infarction pericarditis (Dressler's syndrome). While acute post-infarction pericarditis, also called "epistenocardic pericarditis", has a close temporal relation with the acute event due to the pericardial spread of infarct-related inflammation, Dressler's syndrome has an autoimmune etiology without a close temporal relation with myocardial infarction. Finally, direct or indirect trauma can cause traumatic pericarditis.

In the acute phase, inflammation of the pericardial layers is characterized by formation of young, highly vascularized granulation tissue with fibrin deposition (Taylor et al. 2006). Usually, a variable amount of pericardial fluid is present, and the fibrin deposition may lead to a fibrinous adhesion of the pericardial layers. Chronic inflammation is characterized by a progressive sclerosing pericarditis with fibroblasts, collagen and a lesser amount of fibrin deposition (Francone et al. 2005). This may progress toward an end-stage, chronic fibrosing pericarditis with fibroblasts and collagen, and with a sparse vascularization. The main feature of this end-stage is a stiff pericardium with constriction of the heart (*constrictive pericarditis*). Detection of inflammatory pericarditis has become less challenging with the availability of modern MRI techniques (Kojima et al. 1999; Misselt et al. 2008; Bogaert and Francone 2009). Thickening of the pericardial layers, as well as depiction of associated pericardial effusion can be well depicted on T1w imaging or cine imaging, while T2w imaging allows visualization of edema of the inflamed pericardial layers (Figs. 12, 13). Pericardial enhancement on contrast-enhanced MRI studies is an appropriate way to detect pericardial inflammation (Fig. 12) (Taylor et al. 2006). Both T1w imaging and late Gd imaging are useful (Fig. 14, 15). Addition of a fat-suppression prepulse may be interesting to enhance visualization of pericardial inflammation. Other interesting imaging features are assessment of pericardial layer delineation, which might become more irregular in cases of chronic pericarditis and streaky enhancement of the surrounding fat and enhancement of adjacent myocardial tissue, indicating associated epicarditis or myocarditis, respectively. Today, MRI is considered the non-invasive standard to depict myocarditis (Skouri et al. 2006; Mahrhold et al. 2006). In a recent study, Yelgec and colleagues reported pericardial enhancement in 9 and pericardial effusion in 6 patients in a group of 20 patients studied with MRI for clinical suspicion of acute myocarditis (Yelgec et al. 2007), indicating myopericarditis is not an uncommon presentation (Fig. 16). Tagging MRI techniques may be used to well depict the fibrotic adhesions of pericardial layers (Fig. 17) (Kojima et al. 1999).

6.3 Constrictive Pericarditis

Chronic fibrosing pericarditis is characterized by a thickened, fibrotic and/or calcified pericardium, frequently constricting the heart and impairing cardiac

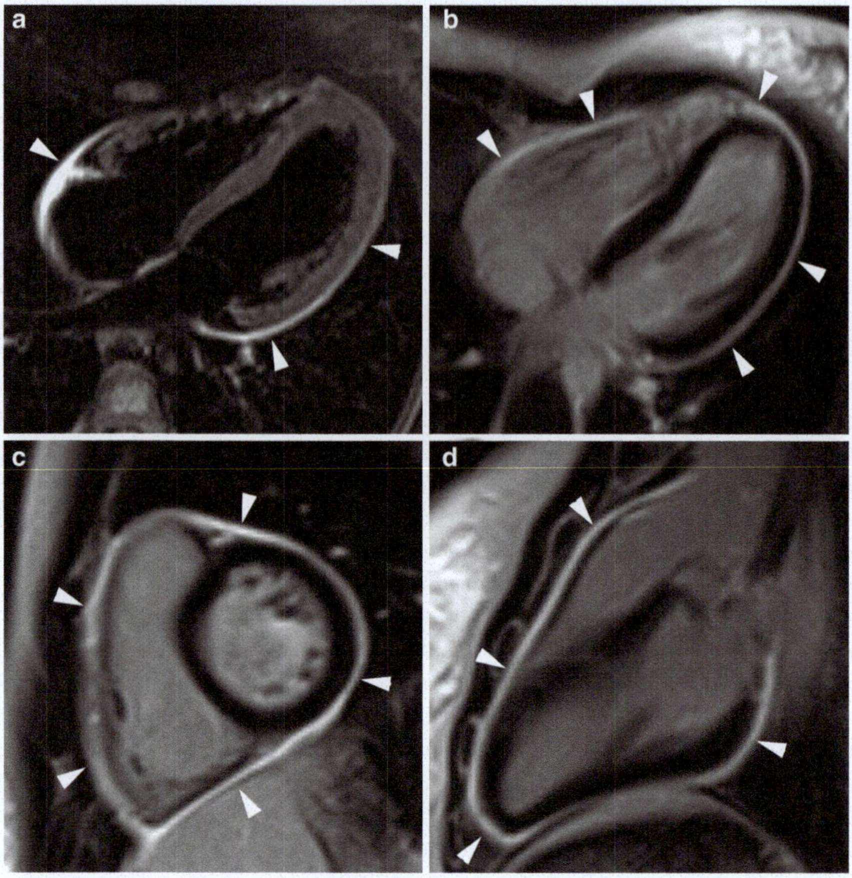

Fig. 12 Acute viral inflammatory pericarditis in 15 year old girl. Horizontal long-axis T2w imaging (**a**), late Gd imaging in horizontal long-axis (**b**), short-axis (**c**) and vertical long-axis plane (**d**). Diffuse hyperintense appearance of the pericardium on T2w imaging (*arrows*)(**a**). Strong, homogeneous enhancement of the entire pericardium following contrast administration (*arrows*) (**b**, **c**, **d**). Courtesy: Marco Francone, MD, PhD, La Sapienza, Rome, Italy

filling ("constrictive" pericarditis) (Myers and Spodick 1999). Patients with pericardial constriction typically present with manifestations of elevated systemic venous pressures and low cardiac output (Ling et al. 1999). The diagnosis should always be considered in patients presenting with predominant right heart failure symptoms (Nishimura 2001). The pathophysiological hallmarks of pericardial constriction, which are caused by confinement of the cardiac chambers by the rigid, fixed pericardial volume, are equalization of end-diastolic pressures in all four cardiac chambers, and increased ventricular coupling which is strongly influenced by respiration (Little and Freeman 2006; Troughton et al. 2004).

Pericardial constriction is most commonly idiopathic but can be the end result of any cause of inflammatory pericarditis. Tuberculosis has become less frequent, while cardiac surgery and radiation-induced pericarditis have also become important (Troughton et al. 2004). In non-tuberculous pericarditis pericardial thickening and calcification may be less prominent. In radiation therapy, systolic dysfunction may accompany constriction and is a marker of poor prognosis after pericardiectomy. Pathology typically shows an avascular collagen-rich, fibrotic tissue, often containing areas of calcification. Moreover, in extensive cases the fibrosing process may be adherent or even involve the myocardium.

Today, despite a wide arsenal diagnostic tools, the diagnosis of constrictive pericarditis often remains a challenge, and the diagnostic approach taken should be individualized for each patient. First, all other causes of (right) heart failure (e.g. pulmonary hypertension, and LV/RV infarction) should be excluded. Second, it should be determined whether the pericardium is causing constriction hereby impeding cardiac filling and thirdly whether the patient will benefit from a pericardial stripping. One of the major dilemmas is that diseases with decreased myocardial compliance, such as restrictive cardiomyopathy, are also characterized by impaired cardiac filling, and may present in a very similar way. Distinction

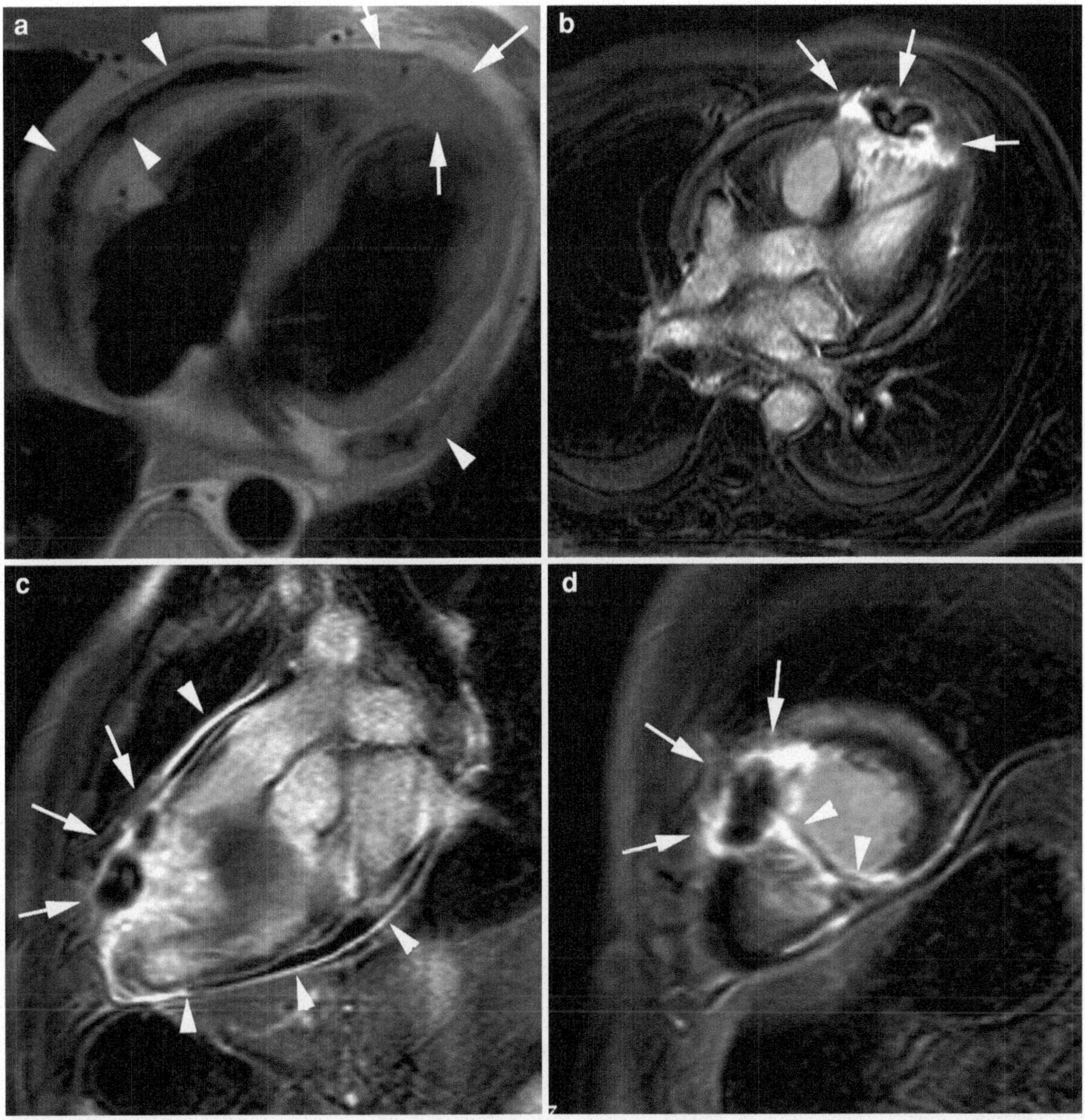

Fig. 13 Acute pericardial inflammation and abscess formation in a patient with a recent myocardial infarction. Axial T1w imaging (**a**), late Gd imaging in horizontal (**b**), vertical (**c**) and long-axis and short-axis plane (**d**). T1w imaging shows diffuse important thickening of both pericardial layers (*arrowheads*, **a**) with a small pericardial effusion. Presence of a soft-tissue structure anteriorly of the right and left ventricle (*arrows*, **a**). Following contrast administration, strong pericardial enhancement occurs (*arrowheads*, **c**). The soft-tissue mass inhomogeneously enhances with central area of non-enhancement (*arrows*, **b**, **c**, **d**). Note the presence of transmural enhancement of the mid anteroseptal wall with central no-reflow zone (*arrowheads*, **d**)

between the two entities is crucial because constrictive pericarditis patients are potentially successfully treated by early pericardiectomy while for restrictive cardiomyopathy medical treatment is recommended (Myers and Spodick 1999; Ling et al. 1999; Nishimura 2001; Kushwaha et al. 1997; Hancock 2001). Several other factors may hamper straightforward diagnosis of constrictive pericarditis. The morphologic pericardial abnormalities classically found in constrictive pericarditis may not be impressive, be absent or have an atypical presentation. Moreover, increased pericardial thickness does not necessarily

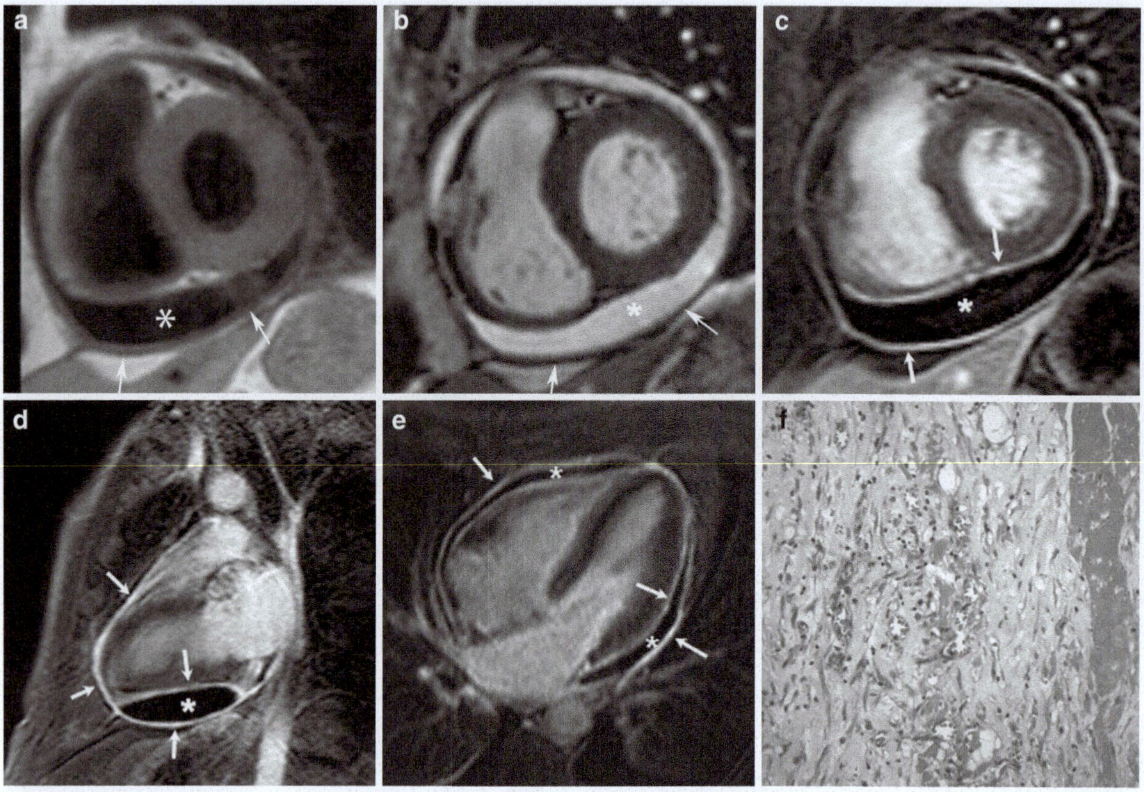

Fig. 14 Chronic inflammatory pericarditis in a patient presenting with pericardial effusion and fever of underdetermined origin. Short-axis T1w imaging (**a**), cine imaging (**b**), late Gd imaging in short-axis (**c**), vertical long-axis (**d**) and horizontal long-axis plane (**e**). Histology (x400) (**f**). On short-axis T1w imaging and cine imaging, a moderate pericardial effusion (*) and thickened pericardial layers (*arrows*, **a**, **b**) is well visible. Following contrast administration the pericardial layers strongly enhance (*arrows*, **c–e**). Histology shows thickened pericardium with young, vascularized granulation tissue and large amounts of fibrin. Adapted from Taylor et al. 2006

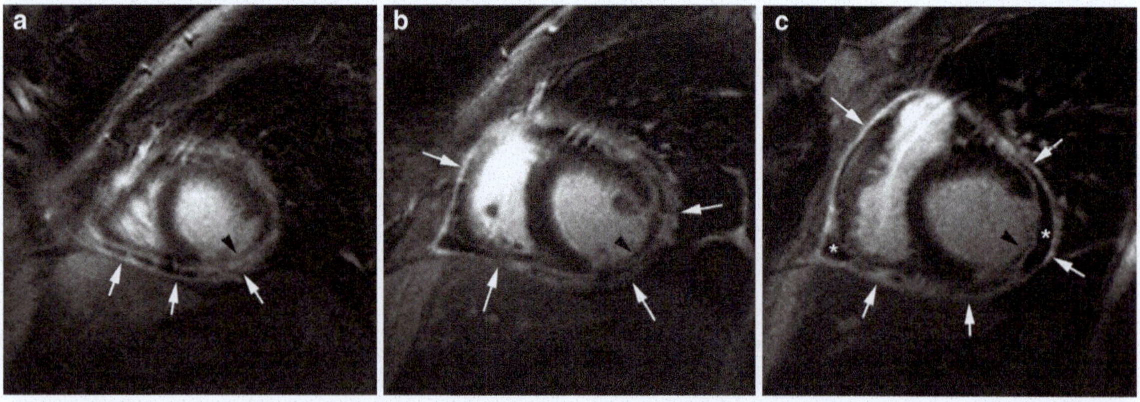

Fig. 15 Chronic inflammatory pericarditis in a patient with history of proximal occluded left circumflex artery and transmural myocardial infarction. Late Gd imaging in cardiac short-axis (**a–c**) shows the infarct as a strongly enhancing thinned lateral LV wall (*arrowhead*, **c**). A diffusely thickened strongly enhancing pericardium (*arrows*) is well visible with a small pericardial effusion along the left ventricle and infero-lateral to the right ventricle (*)

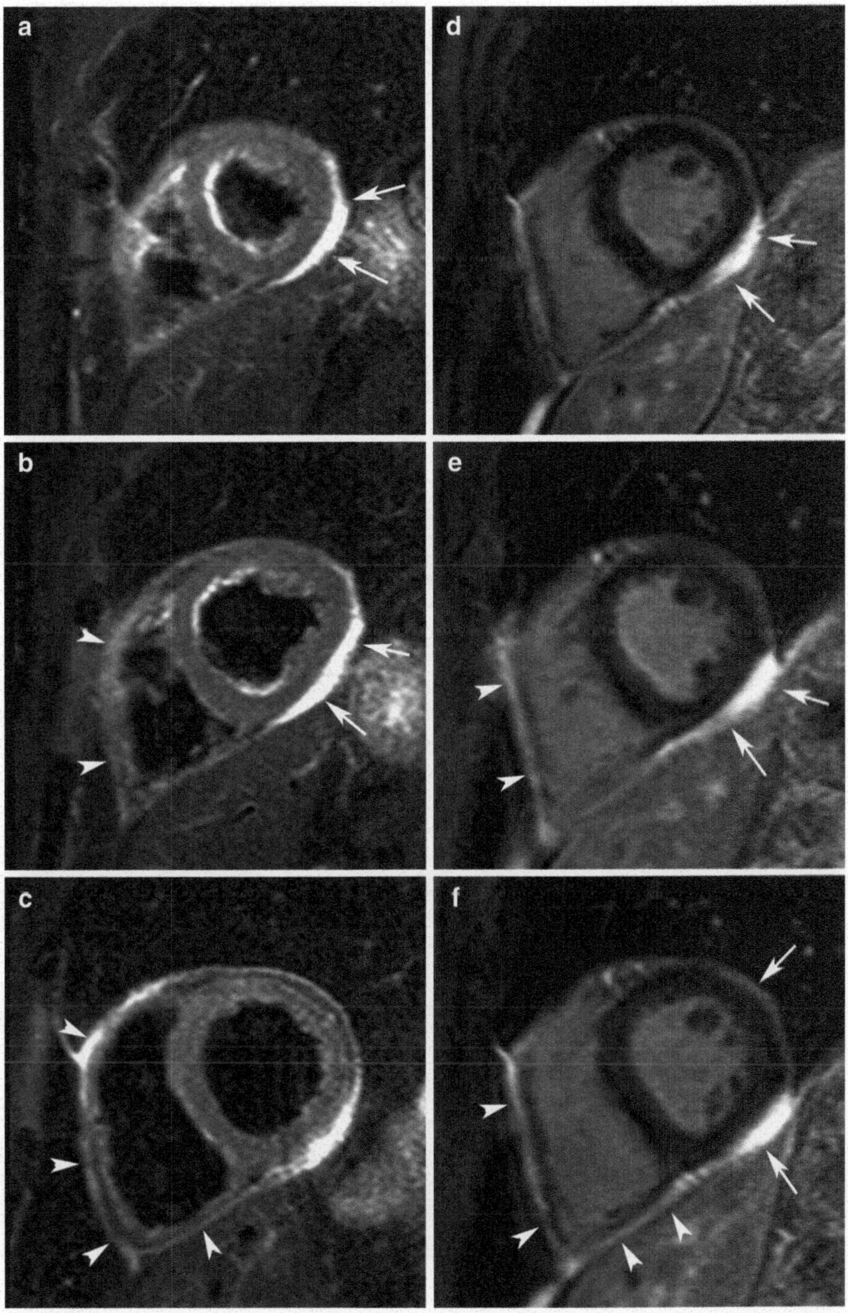

Fig. 16 Inflammatory pericarditis and epi(myo)carditis in a patient presenting with acute chest pain, raised troponins and normal coronary angiogram. Short-axis T2w imaging (**a–c**) and late Gd imaging (**d–f**). T2w imaging shows area of increased signal intensity along the inferolateral border of the LV (*arrows*, **a–c**), less pronounced also over the right ventricle (*arrowheads*, **a–c**). Following contrast-administration these same areas show strong enhancement (*arrows*, and *arrowheads*, **d–f**). These findings are compatible with inflammatory pericarditis with involvement of the epicardial fat (epicarditis). A minor involvement of the adjacent myocardium (myocarditis component) cannot be excluded. Note that there is no pericardial effusion

imply pericardial constriction, and vice versa (Troughton et al. 2004). Finally, for instance in patients with a history of radiation therapy, restrictive cardiomyopathy and constrictive pericarditis may simultaneously occur. This makes the diagnosis of constrictive pericarditis, especially in atypical or complex cases, often challenging. Since no one method is completely reliable, information from more than one imaging should be considered to provide an assessment of anatomical and physiological function (Nishimura 2001).

6.3.1 Morphologic Abnormalities

The typical morphological presentation of constrictive pericarditis is a more or less generalized thickening of the pericardium. This thickening is

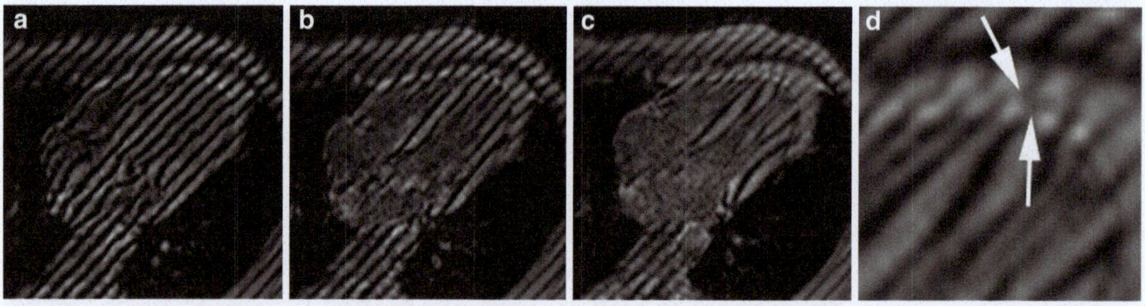

Fig. 17 MRI tagging using the SPAMM (spatial modulation of magnetization) technique in a healthy volunteer in axial plane (**a–c**) and enlarged view at end systole (**d**). The tags are oriented in long-axis direction, and positioned on the heart at end diastole. Because of shear motion between visceral and parietal layer, the continuity of the tags gets lost during cardiac contraction (*arrows*, **d**). Adapted from Bogaert and Francone 2009

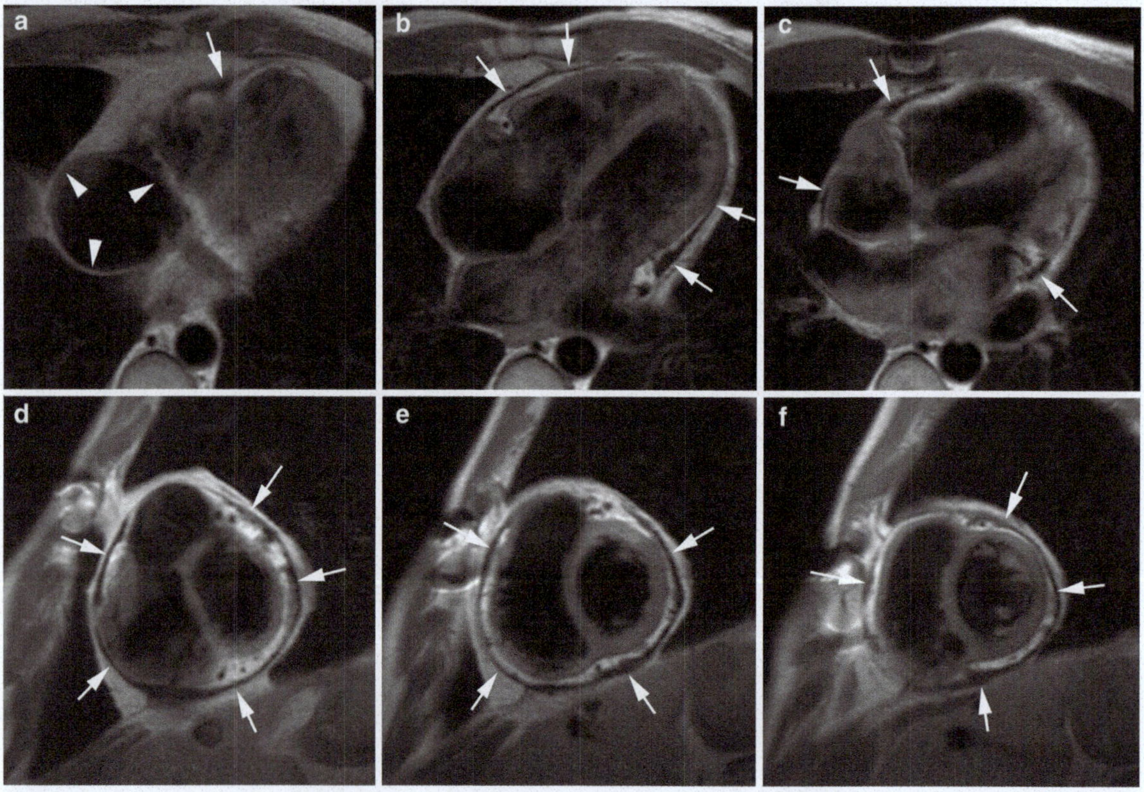

Fig. 18 Classic example of constrictive pericarditis. T1w imaging in axial plane (**a–c**), and short-axis view (**d–f**). Presence of a diffusely thickened and irregularly defined pericardium involving almost the entire pericardium (*arrows*). Presence of a severely dilated inferior caval vein (*arrowheads*, **a**). Slow flow is present in both atria and atrial appendages visible as lack of signal void on T1w imaging (panel **b**, **c**)

usually most pronounced over the right heart side (right ventricle and anterior atrioventricular groove), and the pericardial delineation is often irregular (Fig. 18) (Frank and Globits 1999). The underlying cardiac cavities may be constricted by the abnormal pericardium, having a flattened or tubular-shaped appearance (Fig. 19). Indirectly, as a result of the increased cardiac filling pressures, unilateral or bilateral atrial enlargement, dilatation of caval and hepatic veins, pleural effusion,and ascites are

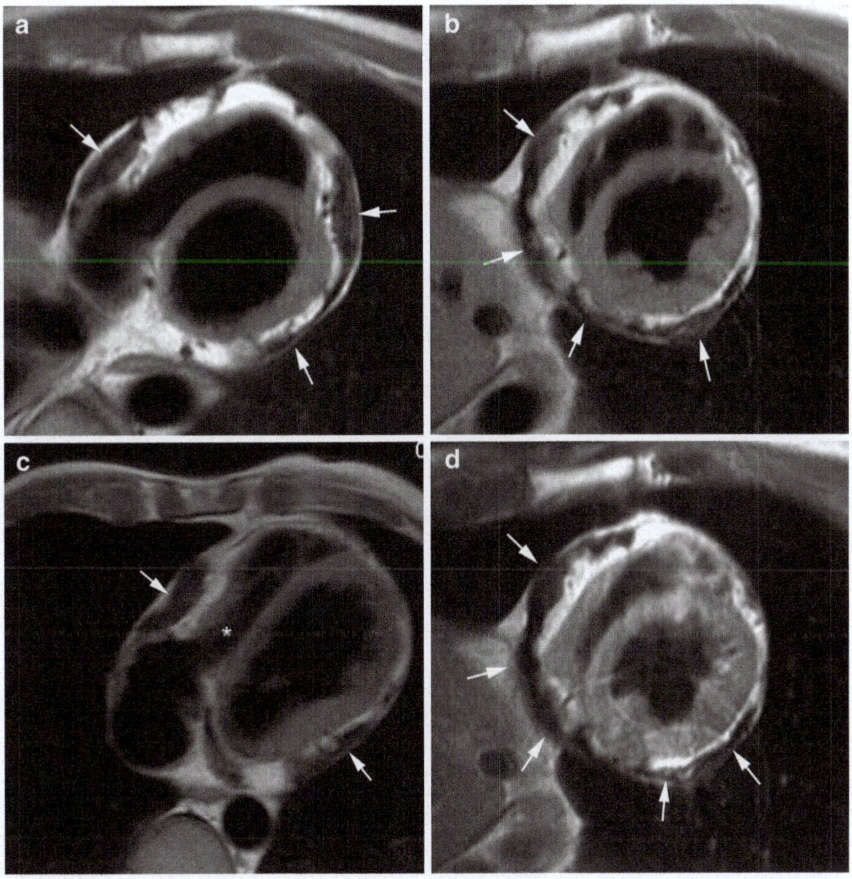

Fig. 19 Calcified constrictive pericarditis with constriction of RV cavity. T1w imaging in short-axis (**a, b**), axial view (**c**), and following contrast administration in cardiac short-axis view (**d**). Extensive, irregular pericardial thickening is present, most pronounced over the basal half of LV and RV and both atrioventricular grooves (*arrows*, **a–c**). Important compression of the RV cavity (**c**, *). No pericardial enhancement occurs following contrast administration (*arrows*, **d**)

encountered. Useful criteria to assess pericardial thickness by MRI are a) pericardial thickness 2 mm or less: normal, b) pericardial thickness greater than 4 mm: suggestive of pericardial constriction in patients with the appropriate clinical presentation, c) pericardial thickness greater than 5–6 mm: high specificity for constriction (Soulen et al. 1985; Maisch et al. 2004; Oh et al. 2001). The thickened fibrotic and/or calcified pericardium has a low signal not only on T1w and T2w imaging but also on cine imaging. In 2006, we mentioned that end-stage chronic fibrosing forms of constrictive pericarditis were characterized by lack of enhancement after contrast administration and that pericardial enhancement in patients with constrictive pericarditis was suggestive of residual inflammation in the pericardium (Figs. 20, 21) (Taylor et al. 2006). Although our findings were in contradiction with the pattern of persistent enhancement in chronic myocardial scars, several recent publications favor our view and focus on the role a CMR in determining which constrictive pericarditis patients may potentially benefit of anti-inflammatory treatment (residual pericardial enhancement) while in others pericardiectomy is the preferred treatment (lack of pericardial enhancement) on late Gd imaging. Differentiation between pericardial thickening and effusion is usually straightforward using a comprehensive MRI approach. Today, CT is the most appropriate technique to depict, even minute amounts of pericardial calcium, whereas significant deposits may be missed by MRI.

In a considerable number of patients the classical morphologic findings are lacking. Pericardial constriction may occur in any condition where the compliance of the pericardium is decreased. *Effusive-constrictive pericarditis* is a condition where the constriction is not relieved after removal of the pericardial fluid (Sagristà-Sauleda et al. 2004; Sagristà-Sauleda 2004; Hancock 2004). This condition was found in 15 of 218 pericarditis patients presenting with cardiac tamponade (Sagristà-Sauleda

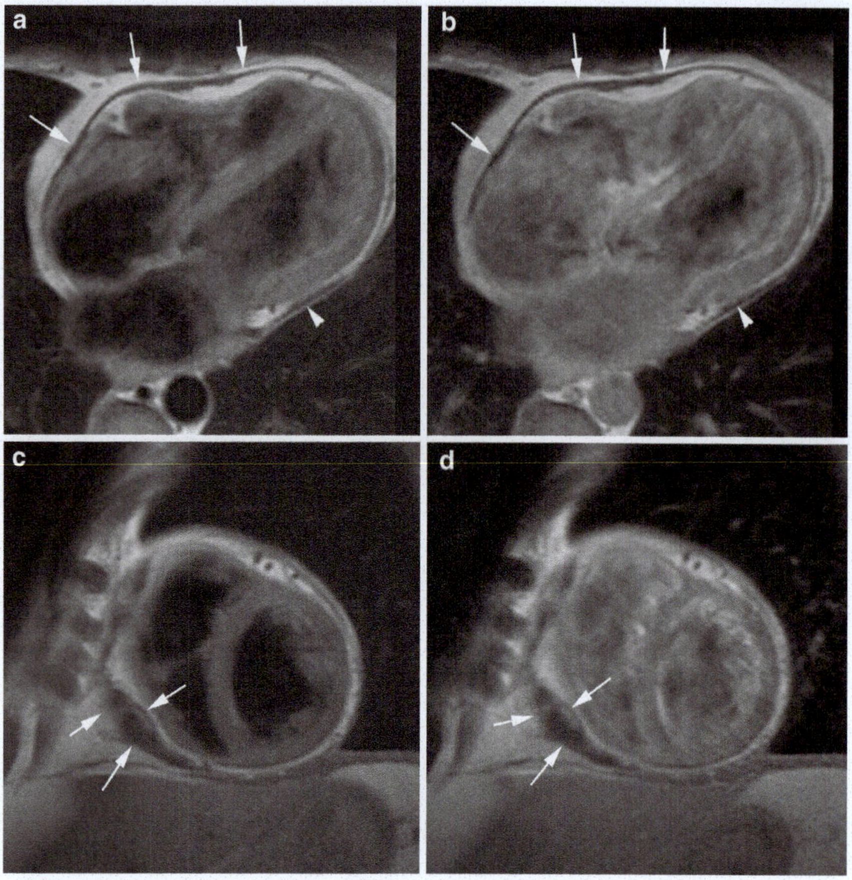

Fig. 20 Calcified constrictive pericarditis. T1w imaging in axial plane (**a**, **b**) and short-axis plane (**c**, **d**), before (**a**, **c**) and after (**b**, **d**) contrast administration. A diffusely thickened, irregularly defined pericardium is present (*arrows*, *arrowhead*, **a–d**). The pericardium exhibitis low-signal intensity on T1w-imaging. No changes in signal intensity occur following contrast administration

et al. 2004). It is believed the non-compliant visceral pericardium is causing the constriction. The diagnosis of effusive-constrictive pericarditis is often challenging because the morphologic abnormalities, even at visual inspection, are not impressive (Hancock 2004). It is believed that effusive-constrictive pericarditis most likely represents an intermediate transition from acute pericarditis with pericardial effusion to pericardial constriction (Hancock 2004). *Transient cardiac constriction* is common in patients with effusive acute idiopathic pericarditis (Sagristà-Sauleda et al. 1987; Haley et al. 2004). Features of constriction may be detected in the phase of resolution of pericarditis, at a time when signs of activity have abated, and residual effusion is minimal or has disappeared entirely. The clinical and hemodynamical features of constriction spontaneously subside after a couple of months (Sagristà-Sauleda 2004). Most likely the inflammatory thickened pericardium has a decreased compliance causing symptoms of temporary constriction (*inflammatory-constrictive pericarditis*) (Fig. 21). Both entities underscore the variable evolution in patients with acute pericarditis, and represent an intermediate between spontaneous resolution and evolution toward constrictive pericarditis. The ability to differentiate fluid from pericardial layer, and to depict pericardial inflammation, makes MRI appealing to assess these atypical forms of constrictive pericarditis (Bogaert and Francone 2009; Klein et al. 2003; Taylor et al. 2006). In some cases pericardial abnormalities might be very localized (*focal constrictive pericarditis*). Symptoms of constriction, will primarily depend on the location of abnormalities and degree of constriction. Focal constriction, for example, at the level of atrioventricular grooves or basal portion of the ventricles, though not visually impressive may significantly impede cardiac filling (Figs. 22 and 23) (Hasuda et al. 1999; Giorgi et al. 2003). This urges for a scrutinized visualization of the entire pericardium with MRI. Since cardiac constriction is caused by decrease in pericardial compliance and not by the pericardial thickness as such, taking the latter parameter as an

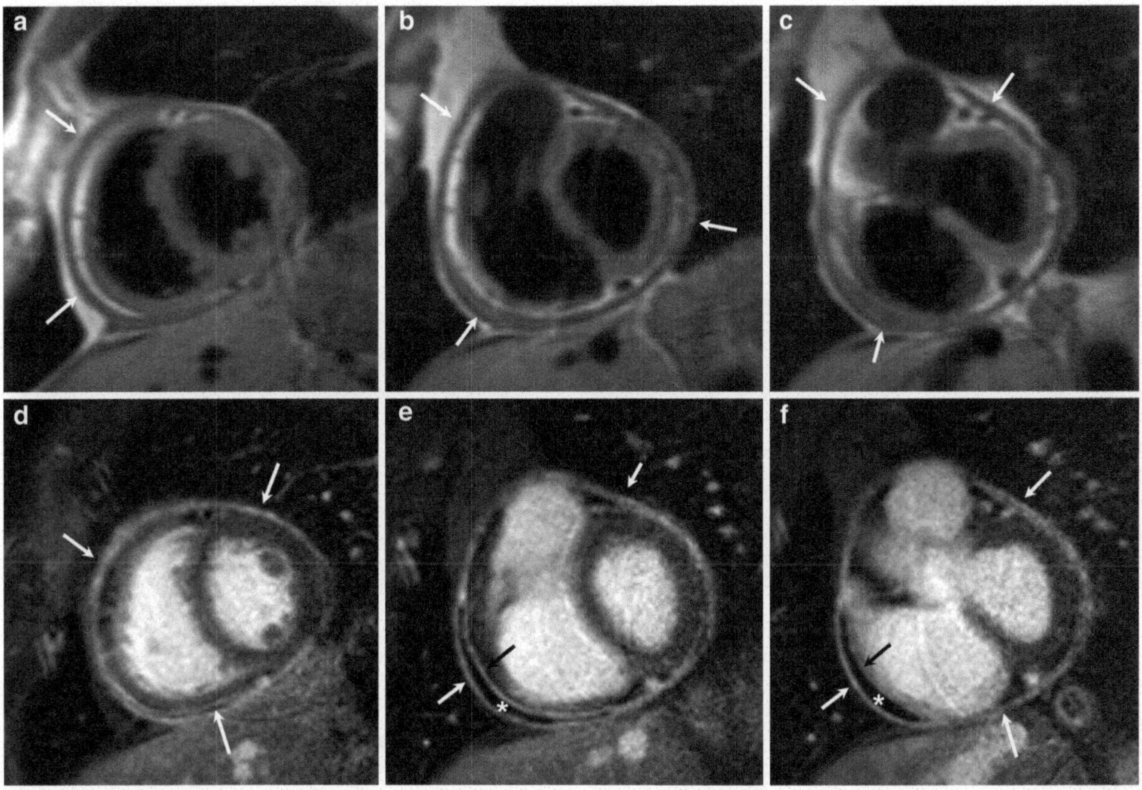

Fig. 21 Inflammatory-constrictive pericarditis. Short-axis T1w imaging (**a–c**) and late Gd imaging (**d–f**). Diffusely thickened pericardium (*arrows*, **a–c**), with strong enhancement of the pericardial layers after contrast administration (*arrows*, **d–f**). Presence of a small pericardial effusion (*) along the inferolateral side of the right ventricle. At surgery, a heavily thickened and inflamed pericardium was found

absolute criterion may create a diagnostic dilemma in patients with hemodynamic findings of constriction without increased pericardial thickness. Up to 18% of patients with histologically proven constrictive pericarditis have a normal or near normal pericardial thickness (i.e., <2 mm) (*non or minimally thickened constrictive pericarditis*) (Talreja et al. 2003) (Fig. 24). Moreover, in some patients physical and hemodynamic features of constriction are not apparent in their baseline state, but when rapidly fluid challenged, they will present a typical hemodynamic constrictive pericarditis pattern. This subgroup is called *occult constrictive pericarditis* (Bush et al. 1977; Sagristà-Sauleda 2004), and shows the close interaction between cardiac filling status and physical properties of the surrounding pericardium.

MRI is an important tool in patients presenting with diastolic heart failure to differentiate those with restrictive cardiomyopathy from those with constrictive pericarditis. As discussed in detail in "Heart Muscle Disease" on heart muscle disease, myocardial enhancement patterns on late-Gd MRI may be strongly indicative of specific myocardial infiltrative or storage diseases, while T2*-weighted MRI may be used to non-invasively depict iron deposition cardiomyopathy.

6.3.2 Functional and Hemodynamic Abnormalities

The consequences of encasement of the heart by a rigid pericardium are basically threefold, (a) dissociation between intrathoracic and intracardiac pressure, isolating the heart from normal respiratory changes in intrathoracic pressure, (b) increased ventricular coupling, and (c) increased cardiac filling pressures with pressure equalization in all four cardiac chambers. Assessment of these effects is usually performed by echocardiography and cardiac catheterization (Hatle et al. 1989; Myers and Spodick 1999; van den Hout et al. 2003; Troughton et al. 2004; Talreja et al. 2003;

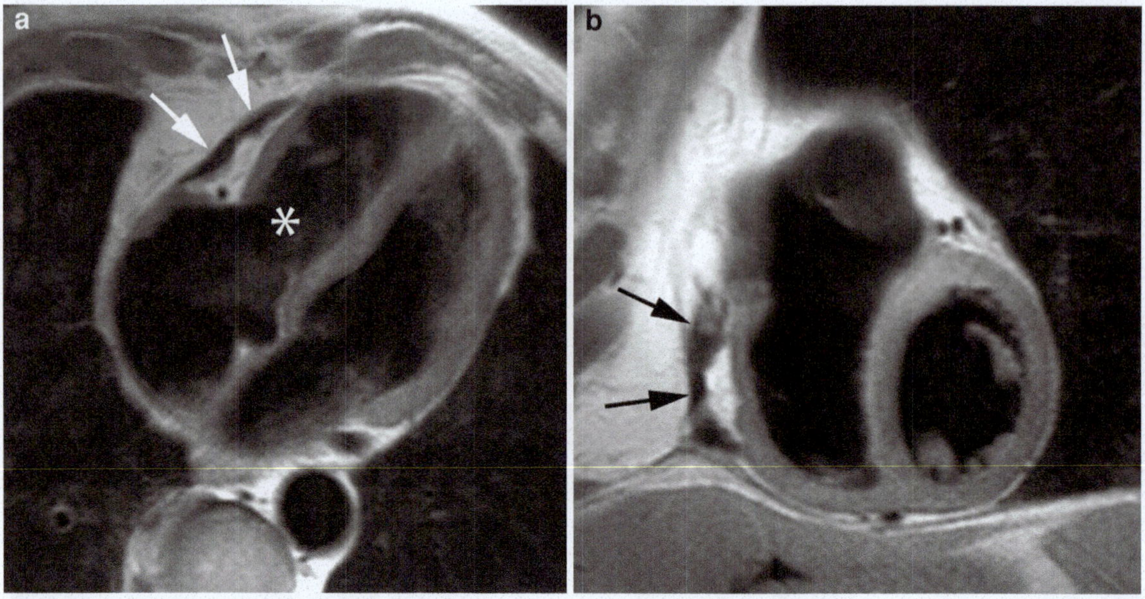

Fig. 22 Focal constrictive pericarditis. T1w imaging in horizontal long-axis (**a**) and short-axis (**b**) plane. Important focal thickening of the pericardium at the level of basal half of the RV and right atrioventricular groove (*arrows*, **a–b**), with partial compression of the RV cavity (*, **a**)

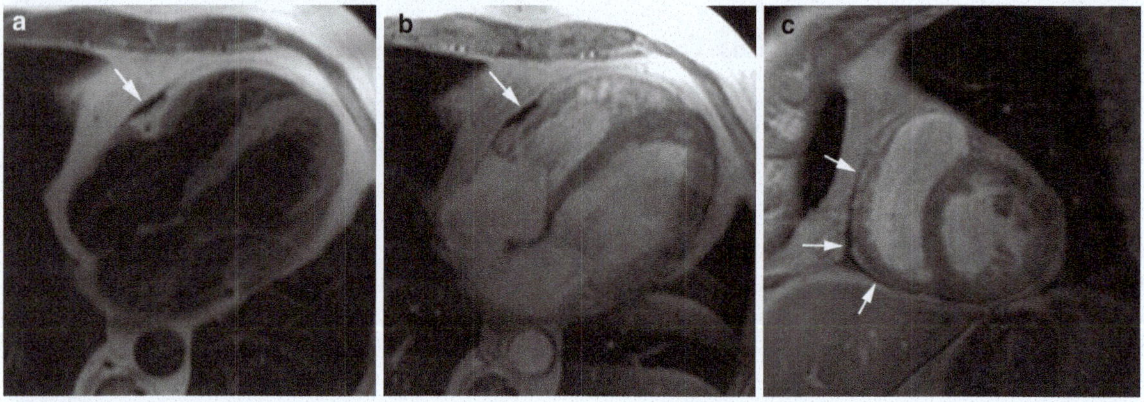

Fig. 23 Focal constrictive pericarditis, axial T1w imaging (**a**) and cine imaging in axial plane (**b**) and short-axis plane (**c**). Focal pericardial thickening (*arrows*) at the level of the right atrioventricular groove and basal part of the free wall of the right ventricle with focal compression of right ventricular cavity (*). The morphologic pericardial abnormalities are not pronounced, but because of their location they have led this patient to symptoms of constrictive pericarditis. Adapted from Giorgi et al. 2003

Little and Freeman 2006). MRI, with the exception of intracardiac pressure measurements, may provide valuable information too, and has the intrinsic advantage that findings may be directly linked to morphologic abnormalities. Phase-contrast MRI typically shows a restrictive filling pattern with an enhanced early filling, and decreased or absent late filling, depending on the degree of pericardial constriction and increased filling pressures. Also the venous flow patterns may show restrictive physiology with diminished or absent forward, or even reversed systolic flow, and increased early diastolic forward flow and late backflow (Fig. 25). Constrictive pericarditis, in contrast with restrictive myocarditis, is typically characterized by a strong respiratory-related variation in cardiac filling (i.e., enhanced RV filling on inspiration, enhanced LV filling on expiration) (Hatle et al. 1989; Talreja et al. 2003). Real-time PC-MRI is a potential

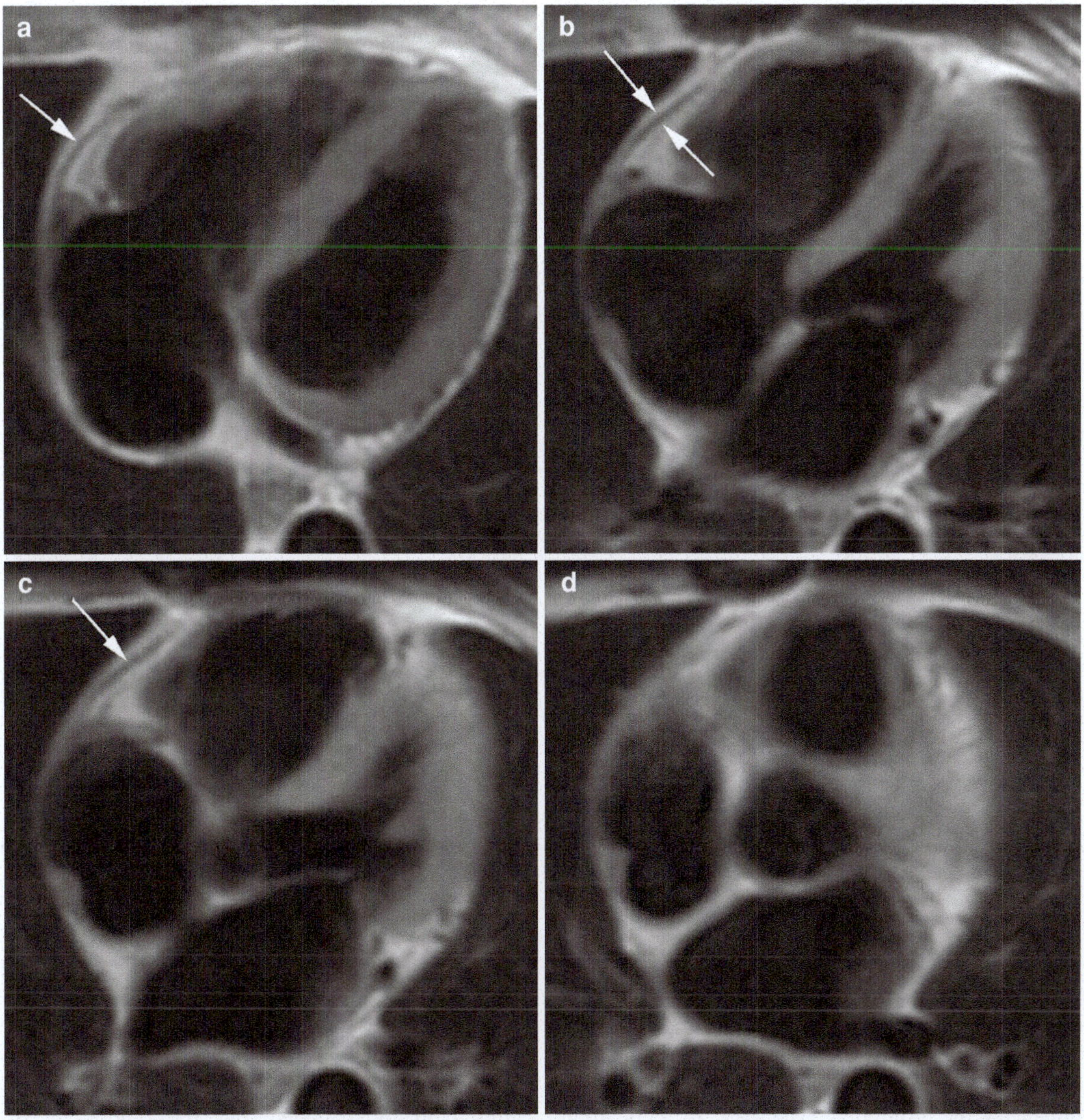

Fig. 24 Non-thickened constrictive pericarditis in a patient with previous CABG surgery presenting with increased right heart filling pressures, dyspnea and peripheral edema. Transthoracic echocardiography shows restrictive physiology. Axial T1w imaging (**a–d**). The pericardium is visible as a thin curvilinear line with a maximal thickness of 1.7 mm (arrows). Real-time cine MRI of the ventricular septal motion shows diastolic septal inversion at the onset of inspiration, and an increased total septal excursion ("pathologic ventricular coupling") (see Fig.11.25). During the pericardiectomy, a non-thickened but very stiff pericardium was found, and the cardiac output increased spectacularly from 1.7 to 7.5 l/min

alternative to echo-Doppler to assess the effects of respiration on cardiac filling, though ideally slice-tracking techniques are needed to compensate for through-plane motion (van den Hout et al. 2003).

Since the pressure difference between the ventricles (or trans-septal pressure gradient) determines the position and configuration of the ventricular septum, this information can be used to determine the degree of ventricular coupling (or ventricular interdependence) (Gibson et al. 1976; Candell-Riera et al. 1978; Janicki and Weber 1980; Freeman and LeWinter 1984; Santamore et al. 1986; Hurrell et al. 1996).

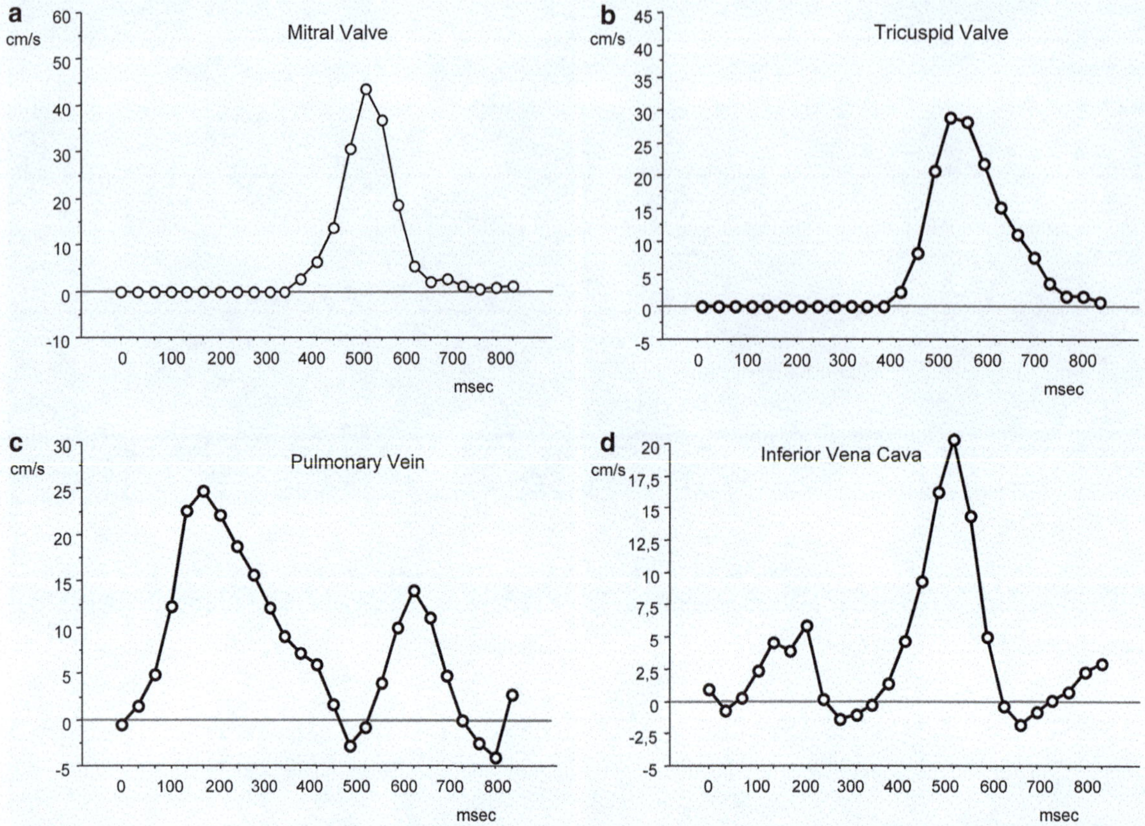

Fig. 25 Inflow curves, using PC-MRI, through the mitral valve (**a**), tricuspid valve (**b**), pulmonary vein (**c**) and inferior vena cava (**d**) in a patient with constrictive pericarditis (same patient as in Fig. 18). Inflow curves show a severe restrictive inflow physiology with absent A-waves through the atrioventricular valves (**a,b**), and absent systolic forward in the inferior vena cava (**d**)

Under normal loading conditions, due to a positive left-to-right trans-septal pressure gradient, the septum has a right-sided convex shape, and this shape is maintained during the cardiac cycle and is minimally influenced by respiration. The lack of pericardial stretch in constrictive pericarditis leads to increased ventricular coupling, characterized by septal flattening or inversion ("septal bounce") on early diastolic ventricular filling (Nishimura 2001) (Fig. 26). Because of the dissociation between intrathoracic and intracardiac pressure, this pattern is strongly influenced by respiration (Troughton et al. 2004; Hurrell et al. 1996). Septal abnormalities are most pronounced at onset of inspiration and rapidly fade away, while at onset of expiration an opposite (right-sided) septal shift occurs. MRI is appealing to functionally study patients with a clinical suspicion of constrictive pericarditis, and to visualize and quantify the degree of ventricular coupling. Giorgi and associates, using breath-hold cine MRI, reported early diastolic septal flattening or inversion in the majority of constrictive pericarditis patients, a pattern that was absent in restrictive cardiomyopathy patients (Fig. 26) (Giorgi et al. 2003). Abnormalities were most evident in the basal septum, leading to a serpentine septal motion on cardiac long-axis view. This pattern was not present if the constrictive pericardium did not involve the right ventricle (Hasuda et al. 1999; Giorgi et al. 2003). With the advent of real-time MRI, the effect of respiration on ventricular coupling could be dynamically exploited (Fig. 27) (Francone et al. 2005). Francone et al. (2005, 2006) analyzed septal shape and position in patients with constrictive and inflammatory pericarditis and restrictive cardiomyopathy patients. Constrictive pericarditis patients showed the typical respiratory pattern of septal

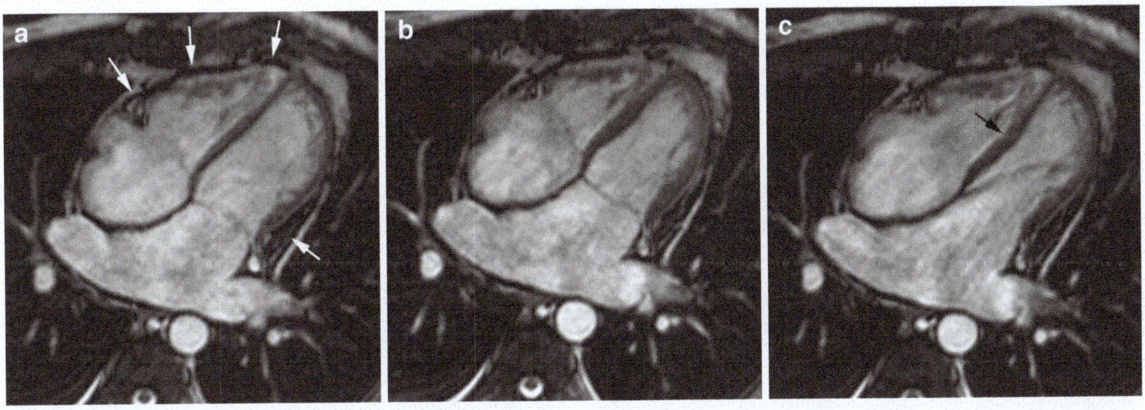

Fig. 26 Early diastolic septal bounce in constrictive pericarditis. Horizontal long-axis cine imaging at end diastole (**a**), end systole (**b**), and early diastole (**c**). The irregularly thickened, hypointense pericardium over the right ventricle and to a lesser extent over the left ventricle (*arrows*, **a**). While the ventricular septum has a normal shape during systole, at the start of diastolic ventricular filling, the non-compliant pericardium impedes RV filling causing a septal inversion (*black arrow*, **c**), visible as serpentine-like motion of the septum during diastole

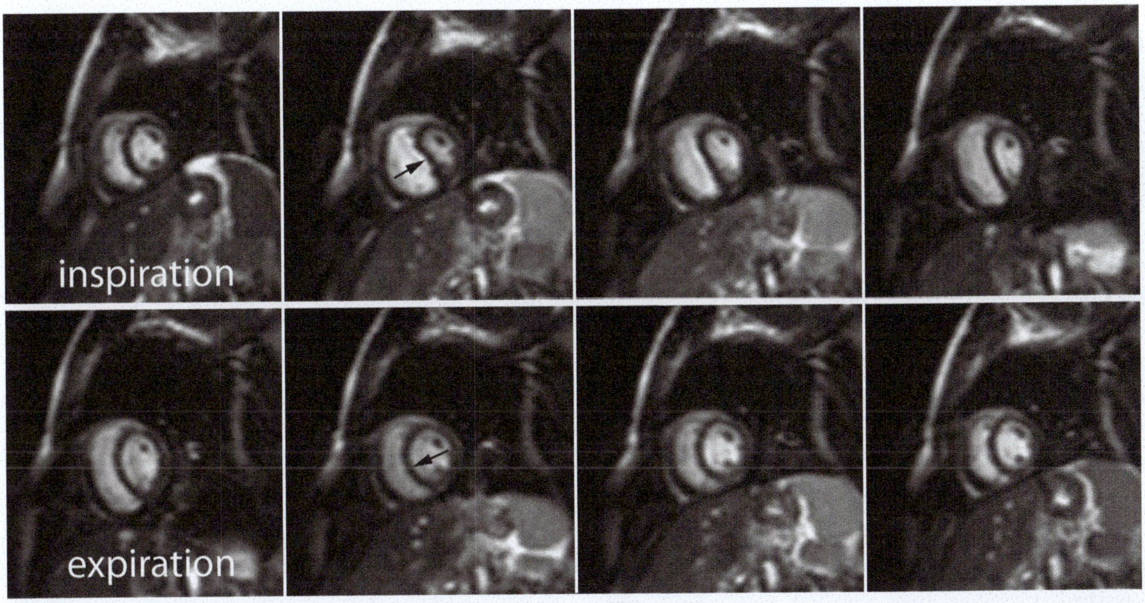

Fig. 27 Assessment of increased ventricular coupling during free breathing using real-time cine MRI in constrictive pericarditis. The figure shows eight short-axis cine panels obtained at early diastole during inspiration (upper row) and during expiration (lower row). Each row shows four consecutive heartbeats. At the onset of inspiration, a septal inversion occurs (*arrow*, upper row). The magnitude is most pronounced during the first heartbeat, and rapidly diminishes during the consecutive heartbeats. During expiration, an opposite phenomenon occurs with a right-sided septal shift (*arrow*, lower row)

abnormalities, while in restrictive cardiomyopathy a pattern similar to healthy volunteers was found (Fig. 28). Quantification of the maximal respiratory septal excursion was helpful to differentiate both groups of patients. Also in patients with inflammatory pericarditis, increased septal excursion was found likely reflecting the decreased compliance of the inflamed pericardial layers. Real-time MRI may be appealing to depict increased ventricular coupling in patients with non or minimally thickened constrictive pericarditis where the morphologic pericardial abnormalities are minimal or absent (Fig. 29) .

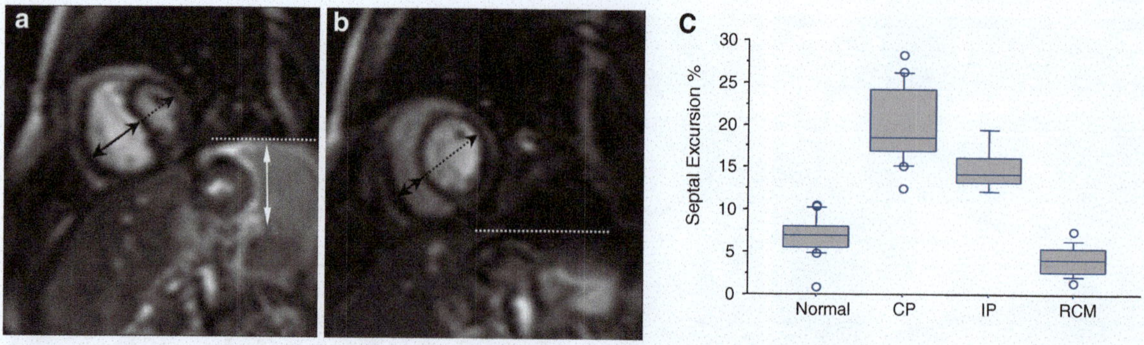

Fig. 28 Assessment of total respiratory septal shift using real-time cine imaging. The difference in early-diastolic position of the ventricular septum between onset of inspiration (**a**) and onset of expiration (**b**) is useful to differentiate between patients with constrictive pericarditis (CP) and patients with restrictive cardiomyopathy (RCM). While, the first group shows a significant increase in septal excursion compared to healthy volunteers, RCM patients have a tendency toward decreased septal excursion. Also note the increased septal excursion in patients with inflammatory pericarditis (IP) which can be explained by the decreased compliance of the inflammatory thickened pericardium. Adapted from Francone et al. 2006

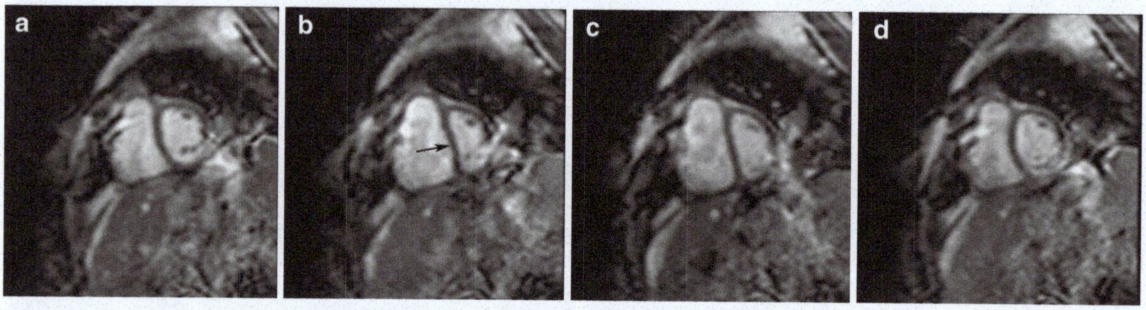

Fig. 29 Real-time cine imaging during free breathing in a patient with non-thickened constrictive pericarditis (similar patient as in Fig. 24). Short-axis cine imaging at early diastole during four consecutive heartbeats (**a–d**). During onset of inspiration a septal inversion (*arrow*, **b**) is seen, rapidly normalizing during the consecutive heart beats

Assessment of pericardial mobility is another potential application of dynamic MRI, and is appealing to differentiate normal from rigid pericardium. The latter exhibits no or at most a limited displacement, while normal pericardium slightly moves during the cardiac cycle, often in synchronicity with the underlying myocardial motion. Moreover, the restricted expansion of the myocardium during cardiac filling abutting against the stiff pericardium can be well appreciated. These issues may be important in diagnosing patients with minimally or non-thickened constrictive pericarditis. MRI tagging may be of help to demonstrate extension of the fibrocalcific process into the underlying myocardium.

6.4 Pericardial Masses

Primary tumors of the pericardium are rare entities, occurring much less frequently than pericardial metastasis (Syed et al. 2008) (see "Cardiac Masses"). Pericardial mesothelioma is the most common primary malignant tumor of the pericardium, and is often associated with hemorrhagic pericardial effusion. Other primary tumors include malignant fibrosarcoma, angiosarcoma and benign and malignant teratoma (Gomes et al. 1987; Lund et al. 1989; Syed et al. 2008). MRI has the advantage to accurately delineate the tumor implantation and determine its relation to contiguous anatomical structures. Tissue characterization of pericardial tumors is often not possible, exceptions being lipoma and liposarcoma, which appear with high-signal intensity due to their fatty content. Pericardial metastases are, in most cases, secondary to lung or breast carcinoma, leukemia or lymphoma (Oyama et al. 2004; Smith et al. 2001). They are often associated with a large and hemorrhagic effusion that is disproportionate in size to the amount of tumor present. Since metastatic pericardial implants are often small, they might be difficult or even not visible on MRI.

Other entities that have a mass-like appearance are pericardial hematoma and pericardial gossypiboma. The appearance and MRI signal characteristics of a pericardial hematoma depends on the age of the collection (Maksimovic et al. 2006). Pericardial gossypiboma or foreign body granuloma should be considered in patients with previous cardiac surgery. In the pericardium, it includes surgical sponges in the pericardial space overlooked after pericardiectomy (Maksimovic et al. 2006; Bogaert and Francone 2009).

7 Conclusions

The added value of MRI compared to the standard techniques used for assessment of patients with pericardial diseases has substantially increased in recent years, questioning whether this technique should not be considered the most appropriate non-invasive modality to study the pericardium (Table 1). Strong points in favor of MRI are the integration of anatomic and functional information within a single examination, the ability for tissue characterization and to determine the presence and degree of inflammation and activity of disease, and the value of MRI to accurately assess the rest of the heart, in particular the myocardium, helpful in the differential diagnosis, which currently often remains a diagnostic challenge.

8 Key Points

- Consider the pericardium as a functional and not purely as a morphological structure. MRI is at present probably the best technique to comprehensively evaluate pericardial abnormalities and their impact on cardiac function and filling.
- Since pericardial pathology may be focal, the entire pericardium should be evaluated for abnormalities, a task that can be best accomplished using MR imaging in different positions (preferably perpendicularly oriented).
- A simple pericardial effusion has smooth contours and no visible pericardial layers.
- Contrast-enhanced MRI is helpful for depicting pericardial inflammation, and for better differentiation between pericardial layers and fluid.
- The main hallmark in constrictive pericarditis is not a thickened pericardium but a non-compliant, stiff pericardium impeding ventricular filling.
- A normal or near-normal thickness of the pericardium does not completely rule out constrictive pericarditis.
- Pathological ventricular coupling is frequently found in constrictive pericarditis and is very helpful in differentiating of restrictive cardiomyopathy.
- Real-time cine imaging during free breathing provides useful information regarding the presence of pathological ventricular coupling, and requires minimal extra measurement time.

References

Abbas AE, Appleton CP, Liu PT, Sweeney JP (2005) Congenital absence of the pericardium: case presentation and review of literature. Int J Cardiol 98:21–25

Aletras AH, Tilak GS, Natanzon A et al (2006) Retrospective determination of the area at risk for reperfused acute myocardial infarction with T2-weighted cardiac magnetic resonance imaging. Circulation 113:1865–1870

Amplatz K, Moller JH (1993) Radiology of congenital heart disease. Mosby year book, St-Louis MO

Bogaert J, Duerinckx AJ (1995) Appearance of the normal pericardium on coronary MR angiograms. J Magn Reson Imaging 5:579–587

Bogaert J, Francone M (2009) Cardiovascular magnetic resonance in pericardial diseases. J Cardiovasc Magn Reson 11:14

Bogaert J, Taylor AM, Van Kerkhove F, Dymarkowski S (2004) Use of the inversion-recovery contrast-enhanced MRI technique for cardiac imaging: spectrum of diseases. Am J Roentgenol 182:609–615

Bush CA, Stang JM, Wooley CF, Kilman JW (1977) Occult constrictive pericardial disease. Circulation 56:924–930

Candell-Riera J, Garcia del Castillo H, Permanyer-Miralda G, Soler–Soler J (1978) Echocardiographic features of the interventricular septum in chronic constrictive pericarditis. Circulation 57:1154–1158

Carretta A, Negri G, Pansera M, Melloni G, Zannini P (2003) Thoracoscopic treatment of a pericardial diverticulum. Surg Endosc 17:158–159

Chako AC, Tempany CM, Zerhouni EA (1995) Effect of slice acquisition direction on image quality in thoracic MRI. J Comput Assist Tomogr 19:936–940

Francone M, Dymarkowski S, Kalantzi M, Bogaert J (2005) Real-time cine MRI of ventricular septal motion. A novel approach to assess ventricular coupling. J Magn Reson Imaging 21:305–309

Francone M, Dymarkowski S, Kalantzi M, Rademakers FE, Bogaert J (2006) Assessment of ventricular coupling with real-time cine MRI and its value to differentiate constrictive pericarditis from restrictive cardiomyopathy. Eur Radiol 16:944–951

Frank H, Globits S (1999) Magnetic resonance imaging evaluation of myocardial and pericardial disease. J Magn Reson Imaging 10:617–626

Freeman GL, LeWinter MM (1984) Pericardial adaptations during chronic cardiac dilation in dogs. Circ Res 54:294–300

Freeman GL, LeWinter MM (1986) Determinants of the intrapericardial pressure in dogs. J Appl Physiol 60:758–764

Freeman GL, Little WC (1986) Comparison of in situ and in vitro studies of pericardial pressure–volume relation in the dogs. Am J Physiol 251:H421–H427

Friedrich MG, Abdel-Aty H, Taylor A, Schulz-Menger J, Messroghli D, Dietz R (2008) The salvaged area at risk in reperfused acute myocardial infarction as visualized by cardiovascular magnetic resonance. J Am Coll Cardiol 51:1581–1587

Gibson TC, Grossman W, McLaurin MP, Moos S, Craige E (1976) An echocardiographic study of the interventricular septum in constrictive pericarditis. British Heart J 38: 738–743

Giorgi B, Mollet NRA, Dymarkowski S, Rademakers FA, Bogaert J (2003) Assessment of ventricular septal motion in patients clinically suspected of constrictive pericarditis, using magnetic resonance imaging. Radiology 228:417–424

Glover LB, Barcia A, Reeves TJ (1969) Congenital absence of the pericardium. Am J Radiol 106:542–548

Gomes AS, Lois JF, Child JS, Brown K, Batra P (1987) Cardiac tumors and thrombus: evaluation with MR imaging. Am J Radiol 149:895–899

Groell R, Schaffler GJ, Rienmueller R (1999) Pericardial sinuses and recesses: findings at electrocardiographically triggered electron-beam CT. Radiology 212:69–73

Gutierrez FR, Shackelford GD, McKnight RC, Levitt RG, Hartmann A (1985) Diagnosis of congenital absence of left pericardium by MR imaging. J Comput Assist Tomogr 9:551–553

Haley JH, Tajik J, Danielson GK, Schaff HV, Mulvagh SL, Oh JK (2004) Transient constrictive pericarditis: causes and natural history. J Am Coll Cardiol 43:271–275

Hancock EW (2001) Differential diagnosis of restrictive cardiomyopathy and constrictive pericarditis. Heart 86: 343–349

Hancock EW (2004) A clearer view of effusive-constrictive pericarditis. N Engl J Med 350:435–437

Hasuda T, Satoh T, Yamada N et al (1999) A case of constrictive pericarditis with local thickening of the pericardium without manifest ventricular interdepence. Cardiology 92:214–216

Hatle LK, Appleton CP, Popp RL (1989) Differentiation of constrictive pericarditis and restrictive cardiomyopathy by Doppler echocardiography. Circulation 79:357–370

Hurrell DG, Nishimura RA, Higano ST et al (1996) Value of dynamic respiratory changes in left and right ventricular pressures for the diagnosis of constrictive pericarditis. Circulation 963:2007–2013

Im JG, Rosen A, Webb WR, Gamsu G (1988) MR imaging of the transverse sinus of the pericardium. Am J Roentgenol 150:79–84

Janicki JS, Weber KT (1980) The pericardium and ventricular interaction, distensibility, and function. Am J Physiol 238:H494–H503

Klein C, Graf K, Fleck E, Nagel E (2003) Acute fibrinous pericarditis assessed with magnetic resonance imaging. Images in cardiovascular medicine. Circulation 107:e82

Kojima S, Yamada N, Goto Y (1999) Diagnosis of constrictive pericarditis by tagged cine magnetic resonance imaging. N Engl J Med 341:373–374

Kushwaha SS, Fallon JT, Fuster V (1997) Restrictive cardiomyopathy. N Engl J Med 336:267–276

Letanche G, Gayet C, Souquet PJ et al (1988) Agenesis of the pericardium: clinical, echocardiographic and MRI aspects. Rev Pneumol Clin 44:105–109

Ling LH, Oh JK, Schaff HV et al (1999) Constrictive pericarditis in the modern era: evolving clinical spectrum and impact on outcome after pericardiectomy. Circulation 100:1380–1386

Little WC, Freeman GL (2006) Pericardial disease. Circulation 133:1622–1632

Lorell BH, Braunwald E (1988) Pericardial disease. In: Braunwald E (ed) Heart disease, a textbook of cardiovascular medicine. W.B. Saunders, Philadelphia, pp 1484–1485

Lund JT, Ehman RL, Julsrud PR, Sinak LJ, Tajik AJ (1989) Cardiac masses: assessment by MR imaging. Am J Radiol 152:469–473

Mahrholdt H, Wagner A, Deluigi CC et al (2006) Presentation, patterns of myocardial damage, and clinical course of viral myocarditis. Circulation 114:1581–1590

Maisch B, Seferovic PM, Ristic AD et al (2004) Guidelines on the diagnosis and management of pericardial diseases executive summary: the task force on the diagnosis, management of pericardial diseases of the European Society of Cardiology. Eur Heart J 25:587–610

Maksimovic R, Dill T, Seferovic PM et al (2006) Magnetic resonance imaging in pericardial diseases. Herz 31:708–714

McMurdo KK, Webb WR, von Schulthess GK, Gamsu G (1985) Magnetic resonance imaging of the superior pericardial recesses. Am J Radiol 145:985–988

Misselt AJ, Harris SR, Glockner J, Feng D, Syed IS, Araoz PA (2008) MR imaging of the pericardium. Magn Reson Imaging Clin N Am 16:185–199

Mulvagh SL, Rokey R, Vick GWD, Johnston DL (1989) Usefulness of nuclear magnetic resonance imaging for evaluation of pericardial effusions, and comparison with two-dimensional echocardiography. Am J Cardiol 64: 1002–1009

Myers RBH, Spodick DH (1999) Constrictive pericarditis: clinical and pathophysiologic chararcteristics. Am Heart J 138:219–232

Nishimura RA (2001) Constrictive pericarditis in the modern era: a diagnostic dilemma. Heart 86:619–623

Oh KY, Shimizu M, Edwards WD, Tazelaar HD, Danielson GK (2001) Surgical pathology of the parietal pericardium. A study of 344 cases (1993–1999). Cardiovascul Pathol 10: 157–168

Oyama N, Oyam N, Komuro K et al (2004) Computed tomography and magnetic resonance imaging of the pericardium: anatomy and pathology. Magn Reson Med Sci 3:145–152

Paelinck BP, Lamb HJ, Bax JJ, Van der Wall EE, de Roos A (2002) Assessment of diastolic function by cardiovascular magnetic resonance. Am Heart J 144:198–205

Psychidis-Papakyritsis P, de Roos A, Kroft LJM (2007) Functional MRI of congenital absence of the pericardium. Am J Radiol 189:W312–W314

Rademakers FE, Bogaert J (2006) Cardiac dysfunction in heart failure with normal ejection fraction: MRI measurements. Prog Cardiovasc Dis 49:215–227

Restrepo CS, Diethelm L, Lemos JA et al (2006) Cardiovascular complications of human immunodeficiency virus infection. Radiographics 26:213–231

Roberts WC, Spray TL (1976) Pericardial heart disease: a study of its causes, consequences, and morphologic features. Cardiovasc Clin 7:11–65

Sagristà-Sauleda J (2004) Pericardial constriction: uncommon patterns. Heart 90:257–258

Sagristà-Sauleda J, Permanyer-Miralda G, Candell-Riera J, Angel J, Soler–Soler J (1987) Transient cardiac constriction: an unrecognized pattern of evolution in effusive acute idiopathic pericarditis. Am J Cardiol 59:961–966

Sagristà-Sauleda J, Angel J, Sanchez A, Permanyer-Miralda G, Soler-Soler J (2004) Effusive-constrictive pericarditis. N Engl J Med 350:469–475

Santamore WP, Bartlett R, Van Buren SJ, Dowd MK, Kutcher MA (1986) Ventricular coupling in constrictive pericarditis. Circulation 74:597–602

Scheuermann-Freestone M, Orchard E et al (2007) Partial congenital absence of the pericardium. Circulation 116: e126–e129

Sechtem U, Tscholakoff D, Higgins CB (1986a) MRI of the normal pericardium. AJR Am J Roentgenol 147:239–244

Sechtem U, Tscholakoff D, Higgins CB (1986b) MRI of the abnormal pericardium. AJR Am J Roentgenol 147: 245–252

Skouri HN, Dec GW, Friedrich MG, Cooper LT (2006) Noninvasive imaging in myoccarditis. J Am Coll Cardiol 48:2085–2093

Smith WHT, Beacock DJ, Goddard AJP et al (2001) Magnetic resonance evaluation of the pericardium: a pictorial review. Br J Radiol 74:384–392

Solomon SL, Brown JJ, Glazer HS, Mirowitz SA, Lee JKT (1990) Thoracic aortic dissection: pitfalls and artifacts in MR imaging. Radiology 177:223–228

Soulen RL, Stark DD, Higgins CB (1985) Magnetic resonance imaging of constrictive pericardial disease. Am J Cardiol 55:480–484

Spodick DH (1992) Macrophysiology, microphysiology, and anatomy of the pericardium: a synopsis. Am Heart J 124:1046–1051

Spodick DH (2003) Acute cardiac tamponade. N Engl J Med 349:684–690

Stark DD, Higgins CB, Lanzer P et al (1984) Magnetic resonance imaging of the pericardium: normal and pathologic findings. Radiology 150:469–474

Syed IS, Feng D, Harris SR et al (2008) MR imaging of cardiac masses. Magn Reson Imaging Clin N Am 16:137–164

Talreja DR, Edwards WD, Danielson GK et al (2003) Constrictive pericarditis in 26 patients with histologically normal pericardial thickness. Circulation 108:1852–1857

Taylor RR, Covell JW, Sonnenblick EH, JJr Ross (1967) Dependence of ventricular distensibility on filling of the opposite ventricle. Am J Physiol 213:711–718

Taylor AM, Dymarkowski S, Verbeken E, Bogaert J (2006) Detection of pericardial inflammation with late-enhancement cardiac magnetic resonance imaging: initial results. Eur Radiol 16:569–574

Troughton RW, Asher CR, Klein AL (2004) Pericarditis. Lancet 363:717–727

van den Hout RJ, Lamb HJ, van den Aardweg JG et al (2003) Real-time MR imaging of aortic flow: influence of breathing on left ventricular stroke volume in chronic obstructive pulmonary disease. Radiology 229:513–519

Wang ZJ, Reddy GP, Gotway MB, Yeh BM, Hetts SW, Higgins CB (2003) CT and MR imaging of pericardial disease. Radiographics 23:S167–S180

Yelgec NS, Dymarkowski S, Ganame J, Bogaert J (2007) Value of MRI in patients with a clinical suspicion of acute myocarditis. Eur Radiol 17:2211–2217

Cardiac Masses

J. Bogaert and S. Dymarkowski

Contents

1	**Introduction**	411
2	**Clinical Presentation**	412
3	**Conventional Imaging Modalities**	412
3.1	X-ray Angiography	412
3.2	Echocardiography	415
3.3	Computed Tomography	415
3.4	Magnetic Resonance Imaging	415
4	**Classification**	418
4.1	Primary Cardiac Tumors	418
4.2	Secondary Cardiac Tumors	433
4.3	Para and Extracardiac Tumors	437
4.4	Nontumoral Cardiac Masses and Mimics	439
4.5	Normal Cardiac Anatomy and Variants	452
4.6	Prosthetic Valves and Other Foreign Devices	456
5	**Conclusions**	458
6	**Key Points**	458
References		459

Abstract

Our look at cardiac tumors and cardiac masses in general has fundamentally changed with the advent of noninvasive cardiac imaging. At present, MRI is probably the technique offering the clinician the most comprehensive approach, even omitting biopsy in a considerable number of patients. Everyone routinely dealing with cardiac imaging will sporadically encounter cardiac masses. Good knowledge of the diversity of pathologies that may present as masses, as well as how cardiac imaging technique should be applied is the best guarantee to correctly diagnose this group of cardiac pathologies. The focus of this chapter is on how MRI can be used to depict cardiac masses, and to differentiate between tumoral and nontumoral conditions. In this chapter, the MRI features of the most common cardiac tumors/masses are summarized and extensively illustrated, providing the reader an useful aid when encountering cardiac tumors/masses in daily clinical practice.

1 Introduction

Before the era of modern cardiac imaging techniques, the diagnosis of cardiac tumors was extremely difficult and often not made antemortem. Nowadays, the availability of transthoracic (TTE) and transesophageal echocardiography (TEE), cardiac computed tomography, and magnetic resonance imaging (MRI) has greatly facilitated their detection. However, because of their rarity and the nonspecific, often misleading, symptomatology that causes them to be

J. Bogaert · S. Dymarkowski (✉)
Department of Radiology and Medical Imaging Research Center (MIRC), University Hospitals Gasthuisberg, Catholic University of Leuven, Herestraat 49, 3000, Leuven, Belgium
e-mail: steven.dymarkowski@uz.kuleuven.ac.be

J. Bogaert et al. (eds.), *Clinical Cardiac MRI*, Medical Radiology. Diagnostic Imaging,
DOI: 10.1007/174_2011_338,

placed at the bottom of the differential diagnostic list, their diagnosis may be considerably delayed. Therefore, a great deal of suspicion is required to direct the clinician toward the proper diagnosis.

The title to this chapter, "Cardiac Masses" was preferred to "Cardiac Tumors" for more than one reason. First, not only are nontumoral cardiac masses much more frequent than true cardiac tumors, but also nontumoral masses usually require a medical (or no) treatment whereas cardiac surgery is still the preferred therapeutic approach for cardiac tumors. Thus, accurate differentiation between the two conditions is a first requirement for each imaging technique dealing with the diagnosis of cardiac masses. Second, precise knowledge of the normal cardiac anatomy and its variants is required since with the advent of modern cardiac imaging techniques, not only are abnormal masses much more easily and frequently detected, but normal cardiac structures may be interpreted as abnormal by inexperienced people. Therefore the major aims of this chapter are to guide the reader in recognizing the diversity of cardiac tumors, nontumoral masses, and normal variants, to discuss their appearance on MRI, and to highlight the role of MRI in the detection and differentiation of cardiac masses, comparing this technique with the other cardiac imaging techniques.

2 Clinical Presentation

The clinical presentation of tumors originating in the heart is often atypical, suggestive more of a systemic illness than a cardiovascular problem (Salcedo et al. 1992; Butany et al. 2006; Maraj et al. 2009). Therefore, a high index of suspicion and a goal-directed diagnostic approach are required. Cardiac tumors can manifest in one of several ways (Table 1). They can be an incidental finding on chest radiography, echocardiography, or another cardiovascular diagnostic test (Fig. 1). The first symptoms can be constitutional, particularly in patients with myxomas, and a high index of suspicion is needed to make the proper diagnosis. Cardiovascular symptoms, specifically congestive heart failure and thromboembolism, can be the presenting manifestations. Since these are rather nonspecific, a great deal of suspicion is required to direct the clinician toward the proper diagnosis. Finally, patients with noncardiac malignancies can have cardiac involvement with or without cardiovascular symptoms.

Table 1 Presentation of cardiac tumors

Systemic illness
Cardiovascular symptoms
Congestive heart failure
Thromboembolism
Arrhythmias/interventricular conduction disturbances
Incidental finding
History of noncardiac malignancy

In patients with cardiac tumors, the history and clinical findings are determined primarily by the anatomic location of the tumor rather than by the histopathology. It can be said that cardiac tumors can be clinically and pathologically benign, but have a "malignant" and fatal outcome, or they can be clinically and pathologically malignant. Generally, tumors manifest symptomatology and clinical signs by virtue of tumor growth that impedes cardiac hemodynamics. Thus, large infiltrative tumors may be clinically silent, while smaller, yet strategically located tumors can produce dramatic symptomatology due to transient obstruction of flow across the valve. Arrhythmias and interventricular conduction defects may also be encountered as a consequence of tumor infiltrating the conduction system.

3 Conventional Imaging Modalities

Whether a cardiac imaging modality is useful in the diagnosis of patients with suspected cardiac masses depends on following requirements: high accuracy (i.e., low rate of false-negative and false-positive results), accurate evaluation of tumor extent and tumor composition (i.e., tissue characterization), and detection of complications (e.g., valvular obstruction). At present, several cardiac imaging techniques are available. Although this chapter is focused on the role of MRI, the advantages and limitations of the other currently available imaging techniques are briefly discussed and summarized in Table 2.

3.1 X-ray Angiography

In many cases, noninvasive imaging (i.e., echocardiography, computed tomography, and MRI) will provide adequate preoperative information on the

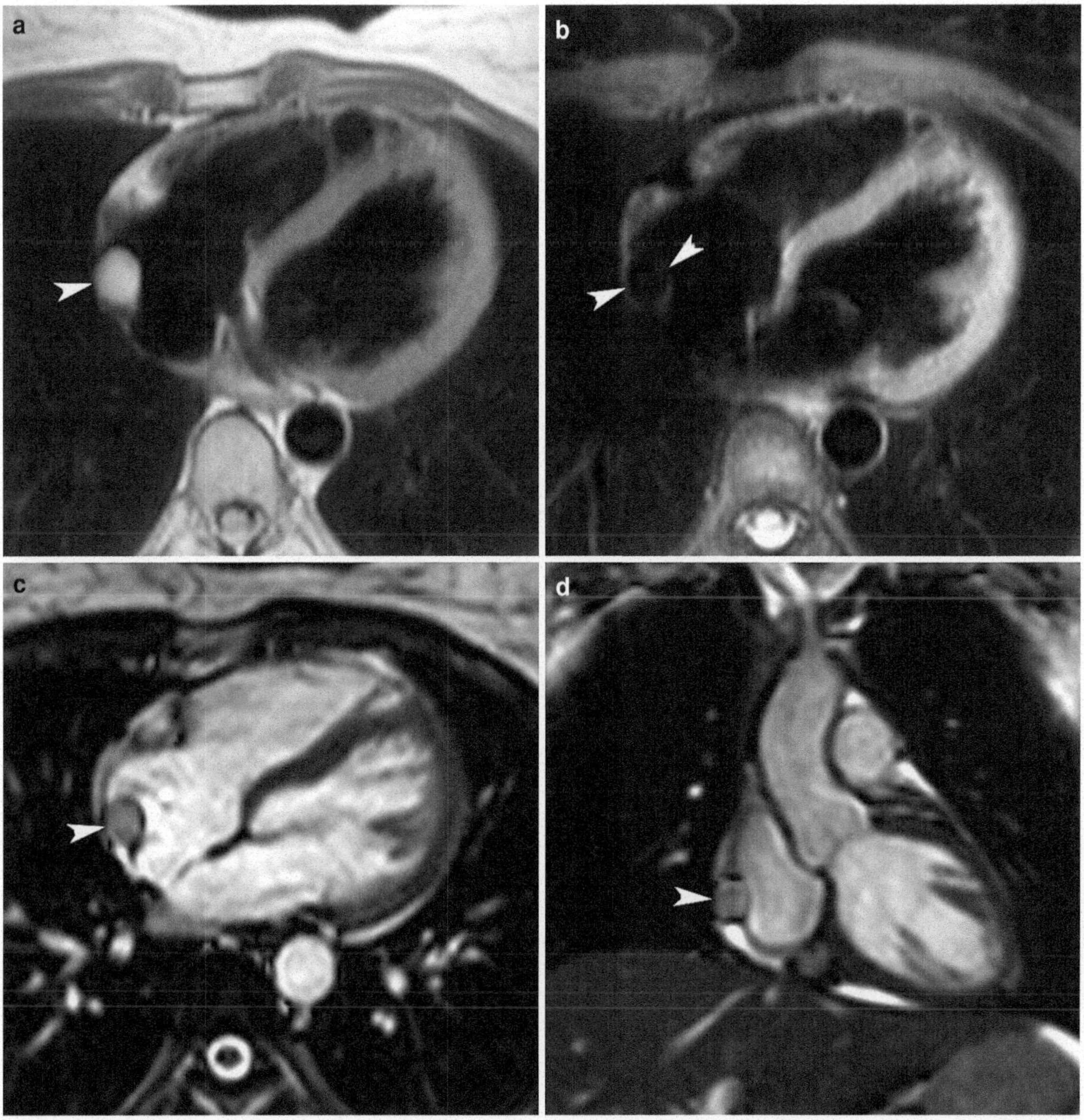

Fig. 1 Incidental finding of RA mass on transthoracic ultrasound in 37-year-old woman presenting with atypical chest pain. For further investigation, a MRI examination was performed showing the presence of a small atrial lipoma. Axial T1w-imaging without (**a**) and with fat suppression prepulse (**b**). Cine imaging in axial (**c**) and coronal (**d**) plane. A rounded, well-defined, homogeneous, hyperintense mass embedded in the RA lateral wall is nicely visible on T1w-imaging (*arrowhead*, **a**). On fat-suppressed T1w-imaging, the signal of the mass is completely suppressed (*arrowheads*, **b**), proving the fatty nature of the mass lesion. Cine imaging enables to well depict the relationship to the atrial wall (*arrowhead*, **c**, **d**). Notice the presence of a small amount of pericardial fluid

location and extent of the cardiac tumor, so that no further cardiac catheterization and selective angiocardiography is required. However, in special circumstances information can be needed (a) when inadequate information on the tumor location, attachment, or extent is obtained by the noninvasive imaging methods, (b) when a malignant tumor is considered likely, and (c) when other cardiac lesions (e.g., coronary artery or valvular lesions) may coexist with a cardiac tumor and possibly dictate a different

Table 2 Advantages and limitations of current cardiac imaging techniques in the detection of cardiac masses

	Advantages	Limitations
X-ray angiography	Tumor size/shape/mobility/location	Radiation/cost
		Invasive
	Tumor vascularity	Dislodgement of tumor fragments
	Nutritive supply	Only indirect information on
		Myocardial masses or invasion
		Pericardial effusions/masses
		False-positive/-negative results
TTE	Widely available/portable	Poor echogenicity in 30% of patients
	Accurate/real-time imaging	No tissue characterization
	Relatively inexpensive	Poor evaluation of pericardium/extracardiac structures
	Tumor size/shape/mobility/location	
TEE	Advantages = those of TTE	Semi-invasive procedure
	Better than TTE in:	Evaluation of pericardium/extracardiac structures may be insufficient
	Defining tumor attachment and tumor extension	No tissue characterization
	Detecting cardiac thrombi	
	Evaluation of pericardium and extracardiac structures	
CT	Noninvasive	Radiation exposure
	High-spatial resolution	Iodinated contrast material required
	High-temporal resolution (ultrafast mode)	No real multiplanar imaging capability
	Possibility of multiplanar reconstruction	
	Tumor size/shape/mobility/location	
	Tissue characterization to a limited extent	
MRI	Noninvasive	Absolute and relative contraindications (such as pacemaker, intracranial vascular clips)
	High-spatial and temporal resolution	Claustrophobia
	Multiplanar imaging capability	
	Large field of view	
	Tumor size/shape/mobility/location	
	Accurate information on tumor extent and tumor vascularity	
	Tissue characterization to a certain extent	

surgical approach (Fueredi et al. 1989). Cardiac tumors present on X-ray angiography as (a) intracavitary filling defects, (b) compression, displacement, or deformation of the cardiac chambers, (c) increased myocardial wall thickness, or (d) local alteration in wall motion. Furthermore, coronary arteriography may provide information on the vascular pattern of the tumor, its vascular supply, and its relation to the coronary arteries (Singh et al. 1984). Differentiation with nontumoral conditions such as thrombus, intramuscular hydatid cyst, and aneurysm may not be possible, which yields a high number of false-positive results. Furthermore, X-ray angiocardiography may be false-negative in patients not suspected for cardiac tumor prior to the catheterization. Finally, the invasiveness of this procedure entails the risk of peripheral embolization due to dislodgement of tumor fragments.

3.2 Echocardiography

Echocardiography is considered the mainstay imaging modality in the diagnosis of cardiac tumors. This technique may provide valuable information regarding size, mobility, shape, and location of cardiac masses, but it cannot describe histologic features. While transthoracic echocardiography is often sufficient for a complete evaluation, transesophageal echocardiography (TEE), or alternatively MRI, may be needed in patients yielding inadequate image quality such as obese patients or patients with obstructive pulmonary disease. Moreover, the transesophageal approach is superior to the transthoracic approach in defining the attachment point of myxomas, in evaluation of compression or infiltration of the cardiovascular system by malignant tumors, and in detecting left atrial thrombi, especially when located in the left atrial appendage (Mugge et al. 1991; Herrera et al. 1992; Engberding et al. 1993). Often, additional noninvasive imaging, using computed tomography or MRI, is required to better characterize the nature and extent of cardiac masses (Altbach et al. 2007; van Beek et al. 2007; Fussen et al. 2011).

3.3 Computed Tomography

Multidetector CT is currently the closest competitor to MRI for morphologic evaluation of cardiac masses enabling to depict very well intra- and extra-cardiac masses, as well as their degree of myocardial or pericardial involvement (Araoz et al. 2000; van Beek et al. 2007; Hoey et al. 2009a; Anavekar et al. 2010). This technique has a very high-spatial resolution, and a sufficiently high-temporal resolution to provide sharp cardiac images, especially if combined with ECG-triggering. It should be emphasized that also on non-ECG triggered “routine” chest CT examinations, cardiac masses are not infrequently depicted. In particular, in patients with a clinical history of malignancy, one should carefully assess the heart for the presence of cardiac metastases (Fig. 2) (Bogaert et al. 2010). For an optimal evaluation of the cardiac structures, administration of intravenous iodinated contrast medium is needed.

3.4 Magnetic Resonance Imaging

Compared to the imaging modalities discussed in previous paragraphs, MRI is probably the most appealing technique to study patients with suspected cardiac masses (Sparrow et al. 2005; Grizzard and Ang 2007; O’Donnell et al. 2009; Fussen et al. 2011). MRI combines high-spatial, temporal, and contrast resolution, free choice of image plane and image size, myocardial motion and perfusion assessment, and this technique is without any doubt the best for tissue characterization. As such highly valuable information can be provided regarding (a) presence, location, size, nature, and extent of cardiac masses; (b) depiction of complications such as valvular entrapment or pericardial effusion; and (c) impact on myocardial contractility and viability. This information is crucial in planning patient’s therapy, particularly if surgical intervention is being considered. Moreover, mimics, such as normal anatomic variants, not infrequently misinterpreted as cardiac mass or tumor by other imaging modalities, are usually well recognized by MRI. A distinct advantage over echocardiography is the large field of view, which allows perfect assessment of both the intracardiac as extracardiac tumor extent. Also, evaluation of the relationship of pericardial, pulmonary, or mediastinal masses to the heart is usually straightforward by MRI. Moreover, MRI may be useful in detecting (early) recurrence postoperatively particularly in patients where surgery has decreased the echo window (Kaminaga et al. 1993). Finally, the evolution toward real-time imaging makes MRI a though competitor with other real-time cardiac imaging modalities in particular echocardiography (Spuentrup et al. 2003).

In contrast to the early days of cardiac MRI where the spin-echo technique was the main sequence to study patients with suspected cardiac masses, nowadays we use a set of different sequences to obtain information regarding morphology and tissue characterization, perfusion and enhancement patterns, mobility and deformation, and to evaluate the impact on cardiac dynamics and integrity (Figs. 3, 4). It is difficult to provide the reader a straightforward, easy-to-use protocol that can be applied in every patient. Instead, one should be well familiar with the arsenal of available MRI sequences that can be used to study this group of patients. A stepwise approach is probably the best guarantee toward a successful examination. Imaging can be started using fast bright-blood or dark-blood

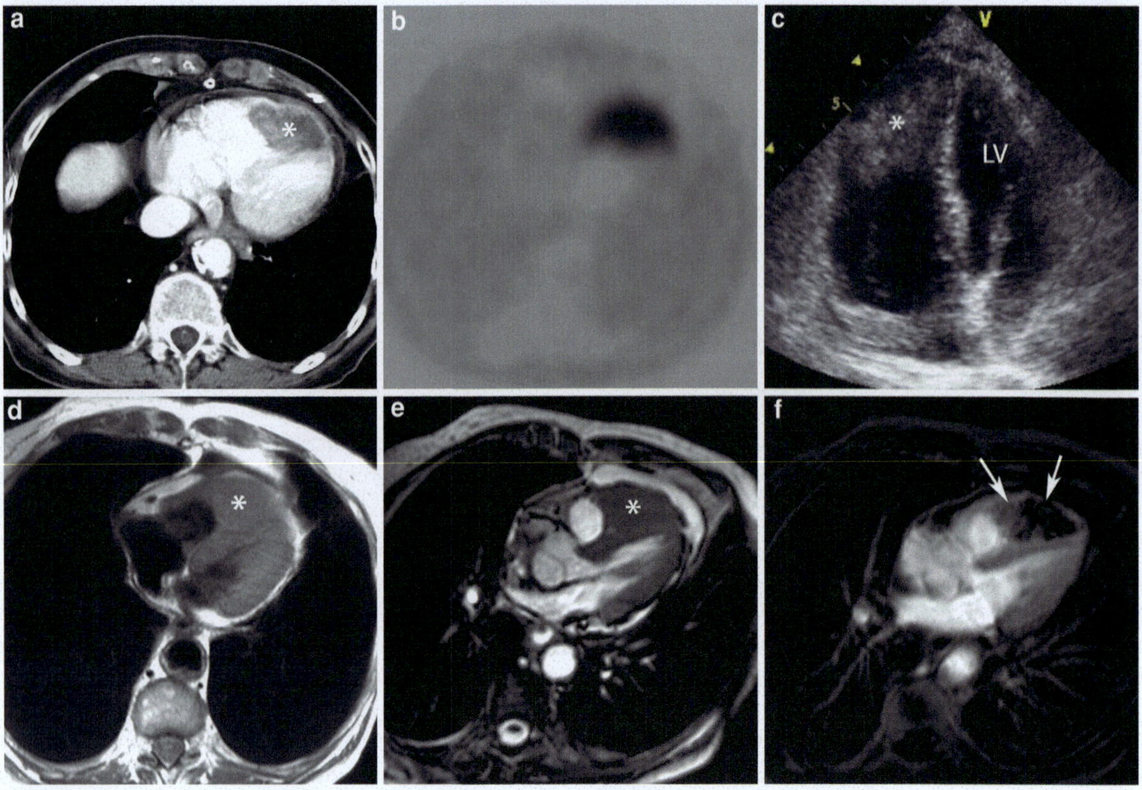

Fig. 2 Multimodality imaging in a 60-year-old woman with esophageal cancer presenting with a metastasis in RV apex. All images are obtained in axial or horizontal long-axis direction. Axial contrast-enhanced CT (**a**) shows irregular defined, slightly inhomogeneous mass in RV apex (*star*), presenting as an area of high tracer accumulation on FDG-PET scan (**b**). Transthoracic echocardiography shows large inhomogeneous mass in apical half of RV (*star,* **c**). On MRI, the structure appears isointense on T1w-imaging (*star*, **d**) and isointense on cine imaging (*star*, **e**). Following contrast administration the metastasis shows an inhomogeneous enhancement on late Gd imaging (*arrows*, **f**)

sequences in one or more imaging planes providing morphologic images of the heart and great vessels that provide a first impression and are used to plan the rest of the examination (Hoey et al. 2009a). A first set of questions that need to be solved is to describe the exact location, presentation and size of the mass, and to define the relationship with the surrounding cardiac structures. This can be approached using a combination of T1w-imaging and cine MRI in one or more imaging planes through the cardiac mass. For example for a mass arising on the interatrial septum (most likely a myxoma), we recommend imaging in both cardiac horizontal and short-axis. Hereby we prefer the dynamic nature of cine MRI above the static T1w images because besides evaluation of the mobility, often the point of attachment and the relation with the heart can be appreciated more appropriately. Also the mass/tumor border is often better visible on cine MRI. To evaluate the tissue characteristics of the cardiac mass a combination of different sequences is used, including T1w- and T2w-imaging, T1w-imaging with fat saturation prepulses, T1w-imaging following contrast administration, and late Gd MRI (Sparrow et al. 2005; Hoey et al. 2009a). First-pass perfusion MRI is of interest to evaluate the vascularity of the lesion. Also tumors with an abundancy of extracellular tissue often show strong enhancement during first-pass imaging. The appearance of the different cardiac masses and tumors will be described in detail in the following paragraphs, though it should be emphasized that the initial hope that the pattern of signal intensity would allow differentiation between benign and malignant neoplasms has not been fulfilled. In general, cystic masses e.g., (pleuro) pericardial cyst, have low-signal on T1w-imaging but a very high signal on T2w-imaging. Masses with a lipomatous composition, e.g.,

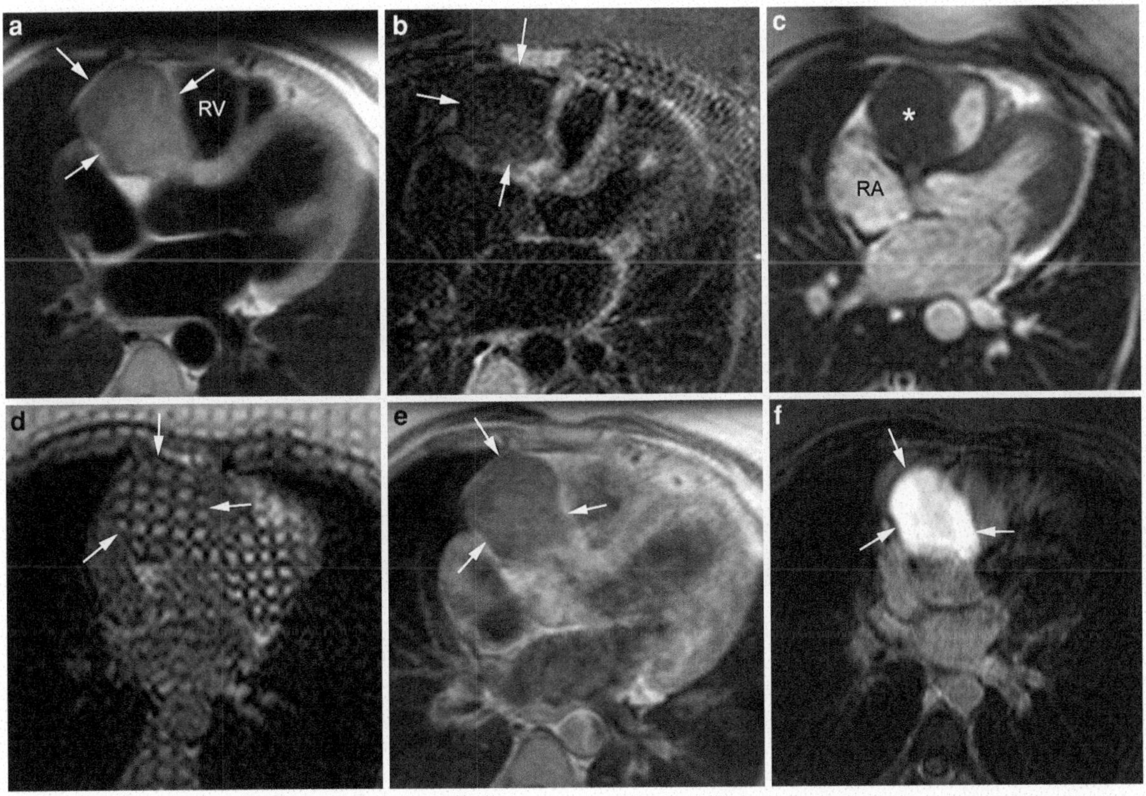

Fig. 3 Contribution of different MRI sequences in the description and characterization of a cardiac mass located in the right atrioventricular groove (*arrows-asterisk*) in a 27-year-old woman with neurofibromatosis. All images are obtained in the axial image plane. T1w-imaging shows a well-defined mass in the right atrioventricular groove partially compressing the RV cavity (**a**). The mass is iso-intense to the signal of myocardial tissue on T1w-imaging, and hypo-intense on T2w-imaging (**b**). Cine imaging (**c**) and SPAMM myocardial tagging (**d**) are highly helpful to evaluate the mobility and absence of deformation of the cardiac mass. Although after administration of paramagnetic contrast agents (gadopentetate dimeglumine) the mass is slightly hypo-intense compared to the myocardium (**e**) it appears strongly hyperintense on late Gd imaging using an inversion time of 250 min (**f**). The *star* and *arrows* indicate the cardiac mass in the right atrioventricular groove. Abbreviations: *RA* right atrium; *RV* right ventricle

lipomas and lipomatous hypertrophy of the interatrial septum, have signal characteristics similar to that of epicardial or subcutaneous fat, with high signal on T1w-imaging and moderate signal on T2w-imaging (Sechtem et al. 1986). Fat suppression techniques are particularly useful for proving the fatty nature of the lesion (see Figs. 1, 2). Most soft-tissue tumors have relaxation times shorter than fluid, but long enough to produce a relatively low-signal on T1w-imaging and a relatively high signal on T2w-imaging (Gamsu et al. 1984). Mineral-rich tissues, containing cortical bone and calcifications, and mature fibrotic tissue have few mobile protons, resulting in low-signal regardless of the type of sequence used. Intralesional hemorrhage will show a low-signal on T2w-imaging (Ganame et al. 2009). Distinction between intramural tumors and surrounding myocardium may be facilitated by administration of paramagnetic contrast agents, hereby assessing differences in first-pass perfusion characteristics and late enhancement patterns (Funari et al. 1991). Contrast-enhanced MRI moreover provides information regarding the internal architecture i.e., presence of nonvascularized, necrotic, or cystic areas. The latter may be of help in the differential diagnosis, and to assess the efficacy of radio- and/or chemotherapy. Another application, in particular of late Gd imaging, is the depiction of intracavitary thrombi, which are visible as hypo-intense structures surrounded by the enhanced blood (Barkhausen et al. 2002; Mollet et al. 2002; Bogaert et al. 2004). Occasionally a chronic thrombus can be vascularized and enhance following contrast administration (Donato et al. 2009). In some

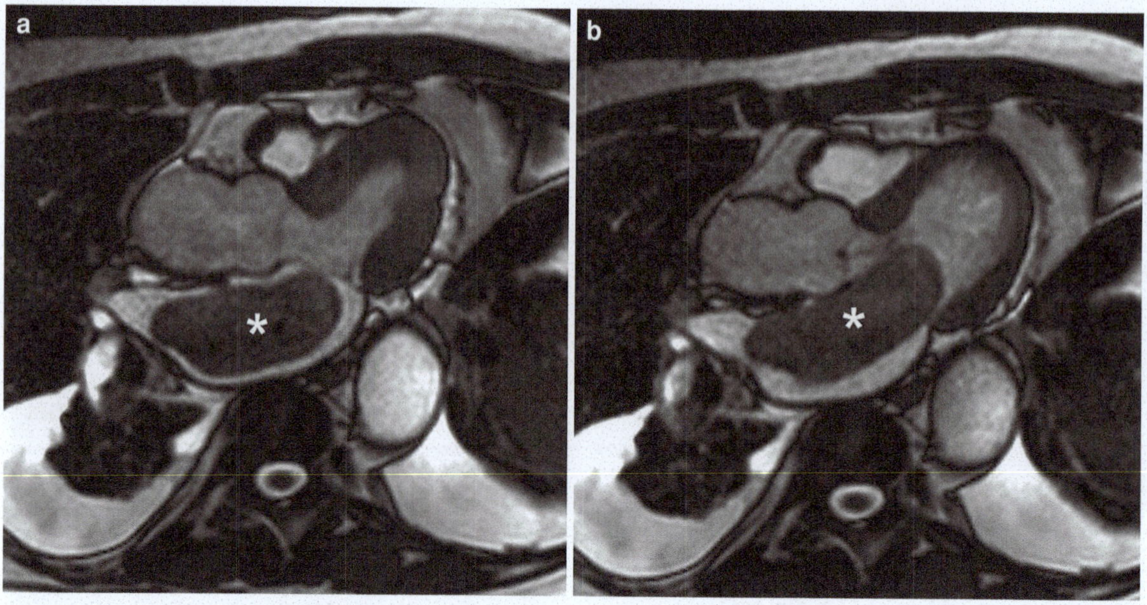

Fig. 4 Use of cine imaging to depict mobility of a giant LA myxoma. Axial cine imaging in systole (**a**) and diastole (**b**). Presence of an elongated, well-defined mass (*) in LA moving during diastole toward LV and causing mitral subobstruction. Note the presence of bilateral pleural fluid

circumstances, other MRI techniques such as myocardial tagging and phase-contrast MRI (PC-MRI) can be of use to improve the differentiation between tumor and myocardium or intracavitary blood, respectively (Rumancik et al. 1988). An interesting application of PC-MRI is the evaluation of valvular entrapment for example of a left atrial myxoma prolabating through the mitral valve during cardiac systole. In a study by Hoffmann et al. (2003) MRI was accurate in the prediction of the lesion type (area under the ROC curve of 0.88 and 0.92). In particular, tumor location, tissue composition, and presence of pericardial or pleural effusion were identified as key predictors of lesion type. In a recent study by Fussen et al. (2011), MRI correctly classified masses as 'benign or malignant' in 95% of cases.

4 Classification

Cardiac masses can be divided into neoplasms and nonneoplastic conditions. Besides primary benign and malignant tumors, the heart can be secondary affected by direct invasion, venous and/or lymphatic extension, or metastatic spread of an extracardiac malignancy. The nonneoplastic group is a heterogeneous entity including all nontumoral cardiac masses and other conditions that may appear "mass-like" on cardiac imaging (Table 3).

4.1 Primary Cardiac Tumors

Primary tumors of the heart and pericardium are extremely rare, with an incidence of between 0.0017 and 0.28% in unselected patients at autopsy, while metastatic tumors to the heart are considered to be 20–40 times more common than primary tumors (Heath 1968; McAllister and Fenoglio 1978). Three-quarters of all primary tumors are benign. Nearly half the benign tumors are myxomas, and the majority of the rest are lipomas, papillary fibroelastomas, and rhabdomyomas (Grebenc et al. 2000). Whereas myxomas are the most common primary tumors in adults, rhabdomyomas, and fibromas clearly predominante in children.

4.1.1 Benign Cardiac Tumors

4.1.1.1 Myxoma

Myxomas are the most frequent primary cardiac tumor typically presenting as intracavitary masses.

Table 3 MRI characteristics of the most common cardiac masses

	Preferential location	T1w-imaging	T2w-imaging	Cine MRI	Contrast enhancement	Appearance
Benign cardiac tumors						
Myxoma	Left atrium (IAS)	Variable	Variable	Low	Yes	Heterogeneous sharp border
Lipoma	No	High	High	Medium	No	Homogeneous, sharp border
Papillary fibroelastoma	Cardiac valves	Medium	Medium	Low	?	Small (less than 1 cm)
Rhabdomyoma	Atrium Intramyocardial/ Intracavitary	Medium/ high	Medium	Low	Similar to myocardium	Infants/Multiple Tendency to disappear
Fibroma	Ventricles Intramyocardial	Medium	Medium	Low	Variable	Infants/Single
Pheochromocytoma	Intrapercardial (roof of left atrium)		High		Yes	
Hemangioma	Ventricles Intramyocardial/ Intracavitary	Medium	Very high	Variable	Yes Variable	Heterogeneous
Malignant cardiac tumors						
Angiosarcoma	Right atrium Pericardial and Myocardial invasion	Variable (mixed)	Variable (mixed)	Low	Yes	Heterogeneous "Cauliflower" appearance
Rhabdomyosarcoma	No	Medium	High	?	Yes	
Malignant fibrous histiocytoma	Left atrium (posterior wall)	Medium	High	?	?	Slightly heterogeneous
Lymphoma	Pericardial effusion Intracardiac masses	Medium	Medium	Low	Yes	Variable
Malignant pericardial Mesothelioma	Pericardium	Medium	High	Low	Yes	Heterogeneous (no myocardial invasion)
Metastases	Variable, pericardial effusion	Low	High	Low	Yes	Often multiple
Nontumoral cardiac masses and mimics						
Thrombus	Atrium/Appendage (valve disease/AF) Ventricles (if diseased)	Medium to high	Medium to high	Low	No (possible if chronic)	Appearance related to age of thrombus
Valvular vegetations	Cardiac valves	Not visible	Not visible	Low	No	
Lipomatous hypertrophy of the interatrial septum	Interatrial septum	High	High	Medium	Low	"Camel hump" or "dumbbell" shaped, sparing the fossa ovalis
Hydatid cyst	Left ventricle (IVS)	Low	Very high		No	Low-signal intensity peripheral border (pericyst)
Pleuropericardial cyst	Right cardiophrenic angle	Low	Very high		No	Sharply defined

The signal intensity of the cardiac masses on SE sequences is compared with the signal intensity of myocardium. The signal intensity of the cardiac masses on GE sequences is compared with the signal intensity of flowing blood

AF atrial fibrillation, *IAS* interatrial septum, *IVS* interventricular septum, *GE* gradient-echo, *SE* spin-echo

Though they can virtually occur anywhere in the heart, about 75% of myxomas occur in the left atrium and the majority is attached to the interatrial septum near the fossa ovalis, either have a broad base, either pedunculated (Hanson 1992; Grebenc et al. 2000, 2002). Another 20% of myxomas is found in the right atrium without predilection for the fossa ovalis (McAllister 1979). The remainder are found in either the right or left ventricle.

The typical patient diagnosed with this condition is a middle-aged female presenting with vague complaints such as atypical chest pains, palpitations, or intermittent shortness of breath with few if any clinical findings. Before the era of diagnostic imaging, the majority of patients were diagnosed late and were moderately or severely symptomatic. Today, myxomas are usually diagnosed in earlier stages or found as incidental finding on routine cardiac imaging.

Depending on their size and mobility, myxomas commonly give rise to signs of obstructed ventricular filling with subsequent dyspnea, recurrent pulmonary edema, and right heart failure. These signs mimic the clinical picture of mitral or tricuspid valve stenosis. Embolism occurs in 30–40% of patients with myxomas. It is suggested that myxomas with high mobility or gelatinous consistency might present a higher incidence of embolization (Engberding et al. 1993; Grebenc et al. 2002). Since most myxomas are located in the left atrium, systemic embolism is particularly frequent. In the majority of cases, the cerebral arteries, including the retinal arteries, are affected. The differential diagnosis of peripheral embolism should therefore include myxoma. The rate of growth of myxomas is unknown but they generally appear to grow rather quickly. Myxomas have a malignant counterpart, "myxosarcomas", which also arise in the left atrium (Klima et al. 1986; Burke et al. 1992).

Myxomas present macroscopically as spherical, oval, or lobular masses. Delineation of the tumor surface may range from firm to gelatinous and irregular. Some myxomas may even have tentacles. Characteristic microscopic features are the typical myxoma cells in combination with an abundant myxomatous stroma. Additionally, intratumoral bleeding as well as calcification and ossification may occur, and the tumor surface may be covered by thrombus (Semelka et al. 1992). It is evident that the presentation of myxoma on MRI is strongly determined by the histological composition. Myxomas with the predominance of myxomatous stroma typically are hyperintense on T2w-imaging (Figs. 5, 6), while the presence of hemosiderin or calcification will lead to a heterogeneous appearance, in particular on T2w-imaging and cine MRI. High intralesional signal is reported to be related to subacute hemorrhage and in patients with abudant presence of hemosiderin the tumor volume may apparently enlarge on gradient-echo-based sequences (Fueredi et al. 1989; Watanabe et al. 1994). Also the enhancement following contrast administration is determined by the tumor histology (Matsuoka et al. 1996). Areas of enhancement correspond with histologic myxoma or inflammation, while unenhanced regions reflect necrosis of cystic changes (Fig. 7). As mentioned, cine MRI is the preferred technique to depict the exact tumor attachment, to differentiate between sessile and pedunculated forms and to depict complications such as atrioventricular tumor entrapment (Figs. 4, 6).

Their predilection to arise near the fossa ovalis facilitates the diagnosis of myxoma. However, when found in another location, differential diagnosis from other primary benign or malignant tumors, metastatic tumors and organized atrial thrombi is much more challenging. Clinical information, such as the presence of central venous catheter, history of cardiac transplantation or extracardiac malignancy, may be of help in making the correct diagnosis. If massive, depiction of the exact position of tumor attachment may be challenging (Fig. 8).

4.1.1.2 Lipoma

Cardiac lipomas account for approximately 10% of all cardiac neoplasms and about 14% of benign cardiac tumors (Hananouchi and Goff 1990). True lipomas are less frequent than lipomatous hypertrophy of the interatrial septum (see Sect. 4.4.4). Lipomas are benign tumors of encapsulated mature adipose cells, and can be found intracavitary, intramyocardial, or intrapericardial (Wolf et al. 1987). The left ventricle and right atrium are the most frequent locations (Fig. 1). Lipomas are usually asymptomatic and in most cases require no treatment or surgical intervention. Symptoms may be produced depending on tumor size and location. On CT, lipomas have a very low density (average -100 Hounsfield units) (Grebenc et al. 2000; Araoz et al. 2000; Gaerte et al. 2002) (Fig. 9). MRI is the most informative imaging technique in that it reveals the nature, size, location, and

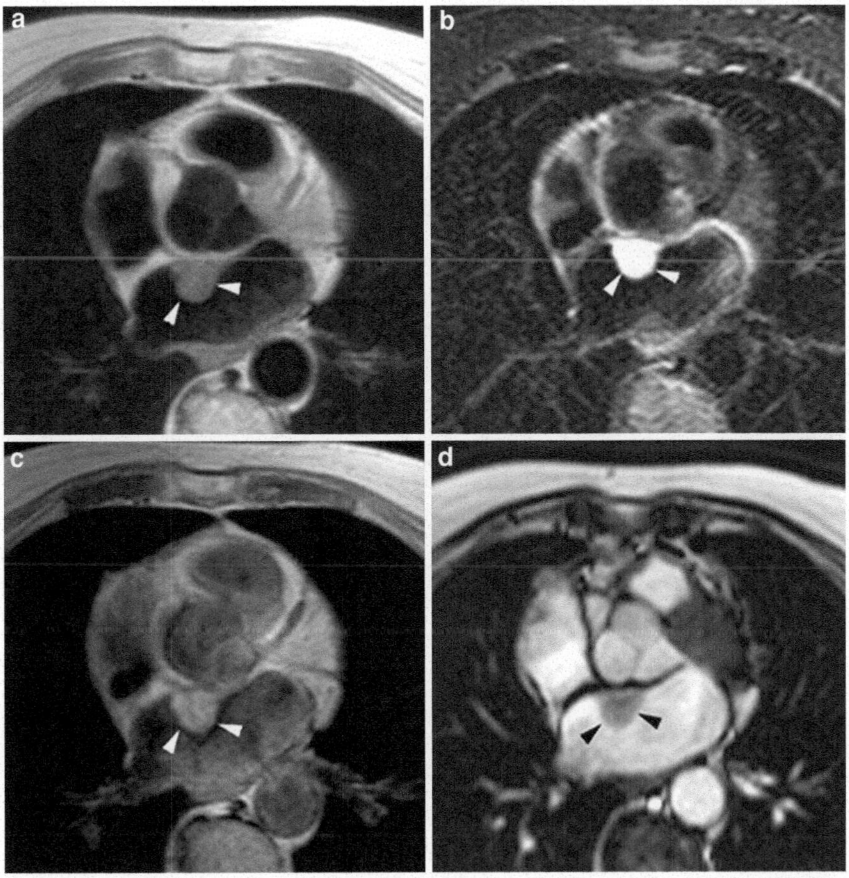

Fig. 5 Sessile myxoma in left atrium in a 81-year-old woman clinically presenting with increasing dyspnea. T1w-imaging (**a**) shows sharply defined mass broadly implanted at the interface between atrial septum and dorsal side of the aortic root (*arrowheads*). T2w-imaging (**b**) shows strongly hyperintense appearance of the mass (*arrowheads*). T1w-imaging post-contrast administration shows moderate enhancement (*arrowheads*) (**c**). The dynamics of the mass can be well appreciated on cine imaging (*arrowheads*) (**d**). All images are obtained in the axial plane

blood flow pattern of the tumor. Lipomas typically have high signal intensity on T1w and T2w-imaging. Addition of T1w-imaging with fat suppression prepulse will selectively suppress the signal of fat, not only proving the nature of the mass, but also allowing to differentiate with other rather 'theoretical' possibilities such as subacute hemorrhage presenting too with high signal on T1w- and T2w-imaging (Figs 1, 9, 10). On cine MRI lipomas typically have a dark-rim because of the opposed phase at the fluid-fat interface (Figs. 10, 11).

4.1.1.3 Papillary Fibroelastoma

Though papillary fibroelastoma are rare benign tumors, they represent the most common primary tumor of the cardiac valves, and the third most common cardiac tumor (Edwards et al. 1991; Araoz et al. 2000; Gowda et al. 2003). They can occur on any of the cardiac valves or on the endothelial cardiac surface, such as the LV apex, tendinous chords, or outflow tract (Shahian et al. 1995). These tumors are usually discovered accidentally or when neurologic or cardiologic complications occur due to emboli with stroke or coronary artery occlusion and myocardial infarction (Kasarskis et al. 1988). Papillary fibroelastomas are small tumors (mean diameter 12 ± 9 mm) that are usually pedunculated and mobile, but they do not cause valvular dysfunction (Klarich et al. 1997) (Fig. 12). Transesophageal echocardiography is the preferred imaging modality (Grote et al. 1995). Although MRI can be used, tumor detection is often challenging because of the small tumor size. The risk of embolic events justifies surgical resection while anticoagulation therapy can be suggested as a substitute for surgery in high-risk patients (Saloura et al. 2009).

4.1.1.4 Rhabdomyoma

Rhabdomyoma is the most common primary cardiac tumor in early childhood, representing 75% of all

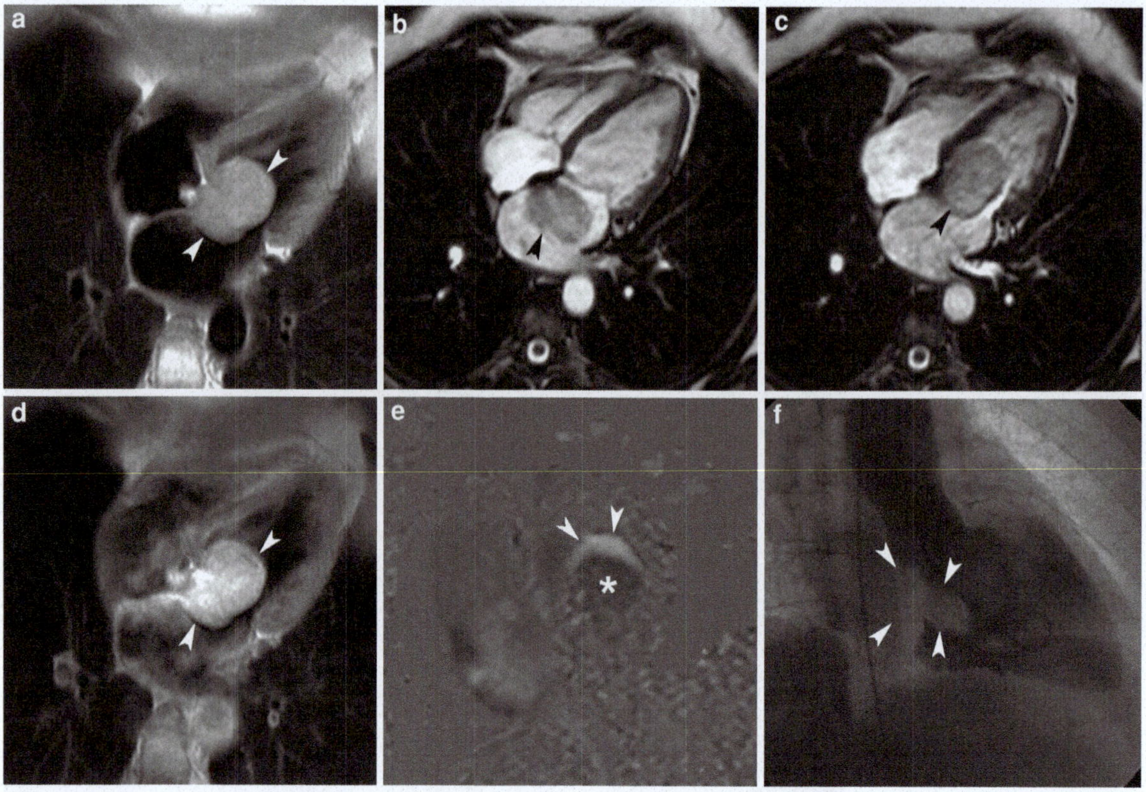

Fig. 6 Large, mobile LA myxoma in 50-year-old woman presenting with palpitations and increasing dyspnea. Axial T1w-imaging shows large (42 × 29 × 31 mm), well-defined mass positioned between LA and LV (*arrowheads*) (**a**). Cine imaging in horizontal long-axis plane at end diastole (**b**) and end systole (**c**) nicely depicts the attachment of the mass to the atrial septum (*arrowhead*, **b**). During systole the mass is displaced in the LV cavity (*arrowhead*, **c**). Axial T2w-imaging show hyperintense appearance of the mass (*arrowheads*) (**d**). PC-MRI obtained in short-axis plane at the level of the mitral valve shows partial obstruction of the mitral valve orifice (*arrowheads*) by the myxoma (*)(**e**). Long-axis ventriculography during cardiac catheterization shows the LA mass with partial displacement into the LV (*arrowheads*)(f)

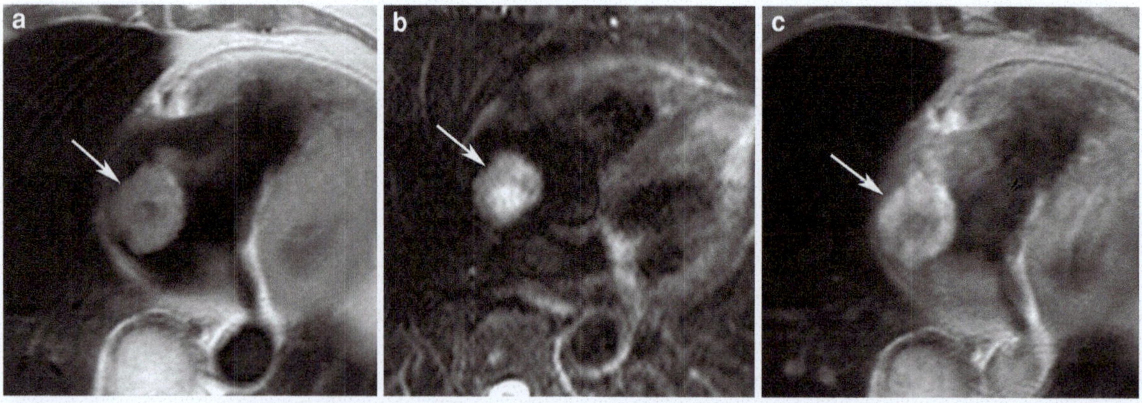

Fig. 7 Right-atrial pedunculated myxoma in 76-year-old woman with a clinical history of CVA, probably due to embolus entering the systemic circulation through a patent foramen ovale. T1w-imaging shows slightly irregularly defined mass in RA (*arrow*) (**a**). The mass has centrally a hypo-intense appearance. T2w-imaging (**b**) shows inhomogeneous hyperintense appearance (*arrow*). Post-contrast imaging shows peripheral enhancement (*arrow*) with central hypointensity (**c**). All images are acquired in axial direction

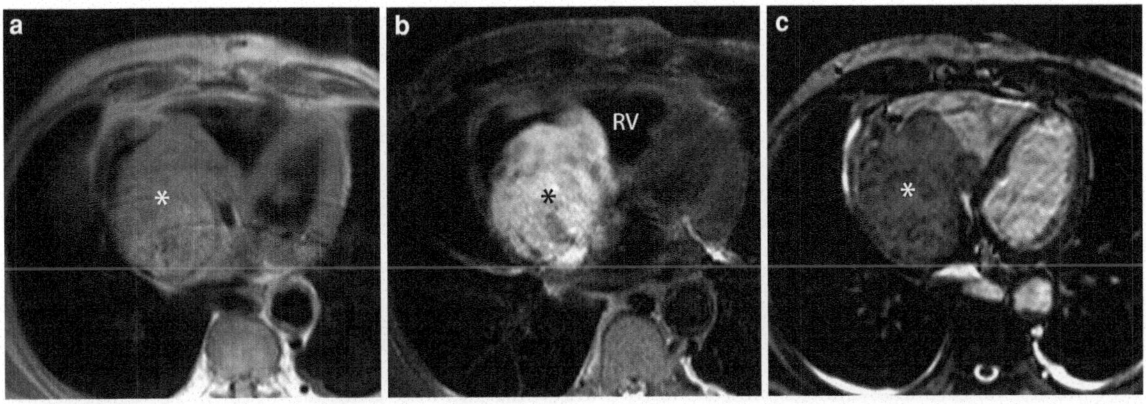

Fig. 8 Giant myxoma in RA in 82-year-old woman. Axial T1w-imaging shows large irregularly defined and slightly inhomogeneous mass (70 × 74 × 53 mm) incompletely filling the RA cavity (*) (**a**). T2w-imaging in the same image plane shows hyperintense inhomogeneous appearance of the mass (*) (**b**). Axial cine imaging allows to better appreciate the contours and movement of the mass (*) (**c**). Abbreviations: *RV* right ventricle

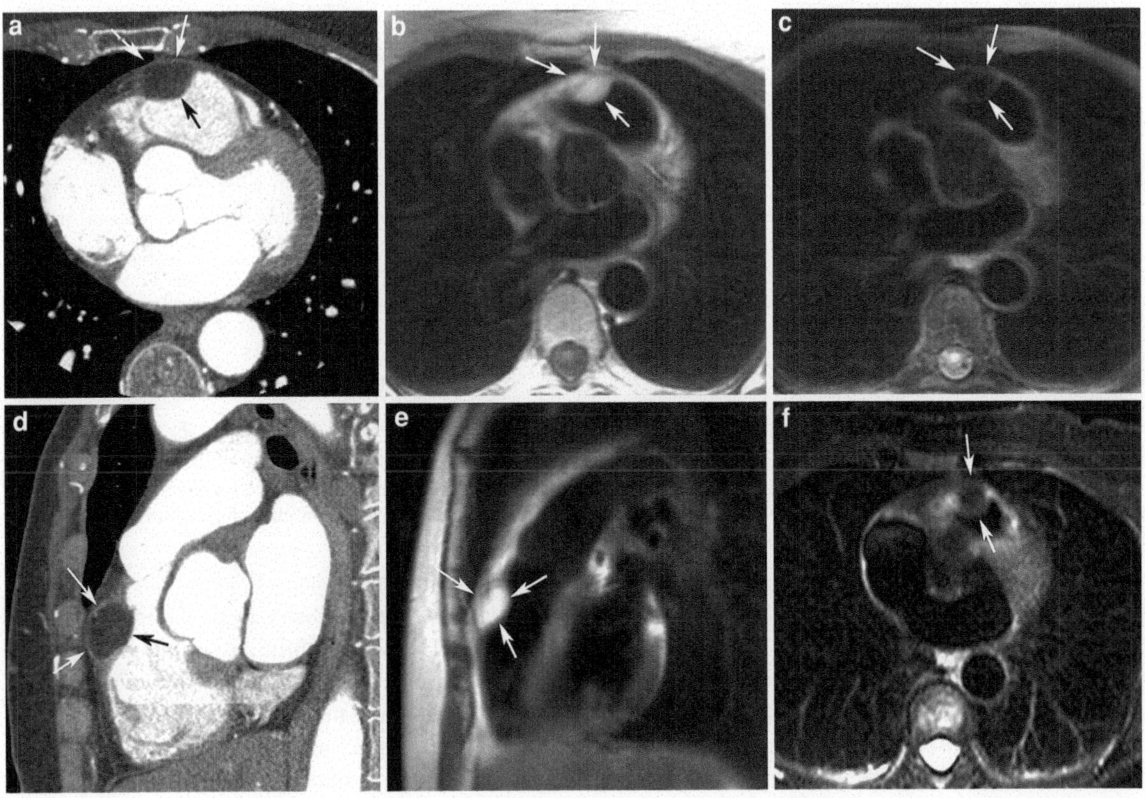

Fig. 9 Presentation of RV lipoma on MDCT and MRI. Axial (**a**) and sagittal (**b**) MDCT image. Axial T1w-imaging without (**c**) and with (**d**) fat suppression prepulse. Sagittal T1w-imaging (**e**). Axial T2w-imaging (**f**). MDCT shows an ovular well-defined mass arising from the free RV wall (*arrowheads*, **a**, **d**). Density measurements show negative Hounsfield Units (-95 HU). The mass appears strongly hyperintense on T1w-imaging (*arrows*, **b**, **e**), and is completely suppressed when using fat-suppressed T1w-imaging (*arrows*, **c**). On T2w-imaging, the mass has a hypo-intense appearance (*arrows*, **f**)

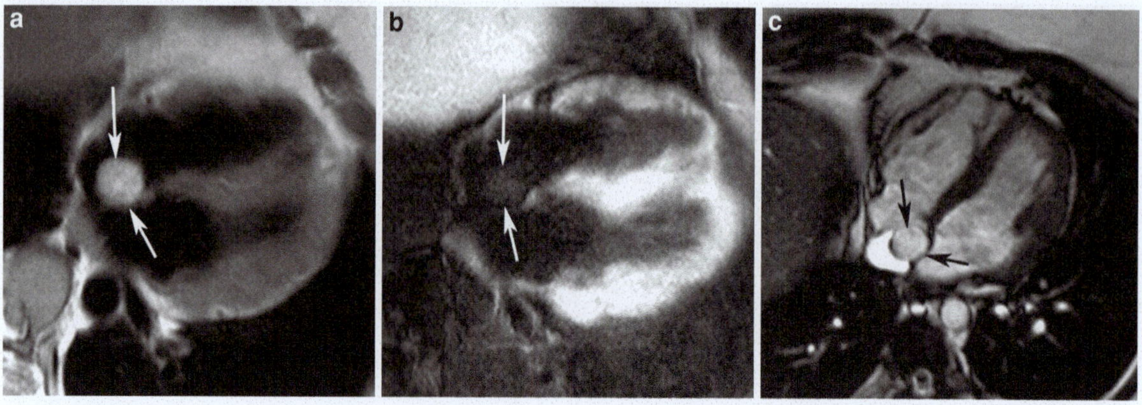

Fig. 10 RA lipoma presenting as cardiac myxoma in a 34-year-old man. Well-defined rounded mass broadly attached to the right side of the atrial septum. Taking into account the location and presentation, a cardiac myxoma is the most likely diagnosis. However, the high signal intensity on T1w-imaging (*arrows*, **a**), completely suppressed on fat-suppressed T1w-imaging establishes the diagnosis of a cardiac lipoma (*arrows*, **b**). Cine imaging enables to evaluate the impact of the tumor on cardiac (in)flow patterns (*arrow*, **c**). All images are acquired in the horizontal long-axis plane

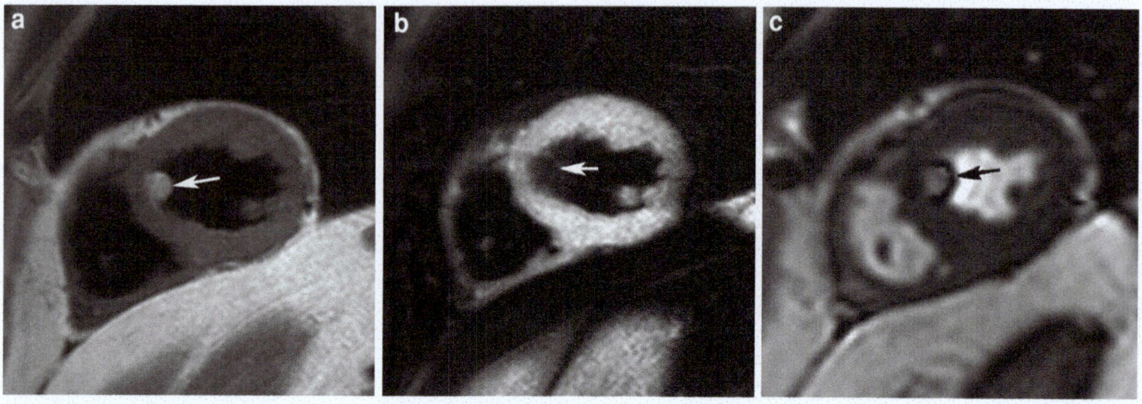

Fig. 11 Cardiac lipoma in LV in 62-year-old man experiencing a transient ischemic attack. T1w-imaging without (**a**) and with fat suppression prepulse (**b**), cine imaging (**c**). All images are acquired in midventricular short-axis plane. The lipoma is clearly visibile as a well-defined nodule broadly attached to the ventricular septum (*arrow*, **a**). It has a high signal intensity on T1w-imaging that is completely suppressed using fat suppression imaging (*arrow*, **b**). A dark-rim artifact at the fat/fluid interface is clearly visible on cine imaging (*arrow*, **c**)

primary tumors arising in the neonatal period (Kiaffis et al. 2002) (Fig. 13). This entity is not infrequently considered as a hamartoma rather than a true tumor, since it may regress spontaneously by the age of 2 years (Matteucci et al. 1997). Cardiac rhabdomyoma should be differentiated from cardiac fibroma, which may have a similar clinical presentation (see 4.1.1.5). Rhabdomyomas are frequently multiple and may involve both the atria and ventricles. They rarely calcify. Fibromas, in contrast, are solitary lesions and infrequently located in the atria. An important feature of rhabdomyomas is their association with Bourneville's tuberous sclerosis, and as mentioned above their tendency to completely disappear with aging (Bader et al. 2003; Rosser et al. 2006). MRI is very helpful in locating and determining the extent of the tumor. Though cardiac rhabdomyomas are mentioned to have an intermediate to high signal intensity on T1w-imaging, an intermediate signal intensity on T2w-imaging and a contrast enhancement similar to the surrounding myocardium (Semelka et al. 1992), in Fig. 13 performed in a one-month-old girl, the rhabdomyoma appears strongly hyperintense on T2w-imaging and shows a strong enhancement. Because rhabdomyomas may be difficult to differentiate from adjacent myocardium, myocardial tagging techniques may be

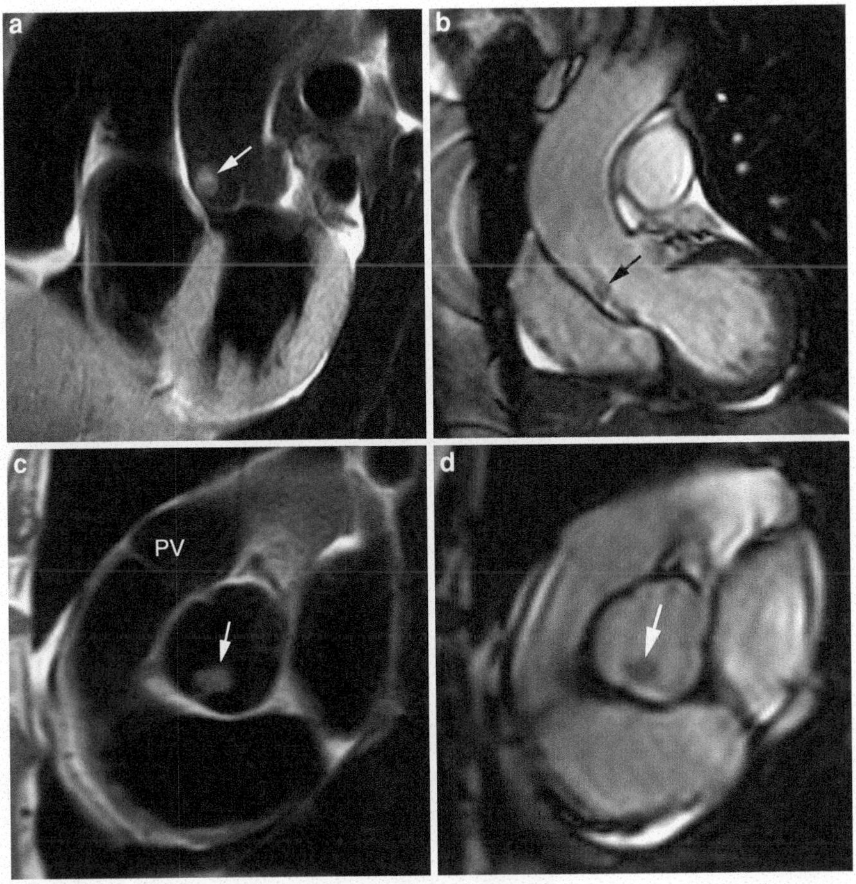

Fig. 12 Papillary fibroelastoma attached on the right coronary cusp of the aortic valve in a 69-year-old woman presenting with systemic emboli. T1w image in the LVOT view (**a**) and a perpendicular view through the aortic root just above the aortic valve (**c**). Cine imaging obtained in similar planes (**b**, **d**). A small (8 mm) nodular structure (*arrow*) is well visible. Because of the small size, assessment of enhancement after contrast administration is often not possible

helpful to make a distinction between contractile and non-contractile tissues (Bouton et al. 1991).

4.1.1.5 Fibroma

In the large series of 533 cases of primary cardiac tumors reported by the Armed Forces Institute of Pathology, cardiac fibromas constituted only 3.2% of the total (McAllister and Fenoglio 1978; Parmley et al. 1988). Fibromas are predominantly found in the pediatric age group, though they may be detected in adolescents and adults too (Burke et al. 1994). Very likely cardiac fibroma is a congenital tumor, since it usually manifest at birth or in early infancy or childhood. Fibromas primarily arise in the ventricles and are commonly located intramurally, i.e., in the anterior wall and intraventricular septum (Figs. 14, 15). These tumors not infrequently calcify. The high frequency of sudden cardiac death and the potential for preventing this occurrence emphasize the need for early diagnosis and appropriate surgical and medical therapy (Parmley et al. 1988). The major tumors requiring differentiation are myxoma, lipoma, and rhabdomyoma. Echocardiography and MRI are very sensitive in the diagnosis and preoperative assessment (Parmley et al. 1988; Burke et al. 1994). The signal characteristics on T1w-imaging are similar to the surrounding myocardium while after contrast administration fibromas demonstrate a heterogeneous enhancement with a lower intensity central area surrounded by a peripheral hyperintense rim (Fig. 14) (Funari et al. 1991). The central area likely corresponds to a poorly vascularized fibrous region.

4.1.1.6 Intrapericardial Paraganglioma (Pheochromocytoma)

Intrapericardial paraganglioma belongs to the group of a catecholamine-secreting tumors (pheochromocytoma) causing persistent or paroxysmal hypertension. In the hypertensive population the incidence of pheochromocytoma is less than 1%. The majority of

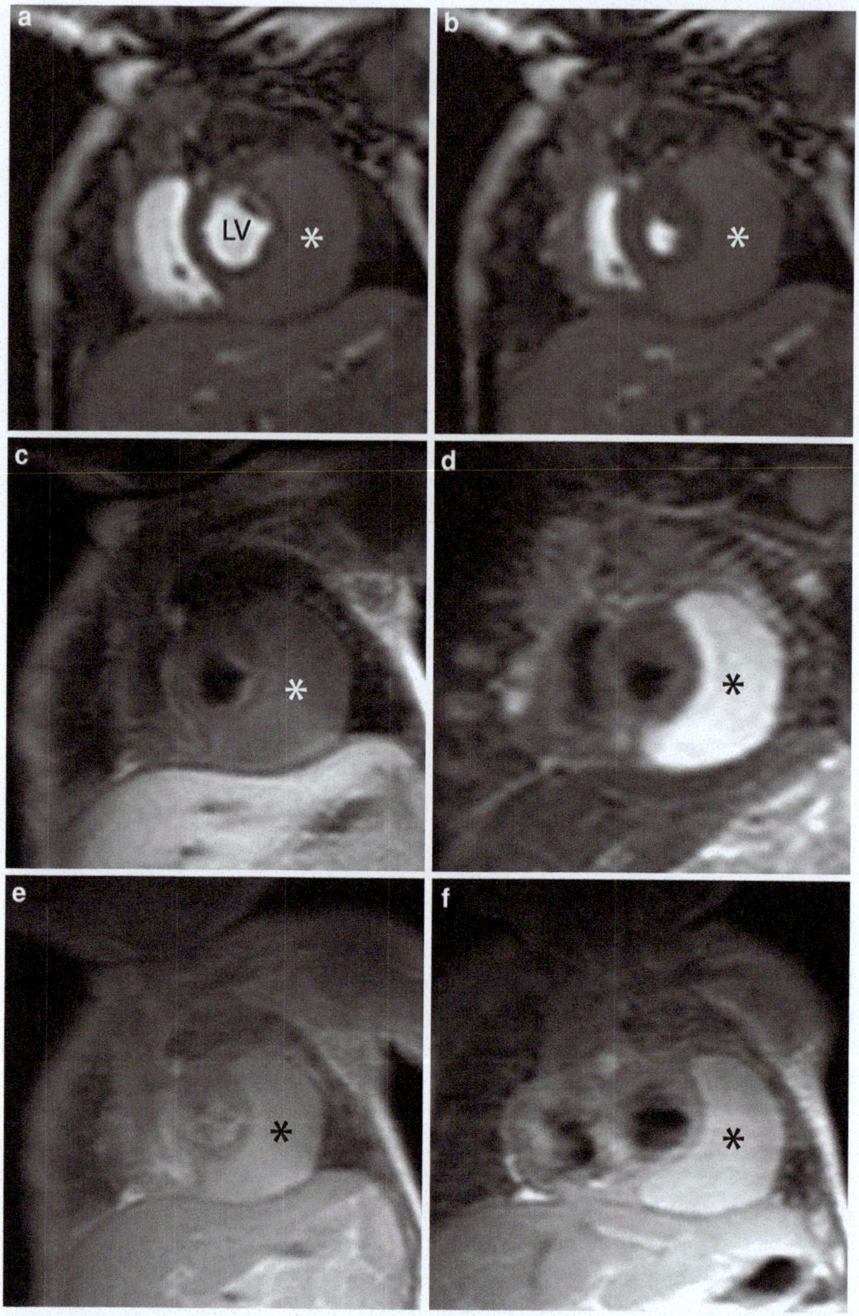

Fig. 13 Cardiac rhabdomyoma in one-month-old girl. Cine imaging at end diastole (**a**) and end systole (**b**). T1w-imaging (**c**) and T2w-imaging (**d**). Post-contrast T1w-imaging (**e**) and late Gd imaging (**f**). All image are acquired in midventricular short-axis. A huge sickle-like soft-tissue mass is present along the LV lateral wall (*). Cine imaging shows that the contractility of the adjacent myocardium is not affected. The mass has a slightly hyperintense appearance on T1w-imaging (**c**) and is strongly hyperintense on T2w-imaging (**d**). Strong enhancement is seen following contrast administration (**e**, **f**). Since the initial diagnosis, 5 years ago, the rhabdomyoma spontaneously decreased in size. Abbreviations: *LV* left ventricle

pheochromocytomas, i.e., 90%, arise from the chromaffin cells of the adrenal medulla. Less than 2% of these tumors are found in the chest (Manger and Gifford 1990). The majority are located in the posterior mediastinum, where they originate from the paravertebral sympathetic ganglia. Cardiac pheochromocytomas are exceedingly rare, and are usually found intrapericardially, most often in relation to the roof of the left atrium, and less frequently arise in the interatrial septum (Kawasuji et al. 1989; Gomi et al. 1994) (Fig. 16). For initial detection, regional location of these extraadrenal tumors and detection of distant metastases by means of metaiodobenzylguanidine (MIBG) scintigraphy is recommended. MRI can then provide detailed anatomic delineation before surgical resection (Ichikawa et al. 1995; Hamilton

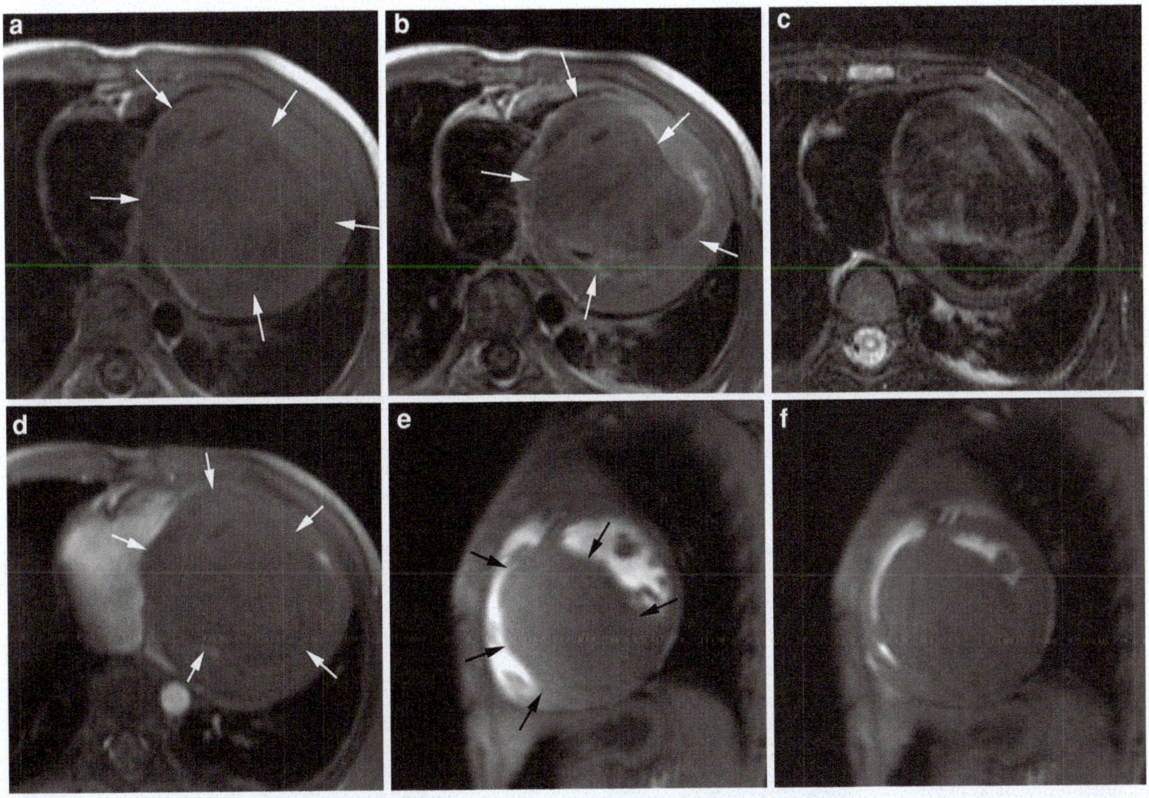

Fig. 14 Huge cardiac fibroma (*arrows*) arising from the ventricular septum in an asymptomatic 7-year-old boy. Axial T1w-imaging before (**a**) and after (**b**) contrast administration, axial T2w image (**c**) and axial cine image (**d**). Midventricular short-axis cine imaging at end diastole (**e**) and end systole (**f**). On the axial image, both ventricular cavities are nearly completely obliterated by a large soft-tissue mass, whose origin and exact location are difficult discernible. The mass, slightly hypo-intense on T1w-imaging does not enhance following contrast administration (except a small peripheral rim of enhancement), and it has a heterogeneous hypo-intense appearance on T2w-imaging. Short-axis cine imaging is helpful to locate the mass, i.e., in the ventricular septum, and to depict the compression of the ventricular cavities mainly during systole. It is worth mentioning that this boy was asymptomatic, and the presence of a cardiac fibroma was detected because of an abnormal murmur during a medical school examination

et al. 1997). Pheochromocytomas usually have a high signal intensity on T2w-imaging (Varghese et al. 1997). These tumors usually strongly enhance on first-pass perfusion MRI and late Gd imaging. Not infrequently, the central portion remains hypo-enhanced likely representing central necrosis or liquefaction (Fig. 16).

4.1.1.7 Hemangioma

Hemangiomas are vascular tumors composed of blood vessels that can be either capillaries, i.e., capillary hemangioma, or large cavernous vascular channels, i.e., cavernous hemangioma. Hemangiomas are most frequently localized in the skin and subcutaneous muscles, and their localization in the heart is extremely rare (Mosthaf et al. 1991; Brizard et al. 1993) (Fig. 17). They most commonly occur in the left ventricular lateral wall, the right ventricular anterior wall, and the interventricular septum (Fig. 18). In 30% of cases multiple locations are found. Half of them grow intramurally while the other 50% have intracavitary localization. On coronary angiography, these tumors have a typical vascular blush. MRI may be helpful in demonstrating the vascular nature of the tumor and in evaluating the surgical resectability (Brizard et al. 1993). Hemangiomas generally present on MRI as heterogeneous masses (Oshima et al. 2003). They have an intermediate signal intensity on T1-weighted images and a high signal intensity on T2-weighted images. Imaging techniques such as first-pass perfusion

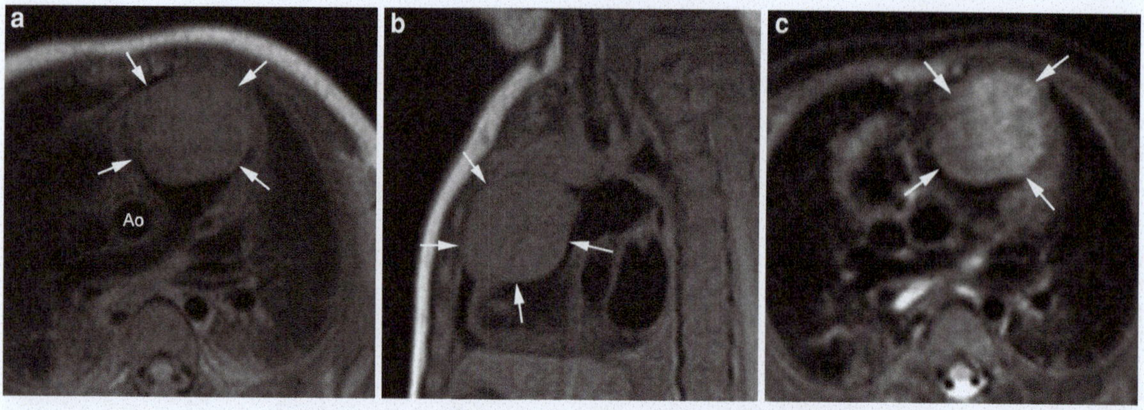

Fig. 15 Cardiac fibroma arising from the anterior RV wall in a 2-month-old boy. Axial (**a**) and sagittal (**b**) T1w-imaging, axial T2w-imaging (**c**). A well-circumscribed mass (*arrows*) is found in the RVOT arising from the anterior wall. This mass is subtotally obstructing the RVOT. On T2w-imaging, the fibroma appears slightly hyperintense (*arrows*, **c**)

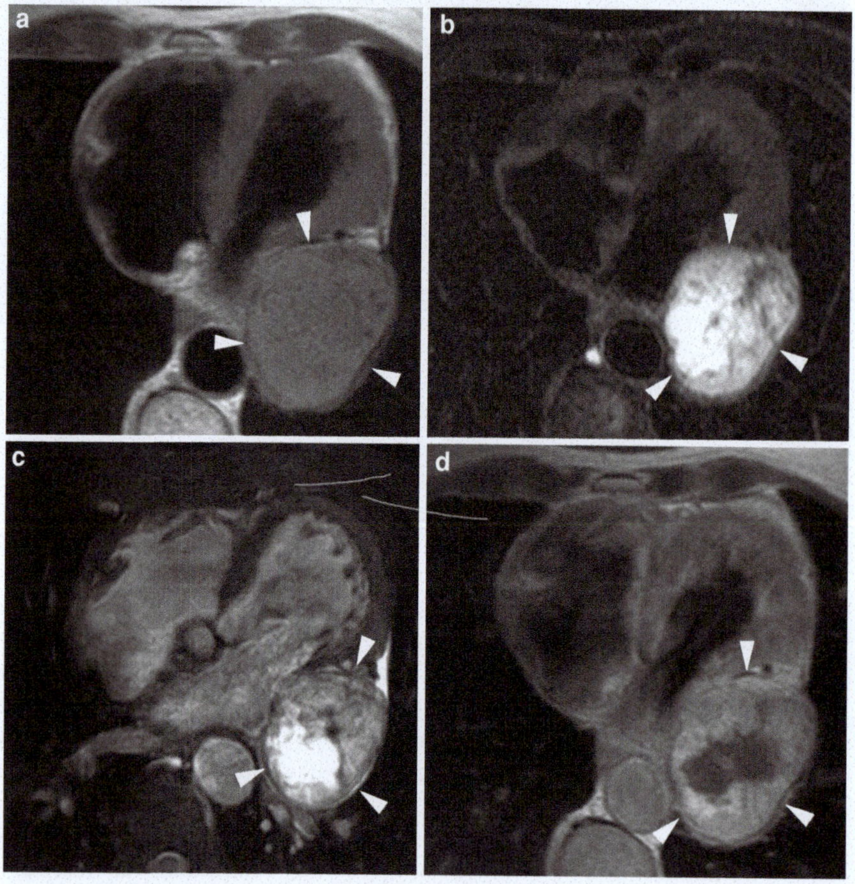

Fig. 16 Cardiac paraganglioma (or pheochromocytoma) (*arrows*) in a 68-year-old man. T1w-imaging (**a**), T2w-imaging (**b**) 3D bright-blood imaging with high-spatial resolution (**c**), post-contrast T1w-imaging (**d**). All images are obtained in the axial plane. A large well-circumscribed mass is shown at the lateral and upper border of the left atrium (*arrowheads*). The appearance is fairly homogeneous on T1w-imaging, but is strongly heterogeneous on T2w-imaging and cine imaging, and the mass shows a strong peripheral enhancement with central nonenhancing zone. Compression of the adjacent cardiac structures by the large mass

imaging and late Gd imaging are helpful to show the vascular nature of the lesion and to discriminate a hemangioma from other cardiac mass or other entities such as hypertrophic cardiomyopathy in case of intra-myocardial location (Fig. 18).

4.1.1.8 Teratoma

Teratomas are generally benign tumors typically occurring in infancy. Not infrequently, they are already detected during intrauterine life by means of fetal ultrasonography. Teratomas are intrapericardially

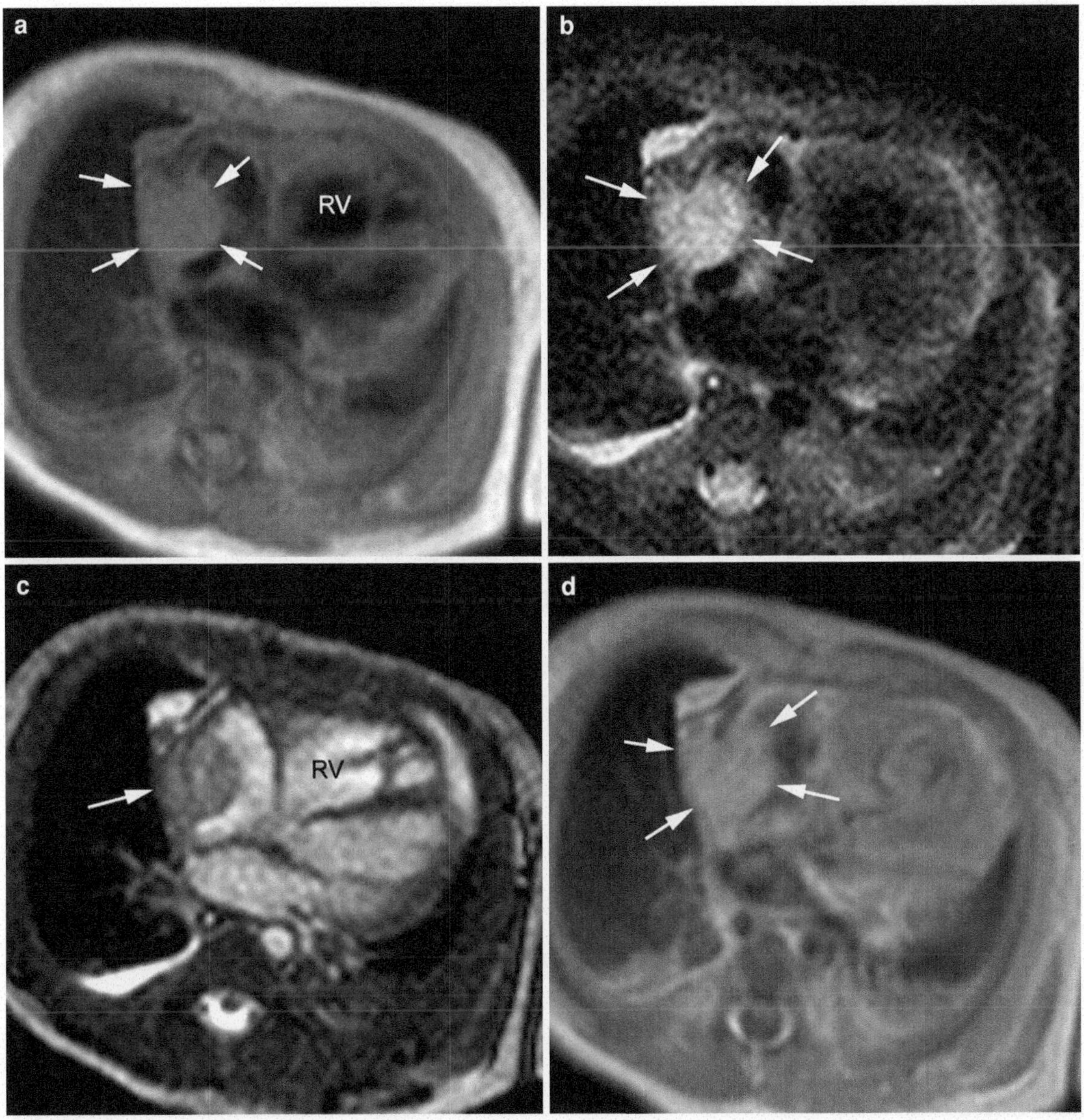

Fig. 17 Cardiac hemangioma (*arrows*) in a one-day old girl. On fetal echocardiography (27 weeks of gestation), a pericardial effusion and a right-atrial mass were detected. At 37 weeks, an urgent delivery was performed because of cardiac tamponade due to an important pericardial effusion. After pericardiocenthesis, she was referred for further evaluation of the RA mass to MRI. All images are obtained in the axial plane. T1w image (**a**) and T2w image (**b**), end-diastolic cine image (**c**), post-contrast T1w image (**d**). A well-defined mass is visible in the RA attached to the lateral wall (*arrowheads*). The mass is homogeneously iso-intense on T1w-imaging, hyperintense on T2w-imaging, and strongly enhances following contrast administration. Besides a small amount of residual pericardial fluid, no pericardial abnormalities are found

located pedunculated tumors, arising from the root of the ascending aorta, and may cause large pericardial effusion with cardiac tamponade (Arciniegas et al. 1980; Benetar et al. 1992). They consist of the three germ layers (i.e., endodermic, mesodermic, and neuroectodermic germinal layers) and may be cystic as well as solid. Early surgical removal is usually curative. Echocardiography generally suggests the diagnosis by showing a heterogeneous intrapericardial mass associated with a pericardial effusion compressing the heart. MRI is advantageous to better define the relationship of large tumoral masses to adjacent structures,

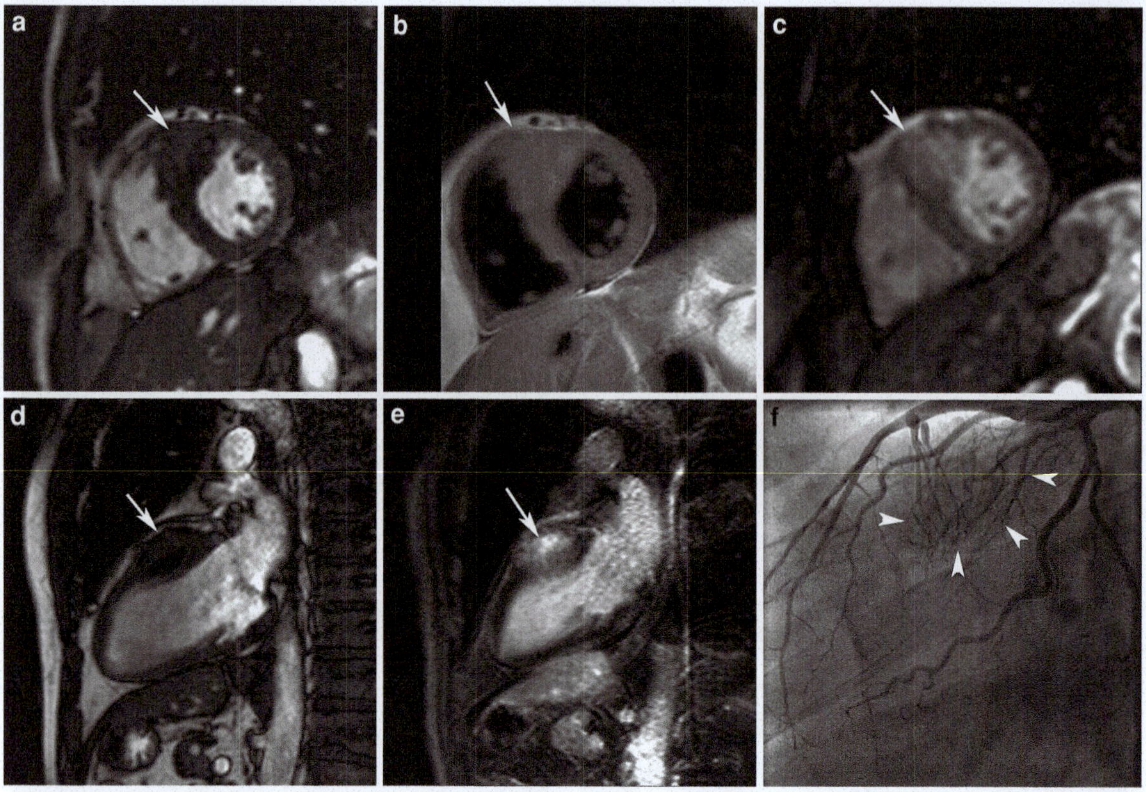

Fig. 18 Cardiac hemangioma in 50-year-old man, presenting as asymmetrical septal hypertrophic cardiomyopathy. Short-axis cine imaging at end diastole (**a**), T1w-imaging (**b**), first-pass perfusion imaging (**c**), vertical long-axis cine imaging at end diastole (**d**), and vertical long-axis late Gd imaging (**e**). Coronary angiography during contrast injection in the left main coronary artery (**f**). Cine imaging and T1w-imaging shows a focally thickened appearance of the LV anteroseptal wall with a maximum thickness of 29 mm (*arrow*, **a**, **b**). The location of the wall thickening can be well appreciated on vertical long-axis cine image (*arrow*, **d**). During first-pass imaging, strong enhancement occurs in the thickened myocardium (*arrow*, **c**) resulting in strong late enhancement (*arrow*, **e**). During coronary angiography, a network of small arterial structures is found in the basal part of the ventricular septum, supplied by branches of the left anterior descending coronary artery (*arrowheads*, **f**). A follow-up MRI study, 6 months later revealed similar findings

in visualizing echocardiographic "blind" spots, and in defining tissue characteristics (Barakos et al. 1989a; Beghetti et al. 1998; Kiaffis et al. 2002).

4.1.2 Malignant Cardiac Tumors

Primary malignant cardiac tumors can be divided into three major groups, i.e., sarcomas, lymphomas, and mesotheliomas (Grebenc et al. 2000).

4.1.2.1 Sarcoma

Soft-tissue sarcomas are the most common malignant neoplasms of the heart, pericardium, and great vessels. Their presentation is usually nonspecific and may mimic other diseases. Noninvasive imaging such as echocardiography, CT, and MRI aid in the diagnosis and preoperative assessment (Raaf and Raaf 1994; Dillman et al. 2010). Overall survival is poor, at present, aggressive and complete surgical resection seems to offer the best hope for palliation and survival in an otherwise fatal disease.

Angiosarcoma. In adults approximately 25% of all primary cardiac tumors are malignant. One-third of these tumors are angiosarcomas (Herrmann et al. 1992; Burke et al. 1992). This highly aggressive malignant tumor can develop from the lymphatic endothelium, i.e., lymphangiosarcoma, or vascular endothelium, i.e., hemangiosarcoma. In a review study by Naka et al. (1995), 12 out of 99 angiosarcomas arose in the heart. Most cardiac angiosarcomas arise in the right atrium (75%), although the reasons for this remain unclear (Janigan et al. 1986). They present as single or multiple nodules, filling the right atrium and/or infiltrating the myocardium and pericardium (McAllister and Fenoglio 1978; Urba and Longo 1986). The pericardial sac is filled by hemorrhage and blood. Since the presentation is often nonspecific, diagnosis is delayed and at the time of the diagnosis cardiac angiosarcomas have usually metastasized, most frequently to the lung (Urba and Longo 1986; Aouate et al. 1988). The pulmonary metastases most frequently have irregular margins due to peripheral hemorrhages. Cardiac angiosarcoma has a dismal prognosis, with a mean survival of 6 months after presentation.

Angiosarcomas usually present on MRI as heterogeneous masses (Best et al. 2003) (Figs. 19, 20, 21). A characteristic presentation of angiosarcomas is the mosaic pattern, consisting of nodular areas of increased signal intensity interspersed with areas of intermediate signal intensity on T1w-imaging. The high signal areas result from intratumoral hemorrhage. T2w-imaging usually shows a clear demarcation of the tumor from the normal myocardium (Sato et al. 1995). Angiosarcomas may have a "cauliflower" appearance on MRI, with focal areas of increased signal intensity probably related to thrombosis or hemorrhage (Kim et al. 1989). Likely the most typical finding of an angiosarcoma on MRI is that of an ill-defined mass arising from the right-atrial wall extending into the pericardium, usually in combination with a pericardial effusion. Not infrequently one or more pericardial metastases may be visible (Figs. 19, 20, 21). Hemangiopericytomas, a much rarer primary cardiac sarcoma, may have a similar appearance on MRI and their distinction relies on pathologic examination (Sato et al. 1995).

Rhabdomyosarcoma. Rhabdomyosarcoma is the second most frequent primary malignant tumor of the heart. These tumors are composed of malignant cells from striated muscle and occur singly or in multiples anywhere in the heart (Szucs et al. 1991). The right and left side of the heart are involved with equal frequency, and in a third to a half of the cases the pericardium is involved by direct extension from the myocardium. The prognosis is generally poor. MRI is not only helpful in quantifying the initial extent of the tumor, but also in evaluating its response to chemotherapy (Szucs et al. 1991). The most common appearance of rhabdomyosarcomas is that of a homogeneous mass, isointense, or minimally hyperintense to muscle on T1w-imaging and hyperintense to muscle on T2w-imaging. After Gd-DTPA administration, these tumors enhance markedly (Yousem et al. 1990).

Malignant Fibrous Histiocytoma. Malignant fibrous histiocytoma is the most common soft-tissue sarcoma in adults, but is distinctly rare as a primary tumor of the heart (Murphey et al. 1994). Malignant fibrous histiocytomas are not infrequently anchored onto the posterior wall in the left atrium while right-sided tumors are extremely rare (Teramoto et al. 1995). This tumor may demonstrate clinical similarities with myxoma, and careful anatomopathologic examination of multiple sections of the tumor is necessary to distinguish it from benign tumors, especially myxomas (Kasugai et al. 1990). However, this tumor is far more aggressive than a myxoma and exhibits a greater tendency for local recurrence and infiltration. The tumors exhibit an intermediate, slightly heterogeneous signal intensity on T1w-imaging and a high signal intensity on T2w-imaging (Mahajan et al. 1989; Kim et al. 1989).

Other Cardiac Sarcomas. The heart is occasionally the primary site of other rare sarcomas, including undifferentiated sarcomas, liposarcomas, osteosarcomas, fibrosarcomas, synovial sarcomas, neuro-fibrosarcomas, intima sarcomas, leiomyosarcomas, chrondrosarcomas, and Kaposi's sarcomas (Figs. 22, 23). In a study by Burke et al. in a total of 75 primary cardiac sarcomas, 18 were undifferentiated sarcomas and nine were osteosarcomas; all of the latter tumors arose in the left atrium (Burke et al. 1991, 1992). Liposarcomas of the heart and pericardium are very rare, while cardiac metastasis of liposarcoma seems to occur more frequently. Most cardiac liposarcomas diffusely involve the heart. The right ventricle is most frequently involved (Papa et al. 1994). In contrast to lipomas, liposarcomas display a signal intensity less than that of fat on T1w-imaging (Conces et al. 1985; Dooms et al. 1985). Metastases are common by the time of diagnosis. Leiomyosarcomas predominate in the muscular arteries and great veins, while primary cardiac involvement is extremely rare (Raaf and Raaf 1994) (Fig. 24). Leiomyosarcomas of the inferior and superior vena cava may directly involve the right atrium. Primary cardiac leiomyosarcomas are usually located in the atria and may invade the pericardium (Takamizawa et al. 1992). Cardiac Kaposi's sarcoma has been found in patients with AIDS and in immunosuppressed organ transplant recipients (Lanza et al. 1983; Raaf and Raaf 1994). Kaposi's sarcoma of the

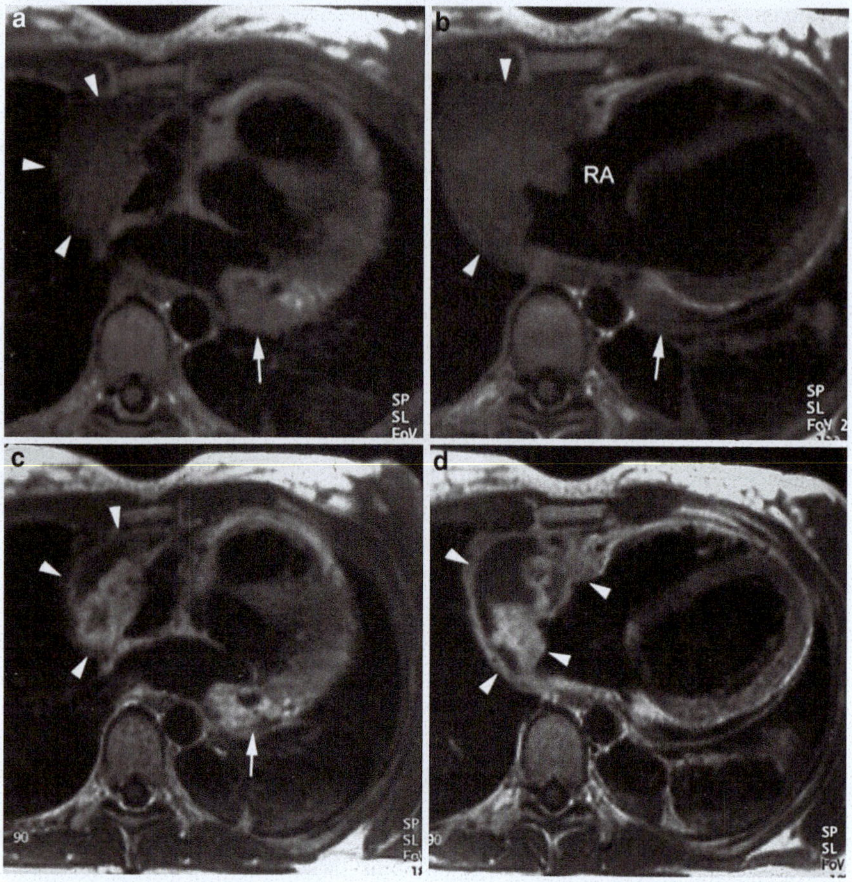

Fig. 19 Cardiac angiosarcoma of the right atrium with massive pericardial invasion in 21-year-old woman. Axial T1w-imaging before (**a**, **b**) and after (**c**, **d**) contrast administration. A large, irregularly defined mass originating in the lateral right-atrial wall is seen broadly invading the pericardium (*arrowheads*, **a**, **b**). Pericardial effusion and malignant pericardial seeding (*arrow*, **a**, **b**, **c**) are present. After contrast administration the tumor borders can be better delineated and the tumor better differentiated from the adjacent pericardial effusion (*arrowheads*, **c**, **d**). The angiosarcoma shows a strong, but inhomogeneous enhancement

heart may present as cardiac masses or as widely disseminated with infiltration of the heart and great vessels (Corallo et al. 1988; Langer et al. 1988).

4.1.2.2 Lymphoma

Primary cardiac lymphomas are extremely rare while metastatic involvement of the heart in patients with malignant lymphoma is far more common and results from retrograde lymphatic spread, hematogenous spread, and direction extension from other primary tumor masses (Roberts et al. 1990; Chiles et al. 2001). However, since primary cardiac lymphoma is associated with AIDS, an increase in primary cardiac lymphomas may be expected (Balasubramanyam et al. 1986). This disease has two definitions, i.e., absence of lymphoma outside the pericardial sac and bulk of the neoplasm within the pericardium or cardiac symptoms from lymphomatous cardiac infiltration at the time of the initial diagnosis (Curtinsinger et al. 1989; Castelli et al. 1989; Butany et al. 2006). The clinical course in most patients with primary lymphoma of the heart is remarkably acute in onset and short in duration, and the diagnosis is often not made antemortem. Primary cardiac lymphoma presents with pericardial effusion, intracardiac masses, arrhythmias, and other nonspecific cardiac manifestations (Bogaert et al. 1995a). In our experience, cardiac lymphomas frequently originate in the right atrioventricular groove and extend to the surrounding structures such as the right-atrial and right-ventricular wall and pericardium (Figs. 25, 26). More extensive cases may involve the atrial septum and inferior left ventricular wall. They may cause significant narrowing of the cardiac chambers. Cytologic examination of the pericardial fluid or pericardial biopsy seems to be the most suitable for diagnosis because of the frequent involvement of the pericardium. MRI provides accurate information on the cardiac masses and the extent of pericardial fluid, and can be repeated at follow-up. Extra-medullary myeloid tumors can occur

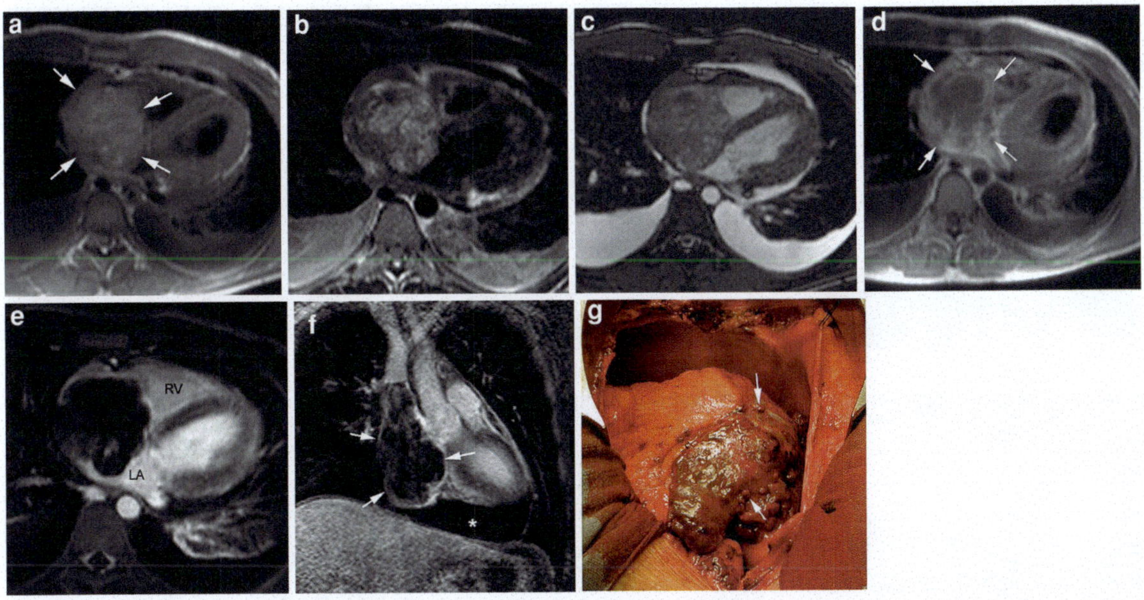

Fig. 20 Right-atrial angiosarcoma in a 20-year-old man experiencing a syncope during a football-game. T1w-imaging before (**a**) and after (**d**) contrast administration, T2w-imaging (**b**), cine imaging (**c**) late Gd imaging (**e**, **f**). Images **a**-**e** are acquired in the axial plane, image **f** in the coronal image plane. Macroscopic view on the opened pericardial sac during surgery (**g**). The angiosarcoma presents as a large mass (*arrows*), nearly completing obstructing the RA cavity extending in the RA appendage. The tumor is attached to the lateral wall and extends into the pericardium. Note the presence of an important pericardial effusion (*star*). The angiosarcoma is diffusely metastasized into the pericardium as shown during surgery (*arrows*, **g**) (Surgical view, Courtesy: P. Herijgers, MD, PhD Leuven Belgium)

after curative treatment for acute myeloid leukemia. This entity, also called *chloroma* or *granulocytic sarcoma*, may sporadically involve the heart, presenting as an intracavitary, intramural, intrapericardial, or paracardiac mass (Fig. 27). Since the imaging features are similar to cardiac lymphoma, differentiation between both entities is not possible without biopsy (Jost et al. 2005; Fritz et al. 2007).

4.1.2.3 Malignant Pericardial Mesothelioma

The incidence of malignant pericardial mesothelioma is approximately 15% of all malignant cardiac tumors, and they account for half of primary pericardial tumors (Salcedo et al. 1992; Butany et al. 2006). Mesotheliomas usually cover diffusely the visceral and parietal pericardium, encasing the heart, but generally do not invade the heart. Unlike malignant pleural mesotheliomas, the cardiac variety has no association with prior exposure to asbestos. Although they may be very extensive, they can sometimes be resected. MRI is helpful in depicting tumor localization and expansion, and in delineating the anatomic extent of malignant pericardial mesothelioma. On T1w-imaging the signal intensity is equal to or sligthly higher than that of the myocardium, and on T2w-imaging it is the same as or higher than that of fat tissue (Gossinger et al. 1988; Lund et al. 1989; Vogel et al. 1989; Kaminaga et al. 1993). A heterogeneous signal on T2w images is related to the presence of intratumoral necrosis. Contrast administration is useful in clarifying the border between the tumor and myocardium (Kaminaga et al. 1993). The location and MRI characteristics of pericardial mesothelioma resemble those of fibrosarcoma and some metastatic tumors in the pericardial space. However, the latter are more invasive than malignant mesothelioma and tend to invade the intracardiac structures (Salcedo et al. 1992; Kaminaga et al. 1993).

4.2 Secondary Cardiac Tumors

Secondary tumors of the heart are 20–40 times more frequent than primary tumors of the heart. They may result from direct extension, hematogenous or venous extension, or retrograde flow by lymphatic vessels (Chiles et al. 2001).

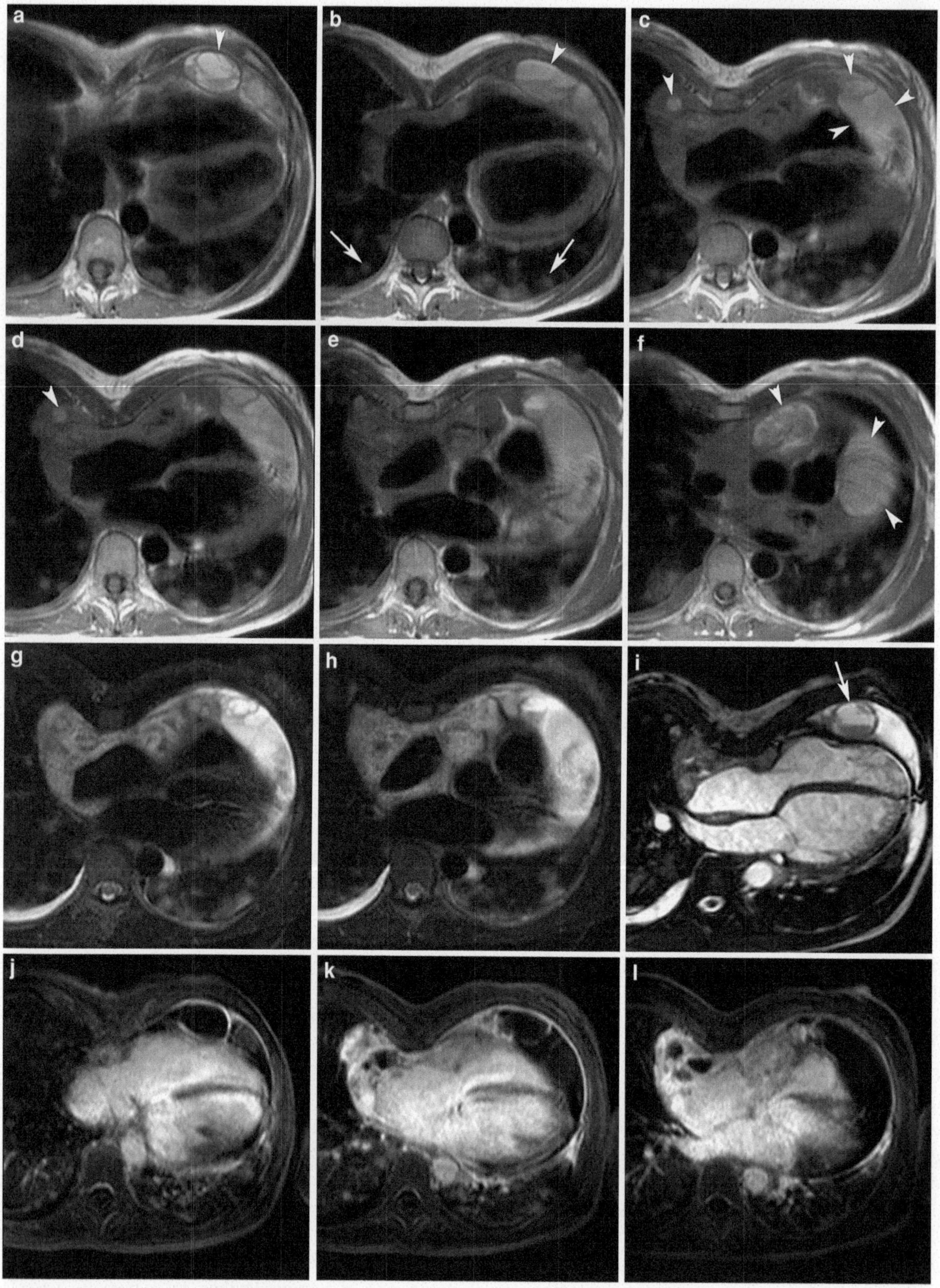
a
b
c
d
e
f
g
h
i
j
k
l

◀ **Fig. 21** Large angiosarcoma arising in RA with diffused pericardial and pulmonary metastases in a 54-year-old woman. T1w-imaging (**a–f**), T2w-imaging (**g–h**), cine imaging (**i**), late Gd imaging (**j–l**). All images are acquired in the axial image plane, except the cine image which is acquired in the horizontal long-axis image plane. Notice the presence of an inhomogeneous mass involving the entire RA wall, extending to the RV free wall and pericardium. Presence of several nodular-appearing pericardial masses (*arrowheads*, **a, b, c, d, f**). Some of these present a fluid–fluid level (*arrow*, **i**). Inhomogeneous enhancement is seen on late Gd imaging (**j–l**). Note the presence of multiple, nodular pulmonary lesions, representing pulmonary metastases (*arrows*, **b**)

4.2.1 Direct Extension

Direct extension of a malignant tumor in the pericardium or in the heart occurs from tumors originating in the lung, mediastinum, or breast. Pericardial invasion of a bronchial carcinoma is characterized by a pericardial disruption associated with focal pericardial thickening and pericardial effusion. Irregular thickening of the atrial or ventricular myocardium is the hallmark of myocardial involvement (Barakos et al. 1989b). As many as 20% of all patients who die of lymphoma are found to have cardiac involvement at autopsy. The vast majority of these patients, however, do not have symptoms referable to cardiac involvement. The most frequent site of involvement is the pericardium, including the subepicardial fat (Chiles et al. 2001). The atrioventricular groove is the most common site of epicardial invasion and often very large deposits occur in it (see Figs. 25, 26). The cardiac chambers are less frequently involved. Not infrequently, the tumor may extend through the entire wall of a cardiac chamber or through the interatrial septum (Roberts et al. 1968). Determination of lymphomatous involvement of the paracardiac spaces, the pericardium, and the heart is important for patients who are treated with radiation therapy. Generally, lung and cardiac blocks are placed to protect normal heart and lung, but these blocks are modified in the presence of pericardial involvement (Jochelson et al. 1983). Also, if the paracardiac disease encompasses a huge area, chemotherapy may be used in addition to radiation therapy.

4.2.2 Hematogenous Extension

The incidence of cardiac metastases ranges from 1.5 to 20.6% (average 6%) in autopsies on patients with malignant diseases (Rosenthal and Braunwald 1992). There has been a gradual increase in the frequency of cardiac metastases, perhaps as a consequence of the rising frequency of cancer plus the existence of reliable noninvasive diagnostic tests (see Fig. 2). Cardiac metastases are usually found in patients with disseminated tumors. In particular, pulmonary metastases are usually present. Despite their frequent occurrence in patients with malignant disease, cardiac metastases are usually clinically silent (Heath 1968). Isolated metastases occurring only in the heart are very unusual. Surgical resection of isolated cardiac metastases can be attempted to improve survival in patients whose primary tumor is well controlled (Lee and Fisher 1989). The most common tumors that metastasize to the heart are of bronchial and breast origin, followed by melanomas, lymphoma, and leukemia (Lagrange et al. 1986; Hallali and Haiat 1987). Malignant melanoma has a peculiar predilection for metastatic cardiac involvement (accounting for 60% of cases of cardiac metastasis). The pericardium is most frequently affected, while isolated involvement of the myocardium is seldom seen (Fig. 28). Intracardiac metastases from neuroendocrine tumors of the carcinoid type may mimic benign cardiac tumors (e.g., myxoma) and this entity has to be differentiated from valvular abnormalities seen in some patients with carcinoid syndrome.

MRI may be of benefit in defining the size, shape, and extent of metastatic cardiac neoplasms (Lee and Fisher 1989; Papa et al. 1994). Metastatic deposits present as focal nodular lesions of the pericardium or myocardium. Myocardial metastases of malignant melanoma tend to be bright on T1w and T2w-imaging, which is attributable to melanin (Chiles et al. 2001). Adjacent pleural effusion or flowing blood provides marked signal contrast, so that myocardial and pericardial lesions are visualized easily, as is the extension of the tumor in the cardiac chamber (Barakos et al. 1989b).

4.2.3 Venous Extension

The caval and pulmonary veins can serve as conduits for tumor extension toward the heart (Fig. 29). Intracaval extension is a well-known but rare complication of benign tumors such as leiomyomatosis arising from a uterine myoma or from the wall of the vessel itself (Rosenberg et al. 1988; Steinmetz et al. 1996) and malignant tumors,

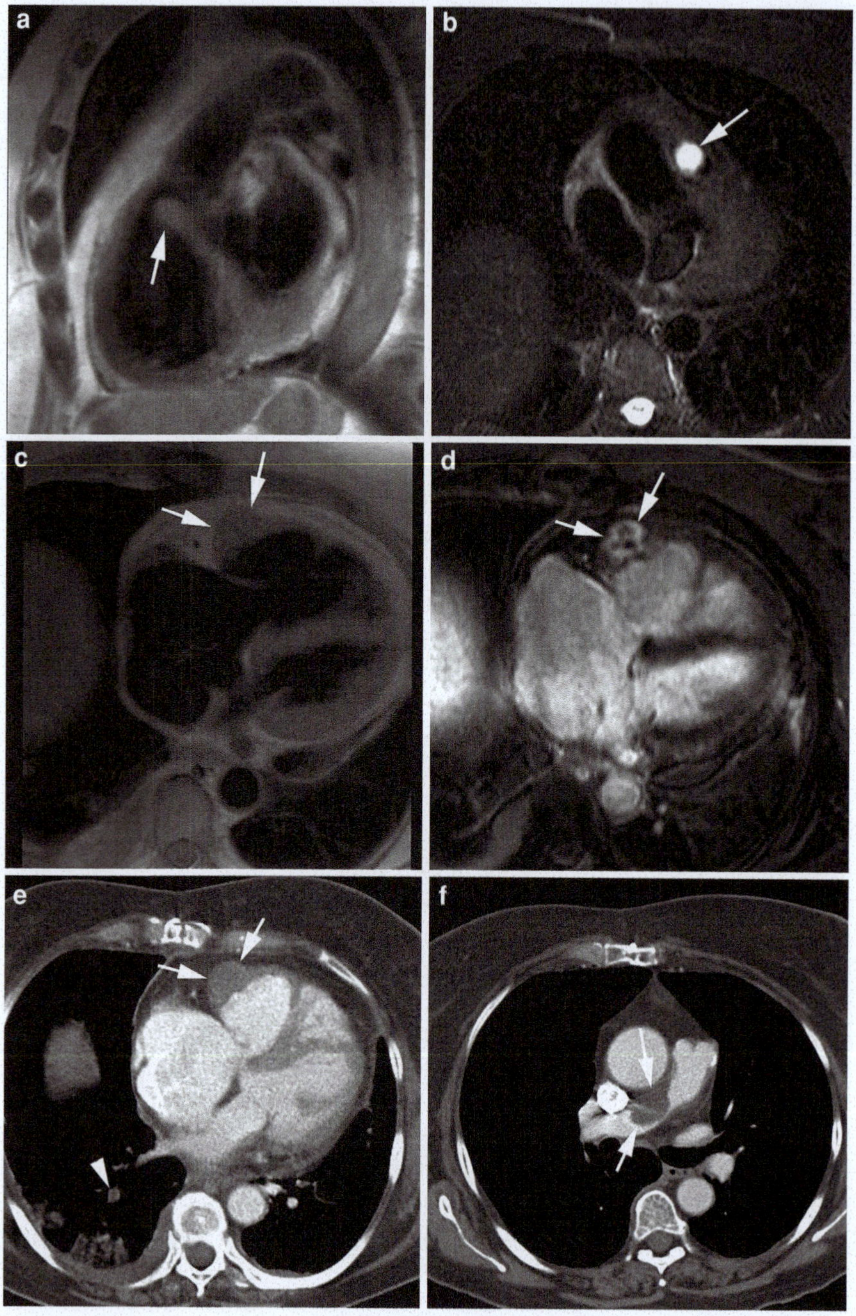

Fig. 22 Incidental finding of intima sarcoma in a 62-year-old woman presenting with cor pulmonale and pulmonary outflow obstruction (peak gradient 35 mm Hg). T1w-imaging in RVOT view (**a**), axial T2w-imaging (**b**). Follow-up MRI and CT one-year post-surgical resection (**c–f**). Axial T1w-imaging (**c**), late Gd imaging (**d**). Axial CT at the level of the ventricles (**e**) and right pulmonary artery (**f**). The intima sarcoma appears as a well-defined mass in the RVOT (*arrow*, **a**, **b**) and is iso-intense on T1w-imaging, strongly hyperintense on T2w-imaging. Tumor recurrence one-year post-surgery, visible as a wall thickening of RV free wall (*arrows*, **c–e**), and metastatic involvement of the right pulmonary artery (*arrows*, **f**). Because of the small, homogeneous, and well-defined appearance at initial presentation on MRI, a tumor with benign characteristics was presumed most likely

e.g., adrenocortical carcinoma (Ritchey et al. 1987; Godine et al. 1990), hepatocellular carcinoma (Kanematsu et al. 1994), Wilms' tumor (Gibson et al. 1990), renal cell carcinoma (Paul et al. 1975), recurrent pheochromocytoma (Rote et al. 1977), endometrial stromal carcinoma (Phillips et al. 1995), and thyroid carcinoma (Thompson et al. 1978). Its presence is potentially hazardous because it can cause caval obstruction, extension of the tumor thrombus into the right atrium causing atrial occlusion, and tumor embolization. Intracardiac leiomyomatosis is a rare complication of right-sided obstruction and should be considered in the differential diagnosis if the patient is of reproductive age

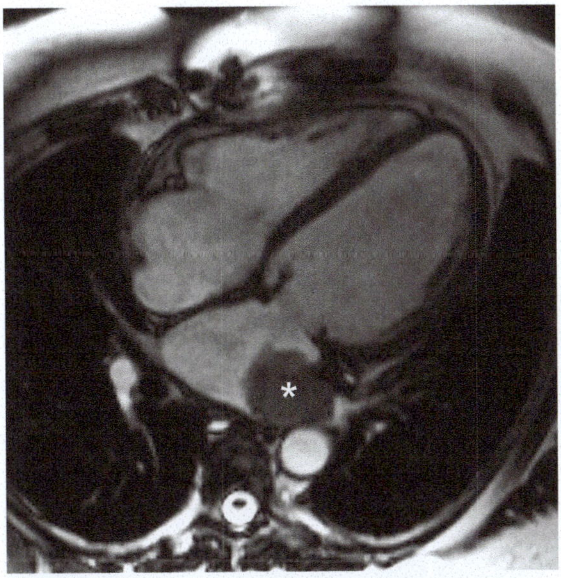

Fig. 23 Recurrence of LA fibrosarcoma in 55-year-old woman six months post-surgical resection. Horizontal long-axis cine image shows irregularly defined soft-tissue mass (*star*) laterally located in left atrium

and is found to have a mass lesion in the right side of the heart.

Complete excision of tumors showing intracaval extension is necessary to avoid recurrence. Preoperative diagnosis of caval involvement is essential for planning the extent of surgery. For instance, intravascular extension of adrenocortical carcinoma is not a contraindication to radical surgery. Accurate identification is essential to plan treatment and to avoid complications. MRI is perfectly suited to detect the presence and extension of an intracaval tumor thrombus. Although differentiation between the tumor component and the accompanying bland thrombus is still difficult with MRI, Nguyen et al. (1996) reported the presence of a patchy flow signal within the cavoatrial thrombus as a pattern of tumoral neovascularity in a patient with a renal granular cell carcinoma.

4.2.4 Retrograde Flow by Lymphatic Vessels

This fourth pathway of cardiac involvement occurs from spread from noncontiguous mediastinal lymph nodes via the lymphatic vessels to the heart with predominant epicardial involvement and variable myocardial invasion. Retrograde spread has been shown to be the most common mechanism in lymphomas and may also be seen in cases of lung and breast carcinoma (DeLoach and Haynes 1953). Disease spreads from the anterior mediastinum to the paracardiac area and pericardium; the hilus may be bypassed and may remain uninvolved, since it is not necessarily part of the drainage (Jochelson et al. 1983).

The lymphatics of the visceral pericardium and the heart drain into larger lymphatic vessels which run within the subepicardial fat and drain either to the nodes situated at the base of the heart, between the transverse part of the aorta and the left pulmonary artery, or directly into the anterosuperior mediastinal nodes. The lymphatics of the parietal pericaridium are scanty and run upward along the phrenic nerve over the lateral aspect of the cardiac silhouette and into the anterior mediastinal nodes. A chain of nodes may also be seen posteriorly, running along the pulmonary ligament to the hilus. Lymph nodes that are sometimes present on the parietal pericardial surface, usually in the right hemithorax, are associated with the lymph drainage from the central part of the diaphragm. Therefore, the nodal areas referred to as pericardiac and paracardiac include the inferior internal mammary, diaphragmatic, paraphrenic, posterior pulmonary ligament, and paraesophageal nodes.

4.3 Para and Extracardiac Tumors

These tumors are not only more frequent than primary cardiac tumors but due to their close relation with the pericardium and heart, knowledge of their presentation is required for those regularly performing cardiac imaging (Lee et al. 2009). Paracardial tumors typically arise within the mediastinum, coming into close contact with the heart by direct growth. Pericardial and myocardial involvement occurs by external compression or tumor invasion. Mediastinal masses (e.g., enlarged lymph nodes) often abut the pericardium without penetration of the pericardium (Fig. 30). The presence of a normal pericardium and pericardial sinuses provides a natural cleavage plane between the heart and the mediastinal mass. In these cases, usually no pericardial effusion is seen (Barakos et al. 1989b). Tumors located in the anterior mediastinum include thymomas, thymo-lipomas, lymphomas, germ cell tumors, and tumor or masses originating from the thyroid gland. Tumors located in

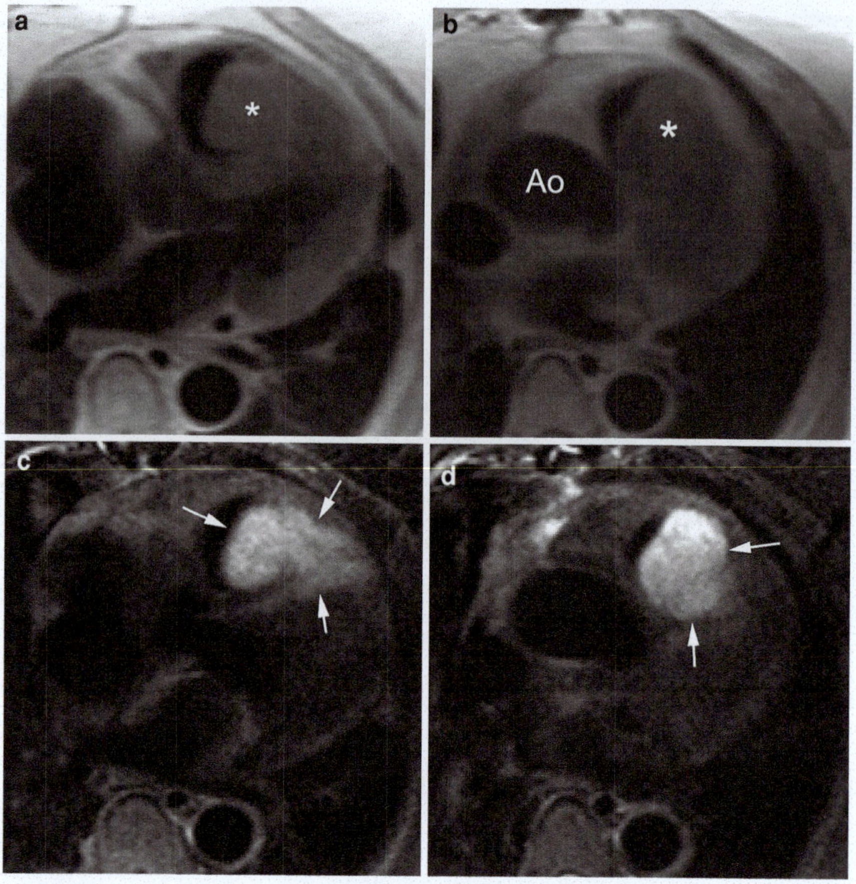

Fig. 24 Leiomyosarcoma of the right ventricular outflow tract in a 64-year-old woman. Axial T1w-imaging (**a**, **b**), axial T2w-imaging (**c**, **d**). The leiomyosarcoma presents a soft-tissue mass subtotally obstructing the RVOT. While iso-intense to the surrounding myocardium on T1w-imaging (*star*), the high signal on T2w-imaging sequences allows a better determination of the tumor borders (*arrows*)

the middle and posterior mediastinum are mostly neurogenic, arise from the esophagus (e.g., esophageal cancer, enteric cyst/duplication), or are related to the trachea or bronchi (e.g., bronchogenic cyst or bronchial cancer).

MRI is perfectly suited to describe the relation of the tumor to the heart, and to evaluate cardiac or vascular compression or invasion by the tumor. Furthermore, the signal characteristics on MRI can be used for tissue characterization. For instance, a bronchogenic cyst has a relatively high signal intensity on T1w-imaging and a very high signal intensity on T2w-imaging (Nakata et al. 1993; Davis et al. 2010) (Fig. 31). A fluid–fluid level in the cyst may be caused by an intracystic hemorrhage or precipitation of calcium in the dependent part of the cyst (Bargallo et al. 1993; Aydingoz et al. 1997). Thymolipomas are anterior mediastinal masses that may conform to the shape of the adjacent structures, and thus may simulate cardiomegaly or diaphragmatic elevation on chest radiographs. MRI typically demonstrates a mixture of fat and soft-tissue signal intensity characteristics (Rosado de Christenson et al. 1994). MRI can be helpful in determining the malignancy of thymomas (Sakai et al. 1992; Kushihashi et al. 1996). Benign thymomas are well-defined round or oval masses in the anterior mediastinum with a homogeneous or slightly inhomogeneous signal on T2w images. On the other hand, invasive thymomas usually have an inhomogeneous signal intensity, a multinodular appearance, and a lobulated internal architecture or fibrous septa, and often display irregular borders. Thymic carcinomas demonstrate low-signal intensities on both T1w and T2w images and irregular margins, but lack fibrous septa or lobutated internal architecture. Although MRI appears promising, histology is still essential to distinguish benign from malignant mediastinal lesions (Massie et al. 1997).

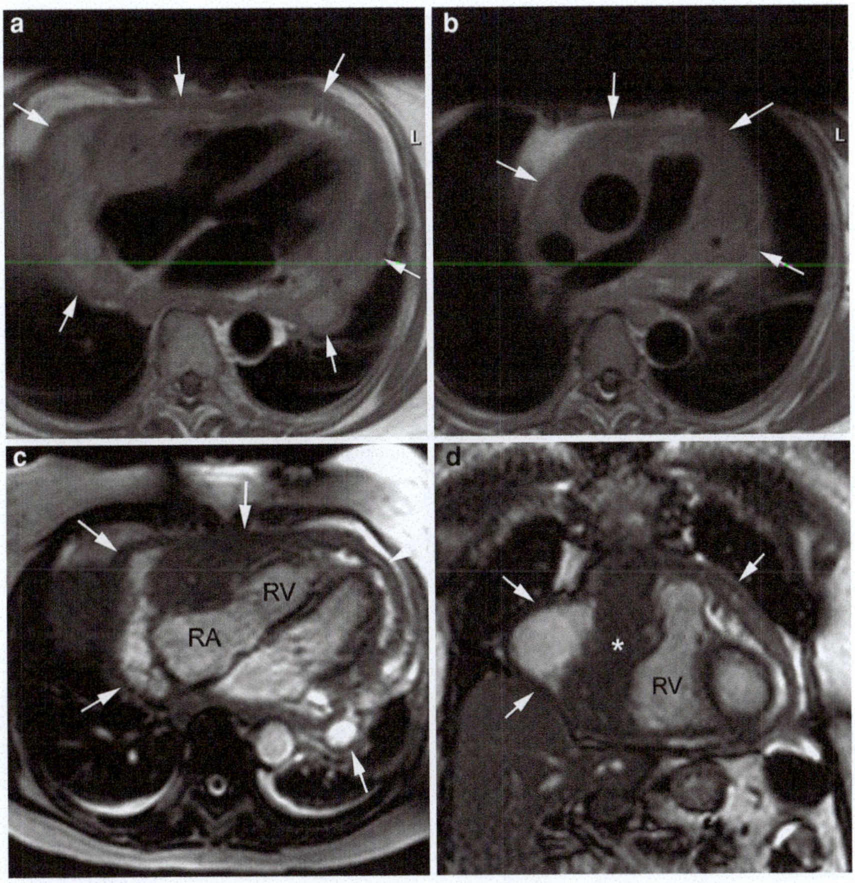

Fig. 25 High-grade non-Hodgkin lymphoma invading the heart in a 68-year-old woman. Axial T1w-imaging (**a**, **b**). Axial (**c**) and coronal (**d**) cine imaging. Although this patient was diagnosed with a pericardial effusion on cardiac ultrasound, cardiac MRI shows a soft-tissue mass diffusely involving the right atrioventricular groove (*star*, **d**). The pericardium is diffusely thickened (*arrows*) with a right-sided localized effusion

4.4 Nontumoral Cardiac Masses and Mimics

4.4.1 Thrombus

Cardiac thrombi are much more frequent than cardiac tumors. Recognition and appropriate treatment remains important because of risk of systemic or pulmonary embolization. The formation of thrombi usually occurs in patients with regional or global wall motion abnormalities, such as those that develop after myocardial infarction and in association with dilated cardiomyopathy or atrial fibrillation, especially if mitral valve disease and enlarged atrium and appendage are present (DePace et al. 1981). In myocardial infarct patients, risk factors for developing left ventricular thrombus are infarct location, i.e., anterior myocardial infarction, infarct size and extent, and impairment in global and regional left ventricular function. Left ventricular thrombi are often attached to the apex or within a discrete aneurysm or dyskinetic ventricular wall (Keeley and Hillis 1996) (Fig. 32). Although ventricular thrombi are exceedingly rare in patients with normal ventricular function, they should be considered in patients with coagulation disorders (DeGroat et al. 1985; Chin et al. 1988) (Fig. 33). Left atrial thrombi are generally attached to the posterior left atrial wall by a broad base, so that they are immobile (Fig. 34). If they are pedunculated and mobile, distinguishing them from a myxoma may be difficult. Right-atrial thrombi (Fig. 35) are usually found in patients with central venous lines or patients having enlarged cavities, e.g., restrictive cardiomyopathy.

The primary screening modality for patients with suspected cardiac thrombus is two-dimensional echocardiography. However, false-negative, false-positive, or equivocal findings are not uncommon, and are related to inadequate echocardiograms caused by anatomic abnormalities of the patients or to certain characteristics or location of the thrombus (Stratton

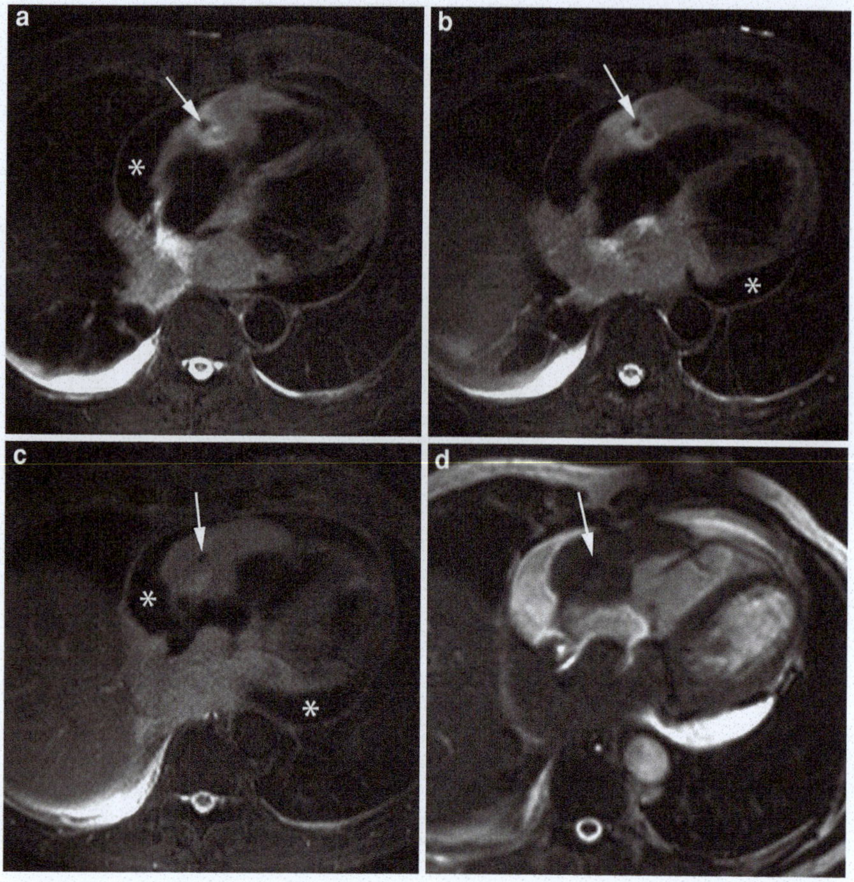

Fig. 26 Cardiac B-cell non-Hodgkin lymphoma in 75-year-old man. Axial T2w-imaging at 3 levels through the heart (**a–c**), axial cine imaging (**d**). An irregularly defined and inhomogeneous mass is diffusely infiltrating the heart. It involves the right atrioventricular sulcus (*arrows*) and extends to the adjacent RV free wall, to the atrial septum, RA dorsal wall, and LA walls. Note the presence of a moderate pericardial effusion (*star*), and right-sided pleural effusion

et al. 1982; Jungehulsing et al. 1992; Weinsaft et al. 2009). For instance, large, echogenic, irregular, mobile mural thrombi are easy to detect on echocardiography, while laminated mural thrombi may be difficult to distinguish from myocardium, and slow flowing blood in aneurysm may be confused with thrombus. Thrombi located in the ventricular apex are often difficult to assess with TTE (near-field probe).

MRI has a great potential in the diagnosis of suspected cardiac thrombi. It was already found in the 1980 s that cardiac thrombi usually have higher signal intensity than normal myocardium on spin-echo MRI (Dooms and Higgins 1986). Differentiation between thrombus and slow-flowing blood on spin-echo MRI, however, may be difficult because of the increased MR signal produced by slow-flowing blood (Fig. 30) (Gomes et al. 1987; Sechtem et al. 1989). Bright-blood MRI, in contrast, permits improved differentiation of thrombi from the surrounding blood pool and myocardium (Jungehulsing et al. 1992). On bright-blood MRI, a thrombus typically has lower signal intensity than blood. Differentiation between thrombus and myocardium on bright-blood MRI is more difficult because the thrombus tends to have a similar signal intensity as the adjacent surrounding myocardium. Since the thrombotic material differs according to its age and degree of organization, the signal intensity of the thrombus will change due to loss of water, condensation of paramagnetic iron complexes, and sometimes calcification (Baumgartner 1973). A major advantage of bright-blood imaging is the capability for dynamic evaluation of cardiac motion and blood flow using cine MRI. With the currently used balanced SSFP cine MRI sequences, high contrast is routinely obtained between blood and surrounding structures, improving detection of mural thrombi (Spuentrup et al. 2003). Alternative methods to cine MRI applicable for the detection of cardiac thrombi are PC-MRI and myocardial tagging (Fig. 32).

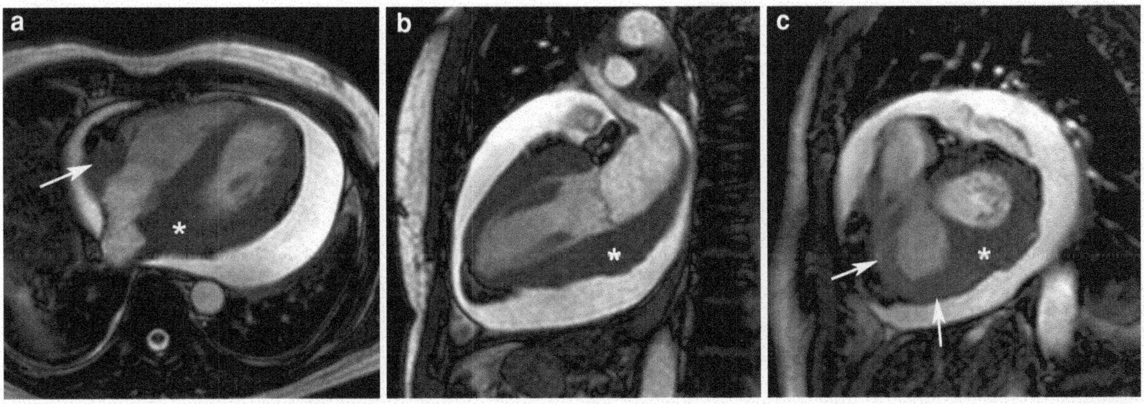

Fig. 27 Chloroma in 56-year-old man with history of acute myeloid leukemia treated with allogenic bone marrow transplantation. Cine imaging in horizontal (**a**), vertical (**b**), and short-axis (**c**), image plane. Presence of a soft-tissue structure (*star*) diffusely involving the right atrioventricular groove. Invasion of the LV inferior and inferoseptal wall that appears thickened and exhibits impaired contractility. Presence of an important pericardial effusion with evidence of cardiac tamponade

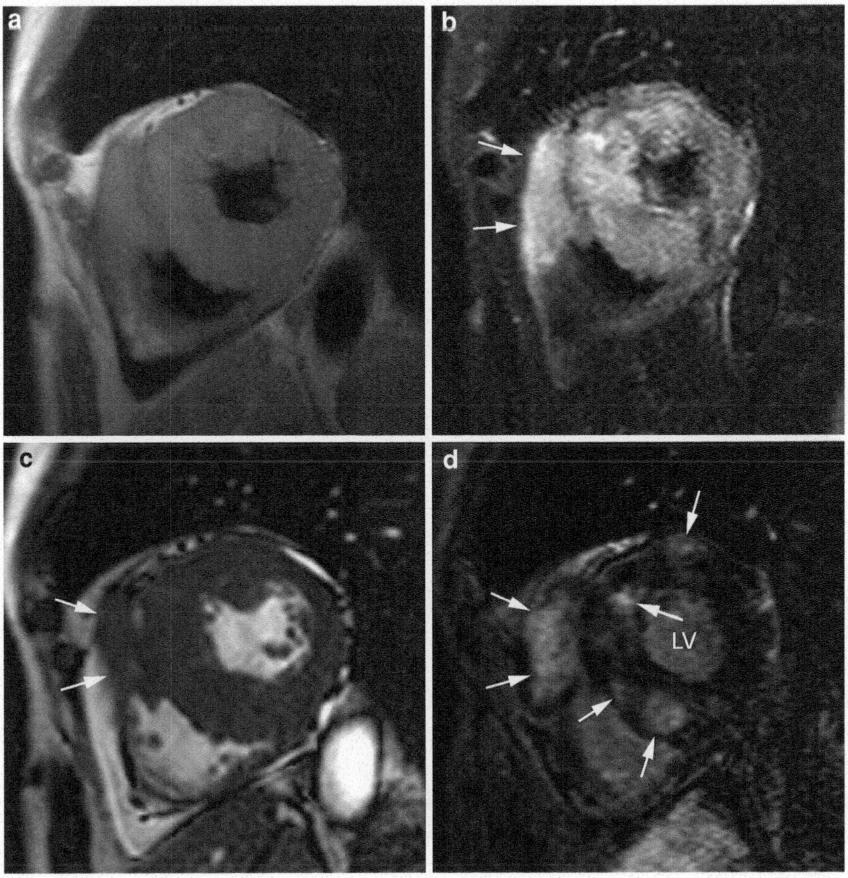

Fig. 28 Pericardial and myocardial metastases in 64-year-old man with malignant melanoma. All images are obtained in the cardiac short-axis at midventricular level, T1w-imaging (**a**), T2w-imaging (**b**), cine imaging (**c**), and late Gd MRI (**d**). The metastastic cardiac involvement presents as a concentric hypertrophy mainly involving the ventricular septum and right ventricular outflow tract (**a**, **c**). On T2w-imaging, the LV wall and the adjacent RV wall (*arrows*) appear inhomogeneously hyperintense. On cine imaging, the ventricular septum appeared diffusely hypokinetic. On late Gd imaging, multiple regions of strong enhancement are found in the thickened LV and RV myocardium (*arrows*)

The late Gd imaging technique has not only lead to a paradigm shift in the way we nowadays look at myocardial infarctions, but this technique showed to be advantageous in many other cardiac diseases, including detection of intracavitary thrombi (Mollet et al. 2002; Barkhausen et al. 2002; Bogaert et al.

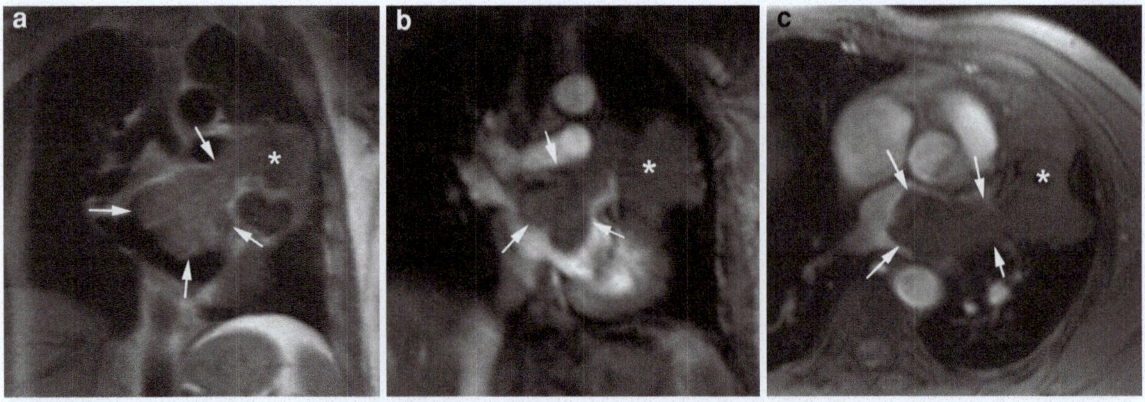

Fig. 29 Venous extension of metastatic fibrosarcoma in the left atrium in a 46-year-old man. Coronal T1w-imaging (**a**). Coronal (**b**) and axial (**c**) cine imaging. Large metastatic mass in the left lung (*star*) invades the left atrium (*arrows*) through left upper lobe pulmonary vein. The left atrial mass is free-floating in the atrial cavity

Fig. 30 Renal cell carcinoma with enlarged (*star*) and hilar (*arrows*) lymph nodes in a 36-year-old man. **a**, **b** Axial T1w-imaging. Bilateral pleural effusion

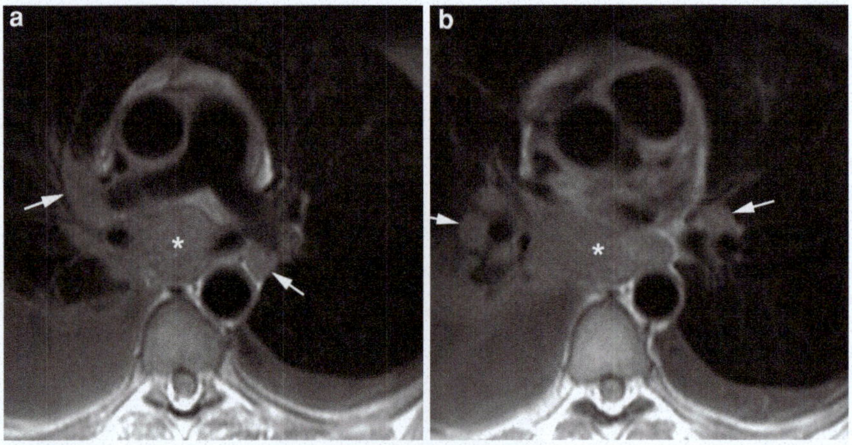

2004; Weinsaft et al. 2008, 2009). The intravenous administration of paramagnetic contrast agents substantially shortens blood T1-relaxation, providing a strong enhancement of the cardiac chambers, hereby facilitating the detection of abnormal intracavitary structures, such as cardiac thrombi, that become visible as 'dark' structures (Fig. 36). The late Gd imaging technique showed to be superior to cine MRI and TTE in detecting left ventricular thrombi in patients with a recent or chronic myocardial infarction (Mollet et al. 2002; Srichai et al. 2006; Weinsaft et al. 2008, 2009, 2011). This technique is particularly beneficial in detecting small thrombi (less than 1 cm^3) for instance when trapped in the endocardial trabeculations, and for apically located thrombi (Fig. 37). While thrombi can often already be suspected on cine MRI, the clear black/white contrast on late Gd imaging usually makes the diagnosis straightforward. As recently proposed by Bekkers et al. (2009), use of a longer inversion time for early late Gd imaging, may not only be beneficial for improved detection of microvascular obstruction in patients with an acute myocardial infarction but may probably improve thrombus detection too, due to an improved contrast difference between thrombus and (normal) myocardium (Weinsaft et al. 2008, 2011). It should be emphasized that the late Gd imaging technique is optimized to nullify signal of normal myocardium, so that it is difficult to evaluate thrombus enhancement and thus to differentiate between subacute and chronic thrombi. Paydarfar et al. (2001) reported, using gradient-recalled-echo MRI and T1w-imaging before

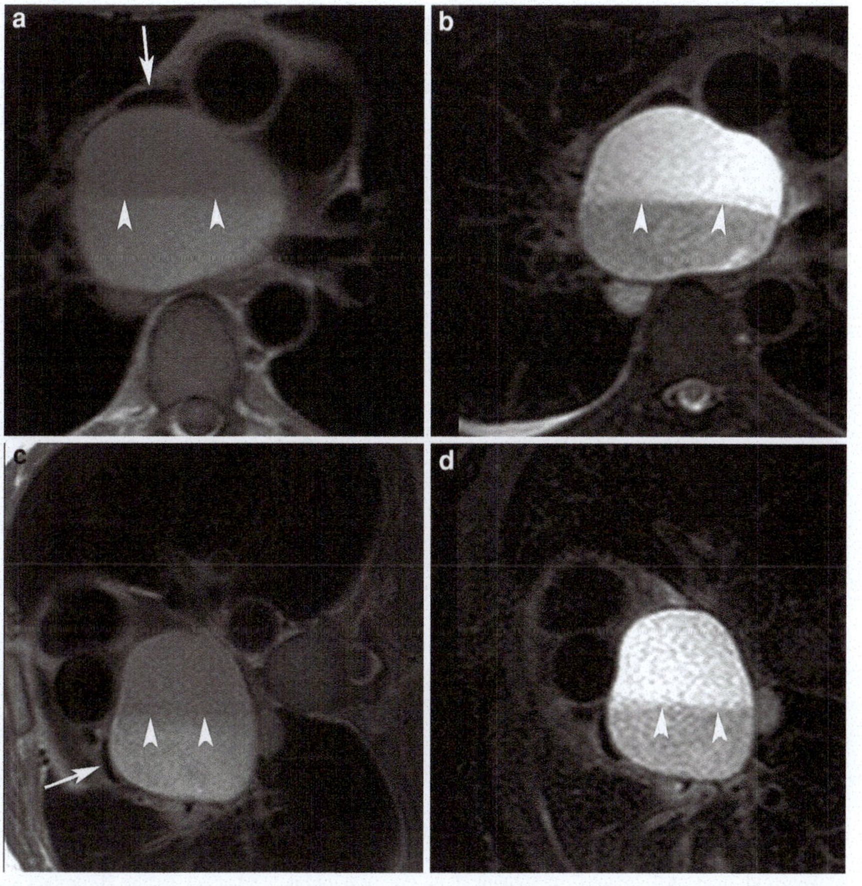

Fig. 31 Bronchogenic cyst. Axial T1w- (**a**) and T2w- (**b**) imaging obtained in debucitus and repeated with the patient positioned in right lateral decubitus position (**c**, **d**). A sharply defined soft-tissue structure is present above the left atrium, compressing the adjacent structures such as the superior vena cava (*arrow*, **a**, **c**). Note the presence of an intralesional fluid–fluid level (*arrowheads*) that remains horizontal independent of patient position. Due the gravity, the lower layer of the cyst has a higher protein content explaining the higher signal intensity on T1w-imaging and lower signal intensity on T2w-imaging compared to the upper layer

and after administration of contrast medium, that subacute clots have an homogeneously low-signal, do not enhance with gadolinium, and exhibit magnetic susceptibility effects while organized clots have a intermediate, heterogeneous signal and whose multiple areas of gadolinium enhancement. Especially the enhancement pattern in organized thrombi might impede differentiation with cardiac tumors, e.g., myxoma.

To summarize, one should be particularly careful for the presence of thrombi in patients with increased risk for thrombus formation. A combination of cine MRI and late Gd imaging with careful analysis of the regions at risk, i.e., the infarct area, (aneurysmatic) ventricular apex and dysfunctional segments for the ventricles, and the appendages for the atria, is probably the best strategy not to miss thrombi. The left atrial appendage on MRI is usually very well evaluable on vertical long-axis images (Fig. 38).

4.4.2 Valvular Vegetations

Valvular vegetations can also be confused as mass lesions by echocardiography. However, in these instances, the echoes generally appear small and movement is limited. Furthermore, the vegetations follow the motion of the valvular cusp to which they are attached. MRI may be useful in clarifying echocardiographic findings and establishing the diagnosis in previously undiagnosed patients. Vegetations may be not or difficulty visible on dark-blood imaging but are well visible on cine MRI, appearing as areas of low-signal at valve leaflets in contrast to the bright flowing blood (Caduff et al. 1996).

Libman-Sacks endocarditis, or the endocardial involvement in patients with systemic lupus erythematosus, is found in up to 50% of hearts at autopsy. It presents as small verrucous vegetations (3–4 mm in size) appearing on the valvular or mural endocardial surface. The posterior mitral valve leaflet is most frequently involved. Infrequently, such vegetations

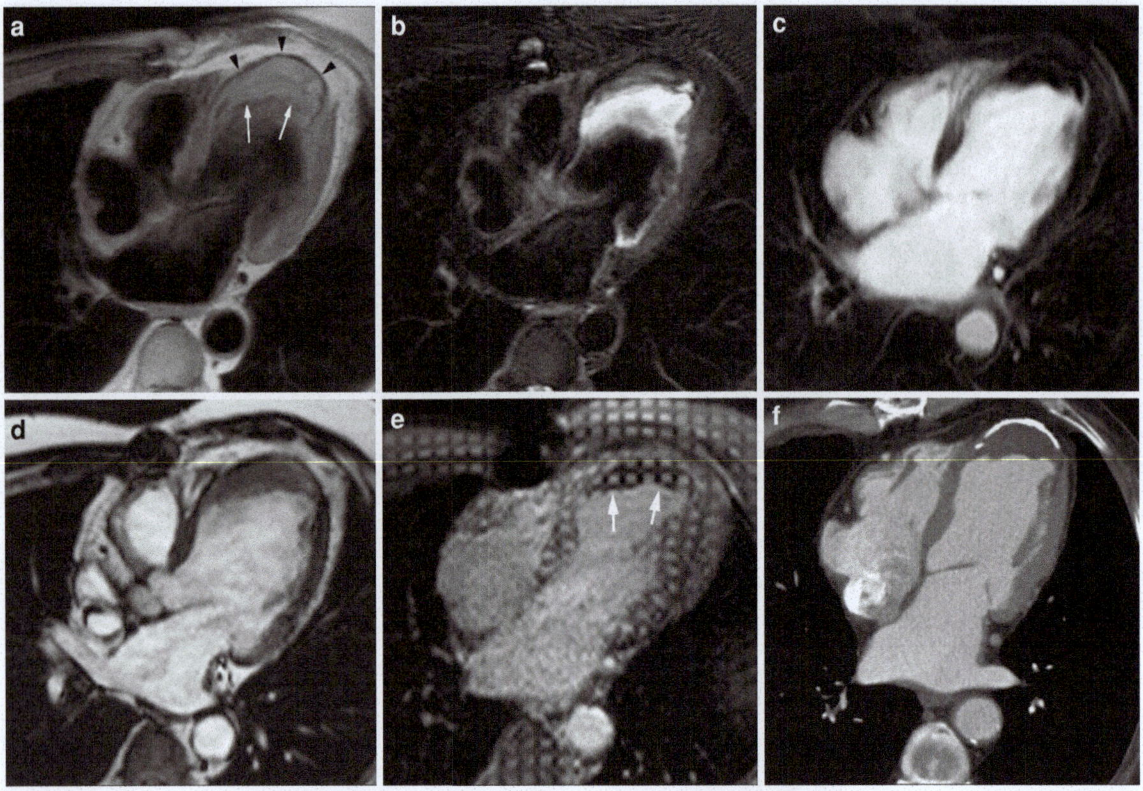

Fig. 32 Comparison of imaging techniques to detect large mural thrombus (*arrows*) in a calcified LV apical aneurysm in a 61-year-old man. All images are obtained in the horizontal long-axis plane. T1w-imaging (**a**), T2w-imaging (**b**), late Gd imaging (**c**) cine imaging (**d**), MRI myocardial tagging performed after contrast administration (**e**), contrast-enhanced CT (**f**). The calcified aneurysm is visible as a curvilinear hypointense line (*arrowheads*) on T1w-imaging (**a**). The appearance and signal intensity of the thrombus is different according the imaging modality used. Note the presence of slow-flow adjacent to the thrombus shown as high signal on the T2w-imaging. The MRI tagging image nicely shows the nondeformation of the tag lines in the thrombus. Moreover, due to contrast administration the signal intensity of the tag lines in the thrombus differs from those in the adjacent myocardium

may become massive thrombotic lesions, up to 10 mm, or even larger (Doherty and Siegel 1985). This entity may predispose to infective endocarditis. As in other causes of valvular vegetations, MRI can be of help in visualization of the valve or mural lesions.

4.4.3 Perivalvular Extension of Infection

Perivalvular extension of infection (i.e., cardiac abscess and pseudoaneurysm) is a not infrequent and potentially fatal complication of bacterial endocarditis (Carpenter 1991). Cardiac abscesses are observed in 20–30% of cases of infective endocarditis and in at least 60% of cases of prosthetic valve endocarditis (Thomas et al. 1993). The aortic valve ring is more frequently affected than the mitral valve ring. The perivalvular extension of infection (usually involving the mitral-aortic intervalvular fibrosa) may present as a closed purulent collection (i.e., cardiac abscess) or as a cavity contiguous with a cardiac chamber (i.e., pseudoaneurysm) (Fig. 39). Subsequent rupture of the infected zone of mitral-aortic intervalvular fibrosa or subaortic aneurysm into the left atrium may occur, a condition which should be differentiated from ruptured aneurysm of the sinus of Valsalva (Bansal et al. 1990).

Although TEE is the imaging method of choice for the diagnosis of valvular vegetations in infectious endocarditis, the diagnosis of an associated ring abscess is sometimes difficult, especially in patients

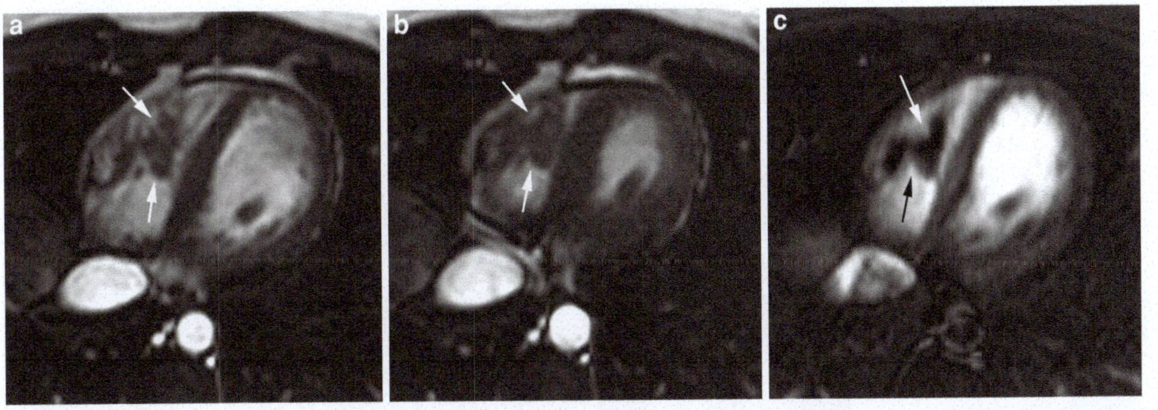

Fig. 33 Right ventricular thrombi (*arrows*) in a 19-year-old man with coagulation disorders. Cine imaging at end diastole (**a**), and end systole (**b**), late Gd imaging (**c**). All the images are acquired in the axial image plane. The thrombus appears as an irregular mass (*arrows*) attached to the endocavitary muscular network in the right ventricle. The thrombus remains hypointense following contrast administration (*arrow*, **c**)

Fig. 34 Mural thrombus in 62-year-old patient presenting with mitral stenosis and dilated LA. Cine imaging in horizontal (**a**) and vertical (**b**) long-axis plane, Late Gd imaging in horizontal (**c**) and vertical (**d**) long-axis image plane. A well-defined soft-tissue mass is visible in broad contact with the posterior LA wall (*arrowheads*, **a**, **b**). No enhancement is found following contrast administration (*arrowheads*, **c**, **d**). The thrombus was surgically resected during mitral valve surgery

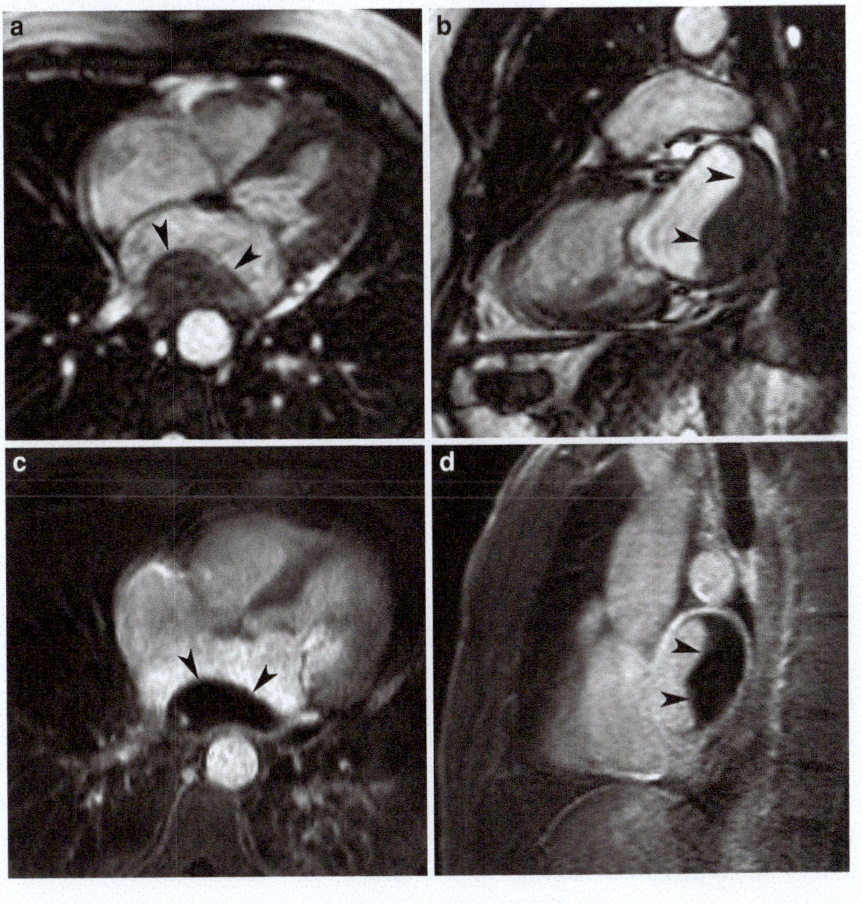

with valvular prostheses or calcifications, which are an important source of artifacts. MRI may be useful to detect the paravalvular abscess and infectious pseudoaneurysms. A cardiac abscess is visible as a heterogeneous low-signal intensity zone on T1w-imaging and as high intensity signal on T2w-imaging. The inflammatory origin is responsible for the increase in signal after injection of paramagnetic

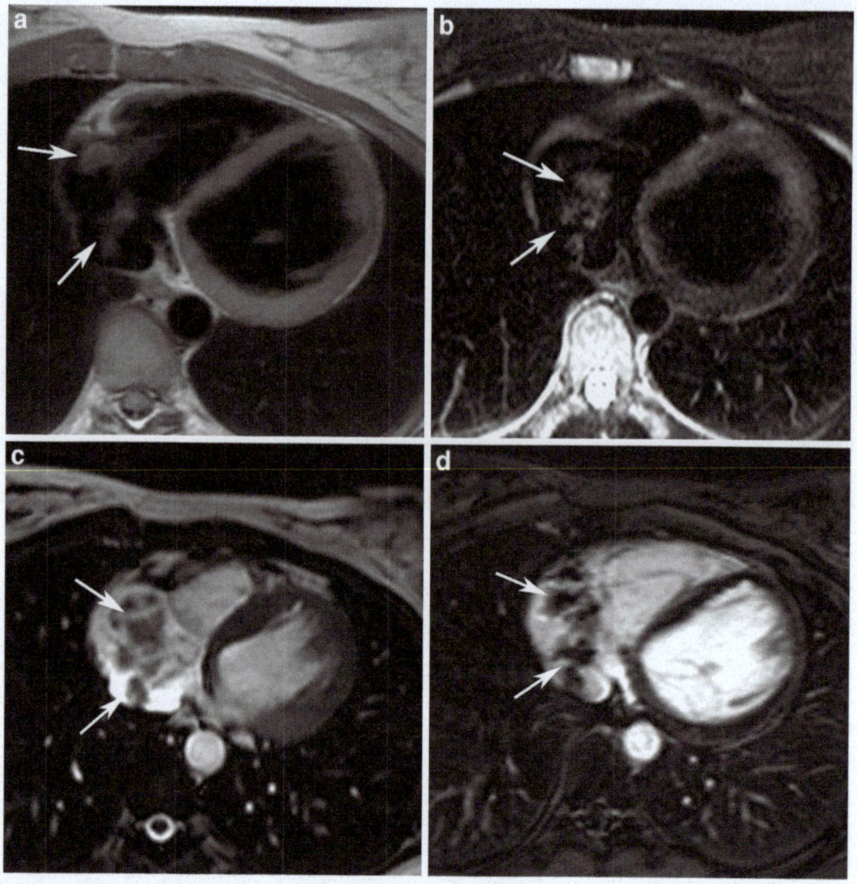

Fig. 35 Right-atrial thrombus in 24-year-old woman with systemic lupus erythematosus and antiphospholipid syndrome. T1w-imaging (**a**), T2w-imaging (**b**), cine imaging (**c**), late Gd imaging (**d**). All images are acquired in the axial image plane. An irregularly defined structure is well visible in the right atrium (*arrow*) without evidence of enhancement following contrast administration (*arrow*, **d**). The thrombus resolved with anticoagulation therapy (echocardiographic follow-up)

contrast agents. Cine MRI is helpful to detect the presence or absence of communication between the abscess cavity and the cardiac chambers. MRI is also recommended in the follow-up of patients with perivalvular extension of infection (Fig. 39).

4.4.4 Lipomatous Hypertrophy of the Interatrial Septum

Lipomatous hypertrophy of the (inter)atrial septum is, pathogenetically, a hypertrophy of preexisting fat, and not a true neoplasm, and it is not infrequently associated with increased epicardial fat (Meany et al. 1997; Cunningham et al. 2006). This poorly recognized, but not rare, benign condition represents a fat accumulation within the interatrial septum in continuity with the epicardial fat. This entity is usually an incidental finding, though some suggest an association with supraventricular arrhythmias and sudden death (O'Connor et al. 2006). Fat acculumation occurs anterior and posterior to the fossa ovalis. Since there is no fat accumulation in the fossa ovalis, lipomatous hypertrophy of the atrial septum often has a typical bilobed "camel-humped" or "dumbbell-shaped" appearance (Fig. 40). Sometimes the fat accumulation can extend in the direction of the entrance of the superior caval vein or toward the right-atrial wall, causing extrinsic compression of these structures (Fig. 41). Because of the typical appearance and the lipomatous nature, presenting as fat attenuation on CT and high signal intensity on T1w-imaging, the lipomatous hypertrophy of the interatrial septum is straightforward, thus obviating biopsy or excision (Levine et al. 1986; Fisher and Edmonds 1988; Gaerte et al. 2002). In addition, selective fat suppression techniques can be used to demonstrate the fatty nature and to differentiate lipomatous hypertrophy of the interatrial septum from other nonlipomatous conditions (e.g., nonacute hematoma, hemangioma, and hemorrhage in a preexisting mass) (Figs. 40, 41). Because of its typical appearance differentiation with a cardiac lipoma usually poses no problem.

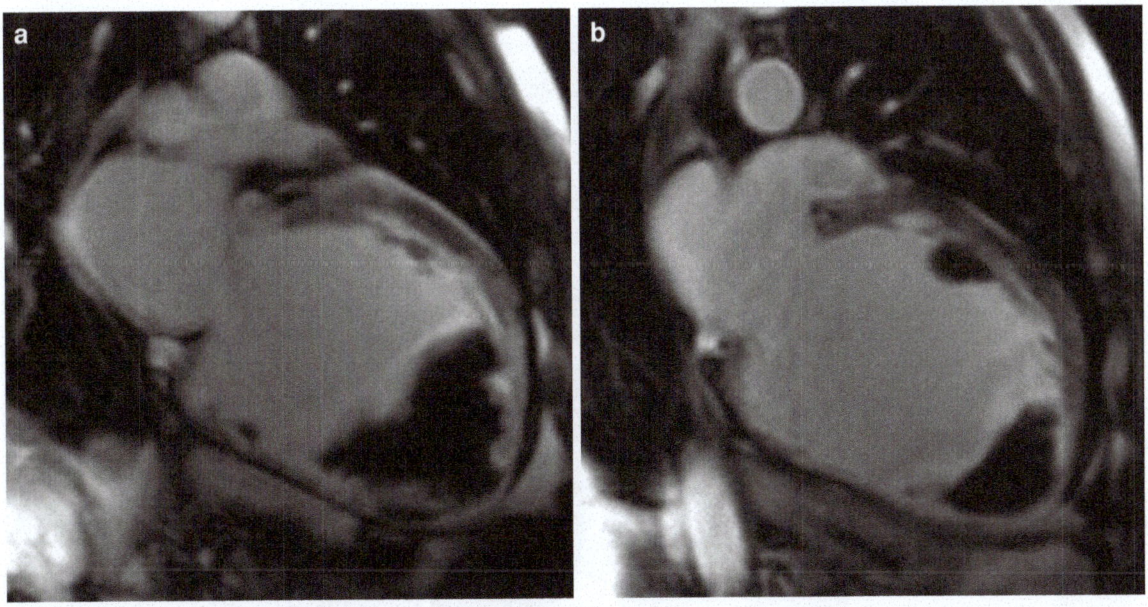

Fig. 36 Extensive thrombus formation in 55-year-old patient with severe ischemic cardiomyopathy (LV end-diastolic volume of 552 ml, and LV ejection fraction of 7%). Vertical long-axis late Gd MRI (**a**, **b**). Note the presence of a large apical thrombus (± 100 g), and a smaller mural thrombus adjacent to the anterior LV wall

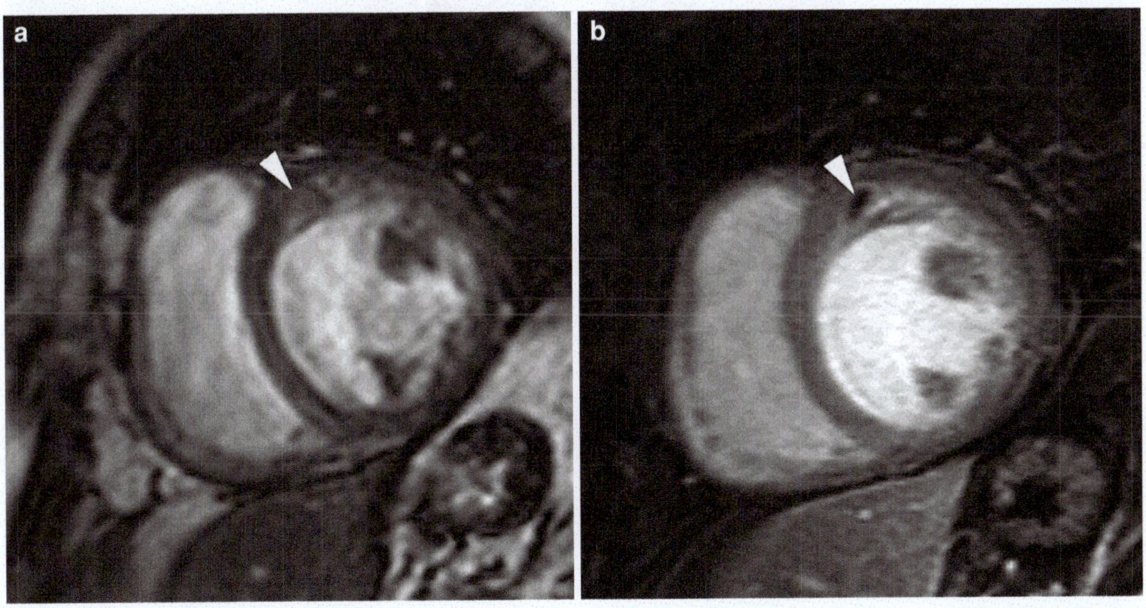

Fig. 37 Small thrombus trapped in anterior muscular trabeculations in a 58-year-old man with ischemic cardiomyopathy. Short-axis cine imaging (**a**), short-axis late Gd imaging (**b**). On late Gd imaging, a small, dark thrombus is well visible (*arrowhead*, **b**). This thrombus was initially not detected on cine MRI because of its small size, and the lack of signal differences with the surrounding myocardium (*arrowhead*, **a**)

4.4.5 Atrial Septal Aneurysm

An aneurysm of the interatrial septum is defined as a diffuse or a localized protrusion of the interatrial septum into the right or left atrium, or both, caused by a bulging of the whole interatrial septum or a bulging of the primary component of the septum through the

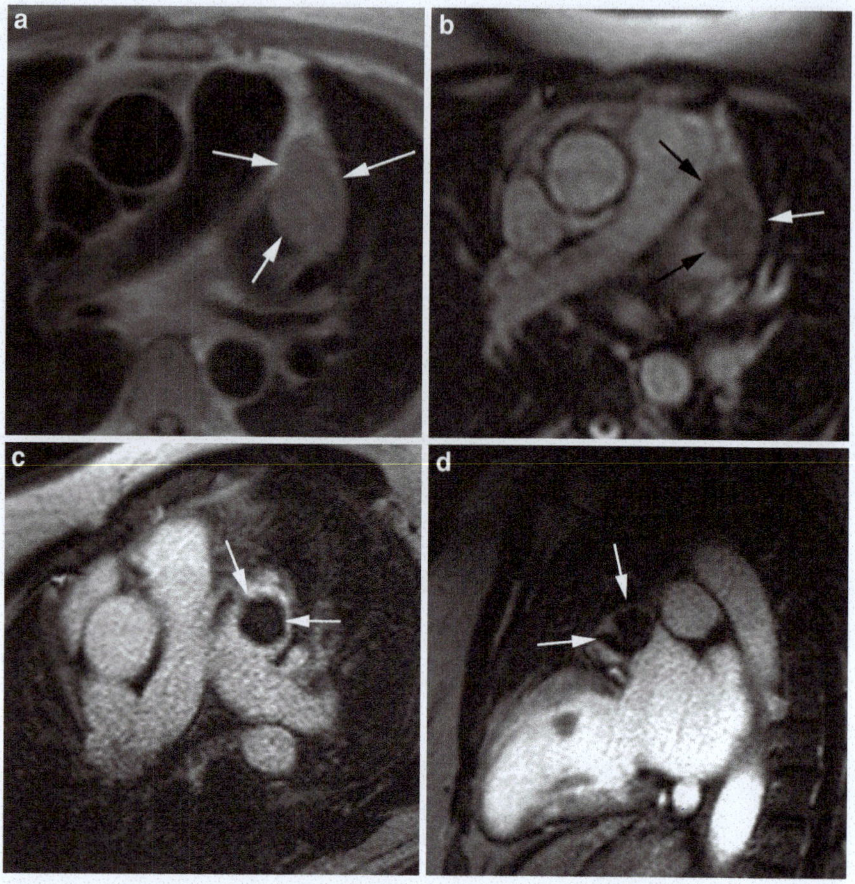

Fig. 38 Thrombus in the left atrial appendage in a 70-year-old woman with chronic atrial fibrillation and history of transient ischemic attacks. TTE (not shown) did not reveal abnormalities. Axial, T1w-imaging (**a**) shows lack of signal void (*arrows*) in dilated left atrial appendage. Is this due to slow flow or thrombus? Axial cine imaging shows gray nodular structure in the left atrial appendage (*arrows*, **b**). Late Gd imaging in axial (**c**) and vertical long-axis plane (**d**) nicely depicts the thrombus as a dark, non-enhancing structure in the appendage (*arrows*)

fossa ovalis. It is an uncommon anomaly and may be associated with other congenital cardiac malformations or with acquired diseases that result in elevated pressures in one atrial chamber with bulging of the septum to the opposite side (Hanley et al. 1985). Atrial septal aneurysms have been associated with septal defects, atrial arrhythmias, systolic clicks, atrioventricular valve prolapse, systemic and pulmonary embolism, and atrial tumors, and they usually occur at the fossa ovalis (Hanley et al. 1985; Gallet et al. 1985, Bogaert et al. 1995b). Hanley et al. (1985) observed three types of fossa ovalis aneurysm and one type of aneurysm involving the entire interatrial septum. Systemic and pulmonary thromboembolic events in the presence of an atrial septal aneurysm are probably due to thrombus formation within the concave aspect of the aneurysm. The frequently associated atrial septal defect may result in paradoxical emboli (Schneider et al. 1990).

Diagnosis is usually made by echocardiography, though stagnant blood flow within the cavity of the aneurysm may mimic a cystic mass (Smith et al. 1990). MRI is helpful in detecting atrial septal aneurysms, though it should be mentioned that low flow or stagnant flow may appear on dark-blood MRI as signal rich rather than signal void, thus mimicking a cardiac mass (Smith et al. 1990). Cine MRI may overcome this shortcoming, and allows a better description of the type and movement of aneurysm (Bogaert et al. 1995b).

4.4.6 Aneurysm of the Sinus of Valsalva

Aneurysms of the sinus of Valsalva are uncommon entities and although they are not truly cardiac masses, it is worth mentioning this condition in the differential diagnostic list of cardiac masses. They usually originate from the right coronary sinus, and much less frequently from the noncoronary and the

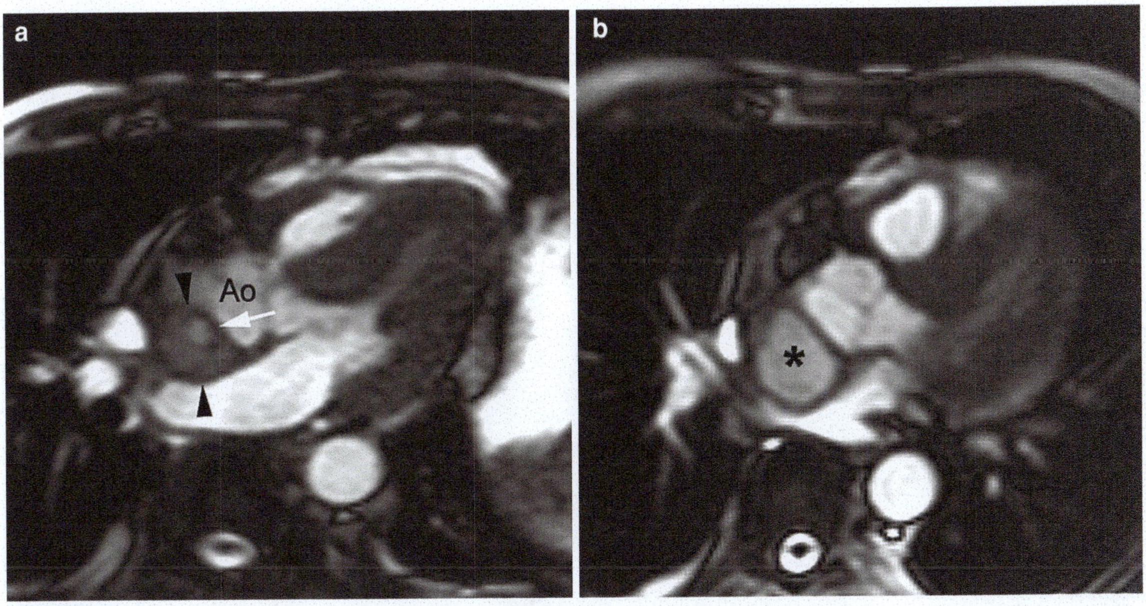

Fig. 39 Perivalvular extension of infection in a 52-year-old man with renal transplant. The patient was admitted with a staphylococcus aureus sepsis. Axial cine imaging at admission (**a**) and 1-week later (**b**). A well-defined soft-tissue structure is visible dorsal of the aorta root (*arrowheads*, **a**). Although highly suspicious of a periaortic abscess because of the presence of a central high signal spot (*arrow*) a pseudoaneurysm should be also be considered. Control study (**b**), one week later, clearly shows a presence of a retro-aortic pseudoaneurysm (*star*) that fills and empties during the cardiac cycle (information obtained on dynamic cine MRI viewing)

left coronary sinus (Dev et al. 1993). The aneurysms are usually congenital but infrequently they can be acquired (usually endocarditis associated). This condition is usually detected in adults as an incidental finding or by virtue of a complication due to the aneurysm (Fig. 42). The most frequent complication is rupture of the aneurysm, usually into the right ventricular outflow tract, right ventricular cavity, or right atrium, and less frequently into the other cardiac chambers or dissecting into the ventricular septum (Dev et al. 1993; Abad 1995). Other less frequent complications are embolization, compression of the coronary arteries by the aneurysm with subsequent myocardial infarction, and thrombosis of the aneurysm (Reid et al. 1990; Wiemer et al. 1996).

Although the diagnosis is usually made by TTE and TEE, MRI may be very helpful to demonstrate the relationship of the aneurysm with the surrounding structures, to depict the presence and to quantify the functional consequences of the aneurysm (Ogawa et al. 1991; Ho et al. 1995; Kulan et al. 1996; Hoey et al. 2010). A ruptured aneurysm will be visible on cine imaging as a continuous hypo-intense jet directed from the aneurysm into one of the cardiac chambers. PC-MRI in the pulmonary trunk and ascending aorta enable to calculate the shunt. Since aneurysms may lead to subobstruction, e.g., of the right ventricular outflow tract, the PC-MRI can be used to calculate the flow gradient.

4.4.7 Liquefaction Necrosis of the Mitral Annulus Calcification

Mitral annulus calcification is common degenerative disorder in the elderly, particularly in women and in patients with kidney disease. Liquefaction necrosis of the posterior mitral annulus, also called *caseous calcification of the mitral annulus*, is a rare and atypical variant of mitral annulus calcification that is usually associated with a benign prognosis and was recently identified as an unusual evolution of mitral annulus calcification. The core of liquefaction necrosis comprises amorphous eosinophilic acellular fluid, and the surrounding rim contains macrophages and lymphocytes as well as multiple areas of calcification and necrotic zones. Both CT and MRI are increasingly

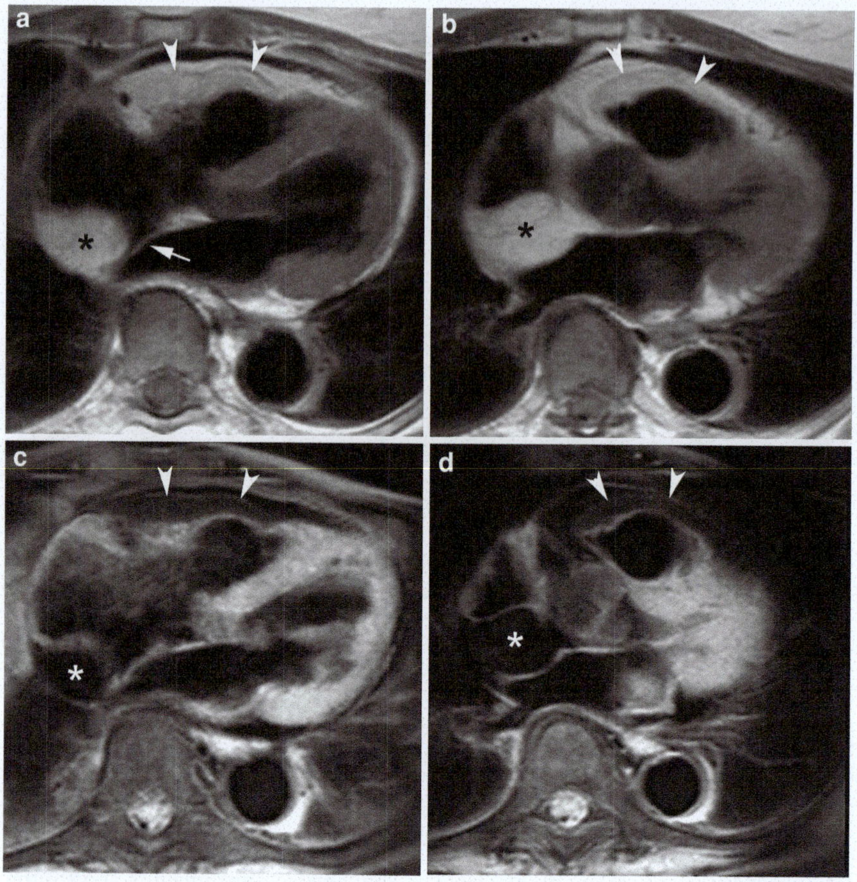

Fig. 40 Lipomatous hypertrophy of the atrial septum. Axial T1w-imaging without (**a**, **b**) and with (**c**, **d**) fat suppression prepulse. Presence of an important thickening of the atrial septum (*star*, **a**, **b**) with the exception of the region of the oval fossa (*arrow*, **a**). The signal intensity is similar as the mediastinal and subcutaneous fat. The signal is completely suppressed using fat-suppressed T1w-imaging (*star*, **c**, **d**). Notice furthermore the fatty infiltration with diffuse thickening of the RV free wall (*arrowheads*, **a**, **b**), which is equally, but to a lesser extent suppressed than the adjacent epicardial fat on fat-suppressed T1w-imaging

used to diagnose this entity and to describe the different components (Yokoyama et al. 2007; DiBella et al. 2008). In our experience, they present as cystic structures with a thickwalled, fibrotic/calcified wall located in the left ventricular (infero)lateral wall in the vicinity of the mitral valve (Fig. 43). Compression of the surrounding myocardium can occur when the lesion is large (Fig. 44). The signal characteristics of the core do not correspond to water but usually they have low-signal intensity on T2w-imaging. Strong enhancement of the thick wall is found on late Gd imaging.

4.4.8 Hydatid Cyst

Echinococcosis is endemic in several countries around the Mediterranean Sea. Cardiac involvement in hydatid disease is rare, representing 0.5–2% of all clinical forms of this condition (Cacoub et al. 1991). Because of the risk of potentially lethal complications (due to cyst rupture and massive embolism), early diagnosis and adequate treatment are very important (Pasaoglu et al. 1994). The diagnosis of cardiac echinococcosis is difficult and is based on a series of findings among which hydatid serology and cardiac imaging are particularly important. Hydatid cysts most frequently involve the left ventricular myocardial wall and ventricular septum (Kardaras et al. 1996). MRI, together with echocardiography and CT, is of considerable importance in the detection of intramyocardial hydatid cysts (Elkouby et al. 1990; Kulan et al. 1995; Kardaras et al. 1996; Macedo et al. 1997). MRI also allows diagnosis of noncardiac lesions, e.g., pulmonary, hepatic, splenic, and renal involvement, and is helpful in planning surgical intervention.

The detection of intramyocardial cystic lesions is virtually pathognomonic for hydatid disease. These hydatid cysts have a fluid content with a homogeneously hypo-intense signal intensity on T1w-imaging and a homogeneously hyperintense signal on

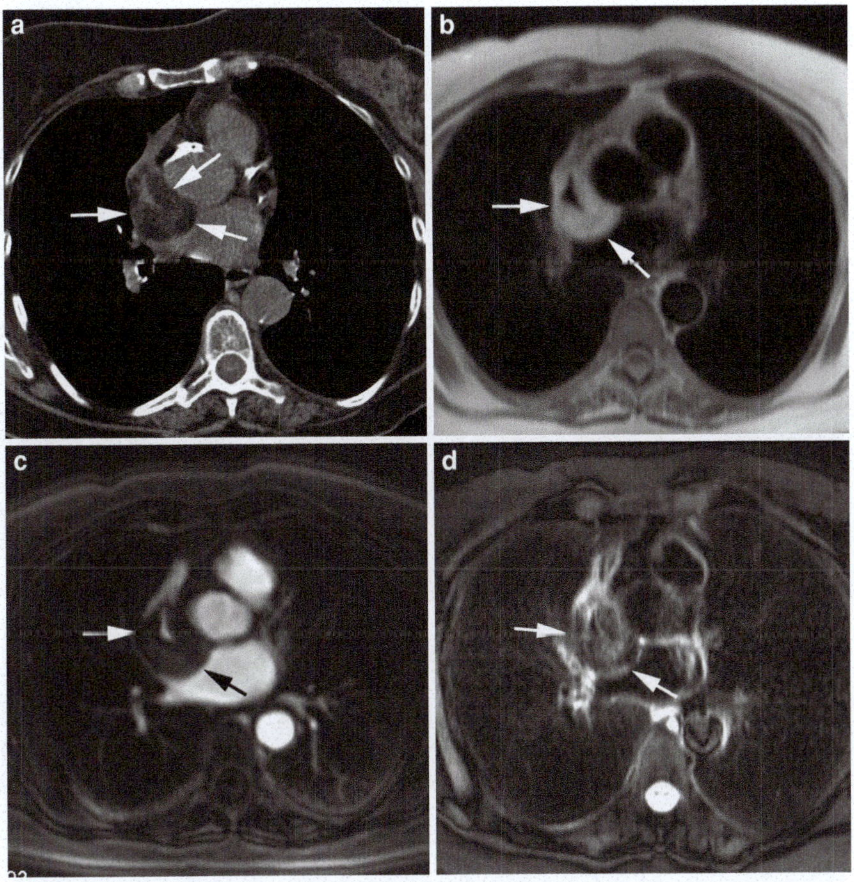

Fig. 41 Atypical presentation of lipomatous hypertrophy of the atrial septum causing compression of the superior caval vein. Contrast-enhanced CT (**a**), T1w-imaging without (**b**) and with fat (**d**) suppression, late Gd imaging (**c**). All images are obtained in the axial plane. Presence of fatty infiltration around the distal part of the superior caval vein causing a triangular luminal narrowing (*arrows*, **a**, **b**). The fatty nature is proven by the lack of signal on fat-suppressed T1w-imaging (*arrows*, **d**). No contrast enhancement occurs following contrast administration (*arrows*, **c**)

T2w-images (Kotoulas et al. 1996). The pericyst, a thick fibrotic membrane surrounding the hydatid cyst, has a low-signal intensity on T1w- and T2w-imaging and this allows differentiation from nonparasitic epithelial cysts (Vanjak et al. 1990; Cacoub et al. 1991; Cantoni et al. 1993).

4.4.9 Pericardial Cyst

Very likely pericardial cysts can be considered as nontumoral masses. They are usually asymptomatic and most frequently arise in the right cardiophrenic angle, followed by the left cardiophrenic angle and, rarely, the anterior or posterior mediastinum. They are usually unilocular and present with a variable diameter. Pericardial cysts are usually discovered during routine radiography. MRI may be very helpful in detecting the water content (Vinee et al. 1992). Pericardial cysts have a low-signal intensity on T1w-imaging and a very high signal intensity on T2w-imaging (Fig. 45). No enhancement following contrast medium is observed. MRI is also helpful in differentiation from other cystic mediastinal structures such as bronchogenic cyst (see Fig. 31), cystic teratoma, cystic neurogenic tumor, and thymus cyst. Differences in signal intensities on T1w-imaging can help in the differentiation since pericardial cysts have a pure water content with low-signal intensities, while the others may have a higher signal intensity due to intracystic hemorrhage or the presence of sebaceous fluid (Murayama et al. 1995) (Fig. 46). Furthermore, cystic teratomas typically contain fat and calcifications.

4.4.10 Gossypiboma or Textiloma

Gossypibomas or textilomas are an iatrogenic cause of cardiac, pericardial, or extracardiac masses. They represent a foreign body reaction surrounding a retained surgical sponge composed of a cotton matrix. Gossypibomas are rare occurrences which are infrequently reported in the literature because of legal

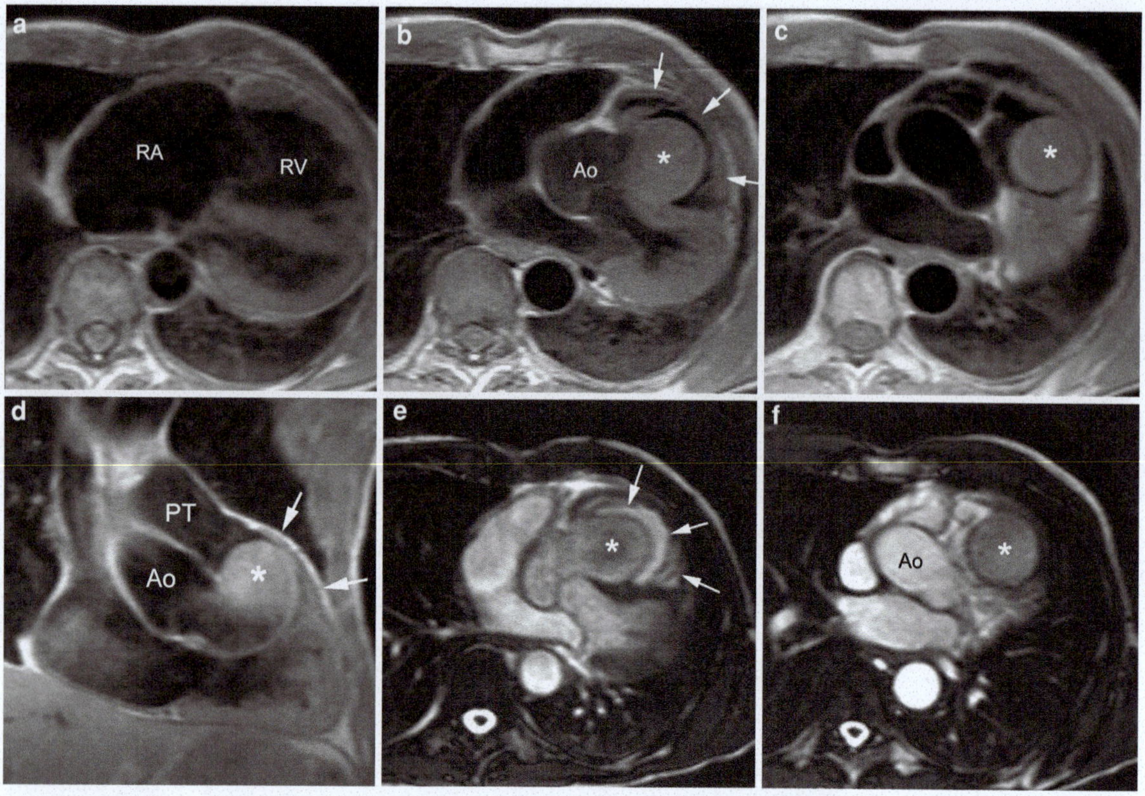

Fig. 42 Aneurysm of the (right) sinus of Valsalva with incomplete RVOTobstruction. Axial T1w-imaging through the right ventricle and RVOT (**a–c**). Oblique T1w-imaging through the RVOT (**d**).Axial cine imaging at two levels through the RVOT (**e–f**). Left-sided lateral rotation of the cardiac axis due to an important dilatation of the right atrium and ventricle (**a**). Presence of a well-defined rounded soft-tissue structure (*star*) with RVOT subobstruction (gradient of 55 mm Hg) (*arrows*) (**b**, **d**, **e**). Especially on cine imaging, the true nature of this "mass" becomes evident: aneurysmal bulging of the right coronary sinus (*star*, **e**) into the RVOT. There was no evidence of any rupture of the aneurysmal wall, leading to the left-to-right shunt

implications (Bhat et al. 1997). Their manifestations and complications are so variable that diagnosis is difficult and patient morbidity is significant. A high index of suspicion in a patient who has previously been operated upon will greatly aid in the diagnosis of this unfortunate complication. Most surgical sponges have radiopaque markers that have a characteristic appearance on plain radiographs (Fig. 47). However, the marker may disintegrate over long periods, or sponges used in some countries may not have markers (Lerner and Dang 1997).

CT, echocardiography, and MRI are particularly important in localizing gossypibomas. Gossypibomas have a typical spongiform pattern on CT; gas bubbles are the most specific sign for the detection of textilomas but do not indicate abscess formation (Kopka et al. 1996). The MRI signal characteristics of gossypibomas are variable depending on the composition of the retained foreign structure, and the degree of associated inflammatory reaction (Mochizuki et al. 1992; Kuwashima et al. 1993; Lerner and Dang 1997). As a result of a pericardial gossypiboma, the heart may be partially compressed.

4.5 Normal Cardiac Anatomy and Variants

Since current cardiac imaging techniques provide a superb anatomic visualization of the heart, adequate knowledge of cardiac anatomy and anatomical variants is required to correctly interpret the images, and

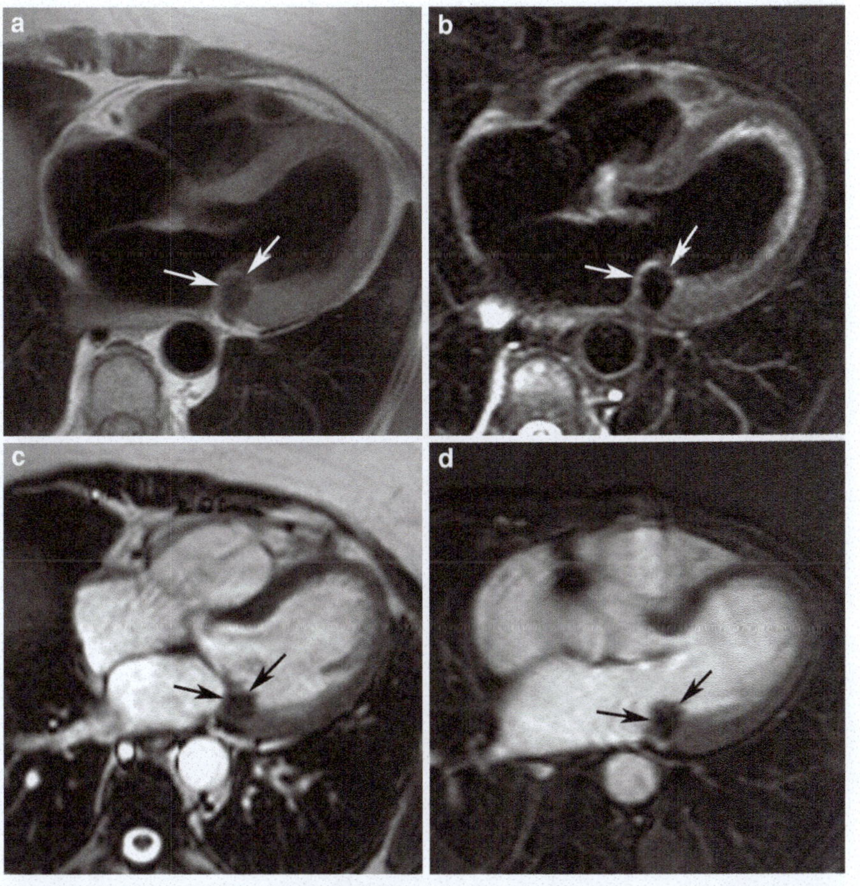

Fig. 43 Liquefaction necrosis of the posterior mitral valve leaflet in a 60-year-old woman. T1w-imaging (**a**), T2w-imaging (**b**), cine imaging (**c**) and late Gd imaging (**d**). All images are obtained in the axial image plane. A hypo-intense rounded nodular structure is visible laterobasally in LV in near contact with the posterior mitral valve leaflet (*arrows*). Following contrast there was some peripheral enhancement

not to misinterpret some structures as pathologic masses. A brief summary per cardiac chamber is given regarding the most common normal variants that may lead to confusion and misinterpretation (see also "Cardiac Anatomy").

4.5.1 Right Atrium

Nodular thickening of the posterior right-atrial wall is a common finding on cardiac MRI and may resemble a mass lesion (Fig. 48) (Mirowitz and Gutierrez 1992). Anatomically this nodular thickening corresponds to the *crista terminalis* or *terminal crest*, which marks the embryologic division between the portion of the right atrium that is derived from the sinus venosus, i.e., smooth-walled sinus venarum, and that which is derived from the embryonic atrium, i.e., trabeculated atrium proper and auriculum. The crista terminalis is a prominent muscular ridge that extends along the posterolateral aspect of the right atrium between the orifices of the superior and inferior venae cavae. Inferiorly, it merges with the valve of the inferior vena cava (*eustachian valve*) and the valve of the coronary sinus (*thebesian valve*). In addition, strand-like fibrous structures, known as the *Chiari network*, may arise from the region of the inferior crista terminalis and/or eustachian valve and extend into the right-atrial chamber. These structures, which are of variable prominence and have a similar signal intensity to myocardial tissue, are routinely observed on cardiac MRI and should not be mistaken for neoplasms, thrombosis, or inflammation (Meier and Hartnell 1994).

4.5.2 Right Ventricle

The *moderator band,* a thin muscular band, is unique for the right ventricle, which can be very helpful in differentiating the right from the left ventricle in congenital heart malformations (see Fig. 16). This muscular structure extends from the mid interventricular septum through the cavity of the right ventricle and attaches near the base of the anterior papillary muscle on the free wall of the right

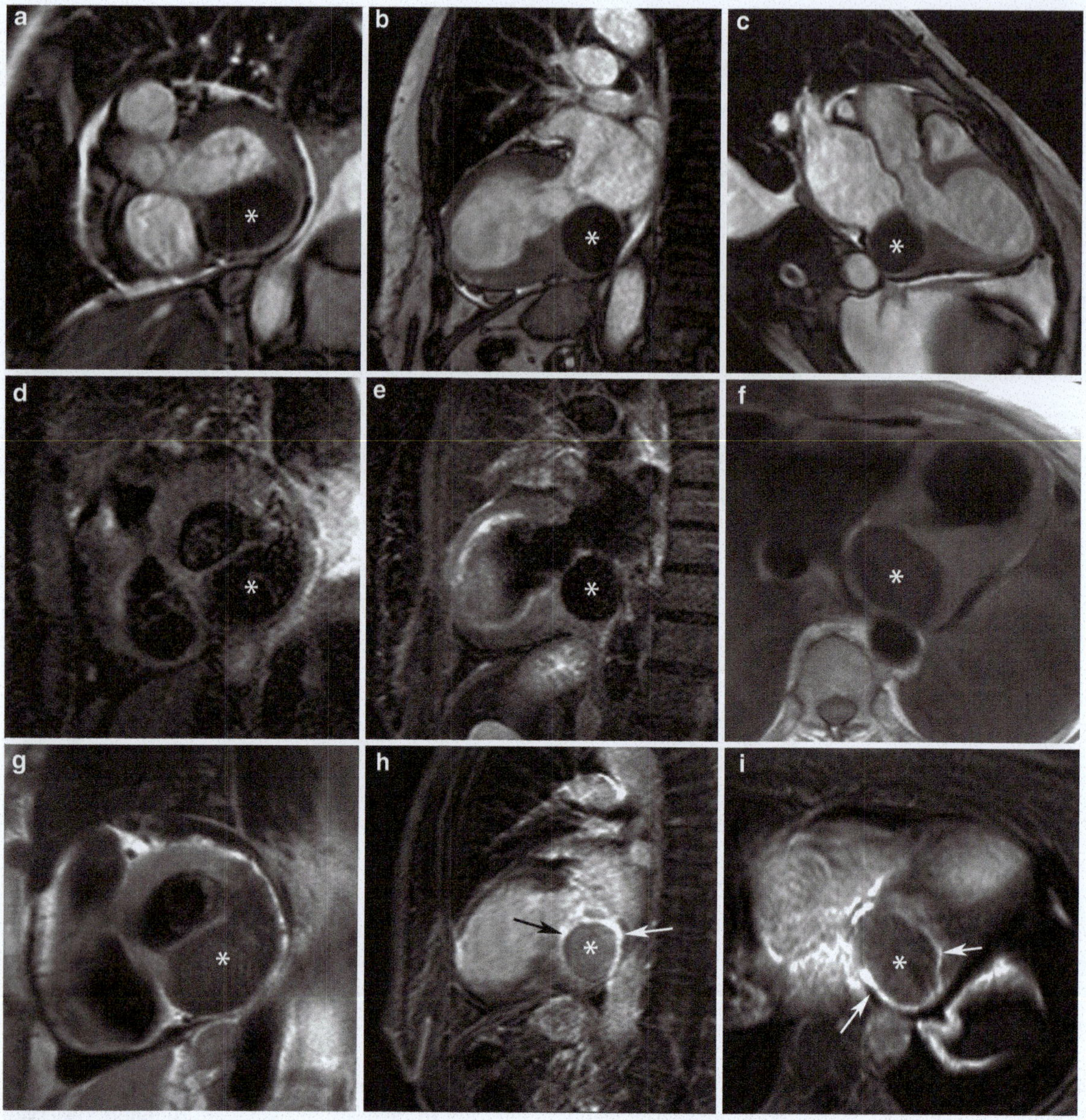

Fig. 44 Liquefaction necrosis of the posterior mitral valve leaflet in a 85-year-old woman. Cine imaging in short-axis (**a**), vertical long-axis (**b**), and along the LVOT view (**c**). T2w-imaging in short-axis (**d**) and vertical long-axis (**e**). T1w-imaging in horizontal long-axis (**f**) and short-axis (**g**). Late Gd imaging in vertical long-axis (**h**) and horizontal long-axis (**i**). An extensive hypo-intense mass is present in the infero- and laterobasal LV wall (*star*), compressing the surrounding myocardium and narrowing the mitral valve area. On pre-contrast imaging the structure seems to have a thin wall that strongly enhances following contrast administration (*arrows*, **h**, **i**)

ventricle. It may become very prominent in patients with right ventricular enlargement or hypertrophy or both, and may be mistaken for a right ventricular thrombus or tumor. MRI allows detection of the muscular nature of the moderator band, with signal intensities similar to the surrounding myocardium.

4.5.3 Left Atrium

While the left atrium has a smooth wall delineation, the left atrial appendage is lined with small, equally spaced muscular pectinate ridges. These pectinate ridges must be distinguished from thrombi. Intracavitary protrusion of the lateral wall at the

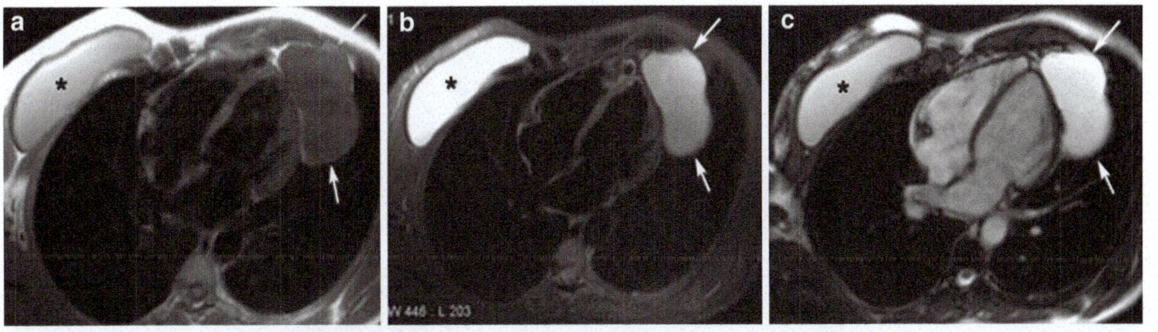

Fig. 45 Pericardial cyst in left cardiophrenic angle in x patient. T1w-imaging (**a**), T2w-imaging (**b**), cine imaging (**c**). Well-defined homogeneous soft-tissue structure (*arrows*) having low-signal intensity on T1w-imaging (**a**) and a very high signal intensity on T2w-imaging and cine imaging (**b**, **c**). Presence of silicone implant in right breast (*star*)

Fig. 46 Large thymic cyst with intralesional bleeding. Axial T1w-imaging before (**a**) and after (**b**) contrast administration. Axial T2w-imaging (**c**). Coronal bright-blood imaging (**d**). Presence of a well-defined right-sided paracardiac structure with partial cardiac compression, showing high signal intensity on both T1w- and T2w-imaging. Presence of several intralesional low-intensity structures (*arrowheads*, **a**, **c**). Surgery showed a benign cyst originating and with vascular supply from the right thymic lobe. The cystic content consisted of old liquefied blood

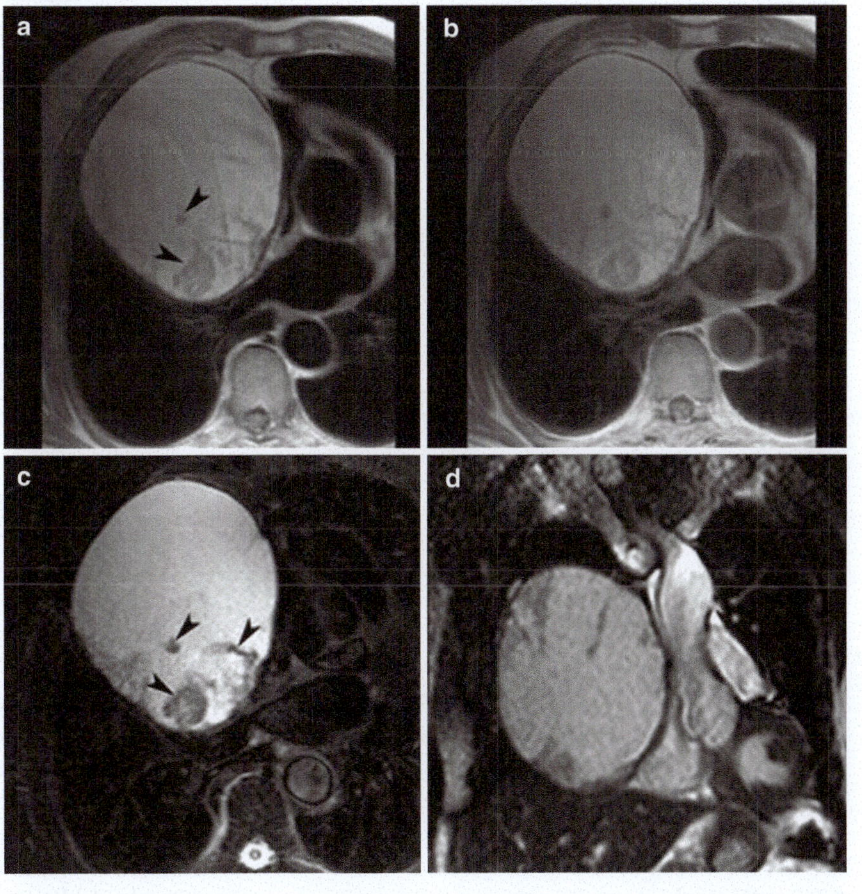

entrance of the left upper pulmonary vein in the left atrium is not infrequently mistaken for a cardiac mass on echocardiography (the so-called "Q-tip sign") (Agostini and Click 2001). This anatomical variant can be easily recognized on MRI (King et al. 1998) Furthermore, a variety of extracardiac abnormalities such as hiatal hernia, esophageal carcinoma, bronchogenic cyst, or tortuous descending aorta can simulate masses in the left atrium on echocardiography (Menegus et al. 1992). The exact location of these "masses" can be determined by means of MRI.

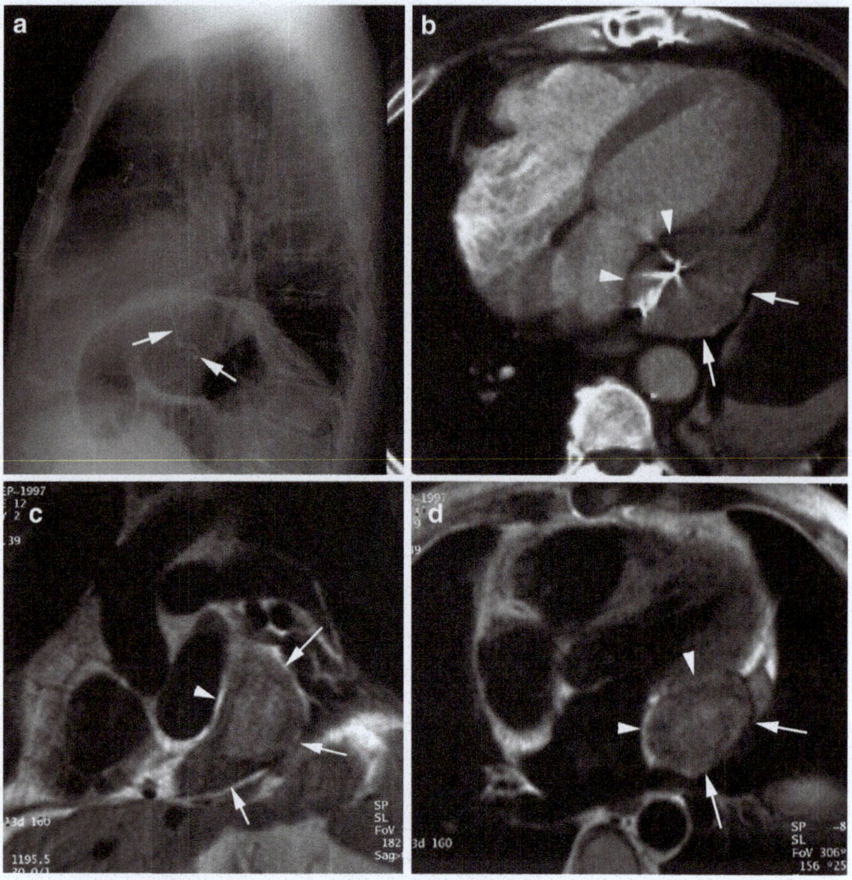

Fig. 47 Gossypiboma. Lateral chest X-ray (**a**); contrast-enhanced CT imaging; (**b**) T1w-imaging in short-axis plane; (**c**) and axial plane (**d**). Intrapericardial gossypiboma or textiloma following coronary bypass graft surgery 25 years previously. The surgical sponge can be easily detected by its radiopaque marker on standard radiographs (*arrows*). Both CT and MRI demonstrate very nicely the foreign tissue granuloma and the compression of the left heart (*arrowheads*). Note the elevation of the left hemidiaphragm

4.5.4 Left Ventricle

Besides the normal papillary muscles and chordae tendinae, in a minority of the population false tendons or false chordae occur as normal variants in the left ventricle (Fig. 49). Rather than connecting the papillary muscles with the valve leaflets, the false chordae are linear structures attached at both ends to the endomyocardium (Keren et al. 1984). They are asymptomatic and usually accidental findings on echocardiography.

4.5.5 Pericardium

Knowledge of the normal appearance of the pericardium on MRI is necessary to adequately interpret cardiovascular MRI studies (see also "Pericardial Disease"). In particular, the superior pericardial sinus may not be mistaken for an aortic dissection, anomalous vascular structure, or a nodular mass on MRI (Black et al. 1993).

4.6 Prosthetic Valves and Other Foreign Devices

Metallic objects, such as metallic heart valves, stents, cardiac occluders, vascular clips, and catheters, may induce artifacts on the MR images (Fig. 50). The artifacts are variable and depend on the type and the amount of metal used in the implant and on the type of MRI sequence (Shellock and Morisoli 1994a, b). Metallic implants induce an alteration of the local magnetic field which leads to loss of signal from the surrounding tissue. For metallic heart valves studied with dark-blood MRI, artifacts are minimal since the prosthetic valves cannot be differentiated from the surrounding dark-blood. Dark-blood MRI is advantageous in the depiction of anatomic structures like paravalvular abscesses (Bachmann et al. 1991). Artifacts, however, are accentuated on (bright-blood) cine imaging. Metallic heart valves are therefore visible as

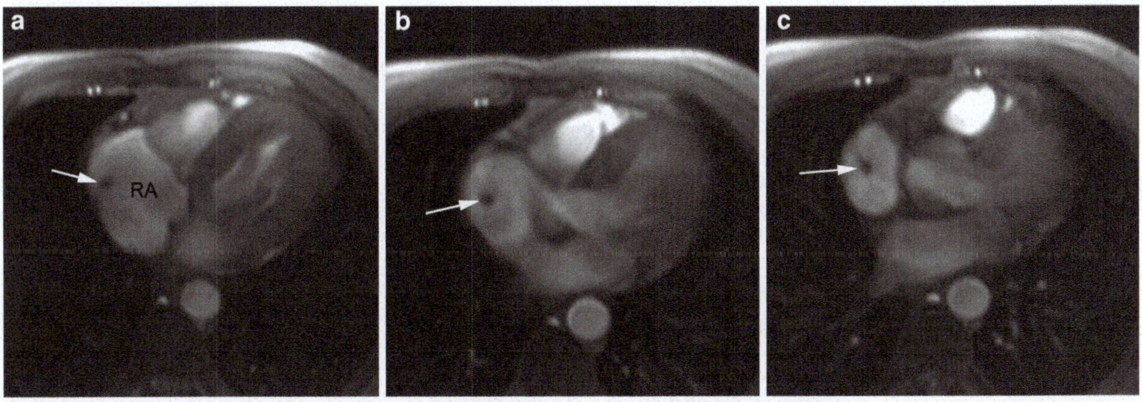

Fig. 48 Crista terminalis (*arrows*), presenting as intracavity nodule in right atrium. **a–c** Axial cine imaging (spoiled gradient-echo imaging). This muscular structure can be easily recognized by its typical location, i.e., posterolateral wall right atrium, connecting the entrances of both caval veins

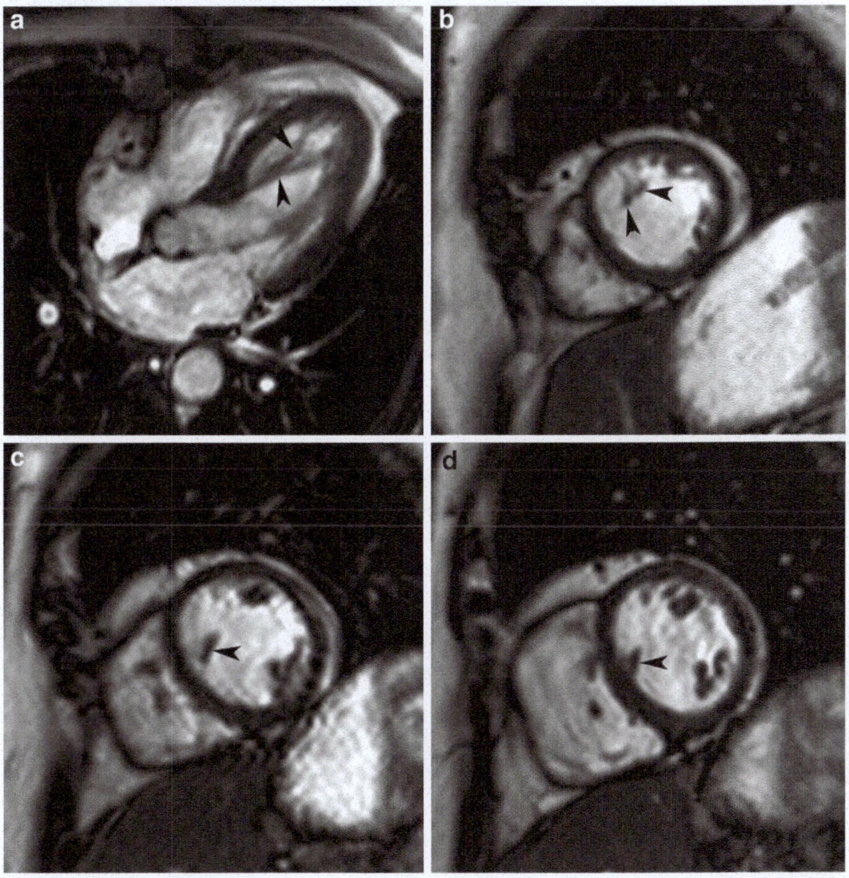

Fig. 49 Extreme form of false tendon in LV. Horizontal long-axis cine imaging (**a**), short-axis cine imaging at 3 levels (**b**, **c**, **d**). Presence of relatively thick-walled muscular bundle in the apical and mid part of the LV (*arrowheads*)

dark areas surrounded by bright-blood. Nevertheless, in a majority of cases qualitative analysis of the valve function and accurate measurement of the blood velocity downstream of the prosthetic heart valve can be performed (Di Cesare et al. 1995; Walker et al. 1995). Physiologic valvular regurgitation can be differentiated from pathologic or valvular regurgitation. Artifacts caused by other foreign cardiac devices, such as intravascular or coronary stents, are similar to those caused by prosthetic valves (Mohiaddin et al. 1995).

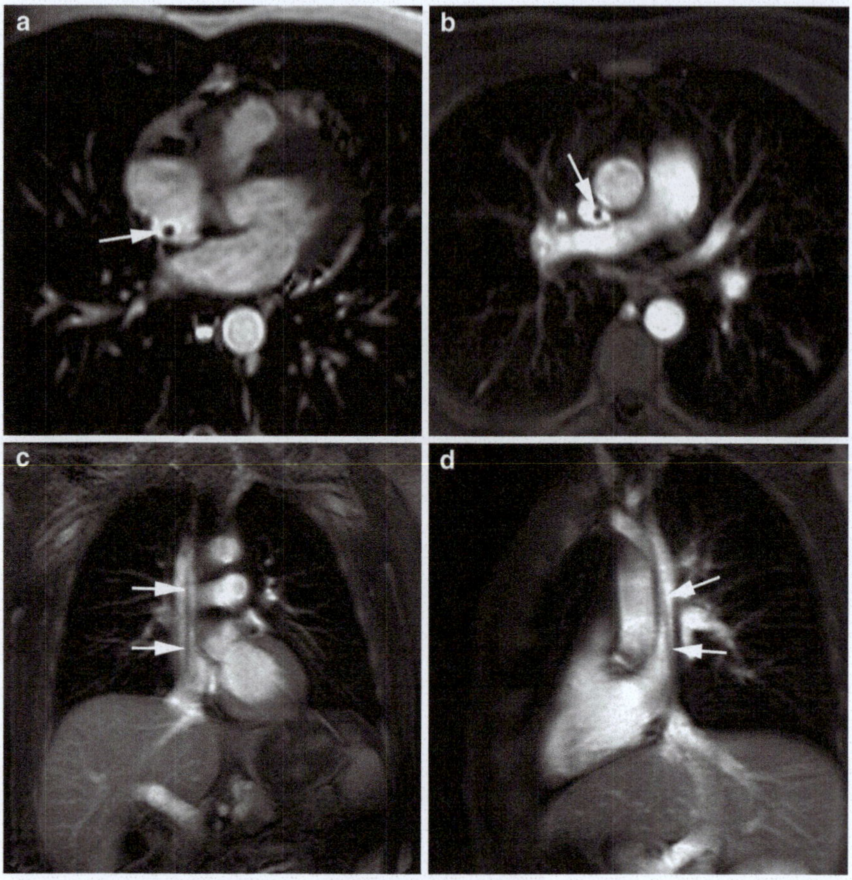

Fig. 50 Hickmann-catheter. Axial cine imaging (**a**, **b**); coronal cine imaging (**c**); sagittal cine imaging (**d**). The presence and position of the central venous line is well visible as a hypo-intense structure using bright-blood imaging (*arrows*)

5 Conclusions

Our look at cardiac tumors and cardiac masses in general has fundamentally changed with the advent of noninvasive cardiac imaging. At present, MRI is probably the technique offering the clinician the most comprehensive approach, even omitting biopsy in a considerable number of patients. Everyone routinely dealing with cardiac imaging will sporadically encounter cardiac masses. Good knowledge of the diversity of pathologies that may present as masses, as well as how cardiac imaging technique should be applied is the best guarantee to correctly diagnose this group of cardiac pathologies.

6 Key Points

- Use a systematic approach to assess cardiac masses:
  - first, determine whether or not the patient has a true cardiac mass.
  - second, determine whether the mass has tumoral or nontumoral characteristics.
  - third, if the mass has features of being a tumor, determine whether the tumor may be benign or malignant.
  - fourth, determine the location, extent, complications, and associated features of the cardiac mass.
  - fifth, use clinical information (e.g., patients' symptoms; history of extracardiac malignancy; heart transplant; restrictive or dilated cardiomyopathy; previous myocardial infarction; …), and knowledge about typical location and appearance of cardiac masses for this analysis.
- For this systematic approach, use a combination of MRI sequences often in different imaging planes.
- Nontumoral conditions are much more frequent cardiac tumors.
- Large infiltrative tumors may be clinically silent, while smaller tumors can produce dramatic symptomatology if strategically located with transient

obstruction of flow across a valve, or when causing systemic emboli.

- A cardiac mass, even small in size, in combination with a pericardial effusion should be suspected of a cardiac malignancy.
- A myxoma has a predilection to arise in the atria near the oval fossa, atrial masses in other locations should be suspected for nontumoral masses or other cardiac tumors (benign/malignant).
- Angiosarcoma, the most common primary cardiac malignancy, typically arises from the right-atrial wall and extends into the pericardium.
- Carefully analyze all cardiac MRI studies, for hidden cardiac thrombi, especially in patients with a predilection for thrombus formation.
- A combination of cine MRI and late Gd imaging is currently the best approach for thrombus detection.

References

Abad C (1995) Congenital aneurysm of the sinus of Valsalva dissecting into the interventricular septum. Cardiovasc Surg 3:563–564

Agostini F, Click RL (2001) More than just the "Q-tip sign". J Am Soc Echocardiogr 14:832–833

Altbach MI, Squire SW, Kudithipudi V, Castellano L, Sorrell VL (2007) Cardiac MRI is complementary to echocardiography in the assessment of cardiac masses. Echocardiography 24:286–300

Anavekar NS, Bonnichsen CR, Foley TA et al (2010) Computed tomography of cardiac pseudotumors and neoplasms. Radiol Clin North Am 48:799–816

Aouate P, Artigou JY, Rovany X et al (1988) Contribution of nuclear magnetic resonance in right atrial angiosarcoma. Apropos of a case (in French). Arch Mal Coeur Vaiss 81:1543–1546

Araoz PA, Mulvagh SL, Tazelaar HD, Julsrud PR, Breen JF (2000) CT and MR imaging of benign primary cardiac neoplasms with echocardiographic correlation. Radiographics 20:1303–1319

Arciniegas E, Hakimi M, Farooki ZQ, Green EW (1980) Intrapericardial teratoma in infancy. J Thorac Cardiovasc Surg 79:306–311

Aydingoz U, Ariyurek M, Selcuk ZT, Demirkazik FB, Baris YI (1997) Calcium within a bronchogenic cyst with a fluid level. Br J Radiol 70:761–763

Bachmann R, Deutsch HJ, Jungehulsing M, Sechtem U, Hilger HH, Schicha H (1991) Magnetic resonance imaging in patients with heart valve prostheses. Rofo Fortschr Rontgenstr 155:499–505

Bader RS, Chitayat D, Kelly E et al (2003) Fetal rhabdomyoma: prenatal diagnosis, clinical outcome, and incidence of associated tuberous sclerosis complex. J Pediatr 143:620–624

Balasubramanyam A, Waxman M, Kazal HL, Lee MH (1986) Malignant lymphoma of the heart in acquired immune deficiency syndrome. Chest 90:243–246

Bansal RC, Graham BM, Jutzy KR, Shakudo M, Shah PM (1990) Left ventricular outflow tract to left atrial communication secondary to rupture of mitral-aortic intervalvular fibrosa in infective endocarditis: diagnosis by transesophageal echocardiography and color flow imaging. J Am Coll Cardiol 15:499–504

Barakos JA, Brown JJ, Brescia RJ, Higgins CB (1989a) High signal intensity lesions of the chest in MR imaging. J Comput Assist Tomogr 13:797–802

Barakos JA, Brown JJ, Higgins CB (1989b) MR imaging of secondary cardiac and paracardiac lesions. Am J Roentgenol 153:47–50

Bargallo J, Luburich P, Garcia Barrionuevo J, Sanchez Gonzalez M (1993) Fluid-fluid level in bronchogenic cysts. Radiology 186:427–428

Barkhausen J, Hunold P, Eggebrecht H et al (2002) Detection and characterization of intracardiac thrombi on MR imaging. Am J Roentgenol 179:1539–1544

Baumgartner HR (1973) The role of blood flow in platelet adhesion, fibrin deposition, and formation of mural thrombi. Microvasc Rev 5:167–179

Beghetti M, Prieditis M, Rebeyka IM, Mawson J (1998) Images in cardiovascular medicine. Intrapericardial teratoma. Circulation 97:1523–1524

Bekkers SCAM, Backes WH, Kim RJ et al (2009) Detection and characteristics of microvascular obstruction in reperfused acute myocardial infarction using an optimized protocol for contrast-enhanced cardiovascular magnetic resonance imaging. Eur Radiol 19:2904–2912

Benetar A, Vaughan J, Nicolini U, Trotter S, Corrin B, Lincoln C (1992) Prenatal pericardiocentesis: its role in the management of intrapericardial teratoma. Obstet Gynecol 79:856–859

Best AK, Dobson RL, Ahmad AR (2003) Best cases from the AFIP. Cardiac Angiosarcoma. Radiographics 23: S141–S145

Bhat HS, Mahesh G, Ramgopal KS (1997) "Gossypiboma": an unusual cause of perinephric abscess. J R Coll Surg Edinb 42:277–278

Black CM, Hedges LK, Javitt MC (1993) The superior pericardial sinus: normal appearance on gradient-echo MR images. Am J Roentgenol 160:749–751

Bogaert J, Rademakers F, Cappelle L, Moerman P, Van de Werf F, Baert AL (1995a) High-grade immunoblastic sarcoma: an unusual type of a primary cardiac non-Hodgkin lymphoma. Rofo Fortschr Rontgenstr 162: 186–188

Bogaert J, De Man F, Rademakers F et al (1995b) Right atrial tumor arising on an atrial septal aneurysm. Assessment by MR imaging. Clin Imaging 19:172–175

Bogaert J, Taylor AM, Van Kerckhove F, Dymarkowski S (2004) Use of the inversion-recovery contrast-enhanced MRI technique for cardiac imaging: spectrum of diseases. Am J Roentgenol AJR 182:609–615

Bogaert J, Centonze M, Vanheste R, Francone M (2010) Cardiac and pericardial abnormalities on chest computed tomography: what can we see? Radio Med 115:175–190

Bouton S, Yang A, McCrindle BW, Kidd L, McVeigh ER, Zerhouni EA (1991) Differentiation of tumor from viable myocardium using cardiac tagging with MR imaging. J Comput Assist Tomogr 15:676–678

Brizard C, Latremouille C, Jebara VA et al (1993) Cardiac hemangiomas. Ann Thorac Surg 56:390–394 (see comments)

Burke AP, Virmani R (1991) Osteosarcomas of the heart. Am J Surg Pathol 51:289–295

Burke AP, Cowan D, Virmani R (1992) Primary sarcomas of the heart. Cancer 69:387–395

Burke AP, Rosado de Christenson M, Templeton PA, Virmani R (1994) Cardiac fibroma: clinicopathologic correlates and surgical treatment. J Thorac Cardiovasc Surg 108:862–870

Butany J, Nair V, Naseemuddin Nair GM, Catton C, Yau T (2006) Cardiac tumours: diagnosis and treatment. Lancet Oncol 6:219–228

Cacoub P, Chapoutot L, Du Boutin LT et al (1991) Hydatid cyst of the interventricular septum. Contribution of magnetic resonance imaging (in French). Arch Mal Coeur Vaiss 84:1857–1860

Caduff JH, Hernandez RJ, Ludomirsky A (1996) MR visualization of aortic valve vegetations. J Comput Assist Tomogr 20:613–615

Cantoni S, Frola C, Gatto R, Loria F, Terzi MI, Vallebona A (1993) Hydatid cyst of the interventricular septum of the heart: MR findings. Am J Roentgenol 161:753–754

Carpenter JL (1991) Perivalvular extension of infection in patients with infectious endocarditis. Rev Infect Dis 13:127–138

Castelli MJ, Mihalov ML, Posniak HV, Gattuso P (1989) Primary cardiac lymphoma initially diagnosed by routine cytology: case report and literature review. Acta Cytol 30:662–664

Chiles C, Woodard PK, Gutierrez FR, Link KM (2001) Metastatic involvement of heart and pericardium: CT and MR imaging. Radiographics 21:439–449

Chin WW, Van Tosh A, Hecht SR, Berger M (1988) Left ventricular thrombus with normal left ventricular function in ulcerative colitis. Am Heart J 116:562–563

Conces DJ, Vix VA, Klatte EC (1985) Gated MR imaging of left atrial myxomas. Radiology 156:445–447

Corallo S, Mutinelli MR, Moroni M et al (1988) Echocardiographic detects myocardial damage in AIDS: prospective study in 102 patients. Eur Heart J 9:887–892

Cunningham KS, Veinot JP, Feindel CM, Butany J (2006) Fatty lesions of the atria and interatrial septum. Hum Pathol 37:1245–1251

Curtinsinger CR, Wilson MJ, Yoneda K (1989) Primary cardiac lymphoma. Cancer 64:521–525

Davis M, Carneiro A, Dymarkowski S, Bogaert J (2010) Bronchogenic cyst masquerading as pericarditis. Circulation 122:e426–e428

DeGroat TS, Parameswaran R, Popper PM, Kotler MN (1985) Left ventricular thrombi in association with normal left ventricular wall motion in patients with malignancy. Am J Cardiol 56:827–828

DeLoach JF, Haynes JW (1953) Secondary tumors of the heart and pericardium. Review of subject and report of 137 cases. Arch Intern Med 91:224–249

DePace NL, Soulen RL, Kotler MN, Mintz GS (1981) Two dimensional echocardiographic detection of intraatrial masses. Am J Cardiol 48:954–960

Dev V, Goswami KC, Shrivastava S, Bahl VK, Saxena A (1993) Echocardiographic diagnosis of aneurysm of the sinus of Valsalva. Am Heart J 126:930–936

Di Bella G, Masci PG, Ganame J, Dymarkowski S, Bogaert J (2008) Liquefaction necrosis of mitral annulus calcification. Detection and characterization with cardiac magnetic resonance imaging. Circulation 117:e292–e294

Di Cesare E, Enrici RM, Paparoni S et al (1995) Low-field magnetic resonance imaging in the evaluation of mechanical and biological heart valve function. Eur J Radiol 20:224–228

Dillman JR, Pernicano PG, McHugh JB et al (2010) Cross-sectional imaging of primary thoracic sarcomas with histopathologic correlation: a review for the radiologist. Curr Probl Diagn Radiol 39:17–29

Doherty NE, Siegel RJ (1985) Cardiovascular manifestations of systemic lupus erythematosus. Am Heart J 110:1257–1265

Donato R, Ganame J, Bogaert J (2009) Contrast-enhancing left ventricular apical thrombus. Eur Heart J 30:1977

Dooms GC, Higgins CB (1986) MR imaging of cardiac thrombi. J Comput Assist Tomogr 10:415–420

Dooms GC, Hricak H, Sollitto RA, Higgins CB (1985) Lipomatous tumors and tumors with fatty components: MR imaging potential and comparison of MR and CT results. Radiology 157:479–483

Edwards FH, Hale D, Cohen A, Thompson L, Pezzella AT, Virmani R (1991) Primary cardiac valve tumors. Ann Thorac Surg 52:1127–1131

Elkouby A, Vaillant A, Comet B, Malmejac C, Houel J (1990) Cardiac hydatidosis. Review of recent literature and report of 15 cases (in French). Ann Chir 44:603–610

Engberding R, Daniel WG, Erbel R et al (1993) Diagnosis of heart tumours by transoesophageal echocardiography: a multicentre study in 154 patients. European Cooperative Study Group. Eur Heart J 14:1223–1228

Fisher MS, Edmonds PR (1988) Lipomatous hypertrophy of the interatrial septum. Diagnosis by magnetic resonance imaging. J Comput Tomogr 12:267–269

Fritz J, Vogel W, Bares R, Horger M (2007) Radiologic spectrum of extramedullary relapse of myelogenous leukemia in adults. AJR 189:209–218

Fueredi GA, Knechtges TE, Czarnecki DJ (1989) Coronary angiography in atrial myxoma: findings in nine cases. Am J Roentgenol 152:737–738

Funari M, Fujita N, Peck WW, Higgins CB (1991) Cardiac tumors: assessment with Gd-DTPA enhanced MR imaging. J Comput Assist Tomogr 15:953–958

Fussen S, De Boeck BWL, Zellweger MJ et al (2011) Cardiovascular magnetic resonance imaging for diagnosis and clinical management of suspected cardiac masses and tumours. Eur Heart J 32:1551–1560

Gaerte SC, Meyer CA, Winer-Muram HT, Tarver RD, conce DJ Jr (2002) Fat-containing lesions of the chest. Radiographics 22:S61–S78

Gallet B, Malergue MC, Adams C et al (1985) Atrial septal aneurysm–a potential cause of systemic embolism. Br Heart J 53:292–297

Gamsu G, Starck D, Webb WR, Moore EH, Sheldon PE (1984) Magnetic resonance of benign mediastinal masses. Radiology 151:709–713

Ganame J, Messalli G, Dymarkowski S et al (2009) Impact of myocardial hemorrhage on left ventricular function and remodelling in patients with reperfused acute myocardial infraction. Eur Heart J 30:662–670

Gibson JM, Hall CM, Dicks MC, Finn JP (1990) Intracardiac extension of Wilms' tumour: demonstration by magnetic resonance. Br J Radiol 63:568–569

Godine LB, Berdon WE, Brasch RC, Leonidas JC (1990) Adrenocortical carcinoma with extension into inferior vena cava and right atrium: report of 3 cases in children. Pediatr Radiol 20:166–168

Gomes AS, Lois JF, Child JS, Brown K, Batra P (1987) Cardiac tumors and thrombus: evaluation with MR imaging. AJR Am J Roentgenol 49:895–899

Gomi T, Ikeda T, Sakurai J, Toya Y, Tani M (1994) Cardiac pheochromocytoma. A case report and review of the literature. Jpn Heart J 35:117–124

Gossinger HD, Siostrzonek P, Zangeneh M et al (1988) Magnetic resonance imaging findings in a patient with pericardial mesothelioma. Am Heart J 115:1321–1322

Gowda RM, Khan IA, Nair CK et al (2003) Cardiac papillary fibroelastoma: a comprehensive analysis of 725 cases. Am Heart J 146:404–410

Grebenc ML, Rosado-de-Christenson ML, Burke AP, Green CE, Galvin JR (2000) Primary cardiac and pericardial neoplasms: radiologic-pathologic correlation. Radiographics 20:1073–1103

Grebenc ML, Rosado-de-Christenson ML, Green CE, Burke AP, Galvin JR (2002) From the archives of the AFIP. Cardiac myxoma: imaging features in 83 patients. Radiographics 22:673–689

Grizzard JD, Ang GB (2007) Magnetic resonance imaging of pericardial disease and cardiac masses. Magn Reson Imaging Clin N Am 15:579–607

Grote J, Mugge A, Schfers HJ, Daniel WG, Lichtlen PR (1995) Multiplane transoesophageal echocardiography detection of a papillary fibroelastoma of the aortic valve causing myocardial infarction. Eur Heart J 16:426–429

Hallali P, Haiat R (1987) Tumeurs malignes du coeur et du péricarde. In: Actualités en Cardiologie. Sandoz, Paris, pp 1–12

Hamilton BH, Francis IR, Gross BH et al (1997) Intrapericardial paragangliomas (pheochromocytomas): imaging features. Am J Roentgenol 168:109–113

Hananouchi GI, Goff WB (1990) Cardiac lipoma: six-year follow-up with MRI characteristics, and a review of the literature. Magn Reson Imaging 8:825–828

Hanley PC, Tajik AJ, Hynes JK et al (1985) Diagnosis and classification of atrial septal aneurysm by two-dimensional echocardiography: report of 80 consecutive cases. J Am Coll Cardiol 6:1370–1382

Hanson EC (1992) Cardiac tumors: a current perspective. N Y State J Med 92:41–42

Heath D (1968) Pathology of cardiac tumors. Am J Cardiol 21:315–327

Herrera CJ, Mehlman DJ, Hartz RS, Talano JV, McPherson DD (1992) Comparison of transesophageal and transthoracic echocardiography for diagnosis of right sided cardiac lesions. Am J Cardiol 70:964–966

Herrmann MA, Shankerman RA, Edwards WD, Shub C, Schaff HV (1992) Primary cardiac angiosarcoma: a clinicopathologic study of six cases. J Thorac Cardiovasc Surg 103:655–664

Ho VB, Kinney JB, Sahn DJ (1995) Ruptured sinus of Valsalva aneurysm: cine phase-contrast MR characterization. J Comput Assist Tomogr 19:652–656

Hoey ETD, Mankad K, Puppala S, Gopalan D, Sivananthan MU (2009a) MRI and CT appearances of cardiac tumours in adults. Clin Radiol 64:1214–123

Hoey ETD, Kanagasingam A, Sivananthan MU (2010) Sinus of Valsvalva aneurysms: assessment with cardiovascular MRI. AJR 194:W495–W504

Hoffmann U, Globits S, Schima W et al (2003) Usefulness of magnetic resonance imaging of cardiac and paracardiac masses. Am J Cardiol 92:890–895

Ichikawa T, Ohtomo K, Uchiyama G, Fujimoto H, Nasu K (1995) Contrast-enhanced dynamic MRI of adrenal masses: classification of characteristic enhancement patterns. Clin Radiol 50:295–300

Janigan DT, Husain A, Robinson NA (1986) Cardiac angiosarcomas. A review and a case report. Cancer 57:852–859

Jochelson MS, Balikian JP, Mauch P, Liebman H (1983) Peri- and paracardial involvement in lymphoma: a radiographic study of 11 cases. Am J Roentgenol 140:483–488

Jost E, Lorenzen J, Haage P et al (2005) Heart and muscle involvement by extra-medullary myeloid leukemia: a case report and review of the literature. Leuk Lymphoma 46:1819–1824

Jungehulsing M, Sechtem U, Theissen P, Hilger HH, Schicha H (1992) Left ventricular thrombi: evaluation with spin-echo and gradient-echo MR imaging. Radiology 182:225–229

Kaminaga T, Yamada N, Imakita S, Takamiya M, Nishimura T (1993) Magnetic resonance imaging of pericardial malignant mesothelioma. Magn Reson Imaging 11:1057–1061

Kanematsu M, Imaeda T, Minowa H et al (1994) Hepatocellular carcinoma with tumor thrombus in the inferior vena cava and right atrium. Abdom Imaging 19:313–316

Kardaras F, Kardara D, Tselikos D et al (1996) Fifteen year surveillance of echinococcal heart disease from a referral hospital in Greece. Eur Heart J 17:1265–1270

Kasarskis EJ, O'Connor W, Earle G (1988) Embolic stroke from cardiac papillary fibroelastomas. Stroke 19:1171–1173

Kasugai T, Sakurai M, Yutani C et al (1990) Sequential malignant transformation of cardiac myxoma. Acta Pathol Jpn 40:687–692

Kawasuji M, Matsunaga Y, Iwa T (1989) Cardiac phaeochromocytoma of the interatrial septum. Eur J Cardiothorac Surg 3:175–177

Keeley EC, Hillis LD (1996) Left ventricular mural thrombus after acute myocardial infarction. Clin Cardiol 19:83–86

Keren A, Billingham ME, Popp RL (1984) Echocardiographic recognition and implications of ventricular hypertrophic trabeculations and aberrant bands. Circulation 70:836–842

Kiaffis MG, Powell AJ, Geva T (2002) Magnetic resonance imaging evaluation of cardiac tumor characteristics in infants and children. Am J Cardiol 89:1229–1233

Kim EE, Wallace S, Abello R et al (1989) Malignant cardiac fibrous histiocytomas and angiosarcomas: MR features. J Comput Assist Tomogr 13:627–632

King MA, Vrachliotis TG, Bergin CJ (1998) A left atrial pseudomass: potential pitfall at thoracic MR imaging. JMRI 8:991–993

Klarich KW, Enriquez-Sarano M, Gura GM, Edwards WD, Tajik AJ, Seward JB (1997) Papillary fibroelastoma: echocardiographic characteristics for diagnosis and pathologic correlation. J Am Coll Cardiol 30:784–790

Klima T, Milam JD, Bossart MI, Cooley DA (1986) Rare primary sarcomas of the heart. Arch Pathol Lab Med 110:1155–1159

Kopka L, Fischer U, Gross AJ, Funke M, Oestmann JW, Grabbe E (1996) CT of retained surgical sponges (textilomas): pitfalls in detection and evaluation. J Comput Assist Tomogr 20:919–923

Kotoulas GK, Magoufis GL, Gouliamos AD et al (1996) Evaluation of hydatid disease of the heart with magnetic resonance imaging. Cardiovasc Intervent Radiol 19:187–189

Kulan K, Tuncer C, Kulan C et al (1995) Hydatid cyst of the interventricular septum and contribution of magnetic resonance imaging. Acta Cardiol 50:477–481

Kulan K, Kulan C, Tuncer C, Komsuoglu B, Zengin M (1996) Echocardiography and magnetic resonance imaging of sinus of Valsalva aneurysm with rupture into the ventricle. J Cardiovasc Surg Torino 37:639–641

Kushihashi T, Fujisawa H, Munechika H (1996) Magnetic resonance imaging of thymic epithelial tumors. Crit Rev Diagn Imaging 37:191–259

Kuwashima S, Yamato M, Fujioka M, Ishibashi M, Kogure H, Tajima Y (1993) MR findings of surgically retained sponges and towels: report of two cases. Radiat Med 11:98–101

Lagrange JL, Despins P, Spielman M et al (1986) Car-diac metastases. Case report on an isolated cardiac metastasis of a myxoid liposarcoma. Cancer 58:2333–2337

Langer E, Mischke U, Stommer P, Harrer T, Stoll R (1988) Kaposi's sarcoma with pericardial tamponade in AIDS. Dtsch Med Wochenschr 29:1187–1190

Lanza RP, Cooper DK, Cassidy MJ, Barnard CN (1983) Malignant neoplasms occurring after cardiac transplantation. JAMA 249:1746–1748

Lee R, Fisher MR (1989) MR imaging of cardiac metastases from malignant fibrous histiocytoma. J Comput Assist Tomogr 13:126–168

Lee W-K, Duddalwar VA, Rouse HC, Lau EWF, Bekhit E, Hennessy OF (2009) Extranodal lymphoma in the thorax: cross-sectional imaging findings. Clin Radiol 64:542–549

Lerner CA, Dang HP (1997) MR imaging of a pericardial gossypiboma. Am J Roentgenol 169:314 (letter)

Levine RA, Weyman AE, Dinsmore RE et al (1986) Noninvasive tissue characterization: diagnosis of lipo-matous hypertrophy of the atrial septum by nuclear magnetic resonance imaging. J Am Coll Cardiol 7:688–692

Lund JT, Ehman RL, Julsrud PR, Sinak LJ, Tajik AJ (1989) Cardiac masses: assessment by MR imaging. Am J Roentgenol 152:469–473

Macedo AJ, Magalhaes MP, Tavares NJ, Bento L, Sampayo F, Lima M (1997) Cardiac hydatid cyst in a child. Pediatr Cardiol 18:226–228

Mahajan H, Kim EE, Wallace S, Abello R, Benjamin R, Evans HL (1989) Magnetic resonance imaging of malignant fibrous histiocytoma. Magn Reson Imaging 7:283–288

Manger WM, Gifford RWJ (1990) Pheochromocytoma. In: Laragh JH, Brenner BM (eds) Hypertension. Raven Press, New York, pp 1639–1650

Maraj S, Pressman GS, Figueredo VM (2009) Primary cardiac tumors. Int J Cardiol 133:152–156

Massie RJ, Van Asperen PP, Mellis CM (1997) A review of open biopsy for mediastinal masses. J Paediatr Child Health 33:230–233

Matsuoka H, Hamada M, Honda T et al (1996) Morphologic and histologic characterization of cardiac myxomas by magnetic resonance imaging. Angiology 47:693–698

Matteucci C, Busi G, Biferali F, Paventi S (1997) Tardive pseudo-ischemic presentation of cardiac rhabdomyoma (in Italian). G Ital Cardiol 27:583–587

McAllister HGJ (1979) Primary tumors and cysts of the heart and pericardium. Curr Probl Cardiol 4:1–11

McAllister HA, Fenoglio JJ (1978) Tumors of the cardiovascular system. Armed Forces Institute of Pathology, Washington, DC, pp 1–39

Meany JFM, Kazerooni EA, Jamadar DA, Korobkin M (1997) CT appearance of lipomatous hypertrophy of the interatrial septum. Am J Roentgenol 168:1081–1084

Meier RA, Hartnell GG (1994) MRI of right atrial pseudomass: is it really a diagnostic problem? J Comput Assist Tomogr 18:398–401

Menegus MA, Greenberg MA, Spindola-Franco H, Fayemi A (1992) Magnetic resonance imaging of suspected atrial tumors. Am Heart J 123:1260–1268

Mirowitz SA, Gutierrez FR (1992) Fibromuscular elements of the right atrium: pseudomass at MR imaging. Radiology 182:231–233

Mochizuki T, Takehara Y, Ichijo K, Nishimura T, Takahashi M, Kaneko M (1992) Case report: MR appearance of a retained surgical sponge. Clin Radiol 46:66–67

Mohiaddin RH, Roberts RH, Underwood R, Rothman M (1995) Localization of a misplaced coronary artery stent by magnetic resonance imaging. Clin Cardiol 18:175–177

Mollet NR, Dymarkowski S, Volders W et al (2002) Visualization of ventricular thrombi with contrast-enhanced magnetic resonance imaging in patients with ischemic heart disease. Circulation 106:2873–2876

Mosthaf FA, Gieseler U, Mehmel HC, Fischer JT, Gams E (1991) Left bundle-branch block and primary benign heart tumor (in German). Dtsch Med Wochenschr 116:134–136

Mugge A, Daniel WG, Haverich A, Lichtlen PR (1991) Diagnosis of noninfective cardiac mass lesions by two-dimensional echocardiography. Comparison of the transthoracic and transesophageal approaches. Circulation 83:70–78

Murayama S, Murakami J, Watanabe H et al (1995) Signal intensity characteristics of mediastinal cystic masses on T1-weighted MRI. J Comput Assist Tomogr 19:188–191

Murphey MD, Gross TM, Rosenthal HG (1994) From the archives of the AFIP. Musculoskeletal malignant fibrous histiocytoma: radiologic-pathologic correlation. Radiographics 14:807–826

Naka N, Ohsawa M, Tomita Y, Kanno H, Uchida A, Aozasa K (1995) Angiosarcoma in Japan. Cancer 75:989–996

Nakata H, Egashira K, Watanabe H et al (1993) MRI of bronchogenic cysts. J Comput Assist Tomogr 17:267–270

Nguyen BD, Westra WH, Zerhouni EA (1996) Renal cell carcinoma and tumor thrombus neovascularity: MR demonstration with pathologic correlation. Abdom Imaging 21:269–271

O'Connor S, Recavarren R, Nichols LC, Parwani AV (2006) Lipomatous hypertrophy of the interatrial septum. An overview. Arch Pathol Lab Med 130:397–399
O'Donnell DH, Abbara S, Chaithiraphan V et al (2009) Cardiac tumors: optimal cardiac MR sequences and spectrum of imaging appearances. AJR 193:377–387
Ogawa T, Iwama Y, Hashimoto H, Ito T, Satake T (1991) Noninvasive methods in the diagnosis of ruptured aneurysm of Valsalva. Usefulness of magnetic resonance imaging and Doppler echocardiography. Chest 100:579–581
Oshima H, Hara M, Kono T, Shibamoto Y, Mishima A, Akita S (2003) Cardiac hemangioma of the left atrial appendage: CT and MR findings. J Thorac Imaging 18:204–206
Papa MZ, Shinfeld A, Klein E, Greif F, Ben AG (1994) Cardiac metastasis of liposarcoma. J Surg Oncol 55:132–134
Parmley LF, Salley RK, Williams JP, Head G (1988) The clinical spectrum of cardiac fibroma with diagnostic and sur-gical considerations: noninvasive imaging enhances management. Ann Thorac Surg 45:455–465
Pasaoglu I, Dogan R, Pasaoglu E, Tokgozoglu L (1994) Surgical treatment of giant hydatid cyst of the left ventricle and diagnostic value of magnetic resonance imaging. Cardiovasc Surg 2:114–116
Paul JG, Rhodes DB, Skow JR (1975) Renal cell carcinoma presenting as right atrial tumor with successful removal using cardiopulmonary bypass. Ann Surg 181:471–473
Paydarfar D, Krieger D, Dib N et al (2001) In vivo magnetic resonance imaging and surgical histopathology of intracardiac masses: distinct features of subacute thrombi. Cardiology 95:40–47
Phillips MR, Bower TC, Orszulak TA, Hartmann LC (1995) Intracardiac extension of an intracaval sarcoma of endometrial origin. Ann Thorac Surg 59:742–744
Raaf HN, Raaf JH (1994) Sarcomas related to the heart and vasculature. Semin Surg Oncol 10:374–382
Reid PG, Goudevenos JA, Hilton CJ (1990) Thrombosed saccular aneurysm of a sinus of Valsalva: unusual cause of a mediastinal mass. Br Heart J 63:183–185
Ritchey ML, Kinard R, Novicki DE (1987) Adrenal tumors: involvement of the inferior vena cava. J Urol 38:1134–1136
Roberts WC, Glancy DL, De Vita VT (1968) Heart in malignant lymphoma (Hodgkin's disease, lymphosarcoma, reticulum cell sarcoma and mycosis fungoides). A study of 196 autopsy cases. Am Heart J 22:85–108
Roberts CS, Gottdiener JS, Roberts WC (1990) Clinically undetected cardiac lymphoma causing fatal congestive heart failure. Am Heart J 120:1239–1242
Rosado de Christenson ML, Pugatch RD, Moran CA, Galobardes J (1994) Thymolipoma: analysis of 27 cases. Radiology 193:121–126
Rosenberg JM, Marvasti MA, Obeid A, Johnson LW, Bonaventura M (1988) Intravenous leiomyomatosis: a rare cause of right sided cardiac obstruction. Eur J Cardiothorac Surg 2:58–60
Rosenthal DS, Braunwald E (1992) Cardiac manifestations of neoplastic disease. Saunders, Philadelphia, pp 1752–1760
Rosser T, Panigrahy A, McClintock W (2006) The diverse clinical manifestations of tuberous sclerosis complex: a review. Semin Pediatr Neuol 13:27–36
Rote AR, Flint LD, Ellis FH (1977) Intracaval extension of pheochromocytoma extending into the right atrium: surgical management using intracorporeal circulation. N Engl J Med 296:1269–1271
Rumancik WM, Naidich DP, Chandra R et al (1988) Cardiovascular disease: evaluation with MR phase imaging. Radiology 166:63–68
Sakai F, Sone S, Kiyono K et al (1992) MR imaging of thymoma: radiologic-pathologic correlation. Am J Roentgenol 158:751–756
Salcedo EE, Cohen GI, White RD, Davison MB (1992) Cardiac tumors: diagnosis and management. Curr Probl Cardiol 17:73–137
Saloura V, Grivas PD, Sarwar AB, Gorodin P, Ledley GS (2009) Papillary fibroelastomas: innocent bystanders or ignored culprits? Postgrad Med 121:131–138
Sato Y, Togawa K, Ogawa K, Hashimoto M, Sakamaki T, Kanmatsuse K (1995) Magnetic resonance imaging of cardiac hemangiopericytoma. Heart Vessels 10:328–330
Schneider B, Hanrath P, Vogel P, Meinertz T (1990) Improved morphologic characterization of atrial septal aneurysm by transesophageal echocardiography: relation to cerebro-vascular events. J Am Coll Cardiol 16:1000–1009
Sechtem U, Tscholakoff D, Higgins CB (1986) MRI of the abnormal pericardium. Am J Roentgenol 147:245–252
Sechtem U, Theissen P, Heindel W et al (1989) Diagnosis of left ventricular thrombi by magnetic resonance imaging and comparison with angiocardiography, computed tomography and echocardiography. Am J Cardiol 64:1195–1199
Semelka RC, Shoenut JP, Wilson ME, Pellech AE, Patton JN (1992) Cardiac masses: signal intensity features on spin-echo, gradient-echo, gadolinium-enhanced spin-echo, and TurboFLASH images. J Magn Reson Imaging 2:415–420
Shahian DM, Labib SB, Chang G (1995) Cardiac papillary fibroelastoma. Ann Thorac Surg 59:538–541 (see comments)
Shellock FG, Morisoli SM (1994a) Ex vivo evaluation of ferromagnetism, heating, and artifacts produced by heart valve prostheses exposed to a 1.5-T MR system. J Magn Reson Imaging 4:756–758
Shellock FG, Morisoli SM (1994b) Ex vivo evaluation of ferromagnetism and artifacts of cardiac occluders exposed to a 1.5-T MR system. J Magn Reson Imaging 4:213–215
Singh RN, Burkholder JA, Magovern GJ (1984) Coronary arteriography as an aid in the diagnosis of angiosarcoma of the heart. Cardiovasc Intervent Radiol 7:40–43
Smith AJ, Panidis IP, Berger S, Gonzales R (1990) Large atrial septal aneurysm mimicking a cystic right atrial mass. Am Heart J 120:714–716
Sparrow PJ, Kurian J, Jones TR, Sivananthan MU (2005) MR imaging of cardiac tumors. RadioGraphics 25:1255–1276
Spuentrup E, Mahnken AH, Kühl HP et al (2003) Fast interactive real-time magnetic resonance imaging of cardiac masses using spiral gradient echo and radial steady-state free precession sequences. Invest Radiol 38:288–292
Srichai MB, Junor C, Rodriguez L et al (2006) Clinical, imaging, and pathological characteristics of left ventricular thrombus: a comparison of contrast-enhanced magnetic resonance imaging, transthoracic echocardiography, and transesophageal echocardiography with surgical or pathological validation. Am Heart J 152:75–84
Steinmetz OK, Bedard P, Prefontaine ME, Bourke M, Barber GG (1996) Uterine tumor in the heart: intravenous leiomyomatosis. Surgery 119:226–229

Stratton JR, Ligthy GW, Pearlman AS (1982) Detection of left ventricular thrombus by two-dimensional echocar-diography: sensitivity, specificity, and causes of uncertainty. Circulation 66:156–164

Szucs RA, Rehr RB, Yanovich S, Tatum JL (1991) Magnetic resonance imaging of cardiac rhabdomyosarcoma. quantifying the response to chemotherapy. Cancer 67:2066–2070

Takamizawa S, Sugimoto K, Tanaka H, Sakai O, Arai T, Saitoh A (1992) A case of primary leiomyosarcoma of the heart. Intern Med 31:265–268

Teramoto N, Hayashi K, Miyatani K et al (1995) Malignant fibrous histiocytoma of the right ventricle of the heart. Pathol Int 45:315–319

Thomas D, Desruennes M, Jault F, Isnard R, Gandjbakhch I (1993) Cardiac and extracardiac abscesses in bacterial endocarditis (in French). Arch Mal Coeur Vaiss 86:1825–1835

Thompson NW, Brown J, Orringer M, Sisson J, Nishiyama R (1978) Follicular carcinoma of the thyroid with massive angioinvasion: extension of tumor thrombus to the heart. Surgery 83:451–457

Urba WJ, Longo DL (1986) Primary solid tumors of the heart. In: Kapoor AS (ed) Cancer and the heart. Springer, New York, pp 62–75

van Beek EJR, Stolpen AH, Khanna G, Thompson BH (2007) CT and MRI of pericardial and cardiac neoplastic disease. Cancer Imaging 7:19–26

Vanjak D, Moutaoufik M, Leroy O et al (1990) Cardiac hydatidosis: contribution of magnetic resonance imaging. Report of a case (in French). Arch Mal Coeur Vaiss 83:1739–1742

Varghese JC, Hahn PF, Papanicolaou N, Mayo-Smith WW, Gaa JA, Lee MJ (1997) MR differentiation of phaechromocytoma from other adrenal lesions based on qualitative analysis of T2 relaxation times. Clin Radiol 52:603–606

Vinee P, Stover B, Sigmund G et al (1992) MR imaging of the pericardial cyst. J Magn Reson Imaging 2:593–596

Vogel HJ, Wondergem JH, Falke TH (1989) Mesothelioma of the pericardium: CT and MR findings. J Comput Assist Tomogr 13:543–544

Walker PG, Pedersen EM, Oyre S et al (1995) Magnetic resonance velocity imaging: a new method for prosthetic heart valve study. J Heart Valve Dis 4:296–307

Watanabe M, Takazawa K, Wada A et al (1994) Cardiac myxoma with Gamna-Gandy bodies: case report with MR imaging. J Thorac Imaging 9:185–187

Weinsaft JW, Kim HW, Shah DJ et al (2008) Detection of left ventricular thrombus by delayed-enhancement cardiovascular magnetic resonance. Prevalence and markers in patients with systolic dysfunction. J Am Coll Cardiol 52:148–157

Weinsaft JW, Kim RJ, Ross M et al (2009) Contrast-enhanced anatomic imaging as compared to contrast-enhanced tissue characterization for detection of left ventricular thrombus. J Am Coll Cardiol Img 2:969–979

Weinsaft JW, Kim HW, Crowley AL et al (2011) LV thrombus detection by routine echocardiography. Insights into performance characteristics using delayed enhancement CMR. J Am Coll Cardiol Img 4:702–712

Wiemer J, Winkelmann BR, Beyersdorf F et al (1996) Multiplicity of clinical symptoms and manifestations of unruptured aneurysms of the sinus of Valsalva. Three case reports. Z Kardiol 85:221–225

Wolf JE, Lambert B, Pilichowski P et al (1987) Value of magnetic resonance imaging in a lipoma of the left ventricle (in French). Arch Mal Coeur Vaiss 80:1801–1805

Yokoyama N, Konno K, Suzuki S, Isshiki T (2007) Serial assessment of liquefaction necrosis of mitral annulus calcification by echocardiography and multislice computed tomography. Circulation 115:e1–e2

Yousem DM, Lexa FJ, Bilaniuk LT, Zimmerman RI (1990) Rhabdomyosarcomas in the head and neck: MR imaging evaluation. Radiology 177:683–686

Valvular Heart Disease

Andrew M. Taylor, Steven Dymarkowski, and Jan Bogaert

Contents

1 **Introduction** 465

2 **Other Imaging Modalities** 466

3 **Magnetic Resonance Imaging of Cardiac Valves** 468
3.1 Morphology 468
3.2 Valvular Regurgitation 469
3.3 Valvular Stenosis 475
3.4 Aortic Valve 476
3.5 Mitral Valve 484
3.6 Pulmonary Valve 487
3.7 Tricuspid Valve 495
3.8 Mixed Valvular Disease 498
3.9 Prosthetic Valves 498
3.10 Magnetic Resonance Spectroscopy 500

4 **Future Directions** 502

5 **Conclusion** 502

6 **Key Points** 502

References 503

A. M. Taylor (✉)
Hospital for Children, Cardio-respiratory Unit,
Great Ormond Street, London, WC1N 3JH, UK
e-mail: a.taylor76@ucl.ac.uk

A. M. Taylor
Centre for Cardiovascular Imaging,
UCL Institute of Cardiovascular Science &
Great Ormond Street Hospital for Children,
Great Ormond Street, London, WC1N 3JH, UK

S. Dymarkowski · J. Bogaert
Department of Radiology, Katholieke Universiteit Leuven,
University Hospital Leuven, Herestraat 49,
3000, Leuven, Belgium

Abstract

The assessment of valvular heart disease by cardiac MRI has changed little over the last decade. However, with the increasing use and development of percutaneous valve interventions (transcatheter and minimally-invasive surgery), there is an increasing need to use cardiac MRI to define which patients will benefit from treatment, which patients are suitable for a specific treatment and how patients will respond to their treatments. As cardiac MRI is the best available in-vivo test to define great vessel flow and ventricular volumes, whilst at the same time providing beautiful, high-resolution 3D/4D anatomical images of the heart, it may become the imaging modalities of choice for these assessments. Importantly, as long-term outcome data is acquired, this ability of cardiac MRI to accurately measure physiological parameters will help us define when to treat patients, in particular asymptomatic patients with valvular regurgitation. Finally, the development and increasing use of high spatio-temporal real-time data for acquiring flow and function information will enable MR scans to be performed over a short time period (e.g. 15 mins) comparable to the time it takes to perform a full echocardiogram!

1 Introduction

Over the last 5 years there has been a dramatic increase in the use of cardiovascular MR to assess valvular heart disease. This has been related not only to the increasing prevalence of valvular heart disease

J. Bogaert et al. (eds.), *Clinical Cardiac MRI*, Medical Radiology. Diagnostic Imaging,
DOI: 10.1007/174_2011_414, © Springer-Verlag Berlin Heidelberg 2012

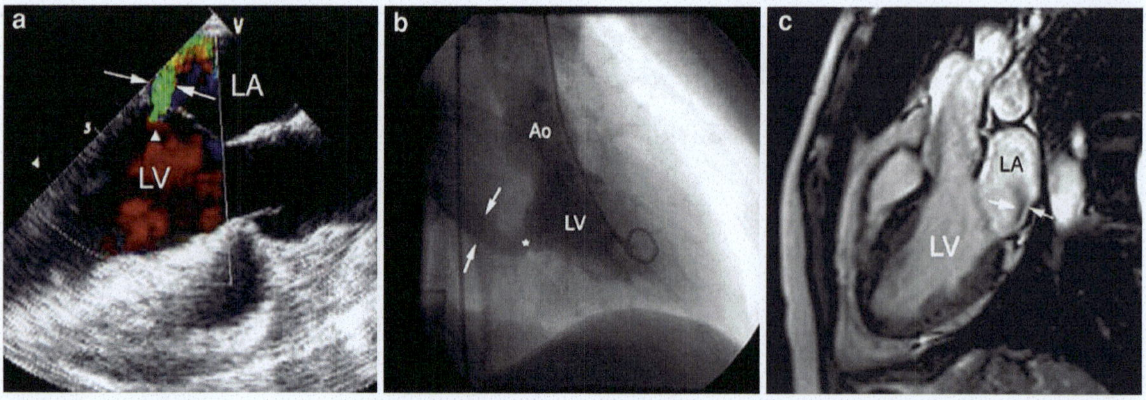

Fig. 1 Eccentric mitral regurgitation. **a** Transesophageal echocardiography shows eccentric jet (*arrows*) directed from left ventricle (LV) into left atrium (LA). The jet impinges on LA wall ("wall jet") dissipating part of its kinetic energy ("jet momentum"), resulting in underestimation of mitral regurgitation severity. **b** Contrast ventriculography, obtained in right anterior oblique view, confirms eccentric regurgitant jet (*) (*arrows*). **c.** Balanced SSFP cine-MRI in LV inflow–outflow view (c) clearly shows eccentric mitral regurgitation (*arrows*). Valve defect was not seen on vertical long and horizontal long axis views (not shown), emphasising the importance of multiplane scanning in eccentric regurgitation

(Nkomo et al. 2006), but also to the introduction of new transcatheter, percutaneous treatment options (Bonhoeffer et al. 2000; Cribier et al. 2002) that require improved pre-procedural imaging assessment to ensure optimal patient selection and safe implantation.

Despite these increased demands, the principles of valve assessment with cardiovascular MR remain little changed over the last decade, though newer sequences, and in particular real-time assessment, now mean that the MR assessment times can be significantly reduced, improving patient throughput and satisfaction. Furthermore, with the increasing acceptance of cardiovascular MR for the assessment of valvular heart disease, there has been an increase in the amount of follow-up and outcome data that enables cardiovascular MR to be used to define when patients should undergo treatment of their valve disease.

When investigating cardiac valves, the information required can be divided into four categories:

- Clarification of the affected valve after auscultation of the heart;
- Definition of the valvular anatomy (valve leaflet number, leaflet thickness, presence of infective endocarditis);
- Assessment of valvular function (degree of valvular stenosis or regurgitation); and
- Definition of the effect of the valvular dysfunction on other cardiac structures and function (ventricular size, function and mass, myocardial perfusion, myocardial fibrosis, pulmonary artery pressure, great vessel anatomy).

These questions can be addressed by combining echocardiography with X-ray angiography. However, cardiovascular MR can provide the required information in a single investigation that is safe, non-invasive and without exposure to X-rays.

In this chapter, we will present an overview of the MR techniques that are currently used in the assessment of valvular heart disease, provide protocols for the cardiovascular MR assessment of valvular heart disease and identify new areas of development in this field. We will also discuss the advantages and limitations of cardiovascular MR with reference to more conventional imaging modalities for investigating valvular heart disease (Fig. 1).

2 Other Imaging Modalities

Transthoracic echocardiography remains the most important and easily accessible investigation for the assessment of valvular heart disease (Carabello and Crawford 1997). The technique is noninvasive, safe, portable and accurate at localising the diseased valve. Quantification of valvular stenosis and valve area can be easily performed (Currie et al. 1985); however, echocardiography is less good at quantifying valvular regurgitation (Hatle and Angelson 1992; Smith and Xie 1998).

A semiquantitive assessment can be achieved by measuring the regurgitant jet length and width, but there is poor correlation to X-ray angiographic measurements (Abbasi et al. 1980; Quinones et al. 1980; Bolger et al. 1988). Several echocardiography methods have been developed in an attempt to quantify valvular regurgitation, but all have their limitations. The regurgitant fraction can be calculated, but this is time consuming, only patients with isolated valvular regurgitation can be readily assessed (Rockey et al. 1987), and echocardiography only provides an estimate of ventricular function (Boehrer et al. 1992). Imaging of the proximal isovelocity surface area has been proposed. However, this technique relies on the assumption that the regurgitant jet orifice is both flat and circular, which is not the case for most patients (Utsunomiya et al. 1991). A final limitation of transthoracic echocardiography is that the imaging plane may be restricted by the lack of good acoustic windows.

Transoesophageal echocardiography is valuable in the assessment of left atrial thrombus (Manning et al. 1993), atrial septal wall defects (Hausmann et al. 1992) and aortic dissection (Tice and Kisslo 1993; Laissy et al. 1995). In the assessment of valvular heart disease, the technique may clarify valvular anatomy in patients with infective endocarditis (Pedersen et al. 1991) or in patients with poor acoustic windows. With regard to functional assessment it is less accurate than transthoracic echocardiography because of difficulties with Doppler alignment and has all the limitations of transthoracic echocardiography in the assessment of valvular regurgitation, in addition to being an invasive procedure. A unique use for transesophageal echocardiography is in the intraoperative assessment of valvular function for monitoring and evaluating surgical and percutaneous interventions (Fix et al. 1993; Bryan et al. 1995).

Importantly, recently advanced with 3D echocardiography (both transthoracic (Tsang et al. 2011) and transoesophageal (Moustafa et al. 2011) mean that the 3D dimensional structure of the valve leaflets can be exquisitely seen, and crucially monitored during valvular interventions (whether surgical or catheter-based) and in real-time. Though 2D echocardiography remains the main stay for valvular assessment, 3D echocardiography offers the potential for a better 3D understanding of the valve leaflets and valve apparatus (Bharucha et al. 2008), that may be crucial for deciding whether patient require valve replacement, valve repair or are suitable for percutaneous transcatheter-based valvular interventions.

X-ray angiography has been regarded as the "gold standard" investigation of valvular heart disease, against which other imaging modalities should be compared (Sandler et al. 1963; Sellers et al. 1964; Carroll 1993). Valvular stenosis can be quantified by calculating the transvalvular gradients and valve areas using the Gorlin formula (Gorlin and Gorlin 1951). However, the grading system used for the assessment of valvular regurgitation is both imprecise and inaccurate. Although generally regarded as safe, the technique is associated with a mortality of approximately 0.1%, and other complications occur such as myocardial infarction, arterial embolization, thrombosis and dissection (Davis et al. 1979). Also the use of ionising radiation during the procedure is not ideal (Razavi et al. 2003). In general, X-ray angiography should only be regarded as necessary if the pulmonary artery pressure needs accurate measurement, if the coronary artery anatomy needs defining, or if there is a discrepancy between the clinical symptoms and the non-invasive investigations.

The main use of radionuclide imaging has been in the monitoring of ventricular function in order to assess when interventions should take place (Rigo et al. 1979; Sorenson et al. 1980). The technique can also be used to calculate the regurgitant fraction, but only when regurgitation in a single valve is present. As with X-ray angiography, the use of ionising radiation is not ideal, especially as serial measurements of ventricular function are necessary. For most centres, radionuclide imaging is no longer used to assess valvular heart disease.

Most recently, advances in computer tomography (CT) have been utilised to assess valvular heart disease (Ketelsen et al. 2010). As with MRI, valve anatomy and structure can be assessed, with the advantage of visualising the 3D structure of the valve leaflets over the cardiac cycle—4D CT (Vitanovski et al. 2009; Schievano et al. 2011) (Fig. 2). However, direct measurement of flow with CT is not possible and though regurgitant volumes can be calculated from differences in right and left ventricular stroke volumes, again this is only applicable when there is regurgitation of a single valve. Radiation dose is also an issue with CT, in particular as many assessments over time are often necessary; however, dose can be kept to a minimum even in the paediatric population (Young et al. 2011).

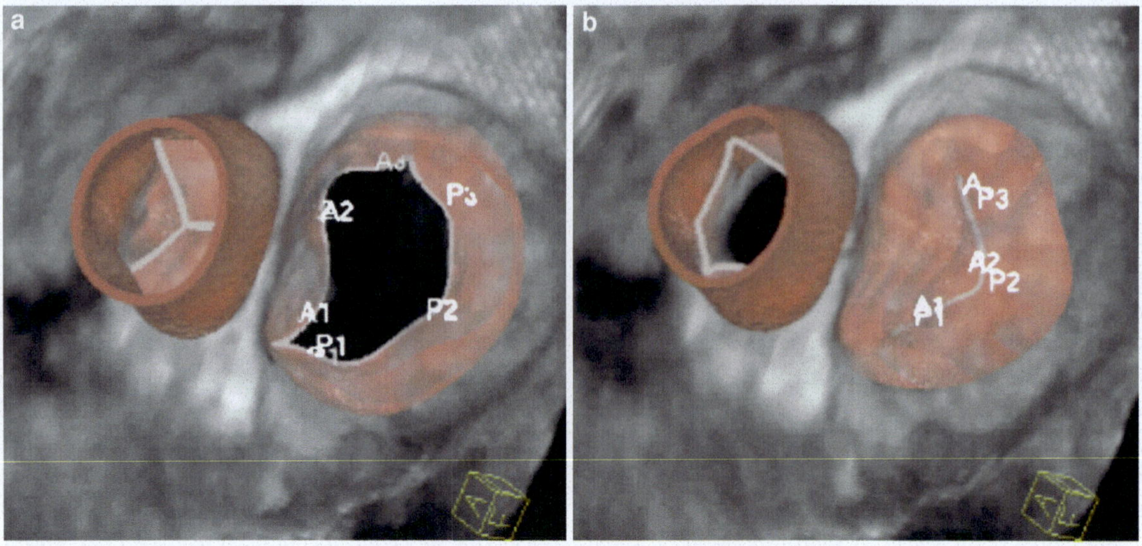

Fig. 2 Four dimension CT data, 2 of 10 frames shown, viewed from with the LV, with the mitral valve on the right of the images, with anterior A1-3 and posterior P1-3 scallops shown. **a** Diastole—open mitral valve, closed aortic valve, **b** systole—open aortic valve, closed mitral valve

3 Magnetic Resonance Imaging of Cardiac Valves

Magnetic resonance imaging can provide good functional information about both valvular stenosis and regurgitation, and allows accurate assessment of ventricular function and relevant cardiac and vascular anatomy. Over the last 5 years, balanced steady state free precession (bSSFP) imaging has replaced spoiled gradient echo (GRE) imaging (Schlosser et al. 2007), though in the dedicated assessment of valve lesions, GRE imaging remains useful. Furthermore, longer free breathing acquisitions used for flow imaging (phase contrast velocity mapping) have been replaced either by rapid breath-hold sequences (Steeden et al. 2011) or real-time flow assessments (Steeden et al. 2010).

3.1 Morphology

3.1.1 Valve Leaflets

Normal valves are fast-moving, low proton density, fine structures that are difficult to visualise with conventional spin-echo (SE) 'black-blood' imaging, due to respiratory motion and averaging. However, turbo spin-echo sequences allow for the acquisition of data at defined points in the cardiac cycle during a single breath-hold (Fig. 3). When thickened and immobile valve leaflet identification is more common.

Using 'white-blood' cine imaging (bSSFP or GRE), the moving leaflets are easily seen as blood flowing over the valve tips leads to signal loss, secondary to eddies and mild turbulence (Kivelitz et al. 2003) (Fig. 4). However, small and mobile lesions can be missed (e.g. vegetations or disruption to chordal anatomy (Stork et al. 2007)). Real-time imaging may help with these issues, in particular when patients have arrhythmias, though reduced temporo-spatial resolution may reduce the imagining sensitivity.

3.1.2 Thrombus

It is important to identify the presence of thrombus in the atria, particularly in the presence of mitral stenosis or valvular disease with atrial fibrillation.

Spin-echo imaging can identify atrial thrombus, but care must be taken to distinguish between slow-moving blood that may appear as increased signal on these images (Dooms and Higgins 1986). Cine imaging and velocity mapping should thus be used to confirm the presence and size of any apparent mass (Fig. 5).

Thrombus can also be distinguished from other atrial masses using gadolinium-based contrast agents (Weinmann et al. 1984). Recently, we have shown

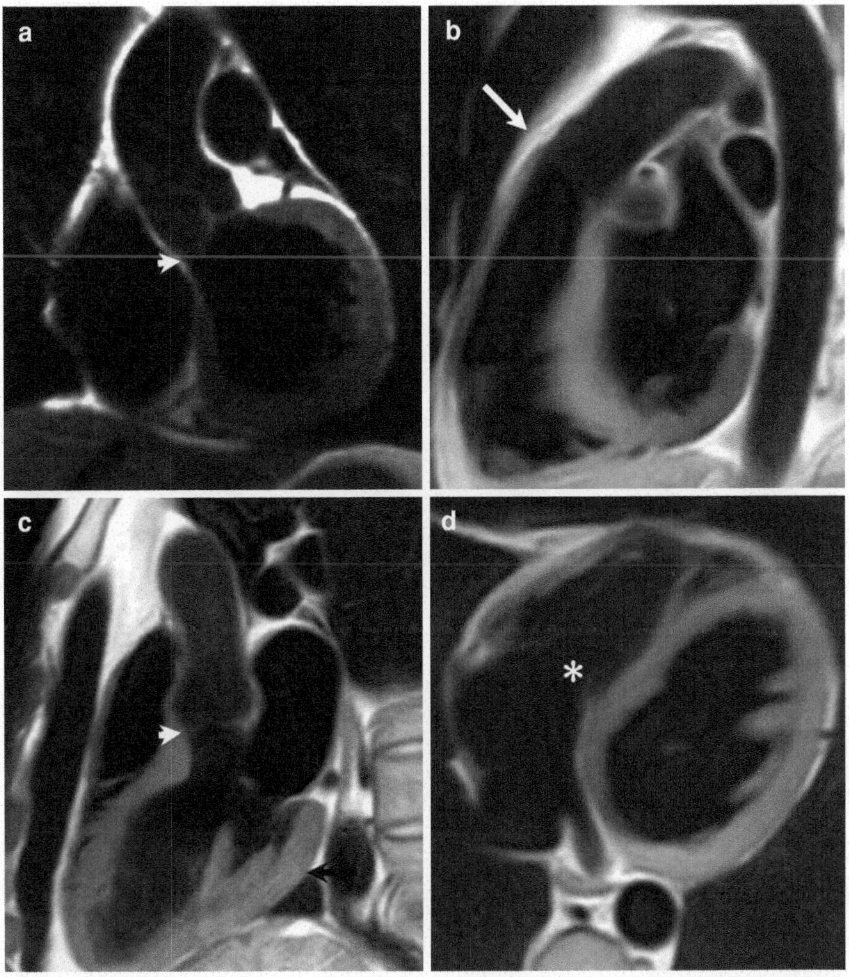

Fig. 3 Turbo spin-echo (TSE) images of the valves. **a** Oblique coronal view of the aortic valve (*arrowhead*). **b** Oblique sagittal view of the pulmonary valve (*white arrow*). **c** Left ventricle inflow/outflow view of the mitral valve (*black arrow*) and aortic valve (*arrowhead*). **d** Axial view (systole) of the tricuspid valve (*)

that late-enhancement MR imaging that has been developed for myocardial infarction imaging (see Chap. 8) can be utilised to image thrombus (Bogaert et al. 2004; Daccarett et al. 2011). Importantly, imaging is best performed early after the administration of gadolinium with a fixed inversion time (TI) of approximately 440 ms. There will be some enhancement of both the blood-pool and myocardium, but no late-enhancement of the thrombus (Fig. 5b).

3.1.3 Endocarditis

Only very large vegetations can be demonstrated by SE MR imaging. Cine imaging has been shown to be helpful in clarifying echocardiographic findings in aortic valve vegetations (Caduff et al. 1996). MR imaging can be invaluable in the identification of abscesses (Jeang et al. 1986) or if infection has spread outside the heart (Fig. 6). Furthermore, sinus of valsalva rupture, secondary to endocarditis can be seen on MR imaging.

3.2 Valvular Regurgitation

None of the other imaging techniques can accurately define valvular regurgitation and it is here that MR imaging has particular value. Cardiovascular MR can image the regurgitant jet in any plane, and thus a 3D appreciation of the jet can be acquired. Furthermore, MR imaging can quantify the regurgitant volume, either as an absolute value or as the regurgitant fraction. Such a non-invasive quantification of the degree of valvular regurgitation, in combination with information about ventricular function, is of particular clinical relevance for the timing of valve replacement.

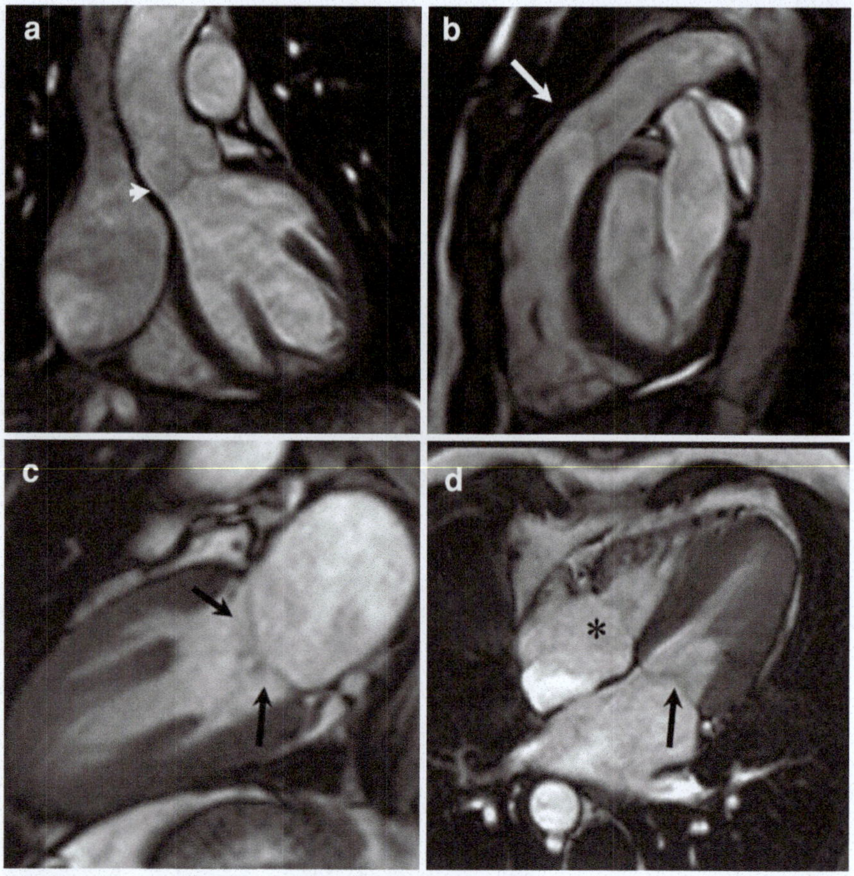

Fig. 4 Balanced steady state free precession (bSSFP) images of the valves. **a** Oblique coronal view of the aortic valve (*arrowhead*). **b** Oblique sagittal view of the pulmonary valve (*white arrow*). **c** Vertical long axis view of the mitral valve. The *black arrows* indicate the insertion points of the chordae tendinae into the tips of the valve leaflets. **d** Four-chamber view (systole) of the tricuspid (*) and mitral valves (*black arrow*)

MR assessment of valvular regurgitation severity can be evaluated by using the following techniques:

- Qualitative assessment of signal loss on cine MR imaging.
- Quantitative assessment by measurement of ventricular volumes.
- Quantitative assessment by phase contrast velocity mapping.

The latter method currently represents the best available in vivo method for the quantification of valvular regurgitation.

3.2.1 Qualitative Assessment With Cine Imaging

In GE cine imaging, dephasing of the proton spins, secondary to turbulent flow, leads to signal loss (Evans et al. 1988). Imaging over multiple frames (20–40) enables accurate assessment of the turbulent flow, throughout the cardiac cycle. For regurgitant lesions the signal loss can be graded in a similar way to X-ray angiography; grade 1 = signal loss close to the valve; grade 2 = signal loss extending into the proximal chamber; grade 3 = signal loss filling the whole of the proximal chamber; grade 4 = signal loss in the receiving chamber throughout the relevant half of the cardiac cycle (Fig. 7) (Underwood et al. 1987a; Sechtem et al. 1987). This qualitative method has been validated, but is unable to separate turbulent volumes when dual valve disease exists (e.g. aortic regurgitation and mitral stenosis), and there remains poor reproducibility of the technique between centres (Sechtem et al. 1988; Wagner et al. 1989; Globits et al. 1991). In addition, signal loss is very dependent on MR parameters such as echo time (TE), and jet size is easily underestimated when it impinges on the myocardial wall, as has been known from echocardiography for some years.

With the increasing dependence on bSSFP cine imaging in cardiovascular MR (Zur et al. 1990), qualitative assessment of signal loss has become less useful. Though bSSFP ‘white blood’ images are much quicker to acquire with better endocardial/blood-pool

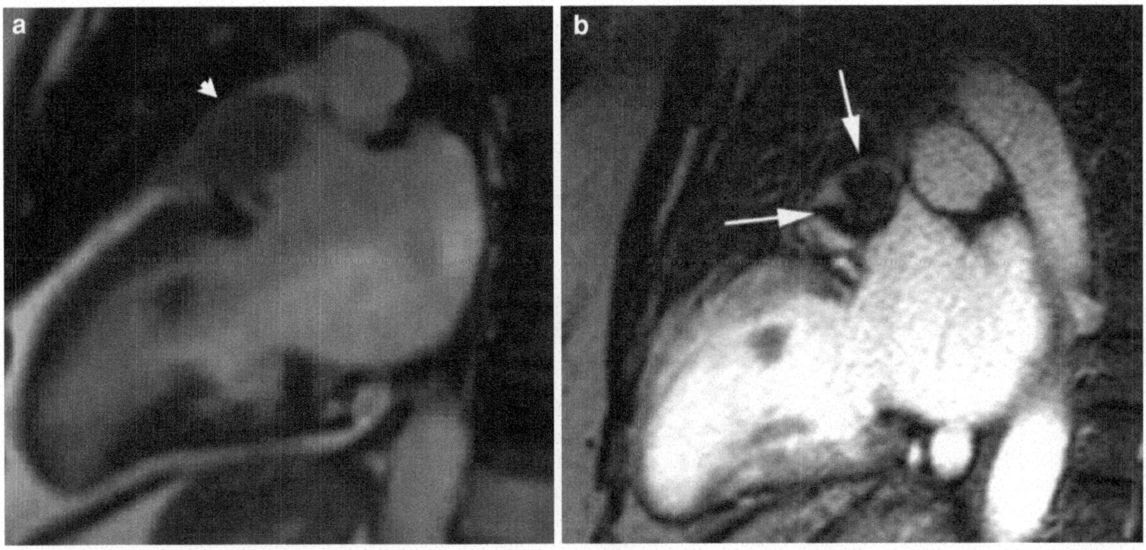

Fig. 5 **a** Vertical long axis bSSFP image showing thrombus in the left atrial appendage (*arrowhead*). **b.** Vertical long axis contrast-enhanced MR image, using T1-weighted 3D fast-field-echo technique (TR: 4.3 ms, TE: 1.3 ms, inversion time: 240), obtained 8 min after injection of 0.2 mmol/kg of Gd-DTPA, showing thrombus in left atrial appendage (*arrows*)

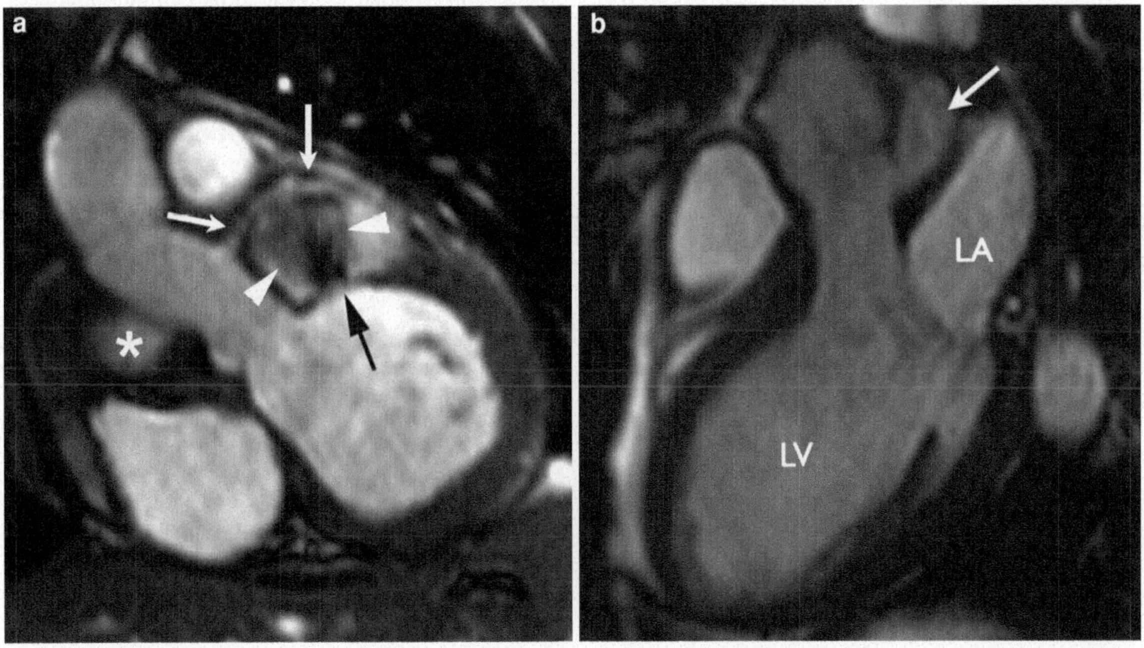

Fig. 6 **a** Aortic root pseudoaneurysm following aortic valve replacement for endocarditis. The pseudoaneurysm surrounds the aorta (* and *white arrow heads*), and displaces the left main stem coronary artery (*white arrows*). *Black arrow* shows communication between LV and pseudoaneurysm, which fills during each cardiac contraction. **b** bSSFP left ventricular inflow/outflow view, in a patient who has undergone the Ross procedure, showing a large aortic root abscess extending between the pulmonary autograft and left atrium—LA (*white arrow*)

definition than conventional GE imaging (Pereles et al. 2001; Barkhausen et al. 2001), the sequence is designed to be relatively flow insensitive. This results in reduced visualisation of flow disturbance secondary to valvular regurgitation, in particular when regurgitation is mild. Thus, in subjects who are being imaged

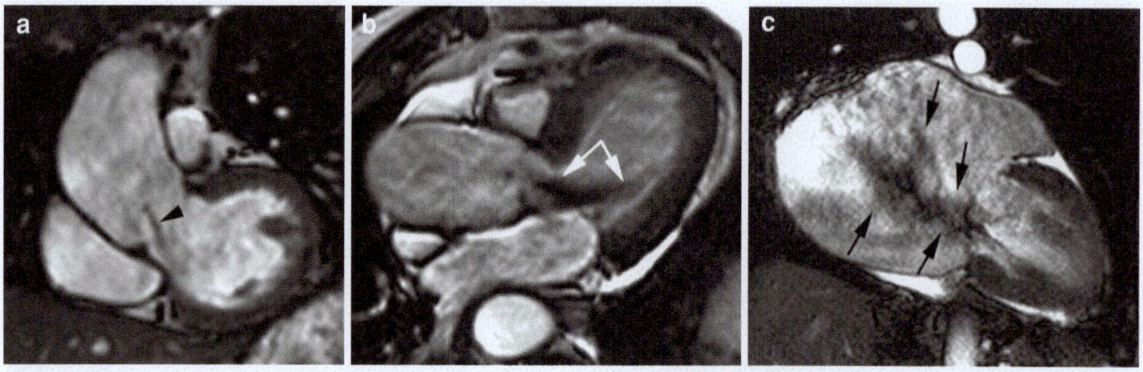

Fig. 7 Balanced SSFP images. **a** Oblique coronal left ventricular outflow tract view. Grade 1 aortic regurgitation (*black arrowhead*) in a patient with aortic root dilatation due to Marfan syndrome. **b** Oblique axial left ventricle inflow/outflow view. Grade 2 aortic regurgitation (*white arrows*). **c** Vertical long axis view. Grade 3 mitral regurgitation (*black arrows*); note the massively dilated left atrium. (Image **c** Courtesy of F. Melonas, R. Truter and G. Wagner, SCP MRI Center, Cape Town, South Africa)

for other reasons, incidental detection of mild valvular regurgitation may not be apparent on bSSFP cine imaging.

3.2.2 Quantitative Evaluation of Ventricular Volume Measurement

Magnetic resonance imaging can now be regarded as the best available in vivo technique for the measurement of ventricular volumes (see Chap. 5) (Grothues et al. 2002). In particular, bSSFP imaging enables good blood-pool/endocardial contrast images to be acquired in a single breath-hold (Moon et al. 2002; Alfakih et al. 2003). Using a set of short axis cuts covering the length of the ventricles, in combination with Simpson's rule, the stroke volumes of both the right and the left ventricle can be measured (Chap. 5, Fig. 3).

In normal individuals there is approximately a 1:1 relationship between these stroke volumes. Any discrepancy between the ventricular volumes in a patient with regurgitation will identify the regurgitant volume. The main limitation of this technique, when used alone, is that only patients with a single regurgitant valve can be assessed. Overall imaging times are now significantly shorter than 5 years ago. In general, 1 or 2 short axis images can be acquired in a single breath-hold, and newer sequence implementations, enable the acquisition of a complete short axis stack in a single breath-hold (Lee et al. 2002; Hori et al. 2003; Taylor et al. 2004). Thus, a complete MR assessment of ventricular volumes can be performed in approximately 20 min (10 min acquisition time; 10 min analysis time (Bellenger et al. 2000). Real-time methods with high temporo-spatial resolution are now available and allow for accurate volumetric assessment without breath-holding (Muthurangu et al. 2008) and even in patients with arrhythmias and at peak exercise (Lurz et al. 2009a).

3.2.3 Quantitative Evaluation With Velocity Mapping

For velocity mapping, phase information and not magnitude information is displayed. The application of short-lived magnetic gradients allows each point in the imaging plane to be encoded with a phase shift that is directly proportional to the velocity at that point. Because phase shifts can arise from other factors, a second velocity-compensated phase image is acquired, and subtraction yields the actual phase relationship of the protons (Nayler et al. 1986; Underwood et al. 1987b). Velocity encoding can be applied in any direction (through plane, left to right, up and down), though for flow quantification through plane imaging is used, and the size of the velocity window defined for increased sensitivity. Stationary material is represented as mid-grey whilst increasing velocities in either direction are shown in increasing grades of black or white (Fig. 8). It is important to define the velocity encode window as close to the peak velocity as possible, to reduce aliasing of peak velocities, whilst maintaining sensitivity for flow measurements.

Measurement of the velocity of all pixels in a region of interest of known area enables the

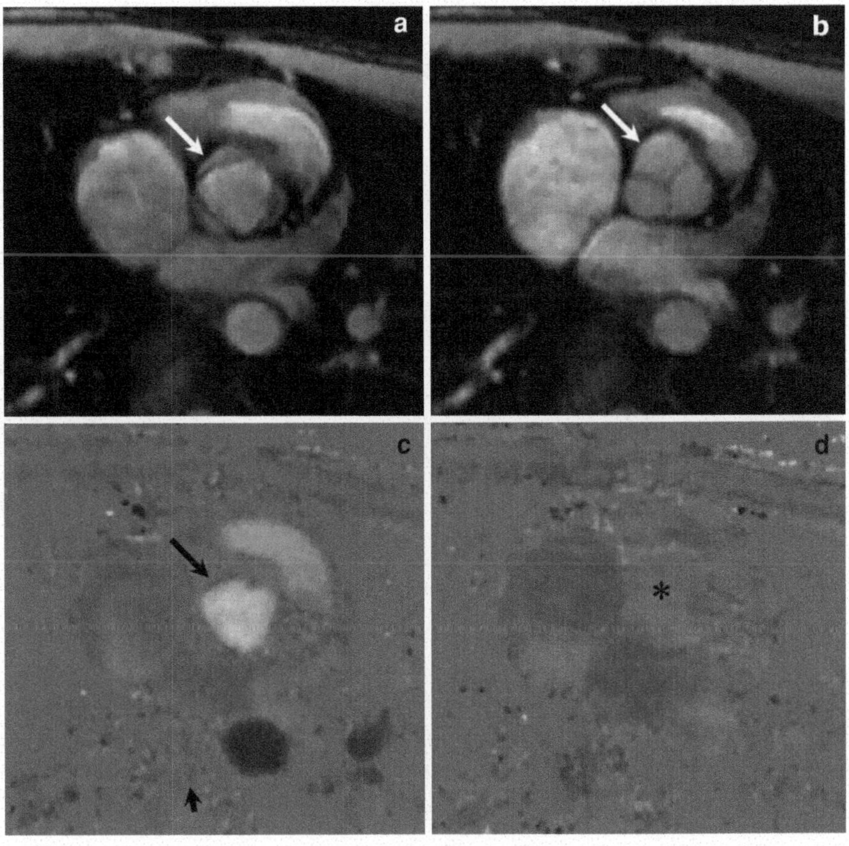

Fig. 8 Phase contrast velocity map, TE 5 ms, velocity encoding window ±1.5 m/s. **a** and **b** Magnitude image at level of aortic root (*white arrow*) during **a** systole and **b** diastole. The opening and closing of the three valve leaflets can be clearly seen. **c** and **d** Velocity image in the same imaging plane during **c** systole and **d** diastole. Stationary material is represented as mid-grey whilst flow towards the head in the aortic root is represented by white pixels (*black arrow* in **c**), and flow towards the feet in the descending aorta (*arrowhead* in **c**) is represented by *black* pixels. There is little flow in the aortic root during diastole (*) during valve closure

calculation of the instantaneous flow volume at any point in the cardiac cycle. Calculation of the flow volume per heart beat can be made by integrating the instantaneous flow volumes for all frames throughout the cardiac cycle. This technique has been validated in vitro and in vivo, and is extremely accurate and reproducible (Firmin et al. 1987; Meier et al. 1988; Bogren et al. 1989a). It now represents the best available in vivo technique for flow measurements. Quantification of the right ventricular (RV) and left ventricular (LV) outputs can be compared using through plane flow measurements from the proximal ascending aorta and pulmonary trunk (1:1 ratio in normal individuals) (Kondo et al. 1991), thus allowing quantification of pulmonary to systemic shunting.

The severity of regurgitation can be defined as follows (Sechtem et al. 1988):

- Mild—regurgitant fraction = 15–20%
- Moderate—regurgitant fraction = 20–40%
- Severe—regurgitant fraction > 40%

3.2.4 Issues Related to MR Functional Measurements

There are several technical issues that must be addressed when performing phase contrast velocity mapping.

First, phase contrast imaging should be performed as close to the centre of the main magnet field (B_0) as possible. This ensures phase errors introduced by eddy currents and Maxwell terms are kept to a minimum. Most MR scanners will now move the patient to the optimal position in the z-direction after prescription of the imaging planes for through plane imaging.

Second, the imaging plane should be perpendicular to the vessel. This ensures that the velocity vectors of the majority of the voxels are perpendicular to the imaging plane. This can be achieved by planning the through plane imaging position from two perpendicular views (e.g. left ventricular outflow tract plane and left ventricular inflow/outflow plane for the aortic valve) (see Figs. 5.5, 5.6, 5.7 and 5.8).

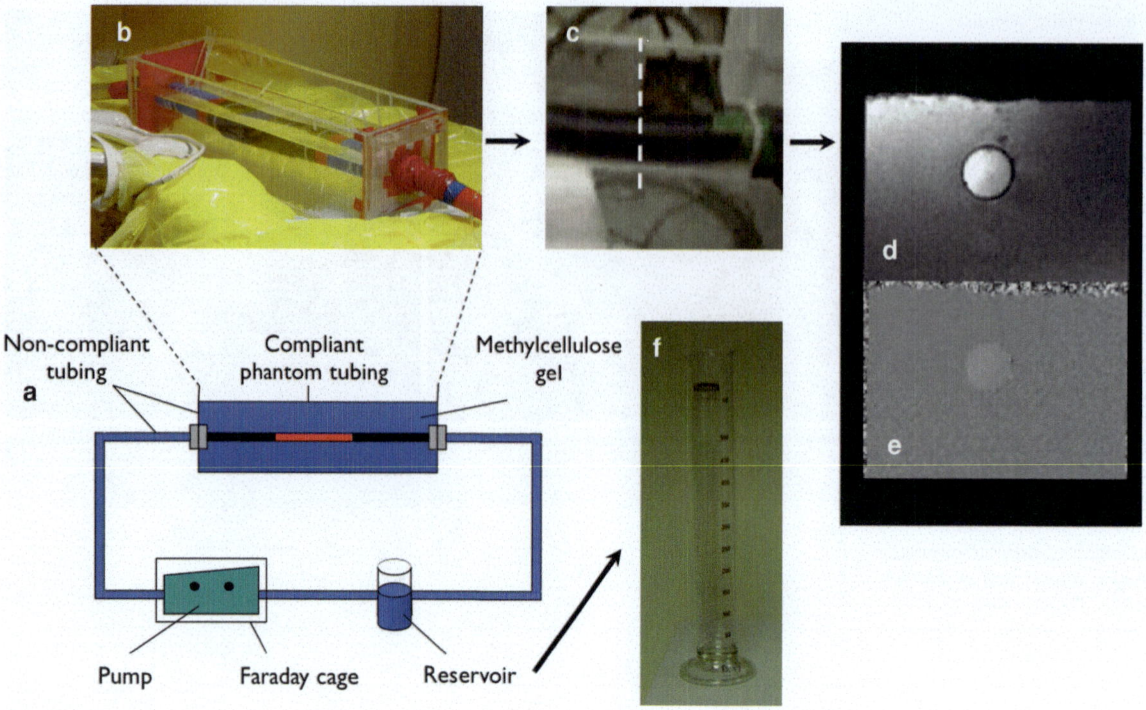

Fig. 9 MR flow phantom. **a** Schematic layout o f the flow phantom. A programmable pump is used to create pulsatile flow for the range of flows seen in the aorta and pulmonary trunk. **b** and **c** Compliant tubing set in methylcellulose gell is used to mimic the compliant vessel. **d** and **e** MR phase contrast imaging is performed to measure flow, through plane, in the compliant tubing (*dotted line*) **d** magnitude image, **e** velocity map. **f** The flowing fluid (water with dilute Gadolinium to give the same T1 as blood) is collected over 1 min to give a flow in mL/min, which is then correlated to the MR flow calculations

Third, the imaging plane should not be at the level of the valve, but just proximal or distal to the valve annulus. This ensures that artefacts secondary to eddy currents and the complex motion of the valve annulus are kept to a minimum. One possible method to compensate for motion of the valve annulus through the imaging plane is to use a moving slice velocity mapping technique (Kozerke et al. 1999). This experimental method enables the imaging slice to follow the valve annulus during the cardiac cycle, reducing velocity offsets and demonstrating discrepancies in conventional measurements of aortic and mitral regurgitation measurements by cardiovascular MR (Kozerke et al. 2001).

Fourth, care needs to be taken when flow in the vessel is not laminar, and is either turbulent or spiral. When flow is spiralling in a great vessel (e.g. dilated pulmonary trunk in pulmonary hypertension, dilated ascending aorta in Marfan syndrome), in order to reduce errors, more distal flow measurements need to be acquired (e.g. in the branch pulmonary arteries and summed or in more distal parts of the aorta, respectively).

Finally, it is important to have a degree of quality control with regard to ventricular volumes and flow measurements, and it is worthwhile performing two validation experiments on one's own scanner. The first validation is to use a flow phantom and compare MR measured flows with those acquired using a bucket and stop watch method (Fig. 9). Such an experiment will only be possible in centres with access to a flow phantom, but will help confirm the accuracy of your own scanner. The second validation can be performed in any centre, and involves assessing ventricular volumes and flow measurements in normal healthy volunteers. In this group of subjects, the stroke volume of the ventricles calculated from the ventricular volume assessment should equal the net forward flow measured by phase contrast velocity mapping. Thus, the normal subjects act as their own control for all the measurements acquired.

Over the last few years, doubt has been raised with regard to the accuracy and reliability of phase contrast velocity flow mapping, with concerns that linear and non-linear phase offsets can occur across the imaging plane (Gatehouse et al. 2010). Sequence optimisation, in particular with regard to gradient eddy currents (Rolf et al. 2011) and the use of phantoms to provide baseline correction of phase contrast images (Chernobelsky et al. 2007) have been proposed; however, strict adherence to the practical imaging solutions mentioned above, and an understanding of when phase contrast flow data may be compromised, should enable accurate, reliable use of phase contrast velocity mapping in routine daily clinical practice.

3.3 Valvular Stenosis

The presence of valvular stenosis can be identified by signal loss seen in MR cine images. Velocity mapping may then be used to establish an accurate peak velocity across the valve to quantify the severity of the stenosis. The use of the mean velocity across the caval veins and mitral valve can be used to describe the inflow curves for the atrioventricular valves (Mohiaddin et al. 1990).

3.3.1 Qualitative Assessment With Cine Imaging

For stenotic lesions, the degree of signal loss is dependent on the degree of stenosis and the echo time used. Thus, for shorter echo times less proton spin dephasing can take place and more signal is recovered (DeRoos et al. 1989; Kilner et al. 1991). Figure 10 demonstrates the relationship between the echo time and the peak velocity across a stenosis. Thus in more severe stenosis, a lower echo time must be used to prevent signal loss in the images.

As with the qualitative assessment of valvular regurgitating, signal loss is less marked on the increasingly used bSSFP cine imaging, due to the design and short TE of this sequence. It is thus much more difficult to get a feel for the peak velocity with SSFP sequences than with conventional GE cine imaging.

Valve area can also be measured on cine images, and this measurement has been shown to correlate well Doppler echocardiography and catheterisation (Sondergaard et al. 1993a; Friedrich et al. 2002).

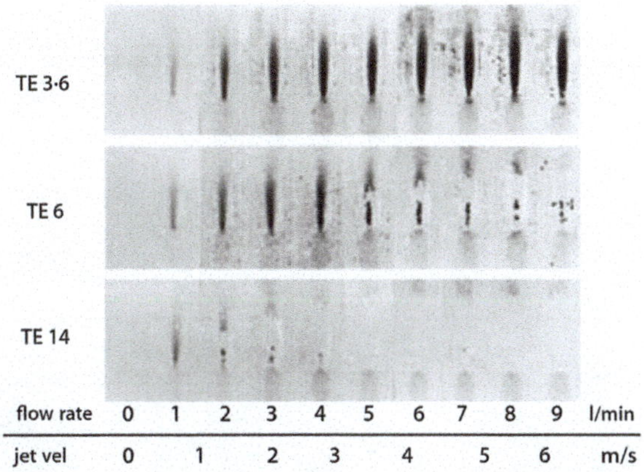

Fig. 10 In vitro jet velocity mapping. Velocity maps obtained with MRI of flow—increased from *left* to *right*—through the test stenosis, showing the significance of shortening the TE from 14 ms (*bottom*) to 6 ms (*centre*) and 3.6 ms (*top*). Only the 3.6 ms TE sequence allows mapping of high-velocity jets, up to a maximum tested velocity of 6.0 m/s [Reprinted with permission from Kilner et al. (1991) Valve and great vessel stenosis: assessment with MR jet velocity mapping. Radiology 178:229–235]

3.3.2 Quantitative Evaluation With Velocity Mapping

Direct measurement from the phase contrast velocity map enables the measurement of the peak velocity across the valve, and application of the modified Bernoulli equation,

$$\Delta P = 4V^2 \quad (1)$$

[where P = the pressure drop across the stenosis (mmHg) and V = velocity (m/s)], enables an estimate of the gradient across the valve. The technique is comparable to Doppler echocardiography valvular stenosis measurements and has an in vitro accuracy of within 4% of the true value (Simpson et al. 1993). The main advantage of the technique over echocardiography is that the velocity jet can be easily aligned in any direction without the limitation of acoustic windows.

Imaging can be performed through plane (velocity jet perpendicular to the imaging plane) or in-plane (velocity jet parallel to the imaging plane). Both strategies have their advantages and disadvantages. For the in-plane method the entire jet can be visualised, and the point within the jet of peak velocity easily identified. However, not all jets are easily aligned in a single 2D plane, and for tight narrow jets, there may be partial volume averaging and motion

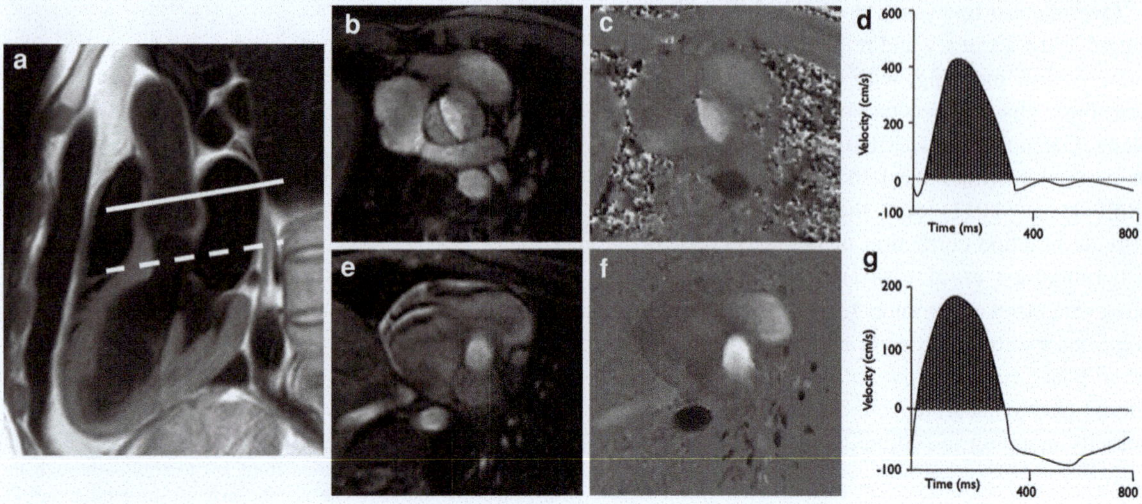

Fig. 11 Calculation of the functional aortic valve area using the VTI continuity equation for aortic stenosis. **a** Imaging planes for the aortic (*solid line*) and left ventricular outflow tract (LVOT, *dotted line*) measurements, prescribed from a left ventricular inflow/outflow view. **b–d** Aortic plane—magnitude image (**b**), velocity map (**c**) and peak velocity versus time curve (**d**) e.g. LVOT plane—magnitude image (**e**), velocity map (**f**) and peak velocity versus time curve (**g**). The summation of the area under the curve (*black shading*) during systole is the velocity time integral (VTI). See Eq. 2

within the imaging slice, and the peak velocity may not be accurately depicted. For through plane imaging, the jet will always pass through the imaging plane, but as only part of the stenotic jet is sampled the peak velocity may not be measured. It is thus best to use a combination of the two strategies with initial definition of the jet in-plane and quantification with through plane imaging at the site of maximum velocity on the in-plane image.

Selection of the correct velocity encode gradient is essential to maintain sensitivity and accuracy of measurements, whilst avoiding aliasing. Most scanners now have a fast phase contrast velocity mapping sequence that can be acquired in approximately 15–20 s or in real-time. This enables an estimate of the peak velocity to be made before progressing to the more time-consuming conventional phase contrast velocity mapping sequence.

Using data acquired from phase contrast flow curves the continuity equation can be used to calculate valve area. For the aortic valve, velocity is measured below the valve in the left ventricular outflow tract (LVOT) and above the valve in the aorta (Ao). The velocity time integral (VTI) is measured for systolic forward flow in both planes (Caruthers et al. 2003) (Fig. 11). The aortic valve area A_{Ao} (cm^2) is given by:

$$A_{Ao} = A_{LVOT}\left(\frac{VTI_{LVOT}}{VTI_{Ao}}\right) \qquad (2)$$

[where A_{LVOT} = LVOT area (cm^2), VTI_{LVOT} = LVOT VTI and VTI_{Ao} = Ao VTI].

3.4 Aortic Valve

3.4.1 Aortic Regurgitation

A protocol for imaging patients with aortic regurgitation is shown in Fig. 12. Table 1 also outlines the important issues that should be addressed during an assessment for aortic regurgitation. Regurgitant aortic jets are best visualised in the coronal or oblique coronal plane. Estimation of the signal void volume is possible (Aurigemma et al. 1991; Nishimura 1992; Ohnishi et al. 1992), but care must be taken to ensure that all the jet has been visualised. The most accurate method for quantifying the regurgitant fraction is with phase contrast velocity encoding in the slice direction, in an oblique axial plane above the aortic valve. In order to ensure that velocity vector for the majority flow is through plane in this image, it is best to use two perpendicular images through the ascending, and prescribe the oblique axial plane perpendicular to both (see also Fig. 5.5).

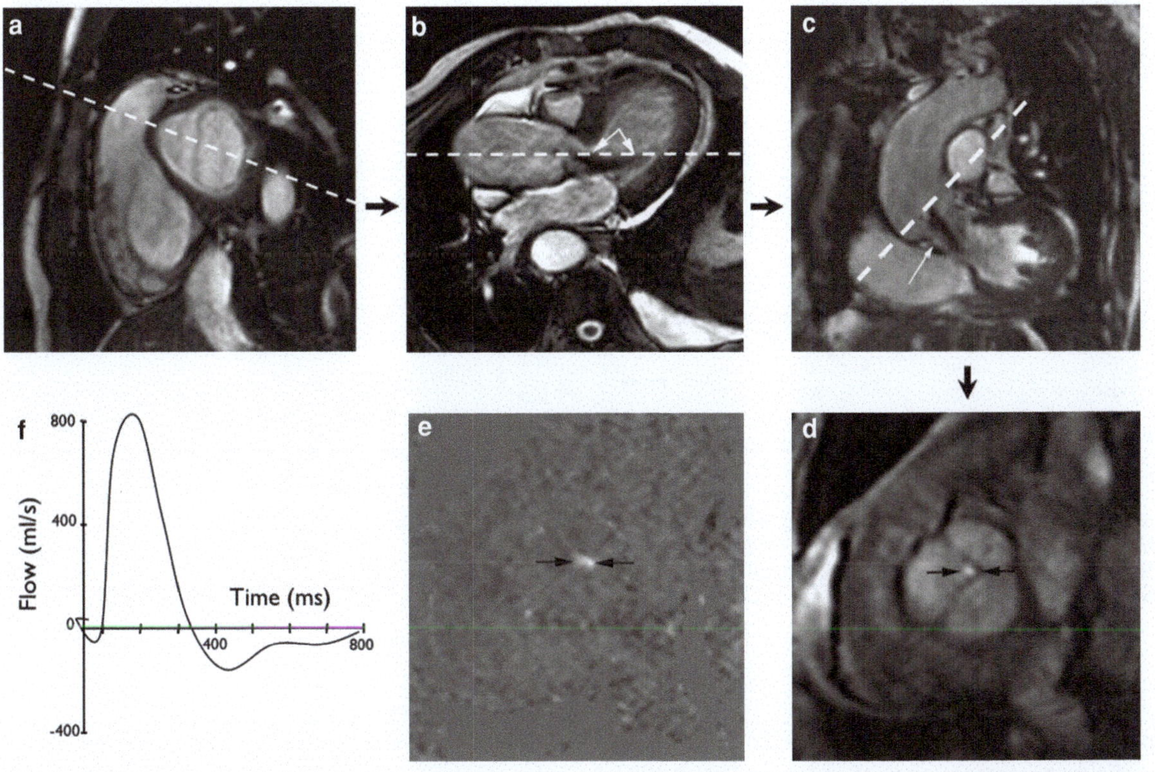

Fig. 12 Aortic regurgitation imaging protocol. **a** Basal short axis bSSFP cine frame. **b** A plane prescribed through the mitral valve and aortic valve on the basal short axis view yields the left ventricular inflow/outflow view, which shows grade 2 aortic regurgitation. **c** A perpendicular plane through the jet of regurgiataion yields an oblique coronal plane through the aortic valve and LV outflow tract. **d** and **e** An oblique axial plane in the aortic root, just above the aortic valve at the level of the coronary artery openings, is then defined from both **b** and **c** for phase contrast velocity mapping. **d** Magnitude image. **e** Velocity map in early diastole shows a narrow jet of aortic regurgitation due to lack of coalition of the valve leaflets centrally (*black arrows*). **f** Flow versus time plot for the ascending aorta. Antegrade flow calculated at 120 ml/beat, retrograde flow 30 ml/beat, and aortic regurgitant fraction 25%

Table 1 Cardiovascular MR assessment of aortic regurgitation

• *Morphology*
Valve leaflet structure e.g. bicuspid valve
Aortic root dilatation-dimensions
Aortic valve prolapse as seen with perimembranous VSD's
• *Function*
Visualise the regurgitant jet using orthogonal planes
Quantify regurgitant fraction with PC-MRI
Grading—mild 10–20%, moderate 20–40%, severe > 40%
Quantify LV volumes, systolic function and LV mass
• *Long-term follow-up* ventricular volumetric quantification
• *Look for* additional pre- and post-surgical causes: Marfan, dissection, infection or vegetation (if large) or abscess

A through plane velocity window of ±1.5 m/s should be set if there is isolated aortic regurgitation. If significant aortic stenosis is present in a dual velocity window, with a high systolic setting of ±5 m/s, changing to ±1.5 m/s for the diastolic frames, may be necessary. Aortic regurgitation volume is the amount of retrograde diastolic flow and is measured in mL/beat or L/min (mL/beat × heart rate) (Fig. 13). The aortic regurgitant fraction (RF) is given by:

$$\mathrm{RF}(\%) = \frac{\mathrm{Aortic\,retrograde\,flow}(\mathrm{mL/beat}) \times 100}{\mathrm{Aortic\ forward\ flow}\ (\mathrm{mL/beat})} \quad (3)$$

A good correlation has been demonstrated between ventricular volume measurements and velocity

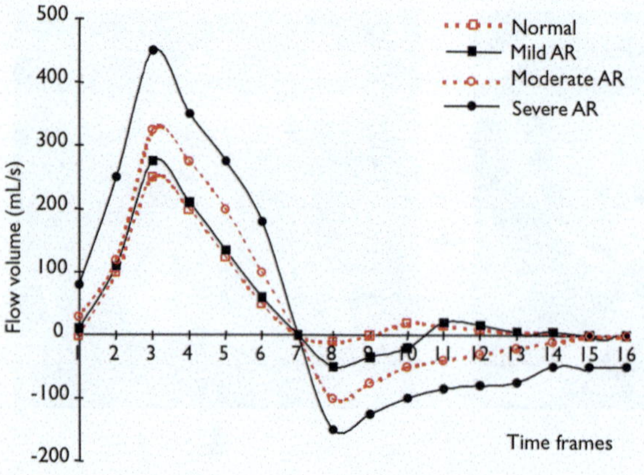

Fig. 13 Plots of flow volume versus time frames per cardiac cycle. Measurements were made in the ascending aorta for a normal subject and patients with increasing severity of aortic regurgitation (*AR*). Each point on the graphs represents the blood flow in the aorta for each image in the cardiac cycle. Negative values represent retrograde flow during diastole. Integration of the area under the curve for antegrade and retrograde flow enables calculation of the regurgitant volume per cardiac cycle (mL/beat)

Table 2 Causes of aortic regurgitation

Valvular causes
Congenital bicuspid aortic valve
Rheumatic heart disease
Bacterial endocarditis
Myxomatous valve associated with cystic medial necrosis
Aortic valve prolapse
Secondary to dilatation of the aortic annulus
Marfan syndrome
Syphilitic aortitis
Ankylosing spondylitis
Reiter disease
Rheumatoid arthritis
Ehlers Danlos syndrome
Secondary to aortic dissection
Deceleration trauma
Hypertension

mapping in the ascending aorta, for the calculation of aortic regurgitant fractions (Sondergaard et al. 1993a, b). Interstudy reproducibility has been demonstrated to be high and thus the technique is ideal for long-term patient follow-up (Dulce et al. 1992).

Some debate still remains as to the positioning of the plane across the aorta. Current in vivo experience suggests that a position between the coronary ostia and the aortic valve may be most accurate (Chatzimavroudis et al. 1997). Positions above the coronary ostia lead to inaccuracies secondary to coronary flow and aortic compliance. Further in vivo studies need to be performed to confirm these findings. The commercial application of moving slice velocity mapping would be a potential aide for slice positioning (Kozerke et al. 2001)

Aortic regurgitation can be caused by abnormalities of the aortic leaflets or annulus or be secondary to dilatation of the aortic root. The aetiologies of aortic regurgitation are given in Table 2. Figure 14 shows rupture of one of the valve leaflets in a patient with bicuspid aortic valve.

In acute aortic regurgitation (bacterial endocarditis, aortic dissection and trauma), ventricular adaptation does not occur and there is a rapid increase in LV filling pressures, reduced cardiac output, increased left atrial pressure, pulmonary oedema and ultimately shock. In chronic aortic regurgitation, the initial response is LV hypertrophy, as compensation for increased wall stress secondary to volume overload. However, over time, the main haemodynamic response to aortic regurgitation is dilatation of the left ventricle and reduction in ventricular function.

Though medical treatments can be used to deal with the symptomatic effects of aortic regurgitation, surgical valvular replacement remains the treatment option for moderate/severe aortic regurgitation. The timing of surgery is important, and the balance between operating too soon (operative risks, insertion of a valve that will not last for ever, life long anti-coagulation) and operating too late (irreversible left ventricular failure). Currently, operative timing depends on symptoms, chest X-ray appearance, echocardiographic findings and the longitudinal changes in these parameters (Bonow et al. 1998). With improving surgical techniques, non-invasive methods of investigation and enhanced knowledge of the natural history and prognosis, there has been progressively earlier application of surgery for both severe aortic and mitral regurgitation (Borer and Bonow 2003).

MR imaging protocols, as outlined above, by providing accurate, quantifiable and reproducible measurements of regurgitant volume may contribute

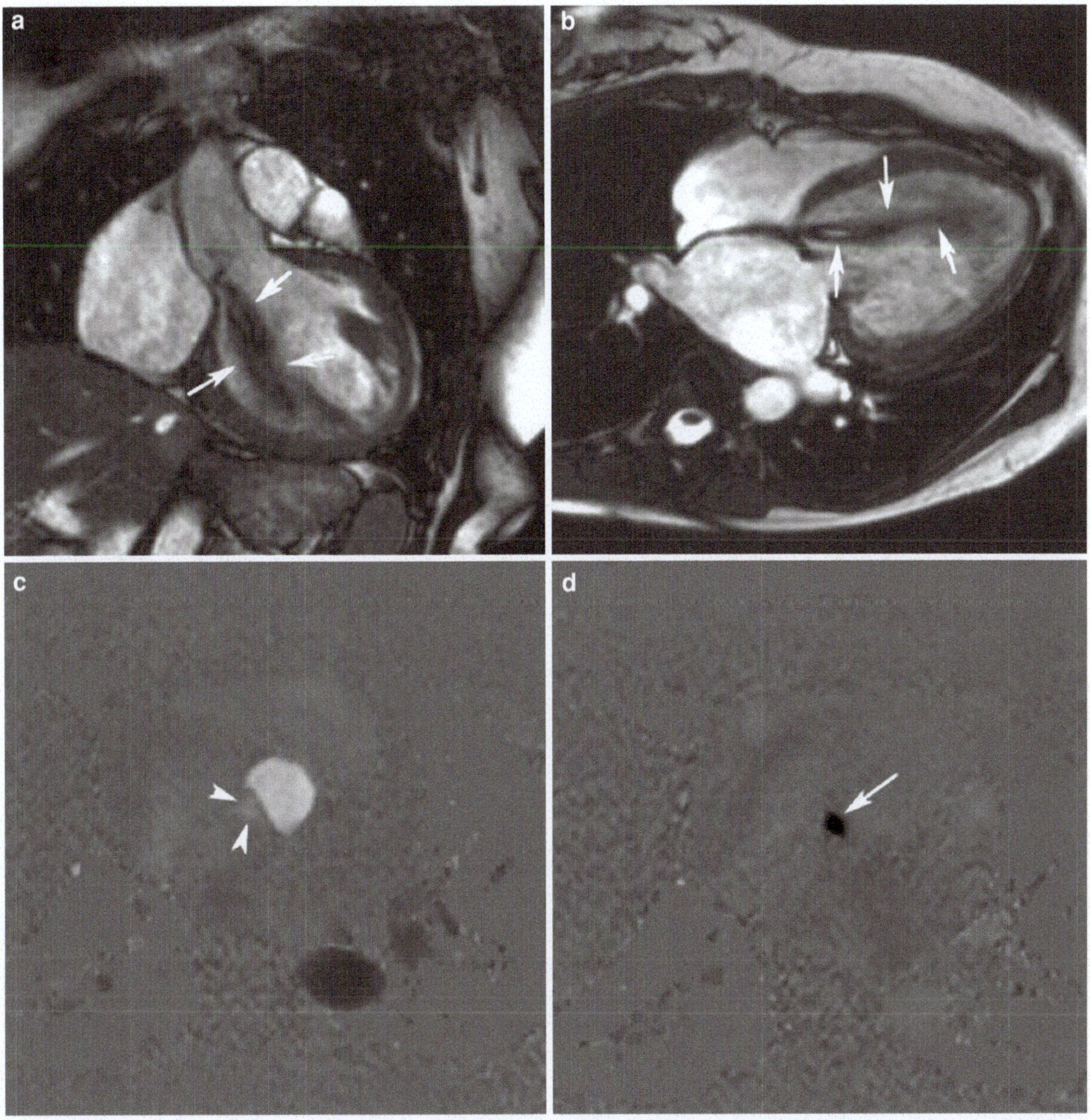

Fig. 14 Severe aortic regurgitation—Bicuspid aortic valve (latero-lateral rim) with rupture of anterior leaflet and severe aortic regurgitation with left ventricular (LV) volume overload. Cine MRI (SSFP sequence) perpendicularly oriented through aortic valve (**a**), along LV outflow tract (**b**). Magnitude (**c**) and phase contrast (**d**) MR image perpendicular through LV outflow tract. In **a**, closure of bicuspid aortic valve (*arrowhead*) but presence of area of signal void (*arrow*) in the middle of anterior leaflet corresponding to the area of rupture. In **b**, anterior leaflet rupture leads to complex and important holodiastolic aortic regurgitation. Severity of aortic insufficiency is quantified using phase contrast imaging, where regurgitation is depicted as a pinpoint dark area (**c** and **d**; *arrows*). Following parameters are derived: regurgitation flow volume: 77 mL; regurgitation fraction: 46%. Chronic volume overload has led to important eccentric LV hypertrophy (end-diastolic volume: 328 mL; ejection fraction: 58%; mass: 195 g)

to the development of more specific criteria for the timing of surgery. In asymptomatic patients with aortic regurgitation, early data suggests that MR assessment of regurgitant fraction and volumes may be better long-term prognosticators than LV volumes and function (Christiansen et al. 2009). As yet, no large-scale cardiovascular MR studies addressing these issue have been published, though velocity

Table 3 Causes of aortic stenosis

Acquired	
	Degenerative (fibrocalcific senile aortic stenosis)
	Rheumatic heart disease
Congenital	
	Subvalvular
	Valvular—bicuspid aortic valve
	Supravalvular

mapping in the ascending aorta has now been performed to analyse the therapeutic effects of ACE inhibition in patients with aortic regurgitation (Globits et al. 1996). MR imaging demonstrated the beneficial effects of the therapy and was able to identify those patients with aortic regurgitation who responded favourably to ACE inhibition.

3.4.2 Aortic Stenosis

Aortic stenosis can be divided into sub-valvular stenosis, valvular stenosis and supra-valvular stenosis. The hemodynamic consequence of all forms of aortic stenosis is concentric left ventricular hypertrophy. The causes of aortic stenosis are outlined in Table 3. Supra-valvular aortic stenosis is discussed in the congenital heart disease chapter (see Chap. 16, Sect. 6.7). Sub-valvular aortic stenosis can be congenital or, more commonly in adults occurs secondary to hypertrophic cardiomyopathy (see Chap. 9, Sect. 4.1.1). The remainder of this section will concentrate on valvular aortic stenosis.

MR imaging of aortic stenosis is outlined in Fig. 15. Table 4 also outlines the important issues that should be addressed during an MR assessment for aortic stenosis. The alignment of the jet and definition of the velocity encode window are important variables. The jet core appears as high signal sandwiched between two jets of low signal. For most scanners, the shortest TE sequence will now be used and manual selection of the TE is less common, in particular as bSSFP sequences will be predominantly used. However, if TE selection is still necessary, the TE and velocity window should be set to aim for greatest signal to noise and velocity sensitivity, though if the shortest TE and largest velocity window are defined, most clinically significant jets will be accounted for.

Good in vivo agreement has been demonstrated for a wide range of pressure gradients across the aortic valve (3–148 mmHg) between MR velocity mapping and Doppler echocardiography and X-ray angiography (Eichenberger et al. 1993). In our own practice, we have found it easiest to interpret velocity maps parallel to the jet, as this reveals the jet length in relationship to pre- and post-stenotic flows (Kilner et al. 1993).

Valve area can also be assessed, using either direct visualisation of the valve area on cine images (Friedrich et al. 2002; John et al. 2003) (Figs. 16 and 17) or the application of the continuity equation to MR data (Caruthers et al. 2003) (Fig. 11). For direct measurement of valve area, the area of flow through plane at the level of the origin of the flow jet is performed. The results of this technique to date have been conflicting. Friedrich et al. (2002) have demonstrated that direct MR measurement of aortic valve area agreed well with aortic area calculated at cardiac catheterisation ($r = 0.78$), and less well with that calculated at echocardiography ($r = 0.52$). Whilst John et al. (2003) have demonstrated good agreement between MR measurements and echocardiography ($r = 0.96$), but poor agreement between MR and cardiac catheterisation ($r = 0.44$). When MR assessment of velocity profiles in the LVOT and aorta was performed and the continuity equation applied (see Eq. 2 above), there was good agreement between the MR method and similar data acquired with echocardiography ($r = 0.83$) (Caruthers et al. 2003). More recently, Debl et al. have demonstrated that planimetry of aortic valve area by MRI can be performed with better image quality as compared with transthoracic echo. However, in the clinical management of patients with aortic stenosis, it has to be considered that MRI slightly overestimates aortic valve area as compared with catheterisation despite an excellent correlation (Debl et al. 2005), and confirmed by others (Reant et al. 2006).

When imaging aortic stenosis it is also important to assess left ventricular mass and aortic root dimensions. Left ventricular mass is increased in aortic stenosis, and can be used as a guide to the significance of the aortic stenosis with a reduction in LV hypertrophy after aortic valve replacement (Rajappan et al. 2000; Sandstede et al. 2000; Lamb et al. 2002; Sensky et al. 2003). The aortic root may be dilated secondary to aortic stenosis, and this is well documented in patients with bicuspid aortic valve (Alegret et al. 2003; Novaro et al. 2003; Nkomo et al. 2003). In patients with angina and aortic stenosis,

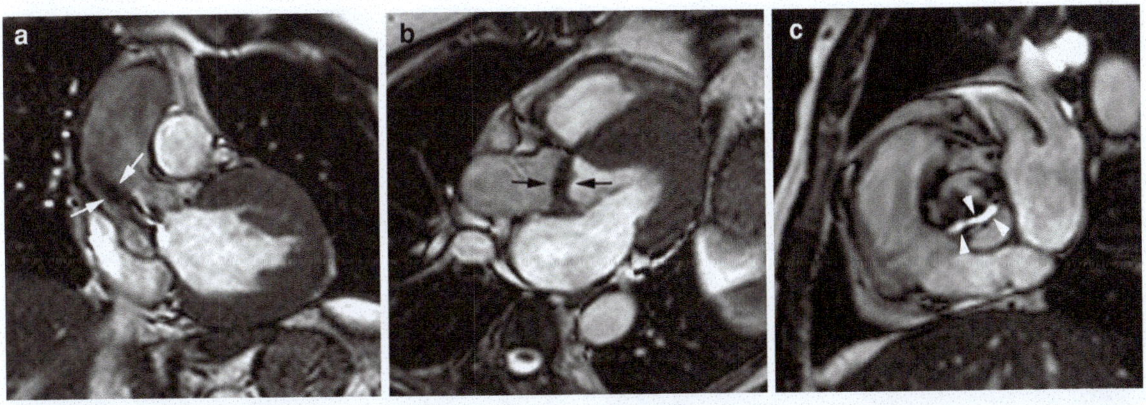

Fig. 15 Balanced SSFP images of severe aortic stenosis. **a** Oblique coronal plane through the aortic valve and LVOT in systole shows a tight jet of signal loss (turbulence) in the ascending aorta (*white arrows*). **b** Left ventricular inflow/outflow view through the aortic valve and LVOT in diastole shows marked thickening of the aortic valve (*black arrows*). **c** Through plane image in the aortic root above the aortic valve in systole. The narrow jet of turbulent flow can be clearly seen (*white arrowheads*)

Table 4 Cardiovascular MR assessment of aortic stenosis

Always consider the aetiology of the valve stenosis—congenital or acquired
• *Morphology*
Lesion site: sub-valvar, valvar or supra-valvar stenosis (see Williams syndrome)
Valve morphology and structure (bicuspid, tricuspid or doming leaflets), presence of leaflet fibrosis ± calcification (*better seen on echo*)
• *Function*
Measure LV mass, volume and systolic function
Planimetry of aortic valve area
MR estimation of valvular gradient (forward velocity is not indicative of degree of stenosis in the presence of impaired LV systolic function)
Aortic valve regurgitation
• *Also look for* post-stenotic dilatation of ascending aorta, coarctation of the aorta
Assess pulmonary valve for suitability for Ross procedure

visualisation of the coronary arteries is often requested to exclude ischaemic heart disease as a contributing factor to the symptoms. At present, this is best performed by direct X-ray cardiac catheterisation, though cardiovascular CT is increasingly used for this role (Pflederer and Achenbach 2010).

More recently, late gadolinium enhanced imaging has shown that up to a third of patients with aortic stenosis have patchy fibrosis (Debl et al. 2006; La Salvia et al. 2006), confirming autopsy findings of fibrosis in areas of maximal hypertrophy (Hein et al. 2003). More interestingly, new methods to assess diffuse myocardial fibrosis (Flett et al. 2010) may yield prognostic information about the clinical response of patients to surgical aortic valve replacement.

Left ventricular contraction can also be assessed using myocardial tagging. In patients with pressure-overloaded hypertrophied ventricles, there is an increase in apical rotation that leads to increased torsion of the left ventricle (Nagel et al. 2000; Sandstede et al. 2002), and delay and prolongation of diastolic untwisting (Nagel et al. 2000). Not only do such studies help improve our understanding of cardiac physiology in aortic stenosis, but may help clinically to distinguish pathological causes of LV hypertrophy from physiological changes that can occur in the 'athlete' heart (see Chap. 9). Furthermore, 1 year after aortic valve replacement for aortic stenosis, there is normalisation of left ventricular torsion, and monitoring such parameters in patients over time may aide in defining the optimal time for operative intervention in aortic stenosis (Sandstede et al. 2002).

3.4.3 Transcatheter Aortic Valve Implantation

Since its introduction in 2002 (Cribier et al. 2002), transcatheter aortic valve implantation (TAVI) has become a routine method of treating aortic valve disease, in particular calcific aortic stenosis in the

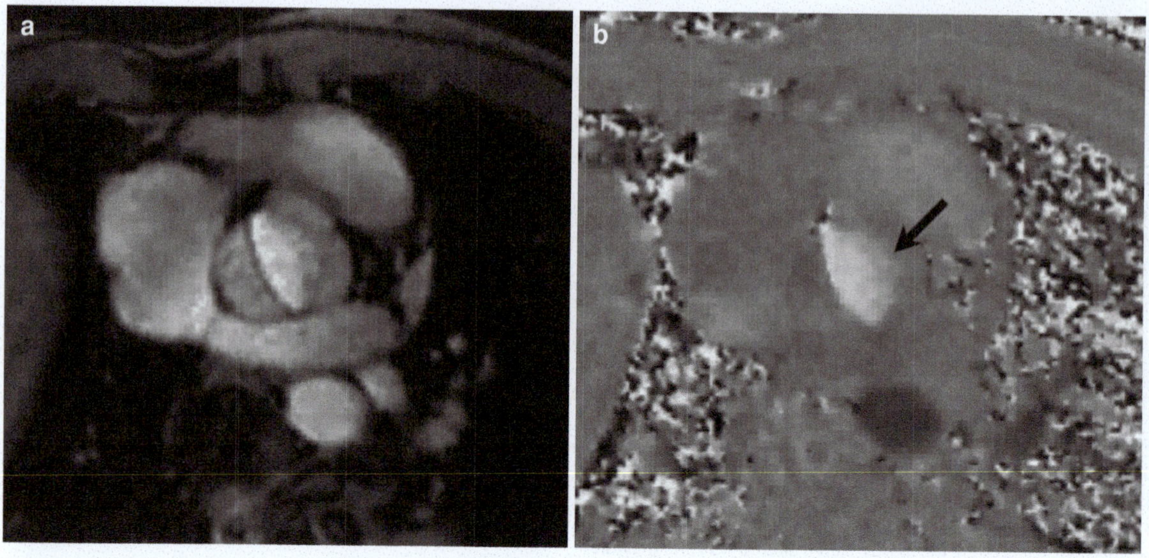

Fig. 16 Bicuspid aortic valve (*arrow*). **a** Magnitude image in systole—note the 'fish mouth' appearance of the aortic valve aperture, when compared with normal valve opening as shown in Fig. 13.6. **b** Velocity map in systole—forward flow is shown as *white*

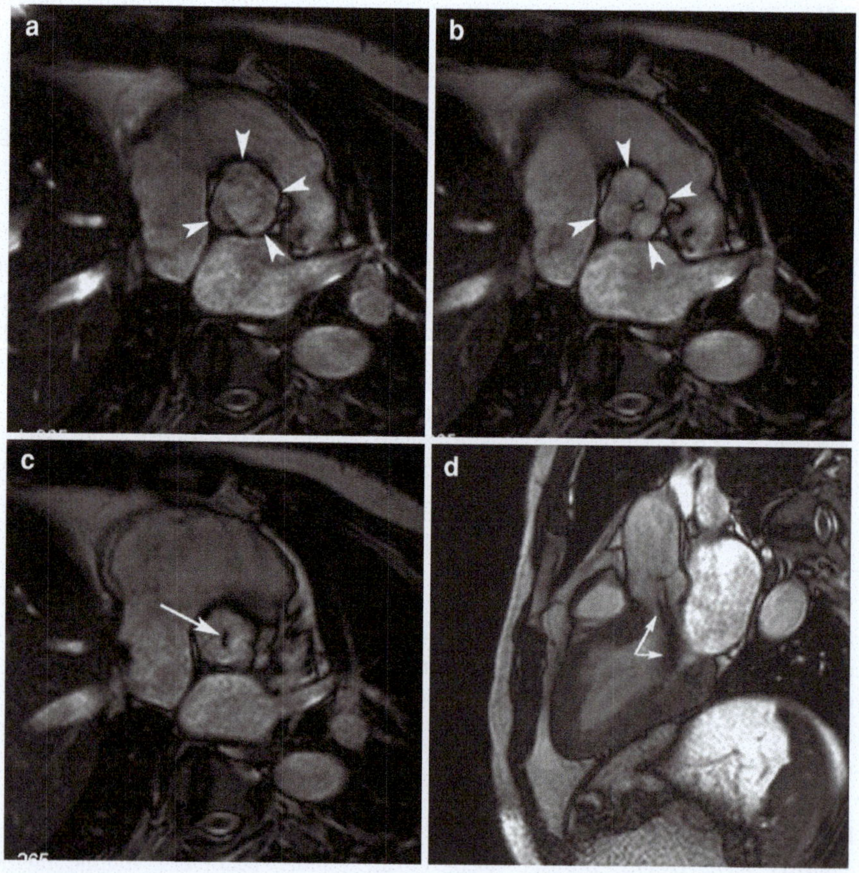

Fig. 17 Quadracuspid aortic valve (*arrowheads*) in systole (**a**) and diastole (**b**)—note the moderate aortic regurgitation (*arrows*) in (**c**) and long axis view (**d**)

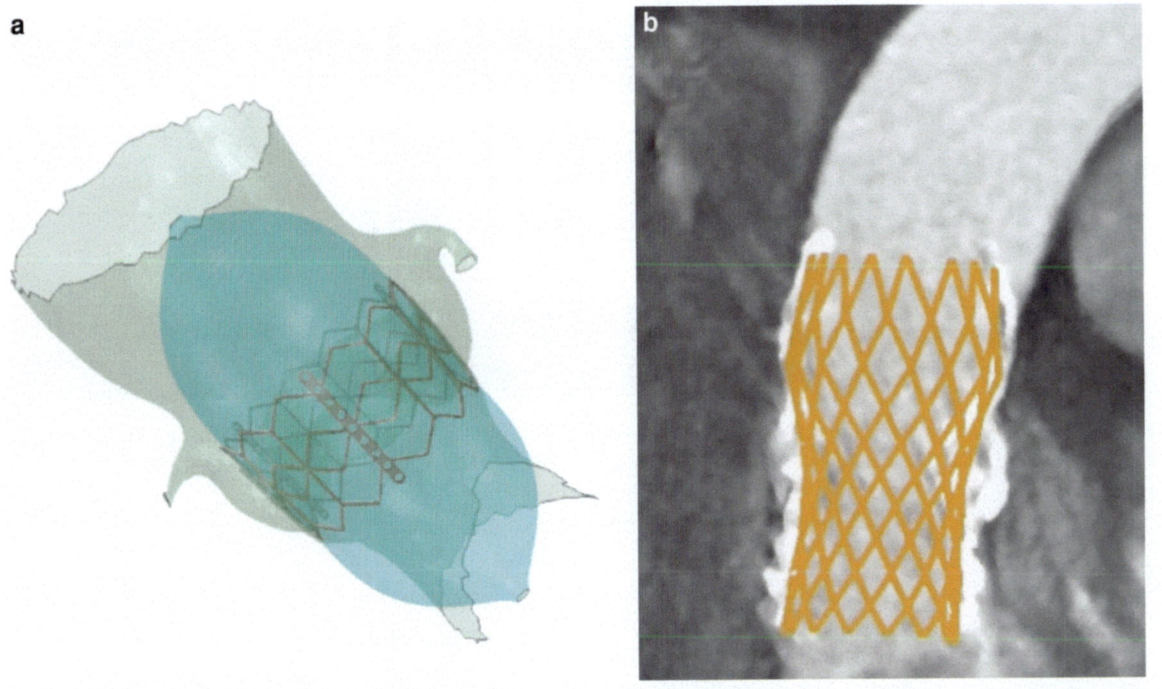

Fig. 18 **a** 3D reconstructions from CT data sets for virtual implantation of a the balloon expandable Edwards SAPIEN device (Edwards Lifesciences, Irvine, CA, USA)—aortic root, device and expanded balloon shown and **b** coronal reformat from a 3D CT data set after implantation of a self expanding CoreValve Revalving System (Medtronic, Minneapolis, MN, USA)—note the marked aortic root calcification

elderly. There is now a good procedural success rate (94–97%) (Webb et al. 2007), with a relatively low complication rate (5–18%) equivalent to that of surgery. There are two CE approved devices, the balloon expandable Edwards SAPIEN device (Edwards Lifesciences, Irvine, CA, USA) and the self expanding CoreValve Revalving System (Medtronic, Minneapolis, MN, USA) (Fig. 18).

Though implantation has been shown to improve qualitative and quantitative measures of patient quality of life, as with all new technologies, there remain several issues that need to be addressed. Importantly, imaging is crucial to many of these issues (Delgado et al. 2010), with regard to:

- Defining pre-procedural issues—patient selection for TAVI, device sizing, and assessment of femoral access;
- Peri-procedural device positioning—avoidance of coronary occlusion or mitral valve entrapment; and
- Post-procedural follow-up—success of treatment from a haemodynmic perspective, exclusion of paravalvular leaks, and assessment of vascular complications including cerebro-vascular events.

Cross-sectional imaging (MRI and CT) can play a role in these assessments (Iozzelli et al. 2009; Ng et al. 2010), though to date the majority of assessments have been performed using cardiovascular CT.Whatever imaging modality is used, the following issues need to be addressed:

- Evaluation of the aortic valve anatomy and morphology (in particular calcifications)—to establish suitability for TAVI;
- Measurement of the aortic valve annulus—to select TAVI device size;
- Evaluation of aortic root and left ventricular outflow tract dimensions and position coronary arteries—to define if aortic root is too dilated, and the coronary arteries are too low;
- Evaluation of peripheral vascular access—define optimal vascular approach; and
- Assessment of LV and mitral valve function.

With increasing numbers of TAVI procedures, MR imaging protocols will become better defined. As the technique becomes used in younger patients with ever lesser degrees of aortic stenosis severity and even pure aortic incompetence, patient selection, to ensure

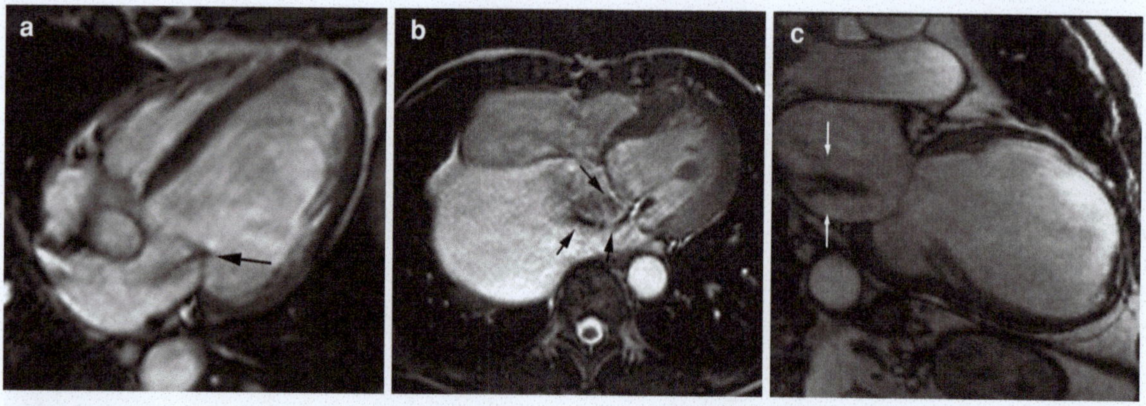

Fig. 19 Balanced SSFP images of mitral incompetence **a** and **b** Horizonal long axis views. Grade 2 mitral incompetence (*black arrows*). **c** Vertical long axis view of grade 3 mitral incompetence (*white arrows*) in a patient with mitral annulus dilatation secondary to ischaemic heart disease. (Image **b** Courtesy of F. Melonas, R. Truter and G. Wagner, SCP MRI Center, Cape Town, South Africa)

low complication rates, will become ever more important. Interestingly, real-time MR imaging may offer the possibility to enable MR-guide TAVI, with MR acting as a useful 3D guide to help in device positioning (Kahlert et al. 2010). Though issues of guide wire and device MR compatibility need to be addressed before MR-guided implantations can become a reality (see Chap. 18).

3.5 Mitral Valve

3.5.1 Mitral Regurgitation

There is good correlation between the signal loss caused by mitral regurgitation on cine MR images and Doppler and X-ray angiographic grading (Aurigemma et al. 1990) (Fig. 19). The regurgitant jet is best visualised in either the horizontal or the vertical long axis plane (Fig. 20). MR imaging has the advantage of being able to define lesions in subjects with poor acoustic windows. For alignment of the optimal imaging planes for the mitral valve see Fig. 5.6.

There are three methods for quantifying mitral regurgitation with cardiovascular MR:

For isolated mitral regurgitation ventricular volume measurements provide an accurate method for quantifying mitral regurgitation (Hundley et al. 1995):

$$\begin{aligned}&\text{Regurgitant volume (mL/beat)}\\&\quad = \text{LVSV (mL/beat)} - \text{RVSV (mL/beat)}\end{aligned} \tag{4}$$

$$\begin{aligned}&\text{Regurgitant fraction (\%)}\\&\quad = \frac{\text{Regurgitant volume(mL/beat)} \times 100}{\text{LVSV (mL/beat)}}\end{aligned} \tag{5}$$

[where LVSV = left ventricular stroke volume and RVSV = right ventricular stroke volume.]

Secondly, when other valvular disease is present, the mitral regurgitant volume can be calculated from the LV stroke volume and phase contrast velocity mapping flow measurements in the aorta:

$$\begin{aligned}&\text{Regurgitant volume (mL/beat)}\\&\quad = \text{LVSV (mL/beat)}\\&\qquad - \text{Aortic forward flow (mL/beat)}\end{aligned} \tag{6}$$

A third proposed method for quantifying mitral regurgitation involves calculation of the difference between ventricular outflow and ventricular inflow (Fujita et al. 1994). Velocity mapping in the ascending aorta can be used to assess ventricular outflow, whilst velocity mapping at the mitral valve annulus during diastole can be used to assess inflow (Fig. 21). Thus:

$$\begin{aligned}&\text{Regurgitant volume (mL/beat)}\\&\quad = \text{LV inflow (mL/beat)}\\&\qquad - \text{Aortic forward flow (mL/beat)}\end{aligned} \tag{7}$$

Using this method, MR is able demonstrate different mitral regurgitant volumes for groups with mild, moderate and severe mitral regurgitation,

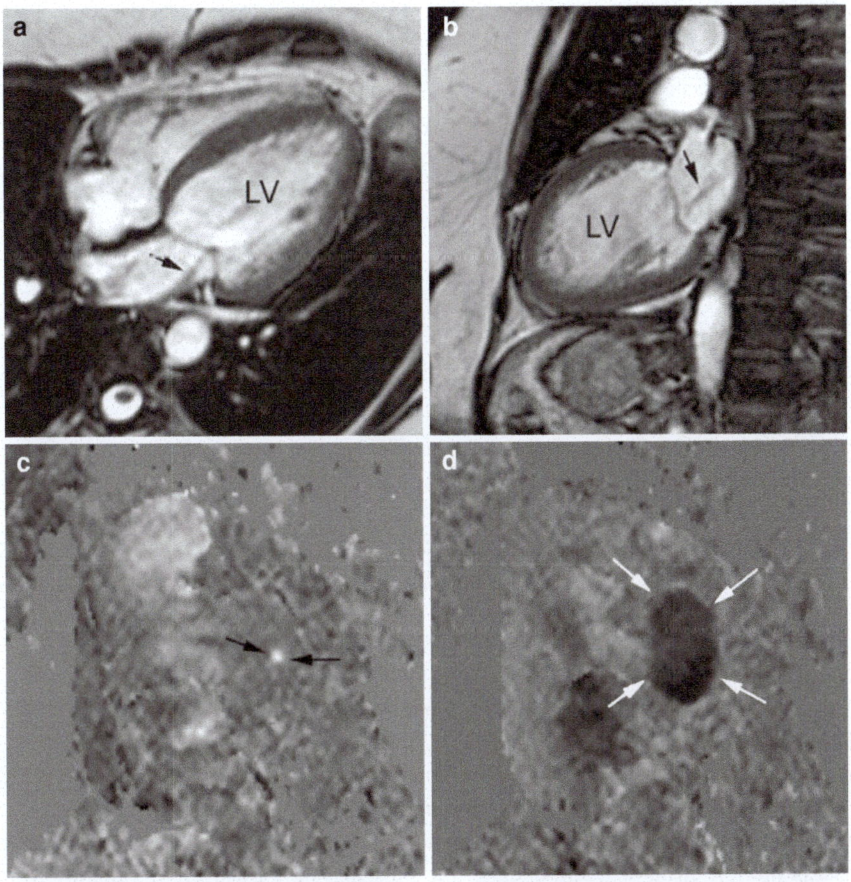

Fig. 20 Functional mitral regurgitation in a 44-year-old woman with idiopathic dilated cardiomyopathy. Functional mitral regurgitation is caused by dilation of mitral ring (loss of sphincter-like function) and tethering of both leaflets due to papillary muscles displacement. Cine MRI (bSSFP sequence) in horizontal long axis (**a**) and vertical long axis (**b**), both at systole. Regurgitant flow appears as stripe-like jet (*arrows*) into left atrium. PC-MRI obtained perpendicularly through the mitral valve. During systole (**c**), regurgitant flow appears as a pinpoint *white* spot (*black arrows*), whereas during diastole (**d**) the inflow through mitral valve is shown as an *oval black* structure (*white arrows*). A regurgitation fraction of 12% was derived

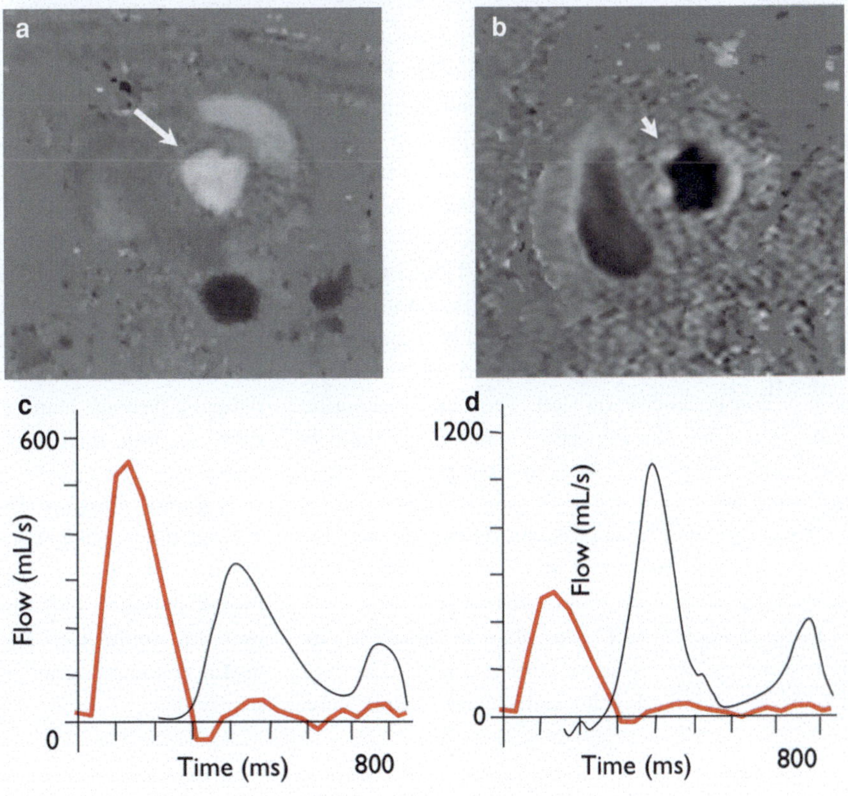

Fig. 21 Measurement of mitral regurgitation by using PC-MRI to measure the difference between outflow across the proximal ascending aorta (**a**) and inflow across the mitral annulus (**b**). Phase images acquired at the level of the proximal part of ascending aorta (*arrow* in **a**) and the mitral annulus (*arrowhead* in **b**). The graphs show the flow volume versus time frame for mitral inflow (*black curve*) and aortic outflow (*red curve*) in a normal subject (**c**) and in a patient with mitral regurgitation (**d**). The difference in the areas under the two curves is the volume of mitral regurgitation

Table 5 Causes of mitral regurgitation

Acute	
	Bacterial endocarditis
	Rupture of chordae tendinae (mitral valve prolapse)
	Myocardial infarction with involvement of the papillary muscle disease
Chronic	
	Rheumatic heart disease
	Mitral valve prolapse syndrome
	Marfan syndrome
	Congenital
	Idiopathic hypertrophic subaortic stenosis
	Persistent ostium primum ASD with cleft mitral valve
	Functional—secondary to dilatation of the mitral annulus in LV dilatation
	Hypertrophic cardiomyopathy

defined at echocardiography. There is also good correlation between the calculated regurgitant fraction and the grading of mitral regurgitation severity at Doppler echocardiography (Fujita et al. 1994), and excellent inter- and intra-observer variability.

When assessing mitral regurgitation with MR imaging it is important to image the left atrium to assess the left atrial size and exclude the presence of thrombi.

As with aortic regurgitation, mitral regurgitation may be acute or chronic (see Table 5). The main haemodynamic consequence of chronic mitral regurgitation is gradual left ventricular dilatation and ultimately left ventricular failure. Importantly, long-term survival is less good if surgical repair is performed when the left ventricular ejection fraction is less than 60% (Enriquez-Sarano et al. 1994). Thus, cardiovascular MR is well placed as an imaging tool that can accurately quantify, and reproducibly monitor the severity of mitral regurgitation and the haemodynamic consequences on left ventricular function. Table 6 outlines the important issues that should be addressed during an MR assessment for mitral regurgitation.

Again, no large-scale clinical studies have assessed the use of MR imaging for defining the timing of surgical repair of mitral regurgitation.

Cardiovascular MR can also to used in the assessment of mitral valve prolapse (Fig. 22), with use of the standard echo criteria for mitral valve prolapse applicable to cardiovascular MR (Gabriel et al. 2008; Han et al. 2008)

Table 6 Cardiovascular MR assessment of mitral regurgitation

• *Anatomy* variable aetiology
Dysfunction of MV apparatus e.g. dysplastic, mitral valve prolapse, papillary muscle ischaemia or infarction, rheumatic change
Dilatation of mitral valve annulus—2° to LV dysfunction (ischaemic DCM, other DCM)
Left ventricular outflow tract obstruction
• *Quantification*
Visualise regurgitant jet (long axis)
(a) Direct quantification with PC-MRI
(b) Indirect with velocity-encoded cine—LV inflow/outflow
Calculate by subtracting Ao forward flow volume (PC-MRI through-plane assessment) from LV stroke volume
Assess other valves
• *Also look for* evidence of endocarditis, myocardial infarction (LGE), cardiomyopathy
• *Assess other* left heart structures (including aortic valve and arch)

3.5.2 Mitral Stenosis

Restrictive opening of the mitral valve in mitral stenosis is most commonly secondary to rheumatic heart disease (Table 7). Elevation of left atrial outflow resistance occurs when the mitral valve area is compromised (see Table 8). This leads to an increase in the diastolic trans-mitral gradient, which can be assessed by measuring the peak velocity across the mitral valve.

Peak velocity measurements at MR across the mitral valve (short axis view below the mitral valve) correlate well with Doppler measurements at echocardiography (Heidenreich et al. 1995). Because of the complicated shape of the stenotic jet in most patients, through plane measurements of velocity are more accurate than in-plane measurements (Fig. 23). Valve area can also be measured.

Velocity mapping flow curves show loss of the normal dual peaks, with high velocities throughout diastole. The flow curves can be used to determine the mitral pressure half-time (the time taken for the pressure gradient to fall to half its peak value), a useful echocardiographic indicator of mitral stenosis severity:

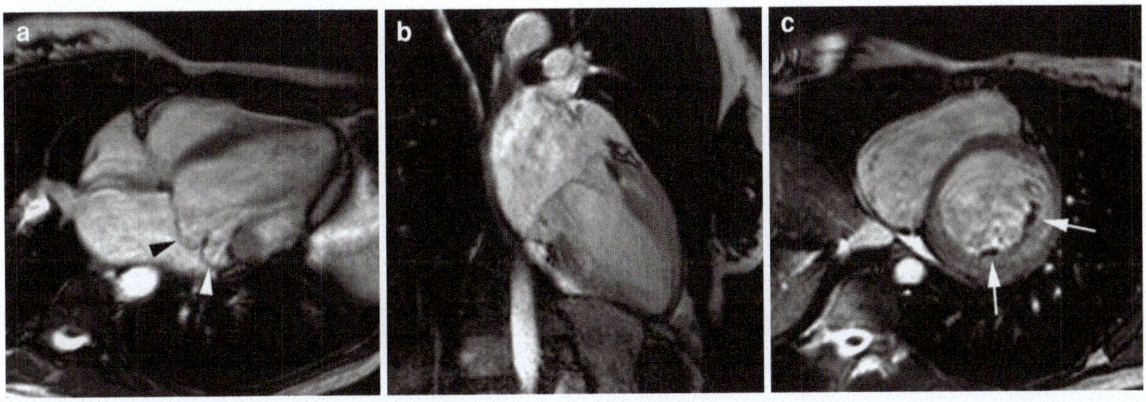

Fig. 22 Mitral valve prolapse shown on horizontal (**a**) and vertical (**b**) long axis bSSFP views of the heart (*arrowheads* in **a**). Note the thinning and low signal of the papillary muscles (*arrows*) in the short axis view (**c**), suggesting fibrosis

Table 7 Causes of mitral stenosis

Congenital
Rheumatic heart disease
Connective tissue disorders
Radiation exposure
Carcinoid
Valve calcification
Obstruction
Thrombus
Myxoma
Tumour

$$\text{Valve area}\ (\text{cm}^2) = \frac{220}{\text{Pressure half time (ms)}} \qquad (8)$$

The severity of mitral stenosis can also be estimated by measuring pulmonary vein flow. In severe mitral stenosis this flow is reversed (Mohiaddin et al. 1991a).

The consequences of mitral stenosis, left atrial enlargement, pulmonary oedema and right ventricular dysfunction and pulmonary regurgitation, secondary to pulmonary hypertension, can all be assessed. In particular, the presence of atrial thrombus should be evaluated in all patients in both atria (secondary to atrial fibrillation). Despite the capability of cardiovascular MR to assess mitral stenosis (see Table 9 for important issues that should be addressed during an MR assessment of mitral stenosis), echocardiography still represents the optimal imaging modality for assessing this valve lesion.

Table 8 Quantitative assessment of mitral stenosis

Degree of mitral stenosis	Valve area (cm^2)	Mean gradient (mmHg)
Normal	4.0–6.0	0
Mild	1.6–3.9	<5
Moderate	1.0–1.5	5–10
Severe	<1.0	>10

3.6 Pulmonary Valve

Difficulties with the alignment of the acoustic window for Doppler echocardiographic investigation have made PC-MRI a useful tool in the investigation of the pulmonary valve and pulmonary arteries (Bogren et al. 1989b; Mohiaddin et al. 1991b; Rebergen et al. 1993). The imaging protocols for aortic regurgitation and stenosis apply for investigation of pulmonary regurgitation (Fig. 24) and pulmonary stenosis (Fig. 25). For the quantification of pulmonary regurgitation, imaging the main pulmonary trunk in cross-section in a coronal or oblique axial plane is most accurate. These images should be prescribed off two perpendicular right ventricular outflow tract (RVOT) views to ensure that the majority of blood flow is perpendicular to the imaging plane (see Fig. 5.8) (Kivelitz et al. 2003).

3.6.1 Clinical Importance of Pulmonary Regurgitation

A trivial amount of pulmonary regurgitation is physiological and can be detected in many healthy individuals. Though significant congenital pulmonary

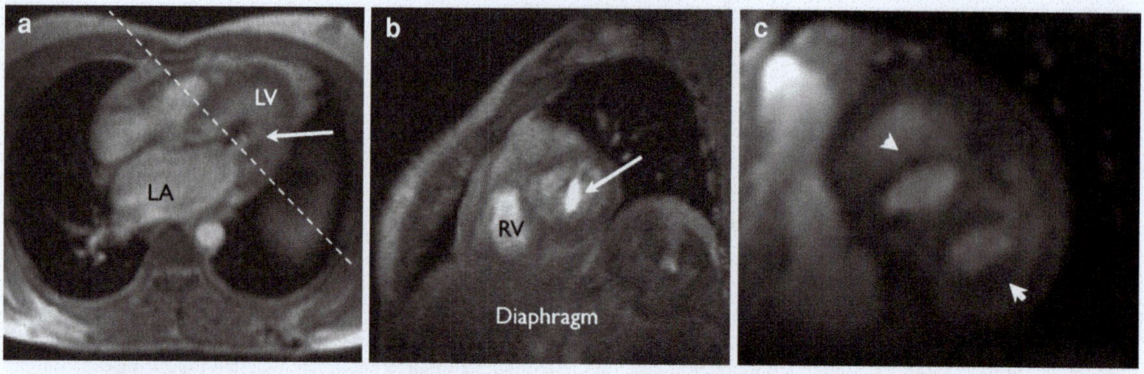

Fig. 23 Mitral stenosis. **a** Axial GE image in mid diastole. Turbulent flow is seen through the mitral valve (*arrow*). *Dotted white lines* represent the image plane for the short axis image. **b** Short-axis GE image in mid diastole. Flow through the mitral valve is shown as bright pixels (*arrow*). The valve orifice area can be easily measured. *LA*, Left atrium; *LV*, left ventricle; *RV*, right ventricle. **c** bSSFP basal short axis view of a rare example of a double mitral valve orifice (*arrowheads*)

Table 9 Cardiovascular MR assessment of mitral stenosis

• *Anatomy*
Abnormalities of valve leaflets—fused, tethered, dysplastic or thickened
Abnormal valvar support structures—shortened chordae, single papillary muscle
Annular hypoplasia (congenital valvar dysplasia)
Presence of supra-mitral membrane
If congenital can be associated with other hypoplastic left heart structures: ventricle, aortic valve, aortic arch, coarctation
Left atrial dilatation (pulmonary veins may also be dilated)
Pulmonary hypertension—RV hypertrophy, PA dilatation
• *Functional significance*
Assess valvar area (planimetry)
Peak velocity, mean gradient (through plane assessment below level of mitral valve).
Quantify mitral regurgitation
LV volumes, systolic function
Aortic valve structure and function
Measure aortic arch dimensions
• *Also look for* 2° pathology—myxoma, atrial thombi, other cardiac valves (rheumatic disease)

regurgitation can occur in absent pulmonary valve syndrome, the majority of pathological pulmonary regurgitation is iatrogenic in nature and is induced by the treatment of pulmonary stenotic lesions (e.g. pulmonary valvuloplasty) or repair of other congenital conditions (e.g. tetralogy of Fallot, transposition of the great arteries, common arterial trunk or Ross operation). Other causes for acquired PR are endocarditis, carcinoid disease or severe pulmonary hypertension. Table 10 outlines the important issues that should be addressed during an assessment for pulmonary regurgitation in the setting of congenital heart disease.

The most commonly encountered complication of severe pulmonary regurgitation is severe RV and RVOT dilatation (Fig. 26) and dysfunction (Fig. 27). The dilemma of when to treat patients with free pulmonary incompetence, presenting late after repair of RVOT obstruction is one that faces all congenital heart disease clinicians. Although there is clear data to suggest that, in the long-term, pulmonary incompetence is detrimental, leading to an increased incidence of adverse events (death, sustained arrhythmias, increasing symptoms) (Yemets et al. 1997; Discigil et al. 2001; Therrien et al. 2002), the conventional thinking has been that the benefit of treating free pulmonary incompetence is outweighed by the potential risk of surgical pulmonary valve replacement and the lack of longevity of this treatment (conduit dysfunction within 10–15 years that exposes patients to multiple operations over their life) (Stark et al. 1998; Oosterhof et al. 2006; Shebani et al. 2006). PVR has therefore often been left until patients develop symptoms; however, once symptoms develop, there is the potential that symptomatic improvement after surgery may be limited due to the fact that the right ventricle has been chronically exposed to pulmonary incompetence.

More recently, there has been a shift in this risk/benefit continuum. Operative mortality and morbidity are now small with modern operative methods and

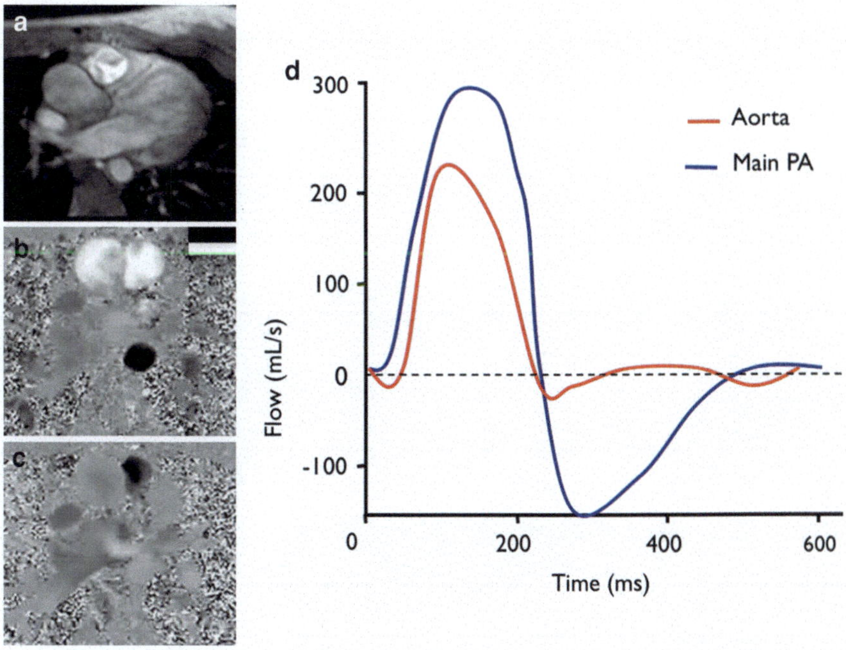

Fig. 24 PC-MRI in pulmonary regurgitation **a** diastolic, modulus image showing non-coaptation of the valve leaflets, **b** systolic phase contrast image with *white* forward flow (note *black* flow in the descending aorta posteriorly), **c** diastolic phase contrast showing pulmonary regurgitation (*black*), **d** flow curve over the cardiac cycle

postoperative care (Oosterhof et al. 2006; Ghez et al. 2007) and conduit life can now be extended using new non-invasive percutaneous approaches to treat conduit dysfunction (Lurz et al. 2008). Thus, the timing of treatment can be based more on the patients' normalisation of parameters in terms of subjective and quantitative measures of outcome and physiological response to pulmonary valve replacement.

Current data from cardiovascular MR assessment of patients with severe pulmonary incompetence have demonstrated elevated RV end-diastolic and end-systolic volumes and reduced RV ejection fraction compared to normals (Roest et al. 2002; Vliegen et al. 2002; Tulevski et al. 2003). Furthermore, there is increasing evidence that RV function may be irreversibly compromised by such long-term changes (Therrien et al. 2000). This is exemplified by three findings that have been demonstrated by CMR. First, RV ejection fraction has been shown to be significantly lower in patients with both RV pressure and volume overload as compared with RV pressure overload alone (Tulevski et al. 2003). Secondly, an abnormal RV response to stress, either physiological (Roest et al. 2002) or pharmacological (Tulevski et al. 2003), has been demonstrated in patients with TOF and pulmonary incompetence. And finally, there appears to be no, or limited, improvement in RV function (ejection fraction at rest) following pulmonary valve replacement (Therrien et al. 2000; Vliegen et al. 2002). Indeed, the only study to demonstrate an improvement in RV ejection fraction following PVR was in patients with moderately dilated right ventricles (Frigiola et al. 2008).

Despite this lack of marked improvement in RV function by correcting pulmonary incompetence, pulmonary valve replacement does reduce RV dimensions (Fig. 28), and if performed before an RV EDV of 160 m/m^2 or an RV ESV of 82 ml/m^2 (Oosterhof et al. 2007) (or RV end-diastolic volume of 170 m/m^2 or an RV end-systolic volume of 85 ml/m^2 (Therrien et al. 2005)) RV dimensions can be normalised (defined as EDV $\leq$ 108 ml/m^2 and ESV $\leq$ 47 ml/m^2). Other supportive data exists (Valsangiacomo Buechel et al. 2005; Frigiola et al. 2008; Knauth et al. 2008), and most centres would consider PVR if the RV EDV is between 150 and 200 ml/m^2. However, these numbers need to be taken with caution as they represent studies done in patients of varying age groups, with varying original operations and varying PVR surgery (RVOT aneurismal reduction or not). Furthermore, as there is no standardisation for the measurement of RV volumes, the quantitative measure of RV dimensions can vary between centres. It may be that as the RV dilates, interaction through the septum reduces LV filling (Lurz et al. 2009b) and reduces LV function.

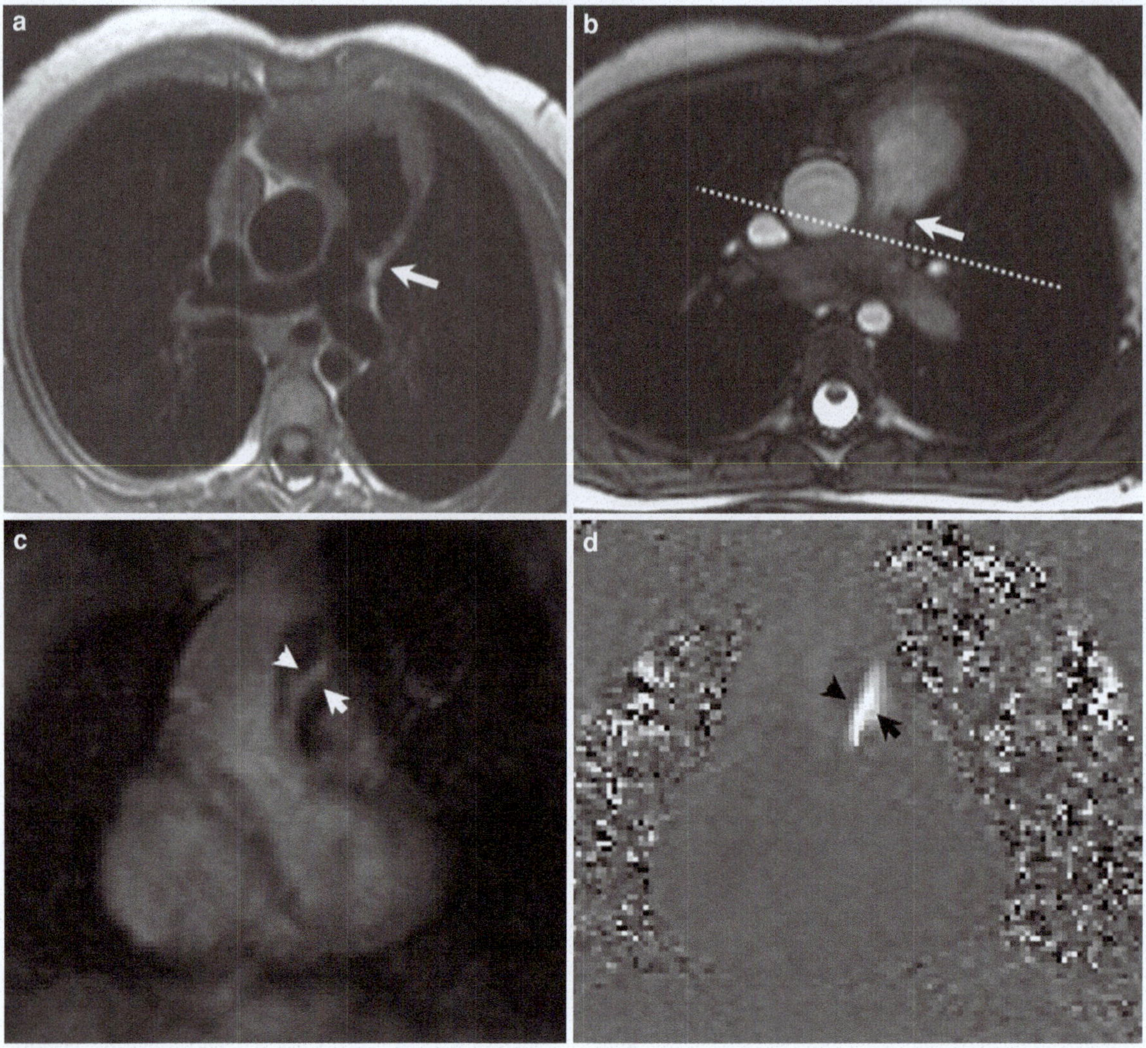

Fig. 25 Severe pulmonary stenosis. **a** TSE 'black-blood' oblique axial view through the pulmonary trunk and pulmonary bifurcation. The thickened, dysplastic pulmonary valve is shown (*white arrow*). **b** bSSFP systolic image in the same plane as (**a**), showing the narrowing at the level of the pulmonary valve (*white arrow*), and the reduced signal of turbulent blood flow at the pulmonary bifurcation. **c** Oblique coronal magnitude image through the distal pulmonary trunk, aligned from (**b**, *dotted line*). Slit-like jet of flow identified (*white arrowheads*). **d** Oblique coronal PC-MRI showing slit-like flow, peak velocity = 4 m/s, which equates to a gradient of approximately 64 mmHg

Importantly, there are suggestions that this may be happening at even moderate RV dilatation, because following PVR, LV EDV increases (Therrien et al. 2000; Therrien et al. 2005; Oosterhof et al. 2007; Frigiola et al. 2008) with a subsequent increase in LV function in some studies (Coats et al. 2007; Frigiola et al. 2008). Further research is required to define cardiovascular MR prognostic factors for pulmonary valve replacement timing, and importantly other information from echocardiography, exercise testing, assessment of neurohormonal activation, ECG data and stress cardiovascular MR may be useful for decision making (Tulevski et al. 2003; Frigiola et al. 2008; van den Berg et al. 2009).

Table 10 Key imaging issues to be assessed in pulmonary incompetence associated with repaired congenital heart disease

Quantify pulmonary valve regurgitation
RV outflow tract and pulmonary trunk anatomy (size, shape and dynamic nature)
RV outflow tract aneurysm
Infundibular, muscular RV outflow tract obstruction
Branch pulmonary artery anatomy (stenoses)
Quantify differential branch PA blood flow
RV and LV volumes and systolic function (indexed to BSA)
Qp:Qs—assess for residual VSD (or ASD)
MAPCAs, (Qs may be > Qp. Increased bronchial blood supply to the lungs. Multiple small vessels may be difficult to see but can lead to a significant Qp:Qs difference)
Aortic root dilation
Coronary artery course (large branch crossing the RVOT, or branches in proximity to potential stents.)

3.6.2 Pulmonary Stenosis

The vast majority of pulmonary valve disease is congenital and results from faulty development of the valve during foetal life. Obstructive lesions—pulmonary valve stenosis and atresia—occur more frequently than regurgitation. According to the site, pulmonary valve stenosis is classified as:

- Valvar,
- Subvalvar (infundibular) or
- Supravalvar.

The involvement of pulmonary stenosis in a range of syndromes together with the fact that there is a risk of recurrence of isolated PS in siblings of 2–4% points to a genetic background. However, non-genetic causative agents as rubella infection have also been reported. Often, no specific cause can be identified.

All forms of congenital pulmonary stenosis can occur as isolated findings, in combination with relatively simple shunt lesions like a ventricular septal defect (VSD), or as part of more complex conditions (see Table 11).

Mild congenital PS usually creates few or no symptoms and often is only detected when a cardiac murmur is heard during routine paediatric investigation. Unless there is an underlying genetic syndrome, patients grow normally. Most patients with mild PS do not show progression to more severe forms. In more than mild congenital PS, however, there is a tendency towards deterioration. Symptoms appear after several years, in moderate cases only in adult life. Reduced exercise tolerance, dyspnoea, respiratory infections, syncope, arrhythmias and ischemic chest pain can develop. If there is a right-to-left shunt via an ASD or PFO, cyanosis occurs. Mortality also depends on the degree of PS and is mostly due to bacterial endocarditis or congestive right heart failure.

For pulmonary stenosis assessment with cardiovascular MR, measurement and visualisation of the pulmonary valve is best performed in a sagittal or oblique sagittal plane (Fig. 29).

3.6.3 Percutaneous Pulmonary Valve Implantation

In patients who develop stenosis of their surgical pulmonary valve replacement (homograft or conduit stenosis) percutaneous transcatheter stenting is possible. This can prolong conduit life and postpone reoperation (Marelli et al. 2007; Meadows et al. 2007). However bare-metal stenting can potentially convert the pressure-overloaded ventricle to one of volume-overload, through relief of obstruction and introduction of free pulmonary incompetence (Lurz et al. 2009c).

In 2000, percutaneous pulmonary valve implantation (PPVI) was described, whereby a new pulmonary valve was placed into a dysfunctional RV-PA prosthetic conduit (Bonhoeffer et al. 2000). Over the following decade, this technology has been accepted into clinical practice, with over 2,000 devices now implanted throughout the world. The Melody^{TM} device (Medtronic Inc., Minneapolis, MN, USA) has CE marking in Europe and Canada and Food and Drug Administration (FDA) approval in the USA. Patients have been successfully treated to relieve both pulmonary stenosis and regurgitation (Khambadkone et al. 2005; Coats et al. 2006, 2007; Lurz et al. 2008; Zahn et al. 2009; McElhinney et al. 2010). This method offers a minimally invasive alternative to open-heart surgery for RVOT/pulmonary trunk dysfunction in children and adults by restoring acceptable RV loading conditions (Lurz et al. 2009c).

The device is composed of a tri-leaflet bovine jugular vein sutured into a platinum–iridium, gold welded, balloon expandable stent (Fig. 30). When expanded, the competence of the valve is maintained at a large range of diameters: 14–22 mm. The device is implanted under general anaesthesia, usually via femoral access.

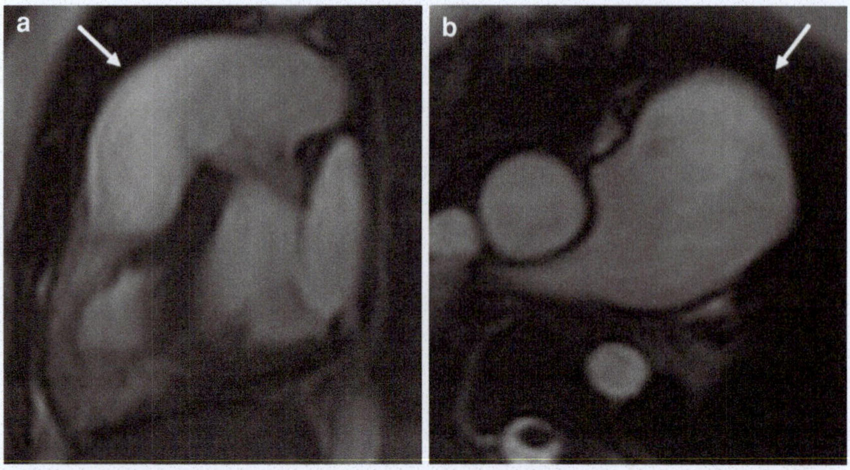

Fig. 26 bSSFP images demonstrating the dilated and aneurismal right ventricular outflow tract (*arrow*) following trans-annular patch repair **a** oblique sagittal, **b** axial

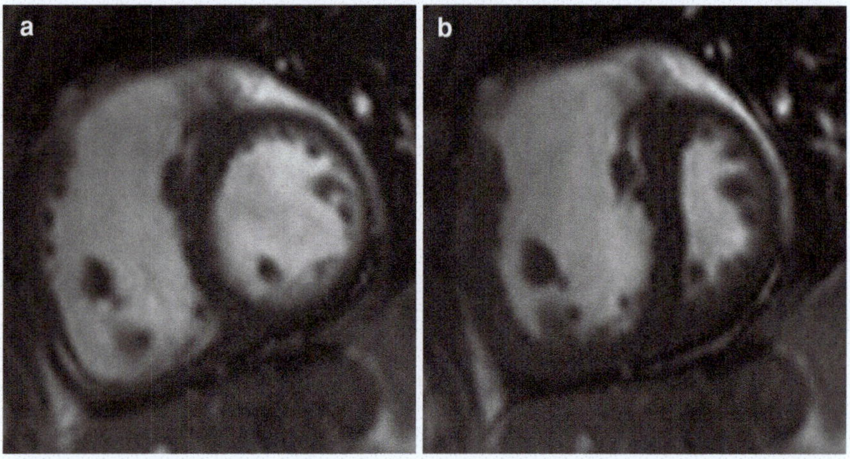

Fig. 27 Balanced SSFP images demonstrating early diastolic flattening of the interventricular septum in a patient with severe pulmonary regurgitation **a** late diastolic **b** early diastolic phases

Once a pulmonary valve replacement has been clinically justified, there is now a choice between surgery and PPVI for approximately 15% of patients with TOF. Technical suitability for PPVI can be defined by cardiovascular MR using in protocol previously defined in Table 10, but with focus on three main areas:

RVOT/pulmonary trunk size and distensibility—PPVI can be performed in RVOT/pulmonary trunks that range from 14 to 22 mm. At the lower end of the spectrum, conduits need to be of an adequate size to allow for sufficient opening without residual gradients. At the upper end, the device can only be expanded to a maximal diameter of 22 mm—any larger and valve leaflet coaptation may fail, or the device may embolise. This precludes PPVI in dilated anatomies (Fig. 16.21). Conduit sizes can be gleaned from operative reports; however, conduits can become smaller (or larger) over time and, in order to have a full understanding of the anatomy of the outflow tract, cardiovascular MR with 3D capabilities is crucial. Although the cardiovascular MR-derived 3D reconstructions can be used to define size, it is important to realise that these reconstructions are performed on data acquired in diastole, or from non-ECG-gated data and, thus, maximal dimensions of very distensible anatomies may be underestimated. Cine imaging of the RVOT/pulmonary trunk in both long and short axes overcomes this problem, enabling the measurement of the maximum diameter of the site at which PPVI may be attempted. If the results of MRI are doubtful or borderline, balloon sizing of the RVOT can be performed at the time of catheterisation.

RVOT/pulmonary morphology—The 3D information from cardiovascular MR can be used to visualise

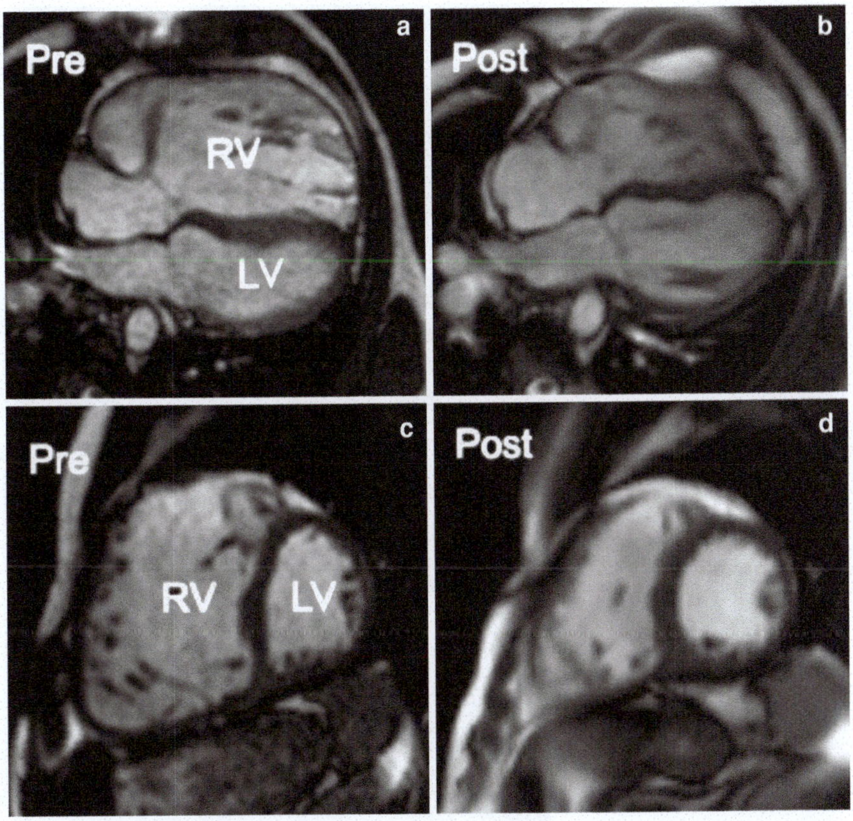

Fig. 28 Response to surgical PVR after 1 year. Four-chamber (**a** and **b**) and short axis (**c** and **d**) views showing marked RV volume reduction and increased LV volumes

Table 11 Conditions associated with pulmonary valve disease

Congenital heart lesions with PS:
Tetralogy of Fallot (ToF)
Double outlet right ventricle
Transposition of the great arteries (TGA)
Absent pulmonary valve syndrome (simultaneous pulmonary regurgitation)
Ebstein's anomaly (functional pulmonary atresia due to weak RV)
Genetic syndromes with PS:
Noonan syndrome (dysplastic valve)
Alagille syndrome (peripheral PS)
Williams syndrome (peripheral PS)
Di George syndrome
Leopard syndrome
Trisomy 18
Marchesani syndrome
Other syndromes associated with PS:
Congenital rubella syndrome

the best site for device anchorage in the RVOT/pulmonary trunk. Furthermore, certain shapes are not suitable for safe implantation of the device (Schievano et al. 2007a). A morphological classification has been created according to measurements of 3D reconstructions of the RVOT (Schievano et al. 2007b). Importantly, a pyramidal morphology, meaning that the RVOT funnels down towards the pulmonary bifurcation, is not suitable for PPVI because of the high risk of device dislodgement. Ideal RVOT/pulmonary trunk shapes comprise conduits with parallel borders or conduits with a narrowing in the mid-portion, since this provides a safe landing zone for the stent (Schievano et al. 2007b).

Proximity of the proximal coronary arteries—The proximity of the proximal coronary arteries to the RVOT/pulmonary trunk has to be assessed (Fig. 31). On cardiovascular MR 3D whole-heart bSSFP images, the anatomical relationship of the coronary arteries and the proposed implantation side can be judged. In addition, aortic root angiography is

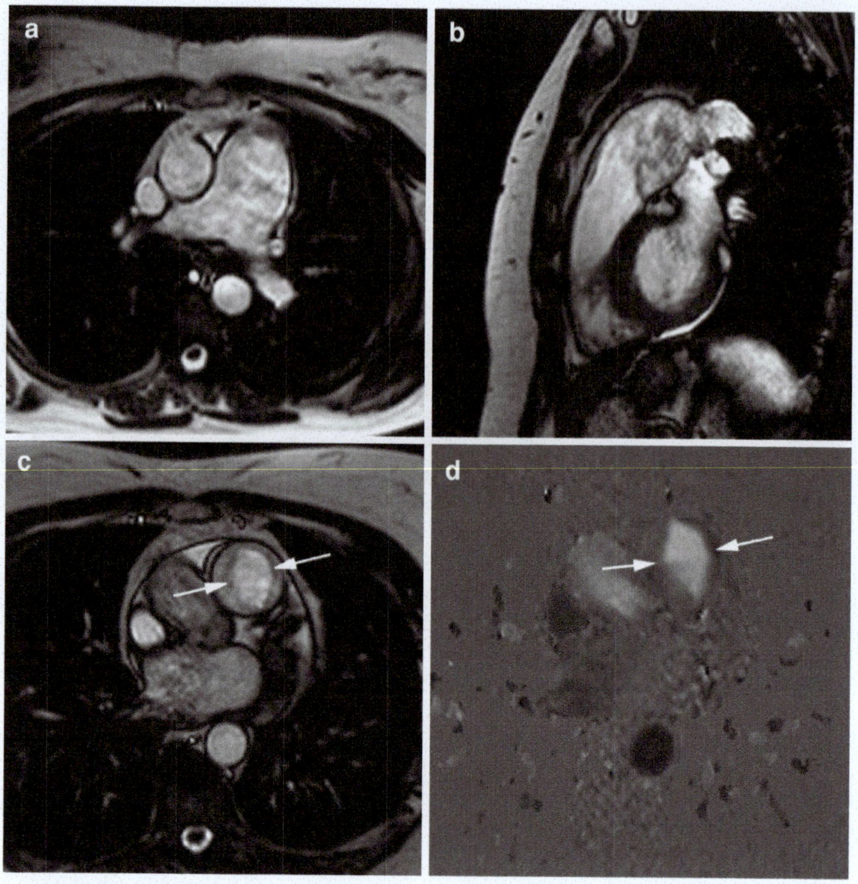

Fig. 29 Congenital pulmonary stenois with marked post-stenotic dilatation of the pulmonary trunk and branch pulmonary arteries, seen on the axial (**a**) and oblique sagittal (**b**) bSSFP images. There is a bicuspid pulmonary valve (*arrows*) in the modulus (**c**) and phase contrast images (**d**) acquired in the pulmonary trunk above the valve leaflets

performed at the time of catheterisation. On biplane projection, the relationship between the coronaries and the pulmonary artery can be judged. In case the cardiovascular MR assessment or aortic root angiography cannot fully rule out the risk for coronary compression, simultaneous high-pressure balloon inflation in the implantation site and selective coronary angiography is performed (Sridharan et al. 2006). Importantly, when angiography and simultaneous balloon inflation is performed, it is crucial to expand the RVOT to a therapeutic size. This manoeuvre is only meaningful, when the conduit is expanded with a high-pressure balloon up to the diameter that will be reached post-PPVI.

3.6.4 Physiological Response to PPVI

Cardiovascular MR performed before and within 1 month of the procedure, with analysis of biventricular function and calculation of great vessel blood flow, has shown an improvement in effective RV and LV stroke volume in both patients with predominantly pulmonary stenosis and those with predominantly regurgitation (Khambadkone et al. 2005; Coats et al. 2006, 2007). Importantly, these effects are maintained at 1 year (Lurz et al. 2011). In patients with predominantly pulmonary stenosis, this is due to decreased RV ESV and improved RV ejection fraction after marked relief of afterload (Coats et al. 2006). By contrast, RV ejection fraction remains unchanged in patients with predominantly pulmonary regurgitation, with the improvement in RV and LV effective stroke volume due to abolishment of pulmonary regurgitation. Whilst relief of RV volume-overload results in a reduction in RV EDV, the total RV stroke volume decreases in patients with predominantly regurgitation (Coats et al. 2007), consistent with the surgical findings presented above.

3.6.5 Development of New Percutaneous Devices

Because of the wide variation in patient morphology, size, and dynamics of the right ventricular

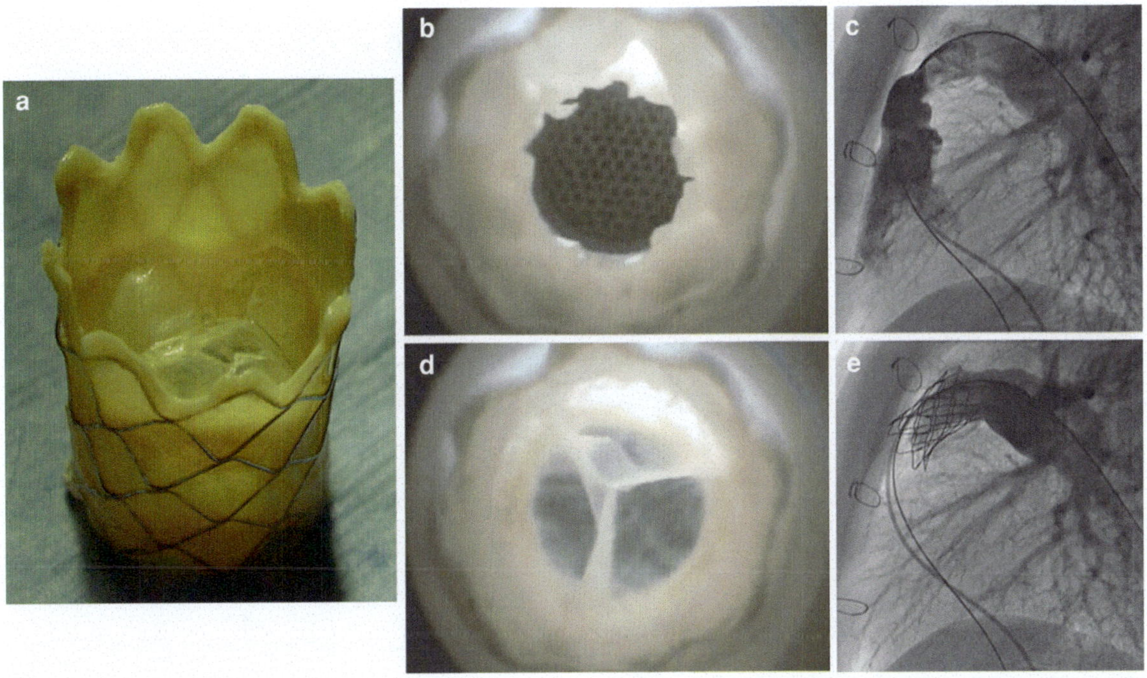

Fig. 30 **a** Percutaneous pulmonary valve implantation (PPVI) device, Melody^{TM} (Medtronic, Minneapolis, MN, USA). Device viewed in water bath showing the valve open during forward flow (**b**) and closed during reverse flow (**c**)—note tri-leaflet morphology of the valve. **c** and **d** Lateral catheter angiogram pre-PPVI (**a**), showing stenosis (*arrow*) and pulmonary reguritation (contrast in RV—*arrowhead*). Post-PPVI (**b**), the stenosis is relieved (note shifted homograft calcification) and no pulmonary regurgitation

outflow tract (RVOT)/pulmonary trunk (Fig. 16.22), only ~15% of patients with a haemodynamic and clinical indication for PPVI can be treated with the current device. Thus, 85% of patients with pulmonary dysfunction still require open-heart surgery for treatment. The majority of these patients are those with dilated, dynamic RVOT/pulmonary trunk anatomy (patients with tetraology of Fallot and previous RVOT patches) in whom the current percutaneous device is too small. Over the last 3 years, we have developed a new device, which can be implanted into the dilated outflow tract (Fig. 32). This device has now undergone a successful 'first-in-man' implantation (Schievano et al. 2010). For this implantation, advanced cardiovascular imaging, in combination with patient-specific computer modelling is crucial to achieve procedural success. We await further human studies of this device in the near future.

3.7 Tricuspid Valve

Examination of the tricuspid valve is as for the mitral valve. The regurgitant jet of tricuspid regurgitation is best visualised in the transverse plane (Fig. 33). PC-MRI in the superior vena cava can demonstrate tricuspid regurgitation. The causes of tricuspid regurgitation are similar to mitral regurgitation. Tricuspid regurgitation of varying degrees is most commonly seen secondary to dilatation of the right ventricle, often due to mitral valve pathology and/or pulmonary hypertension. An important cause of tricuspid regurgitation that should be considered when there is thickening of the valve leaflet is carcinoid syndrome (Fig. 34) (Bhattacharyya et al. 2010). Tricuspid regurgitation can also occur after blunt trauma. It should be noted that trivial tricuspid regurgitation is a common finding in normal subjects (Waggoner et al. 1981). For alignment of the optimal imaging planes for the tricuspid valve see Fig. 5.7.

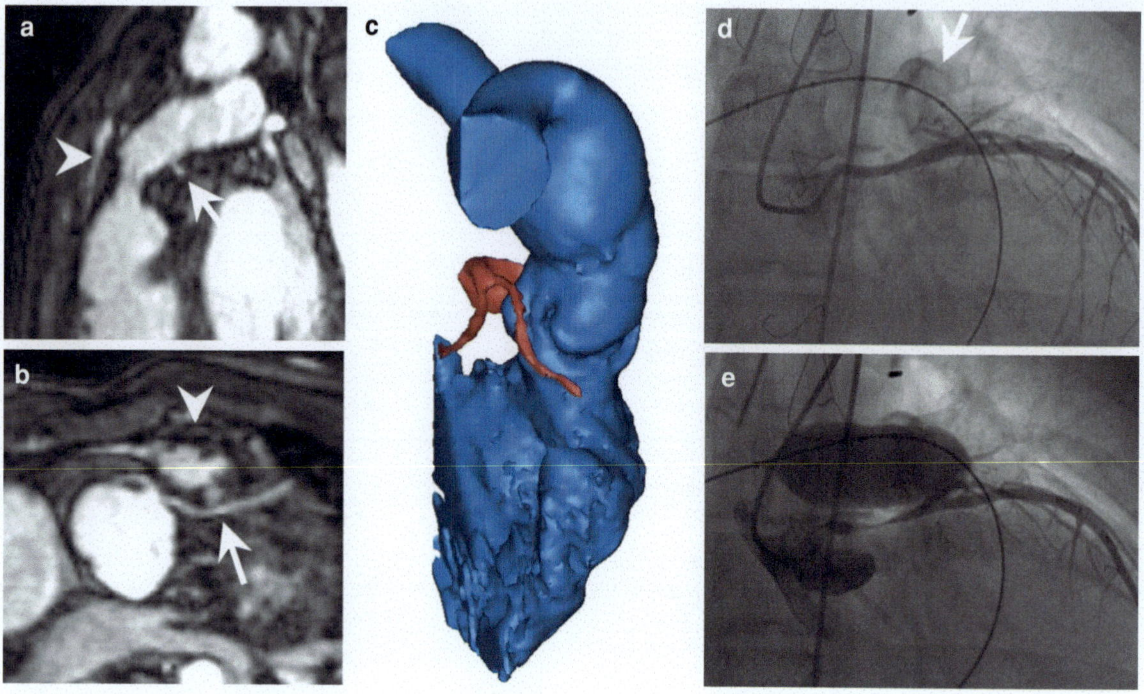

Fig. 31 Sagittal (**a**) and axial (**b**) reformats from a 3D bSSFP whole-heart acquisition. In (**a**) the left coronary artery (LCA—*arrow*) appears to be at some distance from the RVOT/ pulmonary trunk narrowing (*arrowhead*); however in (**b**) the LCA (*arrow*) can be seen to be in very close proximity to the proposed site of PPVI. Test balloon expansion is required in this patient. **c**) Volume rendered 3D contrast enhanced CT showing the relationship of the LCA and the posterior surface of this dilated RVOT/pulmonary trunk. Coronary artery angiogram before (**d**) and after ballon testing (**e**). In (**d**) circular homograft calcification can be clearly seen (*arrow*), and in (**e**) LCA compression. PPVI was not performed in this patient, who was referred for conventional surgical pulmonary valve replacement

As with echocardiography, quantification of the tricuspid regurgitation is possible by measuring the peak velocity within the regurgitant flow jet. If there is no pulmonary valvular or artery stenosis, the addition of an estimate of the right atrial pressure (RA_{Pa}) to the calculated pressure difference between the right atrium and right ventricle (ΔP across the tricuspid valve, calculated using the modified Bernoulli equation), can give an estimate of the right ventricular systolic pressure (RVS_{Pa}) and pulmonary artery pressure (PA_{Pa}).

Thus, tricuspid

$$\Delta P = 4(V_{max})^2 \quad (9)$$

and,

$$RVS_{Pa}(mmHg) = PA_{Pa}(mmHg) = RA_{Pa}(mmHg) + \Delta P\ (mmHg) \quad (10)$$

where RA_{Pa}, the right atrial pressure is estimated at 10 mmHg.

The tricuspid valve orifice is larger than the mitral orifice. Tricuspid stenosis is uncommon, but can be easily diagnosed on cone images. Tricuspid atresia is easily identified on SE images.

3.7.1 Ebstein's Anomaly

Ebstein's anomaly is a congenital abnormality of the tricuspid valve. The septal and mural leaflets are more apically placed than normal, resulting in a malfunctioning, regurgitant tricuspid valve and atrialization of the right ventricle (Anderson et al. 1979). The consequence is gross right atrial enlargement and raised right atrial pressure. The anomaly is usually associated with an ASD and there is thus right-to-left shunting at the atrial level and subsequent cyanosis. Ultimately, Ebstein's anomaly results in gross enlargement of the cardiac contour on the plane chest radiograph. Treatment is problematic, though expert surgical repair of the tricuspid valve is possible in some centres.

MR imaging can be used to assess the valve morphology, quantify ventricular function and size

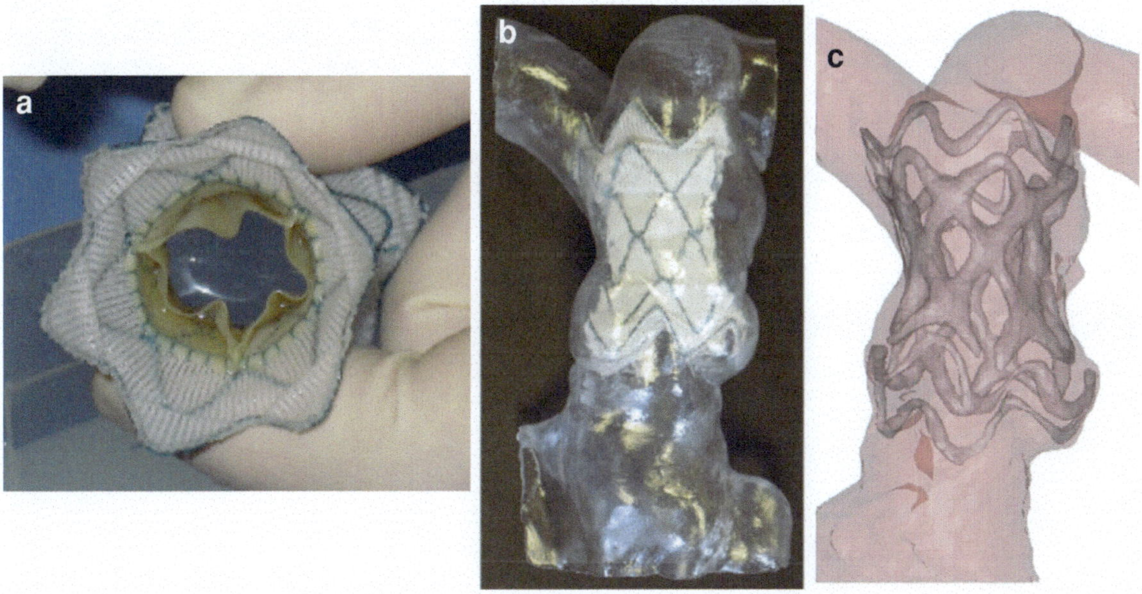

Fig. 32 New percutaneous device for implantation into the dilated outflow tract. **a** Nitinol device, **b** pre-implantation in rapid prototyping model, **c** 3D CT reconstruction post-implantation with device in situ in 'first-in-man' case

Fig. 33 Balanced SSFP four-chamber images of tricuspid regurgitation (*arrowheads*) throughout systole. Time from the R wave. **a** 0 ms, **b** 50 ms, **c** 100 ms, **d** 200 ms

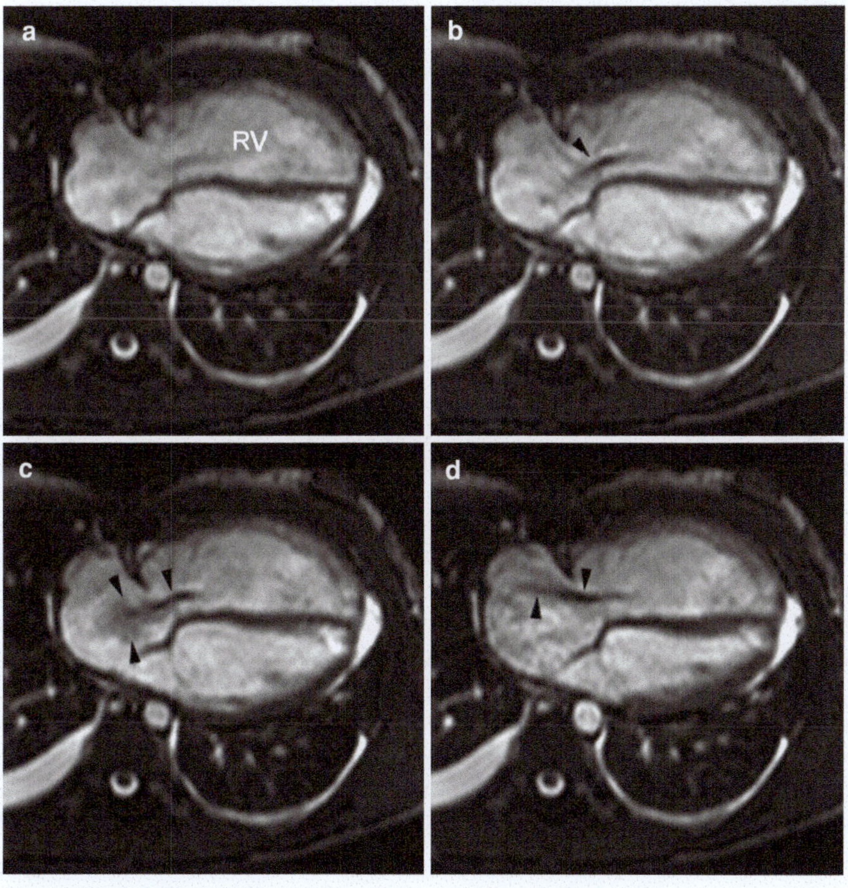

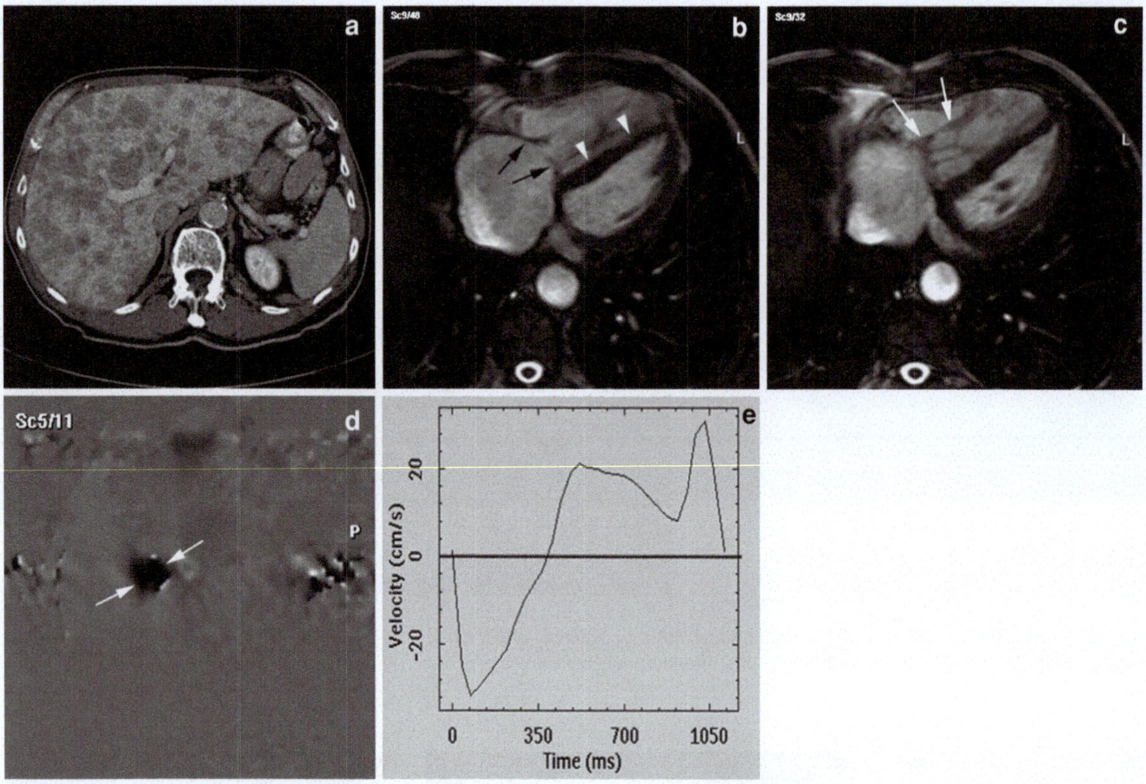

Fig. 34 **a** Carcinoid tumour of small intestine with diffuse liver metastases. Carcinoid syndrome of the heart. **b** and **c** bSSFP four-chamber images in systole (**b**) and diastole (**c**), showing thickened, stiff tricuspid valve (*black arrows* in **b**), and subvalvular apparatus (*white arrows* in **c**). The right ventricle is enlarged with flattening of the septum (*arrowheads* in **b**). **d** and **e** This leads to non closure of tricuspid valve at end systole, with important tricuspid incompetence demonstrated on the basal short a phase contrast velocity map image (**d**, *white arrows*) and tricuspid flow curve (**e**)

the right atrial enlargement (Fig. 35). Differentiation from Uhl's anomaly, which is an extremely rare condition with a partial or total loss of the myocardial muscle in the RV should be considered (Fig. 36).

3.8 Mixed Valvular Disease

The measurement of both RV and LV stroke volumes with MR cine imaging, in combination with velocity mapping measurement of pulmonary and aortic flow, permits the quantification of valvular regurgitation in all four valves, even if aortic, mitral, pulmonary and tricuspid regurgitation are all present. Aortic and pulmonary regurgitation are calculated from the velocity maps and diastolic reverse flow, and subtraction of the systolic forward flow from the LVSV and RVSV yields the amount of mitral and tricuspid regurgitation respectively.

3.9 Prosthetic Valves

For non-biological prosthetic valves and stented biological valves the applied magnetic field is distorted by differences in the local magnetic fields between the prosthesis and the biological tissue, and by eddy currents induced in the valve. These phenomena lead to signal loss around the prosthesis (Fig. 37). These artifacts can be very severe on cine images, and may degrade the image significantly. This makes imaging turbulent jets in the vicinity of the prosthesis difficult; however, velocity mapping distal to the image artefact can still be accurately performed.

Homografts, autografts and stentless porcine valve replacements do not cause signal artefact and can be imaged normally.

All valvular prostheses can be safely imaged, at 1.5T, except for Starr-Edwards mitral pre-6000 series valves used from 1960 to 1964, at field strengths of

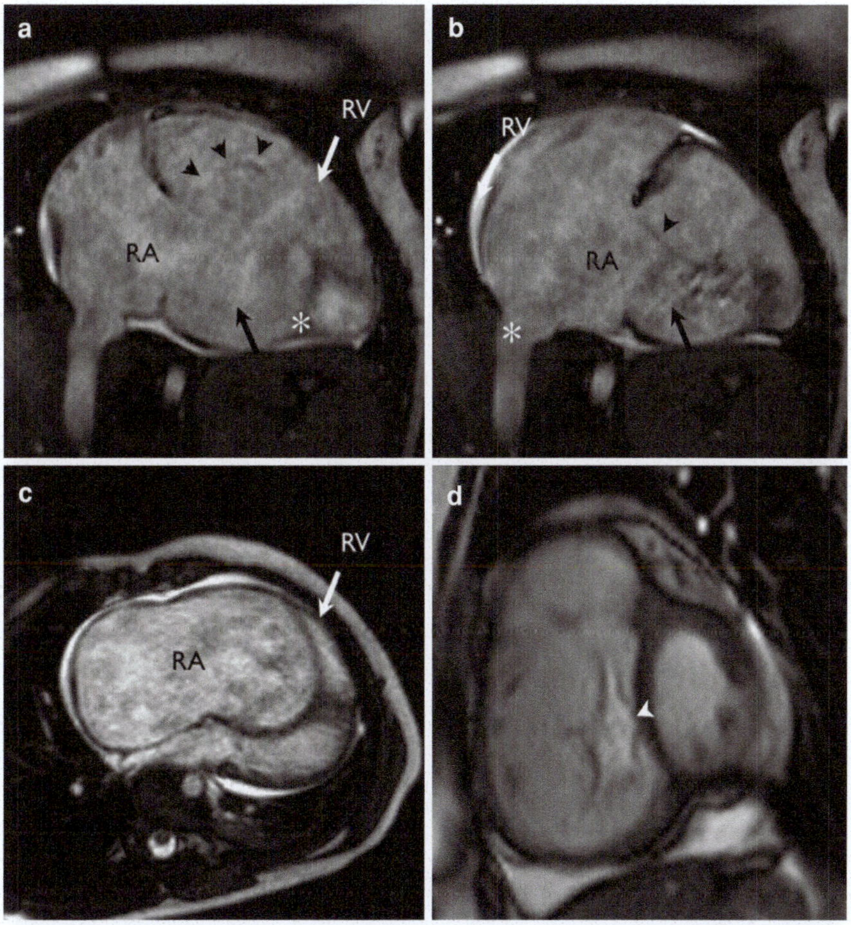

Fig. 35 Ebstein's anomaly. Coronal long axis view through the right atrium (RA) and right ventricle (RV), showing the apical displacement of the mural tricuspid valve leaflet (*), and the septal leaflet in diastole (**a**, *arrowheads*) and systole (**b**, *arrowheads*). **c** Axial plane. In all three images the *black arrow* identifies 'atrialization' of the right ventricle. Short axis view (**d**) in a patient with only mild apical displacement of the septal leaflet, which is plastered to the interventricular septum (*arrowhead*) with resultant severe tricuspid regurgitation, and a severely dilated right atrium

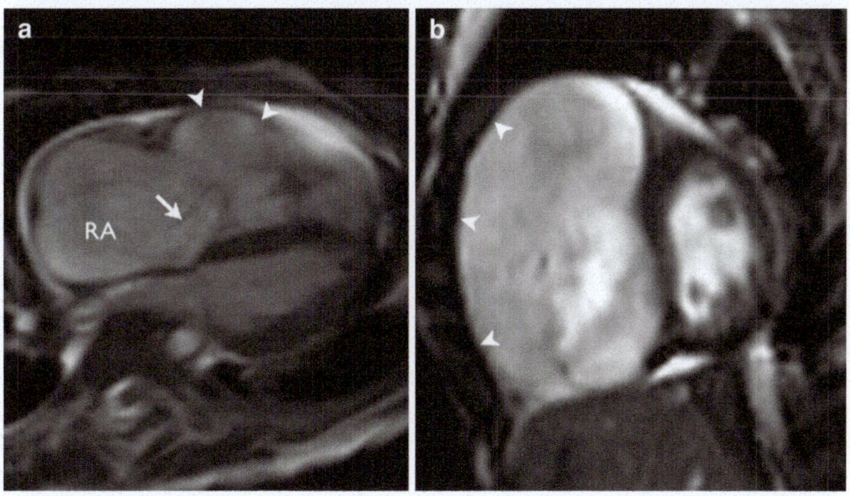

Fig. 36 bSSFP images in a patient with Uhl's anomaly **a** horizontal long axis, **b** short axis views. The right atrium and ventricle are severely dilated, with thinning of the right ventricular wall (*arrowheads*), and tricuspid regurgitation (*arrow*)

greater than 0.35T (Randall et al. 1988; Shellock 1988, 1993). Very few of the aforementioned prosthetic valves still remain in situ. However, with the increased clinical use of high-field MR scanners (3.0–7.0T), safety concerns have again become relevant. In a recent paper, all artificial valves were

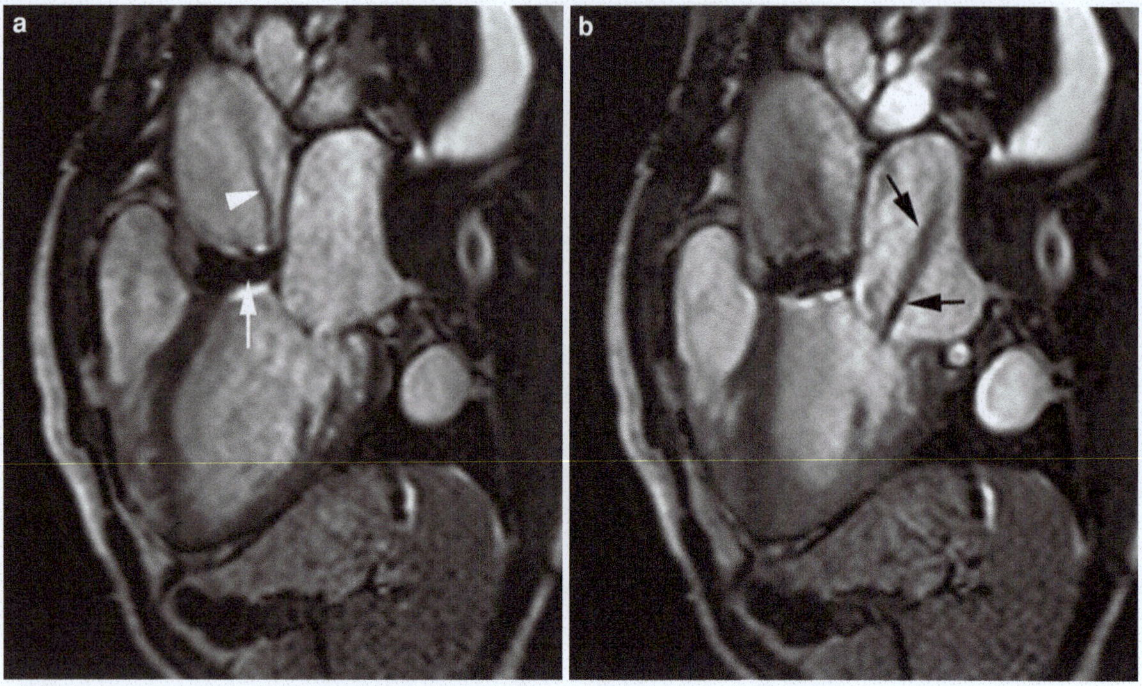

Fig. 37 Aortic prosthetic valve with associated mitral incompetence. **a** bSSFP left ventricular inflow/outflow view showing artifact related to prosthetic valve (*white arrow*), and mild jet of turbulent flow in the aortic root (*white arrowhead*). **b** bSSFP image in a parallel imaging plane to (**a**), but in plane with the mitral valve, reveals grade 2/3 mitral regurgitation (*black arrows*)

considered safe in a static magnetic field up to 4.7 Tesla, except the Carpentier-Edwards Physio Ring containing Elgiloy (Edwards et al. 2005). However, for all patients with devices, we recommend consultation of the most current literature on MRI safety issues (http://www.MRIsafety.com).

MR imaging offers an ideal method for the non-invasive follow-up of patients after valvular surgery (Deutsch et al. 1992). In vitro, the accuracy of MR velocity measurements distal to a wide variety of valvular prostheses has been confirmed by laser Doppler anemometry (Fontaine et al. 1996). The assessment of prosthetic valve function at low field strength (0.2T) has also been demonstrated (DiCesare et al. 1995). Useful clinical follow-up has been reported in patients following aortic root reconstruction, where not only was prosthetic valve function assessed, but also the aortic graft, LV outflow tract and proximal coronary arteries were all evaluated (Lepore et al. 1996). However, the assessment of mechanical valve prosthesis dysfunction may be particularly intricate and small defects can be overlooked by cine MRI. For example, the presence of intra- or peri-prosthetic leaks is often hindered by the signal loss around the prosthesis.

3.10 Magnetic Resonance Spectroscopy

There remains limited experience with MR spectroscopy and valvular heart disease in the clinical setting (Holloway and Clarke 2010). It is known that a reduction in the phosphocreatinine to ATP (PCr/ATP) ratio occurs in patients with heart failure (Conway et al. 1991) and can be a useful predictor of cardiovascular morbidity in patients with dilated cardiomyopathy (Neubauer et al. 1997a). Such changes in the PCr/ATP ratio have been confirmed in patients with aortic valve disease and New York Heart Association class III symptoms of heart failure (Neubauer et al. 1997b). Furthermore, patients with aortic stenosis have been shown to have a reduced PCr/ATP ratio (Neubauer et al. 1997b; Beyerbacht et al. 2001) that normalises following aortic valve replacement (Beyerbacht et al. 2001).

A large-scale prospective study, with measurement of both pre- and post-valve replacement PCr/ATP

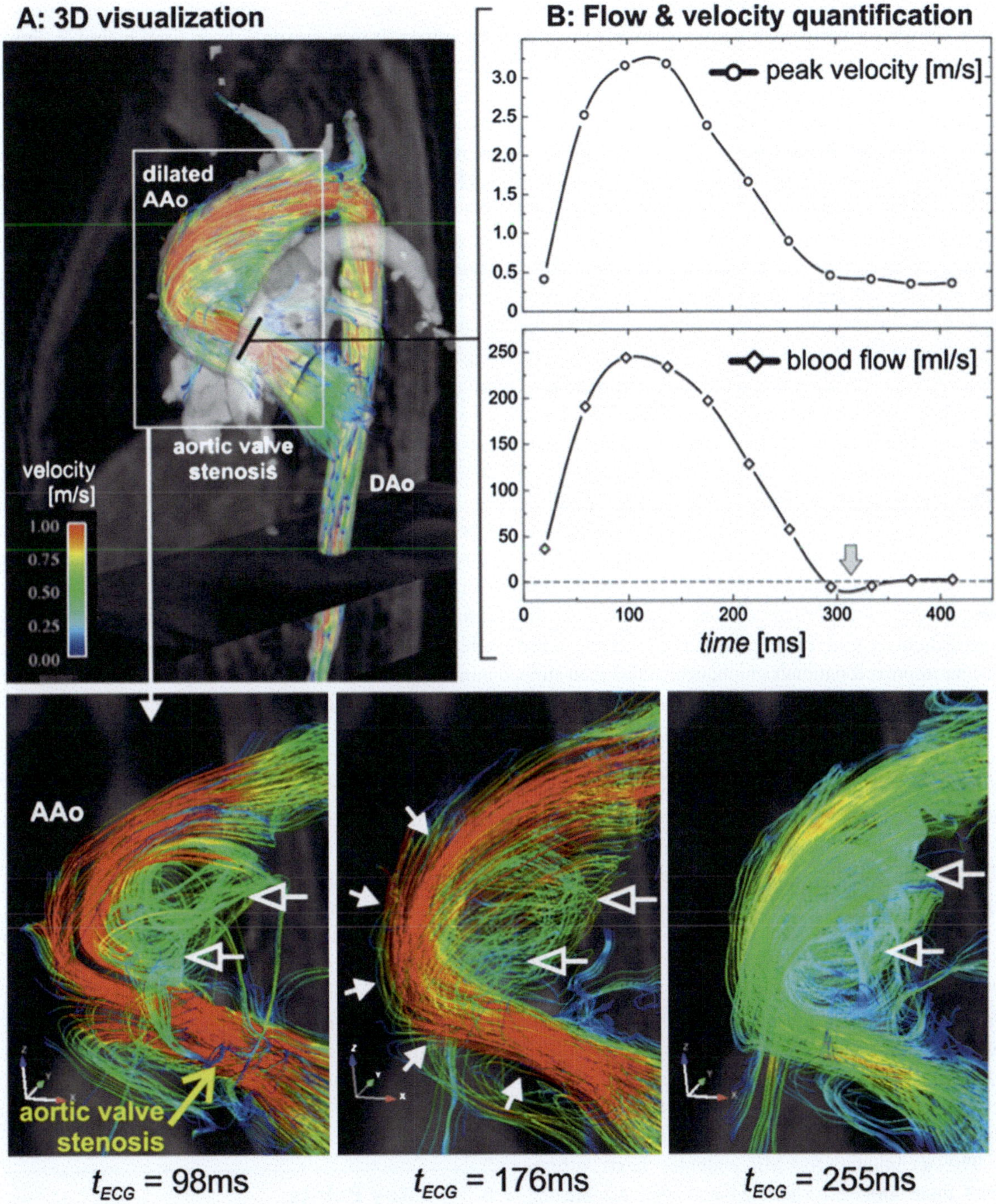

Fig. 38 3D flow visualisation (**a**) and flow quantification (**b**) in a 9-year-old pediatric patient with aortic valve stenosis (aortic valve area = 1.2 cm^2) and dilation of the ascending aorta (maximum diameter = 33 mm). Echocardiography demonstrated normal global cardiac function (ejection fraction EF = 72%) but substantial flow acceleration (peak velocity = 2.8 m/s) and an elevated pressure gradient (maximum pressure = 38 mmHg) at the level of the aortic valve. These findings were confirmed by retrospective quantitative analysis of the 4D PC-MRI data in an analysis plane above the aortic valve which revealed high systolic peak velocities (peak velocity = 3.2 m/s, max pressure gradient = 41 mmHg) but only very mild diastolic retrograde flow (*grey arrow*). 3D flow visualisation using streamlines showed localised flow acceleration along the outer wall of the ascending aorta (*solid white arrows*) which developed into a vortex flow pattern (*open arrows*) occupying the shape of the aneurysm (AAo: ascending aorta, DAo: descending aorta). (Reprinted with permission from Markl et al. 2011)

ratios, needs to be performed to assess the use of MR spectroscopy for optimising treatment of aortic valve disease.

4 Future Directions

Future improvements in MR scanner hardware and sequences will improve the speed of MR assessment of valvular heart disease, with the acquisition of ventricular volume and great vessel flow data in real-time. Improvements in analysis software, in particular the development of robust, automated ventricular volume contour tracking will reduce laborious post-processing. Increasing computer processing unit (CPU) speed will improve data acquisition, but rapid improvements in graphical processing unit (GPU) architecture and speed will ensure that data reconstruction and post-processing can be performed in a timely, instantaneous fashion.

With the acquistion of high temporo-spatial resolution data in real-time, with real-time reconstruction and post-processing, there will be a reduction in the time patients spend in the scanner and hence there will be improved patient compliance (rapid scan time and little patient co-operation) with cardiovascular MR and increased patient throughput. There is no reason why the assessment of a valvular lesion, and its associated issues, can not be performed in 15 min and processed, with a report generated in a further 15 min.

One major area of MR development will be the use of 4D MR flow to assess valvular heart disease (Hope et al. 2011; Markl et al. 2011). 4D flow offers advantages over 2D methods in that retrospective analysis of flow at any location in the imaging volume is possible (Fig. 38), and newer parameters such as shear wall stress and local pressure gradients can be visualised and quantified. At present, acquisition of 4D flow is time consuming, but the technique does promises to improve our understanding of both normal and pathological physiology in the cardiovascular system.

The techniques for MR valvular heart disease assessment are well validated and well established. However, what is still lacking is the large-scale, long-term studies of the physiological natural history of valvular heart disease and the consequences of treatment, either medically or surgically with valve replacement. It is of note that the recently updated guidelines for the management of patient with valvular heart disease (Bonow et al. 2008), did not include cardiovascular MR as a standard assessment. Cardiovascular MR investigations have been included in the ESC guidelines for the management of grown-up congenital heart disease (Baumgartner et al. 2010); however, the evidential basis for cardiovascular MR remains low. Studies with the described accurate MR techniques should enable improved timing for optimal valve replacement to balance the risks of surgery and prosthetic valve insertion and irreversible ventricular dysfunction. As these studies occur, and with the increasing role of imaging for less invasive treatment of valve disease (either catheter-based or surgical valve repair as opposed to valve replacement), cardiovascular imaging protocols will continue to evolve.

5 Conclusion

Cardiac MRI can provide important information about valvular function. Both stenotic and regurgitant lesions can be quantified for all four valves. Quantification can also be performed even when multiple valves are affected. Anatomical information with regard to leaflet number, valve thickness and the presence of endocarditis is still best provided by echocardiography.

Cardiac MRI offers the only non-invasive, accurate and reproducible method for quantifying valvular regurgitation, with no X-ray exposure. In combination with accurate ventricular function assessment, cardiovascular MR imaging is ideal for the long-term follow-up and evaluation of patients awaiting valvular surgery. However, long-term studies using MR imaging in such a role need to be performed to define the optimal timings for these interventions.

As cardiac MRI becomes more cost-effective and easily accessible, its use for the accurate assessment of valvular heart disease in clinical cardiology will increase, and enable physicians to better predict the optimal treatment for their patients with valvular heart disease.

6 Key Points

- Accurate flow and ventricular measurements are the cornerstone of assessment of valvular heart disease
- Confirmation of the accuracy of these technique should be confirmed for each individual scanner using flow phantoms and/or normal healthy subjects

- MR is the best available non-invasive method for quantification of valvular regurgitation
- Accurate quantification of all valves can be performed, even when mixed valvular disease is present
- MR is the best available non-invasive method for the quantification of the consequences of valvular dysfunction, in particular for the assessment of ventricular function and LV mass
- Larger scale studies are required to establish whether MR assessment of valvular regurgitation will be able to optimise treatment timings (surgical or interventional cardiology)
- MR assessment of valve leaflets remains limited
- MR-guided insertion of percutaneous valve device may be a possibility in the future

Acknowledgments We would like to acknowledge the following for their help and support with cardiovascular MR. From Great Ormond Street Hospital for Children, London, UK: Dr. Marina Hughes, Dr. Oliver Tann, Dr. Vivek Muthurangu, Dr. Catherine Owens, Rod Jones, Wendy Norman, and Professor Philipp Bonhoeffer of the Cardiorespiratory Unit; and Dr. Angus McEwan of the Anaesthetic Department.

References

Abbasi AS, Allen MW, Decristofaro D, Ungar I (1980) Detection and estimation of the degree of mitral regurgitation by range-gated pulsed Doppler echocardiography. Circulation 61:143–149

Alegret JM, Duran I, Palazon O et al (2003) Prevalence of and predictors of bicuspid aortic valves in patients with dilated aortic roots. Am J Cardiol 91:619–622

Alfakih K, Plein S, Thiele H, Jones T, Ridgway JP, Sivananthan MU (2003) Normal human left and right ventricular dimensions for MRI assessed by turbo gradient echo and steady-state free precession imaging sequences. JMRI 17: 323–329

Anderson KR, Zuberbuhler JR, Anderson RH, Becker AE, Lie JT (1979) Morphologic spectrum of Ebstein's anomaly of the heart: a review. Mayo Clin Proc 54:174–180

Aurigemma G, Reichek N, Schiebler M, Axel L (1990) Evaluation of mitral regurgitation by cine MRI. Am J Cardiol 66:621–625

Aurigemma G, Reichek N, Schiebler M, Axel L (1991) Evaluation of aortic regurgitation by cardiac cine MRI: planar analysis and comparison to Doppler echocardiography. Cardiology 78:340–347

Barkhausen J, Ruehm SG, Goyen M, Buck T, Laub G, Debatin JF (2001) MR evaluation of ventricular function: true fast imaging with steady-state precession versus fast low-angle shot cine MR imaging: feasibility study. Radiology 219: 264–269

Baumgartner H, Bonhoeffer P, De Groot NM, de Haan F, Deanfield JE, Galie N, Gatzoulis MA, Gohlke-Baerwolf C, Kaemmerer H, Kilner P, Meijboom F, Mulder BJ, Oechslin E, Oliver JM, Serraf A, Szatmari A, Thaulow E, Vouhe PR, Walma E, Vahanian A, Auricchio A, Bax J, Ceconi C, Dean V, Filippatos G, Funck-Brentano C, Hobbs R, Kearney P, McDonagh T, Popescu BA, Reiner Z, Sechtem U, Sirnes PA, Tendera M, Vardas P, Widimsky P, McDonagh T, Swan L, Andreotti F, Beghetti M, Borggrefe M, Bozio A, Brecker S, Budts W, Hess J, Hirsch R, Jondeau G, Kokkonen J, Kozelj M, Kucukoglu S, Laan M, Lionis C, Metreveli I, Moons P, Pieper PG, Pilossoff V, Popelova J, Price S, Roos-Hesselink J, Uva MS, Tornos P, Trindade PT, Ukkonen H, Walker H, Webb GD, Westby J, Task Force on the Management of Grown-up Congenital Heart Disease of the European Society of Cardiology (ESC) (2010) ESC guidelines for the management of grown-up congenital heart disease (new version 2010). Eur Heart J 31(23):2915–2957

Bellenger NG, Francis JM, Davies CL, Coats AJ, Pennell DJ (2000) Establishment and performance of a magnetic resonance cardiac function clinic. JCMR 2:15–22

Beyerbacht HP, Lamb HJ, van der Laarse A et al (2001) Aortic valve replacement in patients with aortic stenosis improves myocardial metabolism and diastolic function. Radiology 219:637–643

Bharucha T, Roman KS, Anderson RH, Vettukattil JJ (2008) Impact of multiplanar review of three-dimensional echocardiographic data on management of congenital heart disease. Ann Thorac Surg 86(3):875–881

Bhattacharyya S, Toumpanakis C, Burke M, Taylor AM, Caplin M, Davar J (2010) Features of Carcinoid Heart Disease Identified By Two- and Three- Dimensional Echocardiography and Cardiac Magnetic Resonance Imaging. Circ Cardiovasc Imaging 3(1):103–111

Boehrer JD, Lange RA, Willard JE, Grayburn PA, Hillis LD (1992) Advantages and limitations of methods to detect, localise and quantitate intracardiac left-to-right shunting. Am Heart J 124:448–455

Bogaert J, Taylor AM, Van Kerkhove F, Dymarkowski S (2004) Use of inversion recovery contrast-enhanced MRI for cardiac imaging: spectrum of applications. AJR Am J Roentgenol 182:609–615

Bogren HG, Klipstein RH, Firmin DN, Mohiaddin RH, Underwood SR, Rees RSO, Longmore DB (1989a) Quantification of antegrade and retrograde blood flow in the human aorta by magnetic resonance velocity mapping. Am Heart J 117:1214–1222

Bogren HG, Klipstein RH, Mohiaddin RH et al (1989b) Pulmonary artery distensibility and blood flow patterns: a magnetic resonance study of normal subjects and patients with pulmonary arterial hypertension. Am Heart J 118: 990–999

Bolger AF, Eigler NL, Maurer G (1988) Quantifying valvular regurgitation: limitations and inherent assumptions of Doppler technique. Circulation 78:1316–1318

Bonhoeffer P, Boudjemline Y, Saliba Z, Merckx J, Aggoun Y, Bonnet D, Acar P, Le Bidois J, Sidi D, Kachaner J (2000) Percutaneous replacement of pulmonary valve in a right-ventricle to pulmonary-artery prosthetic conduit with valve dysfunction. Lancet 356(9239):1403–1405

Bonow RO, Carabello BA, Chatterjee K, de Leon AC Jr, Faxon DP, Freed MD, Gaasch WH, Lytle BW, Nishimura RA, O'Gara PT, O'Rourke RA, Otto CM, Shah PM, Shanewise JS (2008) American College of Cardiology/American Heart Association Task Force on Practice Guidelines 2008 focused update incorporated into the ACC/AHA 2006 guidelines for the management of patients with valvular heart disease: a report of the American College of Cardiology/American Heart Association Task Force on Practice Guidelines (Writing Committee to revise the 1998 guidelines for the management of patients with valvular heart disease). Endorsed by the Society of Cardiovascular Anesthesiologists, Society for Cardiovascular Angiography and Interventions, and Society of Thoracic Surgeons. J Am Coll Cardiol 52(13):e1-142

Bonow RO, Carbello B, DeLeon AC et al (1998) ACC/AHA guideline for the management of patients with valvular heart disease. J Am Coll Cardiol 32:1486–1588

Borer JS, Bonow RO (2003) Contemporary approach to aortic and mitral regurgitation. Circulation 108:2432–2438

Bryan AJ, Barzilai B, Kouchoukos NT (1995) Transesophageal echocardiography and adult cardiac operations. Ann Thorac Surg 59:773–779

Caduff JH, Hernandez RJ, Ludomirsky A (1996) MR visualization of aortic valve vegetations. J Comput Assist Tomogr 20:613–615

Carabello BA, Crawford FA (1997) N Eng J Med 307: 1362–1367

Carroll JD (1993) Cardiac catheterisation and other imaging modalities in the evaluation of valvular heart disease. Curr Opin Cardiol 8:211–215

Caruthers SD, Jiuan Lin S, Brown P et al (2003) Practical value of cardiac magnetic resonance imaging for clinical quantification of aortc valve stenosis. Comparison with echocardiography. Circulation 108:2236–2243

Chatzimavroudis GP, Walker PG, Oshinski JN, Franch RH, Pettigrew RI, Yoganathan AP (1997) Slice location dependence of aortic regurgitation measurements with MR phase velocity mapping. Magn Reson Med 37:545–551

Chernobelsky A, Shubayev O, Comeau CR, Wolff SD (2007) Baseline correction of phase contrast images improves quantification of blood flow in the great vessels. J Cardiovasc Magn Reson 9(4):681–685

Christiansen JP, Edwards C, Armstrong G, Patel H, Scott T, Hart H (2009) Quantitative evaluation of aortic regurgitation in asymptomatic patients using cardiac MRI predicts long-term outcome. Heart Lung Circ 18(Suppl 2):S5–S6

Coats L, Khambadkone S, Derrick G, Sridharan S, Schievano S, Mist B, Jones R, Deanfield JE, Pellerin D, Bonhoeffer P, Taylor AM (2006) Physiological and clinical consequences of relief of right ventricular out- flow tract obstruction late after repair of congenital heart defects. Circulation 113:2037–2044

Coats L, Khambadkone S, Derrick G, Hughes M, Jones R, Mist B, Pellerin D, Marek J, Deanfield JE, Bonhoeffer P, Taylor AM (2007) Physiological consequences of percutaneous pulmonary valve implantation: the different behaviour of volume and pressure overloaded ventricles. Eur Heart J 28:1886–1893

Conway MA, Allis J, Ouwerkerk R, Niioka T, Rajagopalan B, Radda GK (1991) Detection of low phosphocreatinine to ATP ratio in failing hypertrophied human myocardium by P magnetic resonance spectroscopy. Lancet 338:973–976

Cribier A, Eltchaninoff H, Bash A, Borenstein N, Tron C, Bauer F, Derumeaux G, Anselme F, Laborde F, Leon MB (2002) Percutaneous transcatheter implantation of an aortic valve prosthesis for calcific aortic stenosis: first human case description. Circulation 106(24):3006–3008

Currie PJ, Seward JB, Reeder GS et al (1985) Continuous wave Doppler echocardiographic assessment of the severity of calcific aortic stenosis: a simultaneous Doppler-catheter correlative study in 100 adult patients. Circulation 71: 1162–1169

Daccarett M, McGann CJ, Akoum NW, MacLeod RS, Marrouche NF (2011) MRI of the left atrium: predicting clinical outcomes in patients with atrial fibrillation. Expert Rev Cardiovasc Ther 9(1):105–111

Davis K, Kennedy J, Kemp H, Judkins M, Gosselin A, Killip T (1979) Complications of coronary arteriography from the collaborative study of coronary artery surgery (CASS). Circulation 59:1105–1112

Debl K, Djavidani B, Seitz J, Nitz W, Schmid FX, Muders F, Buchner S, Feuerbach S, Riegger G, Luchner A (2005) Planimetry of aortic valve area in aortic stenosis by magnetic resonance imaging. Invest Radiol 40(10):631–636

Debl K, Djavidani B, Buchner S, Lipke C, Nitz W, Feuerbach S et al (2006) Delayed hyperenhancement in magnetic resonance imaging of left ventricular hypertrophy caused by aortic stenosis and hypertrophic cardiomyopathy: visualisation of focal fibrosis. Heart 92:1447–1451

Delgado V, Ewe SH, Ng AC, van der Kley F, Marsan NA, Schuijf JD, Schalij MJ, Bax JJ (2010) Multimodality imaging in transcatheter aortic valve implantation: key steps to assess procedural feasibility. EuroIntervention 6(5): 643–652

DeRoos A, Reichek N, Axel L, Kressel HY (1989) Cine MR imaging in aortic stenosis. J Comput Assist Tomogr 13: 421–425

Deutsch HJ, Bachmann R, Sechtem U et al (1992) Regurgitant flow in cardiac valve prosthesis: diagnostic value of gradient echo nuclear magnetic resonance imaging in reference to transesophageal two-dimensional color Doppler echocardiography. J Am Coll Cardiol 19:1500–1507

DiCesare E, Enrici RM, Paparoni S et al (1995) Low-field magnetic resonance imaging in the evaluation of mechanical and biological heart valve function. Eur J Radiol 20: 224–228

Discigil B, Dearani JA, Puga FJ, Schaff HV, Hagler DJ, Warnes CA, Danielson GK (2001) Late pulmonary valve replacement after repair of tetralogy of Fallot. J Thorac Cardiovasc Surg 121:344–351

Dooms G, Higgins CB (1986) MR imaging of cardiac thrombi. J Comput Assist Tomogr 10:415–420

Dulce MC, Mostbeck GH, O'Sullivan M, Cheitlin M, Caputo GR, Higgins CB (1992) Severity of aortic regurgitation: interstudy reproducibility of measurements with velocity-encoded cine MRI. Radiology 185:235–240

Edwards MB, Ordidge RJ, Hand JW, Taylor KM, Young IR (2005) Assessment of magnetic field (4.7 T) induced forces on prosthetic heart valves and annuloplasty rings. J Magn Reson Imaging 22:311–317

Eichenberger AC, Jenni R, von Schulthess GK (1993) Aortic valve pressure gradients in patients with aortic valve stenosis: quantification with velocity-encoded cine MR imaging. AJR 160:971–977

Enriquez-Sarano M, Tajik A, Schaff H et al (1994) Echocardiographic prediction of survival after surgical correction of organic mitral regurgitation. Circulation 90:830–837

Evans AJ, Blinder RA, Herfkens RJ et al (1988) Effects of turbulence on signal intensity in gradient echo images. Invest Radiol 23:512–518

Firmin DN, Nayler GL, Klipstein RH, Underwood SR, Longmore DB (1987) In vivo validation of MR velocity imaging. J Comput Assist Tomogr 11:751–756

Fix J, Isada L, Cosgrove D, Miller DP, Savage R, Blum J, Stewart W (1993) Do patients with less than "echo-perfect" results from mitral valve repair by intraoperative echocardiography have a different outcome? Circulation 88:39–48

Flett AS, Hayward MP, Ashworth MT, Hansen MS, Taylor AM, Elliott PM, McGregor C, Moon JC (2010) Equilibrium contrast cardiovascular magnetic resonance for the measurement of diffuse myocardial fibrosis: preliminary validation in humans. Circulation 122:138–144

Fontaine AA, Heinrich RS, Walker PG et al (1996) Comparison of magnetic resonance imaging and laser Doppler anemometry velocity measurements downstream of replacement heart valves: implications for in vivo assessment of prosthetic valve function. J Heart Valve Dis 5:66–73

Friedrich MG, Schulz-Menger J, Poetsch T, Pilz B, Uhlich F, Dietz R (2002) Quantification of valvular aortic stenosis by magnetic resonance imaging. Am Heart J 144:329–334

Frigiola A, Tsang V, Bull C et al (2008) Biventricular response after pulmonary valve replacement for right ventricular outflow tract dysfunction: is age a predictor of outcome? Circulation 118:S182–S190

Fujita N, Chazouilleres AF, Hartiala JJ et al (1994) Quantification of mitral regurgitation by velocity encoded cine nuclear magnetic resonance imaging. J Am Coll Cardiol 23:951–958

Gabriel RS, Kerr AJ, Raffel OC, Stewart RA, Cowan BR, Occleshaw CJ (2008) Mapping of mitral regurgitant defects by cardiovascular magnetic resonance in moderate or severe mitral regurgitation secondary to mitral valve prolapse. J Cardiovasc Magn Reson 10:16

Gatehouse PD, Rolf MP, Graves MJ, Hofman MB, Totman J, Werner B, Quest RA, Liu Y, von Spiczak J, Dieringer M, Firmin DN, van Rossum A, Lombardi M, Schwitter J, Schulz-Menger J, Kilner PJ (2010) Flow measurement by cardiovascular magnetic resonance: a multi-centre multi-vendor study of background phase offset errors that can compromise the accuracy of derived regurgitant or shunt flow measurements. J Cardiovasc Magn Reson 12:5

Ghez O, Tsang VT, Frigiola A, Coats L, Taylor A, van Doorn C, Bonhoeffer P, de Leval M (2007) Right ventricular outflow tract reconstruction for pulmonary regurgitation after repair of tetralogy of Fallot. Eur J Cardiothorac Surg 31(4): 654–658

Globits S, Mayr H, Frank H et al (1991) Quantification of regurgitant lesions by MRI. Int J Card Imaging 6:109–116

Globits S, Blake L, Bourne M et al (1996) Assessment of haemodynamic effects of ACE inhibition therapy in chronic aortic regurgitation by using velocity-encoded cine magnetic resonance imaging. Am Heart J 131:289–293

Gorlin R, Gorlin SG (1951) Hydraulic formula for calculation of the area of the stenotic mitral valve, other valves and central circulatory shunts. Am Heart J 41:1–29

Grothues F, Smith GC, Moon JC et al (2002) Comparison of interstudy reproducibility of cardiovascular magnetic resonance with two-dimensional echocardiography in normal subjects and in patients with heart failure or left ventricular hypertrophy. Am J Cardiol 90:29–34

Han Y, Peters DC, Salton CJ, Bzymek D, Nezafat R, Goddu B et al (2008) Cardiovascular magnetic resonance characterization of mitral valve prolapse. JACC Cardiovasc Imaging 1:294–303

Hatle L, Angelson B (1992) Doppler ultrasound in cardiology: physical principles and clinical applications. Lea & Febiger, Philadelphia

Hausmann D, Daniel WG, Mugge A, Ziemer G, Pearlman AS (1992) Value of transesophageal color Doppler echocardiography for detection of different types of atrial septal defect in adults. J Am Soc Echocardiogr 5:481–488

Heidenreich PA, Steffens JC, Fujita N, O'Sullivan M, Caputo GR, Foster E, Higgins CB (1995) The evaluation of mitral stenosis with velocity encoded cine MRI. Am J Cardiol 75:365–369

Hein S, Arnon E, Kostin S, Schonburg M, Elsasser A, Polyakova V et al (2003) Progression from compensated hypertrophy to failure in the pressure-overloaded human heart: structural deterioration and compensatory mechanisms. Circulation 107:984–991

Holloway C, Clarke K (2010) Is MR spectroscopy of the heart ready for humans? Heart Lung Circ 19(3):154–160

Hope MD, Hope TA, Crook SE, Ordovas KG, Urbania TH, Alley MT, Higgins CB (2011) 4D flow CMR in assessment of valve-related ascending aortic disease. JACC Cardiovasc Imaging 4(7):781–787

Hori Y, Yamada N, Higashi M, Hirai N, Nakatani S (2003) Rapid evaluation of right and left ventricular function and mass using real-time True-FISP cine MR imaging without breath-hold: comparison with segmented True-FISP cine MR imaging with breath-hold. JCMR 5:439–450

Hundley WG, Li HF, Willard JE et al (1995) Magnetic resonance imaging assessment of the severity of mitral regurgitation. Circulation 92:1151–1158

Iozzelli A, D'Orta G, Aliprandi A, Secchi F, Di Leo G, Sardanelli F (2009) The value of true-FISP sequence added to conventional gadolinium-enhanced MRA of abdominal aorta and its major branches. Eur J Radiol 72(3):489–493

Jeang MK, Fuentes F, Gately A, Byrnes J, Lewis M (1986) Aortic root abscess—initial experience using magnetic resonance imaging. Chest 89:613–615

John AS, Dill T, Brandt RR et al (2003) Magnetic resonance to assess the aortic valve area in aortic stenosis. How does it compare to current diagnostic standards? J Am Coll Cardiol 42:519–526

Kahlert P, Eggebrecht H, Plicht B, Kraff O, McDougall I, Decker B, Erbel R, Ladd ME, Quick HH (2010) Towards real-time cardiovascular magnetic resonance-guided transarterial aortic valve implantation: in vitro evaluation and modification of existing devices. J Cardiovasc Magn Reson 12:58

Ketelsen D, Fishman EK, Claussen CD, Vogel-Claussen J (2010) Computed tomography evaluation of cardiac valves: a review. Radiol Clin North 48(4):783–797

Khambadkone S, Coats L, Taylor A, Boudjemline Y, Derrick G, Tsang V, Cooper J, Muthurangu V, Hegde SR, Razavi RS, Pellerin D, Deanfield J, Bonhoeffer P (2005) Percutaneous pulmonary valve implantation in humans: results in 59 consecutive patients. Circulation 112:1189–1197

Kilner PJ, Firmin DN, Rees RSO et al (1991) Valve and great vessel stenosis: assessment with MR jet velocity mapping. Radiology 178:229–235

Kilner PJ, Manzara CC, Mohiaddin RH et al (1993) Magnetic resonance jet velocity mapping in mitral and aortic valve stenosis. Circulation 87:1239–1248

Kivelitz DE, Dohmen PM, Lembcke A et al (2003) Visualization of the pulmonary valve using cine MR imaging. Acta Radiol 44:172–176

Knauth AL, Gauvreau K, Powell AJ et al (2008) Ventricular size and function assessed by cardiac MRI predict major adverse clinical outcomes late after tetralogy of Fallot repair. Heart 94:211–216

Kondo C, Caputo GR, Semelka R, Shimakawa M, Higgins CB (1991) Right and left ventricular stroke volume measurements with velocity encoded cine NMR imaging: in vivo and in vitro evaluation. AJR 157:9–16

Kozerke S, Scheidegger MB, Pedersen EM, Boesiger P (1999) Heart motion adapted cine phase-contrast flow measurements through the aortic valve. MRM 42:970–978

Kozerke S, Schwitter J, Pedersen EM, Boesiger P (2001) Aortic and mitral regurgitation: quantification using moving slice velocity mapping. JMRI 14:106–112

La Salvia EA, Gilkeson RC, Dahms BB, Siwik E (2006) Delayed contrast enhancement magnetic resonance imaging in congenital aortic stenosis. Pediatr Cardiol 27:388–390

Laissy JP, Blanc F, Soyer P et al (1995) Thoracic aortic dissection: diagnosis with transesophageal echocardiography versus MR imaging. Radiology 194:331–336

Lamb HJ, Beyerbacht HP, de Roos A et al (2002) Left ventricular remodelling early after aortic valve replacement: differential effects on diastolic function in aortic valve stenosis and aortic regurgitation. J Am Coll Cardiol 40:2182–2188

Lee VS, Resnick D, Bundy JM, Simonetti OP, Lee P, Weinreb JC (2002) Cardiac function: MR evaluation in one breath hold with real-time true fast imaging with steady state precession. Radiology 222:835–842

Lepore V, Lamm C, Bugge M, Larsson S (1996) Magnetic resonance imaging in the follow-up of patients after aortic root reconstruction. Thorac Cardiovasc Surg 44:188–192

Lurz P, Coats L, Khambadkone S, Nordmeyer J, Boudjemline Y, Schievano S, Muthurangu V, Lee TY, Parenzan G, Derrick G, Cullen S, Walker F, Tsang V, Deanfield J, Taylor AM, Bonhoeffer P (2008) Percutaneous pulmonary valve implantation: impact of evolving technology and learning curve on clinical outcome. Circulation 117:1964–1972

Lurz P, Muthurangu V, Schievano S, Nordmeyer J, Bonhoeffer P, Taylor AM, Hansen MS (2009a) Feasibility and reproducibility of biventricular volumetric assessment of cardiac function during exercise using real-time radial k-t SENSE magnetic resonance imaging. J Magn Reson Imaging 29(5): 1062–1070

Lurz P, Puranik R, Nordmeyer J, Muthurangu V, Hansen MS, Schievano S, Marek J, Bonhoeffer P, Taylor AM (2009b) Improvement in left ventricular filling properties after relief of right ventricle to pulmonary artery conduit obstruction—contribution of septal motion and interventricular mechanical delay. Eur Heart J 30(18):2266–2274

Lurz P, Nordmeyer J, Muthurangu V, Khambadkone S, Derrick G, Yates R, Sury M, Bonhoeffer P, Taylor AM (2009c) Comparison of bare metal stenting and PPVI for treatment of RVOT obstruction: utilization of an X- ray/MR hybrid lab for acute physiological comparison. Circulation 119:2995–3001

Lurz P, Nordmeyer J, Khambadkone S, Giardini A, Muthurangu V, Mist B, Schievano S, Derrick G, Taylor AM, Bonhoeffer P (2011) Functional outcome early and late (one year) after percutaneous pulmonary valve implantation as assessed by magnetic resonance imaging and exercise testing. JACC 57(6):724–731

Manning WJ, Silverman DI, Gordon SP, Krumholz HM, Douglas PS (1993) Cardioversion from atrial fibrillation without prolonged anticoagulation with use of transesophageal echocardiography to exclude the presence of atrial thrombi. N Engl J Med 328:750–755

Marelli AJ, Mackie AS, Ionescu-Ittu R, Rahme E, Pilote L (2007) Congenital heart disease in the general population: changing prevalence and age distribution. Circulation 115(2):163–172

Markl M, Kilner PJ, Ebbers T (2011) Comprehensive 4D velocity mapping of the heart and great vessels by cardiovascular magnetic resonance. J Cardiovasc Magn Reson 13:7

McElhinney DB, Hellenbrand WE, Zahn EM, Jones TK, Cheatham JP, Lock JE, Vincent JA (2010) Short- and medium-term outcomes after transcatheter pulmonary valve placement in the expanded multicenter US melody valve trial. Circulation 122(5):507–516

Meadows J, Powell AJ, Geva T, Dorfman A, Gauvreau K, Rhodes J (2007) Cardiac magnetic resonance imaging correlates of exercise capacity in patients with surgically repaired tetralogy of Fallot. Am J Cardiol 100(9): 1446–1450

Meier D, Maier S, Boesiger P (1988) Quantitative flow measurements on phantoms and on blood vessels with MR. Magn Reson Med 8:25–34

Mohiaddin RH, Wann SL, Underwood R, Firmin DN, Rees S, Longmore DB (1990) Vena caval flow: assessment with cine MR velocity mapping. Radiology 177:537–541

Mohiaddin RH, Amanuma M, Kilner PJ, Pennell DJ, Manzara C, Longmore DB (1991a) MR phase-shift velocity mapping of mitral and pulmonary venous flow. J Comput Assist Tomogr 15:237–243

Mohiaddin RH, Paz R, Theodoropolus S et al (1991b) Magnetic resonance characterization of pulmonary arterial blood flow following single lung transplantation. J Thorac Cardiovasc Surg 101:1016–1023

Moon JCC, Lorenz CH, Francis JM, Smith GC, Pennell DJ (2002) Breath-hold FLASH and FISP cardiovascular MR imaging: left ventricular volume differences and reproducibility. Radiology 223:789–797

Moustafa SE, Chandrasekaran K, Khandheria B, Tajik J, Mookadam F (2011) Real-time three-dimensional transesophageal echocardiography assessment of the mitral

valve: perioperative advantages and game-changing findings. J Heart Valve Dis 20(2):114–122
Muthurangu V, Lurz P, Critchely JD, Deanfield JE, Taylor AM, Hansen MS (2008) Real-time assessment of right and left ventricular volumes and function in patients with congenital heart disease by using high spatiotemporal resolution radial k-t SENSE. Radiology 248(3):782–791
Nagel E, Stuber M, Burkhard B et al (2000) Cardiac rotation and relaxation in patients with aortic valvular stenosis. Eur Heart J 21:582–589
Nayler GL, Firmin DN, Longmore DB (1986) Blood flow imaging by cine magnetic resonance. J Comput Assist Tomogr 10:715–722
Neubauer S, Horn M, Cramer M et al (1997a) Myocardial phosphocreatine-to-ATP ratio is a predictor of mortality in patients with dilated cardiomyopathy. Circulation 96: 2190–2196
Neubauer S, Horn M, Pabst T et al (1997b) Cardiac high-energy phosphate metabolism in patients with aortic valve disease assessed by ^{31}P-magnetic resonance spectroscopy. J Investig Med 45:453–462
Ng AC, Delgado V, van der Kley F, Shanks M, van de Veire NR, Bertini M, Nucifora G, van Bommel RJ, Tops LF, de Weger A, Tavilla G, de Roos A, Kroft LJ, Leung DY, Schuijf J, Schalij MJ, Bax JJ (2010) Comparison of aortic root dimensions and geometries before and after transcatheter aortic valve implantation by 2- and 3-dimensional transesophageal echocardiography and multislice computed tomography. Circ Cardiovasc Imaging 3(1):94–102
Nishimura F (1992) Oblique cine MRI for the evaluation of aortic regurgitation: comparison with cineangiography. Clin Cardiol 66:621–625
Nkomo VT, Enriquez-Sarano M, Ammash NM et al (2003) Bicuspid aortic valve associated with aortic dilatation: a community-based study. Arterioscler Thromb Vasc Biol 23:351–356
Nkomo VT, Gardin JM, Skelton TN, Gottdiener J, Scott C, Enriquez-Serano M (2006) Burden of valvular heart diseases: a population-based study. Lancet 368:1005–1011
Novaro GM, Tiong IY, Pearce GL, Grimm RA, Smedira N, Griffin BP (2003) Features and predictors of ascending aortic dilatation in association with a congenital bicuspid aortic valve. Am J Cardiol 92:99–101
Ohnishi S, Fukui S, Kusuoka H, Kitabatake A, Inoue M, Kamada T (1992) Assessment of valvular regurgitation using cine MRI coupled with phase compensating technique: comparison with Doppler color flow mapping. Angiology 43:913–924
Oosterhof T, Meijboom FJ, Vliegen HW, Hazekamp MG, Zwinderman AH, Bouma B, van Dijk AP, Mulder BJ (2006) Long-term follow-up of homograft function after pulmonary valve replacement in patients with tetralogy of Fallot. Eur Heart J 27:1478–1484
Oosterhof T, van Straten A, Vliegen HW et al (2007) Preoperative thresholds for pulmonary valve replacement in patients with corrected tetralogy of Fallot using cardiovascular magnetic resonance. Circulation 116:545–551
Pedersen WR, Walker M, Olson JD et al (1991) Value of transesophageal echocardiography as an adjunct to transthoracic echocardiography in evaluation of native and prosthetic valve endocarditis. Chest 100:351–356
Pereles FS, Kapoor V, Carr JC et al (2001) Usefulness of segmented trueFISP cardiac pulse sequence in evaluation of congenital and acquired adult cardiac abnormalities. AJR Am J Roentgenol 177:1155–1160
Pflederer T, Achenbach S (2010) Aortic valve stenosis: CT contributions to diagnosis and therapy. J Cardiovasc Comput Tomogr 4(6):355–364
Quinones MA, Young JB, Waggoner AD, Ostojic MC, Ribeiro LGT, Miller RR (1980) Assessment of pulsed Doppler echocardiography in detection and quantification of aortic and mitral regurgitation. Br Heart J 44:612–620
Rajappan K, Melina G, Bellenger NG et al (2000) Evaluation of left ventricular function and mass after medtronic freestyle versus homograft aortic root replacement using cardiovascular magnetic resonance. J Heart Valve Dis 11:60–65
Randall PA, Kohman LJ, Scalzetti EM, Szeverenyi NM, Panicek DM (1988) Magnetic resonance imaging of prosthetic cardiac valves in vitro and in vivo. Am J Cardiol 62:973–976
Razavi R, Hill DL, Keevil SF, Miquel ME, Muthurangu V, Hegde S, Rhode K, Barnett M, van Vaals J, Hawkes DJ, Baker E (2003) Cardiac catheterisation guided by MRI in children and adults with congenital heart disease. Lancet 362(9399):1877–1882
Reant P, Lederlin M, Lafitte S, Serri K, Montaudon M, Corneloup O, Roudaut R, Laurent F (2006) Absolute assessment of aortic valve stenosis by planimetry using cardiovascular magnetic resonance imaging: comparison with transesophageal echocardiography, transthoracic echocardiography, and cardiac catheterisation. Eur J Radiol 59(2):276–283
Rebergen SA, Chin JGJ, Ottenkamp J, van der Wall EE, de Roos A (1993) Pulmonary regurgitation in the late postoperative follow-up of tetralogy of Fallot. Circulation 88:2257–2266
Rigo P, Alderson PO, Robertson RM, Becker LC, Wagner HN (1979) Measurement of aortic and mitral regurgitation by gated cardiac blood pool scans. Circulation 60:306–312
Rockey R, Sterling LL, Zoghbi WA, Sartori MP, Limacher MC, Kou LC, Quinones MA (1987) Determination of the regurgitant fraction in isolated mitral regurgitation by pulsed Doppler two-dimensional echocardiography. J Am Coll Cardiol 7:1273–1278
Roest AAW, Helbing WA, Kunz P et al (2002) Exercise MR imaging in the assessment of pulmonary regurgitation and biventricular function in patients after tetralogy of Fallot repair. Radiology 223:204–211
Rolf MP, Hofman MB, Gatehouse PD, Markenroth-Bloch K, Heymans MW, Ebbers T, Graves MJ, Totman JJ, Werner B, van Rossum AC, Kilner PJ, Heethaar RM (2011) Sequence optimization to reduce velocity offsets in cardiovascular magnetic resonance volume flow quantification—a multi-vendor study. J Cardiovasc Magn Reson 13:18
Sandler H, Dodge HT, Hay RE, Rackley CE (1963) Quantification of valvular insufficiency in man by angiocardiography. Am Heart J 65:501–513
Sandstede JJW, Beer M, Hofmann S et al (2000) Changes in left and right ventricular cardiac function after valve replacement for aortic stenosis determined by cine MR imaging. JMRI 12:240–246

Sandstede JJW, Johnson T, Harre K et al (2002) Cardiac systolic rotation and contraction before and after valve replacement for aortic stenosis. AJR 178:953–958
Schievano S, Coats L, Migliavacca F et al (2007a) Variations in right ventricular outflow tract morphology following repair of congenital heart disease: implications for percutaneous pulmonary valve implantation. J Cardiovasc Magn Reson 9(4):687–695
Schievano S, Migliavacca F, Coats L, Khambadkone S, Carminati M, Wilson N, Deanfield JE, Bonhoeffer P, Taylor AM (2007b) Planning of percutaneous pulmonary valve implantation based on rapid prototyping of the right ventricular outflow tract and pulmonary trunk from magnetic resonance imaging data. Radiology 242(2):490–497
Schievano S, Taylor AM, Capelli C, Coats L, Walker F, Lurz P, Nordmeyer J, Wright S, Khambadkone S, Tsang V, Carminati M, Bonhoeffer P (2010) First-in-man implantation of a novel percutaneous valve—A new approach to medical device development. EuroIntervention 5:745–750
Schievano S, Capelli C, Young C, Lurz P, Nordmeyer J, Owens C, Bonhoeffer P, Taylor AM (2011) Four-dimensional computed tomography: a method to assess right ventricular outflow tract and pulmonary artery deformations throughout the cardiac cycle. Eur Radiol 21(1):36–45
Schlosser T, Malyar N, Jochims M, Breuckmann F, Hunold P, Bruder O, Barkhausen J et al (2007) Quantification of aortic valve stenosis in MRI—comparison of steady-state free precession and fast low-angle shot sequences. Eur Radiol 17:1284–1290
Sechtem U, Pflugfelder PW, White RD, Gould RG, Holt W, Lipton MJ, Higgins CB (1987) Cine MR imaging: potential for the evaluation of cardiovascular function. AJR Am J Roentgenol 148:239–246
Sechtem U, Pflugfelder PW, Cassidy MM, White RD, Cheitlin MD, Schiller NB, Higgins CB (1988) Mitral and aortic regurgitation: quantification of regurgitant volumes with cine MR imaging. Radiology 167:425–430
Sellers RD, Levy MJ, Amplatz K, Lillehei CW (1964) Left retrograde cardioangiography in acquired cardiac disease: technique, indication and interpretation. Am J Cardiol 14:437–445
Sensky PR, Loubani M, Keal RP, Samani NJ, Sosnowski AW, Galiñanes M (2003) Does the type of prosthesis influence early left ventricular mass regression after aortic valve replacement? Assessment with magnetic resonance imaging. Am Heart J 146:e13
Shebani SO, McGuirk S, Baghai M, Stickley J, De Giovanni JV, Bu'lock FA, Barron DJ, Brawn WJ (2006) Right ventricular outflow tract reconstruction using Contegra valved conduit: natural history and conduit performance under pressure. Eur J Cardiothorac Surg 29:397–405
Shellock FG (1988) MR imaging of metallic implants and materials: a compilation of the literature. AJR 151:811–814
Shellock FG, Morisoli S, Kanal E (1993) MR procedures and biomedical implants, materials and devices: 1993 update. Radiology 189:587–599
Simpson IA, Maciel BC, Moises V et al (1993) Cine magnetic resonance imaging and color Doppler flow mapping displays of flow velocity, spatial acceleration and jet formation: a comparative in vitro study. Am Heart J 126:1165–1174
Smith MD, Xie GY (1998) Current echocardiography-doppler approaches to the quantification of valvular regurgitation. Cardiol Rev 6:168–181
Sondergaard L, Lindvig K, Hildebrandt P et al (1993a) Valve area and cardiac output in aortic stenosis. Am Heart J 127:1156–1164
Sondergaard L, Lindvig K, Hildebrandt P, Thomsen C, Stahlberg F, Joen T, Henriksen O (1993b) Quantification of aortic regurgitation by magnetic resonance velocity mapping. Am Heart J 125:1081–1090
Sorenson SG, O'Rourke RA, Chaudhuri TK (1980) Noninvasive quantification of valvular regurgitation by gated equilibrium radionuclide angiography. Circulation 62:1089–1098
Sridharan S, Coats L, Khambadkone S, Taylor AM, Bonhoeffer P (2006) Images in cardiovascular medicine. Transcatheter right ventricular outflow tract intervention: the risk to the coronary circulation. Circulation 113(25):E934–E935
Stark J, Bull C, Stajevic M, Jothi M, Elliott M, de Leval M (1998) Fate of subpulmonary homograft conduits: determinants of late homograft failure. J Thorac Cardiovasc Surg 115:506–514
Steeden JA, Atkinson D, Taylor AM, Muthurangu V (2010) Split-acquisition real-time CINE phase-contrast MR flow measurements. Magn Reson Med 64(6):1664–1670
Steeden JA, Atkinson D, Hansen MS, Taylor AM, Muthurangu V (2011) Rapid flow assessment of congenital heart disease with high-spatiotemporal-resolution gated spiral phase-contrast MR imaging. Radiology 260(1):79–87
Stork A, Franzen O, Ruschewski H, Detter C, Mullerleile K, Bansmann PM et al (2007) Assessment of functional anatomy of the mitral valve in patients with mitral regurgitation with cine magnetic resonance imaging: comparison with transoesophageal echocardiography and surgical results. Eur Radiol 17(12):3189–3198
Taylor AM, Dymarkowski S, De Meerleer K et al (2004) Validation and application of single breath-hold cine Cardiac MR for ventricular function assessment in children with congenital heart disease. JCMR 6:409 (abstract)
Therrien J, Siu SC, McLaughlin PR, Liu PP, Williams WG, Webb GD (2000) Pulmonary valve replacement in adult late after repair of tetralogy of Fallot: are we operating too late? J Am Coll Cardiol 36:1670–1675
Therrien J, Marx GR, Gatzoulis MA (2002) Late problems in tetralogy of Fallot—recognition, management and prevention. Cardiol Clin 3:395–404
Therrien J, Provost Y, Merchant N, Williams W, Colman J, Webb G (2005) Optimal timing for pulmonary valve replacement in adults after tetralogy of Fallot repair. Am J Cardiol 95:779–782
Tice FD, Kisslo J (1993) Echocardiography in the diagnosis of thoracic aortic pathology. Int J Card Imaging 9(Suppl 2): 27–38
Tsang W, Lang RM, Kronzon I (2011) Role of real-time three dimensional echocardiography in cardiovascular interventions. Heart 97(10):850–857
Tulevski II, Hirsch A, Dodge-Khatami A, Stoker J, van der Wall EE, Mulder BJM (2003) Effect of pulmonary valve regurgitation on right ventricular function in patients with chronic right ventricular pressure overload. Am J Cardiol 92:113–116

Underwood SR, Firmin DN, Mohiaddin RH et al (1987a) Cine magnetic resonance imaging of valvular heart disease (abstract). Proc Soc Magn Reson Imaging 2:723

Underwood SR, Firmin DN, Klipstein RH, Rees RSO, Longmore DB (1987b) Magnetic resonance velocity mapping: clinical application of a new technique. Br Heart J 57: 404–412

Utsunomiya T, Ogawa T, Doshi R, Patel D, Quan M, Henry WL, Gardin JM (1991) Doppler color flow "proximal isovelocity surface area" method for estimating volume flow rates: effects of orifice shape and machine factors. J Am Coll Cardiol 17:1103–1111

Valsangiacomo Buechel ER, Dave HH, Kellenberger CJ et al (2005) Remodelling of the right ventricle after early pulmonary valve replacement in children with repaired tetralogy of Fallot: assessment by cardiovascular magnetic resonance. Eur Heart J 26:2721–2727

van den Berg J, Strengers JLM, Wielopolski PA et al (2009) Assessment of biventricular functional reserve and NT-proBNP levels in patients with RV volume overload after repair of tetralogy of Fallot at young age. Int J Cardiol 133:364–370

Vitanovski D, Ionasec RI, Georgescu B, Huber M, Taylor AM, Hornegger J, Comaniciu D (2009) Personalized pulmonary trunk modelling for intervention planning and valve assessment estimated from CT data. Med Image Comput Comput Assist Interv Int Conf (MICCAI) 11(Pt1):17–25

Vliegen HW, van Straten A, de Roos A et al (2002) Magnetic resonance imaging to assess the hemodynamic effects of pulmonary valve replacement in adults late after repair of tetralogy of Fallot. Circulation 106:1703–1707

Waggoner AD, Quinones MA, Young JB et al (1981) Pulsed Doppler echocardiography detection of right-sided valve regurgitation. Experimental results and clinical significance. Am J Cardiol 47:279–283

Wagner S, Auffermann W, Buser P, Lim TH, Kircher B, Pflugfelder PW, Higgins CB (1989) Diagnostic accuracy and estimation of the severity of valvular regurgitation from the signal void on cine magnetic resonance imaging. Am Heart J 118:760–767

Webb JG, Pasupati S, Humphries K, Thompson C, Altwegg L, Moss R, Sinhal A, Carere RG, Munt B, Ricci D, Ye J, Cheung A, Lichtenstein SV (2007) Percutaneous transarterial aortic valve replacement in selected high-risk patients with aortic stenosis. Circulation 116(7):755–763

Weinmann HJ, Lanaido M, Mutzel W (1984) Pharmacokinetics of Gd-DTPA/dimeglumine after iv injection. Physiol Chem Phys Med NMR 16:167–172

Yemets IM, Williams WG, Webb GD et al (1997) Pulmonary valve replacement late after repair of tetralogy of Fallot. Ann Thorac Surg 64:526–530

Young C, Taylor AM, Owens CM (2011) Paediatric cardiac computed tomography: a review of imaging techniques and radiation dose consideration. Eur Radiol 21(3):518–529

Zahn EM, Hellenbrand WE, Lock JE, McElhinney DB (2009) Implantation of the melody transcatheter pulmonary valve in patients with a dysfunctional right ventricular outflow tract conduit early results from the US clinical trial. J Am Coll Cardiol 54(18):1722–1729

Zur Y, Wood ML, Neuringer LJ (1990) Motion-insensitive, steady-state free precession Imaging. Magn Reson Med 16:444–459

Coronary Artery Diseases

S. Dymarkowski, J. Bogaert, and A. M. Taylor

Contents

1	**Introduction**	512
2	**Challenges for Non-invasive Coronary Artery Imaging**	512
3	**History of Coronary MR Imaging**	513
4	**Coronary Artery Motion and Acquisition Window**	516
5	**Contrast Generation**	520
5.1	Sequence Design	520
5.2	Magnetization Preparation Techniques	522
5.3	Contrast Agents	523
6	**Spatial Resolution**	525
7	**High Field-Strength (3.0T) Coronary MR Angiography**	526
8	**Coronary Blood Flow Assessment: Strategies**	527
9	**Coronary Artery Bypass Graft Imaging: Strategies**	528
10	**Practical Approach for Coronary MR Angiography**	528
10.1	Patient Setup and Patient Instructions	528
10.2	Cookbook Approach for Free-Breathing Coronary MR Angiography	529
10.3	Practical Approach for Breath-Hold Coronary MR Angiography	531
11	**Post-Processing Techniques for Coronary MR Angiography**	532
12	**Clinical Applications**	534
12.1	Congenital Anomalies of the Coronary Arteries	534
12.2	Coronary Artery Imaging in Congenital Heart Diseases	537
12.3	Coronary Artery Vasculitis	538
12.4	Ischemic Heart Disease	540
13	**Coronary MR Angiography Versus Coronary CT Angiography**	545
14	**Key Points**	545
	References	547

S. Dymarkowski (✉) · J. Bogaert
Department of Radiology,
Gasthuisberg Universitair Ziekenhuis,
Katholieke Universiteit Leuven,
3000 Leuven, Belgium
e-mail: steven.dymarkowski@uz.kuleuven.ac.be

A. M. Taylor
Cardiothoracic Unit, Institute of Child Health
and Great Ormond Street Hospital for Children,
London, UK

Abstract

Although in recent years the image quality, volume coverage, acquisition speed and contrast of coronary magnetic resonance angiography (MRA) have been substantially improved, a technique that merely allows direct visualization of the coronary arteries can be considered a controversial topic. In the following chapter this technique is discussed, stressing the often difficult procedure of acquiring motion-free images, but also the difficulties in of visualizing a diseased artery and the lack of a functional assessment of the severity of ischemic heart disease. Its role against a more functional MRI approach or coronary multislice computed tomography (MSCT) angiography is looked upon and several indications that seem useful in clinical practice are discussed.

J. Bogaert et al. (eds.), *Clinical Cardiac MRI*, Medical Radiology. Diagnostic Imaging,
DOI: 10.1007/174_2011_399, © Springer-Verlag Berlin Heidelberg 2012

1 Introduction

Ischemic heart disease remains the leading cause of morbidity and mortality in the developed countries, and the World Health Organization estimates that it will be the leading cause of morbidity and mortality worldwide in 2020 (Reddy and Yusuf 1998). Catheter-based X-ray coronary angiography remains the technique of choice for detecting, quantifying and treating atherosclerotic coronary lesions. Next to its invasive nature, it has been recognized, since the late 1980s, that coronary catheterization itself does not allow the recognition of the presence or absence of coronary atherosclerosis itself, only significant luminal changes which have occurred as a result of end stage complications of the disease process. Much technical progress and clinical experience in the use of magnetic resonance (MR) imaging and multislice computed tomography (MSCT) in the last decade has opened the door toward non-invasive diagnostic studies of the coronary arteries. Although interest in MR coronary angiography might have waned in the previous years, in the light of the tremendous advances in CT, it still offers diverse strategies for studying coronary artery lesions, the effect of these lesions on the vessel diameter, while MR flow techniques can be applied to assess the severity of a stenotic lesion on the distal vascular bed. Coronary MR imaging techniques can also be part of a broader cardiac investigation, where within a single MR imaging study, valuable and often unique information can be obtained with regard to ventricular function, myocardial perfusion and myocardial viability in patients with ischemic heart disease. In this chapter, several MR strategies currently used will be discusssed. In addition, the current and potential clinical indications, as well as the role of MR imaging compared to MSCT, are highlighted.

2 Challenges for Non-invasive Coronary Artery Imaging

Catheter-based or X-ray coronary angiography is the indisputable reference standard for the detection of coronary artery stenosis. It consists of a photographic approach with selective injection of iodinated contrast material into the left (LCA) and right coronary artery (RCA). Images are obtained with a high temporal resolution (60 images/s) and a high-spatial resolution (0.1×0.1 mm^2). Projectional images of the coronary arteries are obtained without interference of the cardiac chambers in different standardized image planes. Computed techniques are available for quantitative analysis of coronary artery stenoses (QCA techniques). The fluoroscopic approach allows cine viewing and provides information about coronary flow patterns (e.g. TIMI flow patterns after revascularisation of coronary artery stenoses). X-ray coronary angiography is not only a diagnostic technique, but is often used for therapeutic procedures such as balloon angioplasty, coronary artery stenting and more recently the injection of autologous stem cells in patients with an acute myocardial infarction. Nevertheless, X-ray coronary angiography has several shortcomings. For example, since coronary atheromatosis is a diffuse disease, expression of the degree of coronary artery narrowing to the caliber of adjacent "normal" segments yields the risk of underestimation of the severity of coronary artery stenosis. The angiographic or luminographic type of imaging, obtained by X-ray angiography, provides no information about the presence of wall remodeling or about the coronary plaque morphology. Thus, vulnerable plaques, with often a mild or moderate narrowing of the coronary artery lumen, are not detected on coronary angiography. The catheter-based approach has a significant morbidity (e.g. coronary or aortic dissection) and mortality, and because of its invasive nature is not applicable as a screening technique. Also, there are a significant number of negative studies (up to 25%) in patients with a clinical suspicion of coronary artery disease. Other important issues to consider are the X-ray dose, the injection of a considerable amount of iodinated contrast material and the expense of the procedure.

A good non-invasive alternative to conventional coronary angiography has to meet several challenges. Coronary arteries are small, tortuous vessels (size 2–5 mm), embedded in the epicardial fat and located on a curved cardiac surface. Coronary artery anatomy and its branching pattern are highly variable. Coronary artery flow and velocity patterns are complex with differences between LCA and RCA. Furthermore, when significant coronary artery stenosis is present, the contribution of collateral flow should be assessed. Coronary artery motion, due to respiration and cardiac pump function, is a major problem for non-invasive imaging techniques and has a strong impact on image quality. As a consequence, non-invasive coronary artery imaging is a compromise between various parameters: spatial resolution, acquisition window, volume coverage, signal-to-noise ratio (SNR) and contrast-to-noise ratio (CNR). Other issues such as metal artifacts due to coronary stents or bypass clips, or coronary atherosclerotic calcifications should be considered.

3 History of Coronary MR Imaging

The quest for successful MR coronary angiography (MRCA) started in the early 1990s. Since then, huge progress has been made, starting from hardly detectable coronary arteries toward a reliable and reproducible assessment of large portions of the coronary artery tree in a reasonable imaging time in the current era. A brief review of the history of coronary MR angiography gives the reader a good idea of the technical evolution, and the approaches and strategies that have been used to study the coronary arteries. Although most review papers use "generations" to define the major steps in coronary MR angiography, this subdivision in different generations is somewhat artificial and prone to confusion and discussion (Bunce et al. 1999; Wielopolski et al. 2000; Fayad et al. 2000). For example, the navigator-echo ("second" generation) and breath-hold ("third" generation) techniques are two different approaches that are still used for coronary MR angiography, but based on their subdivision "third" generation techniques might be falsely considered as superior to "second" generation techniques.

Although imaging of the coronary arteries by MR was initially described in 1987 (Paulin et al. 1987; Gomes et al. 1987), with mere visualization of small segments of native coronary vessels and bypass grafts, the real start of coronary artery imaging by MR, usually called coronary MR angiography or magnetic resonance coronary angiography (MRCA), coincided with the introduction of ultrafast imaging techniques in 1991. These techniques relied upon a combination of segmental acquisition of data in κ-space to minimize cardiac motion, and the use of a single breath-hold to minimize respiratory motion artifacts (Atkinson and Edelman 1991). Edelman and colleagues used a two-dimensional (2D) ECG-triggered κ-space segmented MR sequence to study coronary arteries (Edelman et al. 1991). Its subsequent value for visualizing the course of the coronary arteries and detecting coronary artery disease has been evaluated by several groups (Manning et al. 1993; Duerinckx and Urman 1994; Mohiaddin et al. 1996; Nitatori et al. 1995; Post et al. 1997; Yoshino et al. 1997) (Fig. 1). For several reasons, this so-called first generation of techniques has been totally abandoned. Two-dimensional imaging techniques are not well suited to the study of the tortuous course of coronary arteries. Only portions of the coronary arteries can be visualized within each breath-hold and the inconsistency of breath-hold position makes coronary artery imaging, even for experienced investigators in the field, a difficult task. The absence of dedicated cardiac receiver coils necessitated the examination of patients in a prone position, which most found uncomfortable and difficult to sustain. Furthermore, the high number of repeated breath-holds was usually too exhausting to study cardiac patients in a comfortable way.

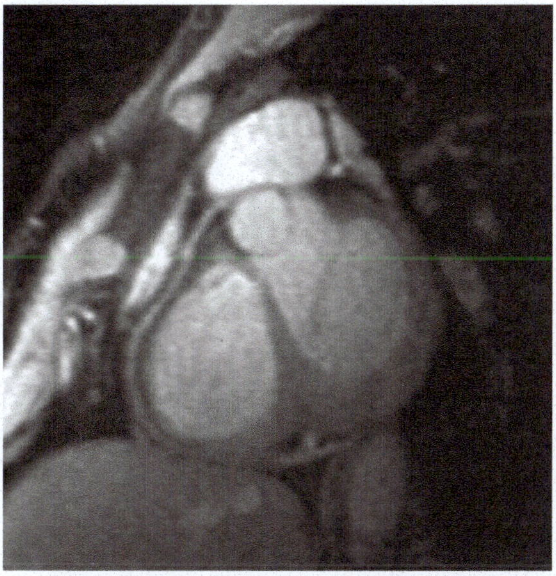

Fig. 1 2D coronary MR angiography of the RCA using the breath-hold segmented κ-space spoiled-GE-technique

Because of the severe limitations of the 2D breath-hold approach, investigators have explored several alternatives to overcome these problems and improve image quality. They can be summarized as: (a) three-dimensional (3D) imaging approaches, (b) techniques

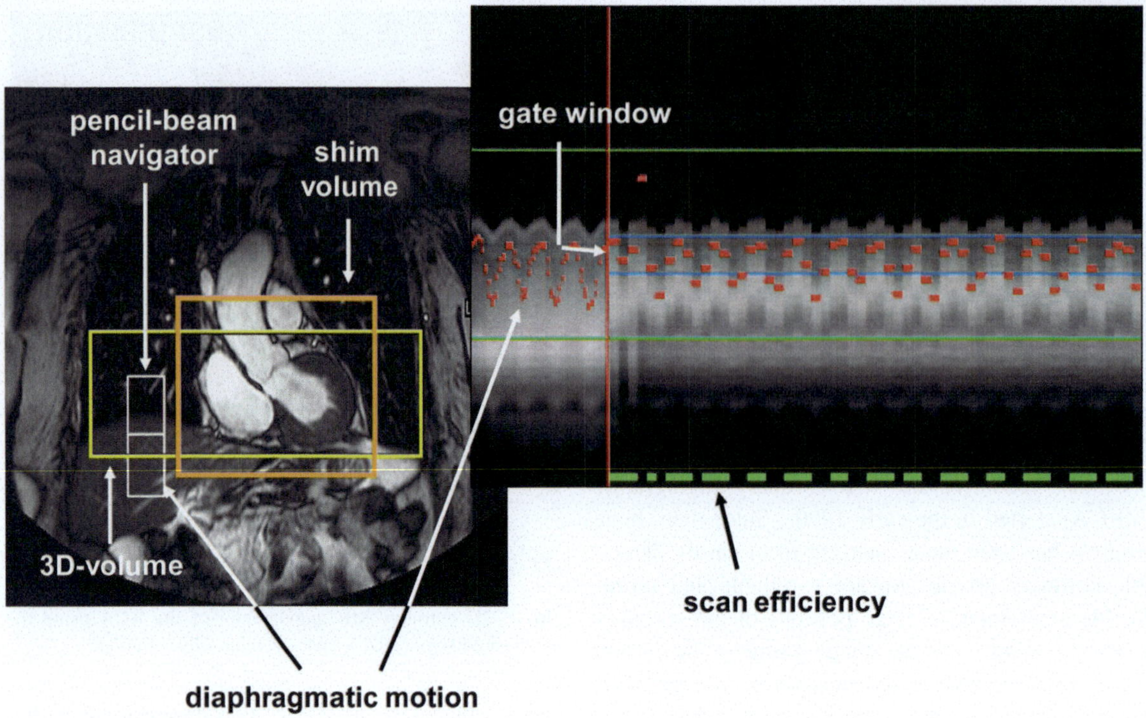

Fig. 2 Real-time prospective NE technique. Coronal scout MR image (*left*). The pencil-beam navigator is positioned on the dome of the right hemidiaphragm. The up and downward motions of the diaphragm is shown as a *red curve* (*right*). The gating window, indicated by the *blue lines*, determines whether or not the shots are accepted for data reconstruction. The scan efficiency is indicated by the *green line*

to suppress respiratory motion either by using navigators or acquisition during breath-hold and (c) use of intravascular contrast agents. Three-dimensional imaging offers the advantages of higher SNR, shorter echo times, more isotropic voxel resolution and the ability to examine the data set with a multiplanar reformatting technique. Moreover, the complex course of the coronary arteries necessitates a 3D-approach. Although, the initial attempts at using signal averaging (without breath-holding) for 3D coronary imaging did not produce very good results (Hofman et al. 1995), Scheidegger and colleagues were the first to use sophisticated 3D imaging display technology (Scheidegger et al. 1994, 1996). This and other pioneering work on 3D coronary MR imaging has formed the basis for the development of currently used 3D coronary MR angiography techniques. More recent improvements in MR imaging technology with stronger gradient systems, shorter rise times and more sophisticated ECG triggering devices have further contributed to current high-quality submillimeter 3D visualization of the coronary arteries.

Navigator echoes (NE) rely upon an MR pulse to determine the motion of the diaphragm (a surrogate of respiratory motion). This enables MR images to be acquired during continuous regular breathing and open the way for higher spatial resolution coronary MR angiography with increased patient comfort. Navigator techniques were first described in 1993–1994 (Wang et al. 1996), but because the initial proposed implementations had severe shortcomings, they have undergone several improvements (Danias et al. 1997; McConnell et al. 1997). Although this technique has been implemented on existing 2D coronary MR angiography techniques, to improve image quality either by providing feedback to the patient for repeated breath-holds (as to when to hold his/her breath), or by feeding information back to the MR computer, NEs have been generally used in combination with 3D coronary MR angiography techniques. The NE pulse most often determines the motion of the diaphragm, but in some implementations it directly monitors the motion of portions of the left ventricular wall. For the repeated breath-

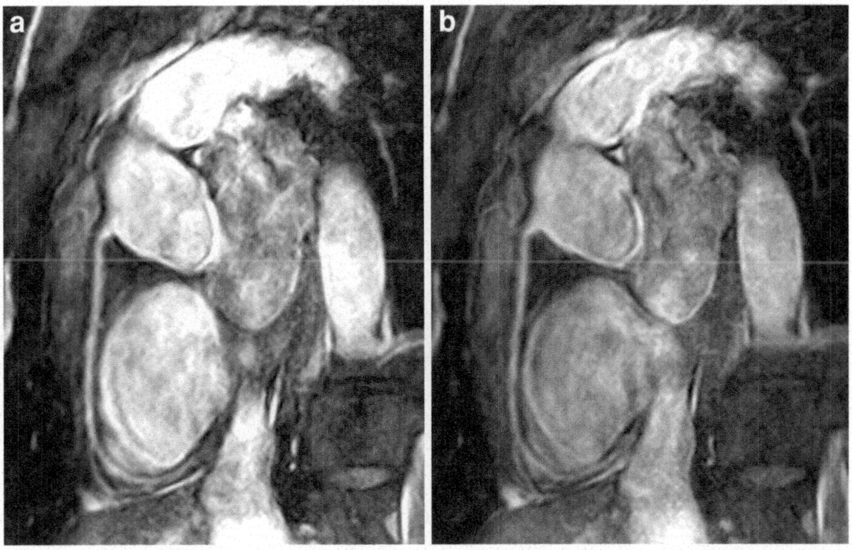

Fig. 3 Comparison between 3D coronary MR angiography (b-SSFP technique) using the breath-hold approach (**a**) and NE approach (**b**). In both approaches the number of shots acquired per cardiac cycle was 32 (acquisition window length: 160 ms)

holding versions, inconsistent breath-holding is no longer a problem, as the patient receives feedback as to when to stop breathing (Fig. 2). For the non-breath-hold versions, the regularity of the breathing pattern during the long scan acquisition (sometimes up to 15 min) is important. It has been recommended that: the navigator-echo window be placed around end-expiratory position; subjects should not sleep; and scan efficiency should be monitored and if necessary the navigator-echo window repositioned (Taylor et al. 1997). Because of these and similar recommendations, many adaptations and improvements to NE schemes have been made to improve their efficacy, including adaptive windowing (to correct for upward creep of the diaphragm in the supine position after 15–20 min) and the use of three orthogonal navigator echoes (to minimize motion in all three directions) (Danias et al. 1997; McConnell et al. 1997; Taylor et al. 1997). Once implemented, this technique requires less expertise and training because a 3D transaxial slab covering the top of the heart and aortic root can be acquired and images can be analyzed later. Potential problems with the NE coronary MR angiography technique are: (a) the length of each acquisition, up to 12–15 min in some cases, versus a single 15–20 s breath-hold, (b) difficulty obtaining a good NE position (up to 50% failure in normal volunteers in initial studies).

Supplements in terms of motion compensating algorithms to navigator-gated acquisitions have also been developed to improve the efficiency, robustness and accuracy of these acquisitions, such as motion adaptive gating (MAG; Langreck et al. 2005). These algorithms improve feasibility and scan efficiency without reduction of image quality and can be routinely used for MR coronary artery imaging with navigator techniques (Fig. 3).

Breath-hold 3D techniques (so-called "third-generation"), are an alternative to NE techniques, and were first described in 1995 by Piotr Wielopolski (Wielopolski et al. 1995). These techniques may provide the ultimate compromise between user-friendliness and acquisition speeds. The entire coronary anatomy can be acquired in a single breath-hold with isotropic resolution (Fig. 4). Using a segmented echoplanar imaging (EPI) technique, with thin slabs oriented along the course of the coronaries, high-spatial resolution images of the coronaries can be obtained in a single breath-hold. This approach using small volume scan acquisitions oriented along the coronaries is called VCATS (volume coronary arteriography using targeted scans) (Wielopolski et al. 1998). Other groups have used a fat-suppressed 3D-segmented ECG-triggered TurboFLASH, with acquisition of small volumes during breath-hold.

Dynamic contrast-enhanced MR angiography (CE-MRA), first described by Martin Prince, has totally changed the way thoracic and body MR angiography are performed today (Prince 1994). Although CE-MRA started out with relatively long acquisition times (over a min), it can now be used within very short breath-hold periods (7–23 s breath-holds to study the aorta or the

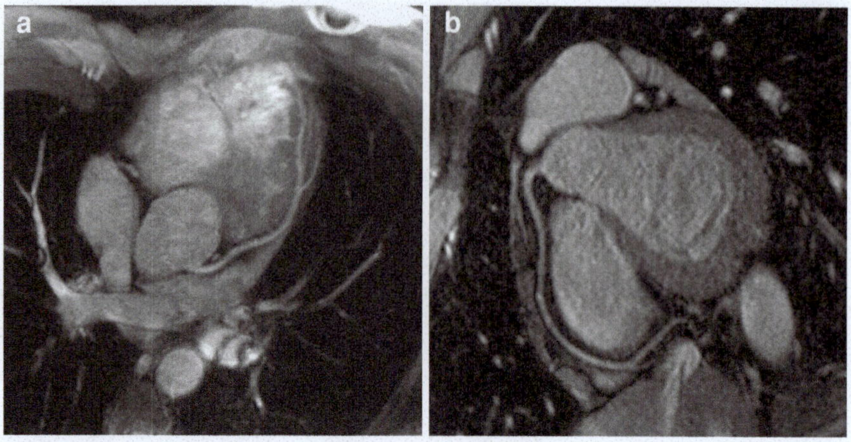

Fig. 4 Breath-hold 3D coronary MR angiography using the b-SSFP (True-FISP technique) (Courtesy: Debiao Li, PhD, Northwestern University, Chicago, USA). LM and LAD (**a**), and RCA (**b**). The length per breath-hold was 24–30 s

pulmonary arteries). The same non-ECG-triggered technique was applied for native coronary artery and CABG imaging (van Rossum et al. 1997; Vrachliotis et al. 1997). In order to acquire ECG-triggered MRA of native coronary vessels, pulse sequences with faster acquisition rates, κ-space data segmentation, data interpolation, and other technical tricks are required.

Initial experience with extravascular MR contrast agents indicated that very high doses of gadolinium would be needed for 2D-breath-hold coronary MR angiography. With bolus arrival timing to catch the first pass of the gadolinium contrast agent, image quality improvements have been obtained (improved SNR and CNR) for the 3D coronary MR angiography techniques.

4 Coronary Artery Motion and Acquisition Window

Another major source of coronary artery motion besides bulk motion of the heart due to respiration is motion induced by cardiac pump activity and pulsatile arterial flow patterns. With an ultrashort acquisition time per image (approximately 15–30 ms for digital images), coronary artery motion is perfectly "frozen" on X-ray coronary angiography. Real-time high-frequency imaging of the coronary arteries during injection of contrast media, allows not only the acquisition of sharp coronary artery images, but also the visualization of coronary artery motion during the cardiac cycle and respiration (Wang et al. 1999). The acquisition length for coronary MR angiography images is unfortunately too long to freeze coronary artery motion. The total measurement time necessary to fill κ-space takes about 2.6 s for a breath-hold 3D coronary MR angiography sequence (using an acquisition length of 120 ms per heart beat and a total of 22 heartbeats), and for the free-breathing approach approximately 13 s (using a data acquisition length or "shot duration" of 80 ms per heart beat, and a total of 164 shots). Different strategies have been developed that cope with these motion problems and attempt to reduce vessel blurring.

Cardiac motion, and thus also coronary artery motion, can be suppressed by synchronizing the image acquisition to the repetitive pattern of cardiac contraction and relaxation. This is usually achieved by ECG triggering (the different currently used ECG-techniques are discussed in "Cardiac MR Physics" and "Practical Set-Up"). Next, the length of data acquisition per heart beat needs to be adjusted to reduce cardiac motion artifacts. This can be done by varying the number of refocusing echoes (for fast spin-echo sequences), or the number of shots (for gradient-echo sequences). Several other methods to reduce the acquisition length will be discussed below. Whereas this adjustment is important for achieving the best image quality for assessment of gross cardiac anatomy or cardiac function, it becomes crucial when studying small structures such as the coronary arteries since the faintest residual motion will lead to image blurring and unsharpness.

Assessment of the coronary artery motion pattern and velocities with biplane conventional angiography, EBCT and MR imaging have shown a highly variable pattern throughout the cardiac cycle, with important differences between the left and right coronary artery systems, and with a large variation between individuals (Wang et al. 1999; Achenbach et al. 2000; Kim et al. 2001). Coronary artery displacement and velocities are much higher for the RCA than for the LAD. This can be explained by the anatomical location of the RCA within the anterior atrioventricular groove, which is prone to larger displacement and higher velocities due to the base to apex contraction of the heart during systole, which is not seen for the LAD in the anterior interventricular groove. Achenbach and colleagues showed that coronary artery motion is most pronounced during early systole, early diastole and atrial contraction; and minimal during isovolumic relaxation and diastasis (Achenbach et al. 2000). Diastasis, or the mid-diastolic period between early ventricular filling and atrial contraction, is a relative rest period with minimal cardiac motion. Diastasis is typically preceded by a gradual slowing of motion, as a result of the normalization of pressures between the atria and ventricles, but is always followed by abrupt motion, due to the onset of atrial contraction. Wang et al. found a huge variation in the length of this rest period, ranging from 66 to 333 ms with a mean of 161 ms for the LCA and from 66 to 200 ms with a mean of 120 ms for the RCA (Wang et al. 1999). The length of this rest period is closely related to the cardiac frequency (Wu et al. 2007). The duration of the rest period decreases as the heart rate increases. For a heart rate less than 45 beats per min, the rest period is approximately 200 and 300 ms for the right and left coronary artery, respectively. As the heart rate increases from 45 to 65 beats per minute, the rest period decreases to about 70 ms for both coronary arteries. For a heart rate greater than 65 beats per minute, the rest period stays at 70 ms. The findings of Wang and colleagues have important implications for coronary MR angiography. First, in patients with a normal heart rate the rest period is short and the data acquisition should be limited and synchronized as best as possible to this brief rest period. Second, in patients with heart rates below 55–60 beats per minute longer acquisition times can be used, thus enabling reduction in the total acquisition time without deterioration in image quality (Tangcharoen et al. 2008).

Precise determination of the timing of the rest period within the cardiac cycle is essential especially in patients with heart rates above 55–60 min. Different approaches have been used to estimate this period of diastasis. Most of the earlier studies on coronary MR angiography used a fixed delay of 500 ms with an adjustment of ±100 ms according to heart rate. Empirical estimations for mid-diastole can be calculated with the Weissler or Stuber formulas (Weissler et al. 1968; Stuber et al. 1999). The trigger delay in the Stuber empirical formula is obtained as: trigger delay (ms) = [(RR interval (ms)–350) × 0.3] + 350. This definition takes advantage of the relatively constant duration of the systolic part of the cardiac cycle (±350 ms). This trigger delay was adjusted to sample the low κ-space profiles in mid-diastole. Empirical formulae have the advantage that they are easy to implement into the coronary MR angiography sequence. However, because these estimations are based on data from heart sounds or electrocardiography, they do or might not represent the actual cardiac motion that is occurring during data acquisition. Direct assessment of the optimal delay for coronary MR angiographic data acquisition window in the cardiac cycle is therefore probably the most correct approach. Direct assessment can be obtained by a breath-hold cine pre-scan at a fixed location (e.g. long-axis scan through the proximal or mid-portion of the RCA and LCx; Fig. 5) with a high temporal resolution (Foo et al. 2000; Kim et al. 2001a; Jahnke et al. 2005) or by an ECG-triggered navigator cardiac motion scan (Wang et al. 2001). The Beth Israel group found a significant improvement in RCA imaging using a subject-specific determination of the diastasis period (compared to the heart-rate-dependent delay) (Kim et al. 2001). Imaging of the RCA vessel wall was only feasible with the subject-specific method, while the coronary wall could not be identified with the heart-rate dependent formula.

Determination of the length of the rest period might be interesting since in patients with long coronary rest periods, extended acquisitions windows can be used with consequently shortened scanning times (Fig. 6). In a study by Plein and colleagues from Leeds, a subject-specific cardiac acquisition window in combination with motion-adapted respiratory gating was used (Plein et al. 2003). On a long-axis cine MR pre-scan through the atrioventricular grooves the timing and duration of the rest period in each subject were determined and the acquisition length was subsequently adjusted. The motion-adapted gating used a 2-mm acceptance window for the central 35% of κ-space and a 6-mm window for the outer 65% of κ-space. Compared to the conventional

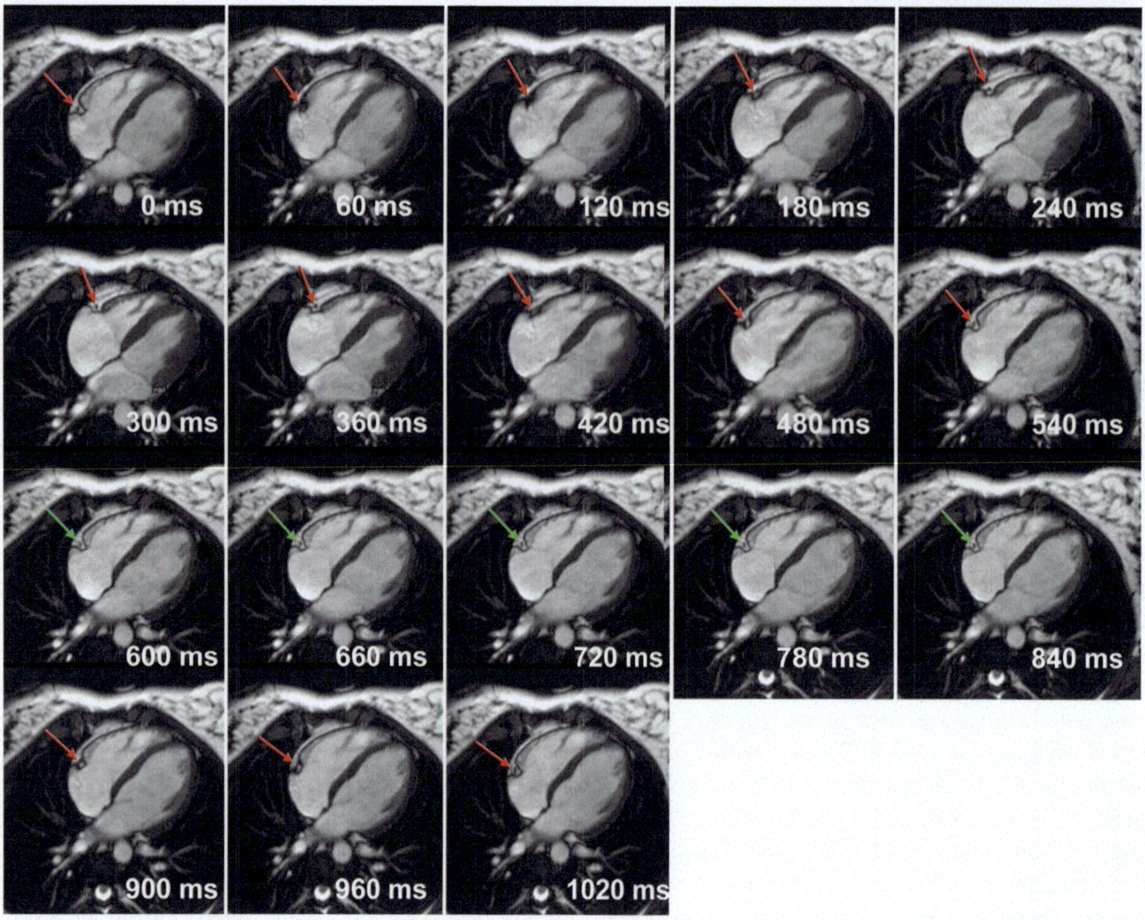

Fig. 5 In-plane motion pattern of the RCA during the cardiac cycle in a normal volunteer with a heart rate of 56 beats per min. Axial cine MRI using the b-SSFP technique (time frame 60 ms). The *arrow* indicates the RCA in the anterior atrioventricular groove. The data acquisition should be adjusted to the period of minimal cardiac motion, i.e. diastasis. In this volunteer the ideal period for imaging is between 600 and 840 ms after the R-wave (*green arrow*). The other cardiac phases are characterized by substantial motion, and are consequently suboptimal for coronary artery imaging (*red arrow*)

technique (consisting of a fixed acquisition window of 73 ms, and a timing of the rest period estimated by the Stuber empirical formula, in combination with a fixed 5 mm gating window at end-expiration with real-time correction for the accepted data within the gating window), scanning times with the adaptive technique were reduced by a factor of 2.3 for the RCA, and by a factor of 2.2 for the LCA without loss in image quality. This was mainly the result of longer rest periods up to 200 ms, usually found in patients with heartbeats less than 60 beats per min.

Another interesting approach to reduce cardiac motion effects is to adjust the κ-space sampling with the motion amplitude (Wang and Ehman 2000). The idea is that the center of κ-space, where the majority of MR signal resides, is sampled during the quiescent mid-diastolic period, and the edge of κ-space is sampled before and after mid-diastole. The traditionally used centric κ-space sampling, in contrast, maximizes signal at the center of κ-space by acquiring it at the beginning of the acquisition window when the spins are fresh. This centric view order can contain substantial cardiac motion effects, because of residual motion of the early, fast filling one. Faster data acquisition not only shortens the scan time, but might be beneficial for the image quality since the acquisition window length can be reduced. The recent introduction of new generation MR scanners with

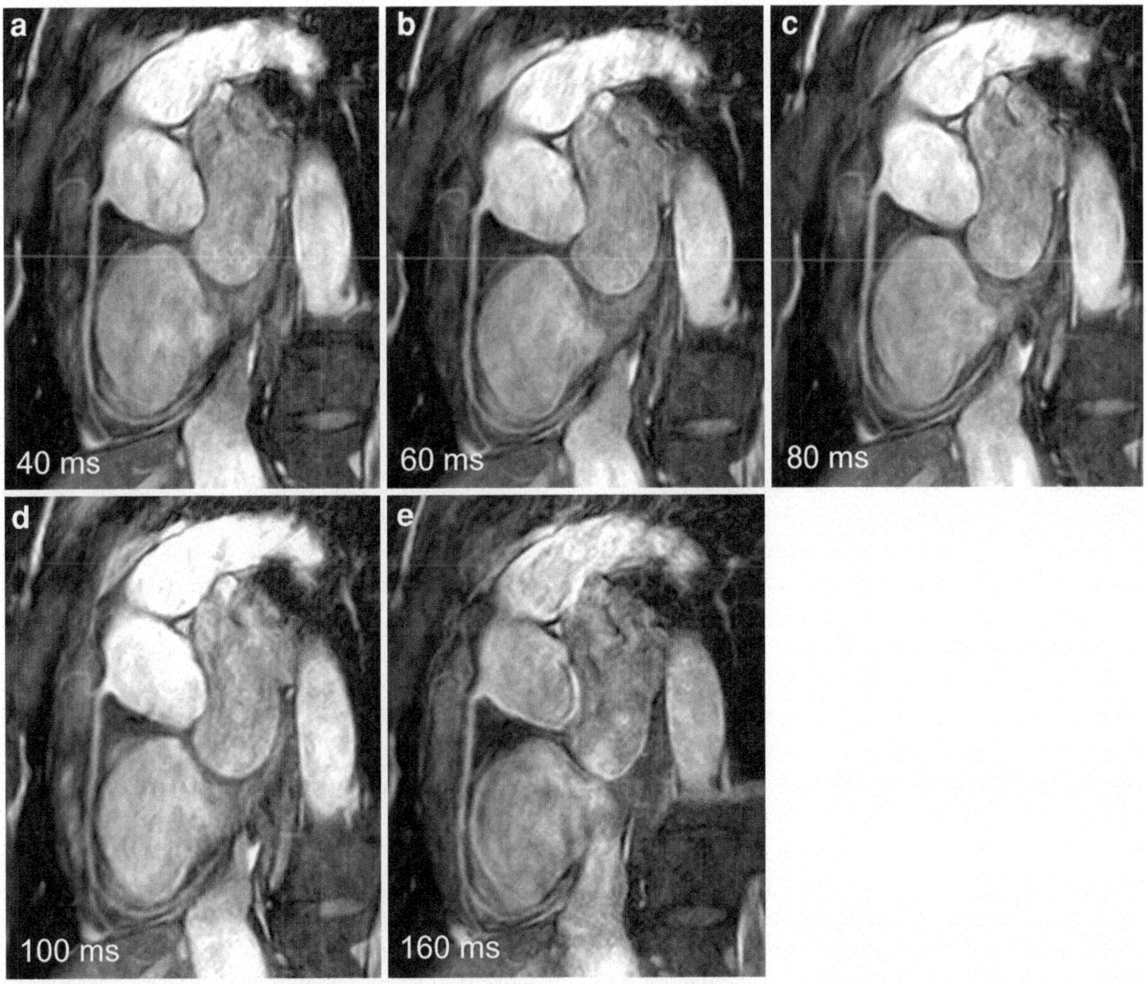

Fig. 6 Impact of acquisition window length. 3D free-breathing coronary MR angiography (b-SSFP technique) of RCA using an acquisition window of 40 ms (**a**), 60 ms (**b**), 80 ms (**c**), 100 ms (**d**), and 160 ms (**e**). The gain in image quality and vessel sharpness is substantial when using an acquisition window length less than 100 ms. However, it should be realized that further reduction in acquisition window length significantly prolongs the total acquisition time

stronger gradients (≥30 mT/m) and faster gradient switching systems have led to a significant shortening of sequence parameters (such as TR and TE).

Hybrid gradient-echo/EPI sequences are an effective method to reduce scan times. However, in the heart the EPI technique is prone to artifacts. Partial Fourier encoding can be used to halve the acquisition time and obtain reasonable coverage and in-plane spatial resolution (Wielopolski et al. 1998). However, partial Fourier acquisitions can produce signal intensity changes and distortions in the image, especially in gradient-echo acquisitions. Another, new and interesting approach to shorten the acquisition time per heartbeat, and therefore to increase image sharpness, is by using parallel imaging (e.g. SENSE, GRAPPA). Sensitivity Encoding (SENSE) uses multiple MR receive coil elements to encode spatial information in addition to traditional gradient encoding (Pruessmann et al. 2001; Van den Brink et al. 2003). Requiring less gradient encodings translates into shorter scan times, which is beneficial for coronary MR angiography. Acceleration of the coronary MR angiography acquisition might be obtained by simultaneous acquisition of multiple rather than one 3D stack (Manke et al. 2001). This approach uses not only diastasis, but also the period of isovolumic relaxation for image acquisition. One 3D stack is positioned through the LCA and measured during isovolumic relaxation, the second stack covering the RCA measured in mid-diastole. This two-stack approach yields a total scan time reduction of 50% with an image quality equivalent to standard single-stack coronary MR angiography.

5 Contrast Generation

One of the most difficult technical issues for coronary MR angiography is the differentiation of the coronary artery lumen from the surrounding tissues, in particular epicardial fat. Different methods to increase the visibility of the coronary arteries have been explored. Nowadays, a combination of techniques is used. In summary, generation of signal in coronary arteries is usually based on differences in physical properties between the coronary artery blood and surrounding structures. This can be related to differences in flow patterns, or to differences in T1- or T2-relaxation behavior between blood and surrounding tissues. Differences in relaxation behavior between tissues can be enhanced by using paramagnetic contrast agents. The visualization of coronary arteries can be indirectly enhanced by suppressing the signal of the surrounding tissues (e.g. fat saturation techniques, magnetization-transfer-contrast techniques, T2-preparation pulse). Other techniques such as spin labeling use another approach to generate contrast in the coronary artery lumen and might be a valuable alternative. The visualization of coronary arteries will also benefit from the use of other dedicated cardiac surface coils and techniques such as CLEAR (i.e. Constant LEvel AppeaRance).

5.1 Sequence Design

The generation of "bright blood" in the coronary arteries can be based on different mechanisms. In 1991, Edelman and colleagues described a segmented κ-space 2D FLASH (fast low angle shot technique) gradient-echo sequence to study the coronary arteries in a single breath-hold (Edelman et al. 1991). Characteristics of this sequence are the small flip angle of the excitation pulse and the use of a gradient spoiler at the end of each repetition time (TR) to destroy the remaining transverse magnetization and thus create T1-weighted contrast ("spoiled-GE" technique). For 2D imaging, the creation of contrast between flowing blood and surrounding stationary tissues is based on the inflow of fully relaxed spins and the progressive saturation of the stationary spins in the image slice—described as "inflow enhancement". The highest contrast is obtained with through-plane flow, while in-plane vessel segments suffer from decreased signal within the vessel. Before the introduction of CE-MRA, 2D-FLASH was a commonly used technique for studying human vessels by MR imaging. As discussed above, the applicability of 2D techniques for coronary artery imaging, however, is limited. The 3D-FLASH technique, as presented by Li and co-workers in 1993, overcomes many of the limitations of the 2D approach for coronary artery imaging, but suffers from inherent problems related to sequence design, especially if acquistion of data is performed during breath-holding. Similar to 2D imaging, for 3D imaging the magnetization of blood has a large signal at the beginning of the 3D acquisition, but is progressively saturated for each subsequent excitation experienced by the blood in the imaging volume. By using a central ordering encoding of the 3D section optimal signal can be achieved (Holsinger and Riederer 1990). To speed up data acquisition for breath-hold coronary MR angiography, the repetition time needs to be shortened at the expense of a larger bandwidth, and as a consequence lower SNR, which may be a limiting factor. Moreover, due to the magnetization recovery during the trigger delay time, the images have limited blood inflow-related signal enhancement. Therefore, the contrast between blood and myocardium is often not adequate for clear visualization of certain coronary segments. T2-preparation or magnetization-transfer contrast (MTC) is necessary to improve contrast but at the expense of reduced SNR. Injection of contrast media is necessary to shorten the blood T1, and thus to improve SNR and CNR (Deshpande et al. 2001). Free-breathing 3D-FLASH or TFE (turbo-field-echo) coronary MR angiography is much less restricted by the need to speed up data acquisition, allowing the use of smaller bandwidths and the creation of higher intra-voxel signal without injection of contrast (Stuber et al. 1999).

Truly balanced steady-state free precession (b-SSFP) acquisition of the heart has become feasible with the recent improvements in gradient (shorter

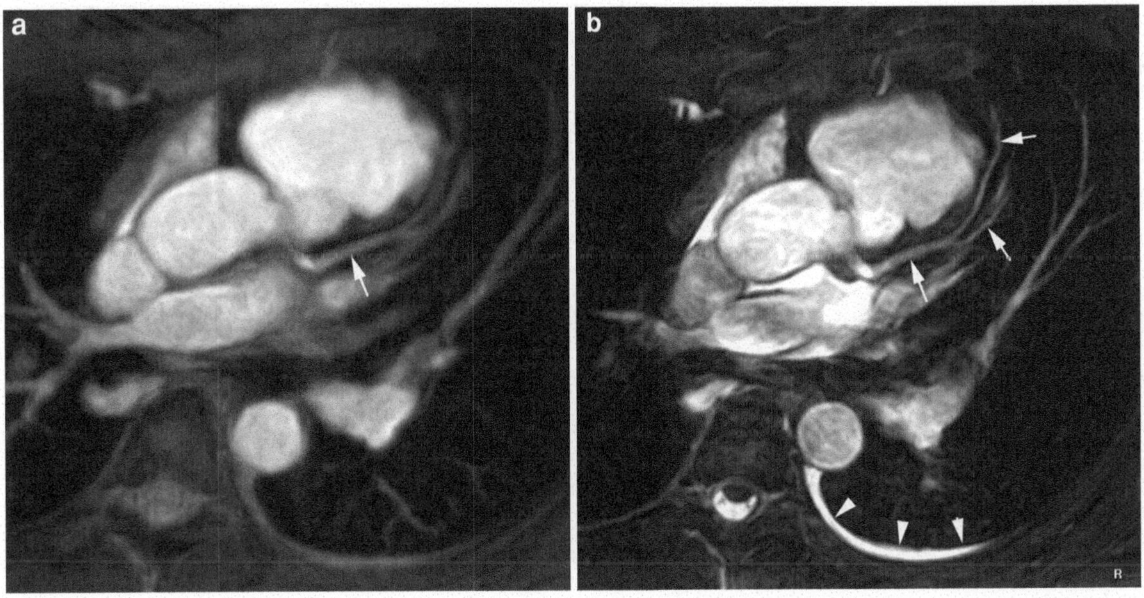

Fig. 7 Coronary MR angiography sequence design, spoiled-GE-technique (**a**) versus b-SSFP technique (**b**). Imaging of the LM and LAD in a normal subject. Improved vessel sharpness and substantially improved visualization of longer portions of LAD and the first diagonal branch (*arrow*) with the b-SSFP technique. Note also the improved depiction of other thoracic vessels such as the pulmonary and mammary arteries. Since the b-SSFP technique is mainly T2-weighted, fluid-containing structures such as pleural effusions (*arrowheads*) show much higher signal intensities and are therefore better depicted than on the spoiled-GE-technique (partially adapted from Giorgi et al. Am J Roentgenol 2003, 179:901–910)

repetition times) and field shimming capabilities (Carr et al. 2001). The commercial name of the balanced-SSFP sequence differs between vendors: True–FISP (fast imaging in steady-state precession—Siemens), balanced-TFE (balanced-turbo-field-echo—Philips), and FIESTA (fast imaging employing steady-state acquisition—General Electric). Because of significant improvement in blood SNR and blood-myocardium CNR as compared to FLASH, these sequences have been recently evaluated for both breath-hold (Deshpande et al. 2001) and free-breathing (Giorgi et al. 2002; Spuentrup et al. 2002) coronary MR angiography. In b-SSFP imaging, the transverse magnetization is maintained between successive RF pulses because the net gradient moments are zero in all three directions and no RF spoiling is implemented. The signal intensity in the b-SSFP sequence is T_2/T_1 weighted, and the contrast between blood and myocardium is therefore enhanced because blood has a much higher T_2/T_1 than myocardium. Higher SNR are obtained than in magnetization-spoiled techniques (FLASH and TFE-technique) because the coherent transverse magnetization contributes to the signal in successive TRs. Giorgi and colleagues compared a 3D-balanced-TFE sequence with a 3D-TFE sequence in volunteers (Fig. 7). The image quality of both the RCA and LCA was significantly better for the balanced sequence, and significantly longer segments of the coronary arteries and more side branches were visualized compared to the TFE sequence (Giorgi et al. 2002). These findings were supported by a study of Spuentrup and colleagues who also reported an improvement in coronary artery border delineation (Spuentrup et al. 2002). Compared to the TFE-technique, the balanced-TFE-technique with "T_2-like" contrast characteristics enables an improvement in differentiation between small epicardial coronary arteries (medium high signal intensity) and adjacent pericardial sac (high signal intensity) (Bogaert and Duerinckx 1995; Giorgi et al. 2002).

As an alternative to the "bright-blood" techniques, Stuber and colleagues recently proposed a free-breathing 3D high-resolution "black-blood" fast spin-echo coronary MR angiography sequence. A modified type of this sequence is also used for

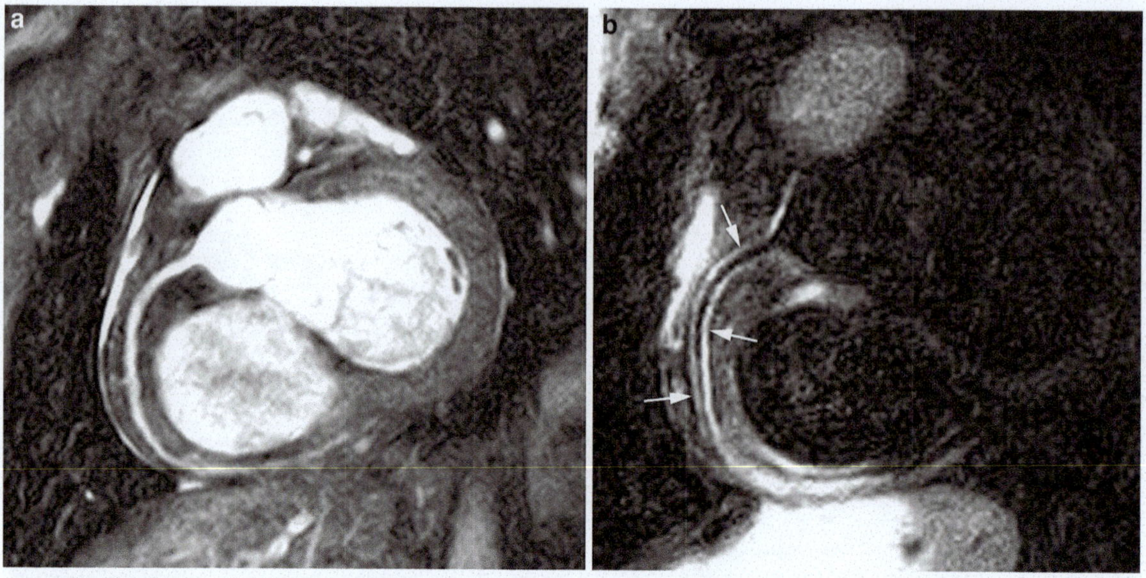

Fig. 8 Coronary artery wall imaging using the dark-blood 4th order local inversion 3D spiral imaging technique. Bright-blood (**a**) versus dark-blood (**b**) technique of the RCA in a normal subject. The CA wall is shown as a thin (curvilinear) line (*arrows*) between the dark CA lumen and hypo-intense epicardial fat. (Courtesy: Matthias Stuber PhD, Johns Hopkins University Medical School, Baltimore, USA)

coronary wall imaging. Three-dimensional spin-echo coronary sequences have intrinsically higher SNR than "bright-blood" sequences, which may be traded for improved spatial resolution. Currently, in-plane-resolutions up to 400 μm are achievable. Other advantages of the spin-echo technique are the reduced susceptibility to turbulent flow in regions of focal stenosis, a reduced sensitivity to artifacts induced by metallic implants and a high CNR. To create "black-blood" a dual inversion-recovery pre-pulse is applied with an inversion properly chosen to null the signal of in-flowing blood at the level of interest (Fleckenstein et al. 1991). The coronary lumens appear as regions of low signal intensity with surrounding high signal intensity from epicardial fat and myocardium (Fig. 8). The length of the coronary arteries visualized with "black-blood" techniques is comparable with currently available "bright-blood" techniques. Its precise role in patients with coronary artery disease needs further research. For instance, it is not known yet whether the "black-blood" technique is suited to studying coronary artery lesions that have low or no signal on spin-echo sequences such as heavily fibrotic and/or calcified stenotic plaques. The different strategies in sequence design for coronary artery imaging are summarized in Table 1.

5.2 Magnetization Preparation Techniques

The epicardial coronary arteries are embedded in the (sub)epicardial fat. By suppressing the fat signal, contrast between coronary blood pool and the surrounding tissue can be enhanced (Manning et al. 1993). Fat suppression can be achieved by pre-saturation of the longitudinal magnetization of fat prior to imaging (Haase et al. 1985) or by using a spectral selective RF-excitation pulse (Meyer et al. 1990). The latter excites only the water signal within the selected slice. Both have advantages and disadvantages. The pre-saturation method is experimentally simple, but the T_1-relaxation process of the fat signal may hamper its relaxation characteristics, particularly for longer sequences. The use of spectral-selective excitation does not have these disadvantages. However, the use of an RF-excitation pulse between each readout limits the shortest available echo time. This in turn leads to a prolonged acquisition window and may be disadvantageous with respect to T_2* effects, secondary to flow and motion problems that can occur during the long RF pulse. In a study by Börnert and colleagues comparing both fat suppression techniques, no significant differences were found

Table 1 Current strategies used for anatomical assessment of coronary arteries

Breathing motion compensation	navigators
	breath-hold
Contrast enhancement techniques	magnetization-transfer contrast (MTC)
	T2-preparation pulse
	steady-state imaging
	(intravascular) contrast agents
	fat suppression techniques
	arterial spin labeling
Fast imaging techniques	echo-planar imaging (EPI)
	parallel imaging
High-spatial resolution techniques	3D spoiled-GE techniques (TFE/FLASH)
	3D balanced-SSFP (b-TFE/true-FISP/FIESTA)
	3D turbo spin-echo (TSE)
κ-Space filling techniques	3D cartesian
	3D radial
	3D spiral
Volume coverage techniques	CA targeted approach (VCATS)
	whole-heart coronary MR angiography
Black-blood imaging	3D TSE
	3D balanced-SSFP

in objective and subjective image parameters (Börnert et al. 2001). It is however, important to realize that fat has a steady-state signal close to that of blood in b-SSFP imaging because of their similar T_2/T_1 ratios. A spectral-selective fat saturation pre-pulse, however, disturbs the steady-state magnetization and lead to magnetization oscillations, and to off-resonance effects during data acquisition. The subsequent signal fluctuations in κ-space lead to image artifacts such as ghosting and blurring (Deshpande et al. 2001). A substantial reduction in image artifacts, higher SNR and better overall image quality is found when using a linearly increasing flip angle series of dummy pre-pulses during the magnetization preparation (Deshpande et al. 2003). Another benefit of the application of a fat saturation pulse is the suppression of the subcutaneous and mediastinal fat, reducing the breathing artifacts in the coronary MR angiography images (Fig. 9).

Magnetization-transfer contrast (MTC) pulses and T_2 preparation pulses are magnetization prepulses that are useful for improving coronary artery visualization by suppressing the signal of the myocardium. This is especially useful for coronary arteries in close contact with the myocardium (e.g. mid and distal portions of the LAD and the side branches).

The MTC technique, described by Wolff and Balaban, consists in the off-resonance application of low-power RF pulses to selectively saturate hydrogen protons with short T_2 (Wolff and Balaban 1989). A 30–60% drop in myocardial signal was found with the use of MTC pre-pulses. As a result, the contrast difference between tissues with a short (myocardium) and long T_2 (arterial blood) can be enhanced, at the expense of SNR.

The T_2-magnetization preparation scheme, as originally proposed by Brittain and coworkers, is based on the fact that the T_2 of myocardium ($\pm$50 ms) is considerably less than that of arterial blood ($\pm$250 ms) (Brittain et al. 1995). The T_2 prep uses a 90° RF pulse to flip the M_z magnetization vector into the M_{xy} plane and is most beneficial in sequences with low inflow contrast [for further sequence details, see work of Brittain and Botnar (Brittain et al. 1995; Botnar et al. 1999)]. Shea et al. found that a T_2-prep length of approximately 40 ms yielded the best CNR between blood and myocardium without compromising the SNR (Shea et al. 2002). Not only the myocardium but also other tissues with a short T_2 relaxation time are suppressed, for example cardiac veins with deoxygenated blood (20% O_2 saturation, T_2 : 35 ms) and epicardial fat (Botnar et al. 1999). Moreover, both MTC and T_2-preparation pulses decrease the signal from the coronary artery wall providing a more realistic measure of the coronary vessel diameter (Botnar et al. 1999). Since the addition of a T_2-prep pulse has a negative influence on SNR, it is mainly the b-SSFP sequence with a higher SNR than the spoiled gradient-echo sequence that benefits from this T_2-prep pulse because adequate SNR is still available for coronary artery visualization.

5.3 Contrast Agents

Although improved sequence design in combination with magnetization preparation techniques has led to a significant improvement in coronary artery

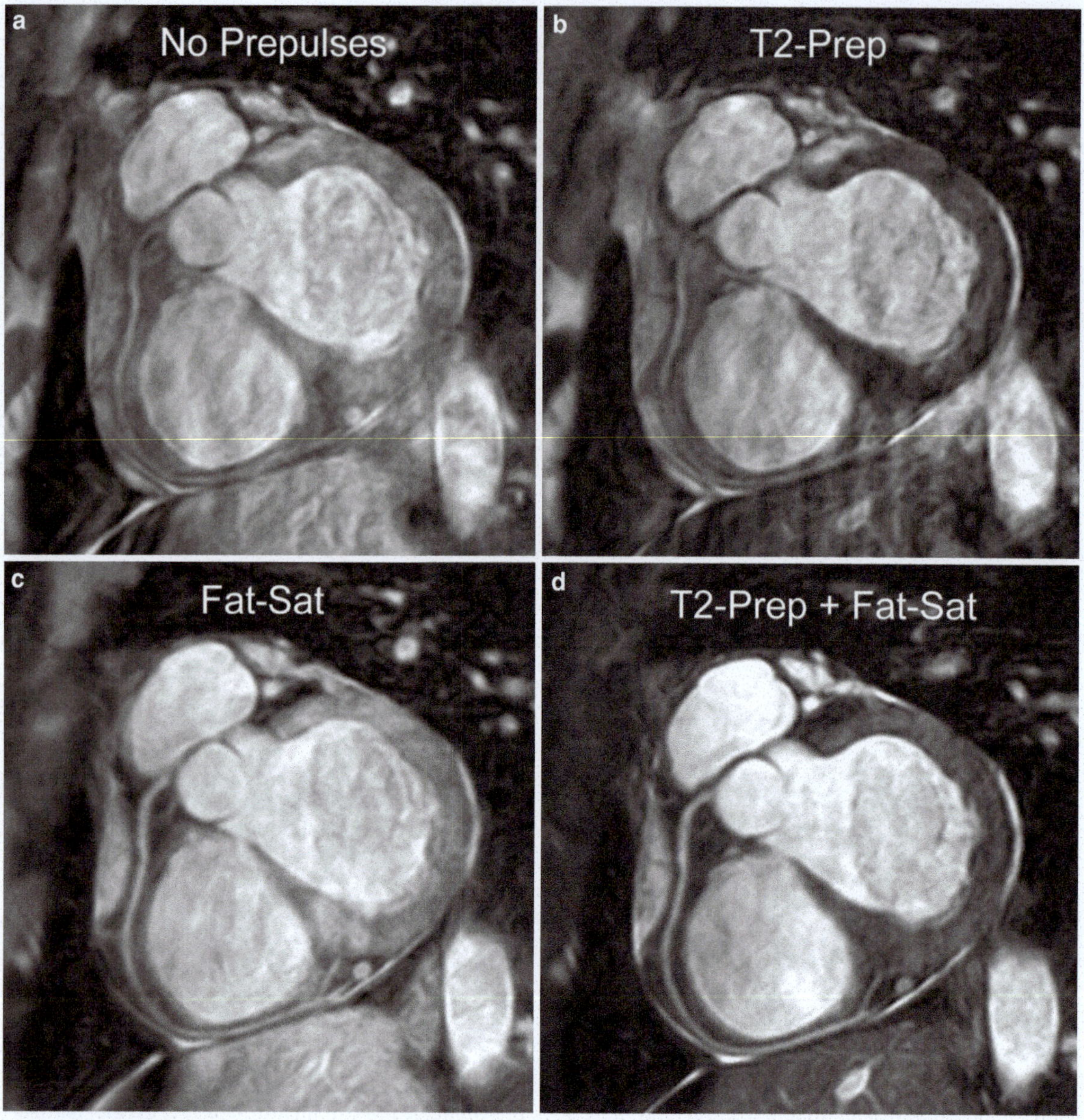

Fig. 9 Beneficial effects of magnetization preparation pulses for coronary artery imaging. 3D free-breathing coronary MR angiography (b-SSFP technique) of the RCA in a normal subject. Compared to the coronary MR angiography sequence without preparation pulses (**a**), use of T2-prep(aration) technique (**b**) suppresses the signal of myocardial tissue, while the fat suppression technique (Fat Sat) (**c**) eliminates the signal of epicardial and mediastinal fat. A combination of both techniques (**d**) substantially improves overall image quality which favours visualization of the coronary arteries

visualization with coronary MR angiography, some issues such as low SNR especially in breath-hold coronary MR angiography are more difficult to solve. Use of T_1-shortening contrast agents in combination with ultrafast 3D MRA techniques, described by Marty Prince in 1994, has become the current standard for MR angiography of the entire body, ranging from the intracerebral vessels to the peripheral arteries (Prince 1994). Also for coronary artery imaging, this technique should be appealing. It provides a flow independent mechanism for blood/background contrast, which is important for visualizing coronary arteries with slow flow and for accurate delineation coronary vessel lumen (Johansson et al. 1999; Lorenz and Johansson 1999; Zheng et al. 2001). Improved blood SNR with efficient T_1-shortening contrast agent may allow for increased spatial resolution and reduced imaging time, which in turn may reduce potential image artifacts caused by cardiac and respiratory motion during a long scan.

In 1998, Goldfarb and Edelman reported an ECG-triggered, breath-hold gadolinium-enhanced 3D-FLASH technique for imaging the coronaries. In a single breath-hold of 24 heartbeats, a 6 cm thick 3D volume positioned transversally at the base of the heart was scanned during the first pass of 40 mL of gadopentate dimeglumine (Goldfarb and Edelman 1998). A pre-scan with a small bolus of contrast is necessary to determine the bolus arrival time. Since only a single slab was obtained in this study, the coverage of the coronary artery tree was limited to its proximal portion. Therefore, Li and colleagues proposed a VCATS technique for better coverage (Li et al. 2001a; Deshpande et al. 2001). Two injections of 20 mL of contrast agent cover the left and right coronary artery system in two breath-holds. The contrast between blood and non-blood tissues (mainly myocardium) can be further improved by the addition of an inversion pulse prior to data acquisition (Hofman et al. 1999). For maximal blood-myocardium contrast, the appropriate length of the inversion time needs to be determined (Li et al. 2001a, b). Zheng and co-workers found a T_1 of blood less than 80 ms optimal for contrast-enhanced MR coronary angiography (Zheng et al. 2001). With an inversion time between 200 and 300 ms, the blood magnetization is almost fully recovered (T_1s less than 100 ms for blood during the first pass of 20–40 mL injections of contrast agent). Conversely, the magnetization of myocardium with T_1s of 400–600 ms is nulled with these inversion times (Nassenstein et al. 2008).

Extracellular contrast agents have a short intravascular half-life because of rapid diffusion through the extracellular space and fast renal excretion. Therefore, data acquisition should be synchronized to the passage of contrast through the coronary arteries, and because of the rapid extravasation contrast need to be (re-)injected for each coronary MR angiography acquisition. Because of dose-related safety reasons and the cost of the contrast agent, the number of (breath-hold) acquisitions is limited and thus also the extended coverage of the coronary arteries. Moreover, breath-hold contrast-enhanced MR coronary angiography, when compared to retrospective free-breathing coronary MR angiography, does not significantly improve coronary artery visualization or stenosis detection. Therefore, contrast-enhanced coronary MR angiography would benefit from the use of "intravascular" or "blood-pool" contrast agents that have a long intravascular half-life. The effectiveness of different new intravascular contrast agents (e.g. iron particles and albumin bound gadolinium) has been tested in animals [MS-325, BSA-(Gd-DTPA) (Hofman et al. 1999), Gadomer-17 (Li et al. 2001b), P792, VSOP-C91] as well as in normal subjects and patients (MS-325 (Stuber et al. 1999), NC100150 (Taylor et al. 1999), AMI-25[Endorem] (van Geuns et al. 1999), Feruglose, SH L 643A. These studies consistently report an improved blood-to-myocardium CNR compared to non-enhanced images and a prolonged and persistent blood-to-myocardium CNR improvement compared to extracellular contrast agents. Their use in assessing patients with coronary artery stenoses needs further evaluation. Deshpande and Li investigated the potential benefits of T1-shortening agents in improving the blood-myocardium contrast using the new 3D b-SSFP coronary MR angiography sequence. Their preliminary results, as well as subsequent studies showed a net increase of 78% in blood-myocardium CNR for post-contrast imaging over pre-contrast imaging (Deshpande et al. 2003; Nassenstein et al. 2009).

6 Spatial Resolution

The issue of spatial resolution becomes increasingly important with decreasing size of the object of interest. For coronary artery imaging, the main challenge is to accurately detect and quantify atherosclerotic stenotic lesions in vessels with a caliber ranging from 5 mm proximally, to 1 or 2 mm in the distal parts and side branches. X-ray coronary angiography, with a pixel size $\sim 0.1 \times 0.1$ mm, allows full coverage of the epicardial coronary arteries and branch vessels. The pixel size in MR imaging is obtained by the ratio of the field-to-view (FOV) to the acquisition matrix. The voxel size is the pixel size multiplied with the slice thickness. Thus, spatial resolution will increase if the FOV decreases, the acquisition matrix increases or the slice thickness is reduced. However, the increase in spatial resolution is inversely related to the SNR. A higher spatial resolution is desired, but can only be acquired if the SNR and CNR are sufficient. In fact, the gain in spatial resolution can be inefficient if the image becomes too noisy as a result of using too small a voxel size. So, for each image, there is an optimal compromise between SNR, CNR and spatial resolution.

The issue of spatial resolution in coronary MR angiography is definitely more complicated than in any other part of the human body, as not only the SNR but other parameters, such as coronary artery motion, acquisition window and total scan time, have a major influence on the achievable spatial resolution. Thus, although spatial resolution similar to X-ray angiography may theoretically be obtained, several parameters pose major technical challenges to a successful high-resolution visualization of the coronary vessels. The large size of the chest has a negative impact on both pixel size and SNR. Use of a rectangular FOV, and foldover suppression techniques are helpful for increasing the pixel size. Moreover, SNR can be increased by using cardiac dedicated phased array surface coils positioned as closely as possible to the coronary arteries. Three-dimensional sequences, not only allow for better depiction of curved and tortuous vessels than 2D sequences, but also provide a higher SNR and therefore enable the acquisition of smaller pixel and voxel sizes. Zero-filling techniques enable the reconstructed slice thickness to be halved (e.g. from 3 mm obtained to 1.5 mm reconstructed slice thickness) and thus reduce partial-volume artifacts (Du et al. 1994). Isotropic scanning is particularly important for coronary artery imaging (Botnar et al. 2000). Since the spatial resolution is equal in all directions in isotropic voxels, the accuracy of imaging coronary arteries becomes independent of the scan positioning, and the coronary artery delineation in the through-plane direction is improved. The risk of creating partial-volume artifacts in tortuous vessels is minimized, and there is a clear benefit for the reconstruction algorithms (MPR, MIP, volume rendering techniques). However, total imaging times are significantly longer than in anisotropic scanning and the smaller voxels yield a lower SNR. Since the available time for coronary artery imaging per heart beat is limited to a small period during the cardiac cycle, increase in spatial resolution will inevitably lead to longer total scan times that may become too long for breath-holding, unless a larger bandwidth is used. The latter, however, significantly reduces the SNR, and necessitates the administration of contrast agents.

7 High Field-Strength (3.0T) Coronary MR Angiography

The recent approval of 3.0T systems for clinical use has opened new perspectives for overcoming some of the limitations encountered on 1.5T systems, in particular, suboptimal SNR which limits spatial resolution and the ability to visualize the distal and branch vessel coronary segments (Stuber et al. 2002). Since SNR is directly related to the strength (β_o) of the static magnetic field, improved SNR and spatial resolution can be expected from 3.0T systems. However, a number of potential adverse affects have been reported at higher field strengths, such as susceptibility artifacts, reduced T_2* and increased T_1 RF field distortions. At high field-strength, reliable ECG triggering becomes more challenging due to the amplified magneto-hydrodynamic effects. Furthermore, the flexibility of sequence design is less because of increased RF deposition. Stuber and colleagues used a free-breathing real-time NE 3D-TFE sequence, adjusted for 3.0T, to study the coronary arteries in volunteers in a 3.0T system (Stuber et al. 2002). The pencil beam of the respiratory NE was positioned at the heart–liver interface. Using vector-ECG, QRS triggering remained accurate despite the enhanced T-wave at 3.0T. Compared to 1.5T coronary MR angiography, using a similar sequence and voxel size, 3.0T yielded visualization of longer segments of the coronary arteries with similar diameters and vessel sharpness, but with an increased SNR and CNR. The increase in SNR and CNR enabled reduction in the voxel size of $\pm$50% (from $1.0 \times 0.7 \times 3$ mm to $0.6 \times 0.6 \times 3.0$ mm), maintaining high image quality and improving visualization of the small-diameter branching vessels. These preliminary studies demonstrate that 3.0T coronary MR angiography is feasible, and with further fine-tuning of the sequence 3.0T might become the preferred field-strength to study the coronary artery lumen and wall.

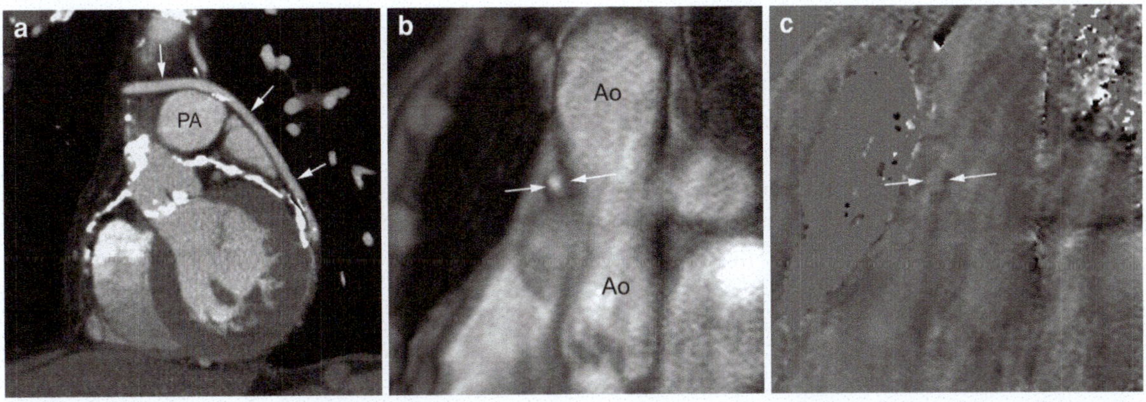

Fig. 10 CABG imaging and flow assessment in a patient with a venous jump graft. Contrast-enhanced ECG-gated CT (**a**), magnitude (**b**) and phase image (**c**) using velocity-encoded cine MRI. The course of the jump vein is well shown on the CT images (**a**). Perpendicular positioned views through the vein graft allow to assess flow patterns and to quantify flow volumes (*arrows*) (**b**, **c**)

8 Coronary Blood Flow Assessment: Strategies

X-ray angiography does not provide accurate information about the physiological significance of a stenosis, in particular stenoses of intermediate severity (40–70%), on the coronary artery flow. In lesions of intermediate severity, assessment of the functional significance is important since this information has a significant influence on patient management (White et al. 1984). Coronary artery flow has a typical biphasic pattern with the highest flow and velocity in mid-diastole. The functional significance of a coronary artery stenosis can be evaluated by measuring the ratio of maximal hyperemic coronary flow to the baseline coronary flow (Gould et al. 1974). Normal coronary arteries are characterized by a threefold augmentation of their blood flow after administration of a coronary vasodilator such as adenosine or dipyridamole. In the presence of a flow-limiting stenosis in an epicardial coronary artery, the downstream vascular bed in the myocardium demonstrates a compensatory dilatation to maintain blood flow, and the ability to achieve augmentation in coronary blood flow is limited. As a consequence, the flow reserve is markedly reduced in a coronary artery with a significant stenosis. Intra-coronary Doppler measurement is an established technique to determine coronary flow and flow reserve, but this technique is available only during cardiac catheterization (Joyce et al. 1994). MR imaging has a unique potential for non-invasive measurement of flow in vessels and across valves. Although highly challenging, MR flow measurements can be performed in the small cardiac vessels (coronary arteries, coronary sinus) and in CABG vessels, during rest and during hyperemia using fast velocity-encoded cine MR imaging techniques (Edelman et al. 1991; Sakuma et al. 1999; (Fig. 10).

A further way to assess coronary perfusion and myocardial blood flow is assessment of blood flow in the coronary sinus, which represents approximately 96% of the total myocardial blood flow. By measuring myocardial mass with cine MR imaging, the average coronary blood flow per gram of myocardial mass can be quantified by using non-invasive MR imaging. A close correlation was found between the estimated myocardial blood flow obtained by coronary sinus flow MR measurement and PET flow data. Bedaux and colleagues applied this technique to quantify the flow velocity and volume flow in the great cardiac vein, which has a close anatomic relationship to the LAD. The flow in the great cardiac vein was found to be mainly systolic and pointing in the inverse direction to the predominantly diastolic flow in the LAD.

To assure accurate coronary flow measurements with MR imaging, at least four important sources of error should be taken into consideration—partial-volume effects, misalignment of flow axis and flow-encoding gradients, intra-voxel dispersion, and through- and in-plane motion (Tang et al. 1993; Marcus et al. 1999; Nagel et al. 1999). With the currently achievable in-plane resolution of approximately 1 × 1 mm, only a few pixels will be effectively located within the coronary artery lumen, while many pixels will be located at the boundary between the lumen and the vessel wall. This may reduce significantly the accuracy of MR measurements, with differences of up to 60% between MR and intravascular Doppler measurements (Tang et al. 1993). Accuracy can be improved when peak velocities (highest at the center of the vessel and thus less dependent on partial-volume effects) are used instead of volume flow. Although Hofman and colleagues have found that with ~3 pixels per vessel diameter, accurate blood volume flow rates can be determined (Hofman et al. 1995), intra-voxel phase dispersion can be reduced by an improvement in spatial resolution, leading to more homogeneous flow velocities within one voxel. Misalignment can be reduced by careful planning of the image plane perpendicular to the coronary vessel of interest. Coronary arteries move significantly during data acquisition. Through-plane motion can be corrected for by measuring and subtracting the velocity of the adjacent myocardium from the flow velocity within the vessel. In-plane velocity cannot be corrected for. In-plane motion is higher for the RCA (6–12 cm/s) (Hofman et al. 1996) than for the LAD (2–5 cm/s) (Sakuma et al. 1999), causing blurring of the vessel boundaries and overestimation of the volume flow. This is most problematic during ejection and early, fast filling. To obtain accurate flow measurements, the acquisition window should be less than 25 ms for the RCA, and less than 120 ms for the LAD (Hofman et al. 1998).

Coronary MR flow measurements can be performed in breath-hold as well during free-breathing with use of the NE technique (Nagel et al. 1999; Sakuma et al. 1999; Keegan et al. 2004). Both approaches have advantages and disadvantages. A higher temporal and spatial resolution can be achieved with the free-breathing technique, but this approach might be problematic due to its longer scan time when using pharmacological stress. It should be noted that coronary blood flow measurement with breath-hold imaging may be different from physiological blood flow during regular breathing, since breath-holding can change the intra-thoracic pressure, which affects the systemic venous return to the heart and thus decrease the cardiac output (29.0 ± 6.3%) when breath-holding at deep inspiration is employed (Ferrigno et al. 1986).

9 Coronary Artery Bypass Graft Imaging: Strategies

In general, the strategies used for coronary artery imaging are also applicable to CABG imaging, but CABG imaging deals with specific problems. Imaging is either focused on angiographic depiction of the bypass graft, or by assessing flow patterns (volume flow and velocities) and flow reserve, or a combination of both techniques. For the angiographic assessment of CABG grafts "black-blood" as well as "bright-blood" techniques have been used in the past (Aurigemma et al. 1989; Galjee et al. 1996). The newer b-SSFP "bright-blood" techniques and for breath-hold ultrafast contrast-enhanced MR angiography have been used for CABG MR angiography (Wintersperger et al. 1998; Kalden et al. 1999; Bunce et al. 2003). Bypass graft flow and flow reserve assessment use the same approach and strategies as applied for coronary artery flow measurement, but should take into account differences in the flow profiles and flow reserves that are related to the type of graft, the position along the graft where the flow is quantified and the flow patterns in the distal run-off vessels.

10 Practical Approach for Coronary MR Angiography

10.1 Patient Setup and Patient Instructions

Patient setup is similar as for other cardiovascular MR indications (see "Practical Set-Up"). Patients are positioned supine with the ECG-leads on the anterior left hemithorax. Although in a recent paper, Stuber and colleagues reported an improved coronary visualization in a prone position, similar to the 2D-approaches used in the early 1990s, this uncomfortable position is not suitable for patient studies (Duerinckx et al. 1995). Patient instructions are important to improve the success of coronary MR angiography. The non-breath-hold sequences are much simpler, as they require virtually no patient instructions besides a recommendation to breathe regularly and to keep still during the scan. For the breath-hold techniques the patient should be instructed on how to hold his/her breath during a non-forced, normal end-expiration for the duration of each scan and these maneuvres should be practiced for several minutes prior to the start of the scan. It is important to work on this with the patient prior to starting the MR scan to obtain breath-holding that is as consistent as possible. For contrast-enhanced coronary MR angiography, the patient needs an intravenous line, preferentially with a continuous perfusion of small amount of physiologic fluid to assure an open line prior to injection.

10.2 Cookbook Approach for Free-Breathing Coronary MR Angiography

The Beth Israel group from Boston was the first to propose a standardized stepwise approach for free-breathing coronary MR angiography. A cookbook offers several advantages:

- It ensures that coronary arteries are always studied in the same way.
- Studies can be performed by technicians with experience in cardiac imaging, and total imaging can be shortened.
- Improvements in sequence designs can be updated in the cookbook without changing the cookbook strategy as such.

The protocol includes 4–5 different scans, all of which are performed during free-breathing. For coronary artery localization and for NE positioning at the right hemidiaphragm, two localizers are utilized (scans 1 and 2). The first localizer is a vector-ECG-triggered, free-breathing, multislice 2D segmented gradient-echo scan with nine transverse, nine coronal and nine sagittal interleaved acquisitions of the thorax (acquisition duration = 1 min). On these images, the NE is positioned at the dome of the right hemidiaphragm. Scan 2 is a low resolution, 3D segmented gradient-echo scout scan (TFE-EPI, or balanced-TFE with parallel imaging) that is used for the localization of the targeted 3D volumes that consitute the final submillimeter MR angiography scans (Bogaert et al. 2003; Giorgi et al. 2002). This low spatial resolution scan is oriented transversely through the origin and course of the RCA and LCA. The scan results in a 3D slab consisting of 40 slices with a reconstructed slice thickness of 2.5 mm and an in-plane resolution of 1.39 × 1.82 mm. T_2-preparation and fat saturation pulses are applied just prior to data acquisition to obtain high contrast between the blood and myocardium and between fat and other structures respectively. This scan, as well as the following scans, are obtained during mid-diastole, using an empirical formula (Stuber et al. 1999), or using a direct assessment of the optimal delay time (Foo et al. 2000; Kim et al. 2001).

To precisely target the scan volumes of the submillimeter scans (scans 3–5), a three-point plan scan is applied to locate the right and left coronary arteries on the low spatial resolution scan. For the RCA (scan 3), the RCA is depicted in three locations (proximal, mid- and a distal segment of the RCA) on transverse images. These 3 points define the geometry of the center plane of the imaged 3D volume, subsequently applied for the submillimeter coronary MR angiography sequence (Stuber et al. 1999). This 3D volume covers not only the anterior atrioventricular groove but also the posterior atrioventricular groove containing the LCx (Fig. 11). For the left coronary tree, two scans are performed. Scan 4 is positioned tangentially to the surface of the left anterolateral part of the heart ("tangential" view), using the LM, the mid LAD and mid LCx as landmarks. The landmarks on the LAD and LCx should be positioned carefully to assure the longest coverage of the left coronary tree, including the diagonal branching vessels (Fig. 12). Scan 5 is a perpendicular view through the LM and entire length of the LAD ("perpendicular" view), using the LM, mid LAD and distal LAD as landmarks. On the perpendicular view, the small, septal branches of the LAD are often visible. In this way, the LM, LCx and LAD (but not the RCA) are scanned in two perpendicular planes. As a result, longer segments of the left coronary artery tree, and more of its branching vessels are visualized (Fig. 13). Also, the visualization and description of stenotic lesions benefits from this approach, since lesions are scanned in-plane (with a better in-plane resolution) at least in one direction. Not unfrequently, the accompanying coronary veins are visible on the MR angiography scans. The American Heart Association classification system to define and number the different CA segments can also be applied on coronary MR angiography (Austen et al. 1975).

The submillimeter coronary scan starts with a flow-insensitive T_2-prepulse for contrast enhancement (60 ms), is followed by an NE (20 ms), a spectrally selective fat saturation pulse (20 ms) and a localized anterior saturation pre-pulse (REST) (8 ms), and finally the high-resolution MR coronary angiography

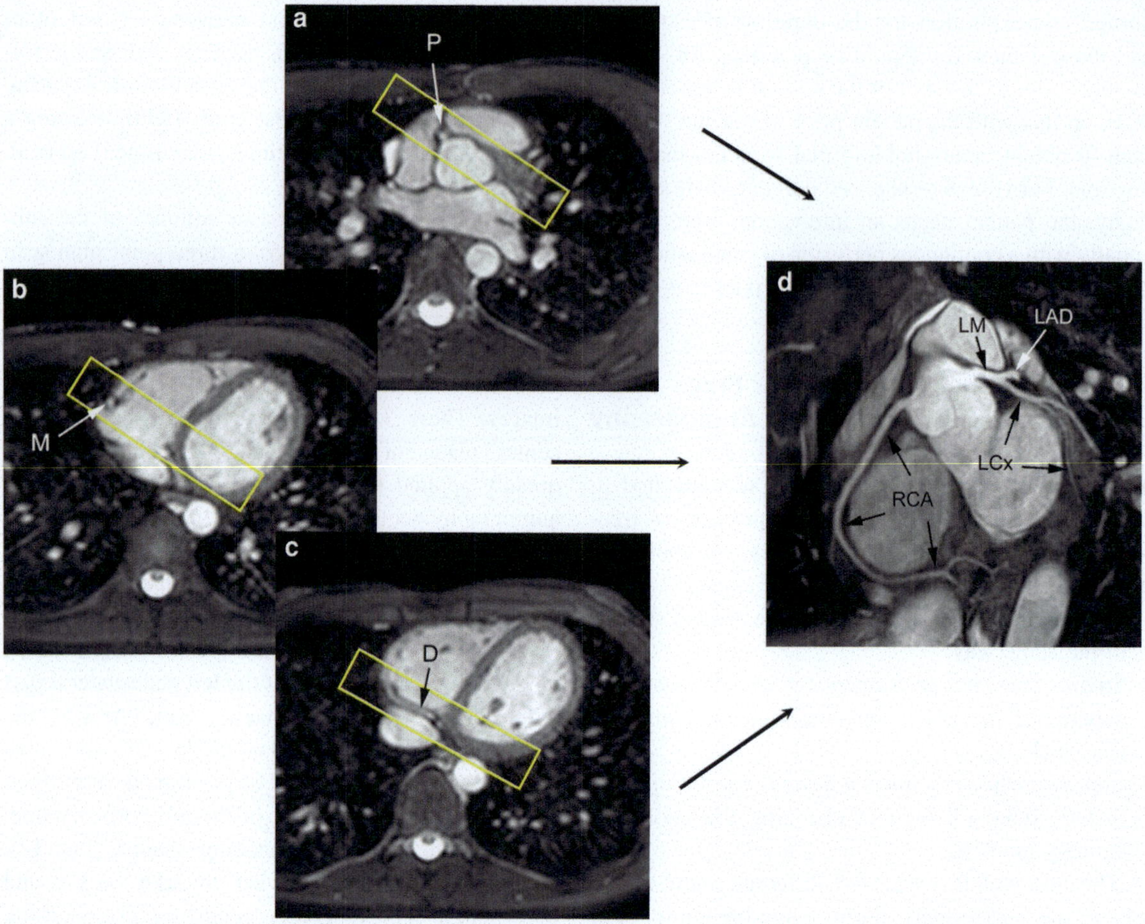

Fig. 11 a–d Positioning of *RCA*. Indication of the position of the proximal (*P*), mid (*M*) and distal (*D*) part of the *RCA* on the low spatial-resolution images allows to determine a small volume (indicated in *yellow*) covering the entirety of the *RCA* in the anterior atrioventricular groove. This small 3D volume usually visualizes also the *LM*, the proximal *LAD* and the *LCx* in the posterior atrioventricular groove

sequence itself. The REST pulse, positioned on the anterior chest wall, is an effective means of suppressing breathing-related artifacts from the anterior chest wall. Different types of high-resolution MR coronary angiography sequences are currently available—3D-segmented κ-space TFE (or FLASH sequence), 3D-segmented SSFP (balanced-TFE or true-FISP). As discussed above, different κ-space sampling strategies can be used (Cartesian, radial, spiral). Usually a low to high fill-in of the κ-space is applied. With a field of view of 360 mm and a 512 × 360 matrix, an in-plane acquisition resolution of 0.7 × 1.0 mm is obtained. The 3D-slab consisted of 20 slices of 1.5 mm reconstructed thickness, resulting in a coverage of 30 mm. Scans are reconstructed to a voxel size of 0.54 × 0.54 × 1.5 mm by additional zero-filling. Image quality can be further improved by using Constant Level AppeaRance (CLEAR) for all scans in order to correct for the non-uniform cardiac coil sensitivity (based on the separate reference scan which determines the coil sensitivity profiles for all cardiac coil elements, the same reference scan which is also used for sensitivity encoding in the scout scan).

A new approach for free-breathing coronary MR angiography, recently described by Oliver Weber and colleagues, is "Whole-Heart" coronary MR angiography (Fig. 14). It represents a simplified version of the cookbook approach, and consists of only two scans. After a localizer (similar to scan 1 in the cookbook), used for positioning of the NE, a transverse-oriented submillimeter high-resolution coronary MR

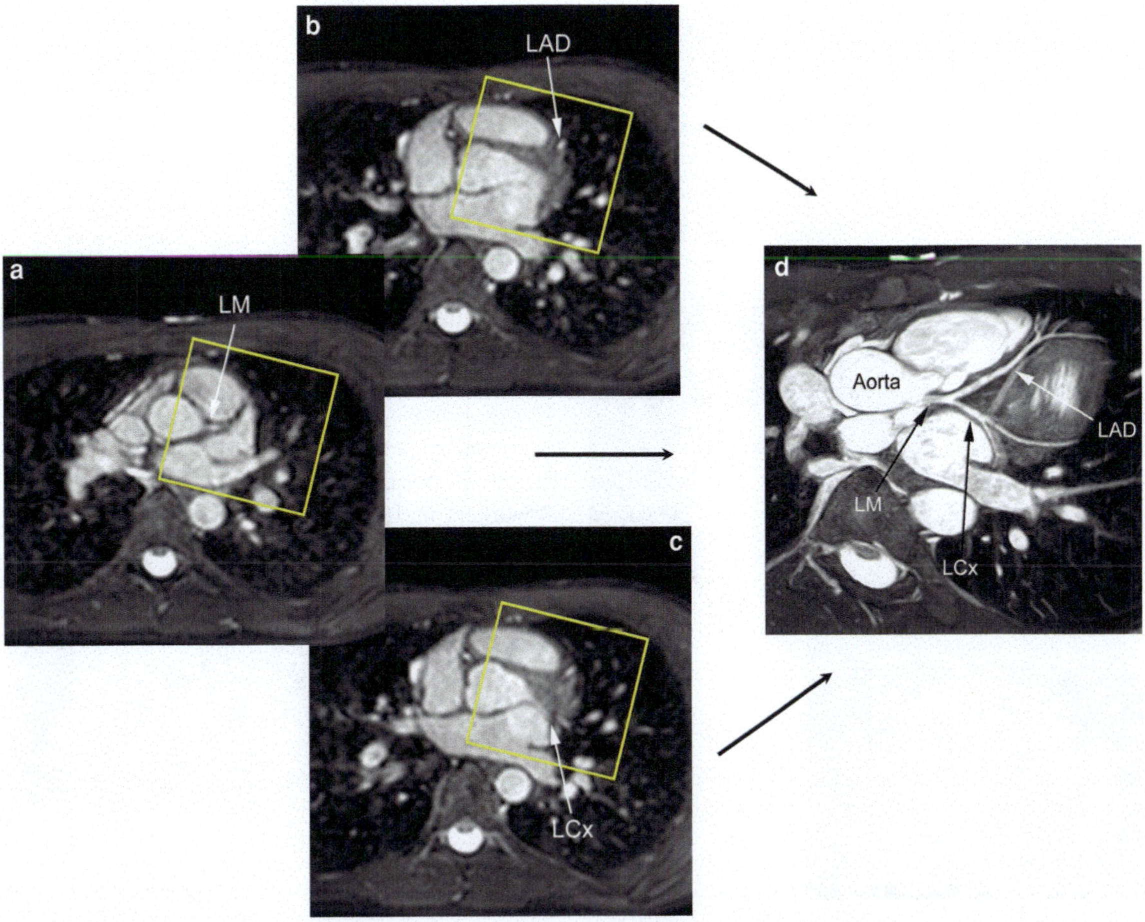

Fig. 12 **a–d** Tangential view to study *LM*, and the proximal and mid portions of the *LAD* and *LCx*. To determine the ideal volume (indicated in *yellow*), the position of the *LM*, mid portions of the *LAD* and *LCx* are indicated on the transverse low spatial-resolution images

angiography scan (balanced-TFE) is obtained which covers the entire heart. With 120–140 axial slices (in-plane reconstructed resolution of 0.54 × 0.54 mm) and a slice thickness of 0.75 mm, the heart is nearly completely, "isotropically" scanned. Advantages of this approach are its simplicity (reduction from 5 to 2 scans without the need to use double-obliquely targeted volumes for optimal coronary artery scanning), and reduction in total scan time. In the study by Weber and colleagues, a scan efficiency of 48% was found. Mean acquisition duration was 5:36 min (range 3:30–11:51 min) for the targeted volumes and 13:48 min (range 7:18–20:18 min) for the whole-heart volume. The near isotropic scanning permits multiplanar reconstruction without loss in image quality, with limited problems related to partial-volume. The efficacy with which different coronary artery segments can be depicted using these different techniques is summarized in Table 2.

10.3 Practical Approach for Breath-Hold Coronary MR Angiography

Wielopolski and colleagues proposed an interactive stepwise approach for 3D breath-hold coronary MR angiography (Wielopolski et al. 1998). The first step involves the acquisition of a scout volumetric data set during end-expiration with a 3D multishot segmented EPI sequence to cover the entire heart. The heart volume localizer data are subsequently loaded into an MPR platform, to interactively compute the optimal orientation for imaging of the different segments of the coronary arteries. The optimal double-oblique

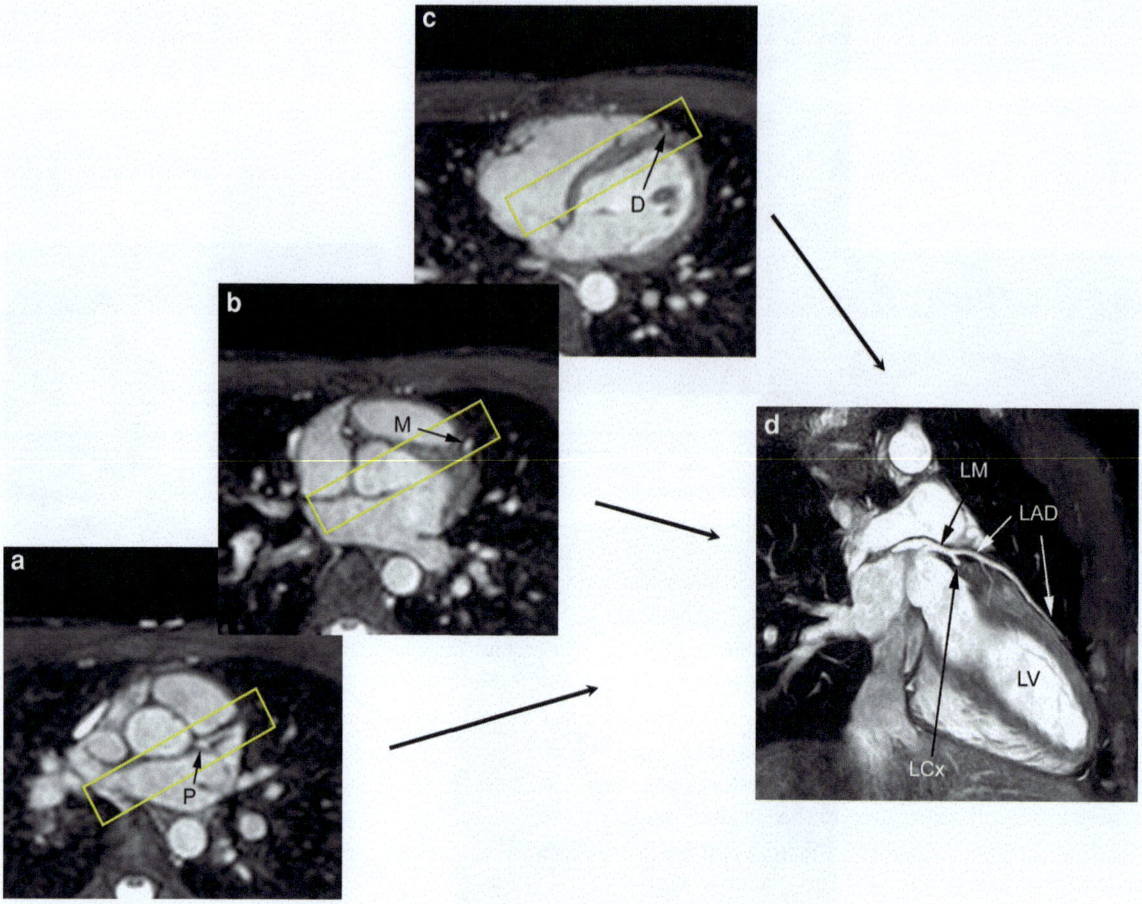

Fig. 13 a–d Perpendicular view to study *LM* and the *LAD* in the anterior interventricular groove. The position of the *LM* (*P*), and the mid (*M*) and distal (*D*) portions of the *LAD* are indicated on the low spatial-resolution images

plane and slab position containing the coronary segment of interest are implemented into an end-expiratory breath-hold 3D segmented Turbo FLASH (or currently the SSFP) sequence (VCATS). This procedure of localization and imaging is continued and repeated until all necessary orientations covering all major coronary segments are interrogated. In just 7 breath-holds, the major coronary segments can be visualized: (1) Plane along LM, proximal LCx, and proximal LAD (transverse); (2) Plane of proximal RCA (transverse); (3) Plane along distal RCA and PDA (oblique); (4) Plane through aortic root and proximal RCA and LM (oblique); (5) Plane along LCx (oblique); (6) Plane along middle and distal LAD (oblique); (7) Plane along middle RCA (oblique) (van Geuns et al. 1999). A detailed description of the optimal positioning of the different volumes can be found in Wielopolski et al. 1998. These VCATS scans obtained in end-expiratory breath-holds of 24 heartbeats have a FOV of 240×320 mm^2, a slab thickness of 24–32 mm, a reconstructed slice thickness of 1.5 mm, an in-plane resolution of $1.4–2.0 \times 1.0–1.2$ mm^2 and an acquisition length of 110 ms (van Geuns et al. 1999; Li et al. 2001a). Magnetization preparation techniques include the use of magnetization-transfer irradiation or a T_2-prepulse for myocardium-blood CNR enhancement and a chemical shift fat suppression pulse.

11 Post-Processing Techniques for Coronary MR Angiography

The coronary arteries have a complex, often tortuous course on the curved surface of the heart. Moreover, especially on the left side, the coronary artery tree

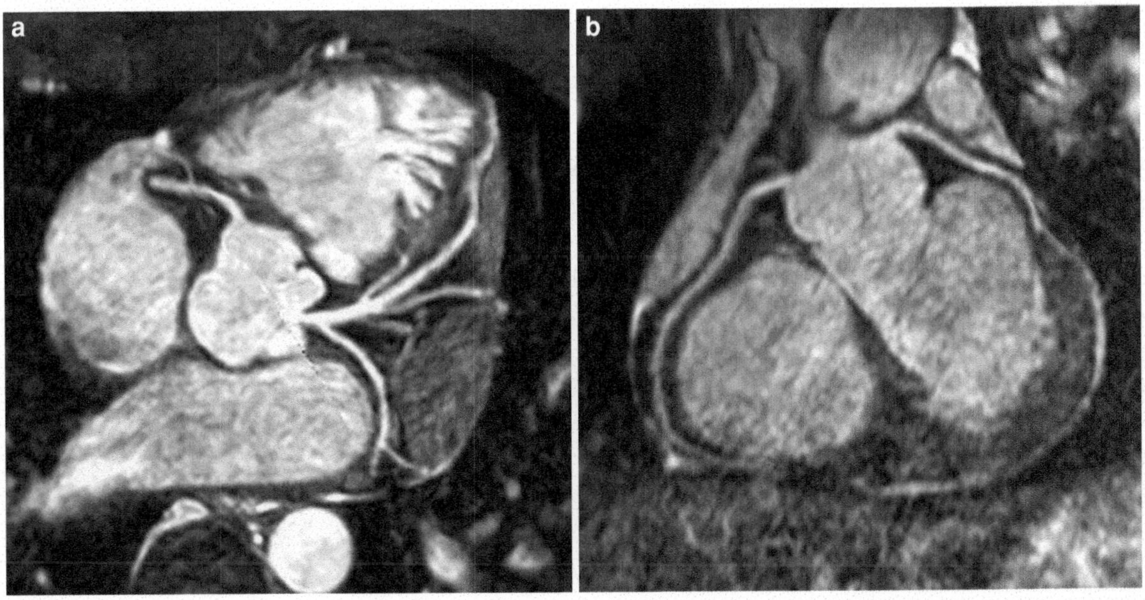

Fig. 14 Whole-heart coronary MR angiography in a normal subject. Reconstruction in an oblique axial image plane of the original data set shows the LM, LAD, LCx, the origin of the RCA and several CA branches (**a**); and reconstruction along the atrioventricular grooves shows the RCA, LM and LCx (**b**). (The post-processing program used for reconstruction was the Soap-Bubble tool, Philips Medical Systems, Best, The Netherlands)

has side branches. Using current 3D volumetric acquisition techniques, the majority of the epicardial coronary arteries can be imaged in a single 3D-volume, only small portions of coronary arteries will be visible on the individual reconstructed images. Therefore, to facilitate coronary arterial depiction, post-processing of the images is necessary. With the advent and wide clinical use of ultrafast contrast-enhanced MR angiography techniques, post-processing techniques, such as maximum intensity projection (MIP), multiplanar reformations (MPR), and surface (SR) and volume rendering (VR) from 3D data sets, are currently available on most clinical MR scanners and offline workstations (van Ooijen et al. 2003). Three-dimensional rendering of coronary arteries is one type of post-processing that requires segmentation of the data (Doyle et al. 1993; Börnert and Jensen 1995). To execute this 3D rendering routine, "seeds" are placed in both the left and right coronary vessels, and thresholds are set to discriminate individual coronary vessels from adjacent structures (Doyle et al. 1993). Segmentation of the left coronary system with its many branches is much more involved than the RCA segmentation. Recently, Etienne and colleagues introduced an elegant "Soap-Bubble" tool for visualization and quantitative analysis of 3D coronary MR angiograms (Etienne et al. 2002). This quantitative software tool facilitates MPR of 3D-volume-targeted coronary MR angiography data sets, while also providing quantitative measures such as SNR, CNR, vessel length and diameter, and local vessel sharpness. The user interactively specifies a curved subvolume, enclosed in the 3D coronary MR angiography data set that closely encompasses the coronary arterial segments and branches that are represented in one 2D representation. All the voxels that are not included in this user-prescribed subvolume are discarded and are not used for subsequent visualization and analysis. Typically 20–60 points are needed for the left coronary system, and 10–20 points for the right coronary system, taking ~3 min and ~8–10 min respectively. Regenfus and colleagues compared the (conventional) MIP versus original source images in patients with coronary artery stenosis (Regenfus et al. 2003). They found no significant differences in overall accuracy for stenosis detection between the processed and unprocessed images. However, the MIP post-processing was compromised by a higher number of images that could not be evaluated due to overlap of coronary arteries with adjacent structures.

Table 2 Effects of coronary MR angiography sequence on length of continuous depiction of coronary arteries

	No.	RCA	LM	LAD	LCx
Breath-hold Approach					
3D Spoiled-GE-Technique (contrast-enhanced)					
Li et al. (2001)	16-V	109 ± 25		78 ± 14[a]	
Free-Breathing with Retrospective Respiratory Gating					
3D Spoiled-GE-Technique					
	12-V	126 ± 19	11 ± 1	116 ± 20	97 ± 13
Free-Breathing with Real-time Prospective Navigator					
3D Spoiled-GE-Technique (volume-targeted)					
Botnar et al. (1999)	12-V	84 ± 14		53 ± 11[a]	
Bunce et al. (2001)	46-P	56 ± 21	12 ± 5	30 ± 11	16 ± 9
Kim et al. (2001)	109-P	91 ± 19		74 ± 10[a]	40 ± 11
Giorgi et al. (2002)	15-V	95 ± 27	8 ± 3	79 ± 24	61 ± 18
Sommer et al. (2002)	107-P	69 ± 26	19 ± 5	55 ± 22	44 ± 17
Weber et al. (2002)	15-V/P	129 ± 19	12 ± 1	117 ± 21	47 ± 5
Bogaert et al. (2003)	19-P	90 ± 31	7 ± 2	72 ± 15	31 ± 15
3D b-SSFP Technique (volume-targeted)					
Giorgi et al. (2002)	15-V	112 ± 27	8 ± 3	92 ± 21	71 ± 18
Spuentrup et al. (2002)	10-V	81 ± 24		61 ± 7[a]	39 ± 11
3D-b-SSFP Technique (whole-heart)					
	12-V	107 ± 32		117 ± 34[a]	69 ± 36
3D-Black-Blood Technique (volume-targeted)					
Stuber et al. (2001)	8-V	112 ± 22		64 ± 6[a]	26 ± 9
3 Tesla					
3D-spoiled-GE-Technique (volume-targeted)					
	9-V	122 ± 35		83 ± 9[a]	52 ± 6

Results are expressed in millimeters, and shown as mean ± standard deviation
Abbreviations *LAD* left anterior descending artery, *LCx* left circumflex artery, *LM* left main stem artery, *No* Number of subjects, *P* patient, *RCA* right coronary artery, *V* volunteer
[a] combined LM—LAD length

12 Clinical Applications

12.1 Congenital Anomalies of the Coronary Arteries

Congenital anomalies of the coronary arteries tend to be primary and are usually not associated in adults with other types of congenital heart diseases. They are, however, associated with an increased risk of sudden cardiac death, infective endocarditis and ischemic cardiomyopathy (Walker and Webb 2001). These anomalies can be classified into three large groups—anomalous origin, anomalous distribution and anomalous drainage of the coronary artery (Anné et al. 2000; Prakken et al. 2010). Of clinical relevance are the haemodynamically significant congenital coronary anomalies.

Although anomalous origin and epicardial course of the coronary arteries is an uncommon entity, it can be the cause of chest pain and sudden cardiac death, often in a younger asymptomatic population (Davis et al. 2001). Together with hypertrophic cardiomyopathy and arrhythmogenic right ventricular dysplasia, anomalous origin of the coronary artery is the most frequent cause of sudden cardiac death in competitive young athletes (Pelliccia 2001). The incidence has been reported to be between 0.3 and

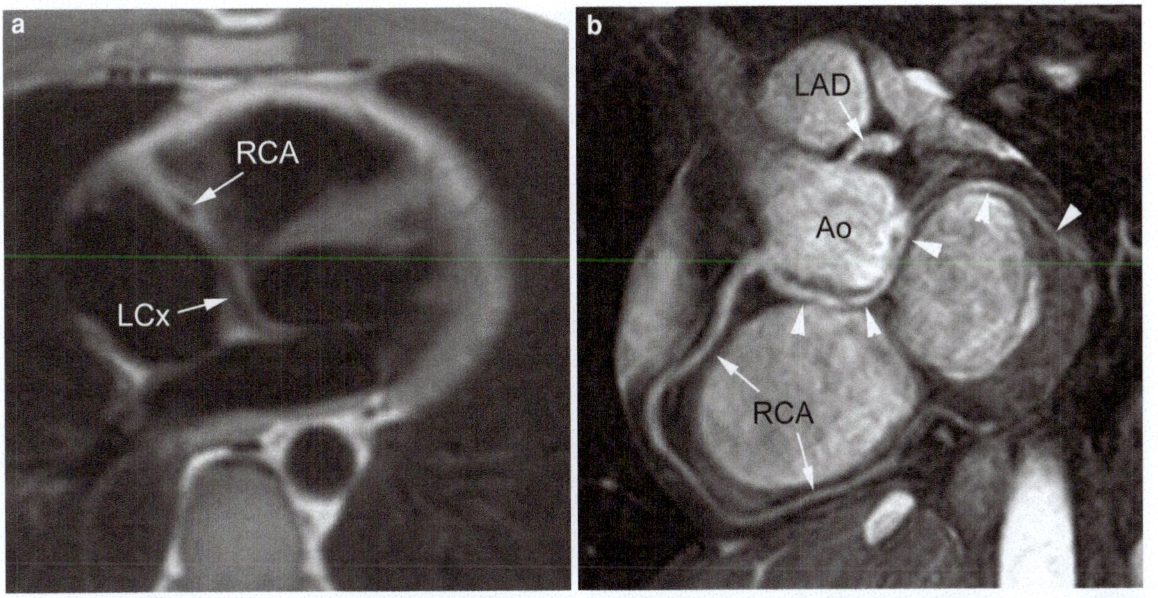

Fig. 15 Abnormal origin of *LCx* from *RCA* with retro-aortic course of the proximal *LCx* in a young male patient referred for MRI to exclude arrhythmogenic right ventricular dysplasia. On the axial spin-echo MR images (**a**), a curvilinear hypointense structure is visible behind the left ventricular outflow tract and aortic root. The vascular anomaly, i.e, an abnormal origin of the *LCx* from the *RCA* with retro-aortic course of the proximal *LCx* (*arrowheads*), is confirmed on 3D free-breathing coronary MR angiography (b-SSFP technique) (**b**)

1.0% of the normal population, although this is likely an underestimate, as many asymptomatic individuals may be unrecognised (Click et al. 1989; Desmet et al. 1992; Garg et al. 2000). From an anatomical point of view, the anomalies are classified according to the coronary artery involved, the origin of the anomalous coronary artery and the anatomic course of the proximal segment. From a clinical point of view, the anomalies are divided into "benign" and "malignant" lesions. The latter have an increased risk for developing myocardial ischemia and sudden cardiac death (Fig. 15).

Anomalous origins represent one third of all coronary artery anomalies. They can present as anomalies in the coronary ostia, e.g. high take-off, multiple ostia, single ostium and congenital hypoplasia, or as anomalies in the origin and proximal anatomic course of the coronary arteries, or as a combination of both. Most of the anomalies in coronary ostia are benign and have normal myocardial perfusion. The commonest type of multiple ostia is separate origins of the RCA and conus branch; less common are separate origins of the LAD and LCx. Single coronary artery is extremely rare and the clinical relevance in adults is limited (Desmet et al. 1992; Walker and Webb 2001). Approximately 60% of all coronary arteries with an anomalous origin and course involve an isolated LCx originating from separate ostium within the right sinus of Valsalva, or as a proximal branch of the RCA This entity has a retro-aortic course and is totally asymptomatic. The remaining 40% involve the right and left coronary arteries (Bunce et al. 2003). The association of coronary artery anomalies and sudden cardiac deaths ("malignant" forms) appears to be exclusively found in patients with an interarterial vessel, in whom the anomalous vessel passes between the aortic root and RV outflow tract or pulmonary artery. This can be the LCA originating form the right sinus of Valsalva or RCA, the LAD originating from the right sinus of Valsalva or RCA with an LCx originating from the left sinus of Valsalva, or the RCA originating from the left coronary artery of left sinus of Valsalva. The precise mechanism leading to myocardial ischemia and sudden cardiac death in these patients is still controversial. Very likely, this long interarterial segment is compressed during exercise or other stress conditions, leading to exertional chest pain, syncope, myocardial ischemia and infarction, and potential sudden death. Other mechanisms causing symptoms can be related to a decrease

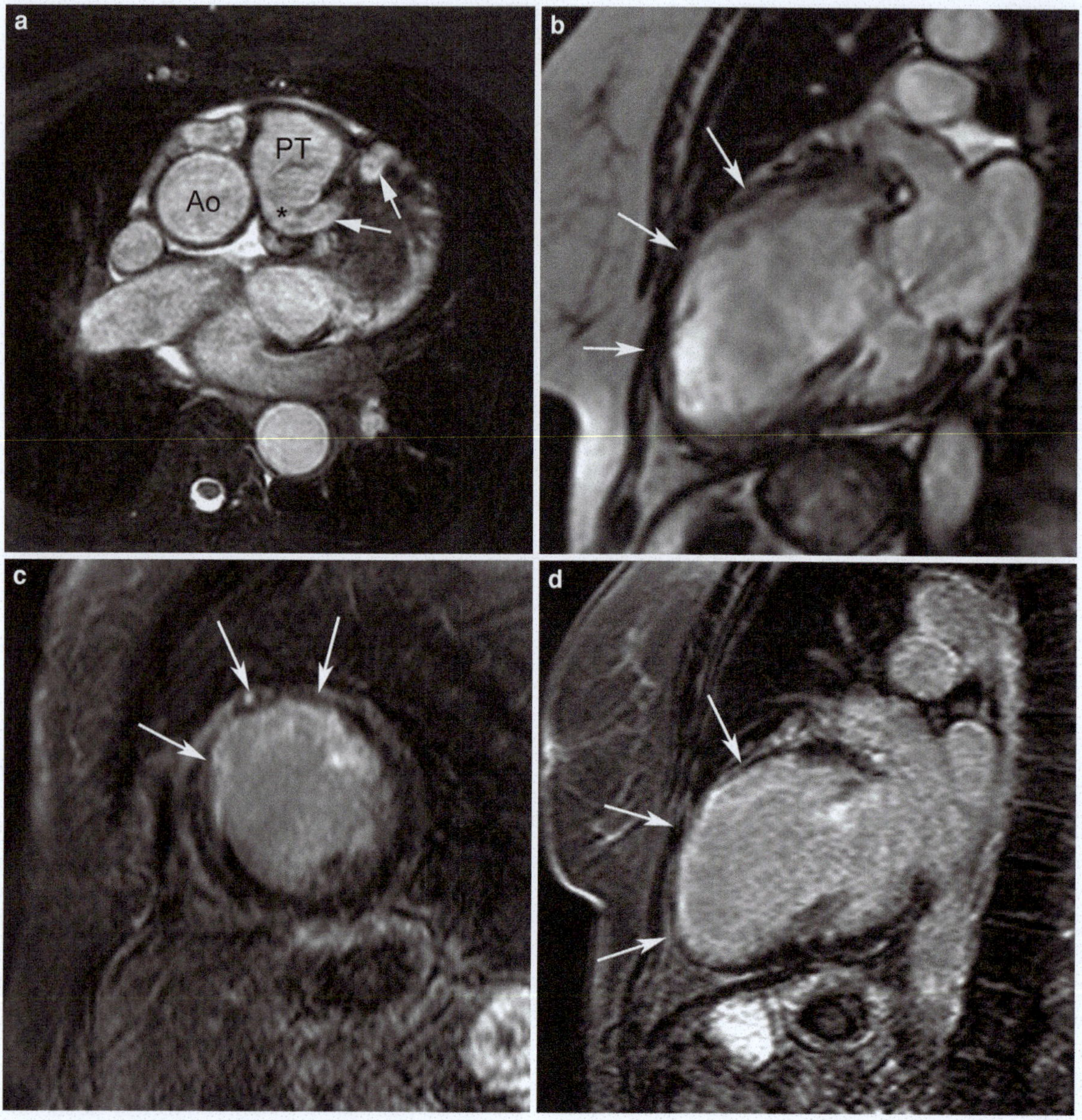

Fig. 16 ALCAPA. In this patient, the left anterior descending coronary artery arises from the pulmonary artery (**a**; *arrows*). Vertical long-axis cine MR shows extensive wall thickening in the anterior wall (**b**; *arrows*). Late Gd-MR shows extenive scarring in the corresponding coronary artery territory (**c**, **d**)

in coronary artery blood flow due to a kinking of the left coronary artery at its origin from the right coronary artery by an increased angulation caused by distension of the aorta during increased cardiac activity (Davis et al. 2001). In young athletes dying from anomalous coronary artery origin and course, the anomalous interarterial segment was most frequently due to an LCA than an RCA (23 and 4 deaths, respectively), presumable due to the more important distribution of LCA blood supply (Walker and Webb 2001). In patients with anomalous coronary artery it is vital to identify the precise anatomic arrangement to enable appropriate management plan to be followed (i.e. surgical reconstruction or bypass graft surgery, medical therapy).

Although very uncommon, another group of coronary artery anomalies not mentioned yet are patients with an origin of the coronary artery from the pulmonary trunk. In 90% of these subjects, the LCA arises from the pulmonary artery ("ALCAPA"). From birth, the myocardium is perfused at low oxygen tension and pressure, stimulating the development of collaterals from the RCA. However, the benefit of collaterals is often offset by a "steal" mechanism whereby blood passing from the RCA to LCA branches flow retrogradely through the LCA back into the pulmonary artery, thus creating a left to right shunt. Without surgical correction this condition is associated with a high mortality in infancy (Fig. 16).

One of the earliest and most widely accepted applications for coronary MR angiography has been the detection of congenital anomalies of the origin and the proximal course of the coronary arteries (Duerinckx et al. 1995; Taylor et al. 2000a; Bunce et al. 2003). Even with multiple projections, the precise location of the proximal course of the vessel in a patient with an abnormal origin of a coronary artery can be difficult to depict with conventional angiography (Bunce et al. 2003). Other techniques such as transthoracic echocardiography fail to visualize the ostium of the RCA in 20% of patients while the more distal parts are often not interpretable (Pelliccia 2001). In contrast, 3D coronary MR angiography provides reliable visualization of the root of the arteries, and the coronary artery tree. Its tomographic approach enables precise description of the origin and course of the different coronary arteries. Moreover, coronary MR angiography can be combined with functional MR studies, rest-stress coronary artery flow studies, rest-stress myocardial perfusion studies and late-enhancement MR studies of myocardium. In this way, a single imaging technique enables assessment of the impact of a proximal coronary artery anomaly on the distal coronary flow, the perfusion and function of the myocardial perfusion territory and to depict myocardial damage, i.e, infarction and fibrosis, as a result of repeated periods of prolonged myocardial ischemia (Bunce et al. 2001; Giorgi et al. 2002).

Anomalous intramyocardial course of the epicardial coronary artery, also known as "myocardial bridging" is a common finding at autopsy and during cardiac catheterization, but the clinical significance remains controversial (Walker and Webb 2001). Myocardial bridges are most commonly localized in the middle segment of the LAD, are at a depth of 1–10 mm with a typical length of ~10–30 mm. The clinical presentation includes angina, myocardial infarction, left ventricular dysfunction, paroxysmal AV blockade and sudden cardiac death. However, considering the prevalence of myocardial bridging, these complications are rare. Myocardial bridges are diagnosed on coronary angiography by the typical "milking effect" induced by systolic compression of the tunneled segment. Non-invasive detection of myocardial bridges with CT and MR imaging should be appealing because these techniques not only visualize the coronary artery lumen, but also the surrounding tissues such as the myocardium. However, it should be stressed that the use of magnetization preparation pulses (MTC pulses and T_2 preparation pulses) to enhance the blood/myocardium CNR, in coronary MR angiography suppresses the myocardial signal and thus will inevitably hamper the visualization of the myocardial bridge. Also, the current acquisition times for cardiac CT are too long to accurately assess the severity of compression of the intramyocardial coronary segment during systole. Other approaches such as MR flow measurements in the LAD might be appealing to assess the severity of myocardial bridging.

12.2 Coronary Artery Imaging in Congenital Heart Diseases

Embryologically, the coronary arterial bed arises from three components: the sinusoids (which go on to develop into myocardium), the in situ vascular endothelial network and the coronary buds (from which the aortopulmonary trunk arises) (Walker and Webb 2001). The coronary ostia form early, but the distal coronary pattern develops later, after formation of the ventricular masses. The ostia arise from the two aortic cusps situated next to the aortopulmonary septum. The origin of the LAD is influenced by the development of the pulmonary conus. Hence, in tetralogy of Fallot (characterized by uneven septation and hypoplasia of the pulmonary infundibulum), an abnormal origin of the LAD from the RCA is not uncommon. Ventricular morphology largely determines the coronary pattern. For example, in ventricular inversion, the coronary arteries are also inverted. The distribution and size of the epicardial coronary vessels are strictly related to the extent of their dependent myocardium. A lack of myocardium would

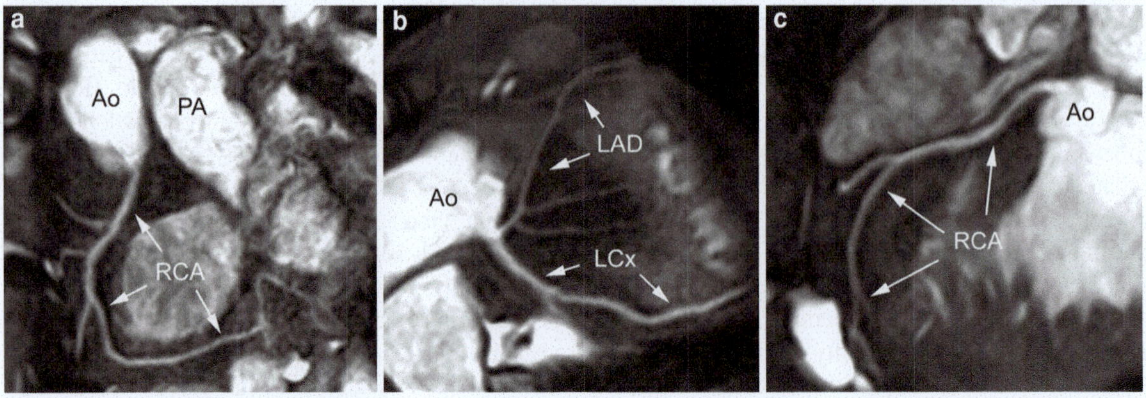

Fig. 17 **a–c** Coronary MR angiography in a patient with transposition of the great arteries, using 3D free-breathing coronary MR angiography (b-SSFP technique). The proximal course of the 3 CAs is well visible. The small caliber of the LAD and its branches is related to the hypoplasia of the morphological left ventricle

induce hypoplasia of the myocardium and conversely, a reduction in myocardium mass would cause a relative hypoplasia of its coronary branch (Angelini 1989). In patients with congenital heart disease, coronary MR angiography has a complementary role to X-ray coronary angiography (Taylor et al. 2000b). Not only is the incidence of anomalous coronary arteries much higher in patients with congenital heart disease (3–36%), but detailed information regarding coronary artery is necessary to avoid damage to the arteries in patients undergoing cardiac surgery (Fig. 17). Since, a high number of these patients have abnormally related great vessels, the identification of the relationship of the coronary arteries with X-ray angiography is much more difficult than it is for normal cardiac anatomy.

Coronary MR angiography may have a role in the postoperative assessment of coronary artery patency in patients who have undergone the arterial switch operation for transposition of the great arteries. This surgical procedure has become the treatment of choice for transposition of the great arteries. Good mid-term prognosis for the operation has been reported recently, with most complications and mortality occurring within the first year of life (Prêtre et al. 2001). The majority of the deaths during this period are secondary to myocardial ischemia/infarction associated with relocation of the coronary arteries at operation. However, little is known about the natural history of the coronary morphology in children as they grow. Due to issues related to repeated X-ray exposure morbidity associated with the procedure itself, and potential toxicity of iodinated contrast agents, screening of this group of subjects with X-ray coronary angiography is not feasible. In a recent study, Taylor and colleagues obtained diagnostic quality images of the coronary artery ostium and proximal coronary in 72% of coronary artery images using free-breathing, real-time NE 3D coronary MR angiography. This figure rose to a 100% in subjects older than 11 years. No ostial stenoses were seen, and in all 16 subjects (mean age, 10.8 ± 1.3 years), the proximal course of the coronary arteries was visualized. In their study, coronary MR angiography was combined with cine MR imaging to evaluate ventricular function, and contrast-enhanced MR imaging to assess myocardial damage. Two subendocardial viability defects were detected, corresponding to known compromise of the artery supplying that territory. Global left and right ventricular function was preserved with no regional wall abnormalities.

12.3 Coronary Artery Vasculitis

Kawasaki disease is an acute vasculitis of unknown etiology that predominantly occurs in young children and produces coronary artery aneurysms in 15–25% of untreated cases. Coronary artery aneurysms may rupture, thrombose or develop stenotic lesions that cause myocardial ischemia. Serial evaluation of the distribution and size of coronary artery aneurysms is necessary for risk stratification and therapeutic management. Although transthoracic echocardiography is

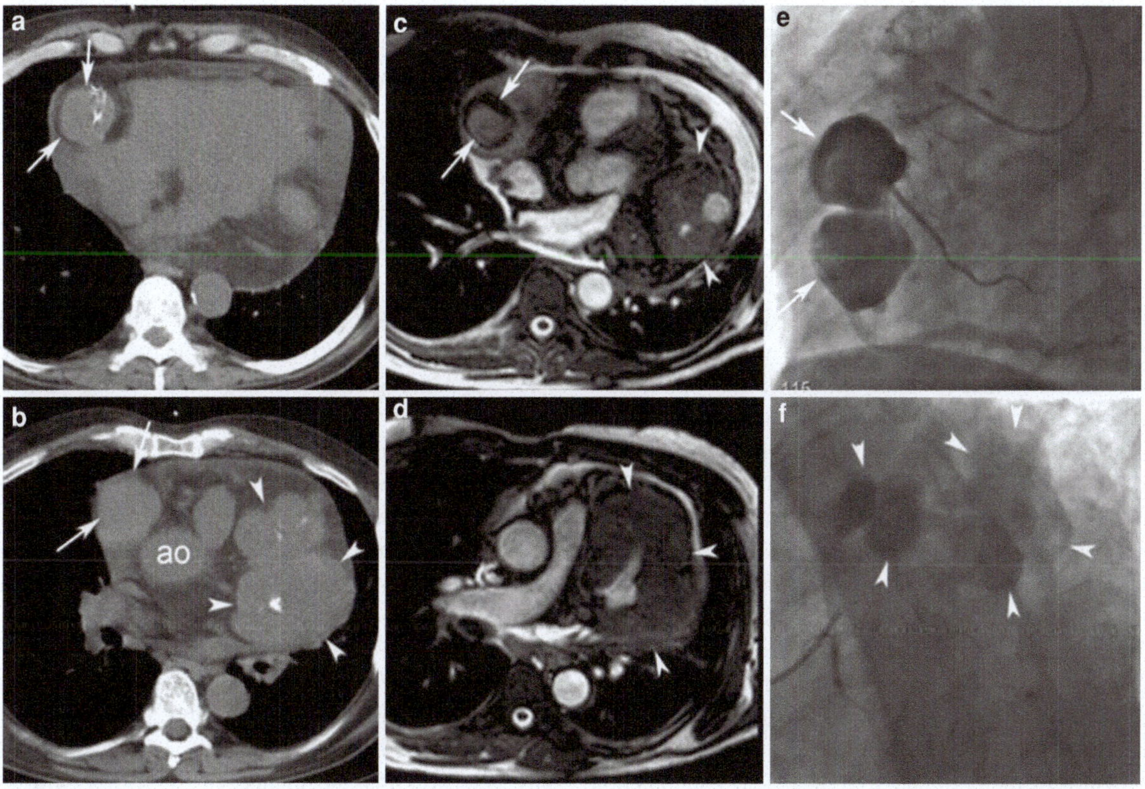

Fig. 18 Churg-Strauss coronary vasculitis. Multiple coronary aneurysms (*arrowheads*) are shown on non-enhanced chest CT (**a–b**), b-SSFP MR coronary angiography (**c–d**) and X-ray angiography (**e–f**)

often sufficient for this purpose initially, visualization and characterization of the coronary arteries become progressively more difficult as children grow. Serial evaluation with X-ray angiography carries risks associated with its invasive nature and exposure to ionizing radiation (Vitiello et al. 1998). Although in a recent paper, Sohn and colleagues reported on the role of MDCT in the detection and follow-up of coronary artery aneurysms due to Kawasaki disease, the considerable X-ray dose of repeated CT investigations will seriously limit its role as a follow-up technique in a pediatric population. Coronary MR angiography on the other hand is totally harmless, and the technique has become sufficiently robust to be used in the pediatric population. In the late 1990s, several groups investigated the use of this technique in a limited number of patients with Kawasaki disease (Flacke et al. 2000; Molinari et al. 2000). More recently, two larger patient studies have been published. Greil et al. compared real-time NE 3D-free-breathing coronary MR angiography with conventional angiography in 6 patients with Kawasaki disease (Greil et al. 2002). They found complete agreement between both techniques in the detection of coronary artery aneurysms (n = 11), coronary artery stenoses (n = 2) and coronary occlusions (n = 2). Moreover, an excellent correlation was found for the maximal diameter and length of the coronary artery aneurysms. In the second study, 14 young patients with Kawasaki disease (mean age: 22 ± 31 months) were studied with MR imaging (Vick et al. 2003). The study protocol included: real-time NE 3D-free-breathing coronary MR angiography, T2-weighted fast spin-echo MR imaging and CE-MRA of the peripheral arteries, with the results compared with echocardiography. Coronary artery diameters were comparable between both techniques but MR angiography demonstrated distal coronary artery regions that were often not well seen echocardiographically. In patients with acute Kawasaki disease, increased signal intensity surrounding coronary artery aneurysm sites on T2-weighted images was found. Moreover, several large aneurysms were found in peripheral arteries with CE-MRA. Further evaluation of MR imaging in patients with Kawasaki disease is now necessary following these initial positive results (Fig. 18). Furthermore, since patients are prone to development of coronary artery stenosis with subsequent development of myocardial ischemia, coronary flow assessment and other MR imaging techniques to detect myocardial ischemia and infarction might be interesting to investigate patients with Kawasaki disease.

Takayasu's arteritis is a chronic vasculitis involving the aorta and its main branches, the pulmonary arteries, and the coronary tree and needs to be considered in a young patient with angina, in particular when pulses are absent. It may lead to stenosis with obstruction caused by fibrosis and thrombus formation or aneurysm formation due to weakening of the vessel wall. Although cardiac features are present in up to 40% of cases, angina pectoris is rarely a presenting feature, reported in 6–16% of cases. Angina pectoris is usually caused by premature coronary disease, in particular involving the ostia of the coronary arteries, but may be related to extrinsic compression of the coronary tree or a steal phenomenon (Malik et al. 2003). At present, the role of coronary MR angiography is not yet defined.

12.4 Ischemic Heart Disease

12.4.1 Coronary Artery Stenosis Detection

As discussed in the previous paragraphs, coronary MR angiography has become an excellent technique for the non-invasive visualization of the origin and course of the coronary arteries. However, the biggest question remains unanswered—What is the current value and clinical role of coronary MR angiography in detecting coronary artery disease (CAD)? And is it an acceptable alternative to X-ray coronary angiography? Moreover, as several recent publications have suggested a promising role for MR imaging of the coronary artery vessel wall and characterization of atherosclerotic plaques, new expectations have been created.

Since the early 1990s, several patient studies using coronary MR angiography for assessing CAD have been published, reporting variable success for imaging coronary artery stenoses with a wide range of sensitivities and specificities (Pennell et al. 1993; Manning et al. 1993; Duerinckx and Urman 1994; Post et al. 1996; van Geuns et al. 1999; Sandstede et al. 1999; Huber et al. 1999; Lethimonnier et al. 1999; Sardanelli et al. 2000; Regenfus et al. 2000; van Geuns et al. 1999; Kim et al. 2001b; Regenfus et al. 2002; Sommer et al. 2002; Weber et al. 2002; Bogaert et al. 2003). Comparison of the different studies is difficult for several reasons. There have constantly been technical improvements in coronary MR angiography techniques over time, and what initially was considered as innovative, is nowadays completely outdated. Although this technical progress has led to a much more reliable and robust visualization of longer coronary arterial segments and side branches, improved coronary artery image quality and vessel sharpness, surprisingly this has not been reflected in an improved accuracy of coronary artery stenosis detection. Most studies used X-ray coronary angiography as reference technique to compare the coronary MR angiography results. The criteria for comparison, however, differed between studies. Some studies included only the segments that were visible on coronary MR angiography for comparison, others used only the proximal segments, or segments with a minimal coronary artery diameter (e.g. $\geq$2 mm) as inclusion criteria. There were inter-study differences between the definitions of a significant coronary artery stenosis, e.g. 50% versus 70% stenosis (Fig. 19).

Statistical analysis has also differed widely between studies. While most studies used a comparison of individual coronary segments, others used the entire coronary artery for comparison or expressed results on a per patient basis. The criteria to include a patient are not always clear, and might lead to bias of results. Although most studies mention a consecutive inclusion of patients (e.g. scheduled for an elective coronary angiography), and a blind reading of the coronary MR angiography studies, these issues are difficult to verify when assessing the published data. Multi-center studies with a central, blinded reading of studies are one way to make results more believable, and only a few studies to date have used receiver operating characteristic (ROC) curves, as a more efficient way to display the relationship between sensitivity and specificity, for expressing their results (Duerinckx et al. 1995; Bogaert et al. 2003). For these ROC-analyses, a degree-of-confidence decision task is used, i.e confidence from 1 (definitely normal) to 5

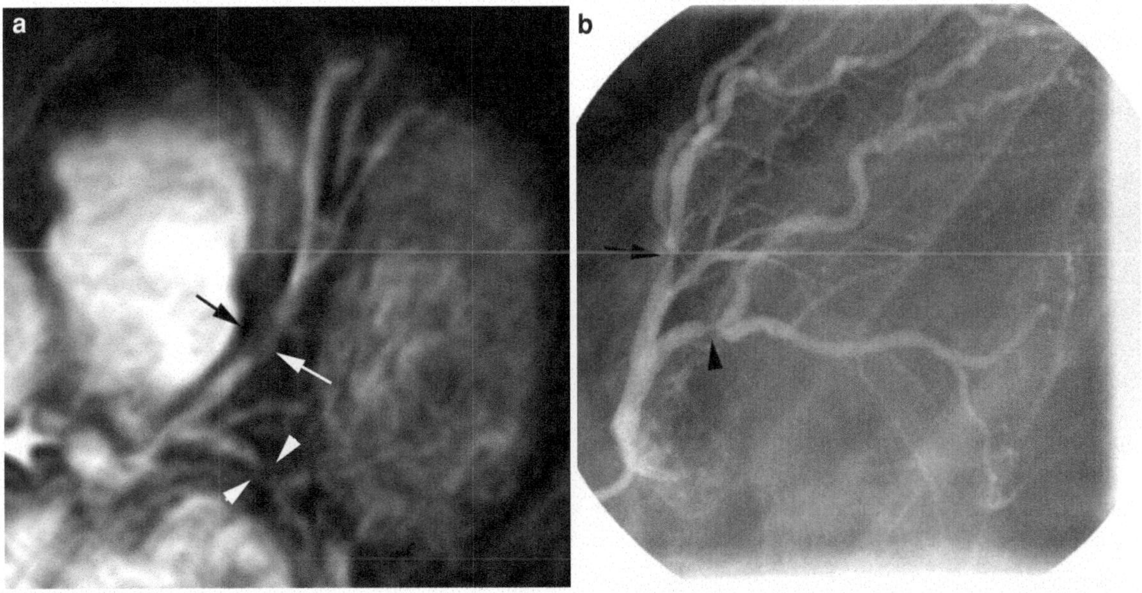

Fig. 19 Hemodynamically significant stenosis of proximal LAD (*arrows*) and proximal LCx (*arrowheads*) on coronary MR angiography (**a**), confirmed by X-ray coronary angiography (**b**). (X-ray coronary angiography, courtesy of Walter Desmet MD, PhD, dept of Cardiology, UZ Leuven, Leuven, Belgium)

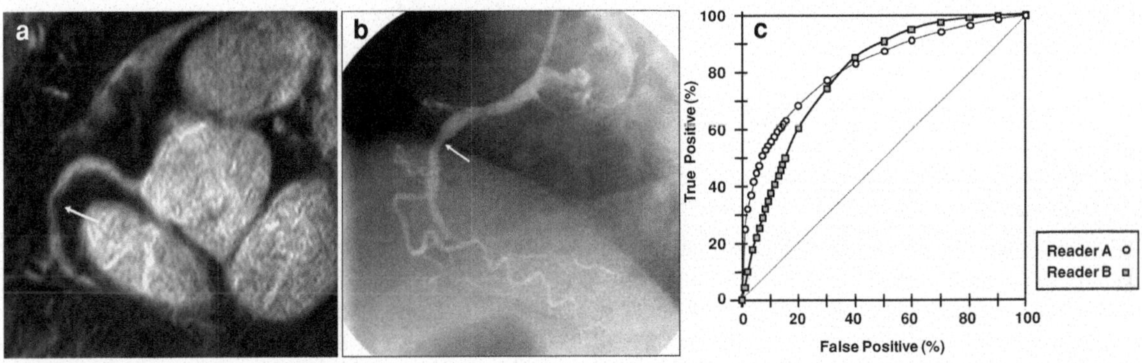

Fig. 20 Hemodynamically significant stenosis in mid-RCA in a 61-year-old male patient on 3D free-breathing coronary MR angiography using spoiled-GE-technique (**a**), confirmed by X-ray coronary angiography (**b**). Corresponding ROC curves (**c**) (area under the curve, reader A: 0.82, reader B: 0.80) for the detection of hemodynamically significant CA stenoses on coronary MR angiography in 21 patients by two independent readers. From Bogaert J et al. (2003) Radiology 226:707–716. Reprinted with permission of Radiology

(definitely abnormal), to define the four cutoffs at which sensitivity and specificity are calculated and the ROC curves are plotted. The closer an ROC is situated to the upper left-hand corner of the graph, the more accurate the coronary MR angiography. Another way to express the clinical feasibility is the assessment of confidence levels between two independent readers, using the kappa statistic to measure the agreement between readers (Fig. 20).

The following points should be considered from the patient studies. The accuracy of stenosis detection is strongly dependent on the image quality (Duerinckx et al. 1995; Wielopolski et al. 2000; Sommer et al. 2002; Bogaert et al. 2003). As soon as the image quality drops, a large number of image artifacts are created which can be misinterpreted as representing lesions (and vice versa), and which inevitably lead to a drop in the degree-of-confidence of lesion assessment. Image quality is often not predictable, but usually there is a drop in image quality between healthy volunteers and patients. Potential explanations for the lower image quality in patients are irregularities in heart rhythm or breathing pattern and breath-hold capacity, patient constitution (such as presence of lung emphysema in elderly patients), or technical issues such as suitability of NE technique in patients.

The more distal a lesion is from the origin the more difficult it is to detect. This is related to the smaller vessel size and less reliable image quality. Assessment of coronary artery stenosis in most studies was limited to the proximal half of the major coronary arteries, excluding the more distal parts and side branches. Although coronary artery stenosis detection is feasible in a considerable number of patients, quantification of the degree of stenosis is not. With the currently available in-plane spatial resolution of 0.7×0.7 mm even in the larger proximal coronary arterial portions distinction between a 40 and 60% stenosis is not possible. Therefore, at present the role of MR imaging as a first-line test that can be used to select patients for cardiac catheterization, seems limited. In diffuse atherosclerotic vessels, stenosis detection is hardly possible. Some other issues such as the influence of plaque composition on stenosis detection are not yet clarified. For example, what is the influence of atherosclerotic plaque calcification on the assessment on the coronary artery stenosis detection? What are the best coronary MR angiography techniques to detect fresh thrombi? New approaches such as combining coronary MR angiography with vessel wall imaging have the advantage that luminographic abnormalities can be directly compared with underlying abnormalities in the arterial wall (Spuentrup et al. 2003). From a clinical point of view, it has to be said that coronary artery wall imaging is still a research topic limited to a few centers. In the coming years, this novel technique will certainly become more widely available for evaluation of its clinical value.

Thus, to conclude, assessment of coronary artery stenosis with coronary MR angiography is promising but is still premature for daily routine clinical use. In some groups of patients, however, MR imaging may be considered for exclusion of coronary artery. For example, to rule out coronary stenosis in patients with a low likelihood of coronary artery disease, scheduled for aortic valve surgery, or, in patients in whom a cardiac catheterization forms a risk (e.g. aortic dissection) or is contraindicated (e.g. renal insufficiency, allergy to contrast media). Moreover, as pointed out in a recent study by Plein and coworkers, coronary MR angiography might be part of a comprehensive MR imaging protocol (Plein et al. 2002). In a one-hour scan, diagnostic information was obtained on cardiac function (short- and long-axis cine imaging), inducible myocardial ischemia (rest and adenosine stress perfusion), coronary artery patency (coronary MR angiography), and myocardial viability (delayed enhancement) in patients with coronary artery disease. From a cost-effective point of view these kinds of comprehensive protocols will become of utmost importance for keeping fast growing medical expenses under control.

12.4.2 Coronary Artery Stent Imaging and Assessment of Coronary Artery Restenosis

To improve the immediate and long-term results of balloon angioplasty, new forms of catheter-based therapies have been developed. Coronary artery stent placement has taken the lead in the treatment of obstructive coronary arterial disease, and is applied in more than 50% of patients undergoing non-surgical coronary artery interventional procedures (Pepine et al. 1996). Coronary arterial stents are typically made of stainless steel or tantalum. After implantation in the artery, they are endothelialized and incorporated into the vessel wall. Initially it was recommended that MR studies should be postponed for 4 to 8 weeks after stent implantation till the endothelialization had occurred, because it was believed that endothelialization opposed possible dislodgement. Several studies, since, have shown that at a field-strength of 1.5T, MR studies <8 weeks after coronary stent placement can be considered to be safe, and the risk of stent heating and stent migration, and subsequent stent thrombosis and myocardial infarction and cardiac death is low (Hug et al. 2000; Schroeder et al. 2000; Gerber et al. 2003a, b). The artifact size, created by the stent, differs according to the type and size of stent, the MR imaging sequence used and the orientation to the main magnetic field (Hug et al. 2000). Fast spin-echo images had minimal artifacts while larger artifacts are seen on the turbo gradient-echo and echo-planar images. Coronary artery stents

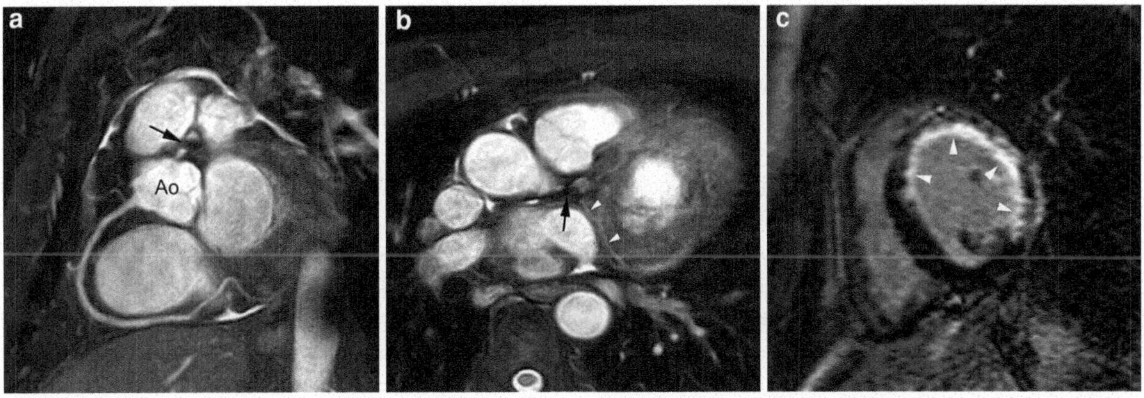

Fig. 21 **a–c** Patient with in-stent restenosis. Stent in LM visible as area of signal void (*arrow*) on MR coronary angiography (**a**, **b**). In contrast to the normal appearance of the (dominant) RCA, the LCx is very thin and the LAD is not visible. On late-enhancement MR imaging using the contrast-enhanced inversion-recovery technique a large infarct is visible involving the anterior and lateral LV walls (LAD and LCx perfusion territory)

typically appear as well-defined areas of signal void on coronary MR angiography (Sardanelli et al. 2002). MR-lucent stents, allowing to assess the CA lumen are currently under development.

Although improved medical treatment regimes have significantly reduced the risk of stent occlusion, this risk is still estimated to be in the range of 20–40%. To date, several MR imaging approaches are under investigation to evaluate patients with suspected stent occlusion or re-stenosis, by either direct assessment of the stent patency (Duerinckx et al. 1998), or indirect evaluation of the distal coronary artery flow (and flow reserve) (Saito et al. 2001; Sardanelli et al. 2002; Nagel et al. 2003). Radiofrequency penetration into the stents is strongly influenced by the stent material. For example, tantalum stents demonstrate minimal intra-luminal signal attenuation, while steel stents show pronounced intraluminal signal voids (Fig. 21). So, future stent design should be focused on the MR imaging characteristics to allow optimal intra-stent imaging. Another new, interesting approach for imaging the stent lumen is to use the stent as a receiver coil itself. Low signal in the distal coronary artery on bright-blood coronary artery MR angiography has been reported to occur in-stent restenosis, in a small group of patients (Sardanelli et al. 2002). Saito and coworkers measured coronary flow reserve repeatedly for 6 months after stent placement and found a significant reduction in coronary flow reserve in patients with an angiographically confirmed re-stenosis at 6 months (2.26 ± 0.49 at 1 month vs. 1.52 ± 0.09 at 6 months). In patients without re-stenosis, coronary flow reserve remained normal (2.31 ± 0.30 at 1 month vs. 2.52 ± 0.25 at 6 months) (Saito et al. 2001). Two other studies found similar results in patients with stent re-stenosis (Nagel et al. 2003). However, the optimal coronary flow reserve threshold for detecting stent re-stenosis differed significantly between the two studies (1.2 vs. 2.0, respectively).

12.4.3 Coronary Artery Bypass Graft Imaging and Patency Assessment

Surgical placement of a coronary artery bypass graft is an effective and frequently performed intervention for patients with coronary artery stenoses. The procedure results in reduced angina symptoms and cardiovascular mortality. However, the 10-year patency rate for saphenous vein grafts is only 40–60% as a result of a combination of early thrombosis, intimal hyperplasia, and accelerated atherosclerosis. For internal mammary artery grafts, survival is better, with up to 90% of grafts patent at 10 years. Conventional angiography is commonly performed to investigate bypass graft and native vessel patency in patients who present with recurrent angina. The altered vascular anatomy and the need to image additional vessels, results in prolonged, more difficult procedures with increased exposure to ionizing radiation and increased renal toxicity to contrast agents. MR imaging has been used to non-invasively assess CABG patency with several techniques; black-blood spin-echo sequences, different bright-blood gradient-echo sequences (Aurigemma et al. 1989; Galjee et al. 1996; Langerak et al. 2002), CE-MRA techniques (Bunce et al. 2003). Coronary artery bypass graft MR angiography has yet to reach the level of reliability required for clinical use. Graft stenosis often occurs at the site of the anastomosis with the native coronary artery, a location where MR imaging encounters spatial-resolution problems, and hence reduced consistency in image quality. Bypass graft angiography encounters similar problems induced by respiratory and cardiac motion as for imaging native coronary artery stenosis.

Metallic clip artifacts remain a problem. Arterial grafts are small, tortuous vessels that are difficult to assess with MR techniques. In a recent study by Langerak and colleagues, diagnostic accuracy of approximately 80% was observed after exclusion of patients with stents and another 11% of patients with insufficient image quality (Langerak et al. 2002). Although the ROC areas under the curve were acceptable for identifying graft occlusion (0.89), significantly lower values were found for assessing ≥50 and ≥70% stenotic lesions. A similar pattern was found for the interobserver agreement. In another recent study, comparing CE-MRA with b-SSFP angiography, 84% of the venous grafts were correctly identified as patent and only 45% correctly identified as occluded with b-SSFP angiography versus 85 and 73% respectively for cardiac-gated CE-MRA (Bunce et al. 2003). Both techniques were unreliable for accurately assessing graft stenosis or stenosis within the distal native vessels.

An alternative to CABG angiography is assessment of flow patterns and flow reserve using the phase-contrast technique (Galjee et al. 1996; Langerak et al. 2003a, b). Defining cutoff or threshold values for different degrees of graft stenoses, however, is complicated. The flow pattern in the bypass graft is influenced by the type of graft used (vein vs. arterial), the number of bypass anastomosis to the coronary arteries (single vs. sequential), the flow pattern in the distal epicardial coronary arteries (i.e, right vs. left coronary artery tree, normal run-off vs. diseased run-off) and microcirculation and the location within the graft where the flow is measured. Moreover, the flow pattern may be influenced by concurrent anterograde flow through native coronary arteries and in collateral vessels. The aorta and mammary arteries have a high systolic forward flow, whereas the coronary arteries (mainly the LAD) have the largest forward flow during diastole. So, proximal measurements in the internal mammary artery preferentially show a systolic pattern, distal measurements a diastolic pattern, while in between a transition pattern will be found. Single and sequential graft are functional different grafts as sequential graft show significantly higher volume flow and velocity values (Galjee et al. 1996; Langerak et al. 2003a, b), a phenomenon likely related to the lower resistance in sequential grafts. Langerak and colleagues found a baseline total flow of 25 ± 9 mL/min and a maximal total flow of 65 ± 33 mL/min during adenosine infusion in normal single grafts, versus 41 ± 15 mL/min and 99 ± 36 mL/min respectively in sequential grafts. The graft flow reserve was 2.7 for both types of grafts, a value that corresponds to those measured with intravascular Doppler flow wires. In another study by the Leiden Group, baseline and stress velocities were measured in different types of bypass grafts and cutoff points were determined to differentiate between grafts with and without stenosis (Langerak et al. 2003a, b). The best results were obtained using velocity reserve to detect bypass stenoses in single vein grafts. MR flow mapping was used by the same group to examine the beneficial effects of percutaneous intervention (PCI) in patients with graft stenosis (Langerak et al. 2003a, b).

Ishida and colleagues measured the flow volumes, and the diastolic-to-systolic peak velocities ratio in internal mammary artery-to-coronary artery bypass grafts. Flow measurements in the midpoint of the internal mammary artery showed a mean flow rate of 80 ± 38 mL/min in the non-stenotic group versus 17 ± 5 mL/min in the stenotic group ($p < 0.01$). Moreover, a reversal in diastolic-to-systolic peak velocity ratios was found in the stenotic group (0.61 ± 0.44) as compared with the non-stenotic group (1.88 ± 0.96) ($p < 0.01$). The flow reserve ratios, however, were not significantly different between the two groups. In another recent study, Bedaux and colleagues used an algorithm combining resting flow (<20 mL/min) and graft flow reserve (<2) for detecting a significant stenosis in the graft or distal run-off vessel. This study combined the approach of previous studies where either flow volumes, graft flow volumes or velocity reserves were independently used to demonstrate significant stenosis in the graft or distal run-off vessels. This algorithm had a sensitivity and specificity of 78 and 80% respectively, for detecting grafts with significant stenosis or diseased run-off. However, it should be stressed that because of significant overlap in values of basal flow and flow reserve ratio between patients with and without a graft or distal run-off vessel stenosis, application of these values in the individual patient should be interpreted with care.

13 Coronary MR Angiography Versus Coronary CT Angiography

Another emerging coronary imaging technique, and at present definitely the closest competitor for coronary MR angiography, is coronary CT angiography. Considerable progress has been achieved in the field of non or minimally invasive coronary imaging with multislice spiral computed tomography (MSCT) (Budoff et al. 2003). Initially, with the use of 4-slice MSCT scanners promising results were published; however, cardiac motion and calcium deposits in the coronary artery wall rendered a substantial number of scans incompletely interpretable (Gerber et al. 2003a, b; Kuettner et al. 2004). Motion artifacts limit proper assessment, particularly at higher heart rates. With the advent of newer generation MSCT scanners, equipped with more (up to 320 slices), thinner detector rows (0.6 mm) and increased rotation speed (up to three rotations per second), some of the previous problems can be solved (Pannu et al. 2003). Cardiac CT largely faces the same constraints as MR imaging for studying the coronary arteries. The strategies used to improve the depiction of the coronary arteries with MR imaging can to a large extent also be applied to coronary CT angiography. However, there are several problems that are specific to coronary CT angiography. The issue of motion remains a potential problem even with newer generation of CT scanners. Acquisition windows have been shortened due to faster rotation times, and improved multisector acquisitions in patients with fast heart rates. However, acquisition windows of 210 ms are still too long to image fast-moving coronary artery segment such as the RCA (Achenbach et al. 2000). Segmented data acquisition in two (or eventual three) heartbeats is feasible as long as the patient has a regular heart rhythm. Breath-hold duration has been considerably shortened with evolutions starting with 64-slice MSCT scanners. A single 10-s breath-hold is feasible for most patients, especially when an oxygen mask is applied. Spatial resolution is currently slightly superior for CT (e.g. 0.6 × 0.6 × 0.6 mm) than for MR angiography. Sub-millimetre, nearly isotropic, volumetric data acquisition enables visualization of almost the entirety of the epicardial coronary artery system. However, the current achievable spatial resolution is insufficient to determine the degree of coronary artery stenoses (Achenbach et al. 2000) (Fig. 22).

Another important issue for CT angiography is the influence of calcium deposition in the coronary wall, which may restrict adequate imaging of the underlying vessel lumen. Two other important issues, which only CT has to face, are the necessity to administer iodinated contrast and the high radiation doses that are currently used in coronary CT angiography. Thus, CT should be considered as being a minimally invasive rather than non-invasive technique.

The main advantages of CT is that simultaneous quantification of the amount of calcium deposition in the coronary arteries—"coronary calcium scoring", and CT angiography. Though, it must be stressed that the role of coronary calcium scoring for assessing the severity of coronary artery disease, and in predicting future cardiac events is still a controversial subject in the literature.

Finally, a possible important role for CT is in the characterization of atherosclerotic plaque composition, assessment of coronary remodeling, and definition of the factors contributing to plaque rupture and cardiac events, and further research is required in this domain (Pouleur et al. 2008; Nunoda et al. 2010).

To date, we do not know whether CT or MR provides the best non-invasive imaging modality for assessing the coronary artery lumen and vessel wall, in particular as neither provides a valuable alternative to conventional X-ray coronary angiography. Both techniques are still emerging, and have great potential to become an alternative or complementary technique for coronary artery imaging.

14 Key Points

Early detection and adequate treatment of CAD is one of the major challenges in current medicine.

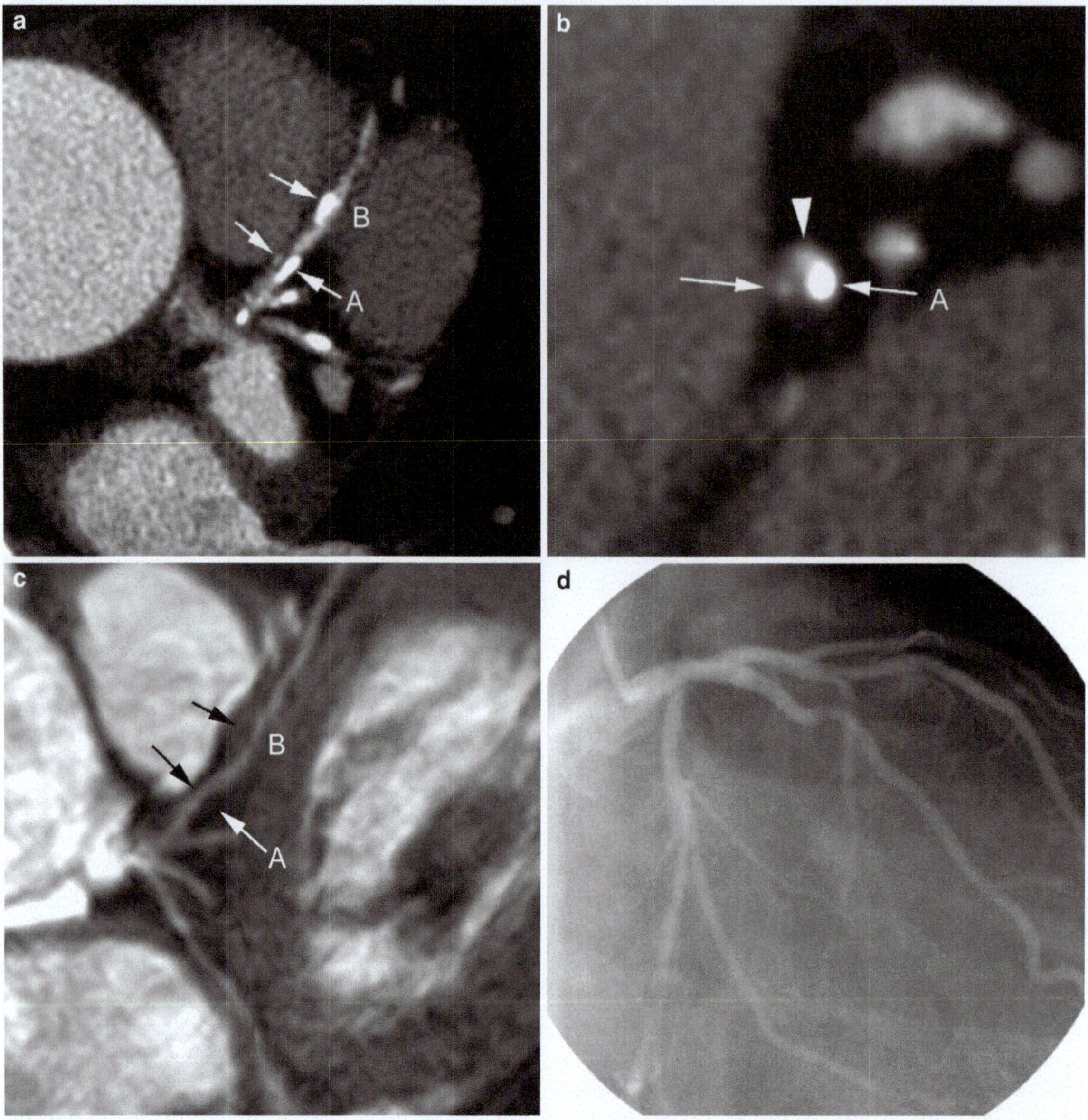

Fig. 22 Influence of CA calcifications and CA caliber in the detection of CA stenoses. Comparison between 16-slice coronary CT (**a**, **b**) and coronary MR angiography (**c**). Reference technique is X-ray coronary angiography (**d**). Coronary artery calcifications (*arrows*) may seriously hamper the detection of underlying CA stenosis on coronary CT angiography. In this patient the proximal and mid LAD are not evaluable on coronary CT angiography. In contrast, coronary MR angiography is much less influenced by atherosclerotic calcifications (*arrows*) (**c**). A cross-sectional reconstruction through A (**b**) shows a peripheral calcification; the CA lumen is indicated by an arrowhead. Taking into account the normal findings on X-ray coronary angiography (**d**), the latter likely represents a plaque with positive remodeling. (X-ray coronary angiography, courtesy of Walter Desmet MD, PhD, dept of Cardiology, UZ Leuven, Leuven, Belgium)

Non-invasive imaging techniques will have a crucial role in determining the “vulnerability index” of atherosclerotic plaques.

MR imaging has the intrinsic strengths to fulfill this role.

Coronary artery imaging with MR has become feasible on routine MR scanners equipped with commercially available cardiac MR hard- and software.

Several approaches for coronary MR angiography are currently available. At present, none of them can be considered as having the gold.

Coronary MR angiography is a perfect example of trading between different parameters that influence image quality.

Large parts of the coronary artery tree can be visualized in a reliable fashion, allowing to determine the origin and course of the epicardial coronary arteries and several of their branches.

Detection of CA stenoses is closely linked to the image quality. Grading of CA stenoses, however, is hampered by the current lack in spatial resolution.

Coronary artery wall imaging and plaque characterization with MR is promising, but these techniques are not yet available for routine clinical applications.

There is a close competition between CT and MR in the field of CA imaging. Although promising results can be found in the literature for both techniques, they are not yet capable to replace catheter-based X-ray coronary angiography.

References

Achenbach S, Ropers D, Holle J, Muschiol G, Daniel WG, Moshage W (2000) In-plane coronary arterial motion velocity: measurement with electron-beam CT. Radiology 216:457–463

Angelini P (1989) Normal and anomalous coronary arteries: definitions and classification. Am Heart J 117:418–434

Anné W, Bogaert J, Van de Werf F (2000) A case report of a patient with a large aneurysmatic coronary artery fistula. Acta Cardiol 55:307–310

Atkinson D, Edelman R (1991) Cineangiography of the heart in a single breathhold with a segmented TurboFLASH sequence. Radiology 178:359–362

Aurigemma GP, Reichek N, Axel L, Schiebler M, Harris C, Kressel HY (1989) Non-invasive determination of coronary artery bypass graft patency by cine magnetic resonance imaging. Circulation 80:1595–1602

Austen WG, Edwards JE, Frye RL et al (1975) A reporting system on patients evaluated for coronary artery disease: report of the Ad Hoc committee for grading of coronary artery disease, Council in cardiovascular surgery, American heart association. Circulation 51:5–40

Bogaert J, Duerinckx A (1995) Appearance of the normal pericardium on coronary MR angiograms. J Magn Reson 5:579–587

Bogaert J, Kuzo S, Dymarkowski S, Becker R, Piessens J, Rademakers FE (2003) Coronary artery imaging using real-time navigator 3D Turbo-field-echo MR coronary angiography technique. Initial experience. Radiology 226:707–716

Börnert P, Jensen D (1995) Coronary artery imaging at 0.5T using segmented 3D echo planar imaging. Magn Reson Med 34:779–785

Börnert P, Aldefeld B, Nehrke K (2001) Improved 3D spiral imaging for coronary MR angiography. Magn Reson Med 45:172–175

Botnar RM, Stuber M, Danias PG, Kissinger KV, Manning WJ (1999) Improved coronary artery definition with T2-weighted free-breathing, three-dimensional coronary MRA. Circulation 99:3139–3148

Botnar RM, Stuber M, Kissinger KV, Manning WJ (2000) Free-breathing 3D coronary MRA: the impact of "isotropic" image resolution. J Magn Reson Imaging 11:389–393

Brittain JH, Hu BS, Wright GA, Meyer CH, Macovski A, Nishimura DG (1995) Coronary angiography with magnetization-prepared T2 contrast. Magn Reson Med 33: 689–696

Budoff MJ, Achenbach S, Duerinckx A (2003) Clinical utility of computed tomography and magnetic resonance techniques for non-invasive coronary angiography. J Am Coll Cardiol 42:1867–1878

Bunce NH, Pennell DJ (1999) Coronary MRA–a clinical experience in Europe. J Magn Reson Imag 10:721–727

Bunce NH, Rahman SL, Keegan J, Gatehouse PD, Lorenz CH, Pennell DJ (2001) Anomalous coronary arteries: anatomic and functional assessment by coronary and perfusion cardiovascular magnetic resonance in three sisters. J Cardiovasc Magn Reson 3:361–369

Bunce NH, Lorenz CH, John AS, Lesser JR, Mohiaddin RH, Pennell D (2003) Coronary artery bypass graft patency: assessment with true fast imaging with steady-state precession versus Gadolinium-enhanced MR angiography. Radiology 227:440–446

Carr J, Simonetti O, Bundy J, Li D, Pereles S, Finn JP (2001) Cine MR angiography of the heart with segmented true fast imaging with steady-state precession. Radiology 219:828–834

Click RL, Holmes DR, Vliestra RE, Kosinski A, Kronmal RA (1989) Anomalous coronary arteries: location, degree of atherosclerosis and effect on survival–a report from the coronary artery surgery study. J Am Coll Cardiol 13:531–537

Danias PG, McConnell MV, Khasgiwala VC, Chuang ML, Edelman RR, Manning WJ (1997) Prospective navigator correction of image position for coronary MR angiography. Radiology 203:733–736

Davis JA, Cecchin F, Jones TK, Portman MA (2001) Major coronary artery anomalies in a pediatric population: incidence and clinical importance. J Am Coll Cardiol 37:593–597

Deshpande VX, Shea SM, Laub G, Simonetti OP, Finn JP, Li D (2001) 3D Magnetization-prepared true-FISP: a new technique for imaging coronary arteries. Magn Reson Med 46:494–502

Deshpande VS, Chung Y-C, Zhang Q, Shea SM, Li D (2003) Reduction of transient signal oscillations in true-FISP using a linear flip angle series magnetization preparation. Magn Reson Med 49:151–157

Desmet W, Vanhaecke J, Vrolix M et al (1992) Isolated single coronary artery: a review of 50000 consecutive coronary angiographies. Eur Heart J 13:1637–1640

Doyle M, Scheidegger MB, De Graaf RG, Vermeulen J, Pohost GM (1993) Coronary artery imaging in multiple 1-sec breath holds. Magn Reson Imaging 11:3–6

Du YP, Parker DL, Davis WL et al (1994) Reduction of partial-volume artefacts with zero-filling interpolation in three-dimensional MR angiography. J Magn Reson Imaging 4:733–741

Duerinckx AJ, Urman M (1994) Two-dimensional coronary MR angiography: analysis of initial clinical results. Radiology 193:731–738

Duerinckx AJ, Bogaert J, Jiang H, Lewis BS (1995) Anomalous origin of the left coronary artery: diagnosis by coronary MR angiography. Am J Roentgenol 164:1095–1096

Duerinckx AJ, Atkinson D, Hurwitz R (1998) Assessment of coronary artery patency after stent placement using magnetic resonance angiography. J Magn Reson Imaging 8:896–902

Edelman R, Manning W, Burstein D, Paulin S (1991) Coronary arteries: breath-hold MR angiography. Radiology 181:641–643

Etienne A, Botnar RM, van Muiswinkel AMC, Boesiger P, Manning WJ, Stuber M (2002) "Soap-Bubble" visualization and quantitative analysis of 3D coronary magnetic resonance angiograms. Magn Reson Med 48:658–666

Fayad ZA, Fuster V, Fallon JT et al (2000) Non-invasive in vivo human coronary artery lumen and wall imaging using black-blood magnetic resonance imaging. Circulation 102:506–510

Ferrigno M, Hickey DD, Liner MH, Lundgren CEG (1986) Cardiac performance in humans during breath-holding. J Appl Physiol 60:1871–1877

Flacke S, Setser RM, Barger P et al (2000) Coronary aneurysms in Kawasaki's disease detected by magnetic resonance coronary angiography. Circulation 101:E516–E517

Fleckenstein JL, Archer BT, Barker BA, Vaughan JT, Parkey RW, Peshock RM (1991) Fast short-tau inversion-recovery MR imaging. Radiology 179:499–504

Foo TKF, Ho VB, Hood MN (2000) Vessel tracking: prospective adjustment of section-selective MR angiographic locations for improved coronary artery visualization over the cardiac cycle. Radiology 214:283–289

Galjee MA, van Rossum AC, Doesburg T, van Eenige MJ, Visser CA (1996) Value of magnetic resonance imaging in assessing patency and function of coronary artery bypass grafts. Circulation 93:660–666

Garg N, Tewari S, Kapoor A, Gupta DK, Sinha N (2000) Primary congenital anomalics of the coronary arteries: a coronary arteriographic study. Int J Cardiol 74:39–46

Gerber TC, Fasseas P, Lennon RJ et al (2003a) Clinical safety of magnetic resonance imaging early after coronary artery stent placement. J Am Coll Cardiol 42:1295–1298

Gerber TC, Kuzo RS, Lane GE et al (2003b) Image quality in a standardized algorithm for minimally invasive coronary angiography with multi-slice spiral computed tomography. J Comput Assist Tomogr 27:62–69

Giorgi B, Dymarkowski S, Maes F, Kouwenhoven M, Bogaert J (2002) Improved visualization of coronary arteries using a new three-dimensional submillimeter MR coronary angiography sequence with balanced gradients. Am J Roentgenol 179:901–910

Goldfarb JW, Edelman RR (1998) Coronary arteries: breath-hold gadolinium-enhanced, three-dimensional MR angiography. Radiology 206:830–834

Gomes A, Lois J, Drinkwater D, Corday S (1987) Coronary artery bypass grafts: visualization with MR imaging. Radiology 162:175–179

Gould KL, Lipscomb K, Hamilton GW (1974) Physiologic basis for assessing critical coronary stenosis: instantaneous flow response and regional distribution during coronary hyperemia as measures of coronary flow reserve. Am J Cardiol 33:87–94

Greil GF, Stuber M, Botnar RM et al (2002) Coronary magnetic resonance angiography in adolescents and young adults with Kawasaki disease. Circulation 105:908–911

Haase A, Frahm J, Hänicke W, Matthaei D (1985) 1H NMR chemical shift selective (CHESS) imaging. Phys Med Biol 4:341–344

Hofman MBM, Visser FC, van Rossum AC, Vink GQM, Sprenger M, Westerhof N (1995) In vivo validation of magnetic resonance volume flow measurements with limited spatial resolution in small vessels. Magn Reson Med 33:778–784

Hofman MB, van Rossum AC, Sprenger M, Westerhof N (1996) Assessment of flow in the right human coronary artery by magnetic resonance phase contrast velocity measurement: effects of cardiac and respiratory motion. Magn Reson Med 35:521–531

Hofman MB, Wickline SA, Lorenz CH (1998) Quantification of in-plane motion of the coronary arteries during the cardiac cycle: implication for acquisition window duration for MR flow quantification. J Magn Reson Imaging 8:568–576

Hofman MB, Henson RE, Kovacs SJ et al (1999) Blood pool contrast agent strongly improves 3D magnetic resonance coronary angiography using an inversion prepulse. Magn Reson Med 41:360–367

Holsinger AE, Riederer SJ (1990) The importance of phase encoding order in ultra-short TR snapshot MR imaging. Magn Reson Med 16:481–488

Huber A, Nikolaou K, Gonschior P, Knez A, Stehling M, Reiser M (1999) Navigator echo-based respiratory gating for three-dimensional MR coronary angiography: results from healthy volunteers and patients with proximal coronary artery stenoses. Am J Roentgenol 173:95–101

Hug J, Nagel E, Bornstedt A, Schnackenburg B, Oswald H, Fleck E (2000) Coronary arterial stents: safety and artifacts during MR imaging. Radiology 216:781–787

Jahnke C, Paetsch I, Nehrke K, Schnackenburg B, Bornstedt A, Gebker R, Fleck E, Nagel E (2005) A new approach for rapid assessment of the cardiac rest period for coronary MRA. J Cardiovasc Magn Reson 7(2):395–399

Johansson LO, Fischer SE, Lorenz CH (1999) Benefit of T1 reduction for magnetic resonance coronary angiography: a numerical simulation and phantom study. J Magn Reson Imaging 9:552–556

Joyce JD, Schulman DS, Lasorda D et al (1994) Intracoronary Doppler guide wire versus stress single-photon emission computed tomography thallium-201 imaging in assessment of intermediate coronary stenoses. J Am Coll Cardiol 24:940–947

Kalden P, Kreitner KF, Wittlinger T et al (1999) Assessment of coronary artery bypass grafts: value of different breath-hold MR imaging techniques. Am J Roentgenol 172:1359–1364
Keegan J, Gatehouse PD, Mohiaddin RH, Yang HZ, Firmin DN (2004) Comparison of spiral and FLASH phase velocity mapping, with and without breath-holding, for the assessment of left and right coronary artery blood flow velocity. J Magn Reson Imaging 19:40–49
Kim WY, Stuber M, Kissinger KV, Andersen NT, Manning WJ, Botnar RM (2001) Impact of bulk cardiac motion on right coronary MR angiography and vessel wall imaging. J Magn Reson Imaging 14:383–390
Kuettner A, Kopp AF, Schroeder S et al (2004) Diagnostic accuracy of multidetector computed tomography coronary angiography in patients with angiographically proven coronary artery disease. J Am Coll Cardiol 43:831–839
Langerak SE, Vliegen HW, de Roos A et al (2002) Detection of vein graft disease using high-resolution magnetic resonance angiography. Circulation 105:328–333
Langerak SE, Vliegen JW, Zwinderman AH et al (2003a) Vein graft function improvement after percutaneous intervention: evaluation with MR flow mapping. Radiology 228:834–841
Langerak SE, Vliegen HW, Jukema JW et al (2003b) Value of magnetic resonance imaging for the non-invasive detection of stenosis in coronary artery bypass grafts and recipient coronary arteries. Circulation 107:1502–1508
Langreck H, Schnackenburg B, Nehrke K, Boernert P, Wahl A, Paetsch I, Bornstedt A, Fleck E, Nagel E (2005) MR coronary artery imaging with 3D motion adapted gating (MAG) in comparison to a standard prospective navigator technique. J Cardiovasc Magn Reson 7(5):793–797
Lethimonnier F, Furber A, Morel O et al (1999) Three-dimensional coronary artery MR imaging using prospective real-time respiratory navigator and linear phase shift processing: comparison with conventional coronary angiography. Magn Reson Imaging 17:1111–1120
Li D, Carr JC, Shea SM, Zheng J, Deshpande VS, Wielopolski PA, Finn JP (2001a) Coronary arteries: magnetization-prepared contrast-enhanced three-dimensional volume targeted breath-hold MR angiography. Radiology 219:270–277
Li D, Zheng J, Weinmann H-J (2001b) Contrast-enhanced MR imaging of coronary arteries: comparison of intra- and extravascular contrast agents in Swine. Radiology 218:670–678
Lorenz CH, Johansson LO (1999) Contrast-enhanced coronary MRA. J Magn Reson Imaging 10:703–708
Malik IS, Harare O Al-Nahhas A, Beatt K, Mason J (2003) Takayasu's arteritis: management of left main stem stenosis. Heart 89:e9–e12
Manke D, Börnert P, Nehrke K, Nagel E, Dössel O (2001) Accelerated coronary MRA by simultaneous acquisition of multiple 3D stacks. J Magn Reson Imaging 14:478–483
Manning WJ, Li W, Boyle NG, Edelman RR (1993) Fat-suppressed breath-hold magnetic resonance coronary angiography. Circulation 87:94–104
Marcus JT, Smeenk HG, Kuijer JPA, Van der Geest RJ, Heethaar RM, Van Rossum AC (1999) Flow profiles in the left anterior descending and the right coronary artery assessed by MR velocity quantification: effects of through-plane and in-plane motion of the heart. J Comput Assist Tomogr 4:567–576
McConnell MV, Khasgiwala VC, Savord BJ et al (1997) Prospective adaptive navigator correction for breath-hold MR coronary angiography. Magn Reson Med 37:148–152
Meyer CH, Pauly JM, Macovski A, Mishimura DG (1990) Simultaneous spatial and spectral selective excitation. Magn Reson Med 15:287–304
Mohiaddin RH, Bogren HG, Lazim F et al (1996) Magnetic resonance coronary angiography in heart transplant recipients. Coronary Artery Dis 7:591–597
Molinari G, Sardanelli F, Zandrino F et al (2000) Coronary aneurysms and stenosis detected with magnetic resonance coronary angiography in a patient with Kawasaki disease. Ital Heart J 1:368–371
Nagel E, Bornstedt A, Hug J, Schnackenburg B, Wellnhofer E, Fleck E (1999) Non-invasive determination of coronary blood flow velocity with magnetic resonance imaging: comparison of breath-hold and navigator techniques with intravascular ultrasound. Magn Reson Med 41:544–549
Nagel E, Thouet T, Klein C et al (2003) Non-invasive determination of coronary blood flow velocity with cardiovascular magnetic resonance in patients with stent deployment. Circulation 107:1738–1743
Nassenstein K, Waltering KU, Kelle S, Schlosser T, Breuckmann F, Maderwald S, Hunold P, Nagel E, Barkhausen J (2008) Magnetic resonance coronary angiography with Vasovist: in vivo T1 estimation to improve image quality of navigator and breath-hold techniques. Eur Radiol 18(1):103–109
Nassenstein K, Breuckmann F, Hunold P, Barkhausen J, Schlosser T (2009) (2009) Magnetic resonance coronary angiography: comparison between a Gd-BOPTA- and a Gd-DTPA-enhanced spoiled gradient-echo sequence and a non-contrast-enhanced steady-state free-precession sequence. Acta Radiol 50(4):406–411
Nitatori T, Hanaoka H, Yoshino A et al (1995) Clinical application of magnetic resonance angiography for coronary arteries: correlation with conventional angiography and evaluation of imaging time. Nippon Acta Radiol 55:670–676
Nunoda S, Machida H, Sekikawa A, Shitakura K, Okajima K, Kubo Y, Ueno E, Otsuka K (2010) Evaluation of cardiac allograft vasculopathy by multidetector computed tomography and whole-heart magnetic resonance coronary angiography. Circ J 74(5):946–953
Pannu HK, Flohr TG, Corl FM, Fishman EK (2003) Current concepts in multi-detector row CT evaluation of the coronary arteries: principles, techniques, and anatomy. RadioGraphics 23:S111–S125
Paulin S, von Schulthess GK, Fossel E, Krayenbuehl HP (1987) MR imaging of the aortic root and proximal coronary arteries. Am J Roentgenol 148:665–670
Pelliccia A (2001) Congenital coronary artery anomalies in young patients. New perspectives for timely identification. J Am Coll Cardiol 37:598–600
Pennell DJ, Keegan J, Firmin DN, Gatehouse PD, Underwood SR, Longmore DB (1993) Magnetic resonance imaging of the coronary arteries: technique and preliminary results. Br Heart J 70:315–326

Pepine C, Holmes DR, Block PC et al (1996) ACC expert consens document. Coronary artery stents. J Am Coll Cardiol 28:782–794

Plein S, Ridgway JP, Jones TR, Bloomer TN, Sivananthan MU (2002) Coronary artery disease: assessment with a comprehensive MR imaging protocol–initial results. Radiology 225:300–307

Plein S, Jones TR, Ridgway JP, Sivananthan MU (2003) Three-dimensional coronary MR angiography performed with subject-specific cardiac acquisition windows and motion-adapted respiratory gating. Am J Roentgenol 180:505–512

Post JC, van Rossum AC, Hofman MBM, Valk J, Visser CA (1996) Three-dimensional respiratory-gated MR angiography of coronary arteries: comparison with conventional contrast coronary angiography. Am J Roentgenol 166:426–433

Post JC, van Rossum AC, Hofman MB, de Cock CC, Valk J, Visser CA (1997) Clinical utility of two-dimensional magnetic resonance angiography in detecting coronary artery disease. Eur Heart J 18:426–433

Pouleur AC, le Polain de Waroux JB, Kefer J, Pasquet A, Vanoverschelde JL, Gerber BL (2008) Direct comparison of whole-heart navigator-gated magnetic resonance coronary angiography and 40- and 64-slice multidetector row computed tomography to detect the coronary artery stenosis in patients scheduled for conventional coronary angiography. Circ Cardiovasc Imaging 1(2):114–121

Prakken NH, Cramer MJ, Olimulder MA, Agostoni P, Mali WP, Velthuis BK (2010) Screening for proximal coronary artery anomalies with 3-dimensional MR coronary angiography. Int J Cardiovasc Imaging 26(6):701–710

Prêtre R, Tamisier D, Bonhoeffer P et al (2001) Results of the arterial switch operation in neonates with transposed great arteries. Lancet 35:1826–1830

Prince MR (1994) Gadolinium-enhanced MR aortography. Radiology 191:155–164

Pruessmann KP, Weiger M, Boesiger P (2001) Sensitivity encoded cardiac MRI. J Cardiovasc Magn Reson 3:1–9

Reddy KS, Yusuf S (1998) Emerging epidemic of cardiovascular disease in developing countries. Circulation 97(6):596–601

Regenfus M, Ropers D, Achenbach S et al (2000) Non-invasive detection of coronary artery stenosis using breath-hold enhanced three-dimensional breath-hold magnetic resonance coronary angiography. J Am Coll Cardiol 36:44–50

Regenfus M, Ropers D, Achenbach S et al (2002) Comparison of contrast-enhanced breath-hold and free-breathing respiratory-gated imaging in three-dimensional magnetic resonance coronary angiography. Am J Cardiol 90:725–730

Regenfus M, Roper D, Achenbach S et al (2003) Diagnostic value of maximum intensity projections versus source images for assessment of contrast-enhanced tree-dimensional breath-hold magnetic resonance coronary angiography. Invest Radiol 38:200–206

Saito Y, Sakuma H, Shibata M et al (2001) Assessment of coronary flow velocity reserve using fast velocity-encoded cine MRI for noninvasive detection of restenosis after coronary stent implantation. J Cardiovasc Magn Reson 3:209–214

Sakuma H, Kawada N, Takeda K, Higgins CB (1999) MR measurement of coronary blood flow. J Magn Reson Imaging 10:728–733

Sandstede JJ, Pabst T, Beer M, Geis N, Kenn W, Neubauer S, Hahn D (1999) Three-dimensional MR coronary angiography using the navigator technique compared with conventional coronary angiography. Am J Roentgenol 172:135–139

Sardanelli F, Molinari G, Zandrino F, Balbi M (2000) Three-dimensional, navigator-echo MR coronary angiography in detecting stenoses of the major epicardial vessels, with conventional coronary angiography as the standard of reference. Radiology 214:808–814

Sardanelli F, Zandrino F, Molinari G, Iozzelli A, Balbi M, Barsotti A (2002) MR evaluation of coronary stents with navigator echo and breath-hold cine gradient-echo techniques. Eur Radiol 12:193–200

Scheidegger MB, Müller R, Boesiger P (1994) Magnetic resonance angiography: methods and its applications to the coronary arteries. Technol Health Care 2:255–265

Scheidegger MB, Stuber M, Boesiger P, Hess OM (1996) Coronary artery imaging by magnetic resonance. Herz 21:90–96

Schroeder AP, Houlind K, Pedersen AM, Thuesen L, Nielsen TT, Egeblad H (2000) Magnetic resonance imaging seems safe in patients with intracoronary stents. J Cardiovasc Magn Reson 2:43–49

Shea SM, Deshpande VS, Chung Y-C, Li D (2002) Three-dimensional true-FISP imaging of the coronary arteries: improved contrast with T2-preparation. J Magn Reson Imaging 15:597–602

Sommer T, Hofer U, Hackenbroch M et al (2002) Submillimeter 3D coronary MR angiography with real-time navigator correction in 107 patients with suspected coronary artery disease. Röfo Fortschr Röntgenstr 174:459–466

Spuentrup E, Manning WJ, Botnar RM, Kissinger KV, Stuber M (2002) Impact of navigator timing on free-breathing submillimeter 3D coronary magnetic resonance angiography. Magn Reson Med 47:196–201

Spuentrup E, Katoh M, Stuber M, Botnar R, Schaeffter T, Buecker A, Gunther RW (2003) Coronary MR imaging using free-breathing 3D steady-state free precession with radial κ-space sampling. Röfo Fortschr Röntgenstr 175:1330–1334

Stuber M, Botnar RM, Danias PG et al (1999) Double-oblique free-breathing high resolution three-dimensional coronary magnetic resonance angiography. J Am Coll Cardiol 34:524–531

Stuber M, Botnar RM, Fischer SE et al (2002) Preliminary report on in vivo coronary MRA at 3 Tesla in humans. Magn Reson Med 48:425–429

Tang C, Blatter DD, Parker DL (1993) Accuracy of phase-contrast flow measurements in the presence of partial-volume effects. J Magn Reson Imaging 3:377–385

Tangcharoen T, Jahnke C, Koehler U, Schnackenburg B, Klein C, Fleck E, Nagel E (2008) Impact of heart rate variability in patients with normal sinus rhythm on image quality in coronary magnetic angiography. J Magn Reson Imaging 28(1):74–79

Taylor AM, Dymarkowski S, Haemaekers P et al (2005) Magnetic resonance coronary angiography and late-enhancement myocardial imaging in children with arterial switch operation for transposition of the great arteries. Radiology 234(2):542–547

Taylor AM, Jhooti P, Wiesmann F et al (1997) MR navigator-echo monitoring of temporal changes in diaphragm position: implications for MR coronary angiography. J Magn Reson Imaging 7:629–636

Taylor AM, Panting JR, Keegan J et al (1999) Safety and preliminary findings with the intravascular contrast agent NC100150 injection for MR coronary angiography. J Magn Reson Imaging 9:220–227

Taylor AM, Keegan J, Jhooti P, Gatehouse PD, Firmin DN, Pennell DJ (2000a) A comparison between segmented κ-space FLASH and interleaved spiral MR coronary angiography sequences. J Magn Reson Imaging 11:394–400

Taylor AM, Thorne SA, Rubens MB et al (2000b) Coronary artery imaging in grown up congenital heart disease. Complementary role of magnetic resonance and x-ray coronary angiography. Circulation 101:1670–1678

Van den Brink J, Watanabe Y, Kuhl CK et al (2003) Implications of SENSE MR in routine clinical practice. Eur J Radiol 46:3–27

van Geuns RJM, de Bruin HG, Rensing Rensing BJWM et al (1999) Magnetic resonance imaging of the coronary arteries: clinical results from three dimensional evaluation of a respiratory gated technique. Heart 82:515–519

van Ooijen PMA, van Geuns RJM, Rensing BJWM, Bongaerts AHH, de Feyter PJ, Oudkerk (2003) Noninvasive coronary imaging using electron beam CT: surface rendering versus volume rendering. Am J Roentgenol 180:223–226

van Rossum AC, Galjee MA, Post JC, Visser CA (1997) A practical approach to MRI of coronary artery bypass graft patency and flow. Int J Cardiac Imaging 13:199–204

Vick GW-III, Muthupillai R, Su JT, Kovalchin JP, Chung T (2003) Magnetic resonance angiography of coronary arteries and peripheral arteries in infants and young children with Kawasaki disease. J Am Coll Cardiol 495A

Vitiello R, McCrindle BW, Nykanen D et al (1998) Complications associated with pediatric cardiac catheterization. J Am Coll Cardiol 32:1433–1440

Vrachliotis TG, Bis KG, Aliabadi D, Shetty AN, Safian R, Simonetti O (1997) Contrast-enhanced breath-hold MR angiography for evaluating patency of coronary artery bypass graft. Am J Roentgenol 168:1073–1080

Walker F, Webb G (2001) Congenital coronary artery anomalies: the adult perspective. Cor Art Dis 12:599–604

Wang Y, Ehman RL (2000) Retrospective adaptive motion correction of navigator-gated 3D coronary MR angiography. J Magn Reson Imaging 11:208–214

Wang Y, Rossman PJ, Grimm RC, Riederer SJ, Ehman RL (1996) Navigator-echo-based real-time respiratory gating and triggering for reduction of respiration effects in three-dimensional coronary MR angiography. Radiology 198:55–60

Wang Y, Vidan E, Bergman GW (1999) Cardiac motion of coronary arteries: variability in the rest period and implications for coronary MR angiography. Radiology 213:751–758

Wang Y, Watts R, Mitchell IR et al (2001) Coronary MR angiography: selection of acquisition window of minimal cardiac motion with electrocardiography-triggered navigator cardiac motion prescanning–Initial results. Radiology 218:580–585

Weber C, Steiner P, Sinkus R, Dill T, Börnert P, Adam G (2002) Correlation of 3D MR coronary angiography with selective coronary angiography: feasibility of the motion-adapted gating technique. Eur Rad 122:718–726

Weissler AM, Harris WS, Schoenfeld CD (1968) Systolic time intervals in heart failure in man. Circulation 37:149–159

White CW, Wright CB, Doty DB et al (1984) Does visual interpretation of the coronary angiogram predict the physiological importance of a coronary stenosis? N Engl J Med 310:819–824

Wielopolski PA, Manning WJ, Edelman RE (1995) Single breath-hold volumetric imaging of the heart using magnetization-prepared 3-dimensional segmented echo-planar imaging. J Magn Res Imaging 5:403–409

Wielopolski PA, van Geuns RJM, de Feyter PJ, Oudkerk M (1998) Breath-hold coronary MR angiography with volume targeted imaging. Radiology 209:209–219

Wielopolski PA, van Geuns RJM, de Feyter PJ, Oudkerk M (2000) Coronary arteries. Review article. Eur Radiol 10:12–35

Wintersperger BJ, Engelmann MG, Von Smekal A et al (1998) Patency of coronary bypass grafts: assessment with breath-hold contrast-enhanced MR angiography–value of a non-electrocardiographically triggered technique. Radiology 208:345–351

Wolff SD, Balaban RS (1989) Magnetization transfer contrast (MTC) and tissue water proton relaxation in vivo. Magn Reson Med 10:135–144

Wu YW, Tadamura E, Yamamuro M, Kanao S, Nakayama K, Togashi K (2007) Evaluation of three-dimensional navigator-gated whole heart MR coronary angiography: the importance of systolic imaging in subjects with high heart rates. Eur J Radiol 61(1):91–96

Yoshino H, Nitatori T, Kachi E et al (1997) Directed proximal magnetic resonance coronary angiography compared with conventional contrast coronary angiography. Am J Cardiol 80:514–518

Zheng J, Li D, Cavagna FM et al (2001) Contrast-enhanced coronary MR angiography: relationship between coronary artery delineation and blood T1. J Magn Reson Imaging 14:348–354

Congenital Heart Disease

Marina L. Hughes, Vivek Muthurangu, and Andrew M. Taylor

Contents

1	**Introduction**	554
2	**Clinical Indications for MRI Evaluation of CHD**	554
3	**MRI Protocols for Congenital Heart Disease**	556
3.1	Scanning Environment for General Anaesthetic Cases	558
4	**Imaging Techniques**	558
4.1	Spin-Echo Imaging	558
4.2	Gradient-Echo Imaging	561
4.3	Two-Dimensional Balanced SSFP Imaging	563
4.4	Real-Time b-SSFP and Radial k–t SENSE Imaging	563
4.5	Phase-Contrast MRI (PC-MRI)	564
4.6	3D Whole-Heart MRA	566
4.7	Contrast-Enhanced Magnetic Resonance Angiography	567
4.8	Imaging Late After Gadolinium Contrast	567
4.9	Stress Perfusion Imaging	569
4.10	Sequence Optimization for the Paediatric Population	569
4.11	Normal Values in Children	569
5	**Sequential Segmental Analysis**	569
5.1	Step 1: Atrial Situs	570
5.2	Step 2: Ventricular Morphology	570
5.3	Step 3: Ventriculoarterial Connection	570
5.4	Step 4: Identification of Other Abnormalities	571
6	**Acyanotic Heart Disease**	571
6.1	Quantifying and Locating a Shunt	571
6.2	Partial Anomalous Pulmonary Venous Return	573
6.3	Total Anomalous Pulmonary Venous Return	573
6.4	Atrial Septal Defect	573
6.5	Atrioventricular Septal Defect	574
6.6	Ventricular Septal Defect	575
6.7	Congenital Aortic Supravalvar Stenosis	577
6.8	Congenital Anomalies of the Aorta	578
7	**Cyanotic Heart Disease**	578
7.1	Tetralogy of Fallot	578
7.2	Pulmonary Atresia with VSD	582
7.3	Pulmonary Atresia with Intact Ventricular Septum	584
7.4	Transposition of the Great Arteries	584
7.5	Double Outlet Right Ventricle	589
7.6	Common Arterial Trunk	590
8	**The Functionally Single Ventricle**	591
8.1	The Borderline Left or Right Ventricle	591
8.2	Hypoplastic Left Heart Syndrome	591
8.3	Evaluating the Circulation Prior to Bidirectional Cavo-Pulmonary Connection (BCPC): "Glenn" Shunt or "hemi-Fontan" Procedure	593
8.4	Evaluating the Cavo-Pulmonary Connection: Glenn or Hemi–Fontan Circulation	594
8.5	Evaluating the Fontan or Total Cavopulmonary Circulation	597
9	**Coronary arteries**	599
9.1	Kawasaki Disease	599
9.2	Anomalous Origin of the Left Coronary Artery (ALCAPA)	599
10	**Role of Cardiovascular CT**	600
11	**Future Directions**	602
12	**Conclusion**	603
13	**Key Points**	603
References		604

M. L. Hughes · V. Muthurangu · A. M. Taylor (✉)
Centre for Cardiovascular Imaging,
UCL Institute of Cardiovascular Science
& Great Ormond Street Hospital for Children,
Great Ormond Street, London,
WC1N 3JH, UK
e-mail: a.taylor76@ucl.ac.uk

J. Bogaert et al. (eds.), *Clinical Cardiac MRI*, Medical Radiology. Diagnostic Imaging,
DOI: 10.1007/174_2011_415, © Springer-Verlag Berlin Heidelberg 2012

Abstract

Cardiac MRI has expanded its role in the diagnosis and management of congenital heart disease in both children and adults. Ongoing technological advancements in both data acquisition and data presentation have enabled cardiac MRI to be integrated into clinical practice with increasing understanding of the advantages and limitations of the technique by cardiologists and congenital heart surgeons. Importantly, the combination of exquisite 3D anatomy with functional physiological data enables cardiac MRI to provide a unique perspective for the management of many patients with congenital heart disease. Cardiac MRI can be challenging in this setting, in particular in neonates and small children, and this chapter will review the technical requirements, imaging protocols and application of cardiac MRI in these complex cardiac conditions.

1 Introduction

Congenital heart disease has an incidence of 6–8 per 1,000 in neonates (Hoffman and Kaplan 2002). Over the past decades, the life expectancy of individuals with congenital heart disease has increased significantly. Improvements in diagnosis and treatment have led to an increasing prevalence of patients with congenital heart disease in the general population. Recent population data from Belgium demonstrates that almost 90% of children born with congenital heart disease have the prospect of surviving into adulthood (Moons et al. 2010).

Imaging is fundamental to the management of these patients, and is required at all stages of patient care, from the fetal stage onwards. Imaging outlines anatomy and physiology, helps to refine management decisions, evaluates the result of interventions and guides prognosis. However, no single available modality fulfils these roles, for all cardiovascular structures and all physiological states. Cardiovascular imaging must involve a variety of modalities that can be used in a complementary manner, and that together are sensitive, accurate and reproducible; all the while minimizing harm.

Echocardiography remains on the imaging frontline for paediatric and adult patients with congenital heart disease, because it is portable, non-invasive and provides immediate, high-resolution anatomical and physiological information. For cooperative patients with clear acoustic windows, echocardiography alone can guide the diagnosis and management of many conditions, particularly in the neonatal period and early childhood. However, echocardiography is highly user-dependent, can be limited by acoustic windows and provides poor images of the distal vasculature.

X-ray-guided cardiac catheterization has traditionally been used to provide haemodynamic information and visualize extracardiac great vessels, but is not without risks due to the invasive nature of the procedure and the exposure to X-radiation. In addition, X-ray fluoroscopy provides a projection image and has limited three-dimensional (3D) capabilities.

Cardiovascular magnetic resonance (MR) imaging is now being used in many centres and with increasing frequency, for the diagnosis and follow-up of infant, adolescent and adult patients with congenital heart disease (Higgins et al. 1984; Warnes et al. 2008; Kilner et al. 2010).

Cardiovascular MR provides a powerful investigative tool, giving morphologic and haemodynamic information that echocardiography and catheterization alone do not provide. Extracardiac anatomy, including the great arteries, systemic and pulmonary veins, can be delineated with high spatial resolution, in any imaging plane, irrespective of body habitus. Vascular and valvar flow patterns and volumes can be assessed (Powell et al. 2000), shunts can be quantified (Beerbaum et al. 2001), and myocardial function can be measured accurately and with high reproducibility, regardless of ventricular morphology (Mooij et al. 2008). Finally, cardiovascular MR surpasses both catheterization and echocardiography in providing high resolution, isotropic, 3D data sets (Fig. 1). This allows for reconstruction of data in any anatomical imaging plane, giving complete visualization of complex congenital cardiac anomalies, without the use of ionizing radiation (Fenchel et al. 2006).

In this chapter, the use of cardiovascular MR in the diagnosis of congenital heart disease is discussed with reference to specific congenital heart defects.

2 Clinical Indications for MRI Evaluation of CHD

The decision to perform a cardiovascular MR examination depends on the information required, the local facilities and resources available for scanning, the

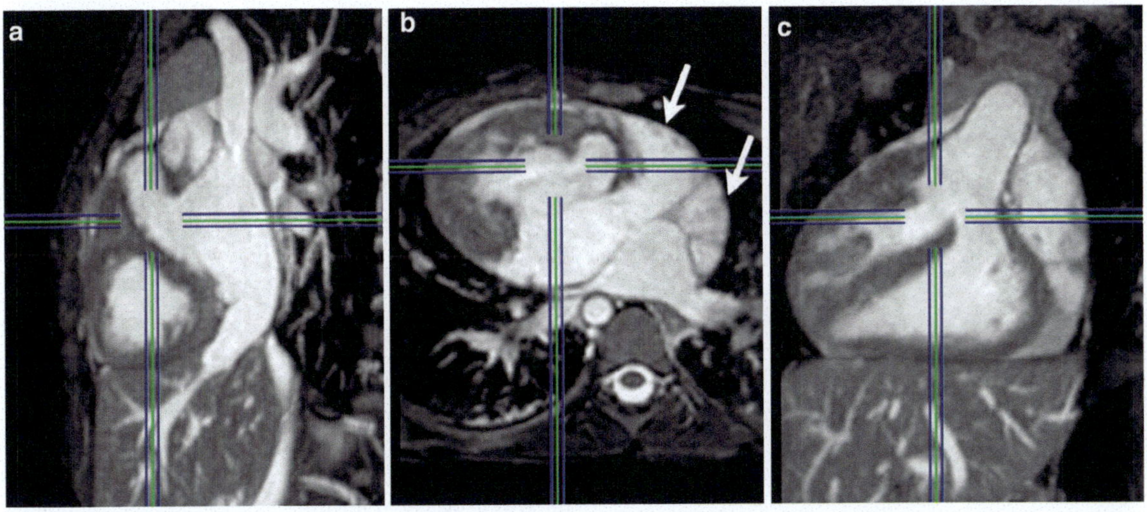

Fig. 1 A navigator-echo respiratory gated, isotropic, 3D bSSFP data set, from a 5-year-old patient, viewed using 3D viewing software (**a** sagittal, **b** axial, **c** coronal), illustrating complex intracardiac anatomy and ventricular relationships. Note juxtaposition of the right atrial appendage in the central panel (*arrows*)

clinical state of the patient, and the risks to the patient of carrying out the examination.

Without the use of sedation or contrast, a comprehensive cardiovascular MR examination in a willing patient carries minimal risk. However, the need for sedation, general anaesthesia or gadolinium contrast changes the balance of risk in some patients.

The technical and diagnostic complexity of paediatric and adult congenital cardiovascular MR is significant. Imaging these patients requires a radiographer and cardiovascular MR physician with expertise in the morphologic and haemodynamic changes in congenital heart disease. Moreover, in paediatric patients, whose body size is small and heart rates are rapid, imaging requires the optimization of pulse sequences in this context.

Additionally, because general anaesthesia is often necessary for the youngest children, a cardiovascular MR unit scanning paediatric patients requires an anaesthetic team trained to care for cardiac patients with unusual and often precarious haemodynamics.

In experienced hands, cardiac anaesthesia is safe for the majority of patients undergoing cardiovascular MR (Odegard et al. 2004; Stockton et al. 2009). Thus, there are many paediatric patients for whom the risk of general anaesthesia is acceptable against the benefit of the accuracy and comprehensiveness of the information gained from CMR. These patient groups are outlined in Table 1.

The older patient groups with congenital heart disease, for whom cardiovascular MR may be indicated, are listed in Table 2. For many of these patient groups the cardiovascular MR is a single, focused study prior to intervention. For others the benefit of cardiovascular MR lies in serial imaging leading up to, or following intervention.

The potential vascular complications of catheterization (Zeevi et al. 1999), and the dangers of exposure to radiation has led to many centres, including ours, to reserve cardiac catheterization for patients in whom haemodynamic data is essential (e.g. high risk Fontan, pulmonary hypertension), or in whom it is known that interventional procedures are highly likely to be necessary.

Some centres are realizing the benefits of a combined cardiovascular MR and cardiac catheterization laboratory, in which patients can be transferred, under the same general anaesthetic, from imaging to interventional procedure and vice versa. This guides the intervention procedure, and gives potential to immediately assess the haemodynamic results of intervention with assessment of flow and ventricular function (Razavi et al. 2003a; Lurz et al. 2009b) (see "MR guided cardiac catheterisation").

Table 1 Common indications for paediatric congenital CMR under general anaesthetic

Patient group	Information sought
Aortic arch abnormalities Coarctation Interrupted arch Pre- and post-repair	Aortic arch morphology LV function and mass LV outflow tract status Aortic valve function and flow assessment
Aortic arch connective tissue disease	Aortic arch morphology Aortic dissection and compliance LV volume, function and mass LV outflow tract
Univentricular heart pre-BCPC (including Norwood I)	Pulmonary artery morphology Aortic arch morphology Ventricular volume and function Valvar function and flow assessment
Univentricular heart pre-TCPC (including Norwood II)	[a]*Jugular venous pressure measurement, under GA* Pulmonary artery morphology Aortic arch morphology Ventricular volume and function Valvar function with flow assessment Quantification of collateral flow
Tetralogy of Fallot with BT shunt	RV outflow tract morphology Pulmonary artery morphology
PA/VSD, DORV, common arterial trunk	RV outflow tract morphology Pulmonary artery morphology Aortopulmonary collateral arteries
TGA—post arterial switch assessment	RV outflow tract morphology Pulmonary artery morphology Aortic arch morphology Ventricular volume and function Valvar function with flow assessment
Pulmonary vein abnormalities	Pulmonary vein morphology and flow Pulmonary artery flow

ASD atrial septal defect, *VSD* ventricular septal defect, *PAPVD* partial anomalous pulmonary venous drainage, *PA* pulmonary artery, *CoA* Coarctation aorta, *BCPC* bidirectional cavo-pulmonary connection, *TCPC* total cavo-pulmonary connection, *BT* Blalock–Taussig shunt, *PA/VSD* pulmonary atresia with ventricular septal defect, *TGA* transposition of the great arteries, *RV* right ventricle

[a] This gives an estimate of pulmonary artery pressure

3 MRI Protocols for Congenital Heart Disease

The imaging protocol outlined in Table 3 is a suggested basic structure for scanning a patient with congenital heart disease. The anatomic emphasis of the protocol, the order of workflow and the sequence choice may be altered, depending on the anatomy, the physiology, the patient's cooperation and their breath-holding capacity. Further optimization of multiple parameters may be necessary for each sequence, depending on heart rate, rhythm and body size. Additional, specific 2D views using bSSFP cine imaging or spin-echo 'black-blood' imaging may be important for accurate delineation of great vessel anatomy.

Understanding the question asked of the scan and being able to quickly interpret each image as it is acquired are essential factors to direct the scan workflow appropriately (Table 4). In this, often complex, patient group there is a high likelihood of previously undiagnosed or unexpected morphological or physiological findings. For this reason, the usual practice is to use a systematic approach, completing a full protocol for most patients, including 3D data. Acquiring a complete image data set gives the opportunity for full delineation of the sequential segmental anatomy in every patient.

Table 2 Common indications for congenital CMR without anaesthetic (usually, older children and adults)

Patient group	Information sought
Regurgitant valves	Outflow tract morphology Valve morphology and function Forward and regurgitant flow quantification Ventricular volume and function
ASD, VSD shunt	Defect position and size Net shunt quantification (arterial flow) Ventricular volume and function
PAPVD	Pulmonary vein morphology Net shunt quantification (arterial flow) Ventricular volume and function
Pulmonary valve stenosis	RV outflow tract morphology Pulmonary artery morphology Valvar function with flow assessment Ventricular volume and function
Branch PA stenosis	RV outflow tract morphology Pulmonary artery morphology Valvar function with flow assessment
Repaired tetralogy of Fallot (including conduit patients—e.g. PA/VSD, post-Rastelli operation)	RV outflow tract morphology Pulmonary artery morphology Ventricular volume and function Valvar function with flow assessment Coronary artery position
Repaired common arterial trunk	RV outflow tract morphology Pulmonary artery morphology Ventricular volume and function Valvar function with flow assessment
TGA—post atrial switch operation (Mustard and Senning operations)	Systemic RV volume and function Atrial baffle morphology and function Valvar function with flow assessment
TGA—post arterial switch operation	RV outflow tract morphology Pulmonary artery morphology Aortic arch morphology Ventricular volume and function Valvar function with flow assessment Coronary artery position
Aortic arch: native or repaired CoA	Aortic arch morphology LV function and mass LV outflow tract status Aortic valve function and flow assessment
Aortic arch: marfan, connective tissue disease	Aortic arch morphology Aortic compliance, dissection LV volume, function & mass LV outflow tract.
Pulmonary vein stenosis—post repair of PAPVD or TAPVD	Pulmonary vein morphology and flow Pulmonary artery flow
Univentricular—post BCPC	Pulmonary artery morphology Aortic arch morphology Ventricular volume and function Valvar function with flow assessment Quantification of collateral flow

(continued)

Table 2 (continued)

Patient group	Information sought
Univentricular—Fontan / TCPC	Fontan pathway morphology Pulmonary artery morphology Aortic arch morphology Ventricular volume and function Valvar function with flow assessment Quantification of collateral flow
Ebstein anomaly	Tricuspid valve leaflet morphology and function Right atrial volume RV volume and function Quantification of net forward flow Quantification of ASD shunt
Complex anatomy—any	3D morphology: connections, outflow tracts Pulmonary artery morphology Aortic arch morphology Ventricular volume and function Valvar function with flow assessment Quantification of net shunt
Anomalous coronary arteries	Coronary morphology Myocardial scar Ventricular volume and function Myocardial perfusion

ASD atrial septal defect, *VSD* ventricular septal defect, *PAPVD* partial anomalous pulmonary venous drainage, *PA* pulmonary artery, *CoA* Coarctation aorta, *BCPC* bidirectional cavo-pulmonary connection, *TCPC* total cavo-pulmonary connection, *BT* Blalock–Taussig shunt, *PA/VSD* pulmonary atresia with ventricular septal defect, *TGA* Transposition of the great arteries, *RV* right ventricle

3.1 Scanning Environment for General Anaesthetic Cases

Performing general anaesthesia in an MR environment is challenging for many reasons: There is limited access to the child and ventilation equipment during the cardiovascular MR scan; care is required for staff and patient safety with regard to ferromagnetic equipment; and there is a potential for RF interference with monitoring. It is therefore very important to have an appropriately trained anaesthetic team (the cardiothoracic operative team in our institution), with excellent monitoring equipment. Several technical factors specific to MR in infants and small children must be taken into consideration. Prolonged, multiple breath-holds are required, thus adequate pauses for ventilation control between breath-holds are required, to ensure that hypoxia and hypercapnoea are avoided. Reliable monitoring of the electrocardiogram, pulse oximetry and expired gas concentrations is necessary. Additionally, patient temperature must be closely monitored. The low ambient temperature in MR scanning room produces a risk of hypothermia, particularly for small infants (Fig. 2).

4 Imaging Techniques

4.1 Spin-Echo Imaging

The earliest MR images of congenital heart disease were acquired using spin-echo 'black-blood' sequences (Higgins et al. 1984; Fletcher et al. 1984; Jacobstein et al. 1984). Although other sequences are now predominantly used in cardiovascular MR, the spin-echo 'black-blood' sequence is still important, particularly for delineation of great vessel anatomy with high spatial resolution. As the name suggests blood appears black, due to the moving spins in the blood producing a signal void. This allows delineation between the blood pool and either vessel wall or myocardium. The use of multiple signal averages allows high through and in-plane spatial resolution, and makes it particularly useful for anatomical

Table 3 Example of the standard sequences and views comprising a cardiac scan for congenital disease, in the approximate order of workflow used in our unit

	Sequence	Planning	Primary purpose	Secondary purpose
Scout/multi-slice	Single shot bSSFP images	Multiple slices in all three radiological planes	Isocentering of the heart in the scanner	Image plane planning
Axial black blood slices	Respiratory-navigated, ECG-gated, 'black-blood' images (HASTE or TSE). Contiguous axial slices	Coverage from liver to neck. Include aortic arch and proximal branches. Include systemic and pulmonary veins	Planning subsequent cine imaging planes	Provides a map of thoracic anatomy
Ventricular long-axis cines (RVLA, LVLA)	Breath-held, ECG-gated, bSSFP cine images	From axial stack. Place perpendicular plane through long axis of ventricle, from mid-atrioventricular (AV) valve to ventricular apex	Planning the true 4-chamber image	Assessment of anterior and inferior myocardium, AV valves, ventricular sizes
AV valve cines	Breath-held, ECG-gated, bSSFP cine image	From axial stack. Place perpendicular plane parallel to, and on apical side of AV. Check orientation is parallel to the vertical axis of the AV valves on RVLA and LVLA views. The image should include base of aortic valve in systole	Planning the four-chamber and LV outflow tract (LVOT) images	Subjective evaluation of AV valve function
4-chamber cine	Breath-held, ECG-gated, bSSFP cine image	From AV valves view. Place perpendicular plane across both AV valve orifices. From LVLA cine check that this plane passes through mid-mitral valve and LV apex. From RVLA check that the plane passes through mid-tricuspid valve and RV apex	Subjective assessment of atrial volumes, biventricular volumes and function, ventricular wall motion, AV valve regurgitation	Planning short axis (SA) stack
Short axis (SAX) or trans-axial cine stack to cover ventricles	Breath-held, ECG-gated, bSSFP cine image	Contiguous slices are placed to cover the entire ventricular mass. For axial coverage plan trans-axial slices from diaphragm inferiorly to outflow tracts superiorly. For SAX coverage, plan from end-diastolic frame of 4-chamber cine. Place image plane perpendicular to interventricular septum, and parallel to both AV valves, in both vertical long axis and 4-chamber views. Extend slices to include the entire basal and apical ventricular blood pool in diastolic frame	Provides the images required for segmentation of ventricular volumes	Assessment of the ventricular septum, ventricular myocardial morphology and wall motion abnormalities, outflow tracts

(continued)

Table 3 (continued)

	Sequence	Planning	Primary purpose	Secondary purpose
ceMRA	Breath-held, not ECG-gated. Gadolinium injection 0.2-0.4 ml/kg. *Infants*: injection rate 2 ml/s with 5 ml flush. *Older children*: injection rate 3 ml/s, 10 ml flush	Isotropic voxels (1.1–1.6 mm). Planned on axial HASTE stack, for coronal-orientated raw data. Include antero-posterior chest wall, lung fields. Image acquisition triggered with bolus-tracking to ensure maximum signal in structure of interest. Two acquisitions acquired, with no interval in young children, or a 15-s interval in older children	Angiographic views of large and small thoracic vessels. Images less subject to artifact caused by low velocity or turbulent flow. The second pass acquisition allows assessment of systemic and pulmonary venous anatomy	Subjective determination of preferential blood flow. Can be expanded to perform time-resolved angiography or 4-dimensional angiography
3D bSSFP whole-heart	[a] Free breathing, respiratory navigated, ECG-gated. Data acquisition optimized to occur in diastole. Signal improved following gadolinium injection Signal improved in tachycardic patients by triggering acquisition with every 2nd heartbeat. Acquisition time 8–15 mins	Planned on axial HASTE stack for sagittal orientation of raw data. Isotropic voxels (1.1–1.6 mm). Respiratory navigator placed mid-dome of diaphragm, avoiding cardiac region of interest	Provides high-resolution images of intracardiac anatomy, including coronary arteries. Allows multiplanar reformatting	Planning further imaging planes in patients with complex anatomy
LV outflow tract cine Long axis views through aortic arch	Breath-held, ECG-gated, bSSFP cine image	From the AV valves cine. Place a perpendicular plane through both basal aortic valve and mid-mitral valve orifice. Check orientation passes through LV apex using LVLA cine. Cross-cut this view to obtain two orthogonal cine views of LV outflow tract. Plan longitudinal views of the aortic arch using a 3-point planning tool from axial stack, or using multiplanar reformatting from 3D data	Outflow tract morphology, subjective assessment of semilunar valve function	Planning phase contrast velocity mapping. Planning "enface" view of semilunar valve
RV outflow tract cine Long axis cines through branch pulmonary arteries	Breath-held, ECG-gated, bSSFP cine image	From axial stack. Place perpendicular plane through the pulmonary trunk. Cross-cut this view to obtain two orthogonal cine views of RV outflow tract. Place perpendicular plane through the right and left pulmonary arteries respectively, or using multiplanar reformatting from 3D data. Cross-cut these views to obtain orthogonal longitudinal PA cines	Outflow tract morphology Subjective assessment of semilunar valve function	Planning phase contrast velocity mapping. Planning "enface" view of semilunar valve

(continued)

Table 3 (continued)

	Sequence	Planning	Primary purpose	Secondary purpose
Great vessel PC-MRI	Through-plane phase contrast velocity mapping. Non-breath held, ECG-gated, phase-contrast sequence. Or Breath-held, prospectively triggered, spiral phase-contrast sequence	From the orthogonal outflow tract images. Place a perpendicular plane across the vessel of interest. Place plane just distal to valve leaflets in systole, to avoid turbulent areas of flow. Optimise velocity encoding to maximize accuracy and prevent aliasing	Vessel flow volume Calculate regurgitant fractions (RF%). Validate ventricular stroke volume measurements	Calculate pulmonary blood flow to systemic blood flow ratio (Qp:Qs), Evaluate presence and location of shunts. Calculate flow velocity
Venous flow PC-MRI	Through-plane phase contrast velocity mapping. Non-breath held, ECG-gated, phase-contrast sequence. Or Breath-held, prospectively triggered, spiral phase-contrast sequence	From the orthogonal venous anatomy images. Place a perpendicular plane across the vessel of interest. Place plane between venous vessel confluence and atrial connection. Velocity encoding in region 60–100 cm/s	Venous flow volume. Calculate net pulmonary blood flow. Calculate pulmonary arterio-venous collateral flow. Calculate veno-veno collateral flow	Portray sites of venous stenoses. Demonstrate direction of flow in venous collateral vessels
In-plane PC-MRI	In-plane phase contrast velocity mapping. Non-breath held, ECG-gated	From 2D cine or multiplanar reformatted image plane. Phase-encode in the predominant direction of flow	Characterise regions of flow acceleration, for CoA, PA, venous stenosis, venous baffle narrowing	Optimise through-plane flow mapping in location of highest velocity

[a] Isometric 3D data is acquired prior to flow assessment, to enable planning of the appropriate image planes for phase contrast flow assessment

delineation. Most spin-echo sequences now acquire multiple echo trains for each set of radiofrequency pulses (e.g. turbo spin-echo), enabling images to be acquired in a single breath-hold.

The main benefit of spin-echo black blood sequences is that contrast improves when the blood flow velocity is high. Thus it is particularly useful when imaging vascular obstructions and valvar stenoses because, unlike gradient-echo and angiographic sequences, it performs better in these situations (Fig. 3). Black blood sequences have been validated successfully for imaging valvular stenosis (Greenberg et al. 1997), conduit stenosis (Martinez et al. 1992) and baffle obstruction (Sampson et al. 1994). It should be noted however that signal loss due to calcification can lead to underestimation of the stenosis.

For the purposes of imaging implanted metallic stents, spin-echo sequences can be helpful because the refocusing pulse compensates for increased T2* effects and field inhomogeneity, however the Faraday cage within stents contributes to poor sensitivity of these images for in-stent stenosis (Nordmeyer et al. 2010a). Sequence development is rapid and ongoing, with 3D black blood techniques showing promise for stent imaging of adults with congenital disease (Winner et al. 2011). However, even in this context, the luminal diameters of stented vessels tended towards overestimation, with this sequence.

4.2 Gradient-Echo Imaging

Gradient echo imaging revolutionized cardiovascular MR, allowing dynamic imaging of cardiac anatomy. The shorter repetition times of gradient echo sequences permit high temporal resolution. Fast acquisition enables multiple phases of the cardiac

Table 4 Suggested imaging protocols for given conditions-for abbreviations see main text

Conditions	Scout	Axial BB	Cines			SA stack	CE-MRA			3D SSFP	RVOT cines	LVOT cines	Flow		LGE	Perfusion	Notes
			VLA	4-Ch	AoV		PA	Ao	SVC				Ao	PA			
Shunts ASD, PAPVD, AVSD, VSD	✔	✔	✔	✔		✔	✔	✔		±	✔	✔	✔	✔			Consider AVSD as Complex CHD. CE MRA ± for PAPVD, SD
Valvar AS, AR, MR, MS	✔	✔	✔	✔	✔	✔		✔			±	✔	±	✔	±		
Aorta Coarctation, aortopathy, vascular rings	✔	✔	✔	✔		✔		✔		✔	±	✔	±	✔			ECG-gated CT may be indicated for coarctaion stent assessment
RVOT/Pulm Arteries PS, ToF, PA/IVS, TGA, Truncus arteriosus	✔	✔	✔	✔	✔	✔	✔	✔		✔	✔	✔	✔	✔	±		ECG-gated CT indicated for stent assessment
Cardiomyopathy HCM, DCM, non-compaction	✔	✔	✔	✔	✔	✔					±	✔	±	✔	✔	±	
Coronary arteries Anomalous, ALCAPA, Kawaski	✔	✔	✔	✔		✔		✔		✔		✔		±	✔	±	Use thin slice 3D SSFP. ECG-gated coronary CT more sensitive for identifying stenoses
Complex CHD DORV, DILV, CCTGA, HLHS, BCPC, Fontan, TCPC, Ebstein	✔	✔	✔	✔	✔	✔	✔	✔	±	✔	✔	✔	✔	✔	±	±	2nd pass ceMRA essential for BCPC, Fontan and TCPC circulations. LGE and stress perfusion may be useful

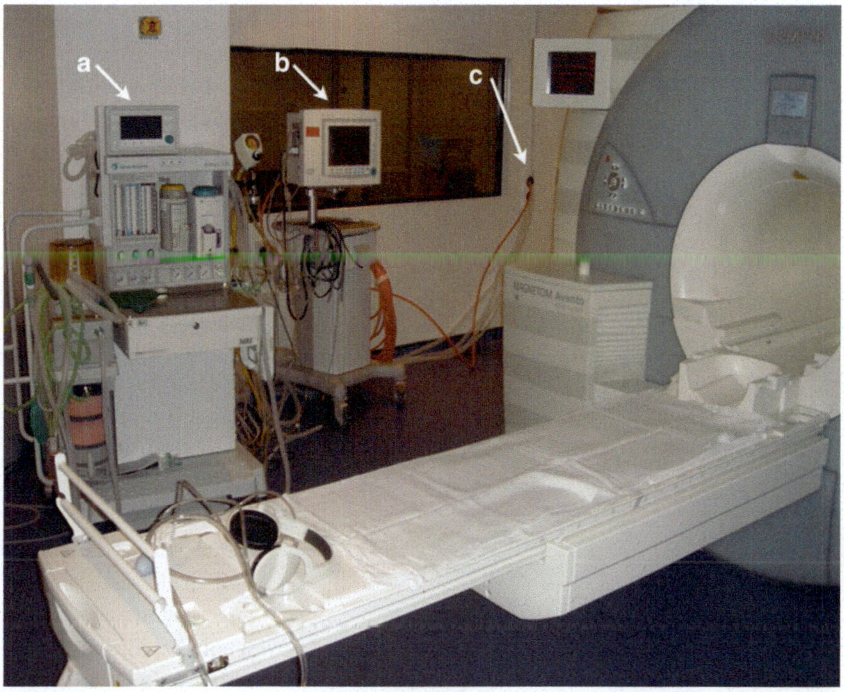

Fig. 2 Cardiovascular MR set-up for paediatric general anaesthetic cases. View of the MR scanner room showing the anaesthetic machine (**a**) and monitoring equipment (**b**). Ventilation tubing and leads from both pieces of equipment pass through a small opening in the wall (**c**) into the control room, so that the anaesthetist can control breath-holding and monitor the patient from within the control room

cycle to be acquired, which can be reconstructed into a cine MR image representing one full cardiac cycle.

Gradient echo sequences have various roles in cardiac imaging as described below.

4.3 Two-Dimensional Balanced SSFP Imaging

Balanced steady-state free precession (b-SSFP) sequences are partially flow compensated and give improved blood pool homogeneity throughout the cardiac cycle. These sequences have the benefit of good myocardial/blood pool contrast and relatively fast acquisition times. However, high velocity blood flow will lead to signal loss, allowing qualitative analysis of blood flow jets (Fig. 4). b-SSFP imaging is the workhouse of congenital heart disease assessment.

Single slice b-SSFP imaging allows qualitative assessment of all cardiac chambers, valvar dysfunction and dynamic vascular anatomy. It proves particularly useful when planning interventions, because accurate measurements of vessel diameter can be made over the whole cardiac cycle.

Multi-slice, two-dimensional b-SSFP imaging provides the best available in vivo assessment for ventricular volumetry (Grothues et al. 2002), as it is not reliant on complex geometric models. This technique has become an integral part of the clinical management for many patients with congenital heart disease, particularly those with disease involving the right ventricle.

Although b-SSFP sequences allow high spatio-temporal resolution imaging of the ventricles, they do require multiple breath-holds. This may not be tolerated in patients, particularly children, with congenital heart disease. In children less than approximately 7 years of age, general anaesthesia may be justified to guarantee no patient movement and enable multiple apnoeic scans. Another approach, not requiring breath-holding, is real-time imaging, discussed below.

4.4 Real-Time b-SSFP and Radial k–t SENSE Imaging

In real-time imaging, k-space is filled rapidly, and therefore the effects of cardio-respiratory motion on image quality are less pronounced. This imaging can be performed during free breathing and without cardiac gating. Furthermore, because each cine loop is acquired in a single heartbeat, acquisition times are short and the image quality is less susceptible to the effects of an irregular heart rate. However, these

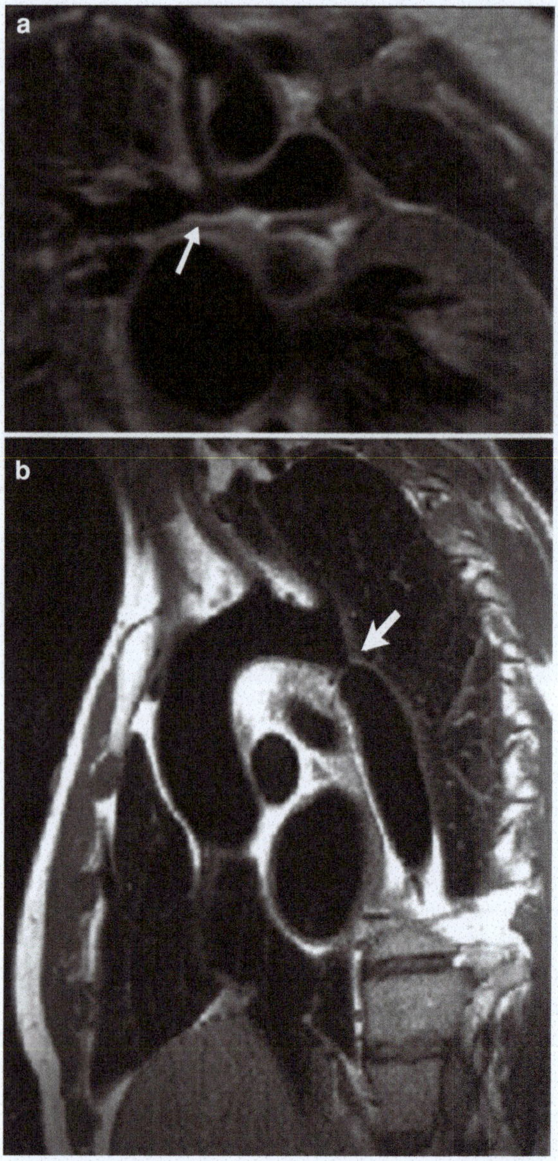

Fig. 3 Black blood turbo spin-echo image of: (**a**) an arterio-pulmonary shunt between the innominate artery and the proximal right pulmonary artery, in an infant. This image illustrates the patency of the shunt, and the focal stenosis of the pulmonary artery (*white arrow*), and (**b**) an aortic coarctation membrane (*arrow*)

benefits come at the cost of lower spatiotemporal resolution, which may affect accuracy.

High spatiotemporal resolution is particularly important for accurate segmentation of the RV, because of its complex trabecular structure. Patients with congenital heart disease often have dilated, heavily trabeculated RVs and quantification of RV end-diastolic volume is important in planning therapy.

Higher spatiotemporal resolution can be achieved through a combination of k-space under-sampling, and reconstruction algorithms that remove the resultant aliasing. One such technique is k-space and time (k–t) sensitivity encoding (SENSE) imaging. When compared with standard real-time volumetric assessment, radial real-time k–t SENSE imaging accurately quantifies ventricular volumes and function in patients with congenital heart disease, and was superior to standard real-time imaging in terms of image quality and better agreement of volume data with ECG-gated MR. (Fig. 5; Muthurangu et al. 2008). Radial k–t imaging more accurately quantified RV end-diastolic volume than other real-time sequences in this population. Therefore, it is a useful tool in the assessment of congenital heart disease in any patient who cannot breath-hold, any patient for whom rapid imaging is desirable and in patients with arrhythmia (Fig. 6).

4.5 Phase-Contrast MRI (PC-MRI)

Quantification of blood flow and velocity adds vital information to the physiological data gained from MRI. Quantification of the pulmonary to systemic blood flow ratio (Qp:Qs), the vavular regurgitation fraction or the flow velocity through a vascular stenosis all contribute to clinical decision making regarding disease progression, suitability for intervention and timing of intervention (Fig. 7).

Traditionally, blood flow has been invasively quantified using indicator dilution methods, which are associated with known morbidity and are less reliable in patients with large intracardiac shunts or valvar regurgitation.

Phase-Contrast MRI enables non-invasive quantification of blood flow in major vessels. Cardiac output and the pulmonary to systemic flow ratio (Qp:Qs) measured using this technique have been shown to be accurate when compared to invasive oximetry (Beerbaum et al. 2001). In addition, PC-MRI has been validated in numerous phantom experiments (Hundley et al. 1995). The quantification of valvar regurgitation is also an important use of this technique (Rebergen et al. 1993; Kang et al. 2003).

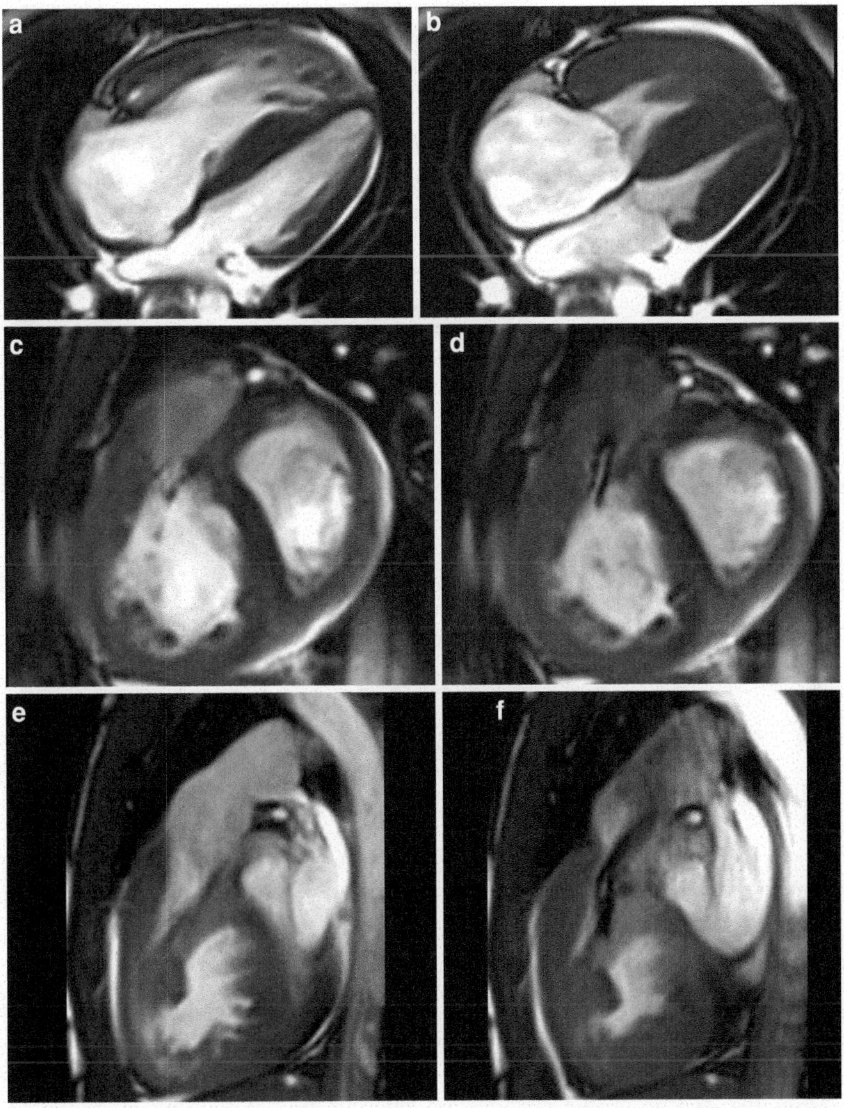

Fig. 4 A set of bSSFP white blood cine views, in diastole and systole from a patient with a type of double-chambered right ventricle. These demonstrate flow acceleration caused by right ventricular outflow tract obstruction in multiple planes: 4-chamber view (**a** and **b**), short-axis view (**c** and **d**), outflow tract view (**e** and **f**)

For all phase contrast flow velocity measurements, careful attention must be paid to planning the image slice position and optimizing the sequence for the patient. When measuring through-plane flow the image plane should be truly perpendicular to the direction of flow in the vessel. This plane should be planned using two orthogonal longitudinal images of the region, or using planes mapped using multi-planar reformatting from the patient's 3D data. The region of interest should be iso-centred in the magnet, and awareness should be maintained about potential inaccuracies caused phase offset effects (Rolf et al. 2011; Gatehouse et al. 2010).

When the mitral and tricuspid valves are competent, arterial flow mapping can be used as an internal quality control or mutual validation for the stroke volume for each ventricle, helping to optimize the accuracy of volumetric data (Devos and Kilner 2010).

Flow mapping, particularly for complex patients for whom measurements of systemic and pulmonary venous flow volumes are required, can be time-consuming and therefore more uncomfortable for the patient. Rapid imaging sequences are now being clinically validated (Steeden et al. 2011). These sequences will give imagers a greater repertoire of PC-MRI sequences for patients in whom long

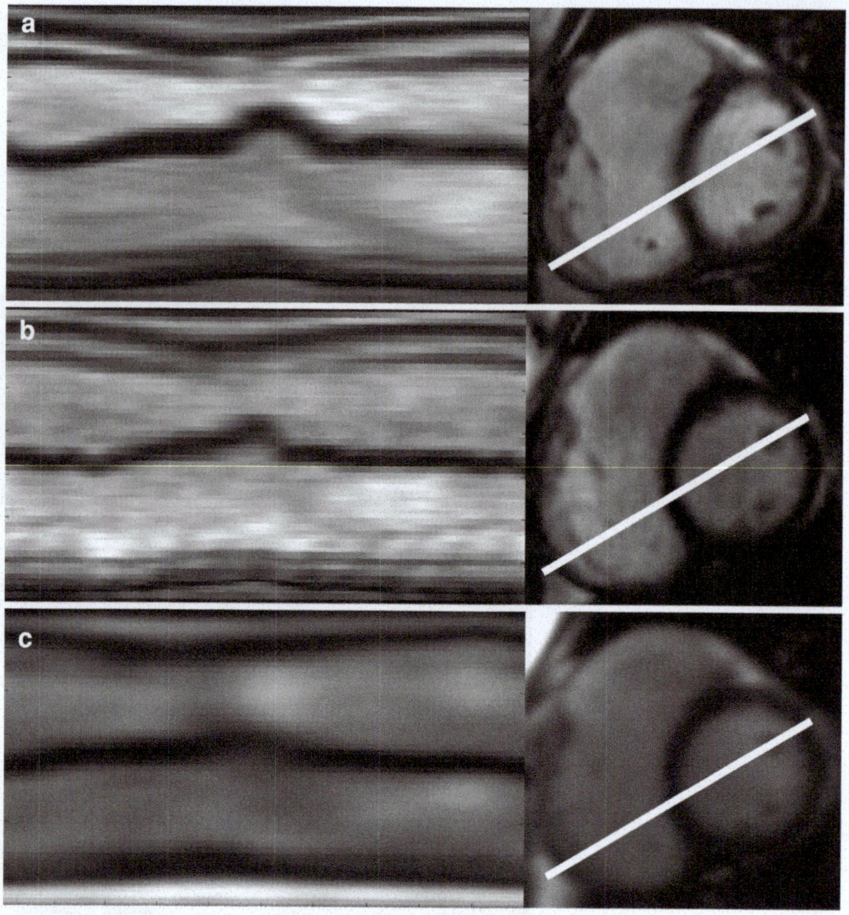

Fig. 5 Pixel profile of a line through both ventricles plotted as a function of time. The geometry of the line is shown on the accompanying short axis image. **a** Cardiac gated profile, (**b**) radial k–t SENSE real-time profile, and (**c**) standard real-time profile. Note the better visualization of the late systolic septal jump (*marked by arrow*) in the gated and radial k–t—good temporal resolution. The visual quality of the radial k–t images is also better than that of the standard real-time images; less blurred—good spatial resolution

breath-holds are difficult, or for whom multiple flow maps are necessary within the workflow.

The techniques of PC-MRI are continuously progressing, and promising methods are entering the clinical arena. 4D PC-MRI can accurately quantify, simultaneously acquired, arterial, pulmonary venous and systemic venous flow data in patients with congenital heart disease (Nordmeyer et al. 2010b). These data are acquired as a 3D volume, which obviates the need for planning 2D imaging planes. In addition, there are a variety of methods for visualizing and analysing the 4D flow velocity data that are not available by conventional 2D PC-MRI (Hope et al. 2010). These methods may help elucidate complex flow patterns in patients with congenital heart disease.

4.6 3D Whole-Heart MRA

3D cardiac MRI acquisition techniques open up the possibility of improved visualization of cardiac and great vessel anatomy, without the requirement for expert planning. The 3D whole-heart sequence is a free-breathing, isotropic, 3D data acquisition, which allows fast imaging of the entire cardiac volume (Razavi et al. 2003b) and gives high-resolution images that can be reconstructed from the raw data in any image plane. This is particularly useful in the assessment of complex congenital disease as it allows offline reconstruction of difficult anatomy.

Data should be acquired during periods when cardiac motion and flow are at a minimum. In most patients this is during mid- to late-diastole, however

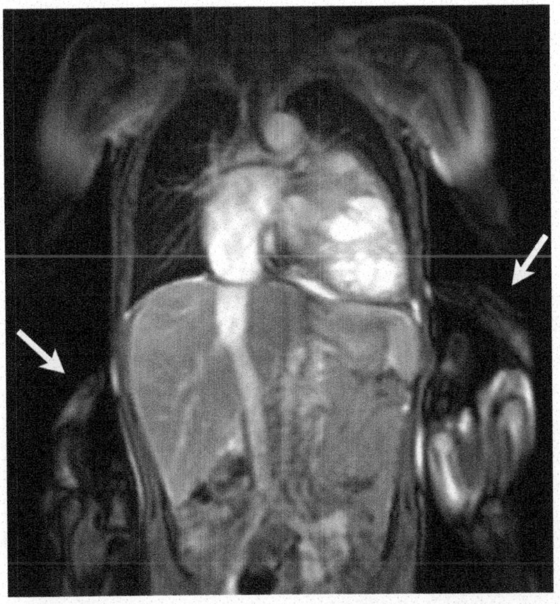

Fig. 6 Coronal white blood "scout" image, illustrating a 2-year-old child in the scanner. A general anaesthetic was considered too high risk for this patient, but arterial flow and ventricular functional data was required. The patient underwent a scan without anaesthetic, using real-time k–t SENSE and free-breathing PC flow imaging, with parent lying on scanner table at the patient's feet, holding the patient's hips for comfort (*arrows to parent's hands*)

in patients with high-heart rates, particularly in children, the mid- to late-diastolic time period is markedly decreased, and imaging is best performed at end systole (Uribe et al. 2011). Systolic imaging is also useful in patients with diastolic flow artefact, often due to regurgitant flow from pulmonary valve incompetence, high volume flow due to shunts, or high velocity flow in the case of tricuspid or mitral valve stenosis.

A specific advantage of 3D whole-heart imaging in patients with congenital heart disease is visualization of the coronary artery morphology and proximal course. Unusual coronary course, coronary proximity to valvar structures or geometric compromise following coronary reimplantation may alter the interventional or surgical management of the patient, though assessment of coronary artery stenoses is best performed either by conventional cardiac catheterization, or more recently CT (Ou et al. 2008). Because this technique provides a complete 3D data set, and can use protocolised acquisition parameters, the raw data allows standardized measurement techniques. This may have significant benefit in minimizing interstudy and interobserver variation. The potential for improved measurement reproducibility is a valuable advantage of this sequence for patients requiring serial assessment, for example of intrathoracic vascular structures (Potthast et al. 2010).

4.7 Contrast-Enhanced Magnetic Resonance Angiography

Contrast-enhanced magnetic resonance angiography (ceMRA) relies on the T1 shortening effect of dilute gadolinium contrast, and has been shown to be valuable in delineating the thoracic great vessels (Leung and Debatin 1997; Dymarkowski et al. 1999; Masui et al. 2000). CeMRA is accurate in the assessment of both dilated and stenotic vessels, and compares well to X-ray angiographic and surgical findings. The techniques and advantages of ceMRA are discussed in more detail in "Imaging of Great Vessels", which describes imaging of the great vessels.

One drawback of ceMRA is image blurring due to cardiac motion (Razavi et al. 2003b). This limits the ability of this technique to visualise intracardiac anatomy and the proximal pulmonary artery and aorta (Fig. 8). In addition, signal drop-out due to flow acceleration can affect ceMRA images, which leads to overestimation of stenosis. Care should be taken when measuring vessel dimensions from ceMRA, as the images are not ECG triggered and thus represent an average of the dimensions throughout the cardiac cycle.

4.8 Imaging Late After Gadolinium Contrast

Late gadolinium enhancement imaging relies on the fact that intravenously injected gadolinium chelate is an extracellular agent and that it remains longer in extracellular tissue spaces than in the blood pool. This imaging provides contrast between healthy myocardium and areas of myocardial scar or increased extracellular space. The techniques for late-gadolinium enhanced imaging are discussed in detail in "Cardiac MRI Physics".

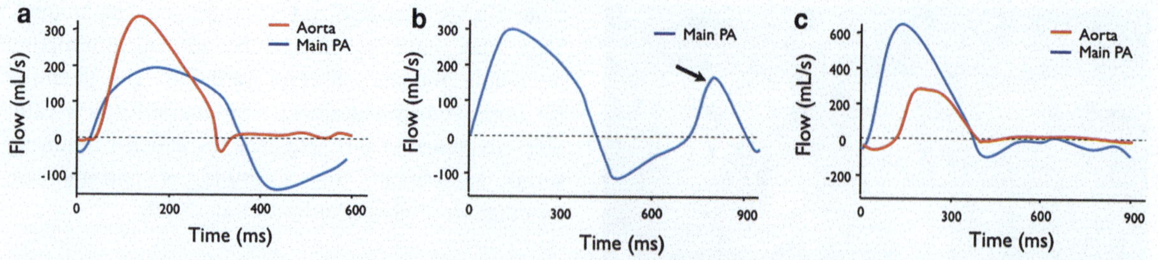

Fig. 7 Plots of instantaneous flow (measured by velocity-encoded phase-contrast MR) as a function of time. **a** Pulmonary valve regurgitation. **b** Pulmonary valve flow demonstrating restrictive right ventricular physiology, note forward flow in diastole (*arrow*). **c** Left-to-right shunting, note greater pulmonary blood flow volume

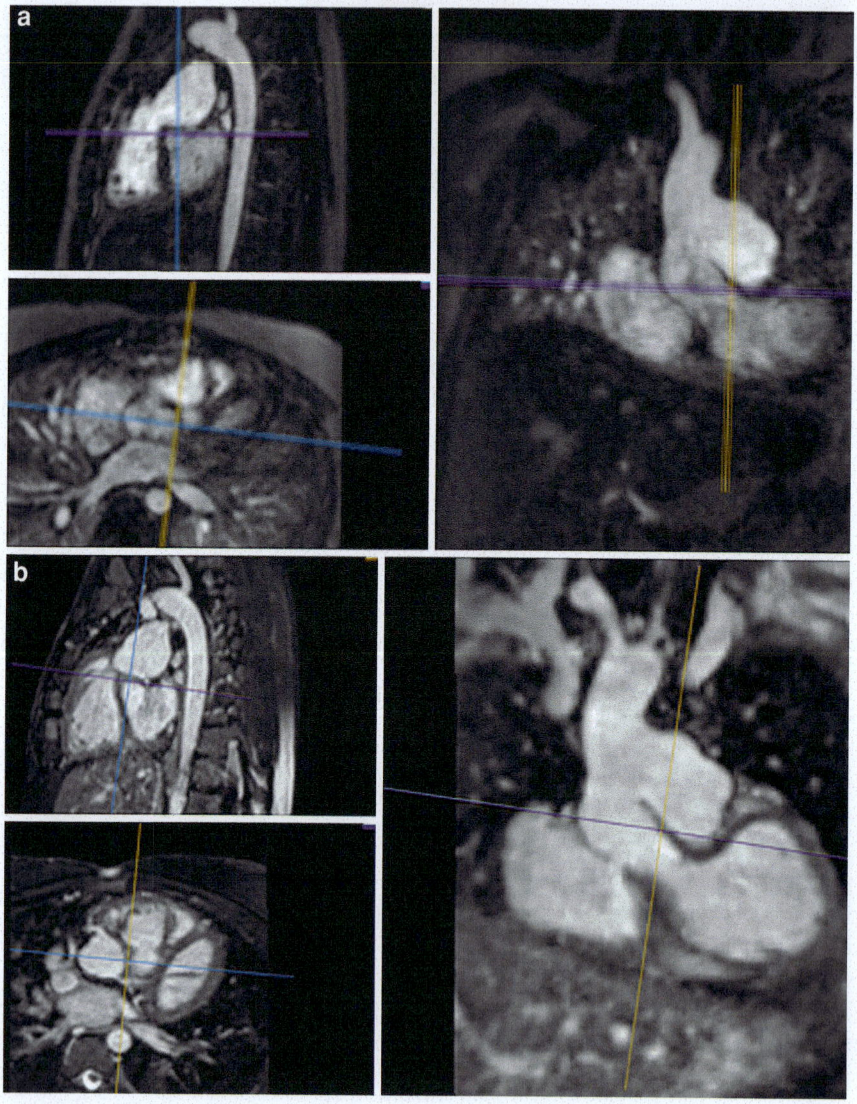

Fig. 8 3D ceMRA images (**a**) and 3D b-SSFP images (**b**) from the same patient with unrepaired aorto-pulmonary window, viewed using 3D viewing software, and demonstrating the differences in visualisation of intracardiac and coronary anatomy (*bottom left-hand panel* in both images)

Following surgery for congenital heart disease, late gadolinium imaging has been shown to document myocardial scarring in patients with repaired tetralogy of Fallot, and in those with a systemic right ventricle after atrial redirection surgery for transposition of the great arteries (Babu-Narayan et al. 2005, 2006).

In both these cohorts, the presence of areas of late gadolinium enhancement in the myocardium related to arrhythmia and ventricular dysfunction. The presence of this type of focal scarring may have a role in risk stratification and clinical decision-making.

The role of MR in elucidation of more diffuse fibrosis affecting the ventricular myocardium, and the clinical implications of this in patients with palliated congenital heart disease, remains a promising field of investigation (Flett et al. 2010; Broberg et al. 2010).

4.9 Stress Perfusion Imaging

MR myocardial perfusion imaging is performed both at rest and during coronary vasodilatation induced by adenosine. This defines myocardial viability and the stress/rest adenosine perfusion deficit, while a bolus of gadolinium contrast agent is being administered. Indications for pharmacological MR perfusion in the paediatric age group include suspected ischemia secondary to acquired coronary artery disease, such as Kawasaki's, or suspected ischemia following surgical transfer of coronary arteries during repair of CHD. The clinical value of adenosine perfusion cardiovascular MR is similar to that of myocardial scintigraphy, with an advantage that adenosine perfusion is performed over a single 45-min session, with no radiation exposure, as compared to two long sessions of scintigraphy. The high specificity and sensitivity of adenosine perfusion studies have been validated in adult patients with coronary artery disease (Nagel et al. 2003; Paetsch et al. 2004).

There is very little data regarding the use of dobutamine stress cardiovascular MR in paediatric patients with congenital disease. The feasibility has been shown in one small study (Strigl et al. 2009). Some centres are utilizing dobutamine stress to provide additional information when making decisions regarding timing for intervention, for example in the population of patients with repaired tetralogy of Fallot (Parish et al. 2010; Valverde et al. 2011).

4.10 Sequence Optimization for the Paediatric Population

Paediatric cardiovascular MR poses various technical challenges that need to be considered in order to obtain optimal images to answer the clinical question being investigated. These include: fast heart rate in neonates and infants (100–150 beats per minute) requiring a high temporal resolution for accurate ventricular volume and flow measurements; small-sized heart and blood vessels requiring greater spatial resolution; and potential arrhythmias as complications surgical procedure or the congenital anomaly itself. These will render cardiovascular MR difficult, and will require adjustments to normal cardiovascular MR imaging protocols.

To meet the needs of successful paediatric cardiovascular MR, some adjustments are as follows. Due to small size of the heart and blood vessels, slice thickness is reduced to 3–7 mm. The field of view is also reduced, but this is at the expense of signal:noise ratio (SNR). Sometimes, smaller size, paediatric radiofrequency coils or the application of multiple signal averages can help to maintain the SNR at high spatial resolution for these small hearts. To avoid image blurring due to fast heart rate in newborns and infants, it is necessary to improve the temporal resolution. Reducing the number of k-space lines to be acquired per segment in the segmented k-space will improve the temporal resolution at the expense of an increase in the total number of heartbeats required. In patients with arrhythmias, real-time imaging can be used. In patients having difficulty with breath-holding, or with respiratory motion artefacts, averaging techniques or a respiratory navigator can be applied.

4.11 Normal Values in Children

The rapid uptake of cardiovascular MR and exponential rise in use for paediatric cardiology accentuates the paucity of CMR data giving normal reference values for paediatric patients. Normal data for ventricular volumes, function and other structural measurements has been published (Lorenz 2000; Buechel et al. 2009) and multicentre data is now being accumulated. It is crucial that these data incorporate, or at least attempt to unify, the multitude of different imaging and post-processing conventions that have evolved in the international centres developing paediatric cardiovascular MR.

5 Sequential Segmental Analysis

The nomenclature of complex congenital heart disease is based on segmental analysis. This requires description of atrial situs, atrioventricular connections, and

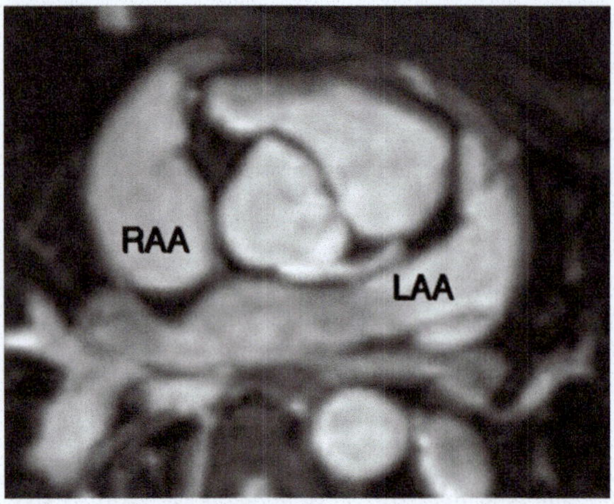

Fig. 9 Post-processed image from 3D b-SSFP data demonstrating the usual position and shape of the atrial appendages, in relation to the aortic root (*centre* of image)

ventriculoarterial connections and other associated lesions (Anderson 2009). Transthoracic and transoesophageal echocardiography are of proven benefit when establishing cardiac diagnosis based on segmental analysis (Rigby and Redington 1989). However, in some cases further imaging is required to fully establish a diagnosis, or to plan the most appropriate management or intervention. Cardiovascular MR represents a non-invasive method of establishing a cardiac diagnosis when the echocardiographic diagnosis remains insufficient.

The descriptions below are not a comprehensive description of the sequential segmental analysis algorithm for congenital heart disease; a more complete explanation can be found in Professor Anderson and colleagues' book (Anderson 2009).

5.1 Step 1: Atrial Situs

The morphology of the atrial appendages are the key to identifying the correct atrial situs, as the venous attachments to each atrial chamber can form a variety of combinations.

The right atrial appendage is a triangular shape, with a wide base and prominent pectinate muscles, whilst the left atrial appendage is a more elongated, tubular structure, and is without trabeculations (Fig. 9).

The most common lesions involve inversion of situs, or isomerism of the left or right atrial appendages. The non-cardiac thoracic and abdominal organs usually (but not always) demonstrate a similar "sidedness" to that of the atrial chambers.

In the normal heart the morphological right atrium is located to the right of the morphological left atrium (situs solitus). The right lung is tri-lobed, with a shorter, early-branching bronchus, and the left lung is bi-lobed. In addition, the inferior caval vein (IVC) is to the right of the abdominal aorta, with a right-sided liver and left-sided spleen.

In situs inversus the mirror image of the normal anatomy is present.

Isomerism of the left atrial appendages is usually associated with bilateral bi-lobed lungs, polysplenia and IVC interruption (Fig. 10). Isomerism of the right atrial appendages is usually associated with bilateral tri-lobed lungs, asplenia and a midline liver (Fig. 11). In isomeric lesions there is often an endocardial cushion defect with varying degrees of atrio-ventricular septal defect (AVSD). Gut malrotation is associated with both right- and left-sided isomerism. All of these abnormalities can be determined with MR, particularly 3D balanced-SSFP techniques (Razavi et al. 2003b).

5.2 Step 2: Ventricular Morphology

Determination of ventricular morphology allows analysis of atrioventricular (AV) and ventriculoarterial concordance. Irrespective of atrioventricular concordance the AV valve is concordant with the ventricle, i.e. the tricuspid valve connects to the morphological right ventricle and the mitral valve connects to the morphological left ventricle. The septal insertion of the tricuspid valve is more apical than that of the mitral valve (apical valve "offset") and allows determination of the ventricular morphology. The muscular structure of the ventricles also differs, the RV being more trabeculated than the LV, with a muscular infundibulum and mid-ventricular 'moderator band'. Although they are different in normal subjects, the size, shape and degree of trabeculation of the ventricles are not good indicators of ventricular origin, as all are dependent on load effects (Fig. 12).

5.3 Step 3: Ventriculoarterial Connection

Description of ventriculoarterial connections represents the final element of sequential segmental analysis. The aorta and pulmonary arteries are defined by

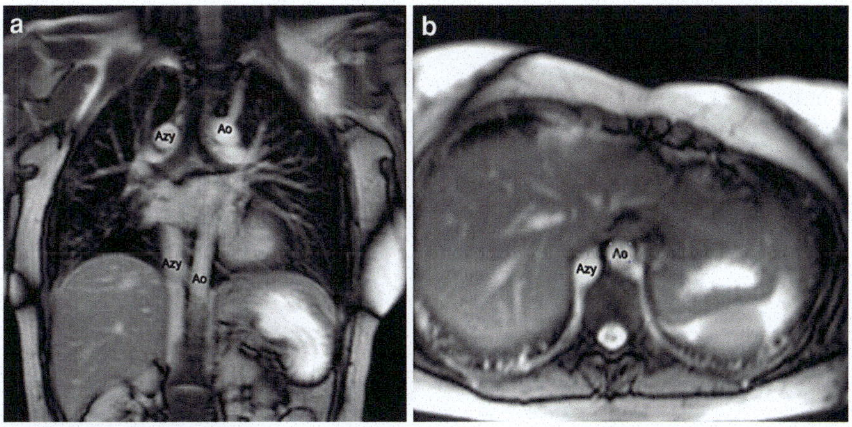

Fig. 10 Coronal (**a**) and axial (**b**) white-blood, "scout" images from a patient with isomerism of the left atrial appendages. Note the azygous continuation of the inferior vena caval vein, and associated bilateral, bi-lobed lungs. This patient had multiple splenic bodies

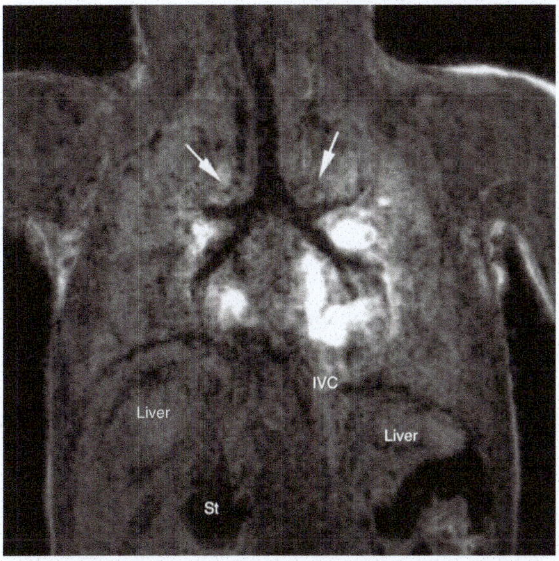

Fig. 11 Minimum intensity projection in the coronal plane, from 3D ceMRA data derived from a 2-year-old patient with asplenia. This demonstrates some extracardiac features associated with isomerism of the right atrial appendages: bilateral tri-lobed lungs (*arrows*), midline liver, IVC on the *left side*, stomach (St) on the *right side*

their typical branching patterns. 3D balanced-SSFP and ceMRA techniques are particularly useful in determining the arrangement of the great vessels and the connections with their respective ventricles.

5.4 Step 4: Identification of Other Abnormalities

Other abnormalities to be considered include: abnormal venous connections, atrial septal defects (ASD), ventricular septal defects (VSD), AVSD and valve abnormalities.

In general, most congenital cardiac lesions are single abnormalities that are easily described. However, almost any combination of abnormalities and connections can occur, and using the sequential segmental analysis method, the description of all conceivable combinations and diagnoses is possible.

6 Acyanotic Heart Disease

6.1 Quantifying and Locating a Shunt

An intracardiac shunt or anomalous pulmonary venous drainage should be suspected if clinical testing reveals asymmetric atrial or ventricular dilatation, or dilatation of the main and branch pulmonary arteries. Cardiac MRI is now the optimum investigation for the identification of the source, or quantifying the degree, of pulmonary venous and intracardiac shunt. However, the accurate diagnosis and quantification of a shunt requires a sound knowledge of the potential technical pitfalls involved in the image acquisition and post-processing. Meticulous techniques and logical physiological reasoning must be maintained.

The accurate quantification of any simple shunt requires assessment of aortic and pulmonary flow volumes. For more complex shunts, or for the assessment of total pulmonary and total systemic blood flow (e.g. Qp:Qs in patients with complex, functionally single ventricles), it is necessary to quantify systemic venous flow volumes and total pulmonary venous flow volumes. The quantification of ventricular stroke volume at the same examination will always serve to

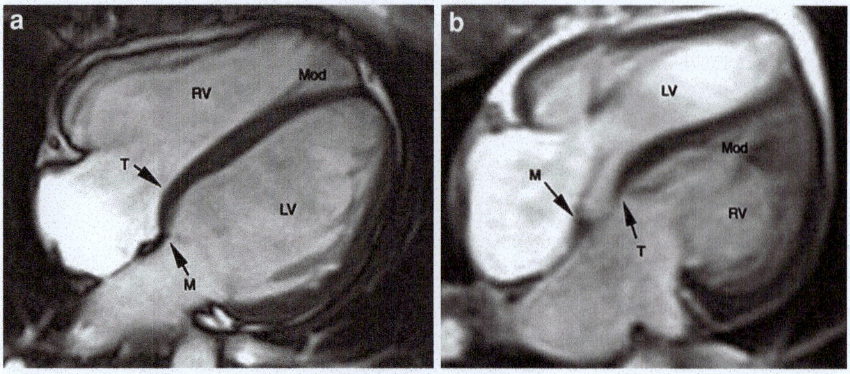

Fig. 12 Single frames from b-SSFP cine images, showing four-chamber views from a normal heart (**a**) *left* hand panel and congenitally corrected transposition of the great arteries (**b**) *right* hand panel. Note the "reversed-offsetting" of the mitral and tricuspid valves in CCGTA

Table 5 Algorithm of relative ventricular stroke volumes and arterial flow volumes for shunts at atrial and ventricular levels

Shunt at atrial level (or PAPVD)	
Pure left to right : Qp > Qs	Pulm FF > Ao FF
Usual pattern	RVSV > LVSV
	RVSV = Pulm FF
	LVSV = Ao FF
Pure right to left : Qp < Qs	Ao FF > Pulm FF
RV low compliance	LVSV > RVSV
	RVSV = Pulm FF
	LVSV = Ao FF
Shunt at ventricular level	
Pure left to right : Qp > Qs	Pulm FF > Ao FF
Usual pattern	LVSV > RVSV
	LVSV = Pulm FF
	RVSV = Ao FF
Pure right to left : Qp < Qs	Ao FF > Pulm FF
RV high pressure	RVSV > LVSV
	RVSV = Ao FF
	LVSV = Pulm FF

Qp total pulmonary flow volume, *Qs* total systemic flow volume, *Pulm FF* pulmonary forward flow volume, *Ao FF* aortic forward flow volume, *RVSV* right ventricular stroke volume, *LVSV* left ventricular stroke volume

confirm the location of a shunt, and to internally validate the flow volume measurements.

Table 5 gives a simple algorithm to assist the diagnostic pathway in locating a shunt. This serves as a simple guide only. The presence of atrioventricular valve regurgitation can confound this simple guide.

Through-plane flow volume assessment is performed using phase-contrast through plane flow mapping. Breath-hold techniques allow higher spatial and temporal resolution images, though free-breathing and rapid acquisition techniques (Steeden et al. 2011) allow flow mapping in younger children or other patients unable to reliably breath-hold.

Detailed instructions for the techniques are given in "Valvular Heart Disease". The image plane for through-plane flow mapping should be placed perpendicular to both orthogonal long axis views of the great vessel. Ideally this plane should be in an area of laminar flow, and during the whole cardiac cycle, should be distal to the semilunar valve tips and proximal to the first aortic or pulmonary artery branches.

Ventricular volumetry and stroke volume quantification is also described in detail elsewhere (see "Cardiac Fuction"). The principles remain the same when imaging patients with congenitally abnormal ventricles, although automated software may be less accurate in this setting. Currently, the cine imaging sequence with optimum blood/myocardial contrast is balanced-SSFP. These images should be obtained with temporal resolution at least 40 ms, using contiguous short axis or horizontal long axis slices. A slice-positioning tool improves the accuracy of segmentation for basal slices. For improved physiological accuracy, the major ventricular trabeculae should be excluded from the blood pool. At the present time, manual tracing of the endocardial border is the most precise processing method for the measurement right ventricular stroke volumes, although the reproducibility of this technique is less robust (Winter et al. 2008).

6.2 Partial Anomalous Pulmonary Venous Return

Imaging techniques for the assessment of partial anomalous pulmonary venous return is discussed in detail in "Imaging of Great Vessels" Sect. 3.3.

6.3 Total Anomalous Pulmonary Venous Return

Imaging techniques for the assessment of total anomalous pulmonary venous return is discussed in detail in "Imaging of Great Vessels" Sect. 3.3.

6.4 Atrial Septal Defect

Atrial septal defects are the most common congenital heart defect detected in adults, with an incidence of 941 per million live births (Hoffman and Kaplan 2002). Irrespective of their type and location, they cause left to right shunting at the atrial level. This leads to atrial dilation, predisposing to tachy-arrythmias, and biventricular volume overload. The presence of an atrial septal defect (ASD) is also an independent risk factor for thrombo-embolic stroke. This is due to the ability of thrombo-emboli, originating either in the right atrium or venous vasculature, to pass through the ASD into the systemic circulation (Mohr and Homma 2003).

Atrial septal defects are, anatomically and developmentally, a heterogeneous group of lesions. The specific nature of the ASD influences the natural history and management of this disease. Ostium secundum defects make up 80% of ASDs and are located in the fossa ovalis (Fig. 13). These defects are due to failure of the septum secundum to form closure of the ostium secundum. The ostium primum defect is actually a component of a common atrioventricular valve ring, also known as an atrioventricular septal defect (AVSD). This defect usually occurs together with some degree of atrioventricular valve abnormality. Finally, the sinus venosus defect is found at the junction of the right atrium and either one of the caval veins. This type of ASD is less common, and is often associated with partial anomalous pulmonary venous drainage.

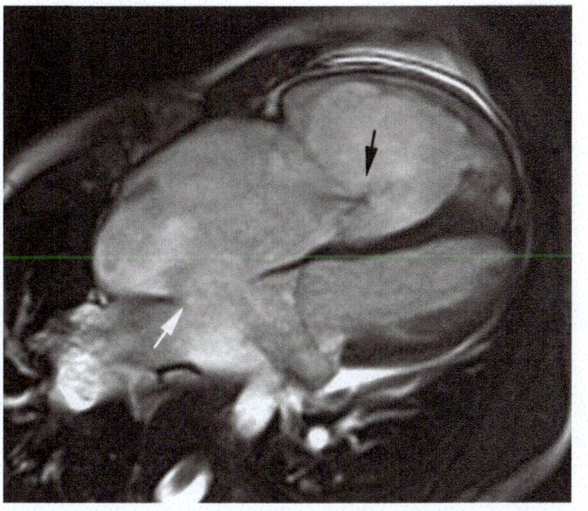

Fig. 13 A systolic frame of a b-SSFP image from a 25-year-old man with a secundum atrial septal defect (*white arrow*). Note the right atrial and right ventricular dilatation and tricuspid valve regurgitation (*black arrow*)

The management of ASDs has changed in the recent years, particularly with the increasing use of transcatheter ASD closure devices. Previously, surgical closure was only considered when a large left to right shunt led to right ventricular volume overload, atrial dilation and symptoms. However, with the advent of transcatheter techniques, management has become aggressive (Fischer et al. 2003). Transcatheter techniques are only viable in patients with small- to medium-sized ostium secundum defects that have adequate margins with which to anchor the device. Deficiency of the anterior or poster–inferior rim of the defect usually precludes transcatheter closure. Patients with large ostium secundum defects, or defects with deficiency of the anterior or postero-inferior rims, or with sinus venosus lesions, usually require operative repair. The clinical aim is to complete ASD closure prior to the development of cardiac failure or atrial dilation, and timing of intervention depends on the haemodynamic status of the patient. Thus, evaluation of ASDs requires definition of type and location of the defect, quantification of the net shunt, detection of any intra-atrial thrombus, assessment of RV volume and systolic function and visualization of the pulmonary venous anatomy. Furthermore, in patients with ostium secundum defects, special attention must be given to delineating the anatomy

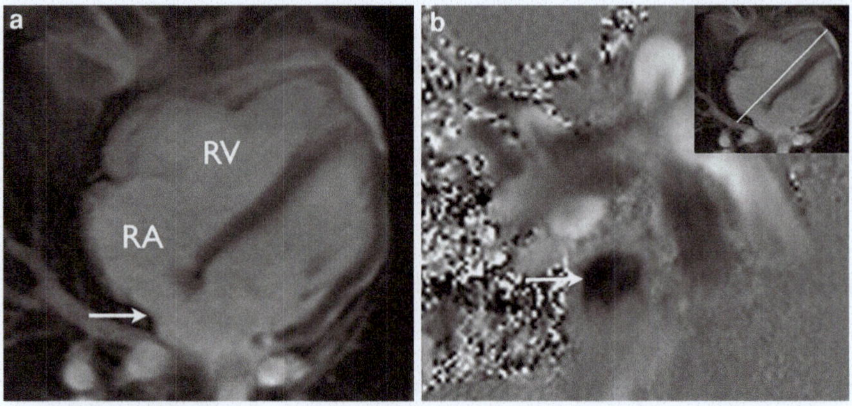

Fig. 14 Balanced-SSFP image, 4-chamber view showing a large secundum ASD, with posterior extension (**a**). The through-plane PC-MRI (**b**) demonstrates significant flow through the ASD. Inset shows the imaging plane in which the flow is performed

of the margins of the defect as this influences planning invasive management.

Transthoracic echocardiography has a limited ability to visualize small ostium secundum and sinus venosus defects. In addition, detection of pulmonary venous abnormalities is technically difficult, using the transthoracic approach. Transoesophageal echocardiography is the main imaging technique used to assess ASDs. However, transoesophageal echocardiography cannot be used to quantify the shunt ($Qp:Q_s$) accurately and it can be difficult to delineate pulmonary venous anatomy. Cardiovascular MR has a significant role to play in the diagnosis and pre-interventional assessment of ASDs.

3D whole-heart techniques, with isotropic resolution, allow accurate multi-planar reformatting with no loss of resolution. These techniques allow 3D rendering of the atrial anatomy. Multi-slice 2D gradient echo techniques can be used to assess the dynamic 3D anatomy of the defect, and phase-contrast through-plane flow techniques can accurately size the cross-sectional dimensions of the defect, or diagnose multiple or fenestrated defects (Fig. 14).

Measurements made using gradient echo techniques compare well with both operative and TTE findings (Beerbaum et al. 2003). It has been shown that MR findings are more powerful predictors of successful catheter closure than transthoracic or oesophageal echocardiographic findings (Durongpisitkul et al. 2004).

Sinus venosus defects are often associated with pulmonary venous abnormalities. Gd-MRA is a sensitive method for detecting pulmonary venous abnormalities (Puvaneswary et al. 2003) and can be useful prior to surgical intervention for sinus venosus defects.

Haemodynamic assessment is also an important part of the evaluation of ASDs. Invasive catheterisation has previously been used to accurately quantify left to right shunts (Beerbaum et al. 2001). Quantification of left to right shunts using velocity-encoded phase-contrast MR compares well to invasive catheterization results (Beerbaum et al. 2001). It has the benefit of being non-invasive and does not require exposure to ionizing radiation. Furthermore, there is some evidence that in certain situations phase contrast MR is more accurate than invasive catheterization (Muthurangu et al. 2004). Ventricular overload can also be accurately assessed using multi-slice balanced-SSFP short axis imaging and can give important information influencing the timing of intervention.

6.5 Atrioventricular Septal Defect

Atrioventricular septal defects are caused by abnormalities of the endocardial cushion and can exhibit a spectrum of abnormalities of the inlet ventricular septum, the atrioventricular valve and the primum atrial septum.

By definition, all atrioventricular septal defects have a common atrioventricular valve ring, losing the usual two-ringed formation of the mitral and tricuspid valves, and resulting in a single, common valve, typically with five leaflets. These are referred to as the superior bridging, right anterosuperior, right mural, inferior bridging and left mural leaflets. The common valve ring can be isolated ("cleft" left AV valve only) or associated with a ventricular septal defect, a primum atrial septal defect, or both. Further anatomical

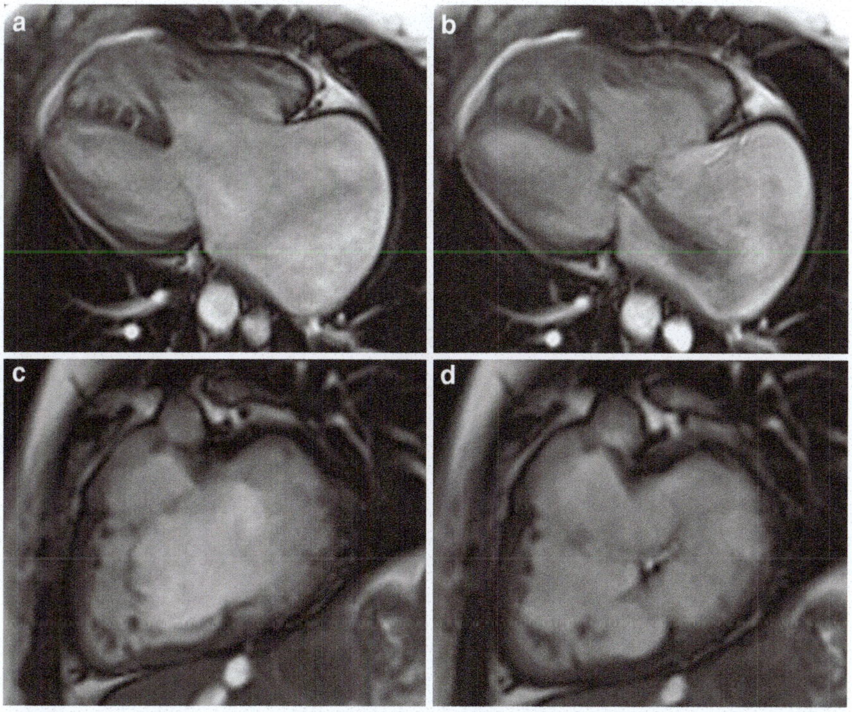

Fig. 15 Balanced-SSFP cine images from patient with isomerism of the left atrial appendages and a functionally single ventricle, involving a balanced AVSD with severe regurgitation. 4-chamber view in diastole (**a**), systole (**b**), short axis view in diastole (**c**), systole (**d**) showing the large coaptation defect

variation involves the variable size of the ventricles and AV valve leaflets, leading to balanced (relatively equal-sized AV valves and ventricles) or unbalanced, when inflow through the AV valves is predominantly into one of the ventricles.

Atrioventricular septal defects can be complex lesions, and can be associated with other complex congenital heart anomalies (e.g. isomerism of the atrial appendages and double outlet right ventricle) (Fig. 15). There is a high incidence of AVSDs in patients with Trisomy 21.

Surgical intervention, with closure of the septal defects and or repair of the AV valves is possible, though some patients with unbalanced AVSDs may be better served with surgical palliation along the single-ventricle pathway.

In the neonatal period, acoustic windows usually allow detailed transthoracic echocardiographic imaging. In this situation, preoperative assessment of AVSDs with MRI is of limited added value. However, improved longitudinal data may show an important role for MR in determining the optimal surgical strategy (biventricular repair or univentricular surgical palliation) for patients with unbalanced AVSD and borderline hypoplasia of the left or right ventricle.

6.6 Ventricular Septal Defect

Ventricular septal defects are the most common congenital heart lesions in the paediatric population, with an incidence of 3570 per million live births (Hoffman and Kaplan 2002). Ventricular septal defects are a heterogeneous group of lesions with the common physiological effect of shunting at ventricular level. The volume of shunt depends on the size of the defect and the relative resistances in the circulations supplied by each ventricle. Thus the haemodynamic effect of VSDs can vary from being insignificant, to causing left-sided heart failure and pulmonary vascular disease. It is this haemodynamic effect that dictates the type and timing of treatment.

Conventionally, invasive catheterization has been used to accurately quantify left to right shunts (Beerbaum et al. 2001). Quantification of left to right shunts using PC-MRI compares well to invasive catheterization results (Beerbaum et al. 2001) and has the benefit of being non-invasive. There is some evidence that in certain situations combining PC-MRI and invasive pressure measurements is more accurate than traditional methods which rely on the Fick principle (Muthurangu et al. 2004).

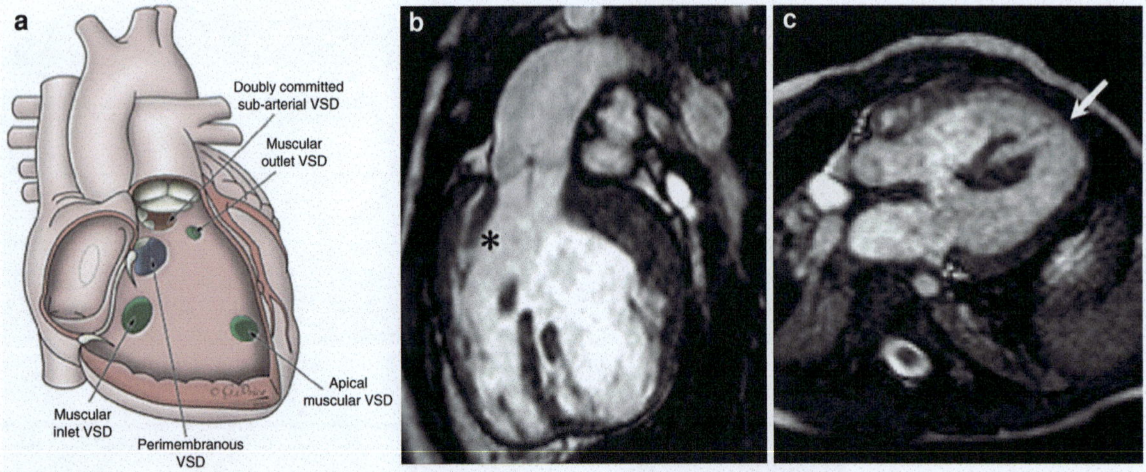

Fig. 16 **a** Schematic drawing showing the categorization used for differentiation of the various types of ventricular septal defects. Viewed from a right ventricular aspect. **b** Balanced-SSFP image of an outlet VSD (*asterisk*) with an overriding aorta. **c** Balanced-SSFP image of an apical VSD (*arrow*) and an inlet VSD

Cardiovascular MR can therefore play an important role in the haemodynamic assessment of VSDs.

The ventricular septum is a complex helical 3D structure (Acar et al. 2002). It is commonly divided into membranous, muscular and apical portions. The location of the VSD influences the natural history of the lesion and the optimum therapy. Perimembranous lesions comprise 80% of all VSDs and the majority of these VSDs, if small, will close spontaneously during childhood. Large, perimembranous VSDs are unlikely to close and if left untreated can lead to the development of pulmonary vascular disease.

Surgical closure with septal augmentation is the accepted treatment for significant perimembranous VSDs and is associated with low mortality and no residual shunting (Thanopoulos et al. 2003). Transcatheter closure of perimembranous VSDs is associated with a high incidence of conduction defects, and is not the intervention of choice. However, transcatheter techniques are becoming increasingly relied upon for some perimembranous VSDs due to their reduced post-operative morbidity (Thanopoulos et al. 2003). Transcatheter VSD closure is safer and more effective for single defects, defects less than 12 mm in size, and defects further than 5 mm away from the aortic or mitral valve (Thanopoulos et al. 2003).

Between 5 and 20% of VSDs occur in the muscular septum (Fig. 16). Muscular VSDs are an extremely heterogeneous group of lesions that can be difficult, from a technical viewpoint, to close surgically. Transcatheter techniques have been used in the closure of muscular VSDs, with some success (Chessa et al. 2002; Chaudhari et al. 2001). Optimum treatment (either operative or transcatheter) depends on accurate demonstration of the VSD anatomy (Sivakumar et al. 2003). Muscular defects often have complex 3D structure with multiple defects ("Swiss cheese" appearance).

Transthoracic echocardiography is used to assess suitability for operative or transcatheter closure, and 3D echocardiographic techniques are proving effective in assessing the VSD morphology, however transthoracic echocardiography is associated with interoperator variability. Cardiovascular MR can provide accurate 2D and 3D images of the defect. Multi-slice 2D gradient-echo techniques can be used to assess the dynamic 3D anatomy of the defect, however, multi-slice techniques suffer from poor through-plane resolution. 3D balanced-SSFP techniques with isotropic resolution allow accurate multiplanar reformatting, with no loss of resolution, allowing 3D rendering of the ventricular anatomy (Razavi et al. 2003b). With image acquisition during the diastolic period, these techniques are particularly useful in assessing the anatomy of a VSD and the relationship of the VSD with valvar structures.

The management of multiple VSDs can be difficult, as both surgical and transcatheter closure can leave residual defects (Seddio et al. 1999). In such situations, palliation with pulmonary artery banding is indicated. Assessment of pulmonary artery band adequacy relies on demonstration of a significant pressure gradient across the band using transthoracic echocardiography. Gradient-echo cine MR has been used to assess band adequacy (Simpson et al. 1993) and has been shown to compare well with surgical and catheter findings. Furthermore, accurate assessment of Qp:Qs ratio can be obtained, and this must represent the optimal method to assess band adequacy.

Approximately 50% of cases patients with a VSD have an associated cardiac or great vessel abnormality. Coarctation of the aorta and aortic stenosis are particularly important and are commonly associated with posterior mal-alignment of the VSD. Cardiovascular MR gives accurate quantification of valvular stenosis and aortic coarctation, and these subjects are dealt with in more detail in the chapters on valvar heart disease (see "Valvular Heart Disease") and imaging of great vessel (see "Imaging of Great Vessels"), respectively.

6.7 Congenital Aortic Supravalvar Stenosis

Congenital supravalvar aortic stenosis is a rare congenital heart defect, the vast majority of cases usually being associated with Williams syndrome (Williams et al. 1961). Williams syndrome is characterized by the presence of supravalvar aortic stenosis, but approximately 80% of patients also have peripheral pulmonary artery stenosis. These vascular phenotypes occur in association with mental retardation, distinctive personality and behavioural traits, elfin facies, and in some instances transient neonatal hypercalcaemia (Beuren et al. 1964). It is now recognized that Williams syndrome is the result of deletion of megabases of chromosome 7q11.23. This deletion involves several genes, including the elastin gene, and the degree and combination of deletions is most likely responsible for the features of the syndrome other than supravalvar aortic stenosis and peripheral pulmonary artery stenosis (Urban et al. 2001). Non-syndromic congenital supravalvar aortic stenosis does occur but is much less common, and occurs in a familial autosomal dominant form and in sporadic isolated cases. These forms lack the cognitive, behavioural and phenotypic abnormalities of Williams syndrome.

The normal presence of elastin is responsible for the distensibility of the aorta during systole and its subsequent recoil during diastole, but the reduced net deposition of arterial wall elastin leads to increased proliferation of arterial wall smooth muscle cells. This results in multilayer thickening of the medial of large arteries and subsequent development of obstructive hyperplastic intimal lesions. A characteristic hour-glass narrowing of the aorta develops at the sinotubular junction, but in approximately 30% of cases there is a diffuse, tubular narrowing of the ascending aorta, often extending to the arch and the origin of the brachiocephalic vessels (Stamm et al. 1997). There may also be localized stenoses in the renal and mesenteric arteries. The aortic valve may also be pathologically involved, and mechanical impairment of coronary blood flow is a frequent and often unappreciated feature of supravalvar aortic stenosis. The possibility of significant coronary obstruction can exist, independent of the degree of arch obstruction.

In these patients, invasive investigation involving anaesthesia and/or X-ray angiography catheterization can be associated with severe complications, usually related to the multitude of reasons for imbalance between myocardial oxygen consumption and perfusion. Therefore non-invasive assessment is important.

The main roles of cardiovascular MR are preoperative anatomical and functional assessment of the aortic arch stenosis, exclusion of commonly associated branch pulmonary artery narrowing and assessment of the results following surgical repair. Cardiovascular MR may also show proximal, anatomical obstruction to coronary flow (Park et al. 2008) however, at present, cardiac catheterization with coronary angiography remains the most sensitive method for delineation of coronary artery lumen caliber in these patients. CeMRA is an accurate method of assessing the type and severity of the supravalvar defect as well as its relationship with the aortic valve. However, if stenosis is severe, signal loss in the ceMRA may lead to overestimation of the severity of the stenosis. In these situations, 2D 'black-blood' imaging (with image data captured in the systolic phase of the cardiac cycle) is useful in assessing both the external and internal diameter of the stenotic region of aorta. PC-MRI can be used to measure peak velocities at the level of the supravalvar aortic obstruction, giving an indication of the pressure

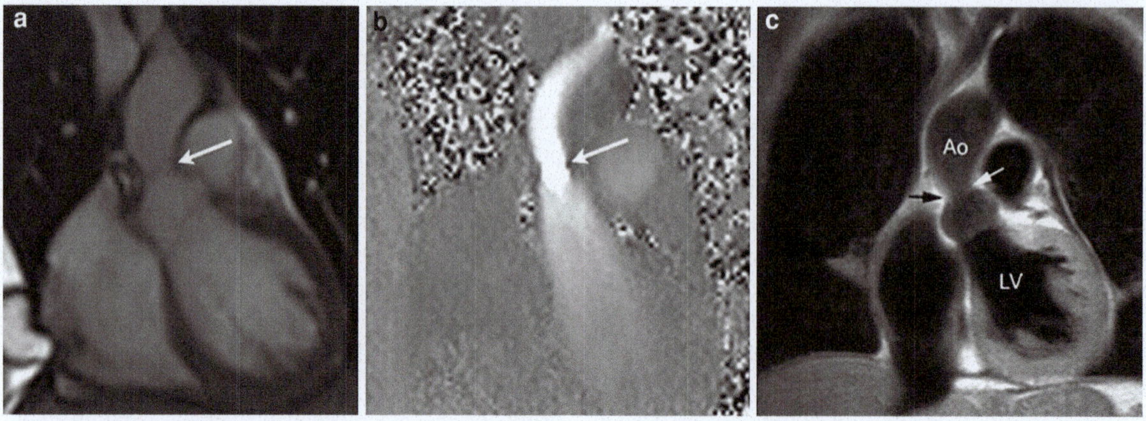

Fig. 17 **a** Balanced-SSFP image of aortic outflow showing supravalvar aortic stenosis (*arrow*). **b** In-plane phase contrast showing flow acceleration (*arrow*) originating at supravalvar level, extending into the aortic arch. **c** Black-blood spin-echo left ventricular outflow tract view of supravalvular aortic stenosis (*arrows*)

gradient and functional significance of a stenosis (Fig. 17).

Balanced-SSFP cine imaging of the LV outflow tract should be performed to evaluate the dynamic nature of the supravalvar stenosis and to subjectively assess the degree of flow turbulence or acceleration. Haemodynamic consequences of arch obstruction should be assessed with volumetric and functional analysis of the ventricles; including LV mass quantification. 3D balanced-SSFP imaging can sensitively display the arch, branch pulmonary artery and coronary artery morphology.

6.8 Congenital Anomalies of the Aorta

Congenital anomalies of the aorta are covered in detail in "Imaging of Great Vessels".

7 Cyanotic Heart Disease

7.1 Tetralogy of Fallot

Tetralogy of Fallot (ToF) is the most common cyanotic congenital heart defect with an incidence of approximately 420 per million live births (Hoffman and Kaplan 2002). The morphological constellation includes malalignment of the infundibular septum, which leads to right ventricular outflow (RVOT) obstruction, a sub-aortic VSD with aortic override, and right ventricular hypertrophy (Fig. 18).

Treatment for this condition was revolutionized by the introduction of the Blalock and Tausig shunt in the late 1940s, and since this time has been undergoing constant evolution. The current management for typical tetralogy of Fallot, consists of single stage reconstructive surgery, usually performed during the first year of life. Many centres are now advocating complete corrective surgery within the first 6 months of life, in an attempt to avoid any palliative shunt surgery. Early repair has the benefit of leaving the patient acyanotic and has good survival rates (Pigula et al. 1999; Bacha et al. 2001). Staged reconstruction may still be required in very small infants and in those with significant hypoplasia of the central pulmonary arteries (Marshall et al. 2003).

Transthoracic echocardiography is the imaging modality of choice for the initial diagnosis and assessment of paediatric patients. However, cardiac MRI does have a role in untreated or shunt-palliated patients, in delineating pulmonary artery anatomy or excluding significant pulmonary artery distortion. It has been shown that pulmonary artery ceMRA findings compare well with both operative and X-ray angiographic findings (Beekman et al. 1997; Holmqvist et al. 2001). MR may in fact be more powerful than X-ray angiography in defining the central pulmonary artery structure (Beekman et al. 1997). MR can also be used to accurately assess the 3D orientation of the VSD and the degree of aortic override (Beekman et al. 1997).

Operative repair of tetralogy of Fallot consists of resection of the infundibular stenosis, enlargement of

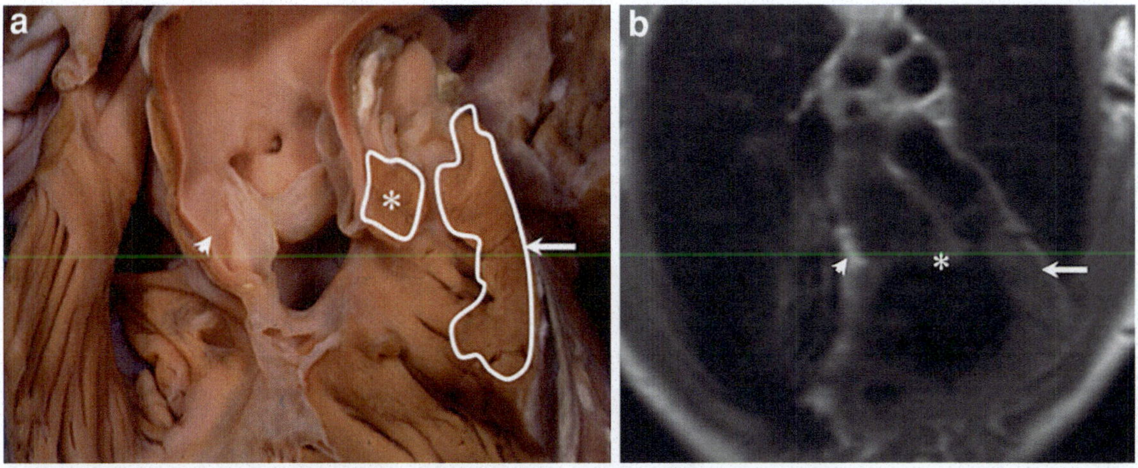

Fig. 18 **a, b** Right ventricular outflow tract coronal view of tetralogy of Fallot. Corresponding morphological (**a**) and black- blood spin-echo images. **b** the deviated outlet septum (*asterisk*), aortic root (*arrowhead*), and hypertrophied septoparietal trabeculations (*arrow*) are shown

the pulmonary valve or valve annulus and closure of the VSD. With current knowledge of the deleterious effects on the right ventricle of chronic pulmonary valve regurgitation, surgical trends are changing, with the aim of preserving pulmonary valve function, possibly permitting more RV outflow tract obstruction.

While early surgical mortality from complete repair of tetralogy of Fallot is very low in the modern surgical era (Pigula et al. 1999), residual anatomic and haemodynamic abnormalities are almost universal. These include RV dilatation from pulmonary regurgitation, RV outflow tract aneurysm, RV outflow tract obstruction, pulmonary artery stenosis, residual atrial or ventricular septal defect, tricuspid valve regurgitation and aortic root dilatation.

Cardiovascular MR has emerged as an essential diagnostic tool in this population because it provides a comprehensive assessment of all the above-mentioned abnormalities and it overcomes many of the limitations of other imaging modalities such as echocardiography, cardiac CT and cardiac catheterization. Cardiovascular MR provides unique quantitative data, accurate definition of the RV outflow tract anatomy, as well as prognostic information (Knauth et al. 2008), and is now the reference standard for imaging of patients late after repair (Warnes et al. 2008).

The main goals of cardiovascular MR in patients with repaired tetralogy of Fallot include the following: (a) a quantitative assessment of left and right ventricular volumes, stroke volumes, ejection fraction and cardiac output, (b) imaging of the RV outflow tract, pulmonary arteries and aorta, (c) quantification of pulmonary valve regurgitation, tricuspid valve regurgitation, relative flow volumes in the branch pulmonary arteries and pulmonary-to-systemic flow ratio, (d) assessment of myocardial viability with specific attention to scar tissue in the ventricular myocardium and in sites of previous surgery (for example in the VSD and RV outflow tract patches).

An example of a comprehensive imaging protocol is given in Table 3 of this chapter.

Balanced-SSFP sequences are used for ventricular functional assessment and should include long and short-axis views of both ventricles. Volumetric analysis is made using contiguous short or long axis slices, with care to prescribe the short axis image planes perpendicular to the ventricular septum in order to minimize through-plane motion (Fig. 19) and with care to include enough slices to incorporate the entire LV and RV at end-diastole.

The offline analysis and quantification of ventricular volumes is described in detail in "Cardiac Fuction". For this population, in whom the predominant pathology involves the RV, and in whom serial data contributes to the decision-making in their clinical care, it is vital to have consistent, systematic post-processing methodology. The current most accurate methodology for quantification of RV volumes involves manual tracing of the endocardial

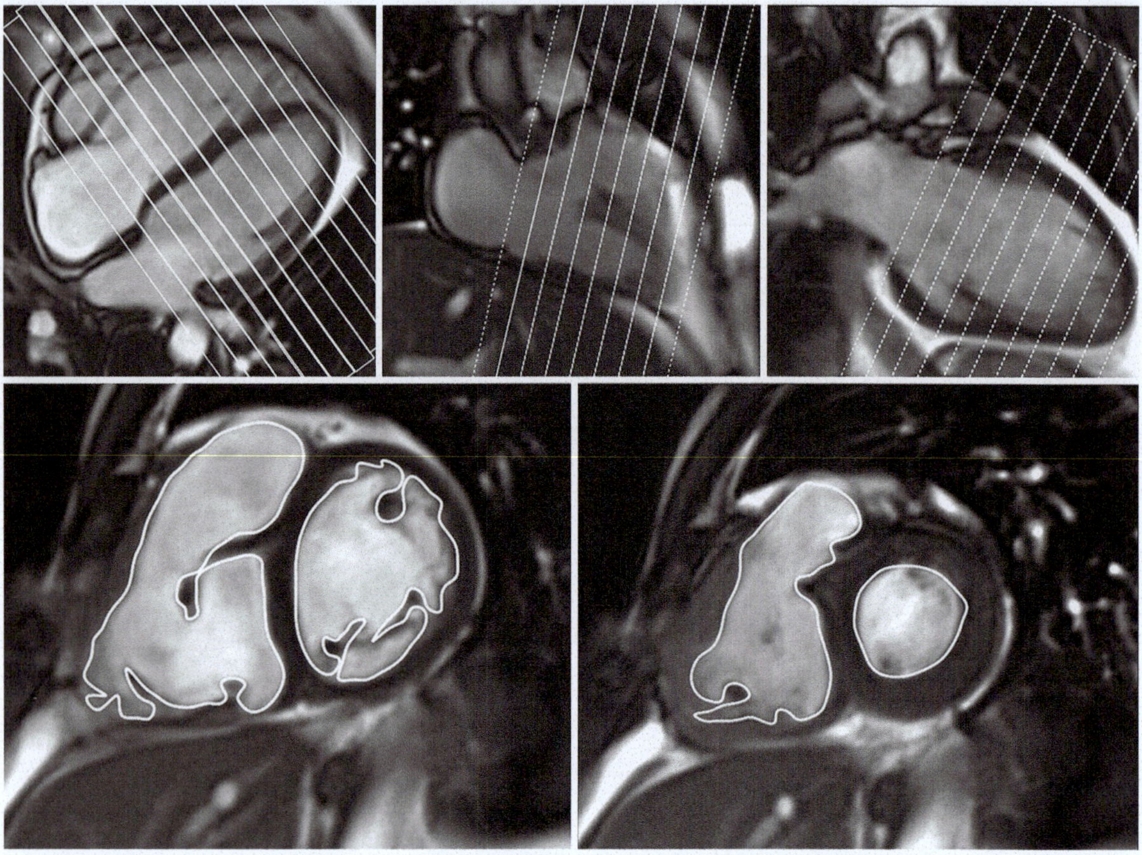

Fig. 19 Cardiovascular MR assessment of biventricular volumes and systolic function in repaired tetralogy of Fallot. Short-axis image planes are planned to cover the entire ventricular volume in diastole, aiming to minimise through-plane motion of the interventricular septal and ventricular free walls. *Lower panel* examples of contour drawings on the *left* and *right* endocardial boundaries, at mid-ventricular level

borders. For optimum physiological accuracy, the major papillary muscles and trabeculations are excluded from the blood pool. However, this involves laborious tracing of complex endocardial borders, with a time cost, and less robust reproducibility. If papillary muscles and trabeculations are included in the blood pool by tracing a smooth, approximated surface of the endocardial border, then the results generally give RV volumes greater than physiologically true, but with rapid post-processing times and less interobserver variability (Winter et al. 2008).

Software that incorporates cross-references between long and short axis images during post-processing greatly reduces the difficulty in determining the valve planes on short axis imaging. In our centre ventricular volumes and mass are measured from short-axis cine images with left and right ventricular long axis and the 4-chamber view facilitating accurate determination of the atrioventricular and semilunar valve planes during systole and diastole.

Balanced-SSFP images planned in oblique planes through the outflow tracts and in axial and oblique coronal planes for the branch pulmonary arteries (Fig. 20), allow views of the dynamic changes in these structures throughout the cardiac cycle.

PC-MRI can allow quantification of the pulmonary valve regurgitant fraction, the velocity of forward flow in obstructed outflow tracts, and the relative distribution of flow in each branch pulmonary artery. For through-plane flow assessment, care must be taken to plan image planes perpendicular to the direction of laminar forward flow, using at least two long-axis planes (Fig. 14.24). Consideration must also be given to the potential for artefact and inaccuracy due to turbulent flow patterns and phase offset phenomena (Gatehouse et al. 2010).

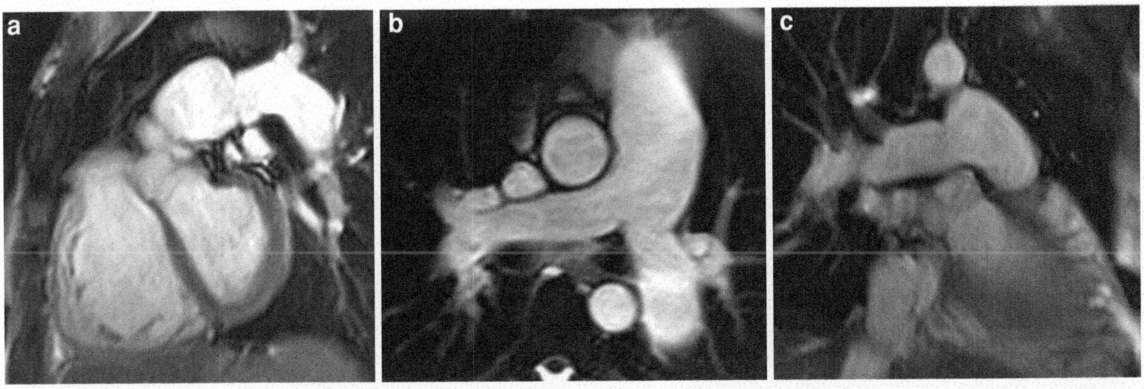

Fig. 20 Balanced-SSFP images of the branch pulmonary arteries allow assessment of the dynamic changes in these structures throughout the cardiac cycle: (**a**) oblique sagittal of the left pulmonary artery, (**b**) oblique axial of both branch pulmonary arteries and the pulmonary trunk, and (**c**) oblique coronal of the right pulmonary artery

CeMRA is particularly useful for 3D depiction of the morphology of the RV outflow tract and branch pulmonary arteries (Fig. 21). This facilitates the planning of interventions on the RV outflow tract, and helps to differentiate patients suitable or unsuitable for percutaneous pulmonary valve replacement (Schievano et al. 2007; Khambadkone et al. 2005). For optimal signal-to-noise ratio, and to facilitate 3D modelling of the outflow tract, bolus-tracking mechanisms can be used to enable image acquisition during the earlier period, when intravenous contrast only fills the right heart and pulmonary arterial structures.

CeMRA is generally acquired without cardiac gating and during breath-hold. This approach must be acknowledged when analysing images. The dimensions represented by the image data are averaged over the cardiac cycle. If dimensions are critical (for example, in planning percutaneous valve replacement), then compliant structures that vary in dimension during the cardiac cycle should also be measured in short and long axis planes, and in systolic and diastole phases, using cine imaging.

The effects of cardiac motion on CeMRA images impair the visualization of intracardiac structures, particularly the coronary arteries. Visualisation of the course of the proximal coronary arteries is often crucial for intervention planning (Nordmeyer et al. 2006). 3D balanced-SSFP imaging is a valuable tool for the assessment of intracardiac structures, particularly coronary arteries in these patients.

Two dimensional spin-echo 'black blood' and SSFP sequences can be used to delineate RVOT anatomy and quantitatively assess RVOT dilation or stenosis, and measurements made from MR data compare favourably with echocardiography and X-ray angiography.

The presence of localized ventricular scarring or fibrosis has been associated with arrhythmia and ventricular dysfunction in patients following repair of tetralogy of Fallot (Babu-Narayan et al. 2006). Late Gd MRI, performed 10–20 min after gadolinium administration can be performed in the long and short axis planes of ventricles and outflow tracts, in areas suspected of scarring. All areas should be imaged in orthogonal planes, with phase direction swapped to facilitate recognition of artefacts.

A plethora of cross-sectional and retrospectively acquired data exists concerning the use of MR data to give decision support with regard to the optimal timing of pulmonary valve replacement in patients with chronic pulmonary regurgitation following tetralogy of Fallot repair. However, there is little longitudinal data, and little data testing the concept of functional "reserve" under physiological or pharmacological stress conditions. With the advent of national collaborative groups (Sarikouch et al. 2010), standardized methodology, and the acquisition of serial, longitudinal data, including data regarding functional reserve (van den Berg et al. 2009), better decision support will be available in the future. The physiological consequences of pulmonary incompetence and pulmonary valve replacement (both surgical and percutaneous) are discussed in "Valvular Heart Disease" Sect. 3.6.1.

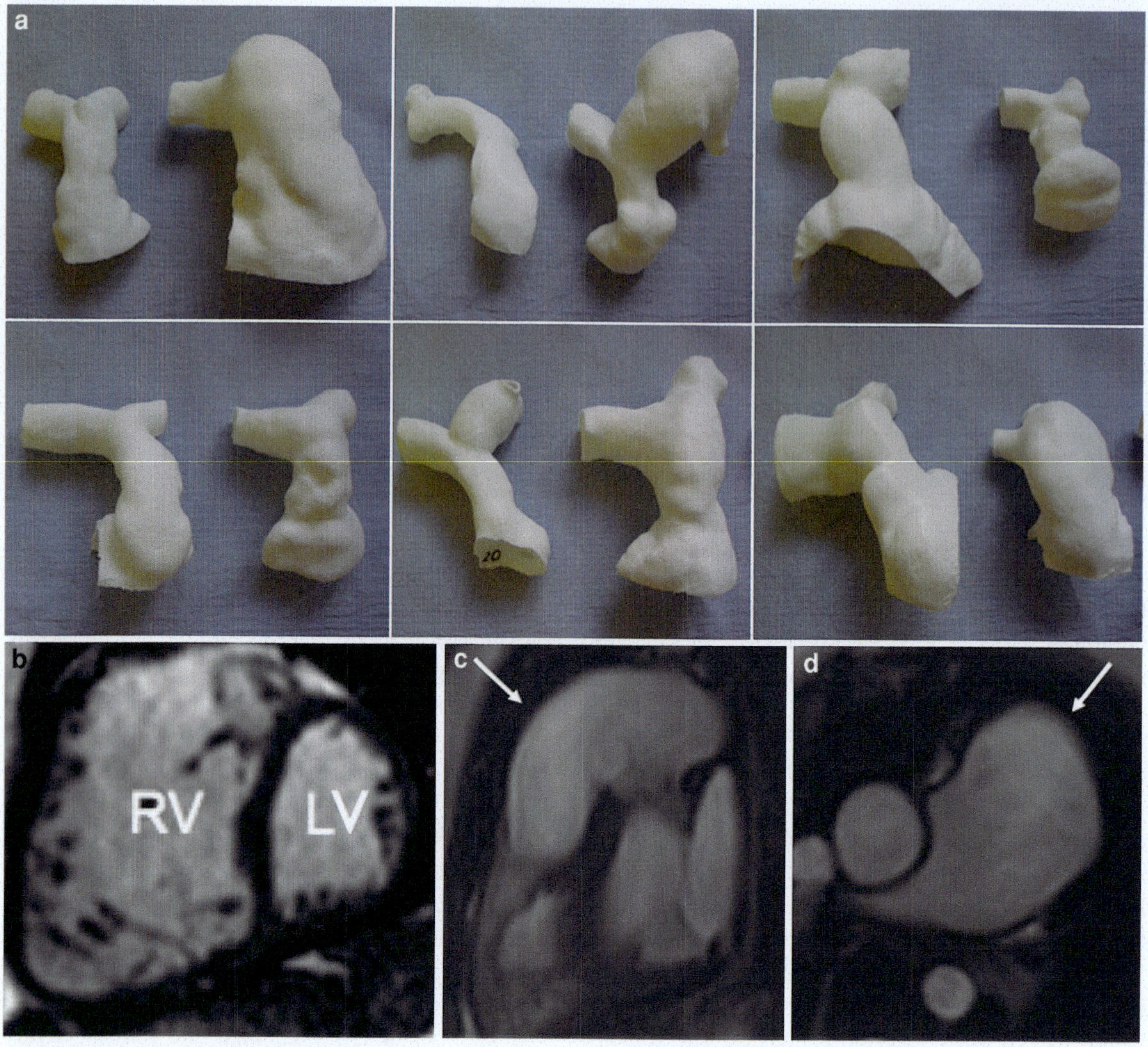

Fig. 21 Repaired tetralogy of Fallot. **a** 3D rapid prototyping models of the right ventricular outflow tract, pulmonary trunk and branch pulmonary arteries (reconstructed from 3D, contrast-enhanced MR angiogram data) from 12 patients with tetralogy of Fallot, all repaired in infancy and imaged 12–15 years later. Note the wide variation in morphology, size and narrowings. **b** End-diastolic, balanced-SSFP, mid-ventricular, short axis view showing severely dilated right ventricle (RV), flattened septum and small left ventricle (LV). **c** (sagittal) **d** (axial), end-systolic, balanced-SSFP images of an aneurismal right ventricular outflow tract (*arrow*)

7.2 Pulmonary Atresia with VSD

Pulmonary atresia is defined as a lack of continuity between the RV outflow tract and the central pulmonary arteries, with a variable degree of hypoplasia of these structures. Pulmonary atresia can be separated into two groups depending on the presence of a ventricular septal defect. As the physiology and clinical management of these two groups is different, it is useful to consider them separately.

Pulmonary atresia with a VSD is the most common variant and is considered by some to be a severe form of tetralogy of Fallot (Fig. 22), with a sub-aortic VSD, overriding aorta, and variable sources of pulmonary blood supply. Patients can be classified into three broad groups, defined by pulmonary blood supply: (1) supply from pulmonary arteries, (2) mixed pulmonary artery and aorto-pulmonary collateral supply, (3) supply solely from aorto-pulmonary collateral arteries (Fig. 23).

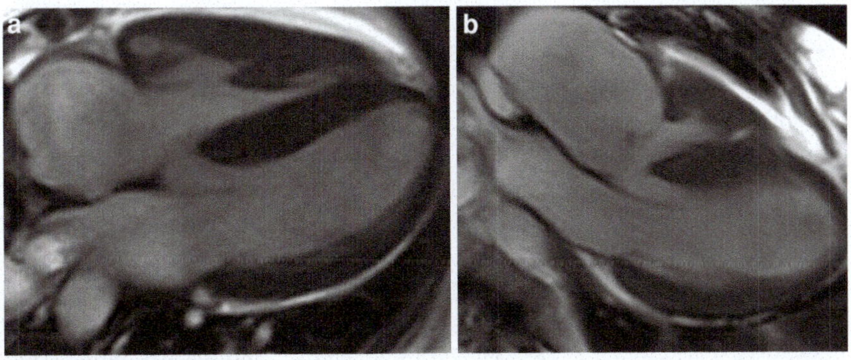

Fig. 22 Balanced-SSFP images from an adult patient with unrepaired PA/VSD, with pulmonary blood flow entirely supplied by aorto-pulmonary collateral arteries. **a** four-chamber view. **b** LV outflow tract view, showing the aorta overriding the VSD and interventricular septum

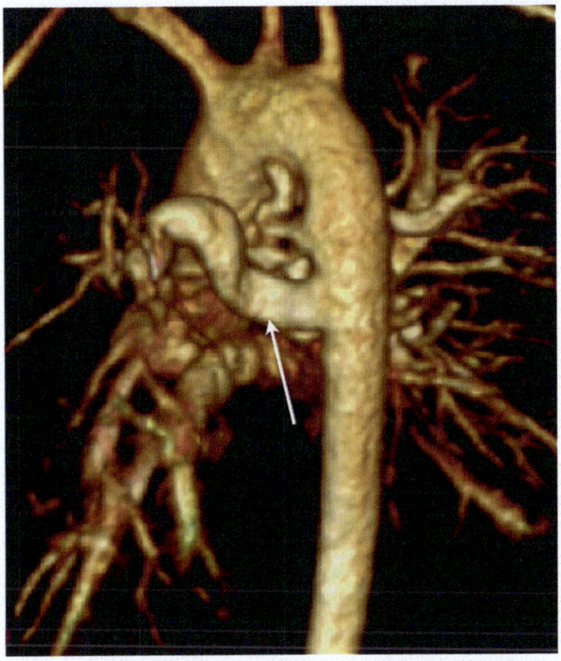

Fig. 23 3D ceMRA viewed from left posterior lateral showing several major aorto-pulmonary collateral arteries (MAPCAs). The *arrow* shows the largest MAPCA to the right lung

These patients can present with cyanosis because of reduced pulmonary blood flow, with reasonably balanced circulation, or with heart failure due to excessive pulmonary circulation. The clinical management from infancy is dependent on the pulmonary blood supply, with the majority of these patients now entering a planned surgical program with the goal of reconstructing the collateral supply onto a valved RV to pulmonary artery conduit, with or without ventricular septal defect closure (Brawn et al. 2009). The outcome of this goal is dependent on the initial accurate anatomical definition of the "true" central pulmonary arteries, and then the result of surgical unifocalisation of any mixed pulmonary supply.

Although, in younger infants, CT angiography is likely to depict small vessels more clearly, ceMRA angiography has a role in preoperative assessment and has been shown to be an excellent method of delineating central pulmonary arteries and MAPCAs prior to surgical or transcatheter procedures in older children (Geva et al. 2002). In addition, the 3D visualization provided by ceMRA, rather than the projection visualization provided by X-ray angiography, allows improved surgical or interventional planning.

Following surgical palliation with the formation of a confluent RV to pulmonary artery communication and VSD closure, the main role of MR in this patient group is the assessment of post-operative complications. The most common long-term complication is homograft failure, usually mixed stenosis and regurgitation leading to RV dysfunction. This is secondary to vavular degeneration and the patient 'out-growing' the non-viable homograft. Current management consists of either homograft replacement or some form of valved stent placement and is dependent on the amount of stenosis and regurgitation, and the dynamic morphology of the homograft (Nordmeyer et al. 2006). As with ToF, PC-MRI is useful in quantifying regurgitation, particularly as Doppler echocardiography of conduits is often technically difficult. PC-MRI can be used to measure peak velocities at the level of the conduit obstruction. Pressure gradients calculated from MR peak velocities compare well with catheter pressure gradients and give some indication of the functional significance of any stenosis (Holmqvist et al. 2001). Such functional data (including ventricular volumetry) is useful in deciding the timing of any invasive procedure. The type of repair undertaken is very dependent on the anatomy of the homograft. Due to the high velocity of blood through most stenosed conduits spin-echo 'black-blood' sequences can be useful for measurement of conduit obstruction, as they are less susceptible to flow artefacts. However, conduit stenosis is often secondary to calcification of the non-viable homograft, and calcified tissue is difficult to visualise using spin-echo 'black blood' imaging.

ceMRA is also useful in assessment of homograft, with the, often complex 3D anatomy of the conduit better appreciated with ceMRAs. One limitation of both these techniques is the inability to assess the dynamic anatomy of the conduit. 2D balanced-SSFP techniques are very useful in assessing the change in conduit architecture during the cardiac cycle, changes which may have a significant effect on the success of interventional procedures. Other long-term complications are similar to those found in patients with ToF and are discussed in the previous section and "Valvular Heart Disease" Sect. 3.6.1.

7.3 Pulmonary Atresia with Intact Ventricular Septum

Pulmonary atresia with intact ventricular septum is the less common variant of pulmonary atresia, and is associated with a variable degree of RV hypoplasia. The type of surgical repair depends on the size and shape of the RV cavity (Shimpo et al. 2000). The presence of an RV infundibulum usually allows a biventricular repair (Sano et al. 2000). Thus, pre-operative assessment of the RV cavity is vital. Spin-echo sequences, balanced-SSFP sequences and ceMRA can all be used to assess the RV cavity. However, no formal trials have yet been done to assess the role of MR in the decision support and the pre-operative management of patients with this lesion.

If biventricular repair has been completed, MR is valuable in assessing postoperative complications. The scanning protocol and plan is similar to that described for tetralogy of Fallot, or PAVSD, with additional specific assessment for the presence of decreased RV compliance, or restrictive RV physiology. This can be demonstrated using through-plane PC-MRI sequences, to assess the tricuspid valve inflow curve profile and the pulmonary valve forward flow profile. The presence of forward flow in the pulmonary artery with atrial contraction, during late diastole, defines poor RV compliance (Fig. 24).

7.4 Transposition of the Great Arteries

Transposition of the great arteries (TGA) is the second commonest cyanotic congenital heart disease in the first year of life with an incidence of 315 per million live births (Hoffman and Kaplan 2002). It is defined as ventriculo-arterial discordance with an anterior aorta arising from the RV, and the pulmonary artery arising from the LV (Fig. 25). Associated with this, 40% of patients with TGA have a VSD and 30% of these patients have sub-pulmonary stenosis (Park et al. 1978). Surgical therapy for this condition was revolutionised in 1958 with the introduction of the Senning procedure in which an intra-atrial baffle was used to divert blood from the right atrium to the left ventricle, and the left atrium to the right ventricle (Senning 1975). A further variation was the Mustard procedure in which a pericardial patch was used to construct the intra-atrial baffle (Mustard 1968). Both procedures produced a physiologically normal but anatomically abnormal circulation (systemic venous return to the left atrium, LV and then pulmonary artery; pulmonary venous return to the right atrium, RV and then aorta).

In 1975, Jatene performed the first arterial switch operation. This had the benefit of producing both a physiological and more anatomically normal circulation (Jatene et al. 1976). For this reason, the arterial switch operation has become the procedure of choice for TGA. In cases of TGA associated with a VSD and sub-pulmonary stenosis the Rastelli procedure is preferred (Rastelli et al. 1969). Transthoracic echocardiography is the imaging modality of choice for neonatal, preoperative diagnosis and assessment. The role of MR is mainly in diagnosis of post-operative complications, particularly those that may progress as the child grows older, and those that become more symptomatic in adulthood.

7.4.1 Arterial Switch Operation

The majority of late complications of the arterial switch operation are related to RV outflow tract or branch pulmonary artery obstruction. The RV outflow tract obstruction is thought to be due to poor growth

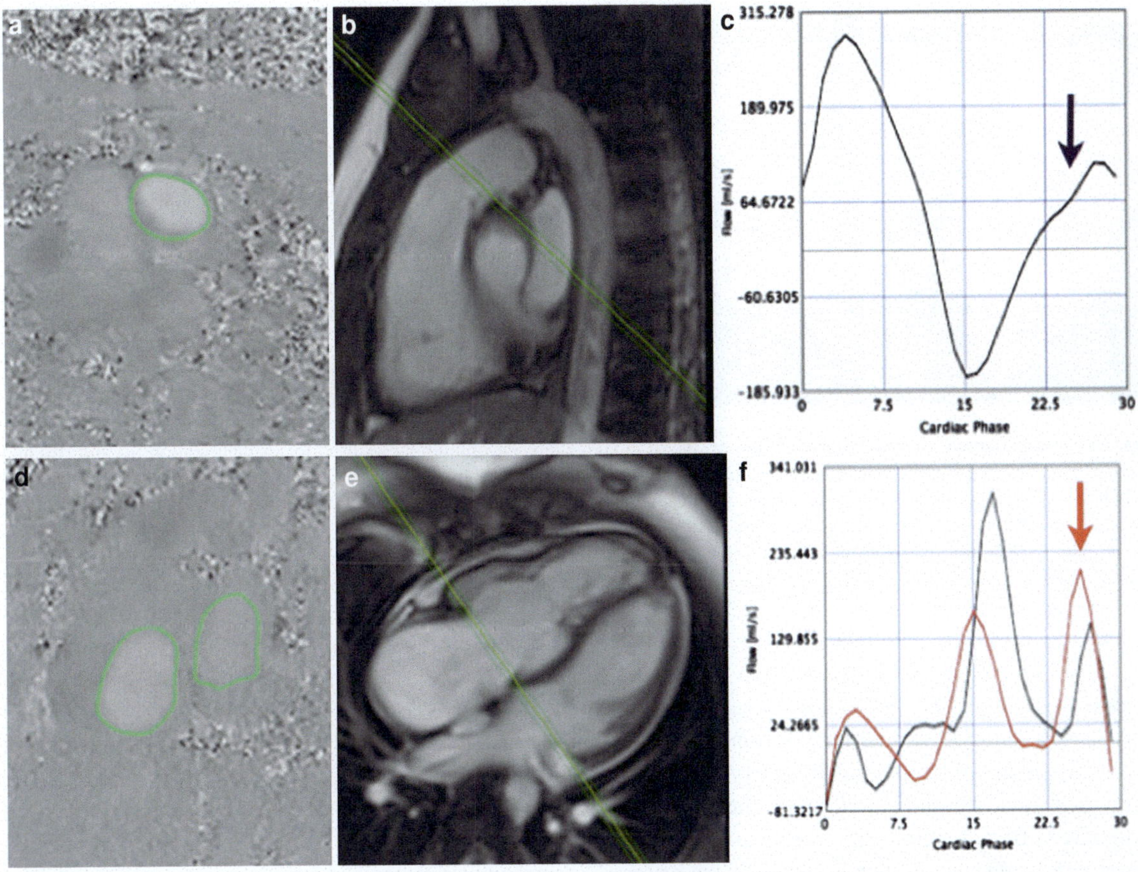

Fig. 24 These images are from an adult patient who has undergone pulmonary valve replacement with an RV-pulmonary trunk homograft, to repair pulmonary atresia/intact ventricular septum. The panels demonstrate the regions of interest on a phase-contrast flow velocity map (**a, d**), the image planes (**b, e**), and the flow volume map generated (**c, f**). The *upper row* illustrates forward flow at end diastole in the pulmonary artery, and the *lower row* illustrates a reversed E/A ratio on tricuspid valve inflow mapping (*red lines and arrow*)

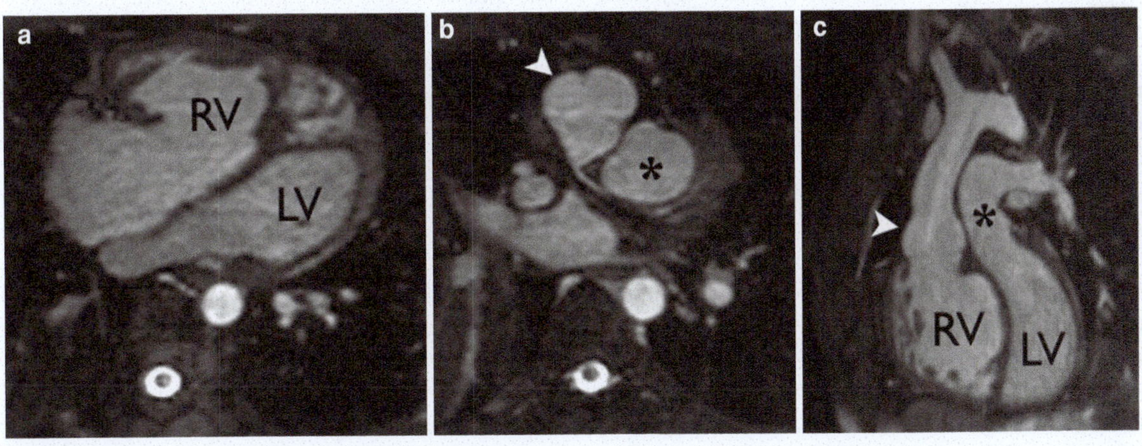

Fig. 25 **a** and **b** Axial balanced-SSFP images of transposition of the great arteries, taken from a 3D whole-heart acquisition. **c** Oblique sagittal balanced-SSFP image through the outflow tracts. Aorta (*arrowhead*) arises anteriorly from the hypertrophied right ventricle (*RV*). The central pulmonary artery (*asterisk*) arises from the left ventricle (*LV*)

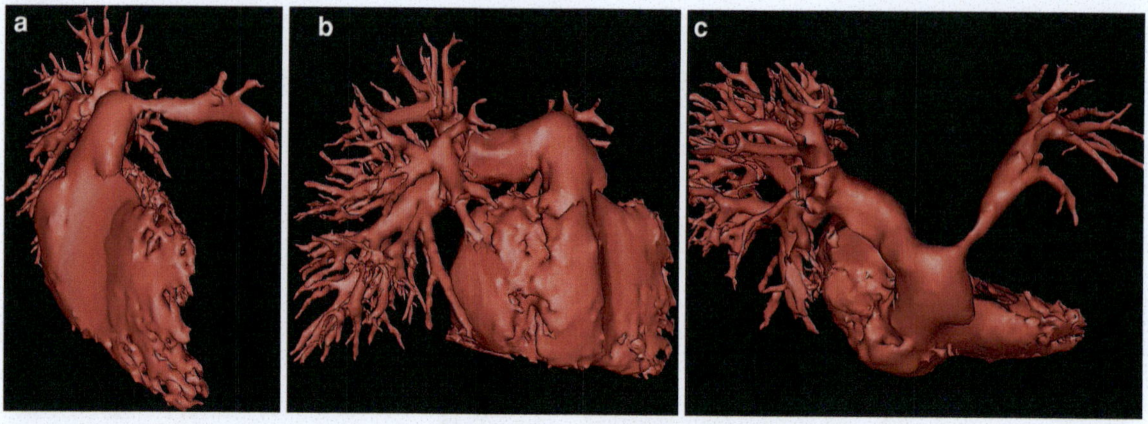

Fig. 26 Volume rendered 3D reconstruction of the RVOT, derived from first-pass ceMRA data, from a patient with arterial switch repair of transposition of the great arteries. These illustrate significant narrowing of the proximal left pulmonary artery. The models are visualized in the alignment of common anterior-oblique views used for catheterization (**a**) and (**b**), and illustrate how this narrowing could be masked on 2D catheter angiographic images. Only with the superior view (**c**) is the morphology clearly seen

of the reconstructed pulmonary artery and may be associated with fibrous tissue formation at the suture lines (Haas et al. 1999). RV outflow tract obstruction may also be due to the anterior position of the tract, and compression of the pulmonary artery between the aorta and the sternum, following the LeCompte manoeuvre. Branch pulmonary artery stenosis is often secondary to stretch and compression of the arteries, related to the posterior aorta. Because of the retrosternal position of the RV outflow tract, transthoracic echocardiography is poor at detecting these lesions. Furthermore, because the narrowing of the branch pulmonary arteries is predominantly in the antero-posterior plane, X-ray angiography lateral and anterior views may not sensitively depict such findings.

Cardiovascular MR is not constrained by the intrathoracic position of vessels and is ideal for imaging the RV outflow tract and branch pulmonary arteries in this group of patients.

CeMRA is used to visualize the 3D anatomy. If acquisition of the sequence is triggered during first-pass through the pulmonary arteries, the enhanced signal in the branch PAs can be used for volume rendering and 3D visualization of any narrowing (Figs. 26 and 27). As previously mentioned, care must be taken with interpretation, as signal loss due to turbulent or high velocity flow can exaggerate the appearance of stenosis on angiographic or cine images. In this situation, spin-echo sequences in carefully positioned longitudinal or cross-sectional planes through the vessel can be used to more accurately assess the degree of stenosis. PC-MRI can be used to measures peak velocities at the level of the obstruction, and calculate pressure gradients. It has been shown that there is greater agreement between MR-derived pressure gradients and invasive pressure measurements than between Doppler ultrasound pressure gradients and invasive measures (Gutberlet et al. 2000). Using such structural and functional information, improved management decisions can be made without resorting to invasive diagnostic procedures.

RV outflow tract narrowing may be associated with regurgitation of the neo-pulmonary valve, or RV dysfunction. As stated in previous sections of this chapter and elsewhere in the text, a combination of balanced-SSFP cine imaging and phase-contrast flow measurements can accurately quantify these parameters.

Less common, but equally important long-term complications of the arterial switch operation involve the LV outflow tract. Regurgitation of the neo-aortic valve, dilatation of the neoaortic root, and narrowing of the ascending aorta can be accurately depicted and quantified using 3D MR angiography, balanced-SSFP cine imaging and phase-contrast flow measurements.

A further complication of the arterial switch operation is coronary stenosis following the reimplantation of the coronary buttons into the neo-aortic root. Although the majority of coronary complications are manifest in the early post-operative period, a

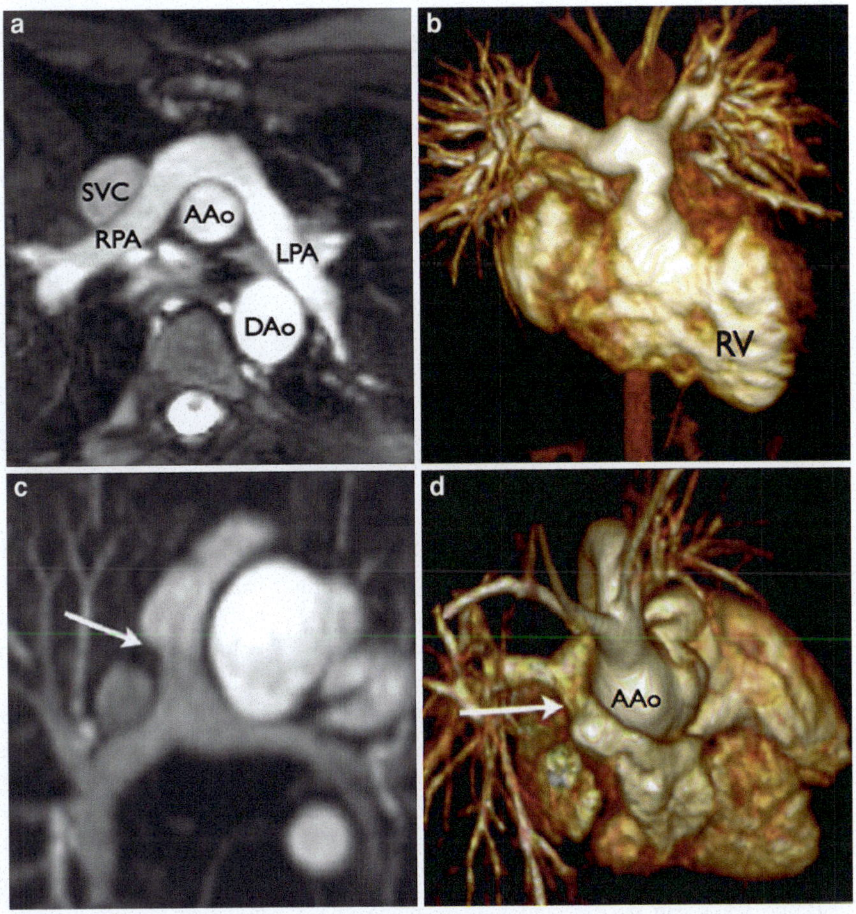

Fig. 27 Transposition of the great arteries—Arterial switch operation, (**a**) Axial reformat from ceMRA. **b** 3D, ceMRA. Both (**a, b**) show Lecompte maneuver with the pulmonary artery anterior to the ascending aorta (*AAo*) with the *right* (*RPA*) and left pulmonary arteries passing either side of the aorta, note descending aorta (*DAo*). **c** Axial reformat from ceMRA. **d** 3D, ceMRA, showing alternative arterial switch operation, with the main pulmonary artery (*arrow*) seen to pass on the right side, between the superior vena cava (*SVC*), and aorta

subset of patients suffer from late coronary events (Legendre et al. 2003). MRCA (either selective or whole heart) is a useful non-invasive method for investigating coronary arteries (Taylor et al. 2005). This is particularly true of the proximal segments, which are usually well visualized (Fig. 28). More recently adenosine stress perfusion techniques have been applied in this population (Manso et al. 2010) and CT to assess the proximal coronary course (Ou et al. 2008). However, in this group of patients, X-ray coronary angiography currently represents the most sensitive modality for investigation of coronary compromise.

7.4.2 Atrial Switch Operation

Although intra-atrial repair has been superseded by the arterial switch operation there is a sizeable population of young adults who have undergone either a Senning or Mustard operation (Fig. 29). The most common complications of intra-atrial repair are baffle obstruction or leak, arrhythmias, and RV dysfunction. Baffle obstruction is more common in the Mustard operation (Sarkar et al. 1999) probably due to calcification and poor growth of the pericardial tissue used to construct the baffle. The venous pathways have a complex 3D structure and are difficult to accurately assess with trans-thoracic echocardiography. It has been shown that ceMRA can fully demonstrate the 3D anatomy of the Senning/Mustard anatomy and detect any luminal narrowing (Fogel et al. 2002). Unfortunately, this is a flow sensitive, non-gated sequence images and is susceptible to signal dropout. Spin-echo sequences and 3D balanced-SSFP are useful in accurately measuring the static baffle obstruction, while 2D balanced-SSFP sequences are able to accurately delineate the dynamic anatomy of intra-atrial baffles (Fig. 29) and qualitatively assess flow.

In the presence of obstruction of either the superior venocaval or inferior veno-caval limb of the intra-atrial baffles, correlative information can be obtained

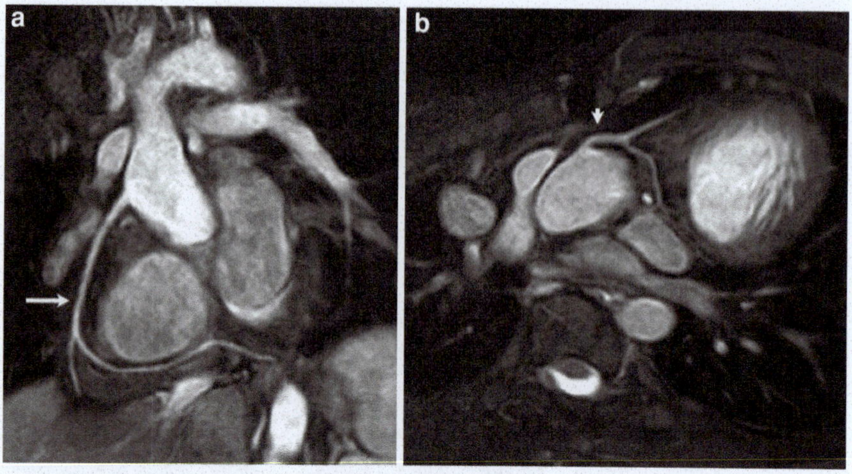

Fig. 28 **a, b** Normal MR coronary angiogram in a patient with arterial switch operation for transposition of the great arteries: (**a**) oblique sagittal view of right coronary artery (*arrow*), (**b**) oblique axial view of the left coronary artery system, left main (*arrowhead*)

from the angiographic or 3D balanced SSFP images regarding the presence of venous collateral formation. Enlargement of the azygous vein or prominent paravertebral venous channels may indicate diversion of systemic venous flow away from a narrowed baffle.

PC-MRI sequences can be used; in-plane to visualize flow turbulence at the site of baffle narrowing, or through-plane to confirm loss of the typical, phasic, venous flow profile. Velocity-encoding should be appropriately low in order to be sensitive for venous flow velocities.

Baffle leaks can be detected with in-plane phase contrast flow velocity mapping, by recording flow volumes in the aorta and pulmonary artery. The pulmonary artery flow profile is often turbulent, because of the acute angulation of the MPA. Thus, more accurate flow volumes may be obtained by measuring the branch pulmonary artery flow volumes and SVC and IVC flow volumes. A combination of all these MR techniques allows comprehensive assessment of intra-atrial baffles.

The aetiology of RV dysfunction in patients with intra-atrial baffles is complex. Deranged AV valve coupling may be important (Tulevski et al. 2002a) and repair of baffle obstruction or regurgitant AV valves can improve RV systolic performance. However, in a significant group, RV dysfunction is present without abnormal AV valve coupling. This may in part be due to the atrial baffle function, and failure to augment RV filling rates during exercise or pharmacological stress, despite appropriate responses in load-independent indices of RV contraction and relaxation (Derrick et al. 2001). RV systolic function has been assessed in patients with intra-atrial repair of TGA using multi-slice balanced-SSFP sequences and it has been shown that RV ejection fraction and end systolic volume are lower than in matched controls (Tulevski et al. 2002a).

Some studies have sought areas of focal myocardial fibrosis using late gadolinium enhancement techniques in adults late after atrial baffle repair of TGA (Giardini et al. 2006; Babu-Narayan et al. 2005; Ladouceur et al. 2009) These studies found a minority of patients with significant focal myocardial fibrosis, however the presence of fibrosis was associated with RV systolic dysfunction, poor exercise tolerance, arrhythmia and progressive clinical deterioration. Further studies characterizing diffuse RV myocardial fibrosis may lead to more knowledge in this area (Broberg et al. 2010).

7.4.3 Congenitally Corrected Transposition

Congenitally corrected transposition (CCTGA) is a rare disorder characterised by atrioventricular and ventricle-arterial discordance (right atrium to left ventricle to pulmonary artery and left atrium to right ventricle to aorta). Thus, although the heart is anatomically abnormal it is physiologically normal in terms of the pulmonary and systemic circuits. This disease is not cyanotic; however, many of the problems are similar to those experienced by patients with simple TGA. Congenitally corrected transposition may be asymptomatic and in some patients is an incidental finding. However, the majority of patients with CCTGA have associated cardiac lesions. The most common associated lesions is a ventricular

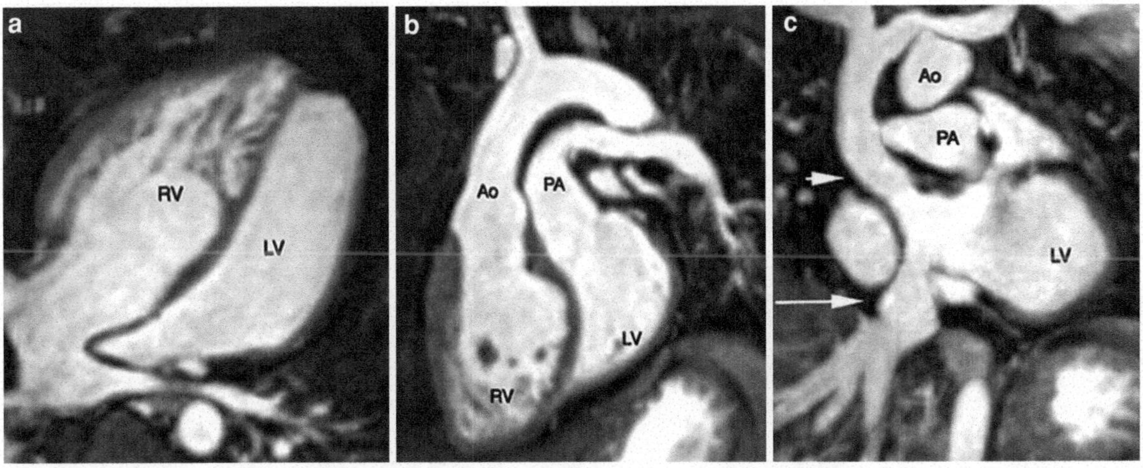

Fig. 29 These are images from a typical adult patient late after the Senning procedure for simple TGA. The images are created from multiplanar reformatting of data acquired using an isotropic 3D b-SSFP sequence. These images are thin maximal intensity projections in three planes: (**a**) through the ventricles, in a 4-chamber view, and showing the pulmonary venous connection to the RV. **b** Through the ventricles in the outflow tract view, showing the aorta arising from the morphological RV and the pulmonary artery arising from the LV. **c** Through the superior and inferior caval baffles (**short* and *long white arrows*, respectively). Ao = aorta, PA = pulmonary artery, RV = morphological right ventricle, LV = morphological left ventricle

septal defect, though pulmonary stenosis is present in approximately 50% of cases, and tricuspid valve abnormalities (i.e. Ebstein abnormality) are found in 20% of cases (Bjarke and Kidd 1976; Fig. 30). Even without associated abnormalities, the majority of patients with CCTGA develop systemic ventricular failure over time.

The main role of MR is in evaluation of associated lesions, quantification of ventricular function and assessment of post-operative complications. The assessment of VSDs and pulmonary stenosis has been dealt with previously in this chapter. Valve abnormalities are be dealt with in the chapter on valvar heart disease ("Valvular Heart Disease"). RV function has been assessed in patients with CCTGA multi-slice SSFP sequences ((Tulevski et al. 2002b) and it has been shown that RV ejection fraction, end systolic volume and response to dobutamine stress are lower than in matched controls (Tulevski et al. 2002b). Late failure of the systemic right ventricle has lead to the increasing use of anatomic repair in CCTGA. This involves either an atrial and arterial switch (Langley et al. 2003) or in the case of CCTGA with an associated VSD, a Rastelli procedure with an atrial switch (Brawn and Barron 2003). The complications of these operative procedures and the role of MR in investigating them have been described in the previous section.

Another management pathway for patients with this cardiac lesion and without pulmonary stenosis, involves forced remodelling of the left ventricle using pulmonary arterial banding, in preparation for a combined atrial and arterial switch procedure. This results in the LV sustaining the systemic circulation (Barron et al. 2011). There is a potential role for MR in assessing the adequacy and performance of the LV related to this procedure, but methods have yet to be validated.

7.5 Double Outlet Right Ventricle

In double outlet right ventricle both great vessels emerge from the right ventricle, with egress from the left ventricle via a VSD. The clinical picture and type of surgical correction depends on the arrangement of the great vessels and the anatomy of the VSD. The most common variant is normal arrangement of the great vessels and a sub-aortic VSD. This variant is often referred to as the Fallot's type, as it is often associated with pulmonary stenosis and has a similar presentation. Double outlet right ventricle can also be associated with an anterior aorta and a sub-pulmonary VSD, known as the Taussig-Bing anomaly. This presents in a similar manner to TGA with VSD. Less

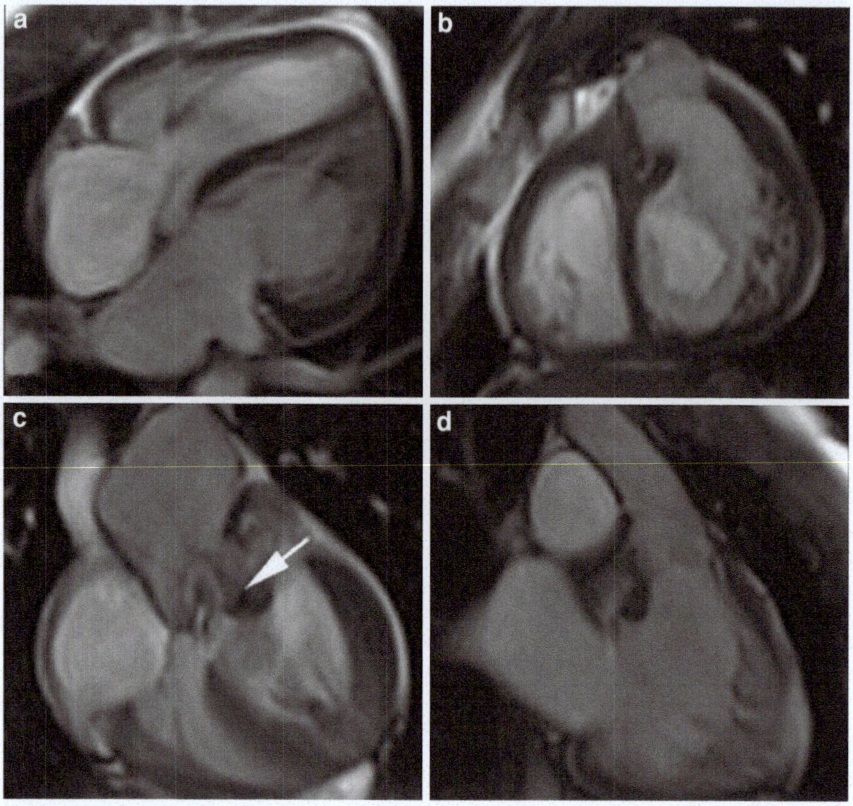

Fig. 30 Balanced-SSFP images from a patient with congenitally corrected transposition (CCTGA), a VSD and subpulmonary stenosis (*white arrow*). **a** Four-chamber view with the subpulmonary LV anterior and the subaortic RV posterior, (**b**) basal short axis view, with the aortic root arising from the posterior, morphologic RV, (**c**) pulmonary outflow tract view, (**d**) systemic outflow tract view

common, are the variants with doubly committed or non-committed VSDs. These patients present with cardiac failure, and some degree of cyanosis. Surgical correction for the Fallot-type variant consists of patch closure of the VSD, which redirects blood to the aorta, and correction of any pulmonary stenosis. For the Taussig-Bing anomaly, the surgical management depends on the presence of pulmonary obstruction. In the absence of pulmonary obstruction, correction consists of patch closure of the VSD and arterial switch (Masuda et al. 1999). In the presence of obstruction, LV flow is tunnelled through the VSD to the aorta, and an RV-PA pathway is established (Wu et al. 2003).

The role of MR in the assessment of post-operative complications of the Fallot-type repair, the arterial switch and the Rastelli procedure have been discussed in the previous sections. However, MR can also play an important role in preoperative assessment in this group of patients. The anatomy of the VSD and the arrangement of the great vessels are particularly important when deciding the type of surgery. Spin echo black blood imaging of the VSD has been shown to compare well with surgical findings and is able to predict the type of repair finally done (Beekmana et al. 2000). 3D balanced-SSFP and 2D balanced-SSFP cine techniques are also useful as they give both anatomical and functional information (Kilner et al. 2002).

7.6 Common Arterial Trunk

Common arterial trunk (truncus arteriosis) is defined as a single arterial trunk that overrides a large misaligned VSD, and therefore arises from both ventricles. The pulmonary, systemic and coronary vessels all originate from this single common arterial trunk, and the classification of common arterial trunk relies on the branching pattern of the pulmonary artery (Fig. 31).

The truncal valve is often abnormal with varying degrees of stenosis and insufficiency. Optimally, the initial surgical repair is performed during infancy, and consists of reconstruction of the trunk to produce a systemic vessel from the LV, patch closure of the VSD and establishment of an RV to pulmonary artery conduit. This conduit is necessarily of low calibre in the infant, and requires intervention or surgical

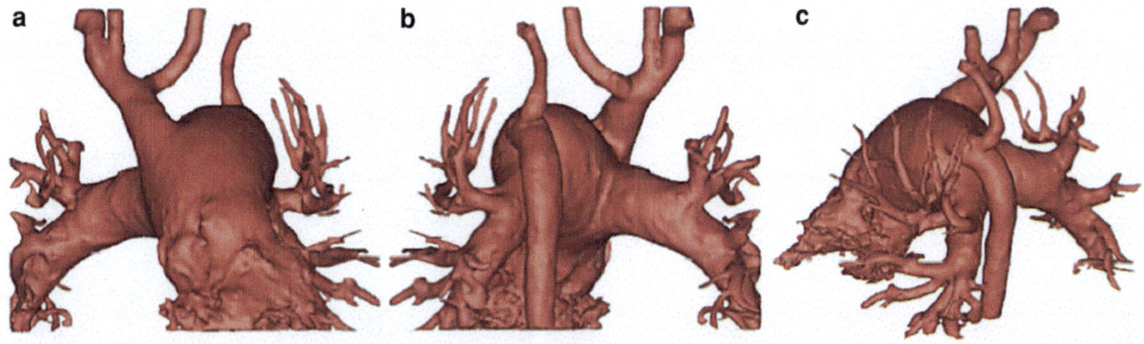

Fig. 31 Volume rendered contrast images of a patient with common arterial trunk, confluence of the pulmonary arteries, and a Type B interruption of the aortic arch (**a**) anterior (**b**) posterior and (**c**) posterior oblique views

replacement as the child grows. The main value of MR lies in assessment of post-operative complications; predominantly those related to the RV outflow tract and the reimplanted branch pulmonary arteries.

The main complications of common arterial trunk repair are RV-PA conduit stenosis or regurgitation, truncal valve insufficiency and VSD patch leak. The role of MR in the assessment of these problems is discussed in other sections of this chapter.

8 The Functionally Single Ventricle

8.1 The Borderline Left or Right Ventricle

Increasing clinical use of cardiac MRI for the assessment of ventricular volumes has led to it being used to help decide the appropriate management of borderline-sized ventricles in infants- suitability for biventricular repair versus functionally single ventricle palliation (Grosse-Wortmann et al. 2008). Because of the difficulty in obtaining high resolution MR reference data from normal neonates and the lack of information about long-term outcome, evidence for the utility of MRI in this context is currently scant, but this is an active area of research.

8.2 Hypoplastic Left Heart Syndrome

Hypoplastic left heart syndrome is specifically discussed in this section, but can also be considered as a prototype example for MR imaging of the infant with a functional single ventricle (Fig. 32). Infants with a functionally single ventricle include those with severe hypoplasia of either the left or the right ventricle, and those in whom straddling atrioventricular valve attachments preclude a biventricular repair.

Hypoplastic left heart syndrome (HLHS) is the fourth commonest cardiac malformation to present in the first year of life, with an incidence of approximately of 266 per million live births (Hoffman and Kaplan 2002). HLHS constitutes a spectrum of congenital heart disease with hypoplasia or atresia of the left heart components, and normal relation of the great vessels. At birth, the right ventricle supplies both the systemic and pulmonary circulations via a patent ductus arteriosus (PDA). After birth, closure of the PDA and the presence of a restrictive patent foramen ovale, lead to increasing cyanosis and heart failure. Surgical treatment has been revolutionized by the introduction of the Norwood procedure in 1980 (Norwood et al. 1980) with subsequent conversion to a total cavo-pulmonary connection (TCPC).

The Norwood procedure, is usually performed during the first week of life, and involves exision of the atrial septum (to enable non-restricted pulmonary venous return to the right atrium via the left atrium) and reconstruction of the aortic arch. Arch reconstruction includes anastomosis of the main pulmonary artery to the hypoplastic aorta. The caliber of the arch is usually augmented with a patch of homograft tissue. Pulmonary blood supply is maintained by a modified Blalock–Taussig (BT) shunt from the innominate artery to the proximal right pulmonary artery (Fig. 33) or by a non-valved, low caliber RV-PA conduit (Sano et al. 2004) (Fig. 34). The advantage of an RV-PA conduit is thought to involve reduced diastolic run off and improved coronary perfusion (Pizarro et al. 2003).

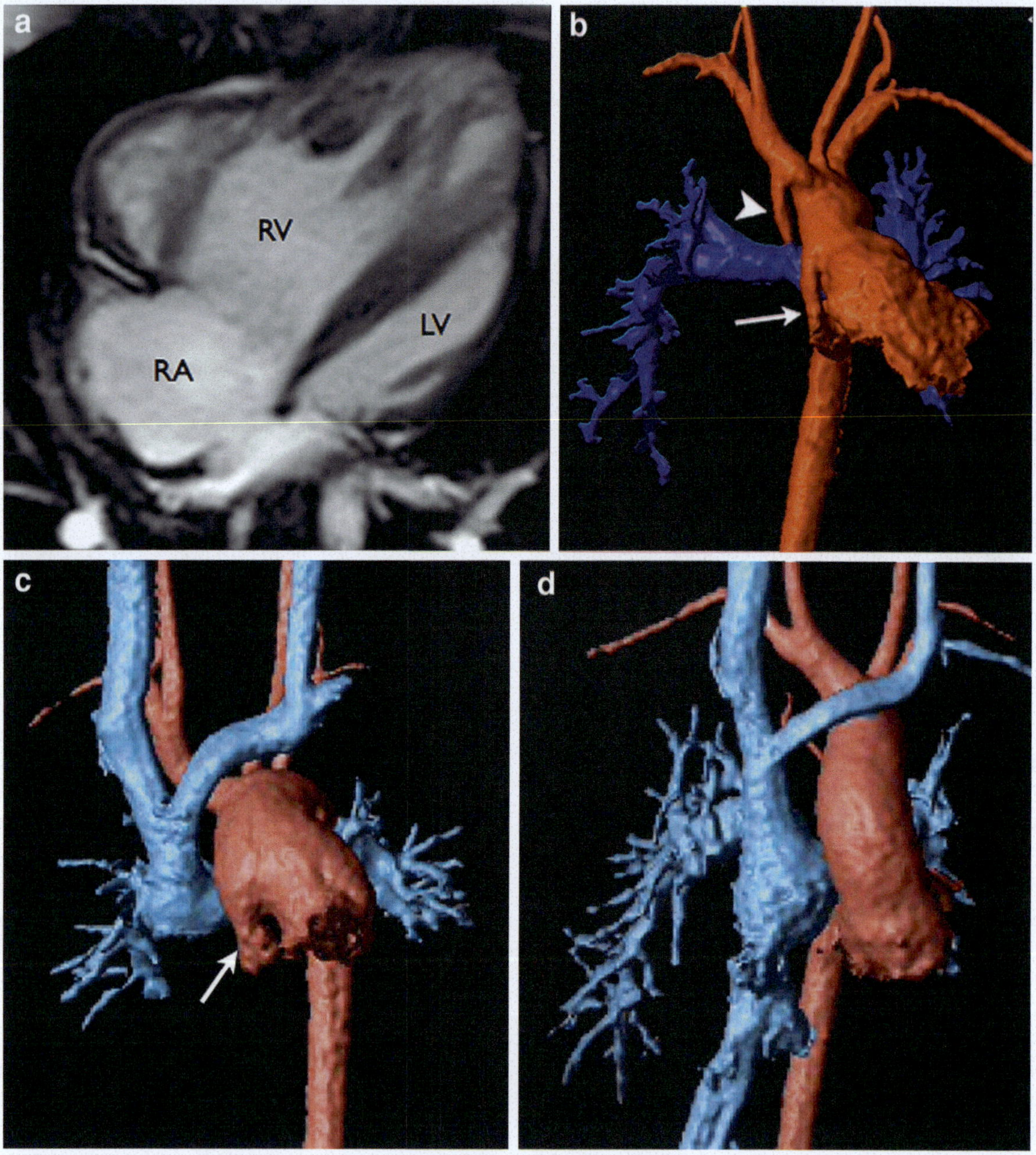

Fig. 32 Hypoplastic left heart syndrome. **a** End-diastolic, balanced SSFP, 4-chamber view showing hypoplastic left ventricle (*LV*). Pulmonary venous return passes from left atrium to the right atrium, via a large atrial septostomy. **b** 3D, ceMRA angiogram after Stage 1, Norward operation, with a modified BT shunt (*arrowhead*) supplying the pulmonary arteries. Note the hypoplastic native ascending aorta (*arrow*). **c** 3D, ceMRA after Stage 2 bi-directional cavo-pulmonary connection operation. This connects the SVC to the branch pulmonary arteries (*pale blue*). Again arrow shows hypoplastic native ascending aorta. **d** 3D, ceMRA after Stage 3, total cavo-pulmonary connection operation. This further connects the IVC into the pulmonary circulation (*pale blue*)

There is improved post-operative stability of infants following a "Sano"-type repair, and a recent prospective, randomized controlled trial of the two procedures showed improved survival and freedom from transplant at 12 months in infants with an RV-PA conduit. However, beyond 12 months there was no difference in transplantation-free survival between the two groups (Ohye et al. 2010).

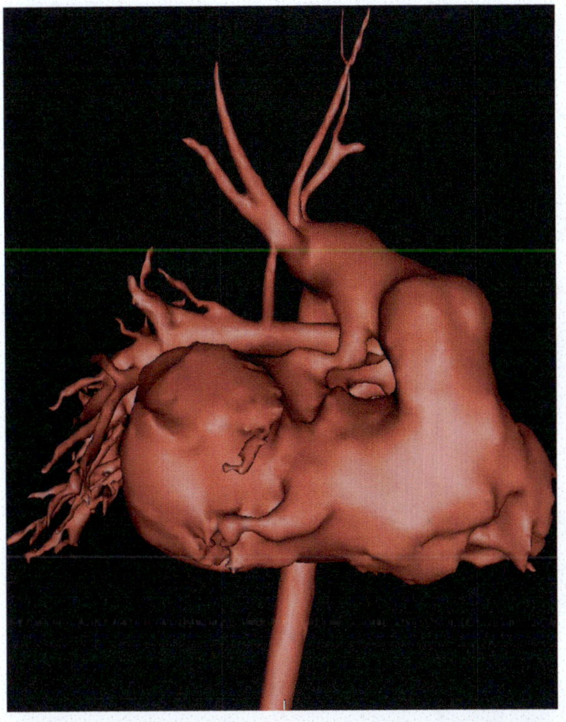

Fig. 33 Volume rendered 3D reconstruction of a ceMRA from a patient with hypoplastic left heart syndrome, following the Norwood I procedure, using a BT shunt. This is viewed from right-anterior, and demonstrates the proximal arch reconstruction, Damus-Kaye–Stansel anastomosis, and arterio-pulmonary shunt from the innominate artery to the right pulmonary artery

The second stage of surgery, involving take-down of the systemic-pulmonary shunt and formation of a bidirectional cavo-pulmonary connection (BCPC) or "Glenn" shunt, is usually scheduled between 3 and 5 months of age, once there has been a natural decrease in pulmonary vascular resistance after the neonatal period. Subsequent to this, the third stage of surgery, conversion to a total cavopulmonary circulation (TCPC), is usually carried out between the ages of 18 months to 5 years.

8.3 Evaluating the Circulation Prior to Bidirectional Cavo-Pulmonary Connection (BCPC): "Glenn" Shunt or "hemi-Fontan" Procedure

Following the first stage Norwood procedure (or any other first-stage palliative surgery for patients with a functionally single ventricle) and prior to the next surgical stage, investigation is required to identify surgical complications that may require additional repair at the time of the BCPC procedure. Traditionally, this investigation consisted of invasive cardiac catheterization, but MRI is increasingly being utilized for this purpose (Muthurangu et al. 2005; Brown et al. 2007).

Following the Norwood stage I procedure, neo-aortic arch obstruction is a recognized problem (Chessa et al. 2000) and is a significant cause of morbidity and mortality. Preoperative recognition of neo-aortic obstruction is vital, to enable aortic reconstruction at the time of conversion to BCPC. Other common complications include narrowing of the systemic—pulmonary shunt, branch pulmonary artery stenosis and tricuspid valve regurgitation.

CeMRA can give excellent 3D images of any obstruction, although carefully planned 2D spin echo images give a more accurate measurement of stenosis (Muthurangu et al. 2005) (Fig. 34). CeMRA is the modality of choice for portraying the often-complex arch configurations in 3-dimensions (Figs. 35, 36).

Balanced-SSFP cine imaging can help to identify the region of narrowing and to visualize the cyclic changes in dimension of the aortic arch and pulmonary arteries. Image planes for 2D cine imaging can be planned using multiplanar reformatted images created using 3D angiographic data (Fig. 37). PC-MRI can also be used to quantify the pressure gradient across any arterial obstruction. The use of MR to detect great vessel stenosis been shown to be a good alternative to invasive cardiac catheterisation in patients prior to BCPC, and the results compare well with operative findings (Muthurangu et al. 2005).

Tricuspid regurgitation is not often present in patients post Norwood procedure; however, in a small proportion, severe tricuspid regurgitation leads to RV failure, and requires surgical valve repair and annuloplasty, often at the time of the stage II or III operation. Echocardiography is the most sensitive modality with which to assess the mechanism of valvar regurgitation, however, with velocity encoded phase contrast MR and multi-slice, balanced SSFP ventricular volumetric data, the volume regurgitation and any associated RV dysfunction can be accurately quantified (Muthurangu et al. 2005). Right ventricular systolic dysfunction in patients following the Norwood procedure has been associated with poor outcome (Hughes et al. 2011).

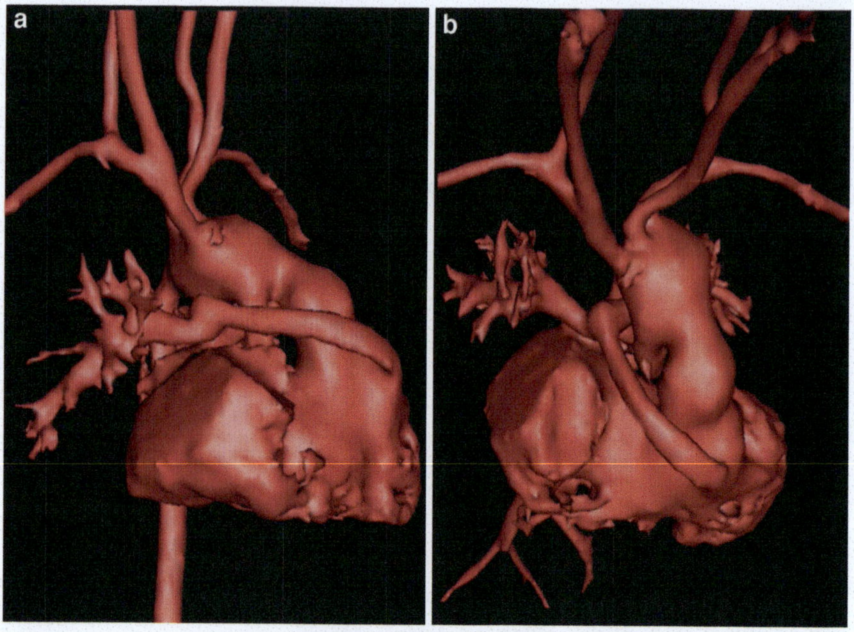

Fig. 34 Volume rendered 3D reconstruction of a ceMRA from a patient with hypoplastic left heart syndrome, following the Norwood I procedure, using an RV-PA ("Sano") conduit. This is viewed from right-anterior (**a**) and superior (**b**)

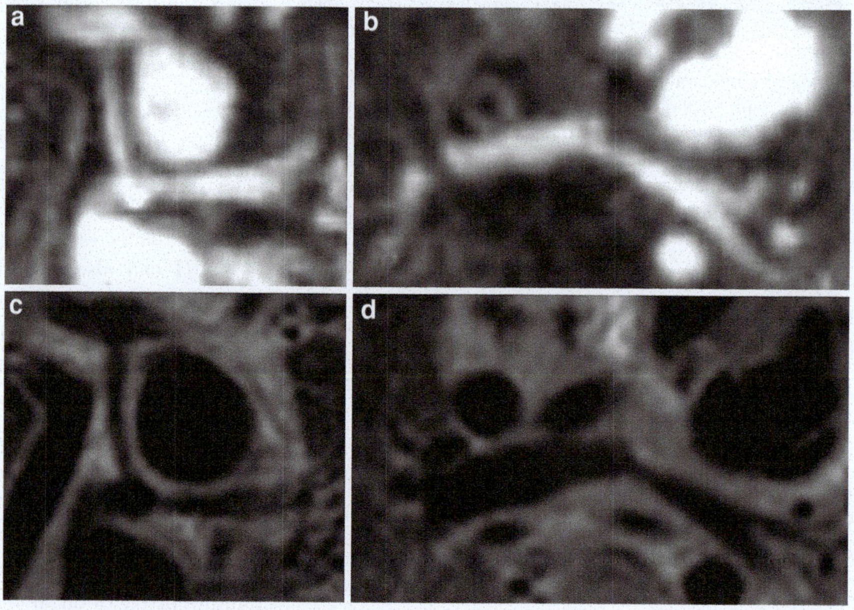

Fig. 35 Corresponding ceMRA and turbo-spin echo black blood images, in oblique coronal (**a, c**) and axial planes (**b, d**) showing the right BT-shunt and proximal pulmonary arteries in a patient with hypoplastic left heart syndrome, following the Norwood Stage I procedure

8.4 Evaluating the Cavo-Pulmonary Connection: Glenn or Hemi-Fontan Circulation

At 3–9 months of age, a stage II procedure, or bidirectional cavo-pulmonary connection (BCPC) is performed. There are two variants of this procedure: the Glenn shunt, which involves a surgical side-to-side anastomosis between the superior vena cava (SVC) and pulmonary arteries, a patch dividing the SVC from the right atrium, and the hemi-Fontan procedure, where the continuity of the SVC and right atrium is maintained when the SVC is connected to the right pulmonary artery, and a patch of homograft tissue is sewn across the superior cavoatrial junction to stop blood flow into the right atrium from the SVC. In both operations, the systemic to pulmonary artery shunt is removed.

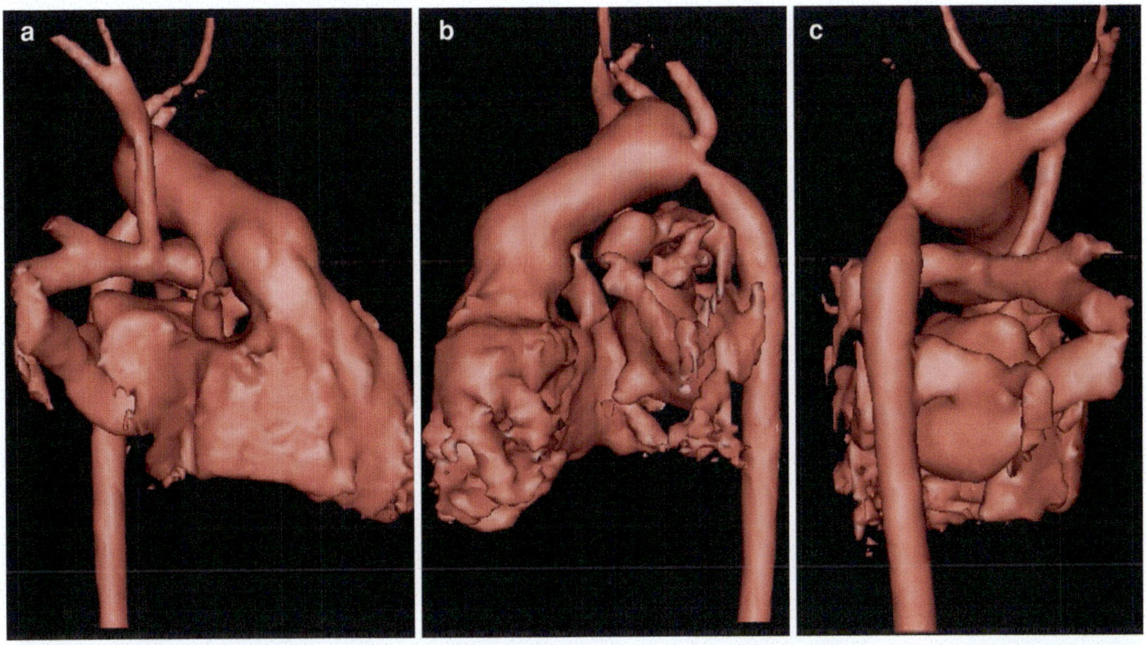

Fig. 36 3D surface-rendered image from a ceMRA, from a patient with hypoplastic left heart syndrome, following the Norwood I procedure. These images show aspects of arch reconstruction, with significant residual coarctation, unobstructed BT shunt and unobstructed branch pulmonary arteries. **a** Viewed from right anterior (**b**) viewed from left side (**c**) viewed from right posterior

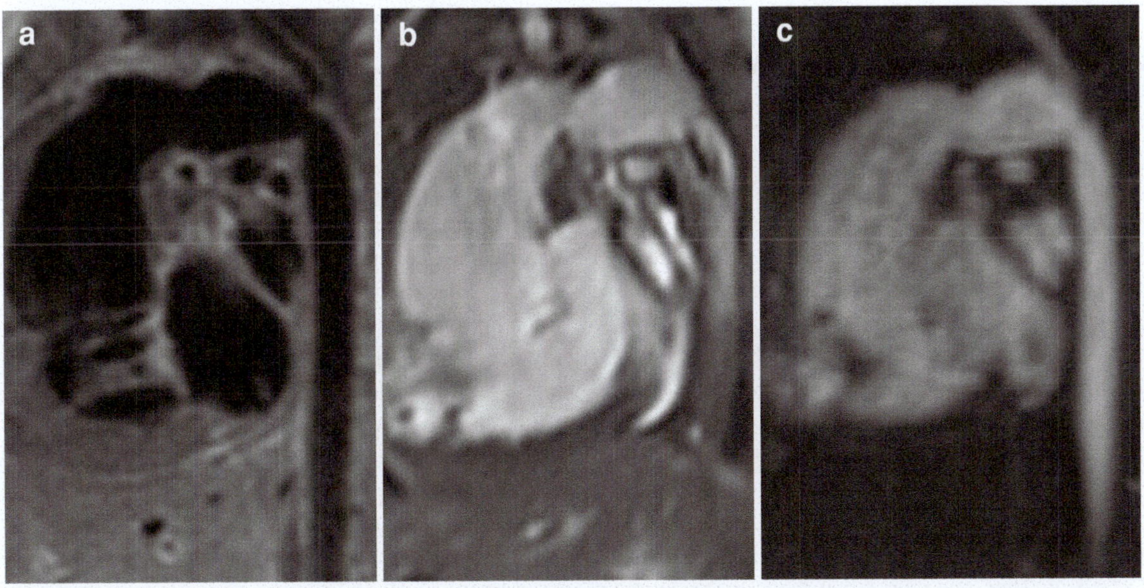

Fig. 37 Reconstructed aortic arch with residual coarctation, following Norwood I procedure for hypoplastic left heart syndrome, demonstrating the appearance with a black blood spin echo sequence (**a**), b-SSFP cine (systolic frame) (**b**), and ceMRA (**c**)

The main complication following this surgery is branch pulmonary artery narrowing; either due to compression by other vascular structures, or due to fibrosis and scarring. Visualization of the BCPC is difficult with echocardiography, and assessment with MR or invasive X-ray catheterisation is necessary.

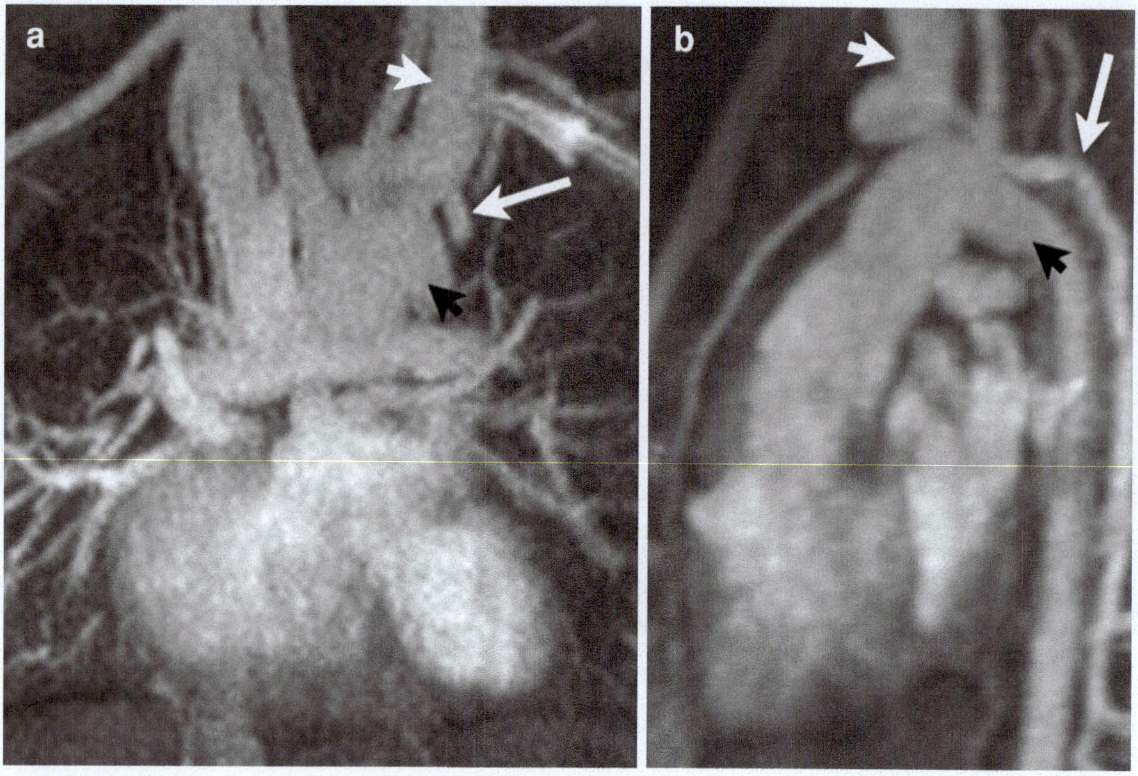

Fig. 38 Thick maximum intensity presentation of ceMRA data (**a** coronal reformat, **b** sagittal reformat), showing hemiazygous re-cannalisation, taking flow from SVC territory to IVC territory in a patient with hypoplastic left heart syndrome, following Norwood I procedure and cavopulmonary shunt. *Short white arrow* = L SVC-innominate vein junction, *long white arrow* = re-canalisation of hemiazgous vein, *black arrow* = aortic arch

In addition, before completion of the total cavo-pulmonary circulation it is important to detect any other causes for increased pulmonary vascular resistance, such as pulmonary venous obstruction or restriction of the interatrial septal defect, as these lead to failure of the total cavo-pulmonary circulation.

Contrast-enhanced MRA can give excellent 3D images of the BCPC and pulmonary venous anatomy and has been shown to compare well with X-ray angiography and operative findings (Julsrud et al. 1989). However, one must remember as the BCPC contains slow-flowing blood, and if normal concentrations of gadolinium are used, signal drop-out will occur due to the T2* effect. Thus, one must either dilute the gadolinium (10%) and administer it slowly (1 mL/sec) or image the gadolinium bolus on the second recirculation through the vasculature. For Glenn imaging 3D balanced-SSFP imaging may have some benefits over ceMRA.

One cause of excessive desaturation following BCPC can be the formation of veno-venous collateral vessels that decompress the SVC-territory circulation by diverting systemic venous flow to IVC-territory. CeMRA may enable visualization of these vessels, and planning of intervention if necessary (Fig. 38).

As well as being the gold standard for the quantification of arterial flow volumes, pulmonary venous flow volumes can be measured accurately using phase-contrast MRI. Some centres are utilizing the comprehensive imaging capability of cardiac MR to assess the presence and significance of aorto-pulmonary collateral flow after BCPC (Grosse-Wortmann et al. 2009).

Most paediatric patients undergoing MR for assessment of BCPC require general anaesthetic for the imaging. In our centre, during anaesthesia, an assessment of venous pressure is made using pressure transduction catheters, via jugular venous puncture. Depending on other risk factors for elevated pulmonary vascular resistance in each patient, this method of assessing pulmonary arterial pressure prior

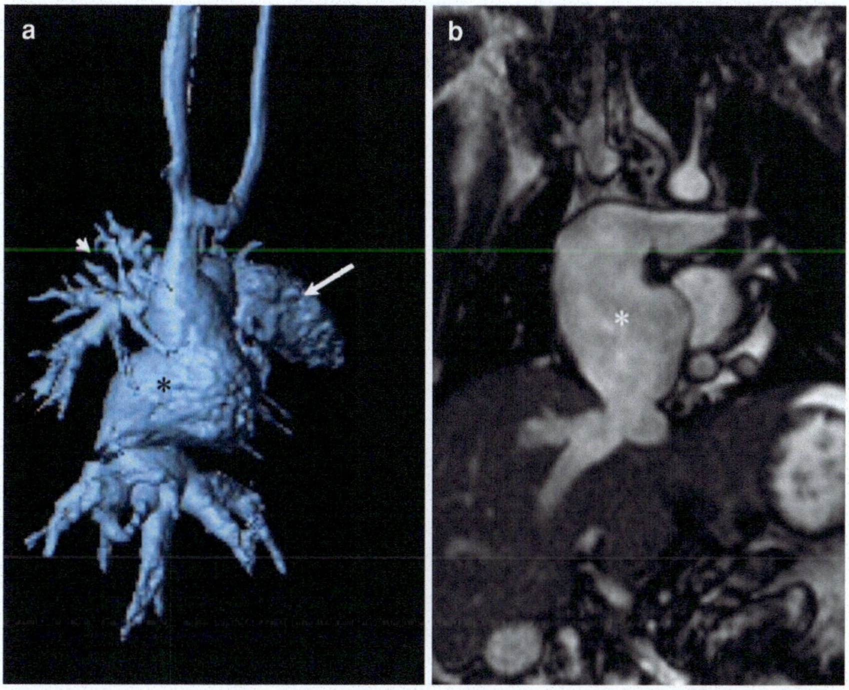

Fig. 39 **a** Volume-rendered 3D reconstruction from ceMRA of a classic Fontan circula- tion showing severe right atrial dilation (*asterisk*): right pulmonary artery (*arrowhead*), right atrial appendage (*arrow*). **b** Balanced-SSFP coronal view through the right atrium (*asterisk*)

to total cavo-pulmonary completion may decrease the need for invasive catheterization.

8.5 Evaluating the Fontan or Total Cavopulmonary Circulation

The total cavo-pulmonary connection (TCPC) of Fontan operation, usually performed in children with a functionally single ventricle, results in a complete departure from normal circulatory dynamics in that the systemic and pulmonary vascular beds are connected in series, downstream of the ventricle. This eliminates shunting at the cost of a critically elevated systemic venous pressure that maintains flow through the lungs. Early Fontan procedures, designed originally for patients with tricuspid atresia (Fontan and Baudet 1971) incorporated the right atrium between the caval veins and pulmonary arteries (Fig. 39). Although long-term results have been good, increased right atrial pressure leads to atrial dilation and predisposes to atrial tachyarrythmias.

The modified Fontan with either an extra-cardiac (Laschinger et al. 1996) or lateral tunnel (de Leval et al. 1988) between the IVC and BCPC was subsequently proposed. These procedures, termed total cavo-pulmonary connection (TCPC), have a lower complication rate than the classical Fontan and have become the procedures of choice, including for the stage III operation in HLHS. In the current era, the TCPC is usually performed between 18 months and 5 years of age.

Cardiovascular MR allows careful assessment of the cavo-pulmonary connections, branch pulmonary arteries and pulmonary veins. The pulmonary veins can be compressed by the dilated right atrium of an atrio-pulmonary connection and lead to failure of the Fontan circulation (Conte et al. 1999). 3D ceMRA has been shown to be useful in assessing pulmonary vein obstruction (Pilleul and Merchant 2000), and using either ceMRA or 3D balanced-SSFP, the 3D anatomy of the atrium can be delineated, and intra-atrial thrombus can be identified.

MR plays a valuable role in the assessment of the modified Fontan procedures (TCPC), particularly assessment of the branch pulmonary arteries and conduits (Figs. 40 and 41) (Fogel et al. 2001).

The method of contrast injection needs to be carefully considered and planned for patients with Fontan circulation. The timing and distribution of contrast arrival in the pulmonary arteries, and its dilution by nonopacified inferior caval flow, need to

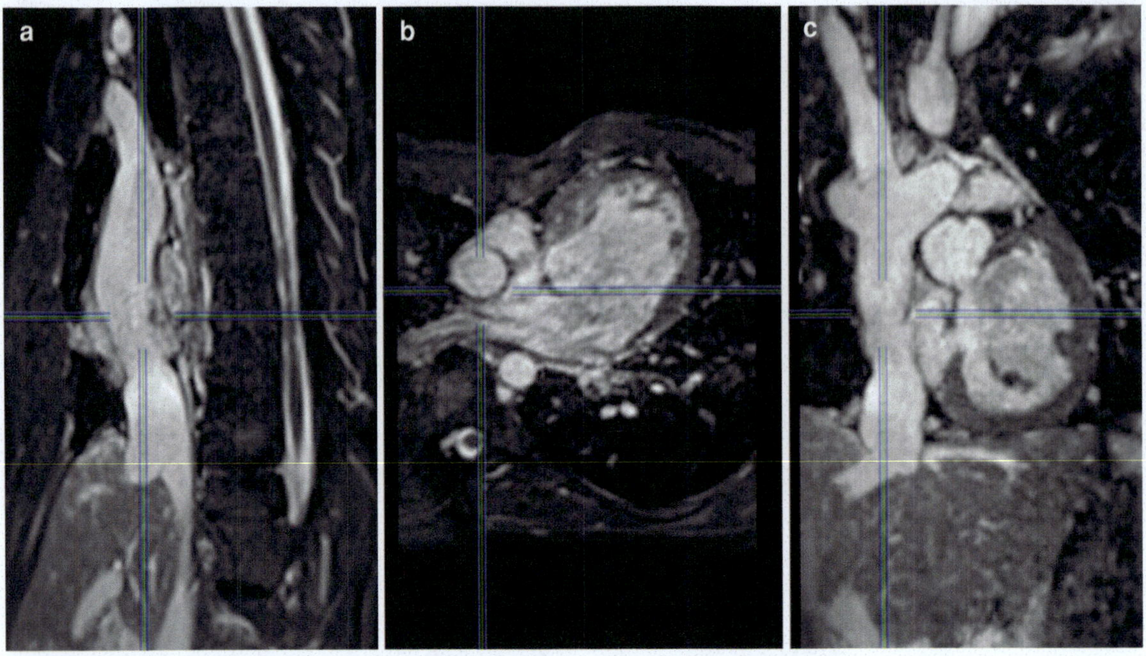

Fig. 40 3D-white blood (b-SSFP) image, viewed using 3D viewing software, (**a**) sagittal, (**b**) axial, and (**c**) coronal. These planes show the intra-atrial baffle from an adult patient with a functionally single ventricle, following surgery to complete the total cavo-pulmonary connection

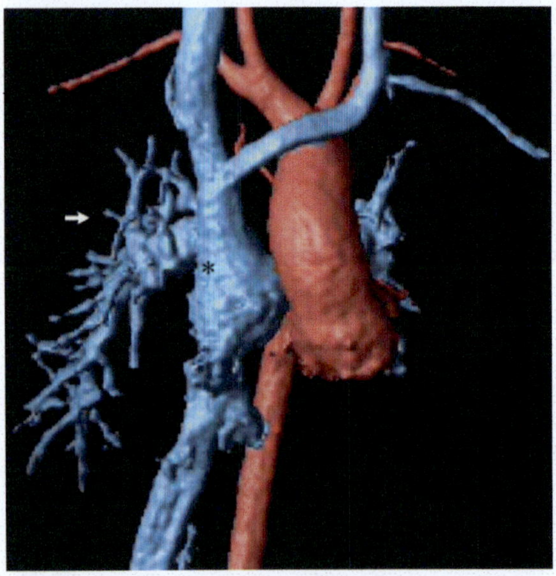

Fig. 41 Volume-rendered 3D reconstruction from ceMRA of a total caval pulmonary connection (TCPC) lateral tunnel Fontan circulation: lateral tunnel (*asterisk*), right pulmonary artery (*arrowhead*)

be factored into the injection parameters. Injection of contrast from a leg may be preferable. Non-contrast, 3D whole-heart imaging avoids some of these issues.

Although artefacts from ferromagnetic occlusion devices may impair image quality during cardiac MR in these patients, imaging can usually be optimized to minimize this artefact.

For comprehensive imaging of the ventricles, the atrioventricular valves and the ventricular outflow tract, then a contiguous stack of transaxial cine images may be most advantageous, and may augment detection of any intra-atrial thrombus or stenosis of the cavo-pulmonary connections. MR can be used to accurately assess ventricular systolic function. It has been demonstrated that ventricular function is impaired in patients with Fontan circulation (Fogel and Rychik 1998), and may ultimately require cardiac transplantation. Multi-slice balanced-SSFP imaging of the ventricle is the most accurate method of assessing global ventricular function and is invaluable in this group of patients.

PC-MRI can be used to assess flow through a suspected cavo-pulmonary narrowing where a peak jet velocity exceeding 1 m/s is likely to represent significant stenosis. Flow assessment will also demonstrate shunt flow through aorto-pulmonary collaterals (Grosse-Wortmann et al. 2009).

Evaluation of myocardial fibrosis by late gadolinium enhancement may be informative in patients with impaired ventricular function. Myocardial fibrosis identified by cardiac magnetic resonance late gadolinium enhancement is associated with adverse ventricular mechanics and ventricular tachycardia late after Fontan operation (Rathod et al. 2010).

9 Coronary arteries

Congenital coronary artery anomalies are rare affecting 0.3–0.8% of the population (Fig. 42) (Davis et al. 2001). CMR is a valuable adjunct for the assessment of anomalous coronary arteries (Post et al. 1995; McConnell et al. 1995; Taylor et al. 2000). 3D mapping of the coronary morphology using respiratory and cardiac-gated balanced SSFP imaging can reveal the proximal course of the coronary arteries and delineate aneurismal dilatation. The definition of the proximal course of the coronary arteries is becoming increasingly important in the assessment of patients who are undergoing interventions to cardiac structures in close proximity to the coronary arteries (e.g. percutaneous pulmonary valve implantation into the pulmonary trunk and compression of the left coronary system (Sridharan et al. 2006), or stenting of the branch pulmonary arteries in ASO and compression of either coronary artery).

9.1 Kawasaki Disease

Kawaski disease is an acute vasculitis that usually occurs in children under 5 years of age. Acutely these children develop myocarditis and pericarditis. Most morbidity is due to the medium-term development of coronary artery aneurysms. These occur in approximately 20% of patients (Park et al. 2002) and predispose the patient to the development of myocardial ischemia and infarction (Burns et al. 1996). Thus long term follow-up into adulthood is important in the management of this condition (Mueller et al. 2009; Fukazawa 2010).

Echocardiography is also useful in the assessment of coronary vascular abnormalities at initial presentation and for later screening, however acoustic windows limit the views beyond the proximal part of the vessels. X-ray coronary angiography has been considered the gold standard in following up coronary abnormalities in Kawasaki disease. Unfortunately it is invasive and exposes the patient to ionizing radiation, which limits its usefulness (Greil et al. 2002). Moreover, neither echo nor catheter angiography can sensitively characterize the segmental myocardial systolic function, perfusion or scar formation, during a single scanning session (Mavrogeni et al. 2006). The MR techniques for this imaging are discussed in other sections of this text (see "Ischemic Heart Disease"). ceMRA and 3D balanced SSFP are of great value in the serial non-invasive evaluation of these patients (Fig. 43). (Mavrogeni et al. 2004), and can include investigation of the peripheral arterial complications of Kawasaki disease (Fig. 44).

9.2 Anomalous Origin of the Left Coronary Artery (ALCAPA)

Anomalous origin of the left coronary artery from the pulmonary artery (ALCAPA), also known as Bland–White–Garland syndrome, is a rare congenital cardiovascular defect that occurs in approximately 1 in 300 000 live births or 0.25–0.5% of children with congenital heart disease. The mortality of untreated ALCAPA has been estimated to be approximately 90% in the first year of life. However, 5–10% of cases can survive past infancy into adulthood. These older patients can present with myocardial infarction, left ventricular dysfunction, mitral regurgitation, or silent myocardial ischaemia, which can lead to sudden cardiac death.

Symptoms and signs usually occur in early infancy (4th-5th month of life) when pulmonary vascular resistance drops and left coronary artery flow is reduced. All blood is now supplied by the right coronary artery and if there are few coronary collateral vessels, this can lead to coronary insufficiency. Patients with better coronary collateralization may present later in life with a 'steal' phenomenon: Blood from the right coronary artery passes to the left system via collaterals, and then directly into the low pressure pulmonary artery (systemic to pulmonary shunt), thus leading to under-perfusion in the left coronary territory. Surgery is the only definitive treatment to restore a dual coronary artery circulation, to correct the shunting and to revert the 'steal' that causes myocardial ischaemia.

Depending on the anatomy, the principle surgical options are direct re-implantation (also known as coronary button transfer technique), Tackeuchi repair

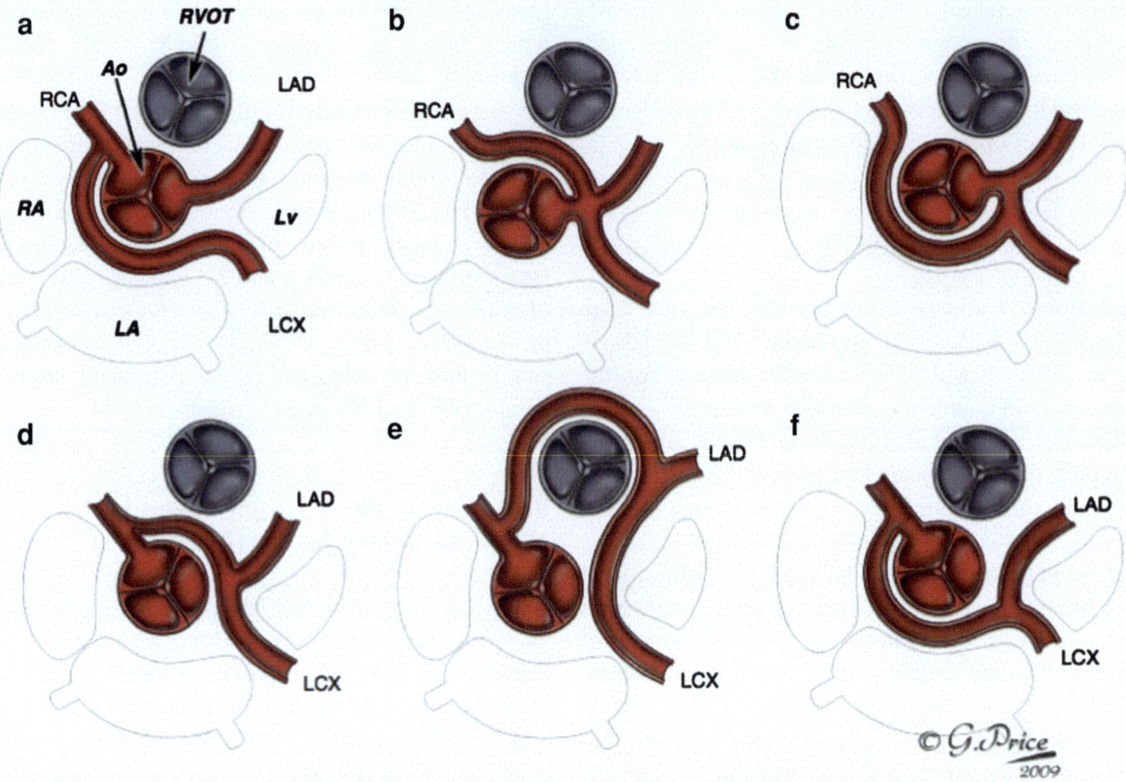

Fig.42 Anatomic representation of the coronary arteries viewed in the oblique axial plane on MRI. RA = right atrium, LA = left atriuim, LV = left ventricle, Ao = aorta, RVOT = right ventricular outflow tract, LAD = left anterior descending artery, RCA = right coronary artery, LCX = left circumflex artery. **a** anomalous LCX from RCA. **b** Anomalous RCA from left main stem (LMS) with interarterial course between pulmonary trunk and aorta. **c** Anomalous RCA from LMS passing posteriorly between aorta and atria. **d** Anomalous left coronary artery arising from RCA with interarterial course between pulmonary trunk and aorta. **e** Anomalous left coronary artery arising from RCA passing posteriorly between aorta and atria. **f** Anomalous left coronary artery arising from RCA passing anterior to pulmonary trunk

(where the pulmonary artery is opened, creating an anterior transverse flap of native pulmonary artery tissue, which creates a baffle to carry the aortic oxygenated blood to the anomalous coronary artery), left coronary artery ligation or coronary artery bypass grafting (CABG). Though a transcatheter closure of ALCAPA has been recently reported as a potentially safe and effective alternative treatment, direct re-implantation is considered as the first line surgical option nowadays, as it yields a more anatomical position by connecting the left coronary artery (LCA) to aorta.

A recent cardiac MRI study of ALCAPA (Secinaro et al. 2011) using cardiac MRI to assess ventricular function at rest, coronary anatomy, adenosine stress myocardial perfusion and late Gd-MRI has shown that at rest, global left ventricular systolic function is normal, though patients have a characteristic sub-endocardial LGE pattern, with fibrosis of the papillary muscles and basal antero-lateral myocardium. Furthermore, a combination of MRCA and adenosine-stress perfusion imaging, can identify patients with significant left coronary artery disease (Fig. 45).

10 Role of Cardiovascular CT

CT imaging also plays an important role in the management of paediatric CHD. This modality provides very high-resolution 3D data sets with an extremely short acquisition period and therefore can usually be performed in infants and small children without general anaesthetic. The expense of this imaging is the exposure of patients to potentially large

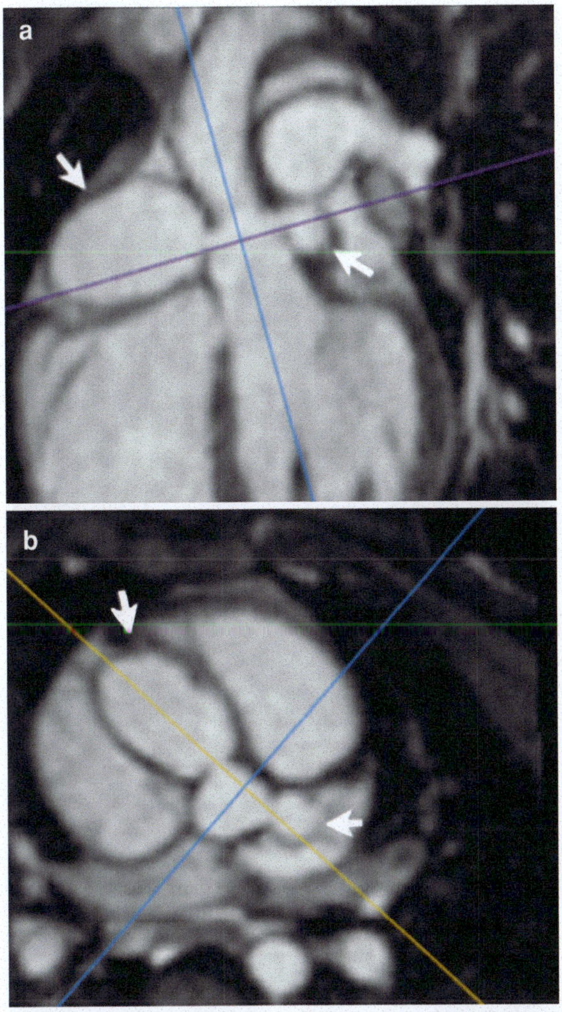

Fig. 43 3D-white blood (b-SSFP) images, from a 5-year-old patient with Kawasaki's disease, viewed using 3D viewing software, (**a**) oblique coronal, (**b**) oblique axial. These planes show giant coronary aneurysms of the proximal right and left coronary arteries (*white arrows*)

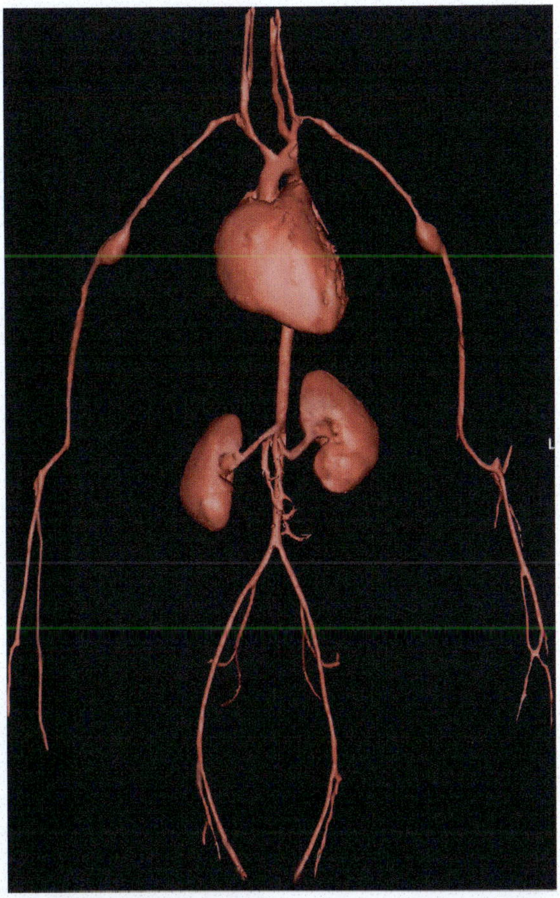

Fig. 44 3D surface-rendered image from a ceMRA, from a 2-year-old patient with Kawasaki's disease, showing bilateral axillary artery aneurysms. The other large and medium-sized arteries in this image are not affected with aneurysm formation

doses of ionizing radiation, particularly for ECG-gated studies, though this continues to fall. Its use for serial evaluations is therefore very limited. CT imaging is useful for patients who are unable to co-operate with cardiovascular MRI or who are too clinically unstable to undergo general anaesthetic. Additionally, when CMR provides inadequate images for clinical decision-making, CT angiography is the modality of choice in:

- Patients with vascular rings, where it is important to visualize the airway anatomy.
- Patients in whom we are investigating pulmonary venous anatomy (in our experience MR imaging of the pulmonary veins can be problematic).
- Patients in whom we are assessing pulmonary atresia with major aorta pulmonary collateral arteries (MAPCAs)—our protocol for assessing these patients is to perform a CT scan prior to cardiac catheterization. The CT scan will identify the number of large aorta pulmonary collaterals and the presence of any central pulmonary arteries, and this information can be used to guide cardiac catheterization. The main purpose of the cardiac catheterization is to identify the temporal distribution of blood flow and define which areas of the lungs the pulmonary arteries, the MAPCAs, or both supply. This significantly aids the surgeons in unifocalisation in these patients.

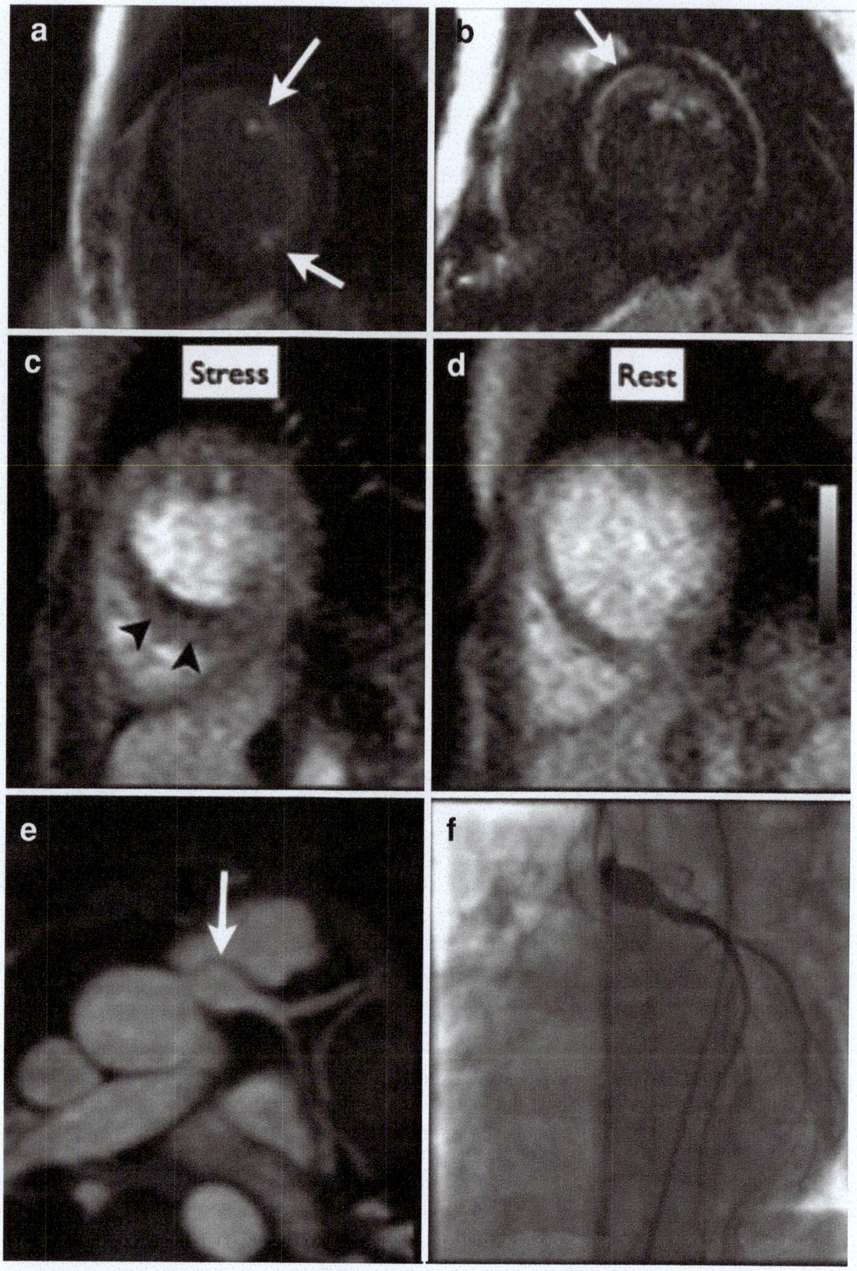

Fig. 45 ALCAPA—**a, b** LGE images from all two patients showing enhancement in both papillary muscles (*arrows*—**a**), and varying degrees of anterior sub-endocardial (*arrow*—**b**). **c, d** Adenosine MR stress perfusion imaging shows reversible sub-endocardial ischaemia of the anterior, septal (*arrowheads*—**c**) and lateral walls and the papillary muscles at the base of the heart—stress and rest images shown. **e** 3D b-SSFP whole heart images, magnetic resonance coronary angiography MRCA shows large patent, reconstructed, reimplanted left coronary artery (*arrow*—**e**) into the left coronary sinus, with confirmatory X-ray coronary angiography (**f**)

- Patients who have metallic implants—e.g. routine CT following aortic coarctation stenting at 3 months to exclude pseudo-aneurysm formation at the distal ends of the stent.
- Patients for the investigation of coronary artery narrowings.
- Patients in whom there is contraindication to MR (e.g. permanent pacemaker).

11 Future Directions

Cardiovascular MR is a rapidly developing field with expanding clinical applications. It provides exceptional visualization of 3D anatomy and reliable measures of cardiovascular function and haemodynamics in patients with congenital heart disease. In the centres producing comprehensive scans, it is becoming an integral part of the management cardiac lesions. The future will see an increasing use of cardiovascular MR in paediatric congenital heart disease, particularly as accelerated imaging techniques allow real-time image acquisition in free-breathing, unsedated patients, without significant compromise of spatial resolution (Muthurangu et al. 2008).

The same accelerated techniques will also permit imaging during exercise (Lurz et al. 2009a) and other pharmacologically altered states, giving better insight into the physiology and functional reserve of many patients with congenital disease.

Time resolved 3D (4D) phase contrast flow velocity acquisition allows the reconstruction of multidirectional flow velocities; measurements for each phase of the cycle being effectively averaged over many heart cycles. Such acquisitions typically take 10 min or more, so beat-to-beat variations related to respiration or flow instabilities are not represented. Besides the visualization of principal multidirectional flow paths, this offers the potential to retrospectively quantify flow through selected planes in the volume covered (Markl et al. 2011). Reported applications include the depiction of large-scale flow patterns in the aortas of patients with bicuspid aortic valves and the retrospective measurements of flow in the presence of more than one shunt (Hope et al. 2009; Valverde et al. 2010). Moreover, this method has also been used in the evaluation of Fontan pathway dynamics (Be'eri et al. 1998; Whitehead et al. 2009).

For all of the above, in order to maintain MR at the forefront of cardiovascular imaging, further work is needed to formally document the clinical added value, relative safety and relative resource efficiency of cardiovascular MR compared to other imaging modalities.

Importantly, the future will see improved collaboration between centres, standardization of techniques and systematic, serial assessment of patients with all types of congenital heart disease. Only with this, will cardiovascular MR contribute significantly to knowledge and management planning for these patients with complex, life-long lesions.

12 Conclusion

Technical advances during the last decade have brought cardiovascular MR into the mainstream of non-invasive imaging for adult and paediatric patients with congenital heart disease. It provides a powerful tool, giving anatomic and haemodynamic information that echo and catheterization alone do not provide. Extracardiac anatomy can be delineated with high spatial resolution, intracardiac anatomy can be imaged in multiple planes, and functional assessment can be made accurately and with high reproducibility. Finally, cardiovascular MR surpasses both catheterization and echo in its ability to create high resolution, 3D reconstructions of complex congenital heart disease. Other well-established clinical applications of cardiovascular MR in patients with congenital heart disease, include measurement of systemic and pulmonary blood flow, quantification of valve regurgitation, identification of myocardial ischemia and fibrosis, and tissue characterization.

The most significant limitations of cardiovascular MR for congenital heart disease are the time and resources required to run a successful scan. A radiographer trained in congenital heart disease is necessary to expedite image planning in the setting of complex disease, often with the added technical challenges of the smaller structures and faster heart rates typical in paediatric patients. During both the acquisition and the reporting stages, a physician with comprehensive experience of the anatomy and physiology of congenital heart disease is required, to guide each scan appropriately. However, with this in place, cardiovascular MR gives a non-invasive, non-irradiative, comprehensive assessment of each patient's morphologic and haemodynamic status, providing valuable decision support for life-long management.

13 Key Points

- Cardiovascular MR assessment is a crucial part of the diagnostic work-up of both paediatric and adult congenital heart disease.
- Cardiovascular MR should be used in conjunction with other imaging methods (echo, CT, cardiac catheterisation) to provide a comprehensive assessment of the patient.
- Protocolisation of MR data acquisition can provide a thorough assessment in all patients.
- A systematic, segmental sequential analysis approach can provide the anatomical connections in all patients.
- Assessment is both anatomical and physiological, with accurate ventricular volume and flow data.

- Newer techniques can provide assessment of coronary artery anatomy, reversible ischaemia and myocardial fibrosis.
- Expert review is necessary in the majority of cases.

References

Acar P, Abdel-Massih T, Douste-Blazy MY, Dulac Y, Bonhoeffer P, Sidi D (2002) Assessment of muscular ventricular septal defect closure by transcatheter or surgical approach: a three-dimensional echocardiographic study. Eur J Echocardiogr J Work Group Echocardiogr Eur Soc Cardiol 3:185–191

Anderson RH (2009) Terminology. In: Anderson RH, Baker EJ, Redington A, Rigby ML, Penny D, Wernovsky G (eds) Paediatric cardiology, 3rd edn. Churchill Livingstone, London, pp 3–16. ISBN-13: 978-0702030642

Babu-Narayan SV, Goktekin O, Moon JC, Broberg CS, Pantely GA, Pennell DJ, Gatzoulis MA, KILNER PJ (2005) Late gadolinium enhancement cardiovascular magnetic resonance of the systemic right ventricle in adults with previous atrial redirection surgery for transposition of the great arteries. Circulation 111:2091–2098

Babu-Narayan SV, Kilner PJ, LI W, Moon JC, Goktekin O, Davlouros PA, Khan M, Ho SY, Pennell DJ, Gatzoulis MA (2006) Ventricular fibrosis suggested by cardiovascular magnetic resonance in adults with repaired tetralogy of fallot and its relationship to adverse markers of clinical outcome. Circulation 113:405–413

Bacha EA, Scheule AM, Zurakowski D, Erickson LC, Hung J, Lang P, Mayer JE, Del Nido PJ, Jonas RA (2001) Long-term results after early primary repair of tetralogy of Fallot. J Thorac Cardiovasc Surg 122:154–161

Barron DJ, Jones TJ, Brawn WJ (2011) The Senning procedure as part of the double-switch operations for congenitally corrected transposition of the great arteries. Seminars Thor Cardiovasc Surg Pediatr Cardiac Surg Annu 14:109–115

Be'eri E, Maier SE, Landzberg MJ, Chung T, Geva T (1998) In vivo evaluation of Fontan pathway flow dynamics by multidimensional phase-velocity magnetic resonance imaging. Circulation 98:2873–2882

Beekman RP, Beek FJ, Meijboom EJ (1997) Usefulness of MRI for the pre-operative evaluation of the pulmonary arteries in Tetralogy of Fallot. Magn Res Imag 15:1005–1015

Beekmana RP, Roest AA, Helbing WA, Hazekamp MG, Schoof PH, Bartelings MM, Sobotka MA, De Roos A, Ottenkamp J (2000) Spin echo MRI in the evaluation of hearts with a double outlet right ventricle: usefulness and limitations. Magn Res Imag 18:245–253

Beerbaum P, Korperich H, Barth P, Esdorn H, Gieseke J, Meyer H (2001) Noninvasive quantification of left-to-right shunt in paediatric patients: phase-contrast cine magnetic resonance imaging compared with invasive oximetry. Circulation 103:2476–2482

Beerbaum P, Korperich H, Esdorn H, Blanz U, Barth P, Hartmann J, Gieseke J, Meyer H (2003) Atrial septal defects in paediatric patients: noninvasive sizing with cardiovascular MR imaging. Radiology 228:361–369

Beuren AJ, Schulze C, Eberle P, Harmjanz D, Apitz J (1964) The syndrome of supravalvular aortic stenosis, peripheral pulmonary stenosis, mental retardation and similar facial appearance. Am J Cardiol 13:471–483

Bjarke BB, Kidd BS (1976) Proceedings: congenitally corrected transposition of the great arteries: a clinical study of 101 cases. British Heart J 38:535

Brawn WJ, Barron DJ (2003) Technical aspects of the Rastelli and atrial switch procedure for congenitally corrected transposition of the great arteries with ventricular septal defect and pulmonary stenosis or atresia: results of therapy. Seminars Thor Cardiovasc Surg. Pediatr Cardiac Surg Annu 6:4–8

Brawn WJ, Jones T, Davies B, Barron D (2009) How we manage patients with major aorta pulmonary collaterals. Semin Thorac Cardiovasc Surg Pediatr Card Surg Annu pp 152–157

Broberg CS, Chugh SS, Conklin C, Sahn DJ, Jerosch-Herold M (2010) Quantification of diffuse myocardial fibrosis and its association with myocardial dysfunction in congenital heart disease. Circ Cardiovasc Imag 3:727–734

Brown DW, Gauvreau K, Powell AJ, Lang P, Colan SD, Del Nido PJ, Odegard KC, Geva T (2007) Cardiac magnetic resonance versus routine cardiac catheterization before bidirectional glenn anastomosis in infants with functional single ventricle: a prospective randomized trial. Circulation 116:2718–2725

Buechel E, Kaiser T, Jackson C, Schmitz A, Kellenberger C (2009) Normal right- and left ventricular volumes and myocardial mass in children measured by steady state free precession cardiovascular magnetic resonance. J Cardiovasc Magn Res 11:19

Burns JC, Shike H, Gordon JB, Malhotra A, Schoenwetter M, Kawasaki T (1996) Sequelae of Kawasaki disease in adolescents and young adults. J Am Coll Cardiol 28: 253–257

Chaudhari M, Chessa M, Stumper O, de Giovanni JV (2001) Transcatheter coil closure of muscular ventricular septal defects. J Interv Cardiol 14:165–168

Chessa M, Dindar A, Vettukattil JJ, Stumper O, Wright JG, Silove ED, Giovanni DE, J. (2000) Balloon angioplasty in infants with aortic obstruction after the modified stage I Norwood procedure. Am Heart J 140:227–231

Chessa M, Carminati M, Cao QL, Butera G, Giusti S, Bini RM, Hijazi ZM (2002) Transcatheter closure of congenital and acquired muscular ventricular septal defects using the Amplatzer device. J Invasive Cardiol 14:322–327

Conte S, Gewillig M, Eyskens B, Dumoulin M, Daenen W (1999) Management of late complications after classic Fontan procedure by conversion to total cavopulmonary connection. Cardiovasc Surg 7:651–655

Davis JA, Cecchin F, Jones TK, Portman MA (2001) Major coronary artery anomalies in a paediatric population: incidence and clinical importance. J Am Coll Cardiol 37(2): 593–597

de Leval MR, Kilner P, Gewillig M, Bull C (1988) Total cavopulmonary connection: a logical alternative to atriopulmonary connection for complex Fontan operations. Experimental studies and early clinical experience. J Thor Cardiovasc Surg 96:682–695

Derrick GP, Josen M, Vogel M, Henein MY, Shinebourne EA, Redington AN (2001) Abnormalities of right ventricular long axis function after atrial repair of transposition of the great arteries. Heart 86:203–206

Devos DG, Kilner PJ (2010) Calculations of cardiovascular shunts and regurgitation using magnetic resonance ventricular volume and aortic and pulmonary flow measurements. Eur Radiol 20:410–421

Durongpisitkul K, Tang NL, Soongswang J, Laohaprasitiporn D, Nanal A (2004) Predictors of successful transcatheter closure of atrial septal defect by cardiac magnetic resonance imaging. Pediatr Cardiol 25:124–130

Dymarkowski S, Bosmans H, Marchal G, Bogaert J (1999) Three-dimensional MR angiography in the evaluation of thoracic outlet syndrome. Am J Roentgenol 173:1005–1008

Fenchel M, Greil GF, Martirosian P, Kramer U, Schick F, Claussen CD, Sieverding L, Miller S (2006) Three-dimensional morphological magnetic resonance imaging in infants and children with congenital heart disease. Pediatr Radiol 36:1265–1272

Fischer G, Stieh J, Uebing A, Hoffmann U, Morf G, Kramer HH (2003) Experience with transcatheter closure of secundum atrial septal defects using the Amplatzer septal occluder: a single centre study in 236 consecutive patients. Heart 89: 199–204

Fletcher BD, Jacobstein MD, Nelson AD, Riemenschneider TA, Alfidi RJ (1984) Gated magnetic resonance imaging of congenital cardiac malformations. Radiology 150:137–140

Flett AS, Hayward MP, Ashworth MT, Hansen MS, Taylor AM, Elliott PM, Mcgregor C, Moon JC (2010) Equilibrium contrast cardiovascular magnetic resonance for the measurement of diffuse myocardial fibrosis: preliminary validation in humans. Circulation 122:138–144

Fogel MA, Rychik J (1998) Right ventricular function in congenital heart disease: pressure and volume overload lesions. Progr Cardiovasc Dis 40:343–356

Fogel MA, Hubbard A, Weinberg PM (2001) A simplified approach for assessment of intracardiac baffles and extracardiac conduits in congenital heart surgery with two- and three-dimensional magnetic resonance imaging. Am Heart J 142:1028–1036

Fogel MA, Hubbard A, Weinberg PM (2002) Mid-term follow-up of patients with transposition of the great arteries after atrial inversion operation using two- and three-dimensional magnetic resonance imaging. Pediatr Radiol 32:440–446

Fontan F, Baudet E (1971) Surgical repair of tricuspid atresia. Thorax 26:240–248

Fukazawa R (2010) Long-term prognosis of Kawasaki disease: increased cardiovascular risk? Curr Opin Pediatr 22:587–592

Gatehouse PD, Rolf MP, Graves MJ, Hofman MB, Totman J, Werner B, Quest RA, Liu Y, von Spiczak J, Dieringer M, Firmin DN, Van Rossum A, Lombardi M, Schwitter J, Schulz-Menger J, Kilner PJ (2010) Flow measurement by cardiovascular magnetic resonance: a multi-centre multi-vendor study of background phase offset errors that can compromise the accuracy of derived regurgitant or shunt flow measurements. J Cardiovasc Magn Res Off J Soc Cardiovasc Magn Res 12:5

Geva T, Greil GF, Marshall AC, Landzberg M, Powell AJ (2002) Gadolinium-enhanced 3-dimensional magnetic resonance angiography of pulmonary blood supply in patients with complex pulmonary stenosis or atresia: comparison with X-ray angiography. Circulation 106:473–478

Giardini A, Lovato L, Donti A, Formigari R, Oppido G, Gargiulo G, Picchio FM, Fattori R (2006) Relation between right ventricular structural alterations and markers of adverse clinical outcome in adults with systemic right ventricle and either congenital complete (after Senning operation) or congenitally corrected transposition of the great arteries. Am J Cardiol 98:1277–1282

Greenberg SB, Crisci KL, Koenig P, Robinson B, Anisman P, Russo P (1997) Magnetic resonance imaging compared with echocardiography in the evaluation of pulmonary artery abnormalities in children with tetralogy of Fallot following palliative and corrective surgery. Pediatr Radiol 27:932–935

Greil GF, Stuber M, Botnar RM, Kissinger KV, Geva T, Newburger JW, Manning WJ, Powell AJ (2002) Coronary magnetic resonance angiography in adolescents and young adults with kawasaki disease. Circulation 105:908–911

Grosse-Wortmann L, Yun TJ, Al-Radi O, Kim S, Nii M, Lee KJ, Redington A, Yoo SJ, Van Arsdell G (2008) Borderline hypoplasia of the left ventricle in neonates: insights for decision-making from functional assessment with magnetic resonance imaging. J Thor Cardiovasc Surg 136:1429–1436

Grosse-Wortmann L, Al-Otay A, Yoo SJ (2009) Aortopulmonary collaterals after bidirectional cavopulmonary connection or Fontan completion: quantification with MRI circulation. Cardiovasc Imag 2:219–225

Grothues F, Smith GC, Moon JC, Bellenger NG, Collins P, Klein HU, Pennell DJ (2002) Comparison of interstudy reproducibility of cardiovascular magnetic resonance with two-dimensional echocardiography in normal subjects and in patients with heart failure or left ventricular hypertrophy. Am J Cardiol 90:29–34

Gutberlet M, Boeckel T, Hosten N, Vogel M, Kuhne T, Oellinger H, Ehrenstein T, Venz S, Hetzer R, Bein G, Felix R (2000) Arterial switch procedure for D-transposition of the great arteries: quantitative midterm evaluation of haemodynamic changes with cine MR imaging and phase-shift velocity mapping-initial experience. Radiology 214:467–475

Haas F, Wottke M, Poppert H, Meisner H (1999) Long-term survival and functional follow-up in patients after the arterial switch operation. Ann Thor Surg 68:1692–1697

Higgins CB, Byrd BF, Farmer D W 3rd, Osaki L, Silverman NH, Cheitlin MD (1984) Magnetic resonance imaging in patients with congenital heart disease. Circulation 70: 851–860

Hoffman JI, Kaplan S (2002) The incidence of congenital heart disease. J Am Coll Cardiol 39:1890–1900

Holmqvist C, Hochbergs P, Bjorkhem G, Brockstedt S, Laurin S (2001) Pre-operative evaluation with MR in tetralogy of fallot and pulmonary atresia with ventricular septal defect. Acta Radiologica 42:63–69

Hope M, Meadows A, Hope T, Ordovas K, Saloner D, Reddy G, Alley M, Higgins C (2009) 4D flow evaluation of abnormal flow patterns with bicuspid aortic valve. J Cardiovasc Magn Res 11:P184

Hope MD, Hope TA, Urbania TH, Higgins CB (2010) Four-dimensional flow magnetic resonance imaging with wall shear stress analysis before and after repair of aortopulmonary fistula circulation. Cardiovasc Imag 3:766–768

Hughes ML, Tsang VT, Kostolny M, Giardini A, Muthurangu V, Taylor AM, Brown K (2011) Lessons from inter-stage cardiac magnetic resonance imaging in predicting survival for patients with hypoplastic left heart syndrome. Cardiol Young 1–8

Hundley WG, Li HF, Hillis LD, Meshack BM, Lange RA, Willard JE, Landau C, Peshock RM (1995) Quantitation of cardiac output with velocity-encoded, phase-difference magnetic resonance imaging. Am J Cardiol 75:1250–1255

Jacobstein MD, Fletcher BD, Nelson AD, Goldstein S, Alfidi RJ, Riemenschneider TA (1984) ECG-gated nuclear magnetic resonance imaging: appearance of the congenitally malformed heart. Am Heart J 107:1014–1020

Jatene AD, Fontes VF, Paulista PP, Souza LC, Neger F, Galantier M, Sousa JE (1976) Anatomic correction of transposition of the great vessels. J Thoracic Cardiovasc Surg 72:364–370

Julsrud PR, Ehman RL, Hagler DJ, Ilstrup DM (1989) Extracardiac vasculature in candidates for Fontan surgery: MR imaging. Radiology 173:503–506

Kang IS, Redington AN, Benson LN, Macgowan C, Valsangiacomo ER, Roman K, Kellenberger CJ, Yoo SJ (2003) Differential regurgitation in branch pulmonary arteries after repair of tetralogy of Fallot: a phase-contrast cine magnetic resonance study. Circulation 107:2938–2943

Khambadkone S, Coats L, Taylor A, Boudjemline Y, Derrick G, Tsang V, Cooper J, Muthurangu V, Hegde SR, Razavi RS, Pellerin D, Deanfield J, Bonhoeffer P (2005) Percutaneous pulmonary valve implantation in humans: results in 59 consecutive patients. Circulation 112:1189–1197

Kilner PJ, Sievers B, Meyer GP, Ho SY (2002) Double-chambered right ventricle or sub-infundibular stenosis assessed by cardiovascular magnetic resonance. J Cardiovasc Magn Res Off J Soc Cardiovasc Magn Res 4:373–379

Kilner PJ, Geva T, Kaemmerer H, Trindade PT, Schwitter J, Webb GD (2010) Recommendations for cardiovascular magnetic resonance in adults with congenital heart disease from the respective working groups of the European Society of Cardiology. Eur Heart J 31:794–805

Knauth AL, Gauvreau K, Powell AJ, Landzberg MJ, Walsh EP, Lock JE, Del Nido PJ, GEVA T (2008) Ventricular size and function assessed by cardiac MRI predict major adverse clinical outcomes late after tetralogy of Fallot repair. Heart 94:211–216

Ladouceur M, Bruneval P, Mousseaux E (2009) Cardiovascular flashlight. Magnetic resonance assessment of fibrosis in systemic right ventricle after atrial switch procedure. Eur Heart J 30:2613

Langley SM, Winlaw DS, Stumper O, Dhillon R, de Giovanni JV, Wright JG, Miller P, Sethia B, Barron DJ, Brawn WJ (2003) Midterm results after restoration of the morphologically left ventricle to the systemic circulation in patients with congenitally corrected transposition of the great arteries. J Thor Cardiovasc Surg 125:1229–1241

Laschinger JC, Redmond JM, Cameron DE, Kan JS, Ringel RE (1996) Intermediate results of the extracardiac Fontan procedure. Ann Thor Surg (62):1261–1267, discussion 1266–1267

Legendre A, Losay J, Touchot-Kone A, Serraf A, Belli E, Piot JD, Lambert V, Capderou A, Planche C (2003) Coronary events after arterial switch operation for transposition of the great arteries. Circulation 108(Suppl 1):II186–II190

Leung DA, Debatin JF (1997) Three-dimensional contrast-enhanced magnetic resonance angiography of the thoracic vasculature. Eur Radiol 7:981–989

Lorenz CH (2000) The range of normal values of cardiovascular structures in infants, children, and adolescents measured by magnetic resonance imaging. Pediatr Cardiol 2000(21):37–46

Lurz P, Muthurangu V, Schievano S, Nordmeyer J, Bonhoeffer P, Taylor AM, Hansen MS (2009a) Feasibility and reproducibility of biventricular volumetric assessment of cardiac function during exercise using real-time radial k–t SENSE magnetic resonance imaging. J Magn Res Imaging 29: 1062–1070

Lurz P, Nordmeyer J, Muthurangu V, Khambadkone S, Derrick G, Yates R, Sury M, Bonhoeffer P, Taylor AM (2009b) Comparison of bare metal stenting and percutaneous pulmonary valve implantation for treatment of right ventricular outflow tract obstruction: use of an X-ray/magnetic resonance hybrid laboratory for acute physiological assessment. Circulation 119:2995–3001

Manso B, Castellote A, Dos L, Casaldaliga J (2010) Myocardial perfusion magnetic resonance imaging for detecting coronary function anomalies in asymptomatic paediatric patients with a previous arterial switch operation for the transposition of great arteries. Cardiol Young 20:410–417

Markl M, Kilner P, Ebbers T (2011) Comprehensive 4D velocity mapping of the heart and great vessels by cardiovascular magnetic resonance. J Cardiovasc Magn Res 13:7

Marshall AC, Love BA, Lang P, Jonas RA, Del Nido PJ, Mayer JE, Lock JE (2003) Staged repair of tetralogy of Fallot and diminutive pulmonary arteries with a fenestrated ventricular septal defect patch. J Thor Cardiovasc Surg 126:1427–1433

Martinez JE, Mohiaddin RH, Kilner PJ, Khaw K, Rees S, Somerville J, Longmore DB (1992) Obstruction in extracardiac ventriculopulmonary conduits: value of nuclear magnetic resonance imaging with velocity mapping and Doppler echocardiography. J Am Coll Cardiol 20:338–344

Masuda M, Kado H, Shiokawa Y, Fukae K, Kanegae Y, Kawachi Y, Morita S, Yasui H (1999) Clinical results of arterial switch operation for double-outlet right ventricle with subpulmonary VSD. Eur J Cardio Thor Surg Offic J Eur Assoc Cardio Thor Surg 15:283–288

Masui T, Katayama M, Kobayashi S, Ito T, Seguchi M, Koide M, Nozaki A, Sakahara H (2000) Gadolinium-enhanced MR angiography in the evaluation of congenital cardiovascular disease pre- and postoperative states in infants and children. J Magn Res Imaging 12:1034–1042

Mavrogeni S, Papadopoulos G, Douskou M, Kaklis S, Seimenis I, Baras P, Nikolaidou P, Bakoula C, Karanasios E, Manginas A, Cokkinos DV (2004) Magnetic resonance angiography is equivalent to X-ray coronary angiography for the evaluation of coronary arteries in Kawasaki disease. J Am Coll Cardiol 43:649–652

Mavrogeni S, Papadopoulos G, Douskou M, Kaklis S, Seimenis I, Varlamis G, Karanasios E, Krikos X, Giannoulia A, Cokkinos DV (2006) Magnetic resonance angiography, function and viability evaluation in patients with Kawasaki disease. J Cardiovasc Magn Res Offic J Soc Cardiovasc Magn Res 8:493–498

McConnell MV, Ganz P, Selwyn AP, Li W, Edelman RR, Manning WJ (1995) Identification of anomalous coronary arteries and their anatomic course by magnetic resonance coronary angiography. Circulation 92:3158–3162

Mohr JP, Homma S (2003) Patent cardiac foramen ovale: stroke risk and closure. Ann Intern Med 139:787–788

Mooij CF, de Wit CJ, Graham DA, Powell AJ, Geva T (2008) Reproducibility of MRI measurements of right ventricular size and function in patients with normal and dilated ventricles. J Magn Res Imaging 28:67–73

Moons P, Bovijn L, Budts W, Belmans A, Gewillig M (2010) Temporal trends in survival to adulthood among patients born with congenital heart disease from 1970 to 1992 in Belgium. Circulation 122:2264 2272

Mueller F, Knirsch W, Harpes P, Pretre R, Valsangiacomo Buechel E, Kretschmar O (2009) Long-term follow-up of acute changes in coronary artery diameter caused by Kawasaki disease: risk factors for development of stenotic lesions. Clinical Res Cardiol Offic J German Cardiac Soc 98:501–507

Mustard WT (1968) Recent experiences with surgical management of transposition of the great arteries. J Cardiovasc Surg 9:532–536

Muthurangu V, Taylor A, Andriantsimiavona R, Hegde S, Miquel ME, Tulloh R, Baker E, Hill DL, Razavi RS (2004) Novel method of quantifying pulmonary vascular resistance by use of simultaneous invasive pressure monitoring and phase-contrast magnetic resonance flow. Circulation 110: 826–834

Muthurangu V, Taylor AM, Hegde SR, Johnson R, Tulloh R, Simpson JM, Qureshi S, Rosenthal E, Baker E, Anderson D, Razavi R (2005) Cardiac magnetic resonance imaging after stage I Norwood operation for hypoplastic left heart syndrome. Circulation 112:3256–3263

Muthurangu V, Lurz P, Critchely JD, Deanfield JE, Taylor AM, Hansen MS (2008) Real-time assessment of right and left ventricular volumes and function in patients with congenital heart disease by using high spatiotemporal resolution radial k-t SENSE. Radiology 248:782–791

Nagel E, Klein C, Paetsch I, Hettwer S, Schnackenburg B, Wegscheider K, Fleck E (2003) Magnetic resonance perfusion measurements for the noninvasive detection of coronary artery disease. Circulation 108:432–437

Nordmeyer J, Coats L, Bonhoeffer P (2006) Current experience with percutaneous pulmonary valve implantation. Semin Thor Cardiovasc Surg 18:122–125

Nordmeyer J, Gaudin R, Tann OR, Lurz PC, Bonhoeffer P, Taylor AM, Muthurangu V (2010a) MRI may be sufficient for noninvasive assessment of great vessel stents: an in vitro comparison of MRI, CT, and conventional angiography. Am J Roentgenol 195:865–871

Nordmeyer S, Riesenkampff E, Crelier G, Khasheei A, Schnackenburg B, Berger F, Kuehne T (2010b) Flow-sensitive four-dimensional cine magnetic resonance imaging for offline blood flow quantification in multiple vessels: a validation study. J Magn Res Imaging 32:677–683

Norwood WI, Kirklin JK, Sanders SP (1980) Hypoplastic left heart syndrome: experience with palliative surgery. Am J Cardiol 45:87–91

Odegard KC, Dinardo JA, Tsai-Goodman B, Powell AJ, Geva T, Laussen PC (2004) Anaesthesia considerations for cardiac MRI in infants and small children. Paediatr Anaesth 14:471–476

Ohye RG, Sleeper LA, Mahony L, Newburger JW, Pearson GD, Lu M, Goldberg CS, Tabbutt S, Frommelt PC, Ghanayem NS, Laussen PC, Rhodes JF, Lewis AB, Mital S, Ravishankar C, Williams IA, Dunbar-Masterson C, Atz AM, Colan S, Minich LL, Pizarro C, Kanter KR, Jaggers J, Jacobs JP, Krawczeski CD, Pike N, Mccrindle BW, Virzi L, Gaynor JW (2010) Comparison of shunt types in the Norwood procedure for single-ventricle lesions. N Engl J Med 362:1980–1992

Ou P, Celermajer DS, Marini D, Agnoletti G, Vouhé P, Brunelle F, Le Quan Sang KH, Thalabard JC, Sidi D, Bonnet D (2008) Safety and accuracy of 64-slice computed tomography coronary angiography in children after the arterial switch operation for transposition of the great arteries. JACC Cardiovasc Imaging 1(3):331–339

Paetsch I, Jahnke C, Wahl A, Gebker R, Neuss M, Fleck E, Nagel E (2004) Comparison of dobutamine stress magnetic resonance, adenosine stress magnetic resonance, and adenosine stress magnetic resonance perfusion. Circulation 110:835–842

Parish V, Bell A, Head C, Rosenthal E, Greil G, Razavi R, Beerbaum P (2010) Dobutamine stress MR in Tetralogy of Fallot with significant pulmonary regurgitation, safety, feasibility and haemodynamic effects. J Cardiovasc Magn Res 12:P3

Park SC, Neches WH, Zuberbuhler JR, Mathews RA, Lenox CC, Fricker FJ (1978) Echocardiographic and haemodynamic correlation in transposition of the great arteries. Circulation 57:291–298

Park YW, Park IS, Kim CH, Ma JS, Lee SB, Yun YS, Lee HJ, Lee SK, Tockgo YC (2002) Epidemiologic study of Kawasaki disease in Korea, 1997–1999: comparison with previous studies during 1991–1996. J Korean Med Sci 17:453–456

Park JH, Kim HS, Jin GY, Joo CU, Ko JK (2008) Demonstration of peripheral pulmonary stenosis and supravalvular aortic stenosis by different cardiac imaging modalities in a patient with Williams syndrome–usefulness of noninvasive imaging studies. Int J Cardiol 128:e95–e97

Pigula FA, Khalil PN, Mayer JE, Del Nido PJ, Jonas RA (1999) Repair of tetralogy of Fallot in neonates and young infants. Circulation 100:II157–II161.

Pilleul F, Merchant N (2000) MRI of the pulmonary veins: comparison between 3D MR angiography and T1-weighted spin echo. J Comput Assist Tomogr 24:683–687

Pizarro C, Malec E, Maher KO, Januszewska K, Gidding SS, Murdison KA, Baffa JM, Norwood WI (2003) Right ventricle to pulmonary artery conduit improves outcome after stage I Norwood for hypoplastic left heart syndrome. Circulation 108(Suppl 1):II155–II160

Post JC, van Rossum AC, Bronzwaer JG, de Cock CC, Hofman MB, Valk J, Visser CA (1995) Magnetic resonance angiography of anomalous coronary arteries. A new gold standard for delineating the proximal course? Circulation 92:3163–3171

Potthast S, Mitsumori L, Stanescu LA, Richardson ML, Branch K, Dubinsky TJ, Maki JH (2010) Measuring aortic diameter with different MR techniques: comparison of three-dimensional (3D) navigated steady-state free-precession (SSFP), 3D contrast-enhanced magnetic resonance angiography (CE-MRA), 2D T2 black blood, and 2D cine SSFP. J Mag Res Imaging 31:177–184

Powell AJ, Maier SE, Chung T, Geva T (2000) Phase-velocity cine magnetic resonance imaging measurement of pulsatile blood flow in children and young adults: in vitro and in vivo validation. Pediatr Cardiol 21:104–110

Puvaneswary M, Leitch J, Chard RB (2003) MRI of partial anomalous pulmonary venous return (scimitar syndrome). Australasian Radiol 47:92–93

Rastelli GC, Mcgoon DC, Wallace RB (1969) Anatomic correction of transposition of the great arteries with ventricular septal defect and subpulmonary stenosis. Journal Thor Cardiovasc Surg 58:545–552

Rathod RH, Prakash A, Powell AJ, Geva T (2010) Myocardial fibrosis identified by cardiac magnetic resonance late gadolinium enhancement is associated with adverse ventricular mechanics and ventricular tachycardia late after Fontan operation. J Am Coll Cardiol 55:1721–1728

Razavi R, Hill DL, Keevil SF, Miquel ME, Muthurangu V, Hegde S, Rhode K, Barnett M, van Vaals J, Hawkes DJ, Baker E (2003a) Cardiac catheterisation guided by MRI in children and adults with congenital heart disease. Lancet 362:1877–1882

Razavi RS, Hill DL, Muthurangu V, Miquel ME, Taylor AM, Kozerke S, Baker EJ (2003b) Three-dimensional magnetic resonance imaging of congenital cardiac anomalies. Cardiol Young 13:461–465

Rebergen SA, Van der Wall EE, Doornbos J, de Roos A (1993) Magnetic resonance measurement of velocity and flow: technique, validation, and cardiovascular applications. Am Heart J 126:1439–1456

Rigby ML, Redington AN (1989) Cross-sectional echocardiography. British Med Bull 45:1036–1060

Rolf MP, Hofman MB, Gatehouse PD, Markenroth-Bloch K, Heymans MW, Ebbers T, Graves MJ, Totman JJ, Werner B, van Rossum AC, Kilner PJ, Heethaar RM (2011) Sequence optimization to reduce velocity offsets in cardiovascular magnetic resonance volume flow quantification–a multivendor study. J Cardiovasc Magn Res Off J Soc Cardiovasc Magn Res 13:18

Sampson C, Kilner PJ, Hirsch R, Rees RS, Somerville J, Underwood SR (1994) Venoatrial pathways after the Mustard operation for transposition of the great arteries: anatomic and functional MR imaging. Radiology 193: 211–217

Sano S, Ishino K, Kawada M, Fujisawa E, Kamada M, Ohtsuki S (2000) Staged biventricular repair of pulmonary atresia or stenosis with intact ventricular septum. Ann Thor Surg 70:1501–1506

Sano S, Ishino K, Kawada M, Honjo O (2004) Right ventricle-pulmonary artery shunt in first-stage palliation of hypoplastic left heart syndrome. Seminars in thoracic and cardiovascular surgery. Pediatr Cardiac Surg Annu 7: 22–31

Sarikouch S, Peters B, Gutberlet M, Leismann B, Kelter-Kloepping A, Koerperich H, Kuehne T, Beerbaum P (2010) Sex-specific paediatric percentiles for ventricular size and mass as reference values for cardiac MRI: assessment by steady-state free-precession and phase-contrast MRI flow Circulation. Cardiovasc imaging 3:65–76

Sarkar D, Bull C, Yates R, Wright D, Cullen S, Gewillig M, Clayton R, Tunstill A, Deanfield J (1999) Comparison of long-term outcomes of atrial repair of simple transposition with implications for a late arterial switch strategy. Circulation 100:II176–II181

Schievano S, Coats L, Migliavacca F, Norman W, Frigiola A, Deanfield J, Bonhoeffer P, Taylor AM (2007) Variations in right ventricular outflow tract morphology following repair of congenital heart disease: implications for percutaneous pulmonary valve implantation. J Cardiovasc Magn Res Off J Soc Cardiovasc Magn Res 9:687–695

Secinaro A, Ntsinjana H, Tann O, Schuler PK, Muthurangu V, Hughes M, Tsang V, Taylor AM (2011) Cardiovascular magnetic resonance findings in repaired anomalous left coronary artery to pulmonary artery connection (ALCAPA). J Cardiovasc Magn Res Off J Soc Cardiovasc Magn Res 13:27

Seddio F, Reddy VM, Mcelhinney DB, Tworetzky W, Silverman NH, Hanley FL (1999) Multiple ventricular septal defects: how and when should they be repaired? J Thor Cardiovasc Surg 117:134–139, discussion 39–40

Senning A (1975) Correction of the transposition of the great arteries. Ann Surg 182:287–292

Shimpo H, Hayakawa H, Miyake Y, Takabayashi S, Yada I (2000) Strategy for pulmonary atresia and intact ventricular septum. Ann Thor Surg 70:287–289

Simpson IA, Valdes-Cruz LM, Berthoty DP, Powell JB, Hesselink JR, Chung KJ, Sahn DJ (1993) Cine magnetic resonance imaging and color Doppler flow mapping in infants and children with pulmonary artery bands. Am J Cardiol 71:1419–1426

Sivakumar K, Anil SR, Rao SG, Shivaprakash K, Kumar RK (2003) Closure of muscular ventricular septal defects guided by en face reconstruction and pictorial representation. Ann Thor Surg 76:158–166

Sridharan S, Coats L, Khambadkone S, Taylor AM, Bonhoeffer P (2006) Transcatheter right ventricular outflow tract intervention: The risk to the coronary circulation. Circulation 113(25):e934–e935

Stamm C, Li J, Ho SY, Redington AN, Anderson RH (1997) The aortic root in supravalvular aortic stenosis: the potential surgical relevance of morphologic findings. J Thor Cardiovasc Surg 114:16–24

Steeden JA, Atkinson D, Hansen MS, Taylor AM, Muthurangu V (2011) Rapid flow assessment of congenital heart disease with high-spatiotemporal-resolution gated spiral phase-contrast MR imaging. Radiology 260(1):79–87

Strigl S, Beroukhim R, Valente AM, Annese D, Harrington JS, Geva T, Powell AJ (2009) Feasibility of dobutamine stress cardiovascular magnetic resonance imaging in children. J Magn Res Imag 29:313–319

Stockton E, Hughes ML, Taylor AM, Mcewan A (2009) A prospective assessment of paediatric cardiac mri under general anaesthesia; practise and problems. J Cardiovasc Magn Reson, 11(Suppl 1):P249 (http://jcmr-online.com/content/11/S1/P249)

Taylor AM, Thorne SA, Rubens MB, Jhooti P, Keegan J, Gatehouse PD, Wiesmann F, Grothues F, Somerville J, Pennell DJ (2000) Coronary artery imaging in grown up congenital heart disease: complementary role of magnetic resonance and X-ray coronary angiography. Circulation 101(14):1670–1678

Taylor AM, Dymarkowski S, Hamaekers P, Razavi R, Gewillig M, Mertens L, Bogaert J (2005) MR coronary angiography and late-enhancement myocardial MR in children who underwent arterial switch surgery for transposition of great arteries. Radiology 234:542–547

Thanopoulos BD, Tsaousis GS, Karanasios E, Eleftherakis NG, Paphitis C (2003) Transcatheter closure of perimembranous ventricular septal defects with the Amplatzer asymmetric ventricular septal defect occluder: preliminary experience in children. Heart 89:918–922

Tulevski II, Romkes H, Dodge-Khatami A, van Der Wall EE, Groenink M, van Veldhuisen DJ, Mulder BJ (2002a) Quantitative assessment of the pressure and volume overloaded right ventricle: imaging is a real challenge. Int J Cardiovasc Imaging 18:41–51

Tulevski II, van Der Wall EE, Groenink M, Dodge-Khatami A, Hirsch A, Stoker J, Mulder BJ (2002b) Usefulness of magnetic resonance imaging dobutamine stress in asymptomatic and minimally symptomatic patients with decreased cardiac reserve from congenital heart disease (complete and corrected transposition of the great arteries and subpulmonic obstruction). Am J Cardiol 89:1077–1081

Urban Z, Zhang J, Davis EC, Maeda GK, Kumar A, Stalker H, Belmont JW, Boyd CD, Wallace MR (2001) Supravalvular aortic stenosis: genetic and molecular dissection of a complex mutation in the elastin gene. Hum Genet 109:512–520

Uribe S, Hussain T, Valverde I, Tejos C, Irarrazaval P, Fava M, Beerbaum P, Botnar RM, Razavi R, Schaeffter T, Greil GF (2011) Congenital heart disease in children: coronary MR angiography during systole and diastole with dual cardiac phase whole-heart imaging. Radiology 260(1):232–240

Valverde I, Simpson J, Schaeffter T, Beerbaum P (2010) 4D Phase-contrast flow cardiovascular magnetic resonance: comprehensive quantification and visualization of flow dynamics in atrial septal defect and partial anomalous pulmonary venous return. Pediatr Cardiol 31:1244–1248

Valverde I, Parish V, Tzifa A, Head C, Sarikouch S, Greil G, Schaeffter T, Razavi R, Beerbaum P (2011) Cardiovascular MR dobutamine stress in adult tetralogy of fallot: Disparity between CMR volumetry and flow for cardiovascular function. J Magn Res Imaging 33:1341–1350

van Den Berg J, Strengers JL, Wielopolski PA, Hop WC, Meijboom FJ, de Rijke YB, Boomsma F, Bogers AJ, Pattynama PM, Helbing WA (2009) Assessment of biventricular functional reserve and NT-proBNP levels in patients with RV volume overload after repair of tetralogy of Fallot at young age. Int J Cardiol 133:364–370

Warnes CA, Williams RG, Bashore TM, Child JS, Connolly HM, Dearani JA, Del Nido P, Fasules JW, Graham T P Jr, Hijazi ZM, Hunt SA, King ME, Landzberg MJ, Miner PD, Radford MJ, Walsh EP, Webb GD (2008) ACC/AHA 2008 guidelines for the management of adults with congenital heart disease: executive summary: a report of the American College of Cardiology/American Heart Association Task Force on practice guidelines (writing committee to develop guidelines for the management of adults with congenital heart disease). Circulation 118:2395–2451

Whitehead KK, Sundareswaran KS, Parks WJ, Harris MA, Yoganathan AP, Fogel MA (2009) Blood flow distribution in a large series of patients having the Fontan operation: a cardiac magnetic resonance velocity mapping study. J Thorac Cardiovasc Surg 138:96–102

Williams JC, Barratt-Boyes BG, Lowe JB (1961) Supravalvular aortic stenosis. Circulation 24:1311–1318

Winner MW III, Raman SV, Chung YC, Simonetti OP, Mihai G, Cook SC (2011) Post-interventional three-dimensional dark blood MRI in the adult with congenital heart disease. Int J Cardiol 65(6):1786–1792

Winter MM, Bernink FJ, Groenink M, Bouma BJ, van Dijk AP, Helbing WA, Tijssen JG, Mulder BJ (2008) Evaluating the systemic right ventricle by CMR: the importance of consistent and reproducible delineation of the cavity. J Cardiovasc Magn Res Off J Soc Cardiovasc Magn Res 10:40

Wu Q, Yu Q, Yang X (2003) Modified Rastelli procedure for double outlet right ventricle with left-malposition of the great arteries: report of 9 cases. Ann Thor Surg 75:138–142

Zeevi B, Berant M, Fogelman R, Galit BM, Blieden LC (1999) Acute complications in the current era of therapeutic cardiac catheterization for congenital heart disease. Cardiol Young 9:266–272

Imaging of Great Vessels

Oliver R. Tann, Jan Bogaert, Andrew M. Taylor,
and Vivek Muthurangu

Contents

1 **Introduction** ... 611

2 **Magnetic Resonance Imaging Techniques** ... 612
2.1 Contrast-Enhanced Magnetic Resonance Angiography ... 612
2.2 3D Whole-Heart MRA ... 616
2.3 Cine Imaging ... 616
2.4 Black-Blood Imaging ... 617
2.5 Phase-Contrast Imaging ... 619

3 **Disease of the Great Vessels** ... 619
3.1 Aorta ... 619
3.2 Pulmonary Arteries ... 640
3.3 Pulmonary Veins ... 644
3.4 Systemic Veins ... 649

4 **Conclusion** ... 650
4.1 The Future ... 650

5 **Keypoints** ... 651

References ... 651

A. M. Taylor · V. Muthurangu (✉)
Cardio-Respiratory Unit, Hospital for Children,
Great Ormond Street, London, WC1N 3JH, UK
e-mail: v.muthurangu@ucl.ac.uk

O. R. Tann
Consultant in Cardiovascular Imaging,
Cardio-Respiratory Unit, Great Ormond Street Hospital
for Children, London, WC1N 3JH, UK

J. Bogaert
Deptartment of Radiology,
Katholieke Universiteit Leuven,
University Hospital Leuven, Herestraat 49,
3000 Leuven, Belgium

Abstract
Imaging the great vessels is important in the clinical management of many forms of cardiovascular disease. Cross-sectional imaging has many advantages when assessing the great vessels and in this chapter the role of MRI will be reviewed. Specifically, the uses of different MRI sequences will be discussed in relation to different great vessel diseases. This will be followed by an in-depth discussion of important great vessel diseases and the most suitable types of MRI. By the end of this chapter the reader should have a better idea of how to use MRI when assessing the great vessels.

1 Introduction

The great vessels is a collective term for the large vessels that enter and leave the heart, and includes the aorta, pulmonary arteries and pulmonary veins, and the caval veins. Assessment of the great vessels is highly reliant on imaging.

In pediatric and adult practice the mainstay of cardiac imaging is echocardiography. While echocardiography provides excellent delineation of intracardiac anatomy and function, it remains limited at assessing the extracardiac vascular tree. In order to assess these structures more accurately, a second-tier of investigations is required. Cross-sectional imaging such as computed tomography (CT), and magnetic resonance imaging (MRI) are increasingly being used. One of the main advantages of CT and MRI is the acquisition of isotropic 3D datasets that can be reconstructed in any imaging plane, and therefore

J. Bogaert et al. (eds.), *Clinical Cardiac MRI*, Medical Radiology. Diagnostic Imaging,
DOI: 10.1007/174_2011_422,

allow complete visualization of complex great vessel pathology. The choice of modality is currently dependent on local expertise and availability.

As well as excellent anatomical definition, MRI is able to assess complex hemodynamics; associated valve anomalies; and cardiac anatomy and function in one examination. MRI is multiplanar, and crucially, does not use ionizing radiation, and can therefore be used confidently for long-term follow-up. MRI continues to advance with faster sequences, improved spatial and temporal resolution, and better post-processing techniques. This means that not only are examinations becoming quicker, but that the information acquired is better, and can be displayed in increasingly sophisticated ways to aid clinical decision-making. Because of this, MRI is widely considered to be the modality of choice for both pre- and post-operative evaluation of diseases that affect the great vessels.

X-ray guided cardiac catheterization is still important, but is reserved for when there remains diagnostic uncertainty, for when pressure measurement is essential, and for when other imaging suggests that a lesion may require catheter intervention.

In clinical practice, the primary focus of great vessel assessment is on anatomy, including pathological changes, and their hemodynamic consequences. Increasingly, attention is turning toward assessment of the biomechanical properties of the great vessels, including the evaluation of cardiovascular responses to stress. As these MRI techniques develop, it is possible that we may be able to noninvasively identify asymptomatic at-risk individuals, and have a more sensitive way of monitoring disease progression and response to treatment.

In this chapter, the use of MRI in the diagnosis and management of patients with congenital and acquired diseases of the great vessels is discussed.

2 Magnetic Resonance Imaging Techniques

2.1 Contrast-Enhanced Magnetic Resonance Angiography

Contrast-enhanced magnetic resonance angiography (ceMRA) is the most widely used and valuable technique for imaging the great vessels (Leung and Debatin 1997; Dymarkowski et al. 1999; Razavi and Baker 1999; Masui et al. 2000) (Table 1). The bright intravascular signal visualized relies on the T1-shortening properties of dilute gadolinium. ceMRA has been shown to be accurate in the assessment of both dilated and stenotic vessels, and compares well to X-ray angiographic and surgical findings. However, it should be used in conjunction with other sequences to avoid missing important pathology.

Table 1 Indications for ceMRA

Aortic aneurysm
Aortic dissection
Congenital anomalies of great vessels
Vasculitis evaluation
Central thoracic veins
Pulmonary artery anatomy
Post-surgical follow-up
Contraindications to CT

It is important to time the ceMRA accurately such that data acquisition occurs when contrast is within the area of interest. Timings will vary between different patients, and even in the same patient performed at different times (Francois et al. 2003). The bolus-track technique is now recognized as the optimal solution with reliability of 98.5% for bolus detection (Riederer et al. 2000) (Fig. 1). Other timing methods include using a test bolus (Earls et al. 1996) and moving-table MRA (Ho et al. 1999). An automated bolus detection algorithm has also been developed for optimization of ceMRA (Ho and Foo 1998).

With the bolus-track technique, contrast is visualized by a 2D fluoroscopic preview scan which displays the bolus arrival in real-time. The 3D ceMRA is triggered when the contrast is visualized in the area of interest. Using a suitable MRI compatible injector, 0.2–0.4 mL/kg of gadolinium is injected at 2–4 mL/s by way of an intravenous cannula. The bolus-track technique should be combined with a centric-order phase-encode MRA sequence, such that central phase-encode steps that encode for bulk contrast are acquired first, and peripheral phase-encode steps that encode for edge definition are acquired at the end of the sequence. Not only does this ensures high contrast, but it also minimizes image blurring if the patient is unable to maintain the breath-hold for the entire scan duration (Fig. 2). It should be noted that on most scanners, there is a small delay when

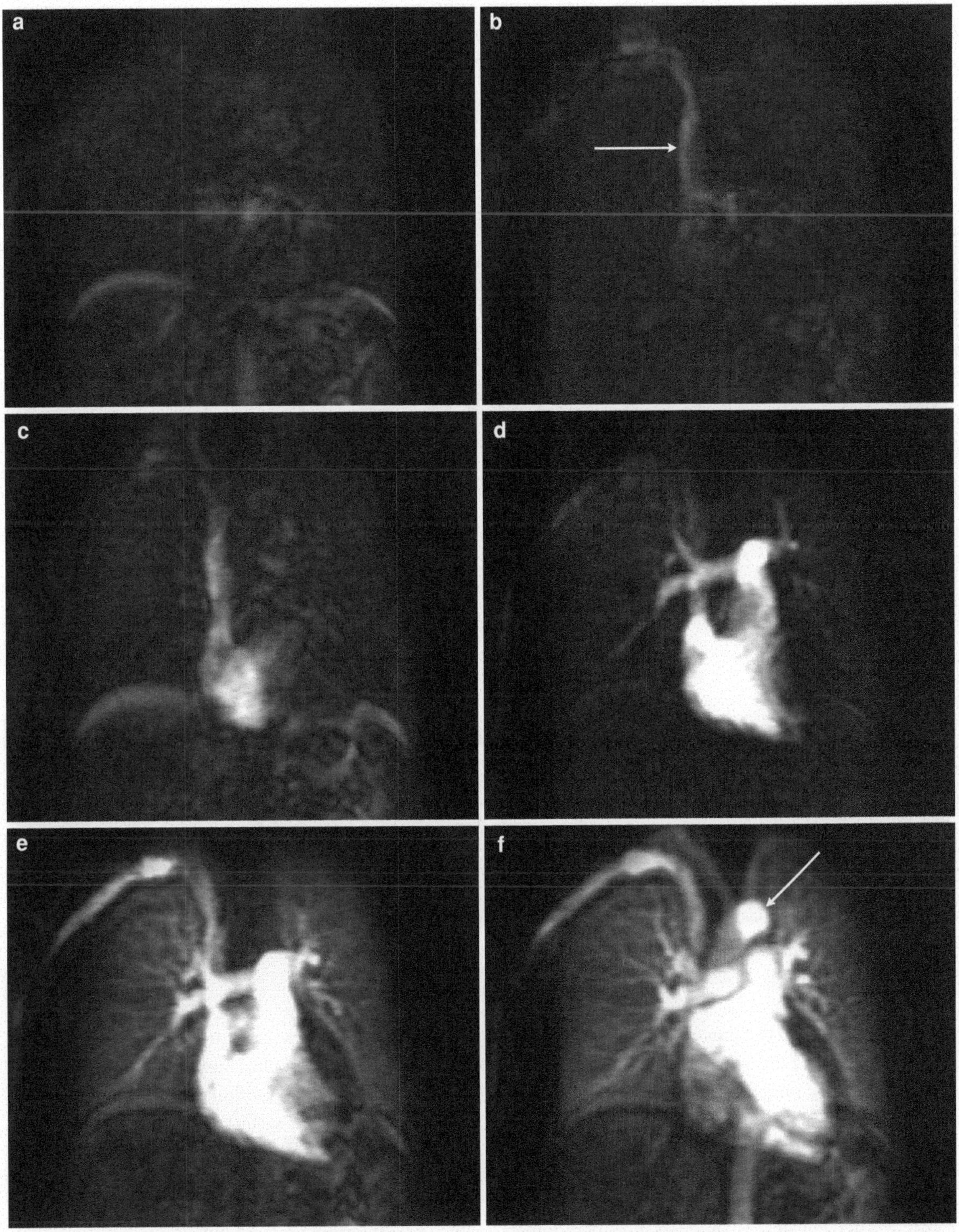

Fig. 1 Selected coronal 2D 'bolus-track' images from a 20 s (20 image) sequence. **a** Image before gadolinium contrast administration, **b** contrast arriving in the superior vena cava (*arrow*), **c** contrast in the right atrium, **d** contrast in the pulmonary trunk (trigger for pulmonary MRA at this time point), **e** contrast passing through the pulmonary parenchyma, **f** contrast reaching the aortic arch (*arrow*) (trigger for aortic MRA at this time point)

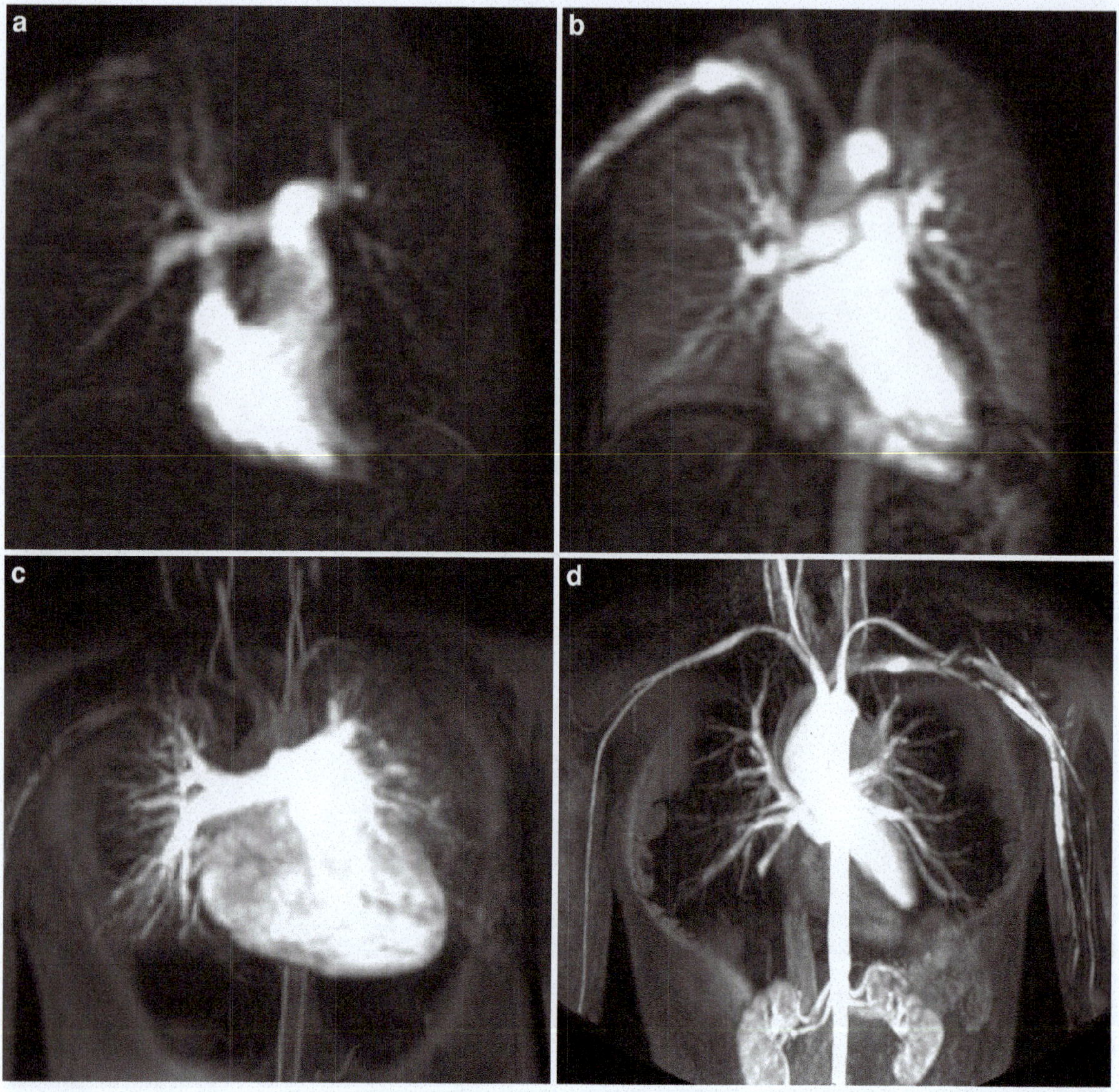

Fig. 2 Triggers for pulmonary (**a**) and aortic (**b**) angiograms. Coronal pulmonary (**c**) and systemic (**d**) arterial maximum-intensity projection images viewed from anterior

switching from the 2D bolus-track sequence to the MRA sequence, and this should be taken into account for optimal MRA imaging. However it is important not to trigger too early, as this will produce a characteristic tramline effect along the vessel wall.

ceMRA images can be acquired in approximately 10–14 s (using parallel imaging techniques, see "Cardiac MRI Physics"), and thus two angiograms can be acquired in a single 20s breath-hold. In our own experience, this enables the acquisition of an optimal pulmonary ceMRA (triggered as contrast enters the main pulmonary artery), and an optimal aortic ceMRA, which is acquired after the transit of contrast through the pulmonary vasculature.

Post-processing algorithms such as maximum-intensity projection, surface and volume rendering, and multi-planar reformatting provide very useful images that help to delineate and better understand complex vascular anatomy. However these should always be interpreted in conjunction with the raw data (Fig. 3). Care needs to be taken when measuring vessels using ceMRA since the images are not ECG-gated, with image blurring due to cardiac motion. In addition, signal dropout will occur in

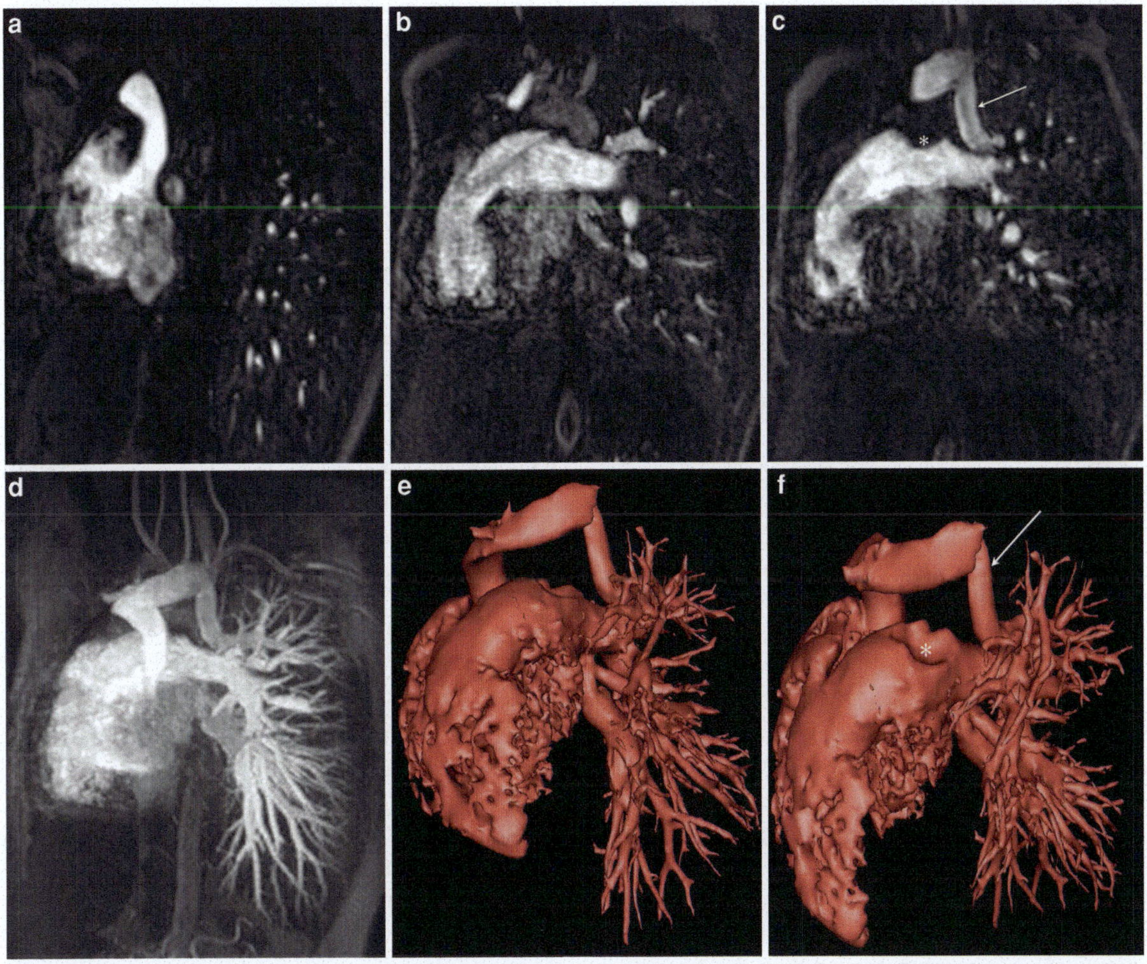

Fig. 3 A 45-year-old woman who had a right pneumonectomy for right lung dysplasia was sent for investigation of progressive breathlessness—reconstruction of the ceMRA data. **a–c** Selected coronal pulmonary ceMRA raw data (three images from 144). **d** maximum-intensity projection reconstruction of the ceMRA raw data viewed from anterior. **e**, **f** Volume-rendered 3D reconstruction viewed from anterior, and anterior with superior angulation. Images demonstrate unexpected partial anomalous pulmonary venous drainage of the left upper lobe pulmonary vein (*arrow*), and also an unexpected filling defect (*asterisk*) in the left pulmonary artery due to a chronic laminated thrombus

regions of flow acceleration, with resultant overestimation of stenosis. In our experience, ceMRA should be performed early within any protocol assessing the great vessels. This has the advantage of being able to use the ceMRA data to plan image planes for subsequent sequences, (by performing and saving multiplanar reformatted images to the scanning console), and also alerts the imager to any unexpected findings.

An alternative technique to standard ceMRA is time-resolved ceMRA (Korosec et al. 1996; Finn et al. 2002). The developments of ultrafast pulse sequences, phased multi-array surface coils, and parallel data acquisition techniques, have increased the clinical applicability of time-resolved MRA (Lohan et al. 2008). Time-resolved ceMRA is dynamic, and displays vascular filling in a manner similar to conventional X-ray angiography by rapidly acquiring sequential images. This eliminates the need to time the contrast bolus, it ensures peak vascular contrast is acquired, and provides temporal information on the dynamics of blood flow. The rapid frame rates means there is no appreciable reduction in image quality in patients who cannot hold their breath. Hence, this scanning method is suitable for scanning critically ill patients

(Carr and Finn 2003). Additionally, time-resolved MRA requires substantially less intravenous contrast than standard ceMRA, which is particularly advantageous when imaging patients with impaired renal function (Kim et al. 2008). The main drawback of time-resolved angiography is reduced spatial resolution.

Time-resolved ceMRA has been shown to be useful for a range of abnormalities involving the great vessels including delineation of complex vascular anatomy, arteriovenous malformations, aortic dissections, subclavian steal syndrome, defining flow direction, delineation of collateral pathways, and mapping of altered lung perfusion associated with pulmonary artery occlusion (Krishnam et al. 2008).

2.2 3D Whole-Heart MRA

3D whole-heart imaging is an excellent technique for both great vessel assessment and depiction of intracardiac anatomy, as it provides a high contrast between the blood-pool and surrounding tissues without the necessity of contrast agents (Razavi et al. 2003). Despite this, ceMRA is often performed before 3D whole-heart imaging as it provides complementary information, and the T1 shortening effect of gadolinium increases the intravascular signal observed in bright-blood imaging techniques.

The 3D whole-heart sequence is a free-breathing, isotropic, 3D data acquisition, which allows high-resolution images to be reconstructed from the raw data in any image plane (Sorensen et al. 2004). In patients who are unable to breath-hold, whole-heart imaging can still produce excellent anatomical depiction of the great vessels, since a respiratory navigator tracks diaphragmatic movement. Data should be acquired during periods when cardiac motion and flow is at a minimum. In most patients this is during mid to late diastole. This will vary between patients, even in those with the same heart rate, and can be assessed by visualizing a four-chamber cine image. However in patients with high heart rates, particularly in children, the mid to late diastolic time period is markedly decreased, and imaging is best performed at end systole. The end systolic rest period in these circumstances is of a more constant duration and position in the cardiac cycle (Tangcharoen et al. 2011). Systolic imaging is also useful in patients with diastolic flow artifact, either due to high volume flow in the case of shunts, or high velocity flow in the case of tricuspid or mitral valve stenosis. This is also best assessed on the four-chamber cine image.

2.3 Cine Imaging

Cine imaging of the great vessels can be used to highlight regions of abnormal flow acceleration or turbulence, and should be accompanied by cine imaging of the heart to detect accompanying lesions (Higgins and Sakuma 1996), and assess ventriculo-arterial interaction. Cine imaging can also be used to assess regional vessel wall compliance (Chien et al. 1994; Forbat et al. 1995).

The most common form of cine imaging used is 2D-balanced steady state free precession (b-SSFP) (Oppelt et al. 1986; Carr et al. 2001; Pereles et al. 2001). Again, it provides a high contrast between the blood-pool and surrounding tissue without the use of contrast agents. Usually, it is a breath-hold, retrospectively gated, segmented *k*-space acquisition technique with an average imaging time of 8–12 s/slice. Changing the number of lines acquired per segment of *k*-space alters the temporal resolution of the image. Each cine image can be optimized such that a temporal resolution of 30–40 ms is achieved in patients scanned without sedation, and 20–30 ms in anesthetized patients with rapid heart rates. These cine images can be acquired in any orientation to depict the relevant anatomy. A sagittal oblique image through the upper chest is particularly useful for demonstrating the aortic arch (Carr and Finn 2003) (Fig. 4).

Another form of cine imaging used is spoiled gradient echo (GRE) imaging. This has lower contrast than b-SSFP, and hence it is not used routinely. Nevertheless, it is also less susceptible to artifact, and can be particularly useful when artifact from metal clips or coils in the chest obscures important detail on b-SSFP imaging. It is also useful and in the case of stent imaging (Nordmeyer et al. 2010a).

An alternative cine technique in patients who cannot hold their breath is standard real-time imaging, as it does not require breath holding or ECG triggering (Lee et al. 2002). Diagnostic images of the great vessels can usually be obtained at reduced spatial and temporal resolution. Newer real-time techniques with greater undersampling and thus greater temporal and spatial resolution are also available such as radial *k-t* SENSE (Muthurangu et al. 2008).

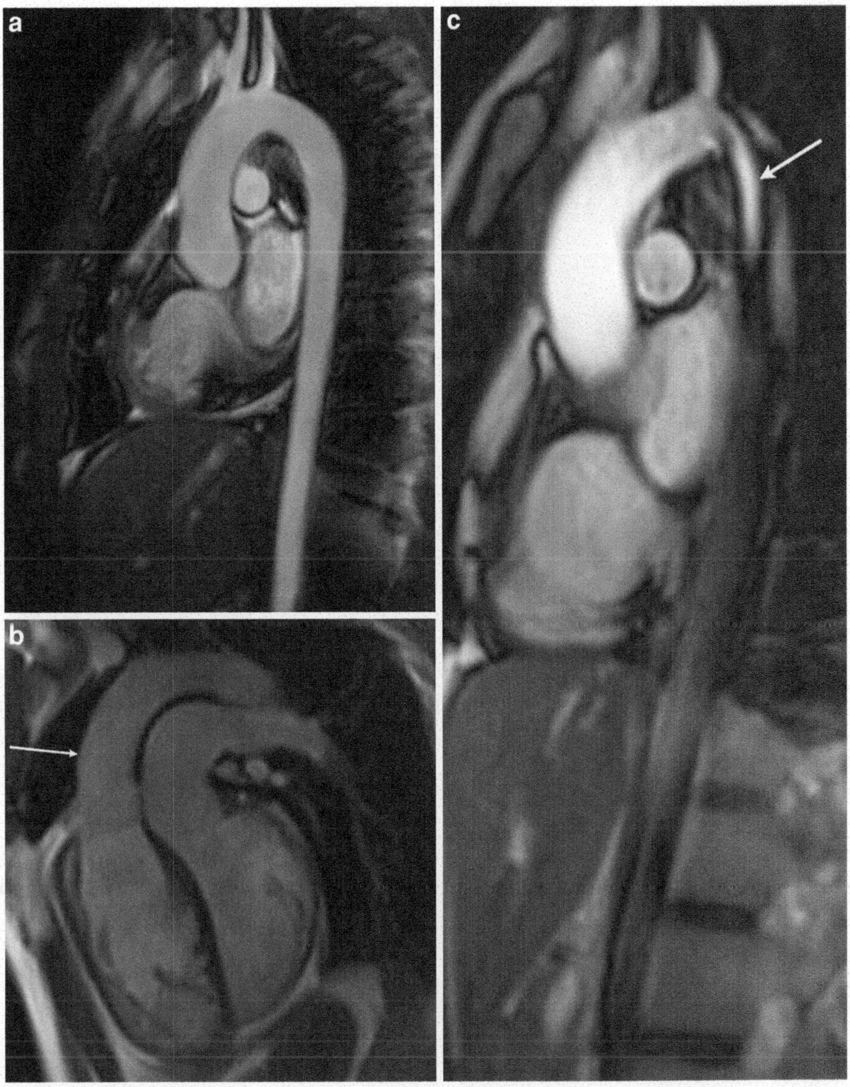

Fig. 4 Oblique sagittal cine images through the aorta. **a** Normal aorta, **b** normal aortic anatomy in transposition of great arteries. The aorta (*arrow*) lies anterior to the pulmonary trunk. **c** Accelerative flow across a coarctation repair site (*arrow*)

2.4 Black-Blood Imaging

Black-blood pulse sequences remain an essential component of great vessel imaging for evaluation of the lumen, vessel wall and for the mediastinum (Simonetti et al. 1996; Stemerman et al. 1999) (Fig. 5). Black-blood images appear black because of signal loss from moving spins in the blood pool. Contrast is improved by high velocity blood flow as is seen in regions of vascular and valvular stenosis. For this reason, images are best acquired during systole.

The use of multiple signal averages increases the spatial resolution making it excellent for anatomical delineation. Black-blood imaging is particularly good at assessing vessel wall thickening associated with arteritis, for looking at vascular membranes as seen in aortic coarctation, and visualizing dissection flaps.

It should be noted that signal loss is seen in areas of calcification (Martinez et al. 1992), and within metallic stents (Nordmeyer et al. 2010b), and therefore stenosis can be missed.

A single-shot ECG-triggered black-blood half-Fourier acquisition can also be used, (Stehling et al. 1996) and allows acquisition of an entire image in a single heartbeat. This is useful for both planning imaging planes when acquired at the beginning of the scan, and also for patients who cannot hold their breath (Carr and Finn 2003).

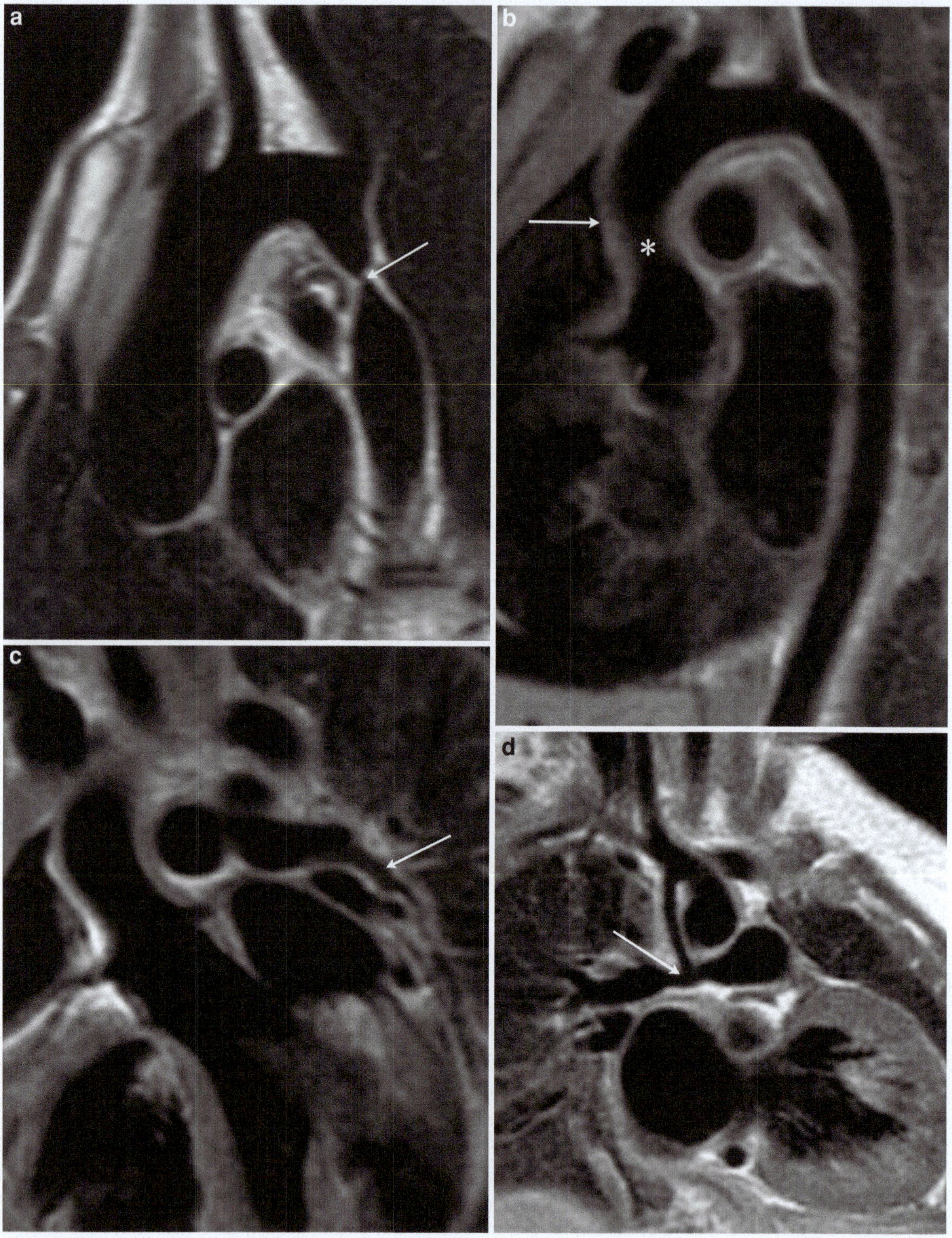

Fig. 5 Black-blood images. **a** Oblique sagittal image through the aorta showing a severe circumferential waist-like coarctation (*arrow*). **b** and **c** Selected images in a patient with Williams syndrome. **b** Oblique sagittal image through the aorta showing supravalvar aortic stenosis (*asterisk*), arterial wall thickening (*arrow*), and long-segment narrowing of the descending aorta. **c** Oblique coronal image through the left pulmonary artery showing severe stenosis of the left lower lobe branch pulmonary artery (*arrow*). **d** Right modified Blalock-Taussig shunt in a 4-month-old child with Tetralogy of Fallot. There is moderate narrowing of the right pulmonary artery at the site of anastomosis (*arrow*)

2.5 Phase-Contrast Imaging

Calculation of blood flow and velocity is important in the complete assessment of the great vessels. Phase-contrast MRI (PC-MRI) is the gold standard for quantifying flow volume, making it invaluable for quantification of shunts in the case of anomalous pulmonary venous drainage. The pulmonary to systemic blood flow ratio (Qp:Qs) can be calculated by measuring flow in the main pulmonary artery and comparing it to the flow in the ascending aorta. In aortic coarctation, PC-MRI can be used to calculate the amount of collateral flow present by measuring blood flow proximal and distal to the region of narrowing.

PC-MRI can be used to measure peak velocity across stenoses, and give an estimated pressure gradient. Analysis of the curve shape and slope can also help determine whether stenoses are significant (Carr and Finn 2003). This enables the monitoring of diseases for evidence of progression and suitability for intervention.

It is important to be aware that PC-MRI accuracy depends on laminar flow. In regions of turbulence, flow calculations can be inaccurate (Fatouraee and Amini 2003). In these circumstances surrogate flow measurement can be used. Combined branch pulmonary artery flow can be used as a marker of main pulmonary artery flow in patients with pulmonary regurgitation. Pulmonary venous return can be used to determine net pulmonary flow, which is particularly useful in patients with systemic to pulmonary artery shunts, and in the total cavo-pulmonary circulation. SVC and IVC flow can be used to measure systemic flow in patients with aortic valve disease.

PC-MRI can be performed using either through-plane or in-plane techniques. Through-plane imaging provides accurate assessment of velocity, and flow volume. The in-plane technique provides direct visualization of the flow acceleration, maximum velocity, and direction within a prescribed 2D plane. Using PC-MRI with either through-plane or in-plane techniques, blood flow mechanics can be mapped in every dimension of the great vessels (Kilner et al. 1993).

An alternative method of flow imaging is to use 4D flow. This technique can accurately quantify, simultaneously acquired, great vessel blood flow including pulmonary venous and systemic venous flow (Nordmeyer et al. 2010b). Using 4D flow imaging data is acquired as a 3D volume, which obviates the need for planning 2D-imaging planes. In addition, there are a variety of methods for visualizing and analyzing the 4D flow velocity data that are not available by conventional 2D PC-MRI (Hope et al. 2010). 4D flow (Markl et al. 2003a; Bammer et al. 2007) has also been used to characterize multidirectional flow patterns in the normal and diseased aorta furthering our understanding about the complex interaction of flow patterns, and the development of aortic pathology (Weigang et al. 2008; Hope et al. 2007).

3 Disease of the Great Vessels

3.1 Aorta

The aorta serves two important functions both structural and functional. Firstly it acts as a conduit through which blood is distributed around the body. Secondly, through the 'windkessel' effect, it acts as an elastic reservoir, converting the pulsatile ejection of blood into a steady stream of flow. In addition, the vascular endothelium maintains vascular homeostasis by the release of vasoactive substances.

While CT provides excellent structural assessment of the aorta, MRI can provide additional complex hemodynamic information to complement excellent visualization of the vessel lumen and wall, and can also be used to assess endothelial responses to stimuli (Leeson et al. 2006). Furthermore, MRI provides accurate assessment of associated valve anomalies, and cardiac anatomy and function. It is important to note that the function of the systemic vasculature, and systemic ventricle is intertwined, with dysfunction of one affecting the other through their ventriculo-arterial interactions. Thus, MRI has a vital role to play in the evaluation of both congenital and acquired anomalies of the aorta.

There is increasing interest in measuring the biomechanical properties of the aorta. In the adult population, arterial compliance is reduced in normal aging, hypertension, atherosclerosis, diabetes, and heart failure. In children, reduced compliance is seen in patients with congenital heart disease in particular conotruncal anomalies (Senzaki et al. 2008), connective tissue disease (Groenink et al. 2001), and following aortic arch repair and reconstruction (Ou et al. 2008; Voges et al. 2010). Early detection of arterial dysfunction could be useful in the identification of early disease in asymptomatic individuals, for monitoring disease progression and assessing response to treatment.

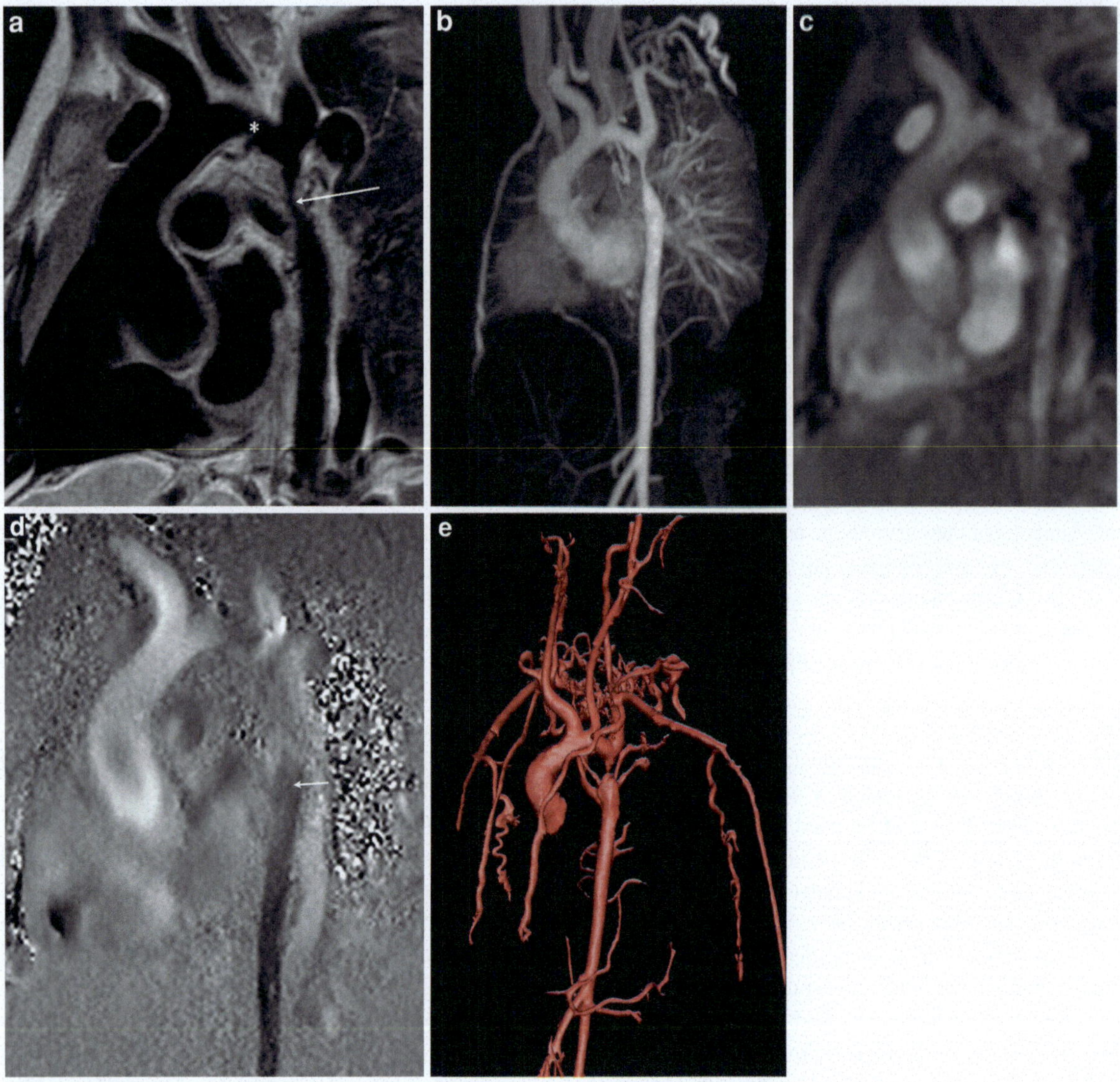

Fig. 6 A 10-year-old girl with unrepaired aortic coarctation—selected images from a single MRI study. **a** Black-blood oblique sagittal image through the aorta showing a severe long-segment aortic coarctation involving the aortic isthmus (*arrow*). Note also the hypoplasia of the aortic arch (*asterisk*). **b** maximum-intensity projection image from the ceMRA—multiple collateral vessels can be seen. Magnitude **c** and phase **d** images demonstrate flow acceleration in the descending thoracic aorta (*arrow*). **e** Volume-rendered 3D reconstruction of the ceMRA—the collateral vessels are clearly demonstrated

3.1.1 Congenital Anomalies of the Aorta

3.1.1.1 Aortic Coarctation

Aortic coarctation represents a narrowing of the aorta typically occurring just distal to the origin of the left subclavian artery in the region of the ductus arteriosus. It accounts for 6–8% of live births with congenital heart disease (Samanak et al. 1989), and there is an increased incidence in patients with Turner syndrome (Gotzsche et al. 1994). It represents a spectrum of lesions ranging from a discrete shelf-like lesion or waist, through long-segment tubular hypoplasia, to, at the extreme end of the spectrum, complete interruption of the aortic arch (Hoschtitzky et al. 2009) (Fig. 6).

Most patients present within the first three months of life, when arterial duct closure critically limits blood flow to the lower body. In these circumstances,

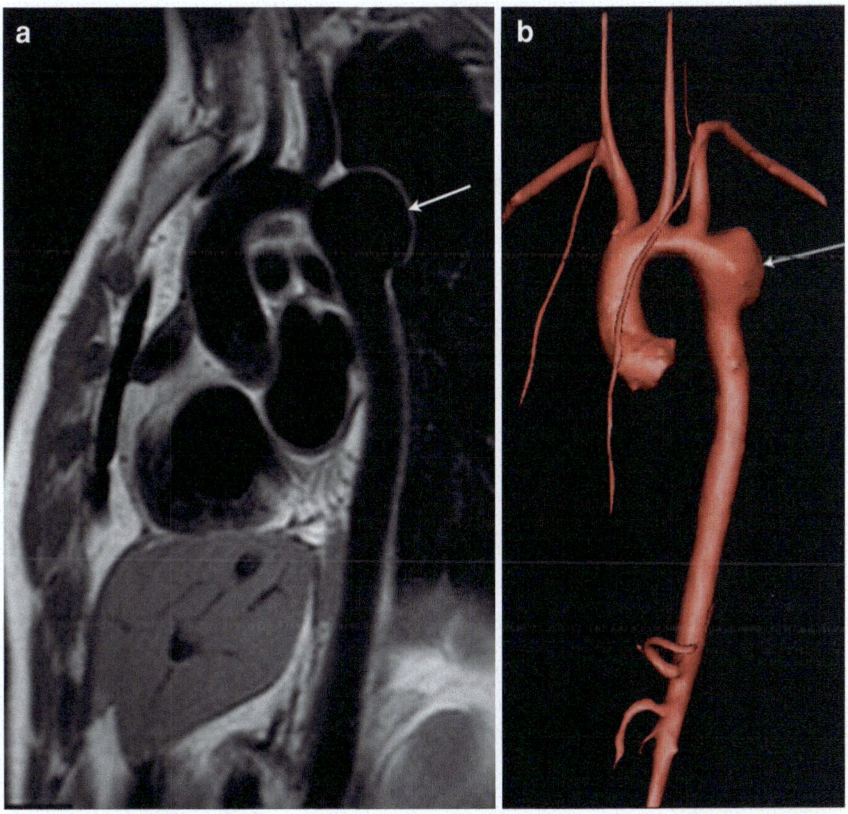

Fig. 7 Large proximal descending aorta psuedoaneurysm, complicating a previous patch aortoplasty repair. **a** Black-blood oblique sagittal view and **b** volume-rendered 3D reconstruction from ceMRA showing a large pseudoaneurysm (*arrow*)

echocardiography usually suffices in terms of pre-operative assessment. Occasionally, coarctation presents much later because of unexplained systemic arterial hypertension or as an incidental finding when evaluating a murmur in a patient with bicuspid aortic valve disease or a VSD. Current guidelines suggest that all these patients should be examined with MRI or CT (ACC/AHA 2008 Guidelines for the Management of Adults with Congenital Heart Disease) (Warnes et al. 2008).

However the main role of cross-sectional imaging is in the long-term follow-up of treated patients because despite relief of the initial obstruction, long-term complications are common. Systemic hypertension develops in a group of patients at rest and a majority are hypertensive during exercise (Daniels et al. 1987). Re-coarctation occurs in 3–35% of patients (Roos-Hesselink et al. 2003; Dietl et al. 1992), and aneurysm formation occurs in 5% of patients (Knyshov et al. 1996; Giordano et al. 2005; Bogaert et al. 1995; Kaemmerer et al. 1993). This is a serious complication because of the risk of rupture (Fig. 7).

The diagnostic strategy for evaluation of aortic coarctation falls into three main areas:

- Anatomical assessment of the lesion itself;
- Functional assessment of the lesion and its effects; and
- Assessment of treatment complications.MRI where available should be considered the investigation of choice for both pre-operative assessments in the older patient, and the long-term follow-up of patients with coarctation repair (Bogaert et al. 2000, 2001), as it can provide complete assessment in one examination (Gomes et al. 1987; von Schulthess et al. 1986).

3D ceMRA is an excellent first-line technique, and can show the location, length, relationship to the left subclavian artery, associated arch hypoplasia, and assess for post-stenotic dilatation. More than any other technique, ceMRA is particularly good at visualization of the collateral circulation. It should be remembered that signal dropout occurs in regions of flow acceleration, with resultant overestimation of stenosis, and therefore ceMRA should not be used alone. ceMRA is also good at assessing complications

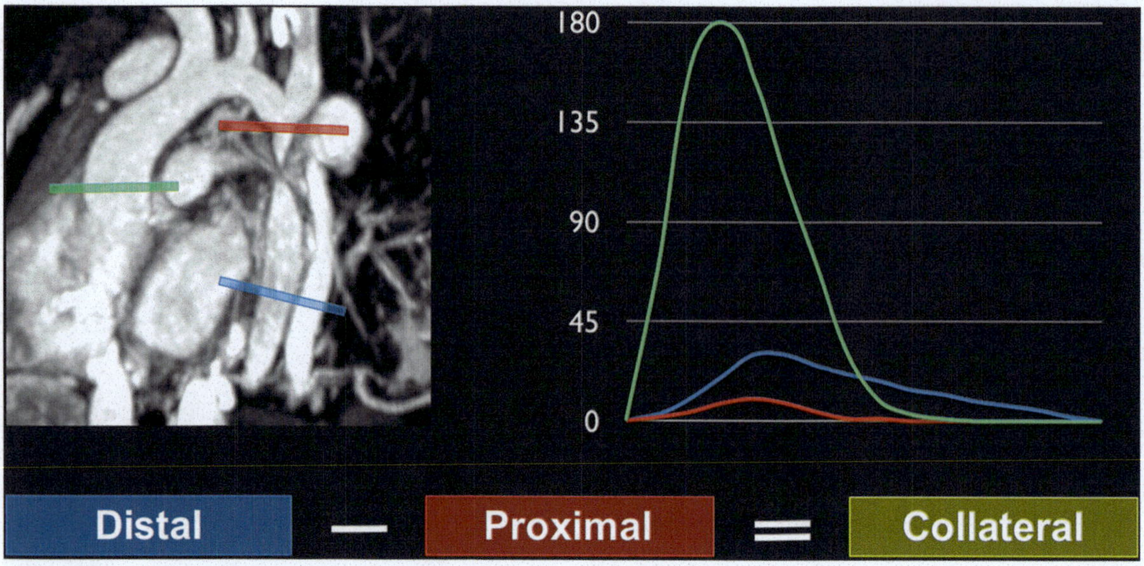

Fig. 8 Collateral flow assessment in aortic coarctation. Flow is measured just prior to the coarctation (*red bar*, and *red curve*) and in the descending aorta at the level of the diaphragm (*blue bar*, and *blue curve*). Planes prescribed of an oblique sagittal maximum-intensity projection image from a 3D whole-heart. Collateral flow is calculated, by taking proximal flow away from distal flow. In this example, flow at the diaphragm is higher than that in the proximal descending aorta, indicating extensive collateral flow to the descending aorta, and a significant coarctation. This method is best used for follow-up of treated aorta coarctation to assess the success (reduced collateral flow) in individual subjects. Flow above the aortic valve (*green bar*, and *green curve*) is shown for comparison

of treatment such as true aneurysms and pseudoaneurysm formation (see Sect. 3.1.2).

3D whole-heart imaging is a good technique to follow the ceMRA because the T1 shortening effect of gadolinium increases the intravascular signal of the whole-heart sequence. It is excellent for accurate aortic measurement, and assessment of associated abnormalities, in particular in the aortic root and proximal ascending aorta, which are often affected by cardiac motion blurring during ceMRA (non-ECG-gated technique). However, signal loss in regions of flow acceleration may limit assessment of the region of coarctation itself. This is reduced but not eliminated by performing the sequence during diastole.

It is important to perform cine images in the region of coarctation, or sites of previous repair. These can identify regions of narrowing and flow acceleration, which are occasionally unsuspected on 3D imaging. In particular it is important to look at the width of the jet of acceleration in comparison to the perceived true lumen. Narrower jets may indicate intraluminal webs or membranes. These can then be confirmed with high-resolution black-blood imaging along the planes the cine images were performed (Holmqvist et al. 2002). Black-blood imaging is improved by high flow, and is therefore particularly suited to the assessment of coarctation, when other sequences suffer from signal loss.

The functional assessment of coarctation relates to the effect on the ventricle, and estimation of the pressure gradient across the region of narrowing. Cine imaging should be used to perform volumetric analysis of the ventricles, and assess for left ventricular hypertrophy by measuring left ventricular mass.

Both through-plane and in-plane PC-MRI can define the severity of the stenosis by measuring the maximum flow velocity across the coarctation, although in tortuous coarctation segments estimation of the velocity may be difficult (Mohiaddin et al. 1993; Fattori and Nienaber 1999). It is important to note that in-plane measurements can underestimate maximum flow velocity if they are not orientated exactly along the plane of the highest velocity. The maximum velocity can be used to estimate the pressure gradient across the region of narrowing. The combination of anatomical and flow can then be used to determine the need for intervention (Nielsen et al. 2005).

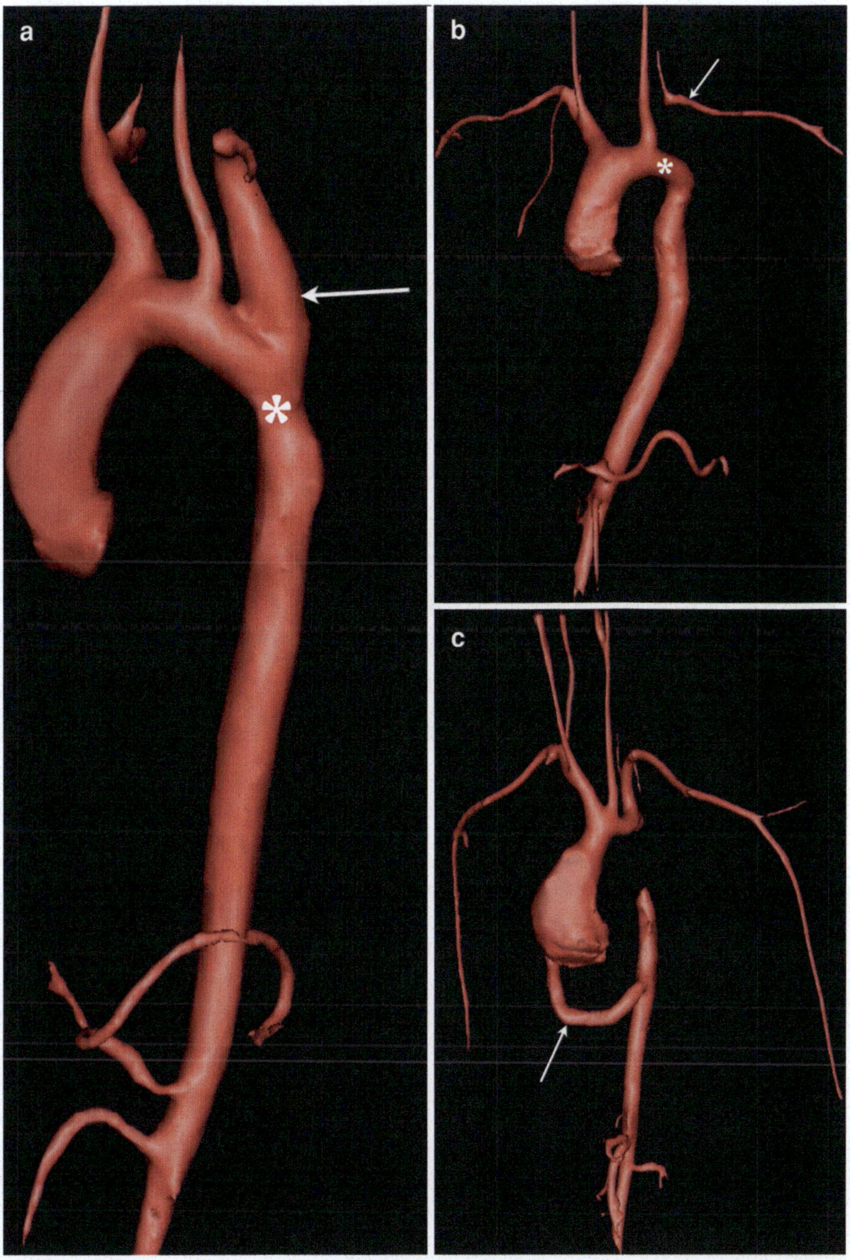

Fig. 9 Volume-rendered images from ceMRAs showing appearances of different types of coarctation repair. **a** End-to-end anastamosis with mild residual aortic narrowing (*asterisk*), and dilatation of the left subclavian artery (*arrow*). **b** Left subclavian flap repair with mild hypoplasia of the aortic arch and proximal descending thoracic aorta (*asterisk*), and retrograde filling of the left subclavian artery from the left vertebral artery (*arrow*). **c** Extra-anatomic conduit (*arrow*) in a patient with a long-segment severe coarctation

PC-MRI can also determine the amount of collateral flow present. This can be calculated, by measuring flow in the proximal and diaphragmatic descending aorta (Holmqvist et al. 2002; Szolar et al. 1996). Reassessment of collateral flow following treatment can be used to assess the success of the treatment option (Araoz et al. 2003) (Fig. 8).

Associated cardiovascular abnormalities are common, and need to be looked for. Up to 75% of patients with coarctation have a bicuspid aortic valve, which may become stenotic and or regurgitant, and long-term, there is a risk of aortic dilatation, and subsequent dissection (Smith and Matthews 1955; Becker et al. 1970). An en-face cine of the aortic valve is essential to look at valve morphology, and in the case of stenosis to measure the orifice area by direct planimetry.

Treatment for coarctation may be achieved by surgery, or by interventional catheterization either using angioplasty or stent implantation. Several

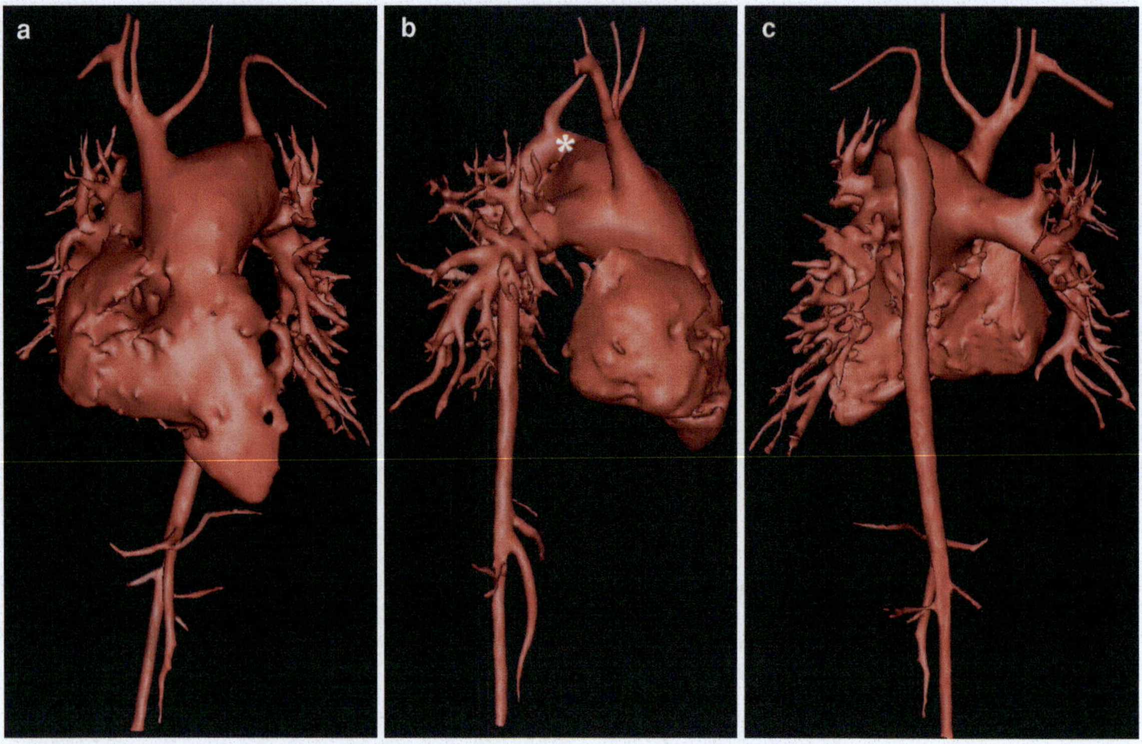

Fig. 10 A 3-year-old girl with an unrepaired common arterial trunk, type B interruption of the aortic arch, and pulmonary hypertension—selected volume-rendered 3D reconstruction from **a** ceMRA—a anterior, **b** lateral, and **c** lateral. The branch pulmonary arteries arise posteriorly from the common arterial trunk, and are dilated centrally, with peripheral pruning and tortuosity in keeping with pulmonary hypertension. The descending aorta is connected to the common trunk via a patent arterial duct (*asterisk*). The left subclavian artery arises distal to the arterial duct

Table 2 Classification of interrupted aortic arch (Van Praagh et al. 1971)

Type A (44%)
• Discontinuity of the aortic arch distal to the left subclavian artery
Type B (55%)
• Discontinuity between the left subclavian and the left common carotid arteries
Type C (5%)
• Interruption between the left common carotid and the innominate arteries

surgical techniques have been developed to treat aortic coarctation. These have different appearances on cross-sectional imaging, and it is important to be aware of them in order to interpret the findings correctly (Fig. 9). The decision to perform either surgery or treat by percutaneous intervention can be complex. However, high-resolution MRI may help define the most appropriate treatment algorithm.

3.1.1.2 Interrupted Aortic Arch

Interrupted aortic arch results from a structural discontinuity between the ascending and descending aorta. The site of interruption relative to the brachiocephalic arteries is the basis of classification (Table 2) (Fig. 10). There is a high incidence of DiGeorge syndrome (Van Mierop and Kutsche 1986), and therefore, the presence of a thymus should be looked for.

The site and length of interruption and any associated anomalies can be demonstrated well by MRI. It is important to interrogate the repair site for residual narrowing, assess for the presence of LVOT obstruction due to posterior deviation of the outlet septum, and look for residual intracardiac shunts. 3D ceMRA (Roche et al. 1999), and 3D whole-heart imaging are extremely useful as well as cine imaging to look for regions of flow acceleration, and flow evaluation in the aorta and pulmonary arteries to check for residual shunts. Black-blood imaging in the sagittal oblique plane can be used to look for a raised

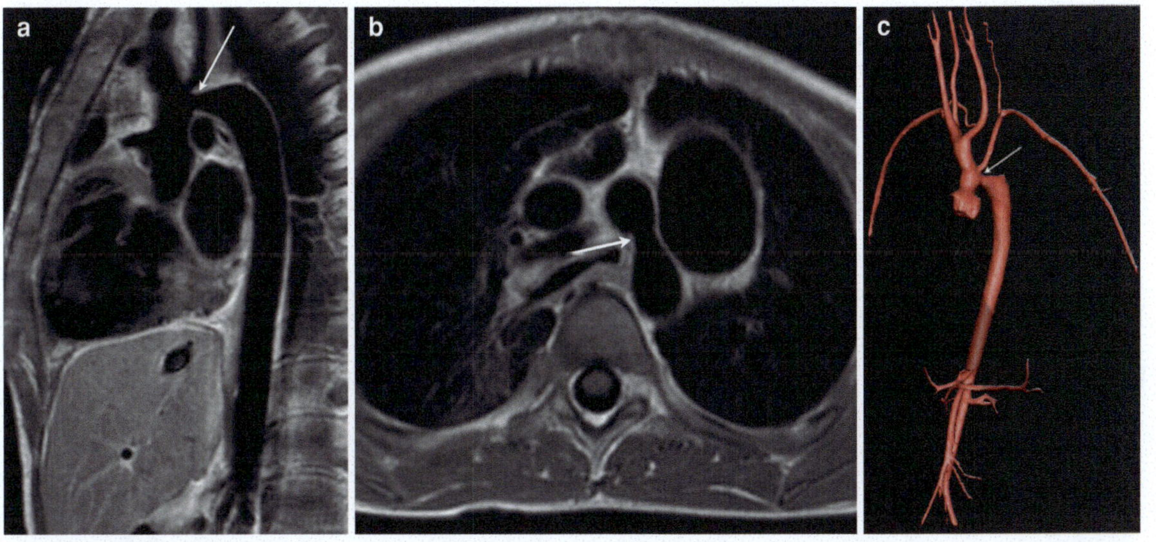

Fig. 11 Selected images from an MRI study in a patient with a repaired type A interruption of the aortic arch. **a** sagittal oblique black-blood through the aortic arch, **b** axial oblique cross-cut through the narrowest point, and **c** volume-rendered 3D reconstruction from a ceMRA showing persistent narrowing at the site of end-to-side anastamosis (*arrow*)

intraluminal ridge as a cause for narrowing at the site of surgical end-to-side anastamosis (Fig. 11).

3.1.1.3 Anomalies of the Aortic Arch

The aortic arch, ductus arteriosus, and branch pulmonary arteries have a close spatial relationship with the esophagus and major airways. Alterations in the branching pattern of the great vessels may cause significant obstruction to swallowing and breathing, due to encirclement of the esophagus and major airways, and the creation of so-called vascular rings and slings. Normal and abnormal aortic arch development is best understood using the hypothetical model of arch development proposed by Edwards (1948) (Fig. 12).

Diagnostic imaging strategies are focused on anatomical depiction, with delineation of the vascular configuration of the great vessels, and also the demonstration of compression of the surrounding structures. Both CT and MRI are equally good at demonstrating great vessel anatomy, although CT is better at visualizing the airways, and associated lung parenchymal abnormalities (Fig. 13). However there is concern about the long-term risks of radiation in children, and for this reason many centers prefer to use MRI. The functional degree of esophageal compression is best assessed separately with a barium swallow, as the degree of esophageal compression is over estimated with both CT and MRI.

3D ceMRA is the best technique for demonstrating abnormal patterns of arch development. Triggering the first run of the angiogram when there is maximum aortic contrast makes post-processing of aortic anatomy easier, and also usually shows the pulmonary arterial anatomy, with respect to clues for possible ligamentous attachments (as will be described later). A second run should also be interrogated, as occasionally it will show delayed filling of the branches, for example in the case of the isolated subclavian artery (Van Grimberge et al. 2000) (Fig. 14). In younger children who cannot hold their breath, time-resolved angiography is useful. By performing a minimum-intensity projection on the 3D data set, the airways can be visualized, although further sequences are also needed for a complete airway assessment.

The 3D-whole-heart technique is also useful, and provides improved contrast between the airway and esophagus, and the great vessels (Greil et al. 2005). Associated cardiovascular abnormalities are common, and these are also well demonstrated with this technique.

Where airway compression is suspected, high-resolution black-blood imaging is extremely good at depicting regions of narrowing. A combination of axial and coronal images can be performed in both inspiration and expiration to assess for

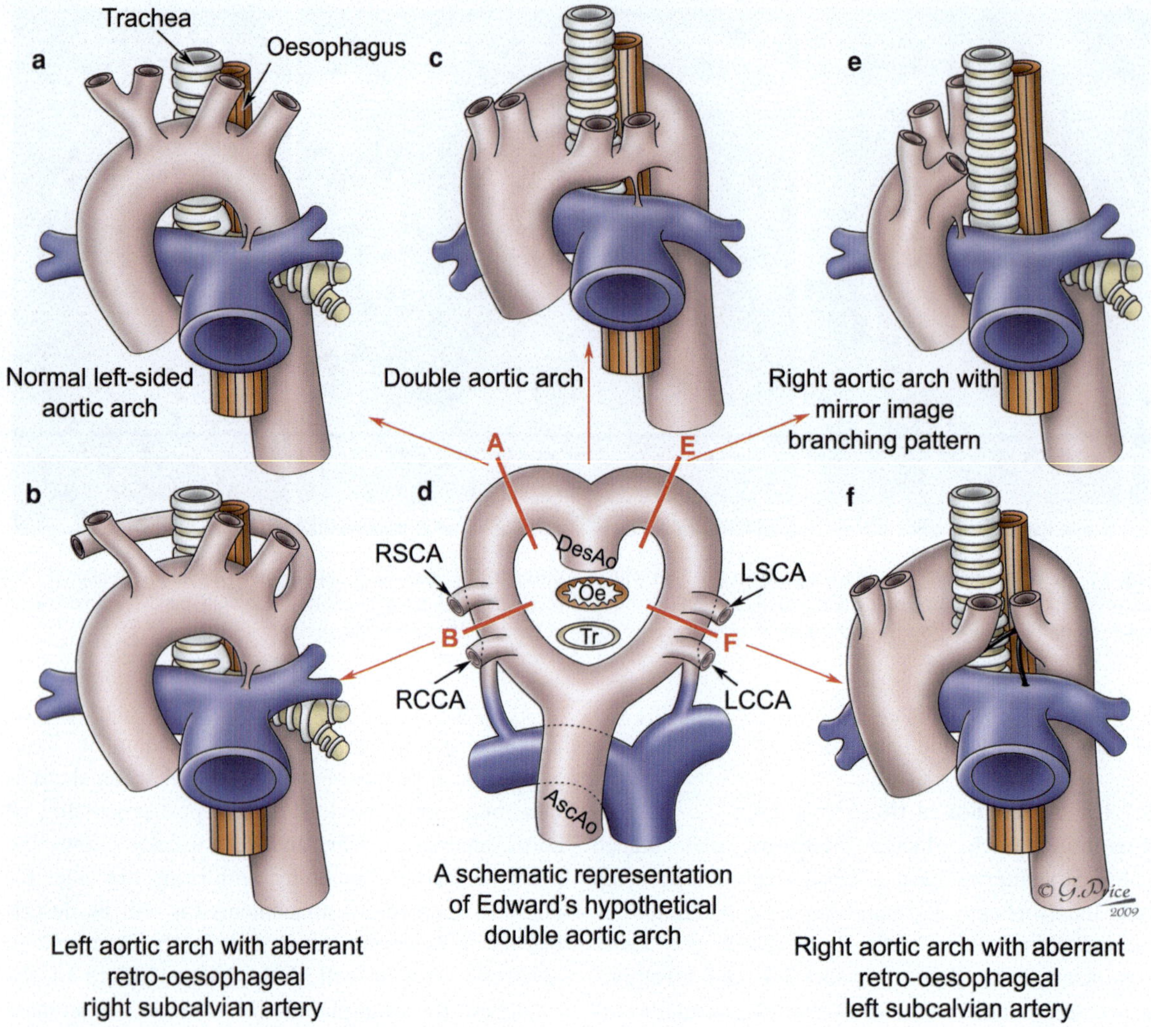

Fig. 12 **d** A schematic representation of Edward's hypothetical double aortic arch, showing right and left aortic arches and bilateral arterial ducts. Failure of arch division results in **c**, a double arch with the ringed trachea and striated esophagus within the vascular ring. Division of the double arch along the line A gives **a**, and a normal left-sided arch; ringed trachea and striated esophagus posteriorly. Division of the double arch along the line B gives **b**, a left aortic arch with aberrant, retro-esophageal right subclavian artery. Division along the line E, gives **e**, a right-sided aortic arch, with mirror-image branching. Division along the line F gives **f**, a right arch with aberrant retro-esophageal left subclavian artery. On image f, the black lines represent potential complete vascular rings of an atretic left arch (*superior line*) and a fibrotic left arterial duct (*inferior line*) [All images reproduced with permission of Gemma Price, Cardiac Unit, Institute of Child Health, who also retain full copyright.]

tracheo-bronchial malacia, and in both systole and diastole to look for dynamic compression. Another technique to assess dynamic airway compression is with real-time cine imaging (Faustet al. 2001) although the airways are not always well seen.

In the neonate, MRI can be used to diagnose arch anomalies with a feed-and-wrap technique. Using a combination of axial and coronal oblique single-shot bright-blood images, combined with black-blood imaging of the trachea, an examination can be performed in 5–10 min (Weinberg and Whitehead 2010).

The easiest arch anomaly to conceptualize, and also the commonest cause of tracheo-esophageal compression, is the double-aortic arch (Van Son et al. 1993) (Fig. 15). This represent a persistence of both left and right dorsal aortic arches, which pass either side of the trachea, before joining posteriorly to form the descending aorta.

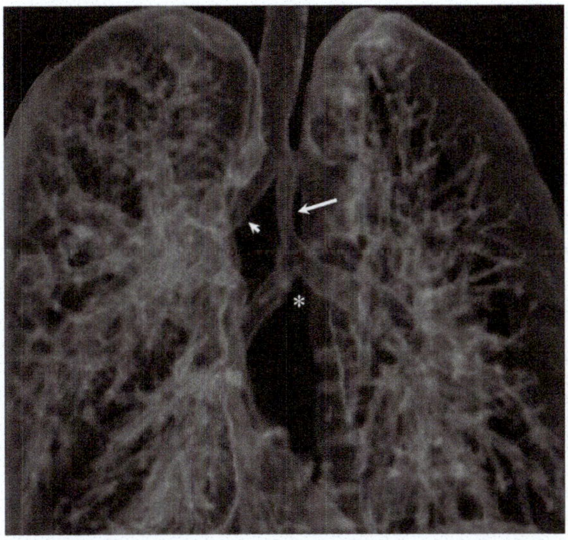

Fig. 13 Volume-rendered 3D reconstruction from a CT scan through the chest of the proximal airways in a patient with pulmonary artery sling (see Fig. 33 in "Congenital Heart Disease"). The image shows an accessory right upper lobe 'pig' bronchus (*short arrow*), and a narrowed 'stove pipe' distal trachea (*long arrow*) prior to the carina (*star*). This tracheo-bronchial anatomy is associated with the left pulmonary artery sling. Care should be taken when bronchoscopy is performed in such patients, as it is often mistaken that the carina has been visualized, when in fact the first bifurcation is at the origin of the accessory right upper lobe bronchus. [Figure courtesy of Dr. Cathy Owens, Department of Clinical Radiology, Great Ormond Street Hospital for Children, who maintains copyright]

The dominance (largest) of the arches is important, because at surgery, the surgeon will divide the smaller arch.

However, it is only the minority of rings that are entirely vascular, most are completed by atretic or ligamentous structures, which are rarely visualized. If we return to the Edwards hypothetical arch model, any embryological structure that regresses can leave behind a ligament, and this is as true for arch regression as it is for arterial ducts that close. We therefore have to look for at least two possible rings—the presumed site of the arterial duct, and between the first and last head and neck branches from the aortic arch (Fig. 16).

Any arch anomaly can give rise to a vascular ring, even a right arch with mirror-image branching pattern, in the rare circumstances of a duct from the descending aorta to the left pulmonary artery (De Leval and Elliott 2006). It is best to assume the presence of a ring until all images have been carefully scrutinized. These signs can be subtle, and volume rendering the 3D ceMRA or 3D whole-heart data sets can be extremely useful. What is commonly seen is the stenting or traction effect on the aorta, subclavian and pulmonary arteries caused by the ligamentous structures themselves. Occasionally, a ligament is suggested by a region of narrowing being simply in the region of the presumed site of the arterial duct.

In the case of a double arch completed by an atretic or ligamentous segment (Figs. 17, 18) there are several features that would suggest a vascular ring. The first is the presence of a Kommerell's diverticulum (Fig. 19). This is thought to represent the remnant of the atretic arch, and is often seen at the origin of an aberrant subclavian artery, although it can also occur in a right arch with mirror-image branching pattern. Secondly, a double arch is suggested by symmetric arrangement of the common carotid and subclavian vessels arising from the aortic arch—two either side of the trachea. Thirdly, in the case of a double arch with an atretic left arch, the proximal patent part of the atretic left arch follows a more posteriorly directed course, than the left brachiocephalic artery in the setting of a right-aortic arch with mirror-image branching pattern (Schlesinger et al. 2005). Lastly, in patients with a retro-esophageal proximal descending thoracic aorta, with the descending aorta seen to course down the opposite side of the trachea to the aortic arch (Fig. 20).

In the presence of these findings, the surgeon can be asked to operate with a high degree of certainty, identifying and transecting the fibrous connection, with immediate relief of the vascular ring.

3.1.2 Aortic Aneurysm

Aortic aneurysms are areas of focal dilatation of the aortic wall and can be classified as true aneurysms or pseudo-aneurysms. True aneurysms involve all three layers of the aortic wall (intima, media, and adventitia) and exceed the expected aortic diameter by a factor of 1.5 or more (Fattori and Nienaber 1999). Pseudo-aneurysms tend to occur because of trauma to the aortic wall, usually iatrogenic, and represent a contained leak of blood by adventitial, and peri-adventitial tissue. Importantly, there is a residual communication with the damaged vessel. The size of the communication or neck may determine the treatment strategy. Small pseudoaneurysms may spontaneously clot; those with a narrow neck may be

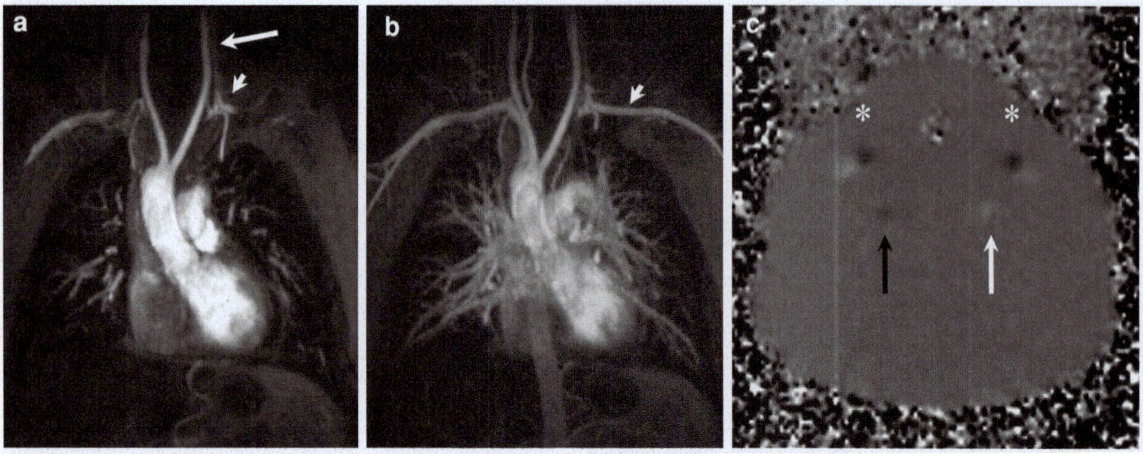

Fig. 14 Right-aortic arch with isolated left subclavian artery. **a** Coronal maximum-intensity projection of early phase of a ceMRA. The proximal left subclavian is seen (*white short arrow*), but is not directly connected to the aortic arch. The left subclavian is supplied by the left vertebral artery (*long arrow*). **b** Coronal maximum-intensity projection of late phase of a ceMRA. The left subclavian artery is now completely filled with contrast (*arrowhead*). **c** PC-MRI of arterial flow in the neck; 'black' is flow to the head in both carotid arteries (*star*) and the right vertebral artery (*black arrow*), and 'white' is retrograde flow from the left vertebral artery to the left subclavian artery. This raises the potential for a subclavian steal syndrome

suitable for embolization, whereas wide communications may necessitate stenting or surgery. Left untreated, pseudoaneuryms have the potential to grow, and cause local mass effect on adjacent structures, and also rupture.

True aortic aneurysms are common, although the true incidence is unknown because of their silent nature (Elefteriades and Farkas 2010). However, certain conditions are known to predispose to aneurysm development (Table 3). Atherosclerosis is the commonest cause in adults, yet there are also many patients with congenital cardiac disease who are at risk of progressive aortic dilatation. In children, aneurysms are usually associated with connective tissue disease, and as such there are usually phenotypic clues to identify patients at risk. Marfan syndrome, Loeys Dietz syndrome, and bicuspid aortic valve account for the majority of these aneurysms (Zanotti et al. 2008). Aneurysms of the thoracic aorta are important because of their potential for aortic valve insufficiency, aortic dissection, and rupture (Pitt and Bonser 1997) (Fig. 21).

Evaluation of the size and location of the aneurysmal segment is critical, as well as the relationship with surrounding structures. It is important to quantify the degree of dilatation in relation to uninvolved segments of the aorta. To produce consistent results, vessel dimensions should be measured at the same anatomic location and be performed in the true short axis plane of the aortic section in question (Fig. 22). The multi-planar ability of MRI and the availability of multiple pulse sequences are ideal for evaluation of aneurysms and provide a better understanding of pathology (Schmidta et al. 2000). 3D ceMRA, and 3D whole-heart imaging are the most useful for depicting location, extent, and exact diameter. Black-blood sequences are also helpful in the evaluation of changes to the aortic wall and peri-aortic space.

To perform accurate measurements, 3D data sets are needed. 3D whole-heart MRA is preferred to 3D ceMRA because it is gated and therefore not susceptible to blurring from cardiac motion, which is particularly important for evaluating the dimensions of the aortic root. By using a 3D multiplanar reformatting tool, it is possible to ensure that the short axis of the vessel being measured is perpendicular to the long axis of the vessel in two other planes.

MRI is very useful for the detection of the characteristic morphology of aneurysms such as; annulo-aortic ectasia of aortic root as seen in Marfan syndrome; isolated fusiform dilation of the ascending aorta seen in bicuspid aortic valve disease; fusiform aneurysm of descending aortic segment due to atherosclerosis, and saccular out-pouching of under surface of aortic isthmus due to post-traumatic pseudoaneurysm formation.

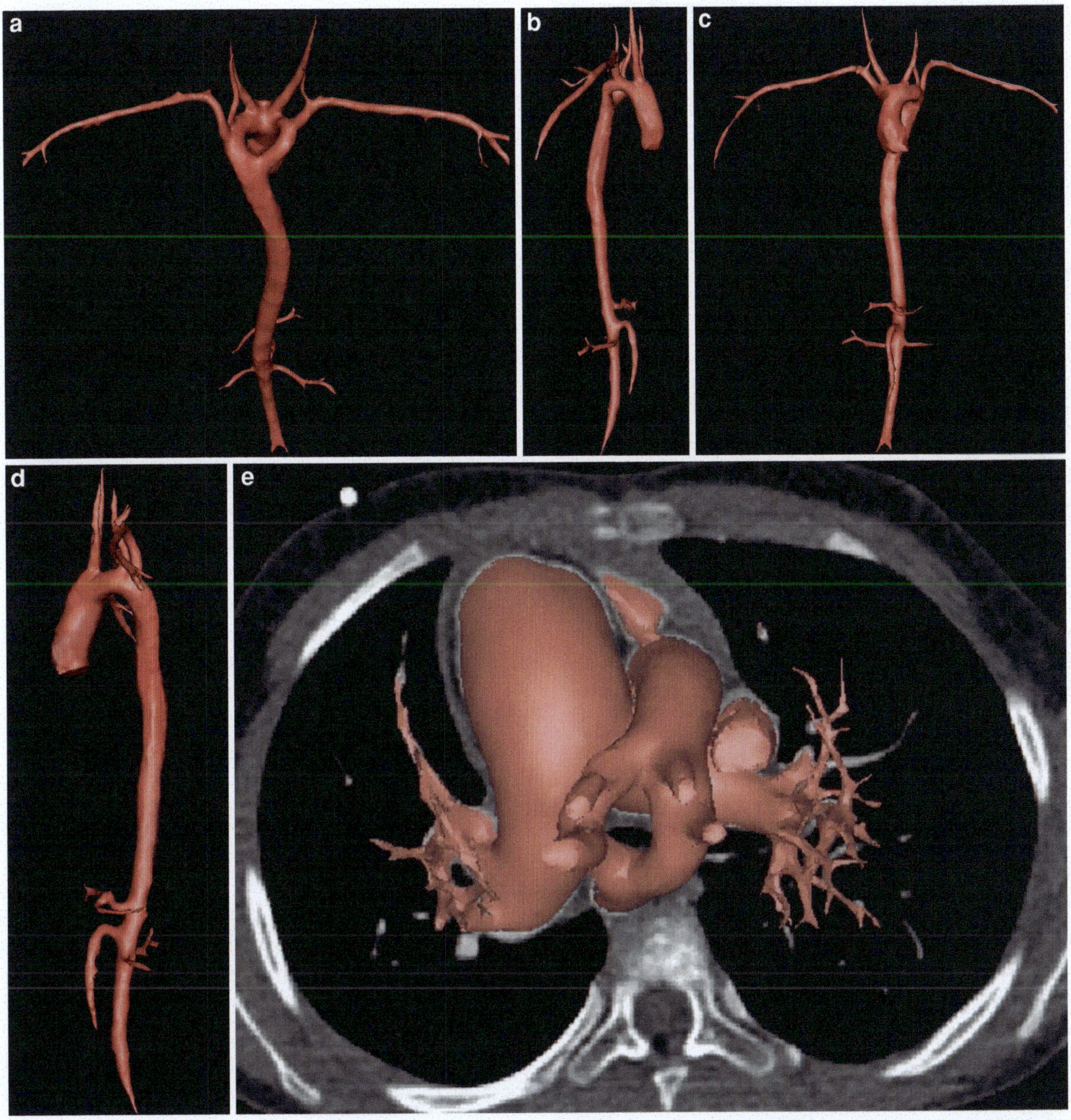

Fig. 15 Selected images from two different patients with a double aortic arch. Volume-rendered images from a ceMRA **a** superior oblique view **b** right-sided view **c** anterior view **d** left-sided view **e** volume-rendered image from a contrast-enhanced CT which has been superimposed upon the background of the axial CT data set to show the relationship of the arch to the trachea

MRI is frequently used as a follow-up tool for monitoring the progression of disease. Where aneurysms involve the ascending aorta or sinuses of Valsalva, concomitant aortic valve disease can be evaluated using cine and flow imaging. In addition it is important to assess ventricular function as increased stiffness of the aorta associated with dilatation has been shown to adversely affect left ventricular ejection fraction (Senzaki et al. 2008).

3.1.3 Marfan Syndrome

Marfan Syndrome is a connective tissue disorder caused by defects in the FBN1 gene, which is characterized by abnormalities in the cardiovascular,

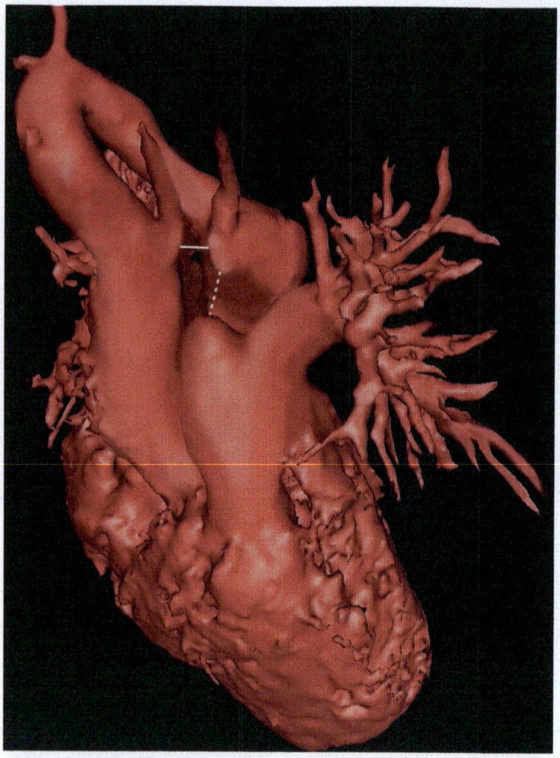

Fig. 16 Potential vascular rings in a patient with a double-aortic arch with atretic left arch and an aberrant left subclavian artery. A *white line* marks the atretic left-sided arch, and a *dashed line* marks the position of the ductal ligament

ocular, and skeletal systems. Recently, the diagnostic criteria for Marfan syndrome were revised to give more weight to aortic root dilatation (Table 4) (Loeys et al. 2010). MRI provides definitive measurements of aortic dimensions, which is essential for the diagnosis of aortic involvement and monitoring the course of aortic enlargement (Kersting-Sommerhoff et al. 1987). In this respect, 3D whole-heart imaging is the best technique, although 3D ceMRA can also be used. The dilatation usually starts at the sinuses of Valsalva, and hence this measurement is critical in monitoring the early evolution of this condition (Fig. 23). Diameters must however be related to normal values for age and body surface area (Roman et al. 1987; Mohiaddin et al. 1990). It is extremely important to carefully scrutinize the aortic images for signs of dissection. Dilatation of the main pulmonary artery is also recognized, although dissection of the pulmonary artery is extremely rare. Cine imaging and PC-MRI can be used to assess the aortic, mitral, and tricuspid valves, as there is often prolapse with associated regurgitation.

MRI also enables the assessment of aortic biophysical properties in patients with Marfan syndrome (Groenink et al. 2001; Fattori et al. 2000). A number of studies have shown that significantly decreased aortic distensibility and increased pulse wave velocity can be detected in the undilated aorta distal to the aortic root in these patients.

3.1.4 Aortic Dissection

Aortic dissection is diagnosed if two separate lumens, the true and a false lumen separated by an intimal flap, are identifiable (Table 5) (Nienaber et al. 1993). Classification of aortic dissections has been based traditionally on anatomical location (Stanford or Debakey) and time from onset (Table 6, Fig. 24) (Debakey et al. 1965). A more recent classification includes intramural hematoma, and aortic ulcers, since these may represent signs of evolving dissections or dissection subtypes (Svensson et al. 1999; Erbel et al. 2001). The 14-day period after onset has been designated as the acute phase because morbidity and mortality (15–25%) rates are highest, and surviving patients typically stabilize during this period. Early diagnosis is crucial as the presenting clinical features are diverse and serious complications occur rapidly (Hagan et al. 2000).

It is important to look for the presence of the intimal flap, which identifies the origin of the dissection, and also the re-entry point as this can affect management. In the rare situation of a retrograde dissection from the descending to ascending aorta, stenting of the intimal flap in the descending aorta may treat the dissection.

CT remains the most widely available imaging modality for patients with aortic dissection, but the findings from static imaging can be misleading. The images acquired with CT represent a single moment in the cardiac cycle and may not demonstrate the complex anatomical and functional changes occurring in aortic dissection. The dimensions of the true and false aortic lumens vary with systole and diastole and this will affect device sizing and determination of dynamic from static obstruction. MRI is able to give both static and dynamic high-resolution information in a single examination and is increasingly regarded as the best available imaging modality (Clough et al. 2010) (Figs. 25, 26). In addition, MRI provides comprehensive information of important complications of dissections such as aortic valve insufficiency,

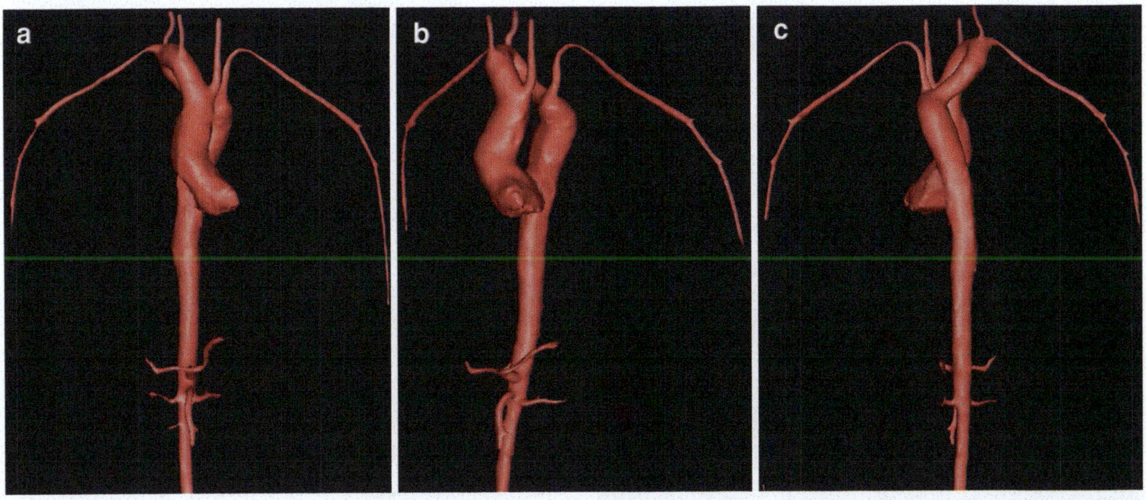

Fig. 17 Volume-rendered 3D reconstruction from a ceMRA of a double-aortic arch with atretic left arch and an aberrant left subclavian artery. **a** Anterior view, **b** left lateral view, **c** posterior view

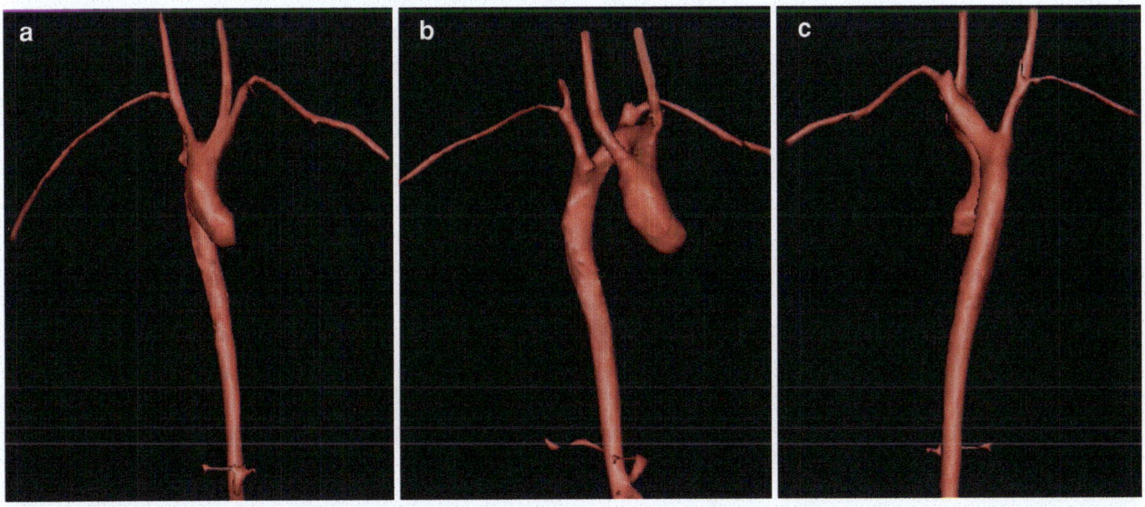

Fig. 18 Volume-rendered 3D reconstruction from a ceMRA of a double-aortic arch with atretic right arch and an aberrant right subclavian artery. **a** Anterior view, **b** left lateral view, **c** posterior view

myocardial infarction from coronary artery compromise, aortic wall rupture, arterial branch vessel dissection or occlusion, and pericardial effusion (Summers et al. 1996; Nienaber et al. 1993).

3D whole-heart imaging is an excellent technique for imaging aortic dissection with high natural contrast between the bright-blood-pool, and low signal intimal flap. It allows accurate delineation of the true and false lumen, and can be used to visualize the relationship of the lumen with the visceral branches. Note that in the early stages of aortic dissection, the true lumen is most often the smaller of the two lumens seen on MRI (see Fig. 26).

ceMRA is also accurate in diagnosing aortic dissections. ceMRA is useful for assessing the proximal and distal extent of the dissection and its involvement of branch vessels (Bogaert et al. 1997). A separate ceMRA study of the abdomen may be required to assess distal dissections extending into the abdominal aorta (Carr and Finn 2003). Time-resolved angiography is an alternative method, and allows dynamic information about the true and false lumen filling

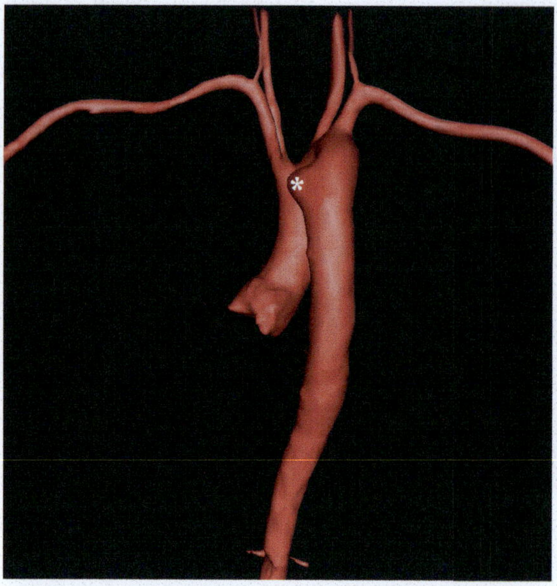

Fig. 19 Posterior view of a volume-rendered 3D reconstruction from ceMRA of a right arch with mirror-image branching head and neck vessels, and a large Kommerell's diverticulum (*asterisk*)

patterns, with the true lumen filling earlier than the false lumen (Krishnam et al. 2008).

Thrombosis of the false lumen is an important factor in determining the prognosis of patients presenting with dissection (Bernard et al. 2001). Using CT, the diagnosis is made when contrast fails to opacify the false lumen on first-pass imaging. A delayed second scan may detect late enhancement of the false lumen, but the ideal timing for this is unpredictable and dependant on both the cardiac output and local flow conditions. By using time-resolved angiography and or PC-MRI techniques, it is possible to distinguish thrombosis of the false lumen from slow flow on MRI. It may be difficult to distinguish a thrombosed false lumen from an intramural hematoma, although an intramural hematoma tends to have a more cresentic appearance.

Cine imaging can be useful in the plane of the dissection to assess the dynamic nature of the true and false lumen size, and also in the identification of the dissection flap. Furthermore cine imaging can be used to assess for complications such as aortic regurgitation, and look for wall motion abnormalities of the myocardium in myocardial infarction. Occasionally, flow artifact related to cine imaging and 3D whole-heart imaging can mimic a dissection. In these circumstances black-blood imaging can be extremely helpful.

MRI remains important in the post-operative assessment of aortic dissection. Complications include anastamotic leakage, the development of false channels, anastomotic aneurysms and dilatation and dissection of the residual aorta (Fig. 27) A slight thickening around the graft due to peri-graft fibrosis is a common finding (Gaubert et al. 1995), but large or asymmetric thickening suggests localized hematoma due to an anastomotic leakage (Fattori and Nienaber 1999).

Real-time cine imaging, single-shot black-blood, and single-shot bright-blood, and time-resolved MRA can be used for imaging critically ill patients who cannot hold their breath (Pereles et al. 2001; Lee et al. 2002), although CT may be more appropriate in these circumstances.

3.1.5 Penetrating Aortic Ulceration and Intramural Hematoma

The term acute aortic syndrome encompasses a range of conditions, with a similar clinical profile the most prominent symptom being aortic pain, and includes penetrating aortic ulcer, intramural hematoma and aortic dissection. These conditions have become grouped together because of the propensity of penetrating aortic ulcers, and intramural hematomas to develop into overt aortic dissection in some patients, and the coexistence of these different pathologies in other patients (Vilacosta et al. 2009).

A penetrating aortic ulcer occurs, when there is corrosion of an atherosclerotic plaque through the internal elastic lamina into the aortic media. It may rupture into the media to form an intramural hematoma, or penetrate to the adventitia to form a saccular pseudoaneurysm, or even lead to complete transmural rupture into the mediastinum. The ulcer may also give rise to an aortic dissection either directly, with the ulcer providing the leading edge for the intimal tear, or through intramural hematoma and then dissection. Aortic ulcers predominantly occur in the descending aorta, less frequently in the aortic arch and rarely in the ascending aorta (Lansman et al. 2010) (Fig. 28). The ulcer appears as an out-pouching that extends beyond the expected aortic wall boundaries and generally occurs in the presence of severe atheromatous disease. With 3D ceMRA the out-pouching fills with contrast and can be seen to connect to the aortic lumen

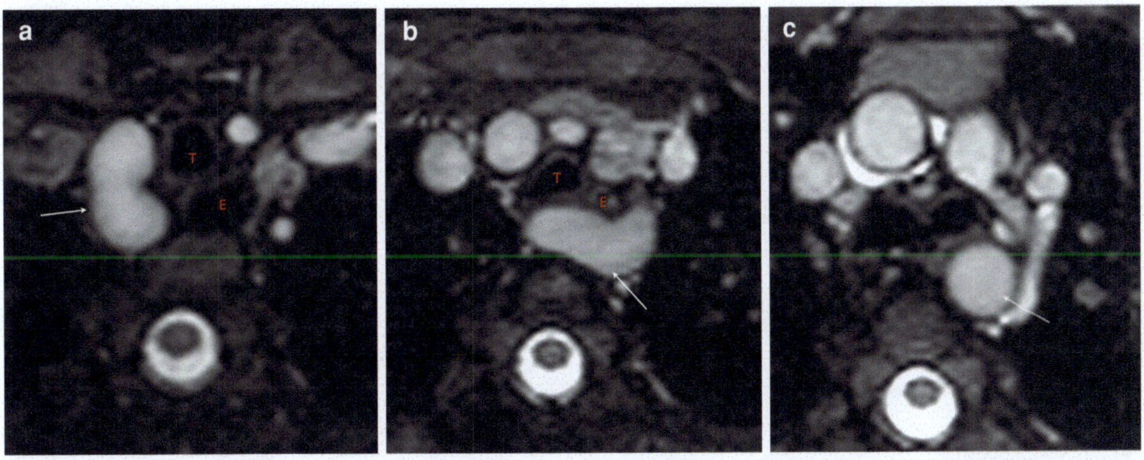

Fig. 20 Selected images from a 3D whole-heart MRA in a patient with features suggestive of a double arch. **a** Right-sided aortic arch (*arrow*), **b** proximal descending thoracic aorta passes behind the esophagus (*arrow*), **c** descending aorta now continuing its' course to the left of the spine (*arrow*). T=Trachea, E=esophagus

Table 3 Causes of aortic aneurysm

Atherosclerosis
Marfan syndrome
Ehlers danlos syndrome
Syphilis
Infectious aortitis
Giant cell arteritis
Aortic trauma
Aortic dissection
Secondary to aortic valve pathology (stenosis or regurgitation)
Post-operative

(Mohiaddin et al. 2001). 3D whole-heart imaging is also useful, and excellently depicts aortic wall irregularity. Black-blood imaging can be used to examine the aortic wall in more detail because of its high spatial resolution. MRI however, cannot detect dislodgement of the intimal calcification commonly associated with this condition (Fattori and Nienaber 1999).

The natural history of penetrating aortic ulcers is not known, which has led to opposing management strategies. Those occurring in the ascending aorta, arch, and proximal descending aorta have a more malignant course, probably as a result of increased wall shear stress. Should medical management be advocated, careful follow-up with repeat imaging is essential. Surgery is then suggested if there is increasing size of the ulcer, an increasing pleural effusion, or if there is recurrent pain (Ganaha et al. 2002).

Intramural hematoma accounts for 10–30% of all acute aortic syndromes (Vilacosta et al. 2009). The most likely cause of intramural hematoma is from rupture of the vasa vasorum at the medial adventitial junction of the aortic wall, although it may also occur from rupture of a penetrating aortic ulcer. The major risk of intramural hematoma is that it may evolve into an overt aortic dissection and aortic rupture (von Kodolitsch et al. 2003).

On cross-sectional imaging, intramural hematoma appears as smooth, cresentic, and occasionally circumferential thickening of the aortic wall. With expansion, the hematoma may encroach on the aortic lumen (Lansman et al. 2010). This can be associated with infiltration of the adjacent mediastinal fat and/or pericardial effusion, caused by leakage of blood. A combination of bright-blood (using 3D whole-heart sequence), and black-blood imaging is needed to characterize the blood within the aortic wall. Acutely, blood will have a bright signal on black-blood imaging, but will become dark with chronic intramural hematoma. Importantly, there is no entrance tear visualized. Cine imaging may also be useful to differentiate hematoma from aortic dissection with thrombosed lumen (Fig. 29) (Sonnabend et al. 1990).

As with penetrating aortic ulceration, there is divergent opinion as to how to treat intramural hematoma, with some advocating surgery for intramural hematoma involving the ascending aorta, and

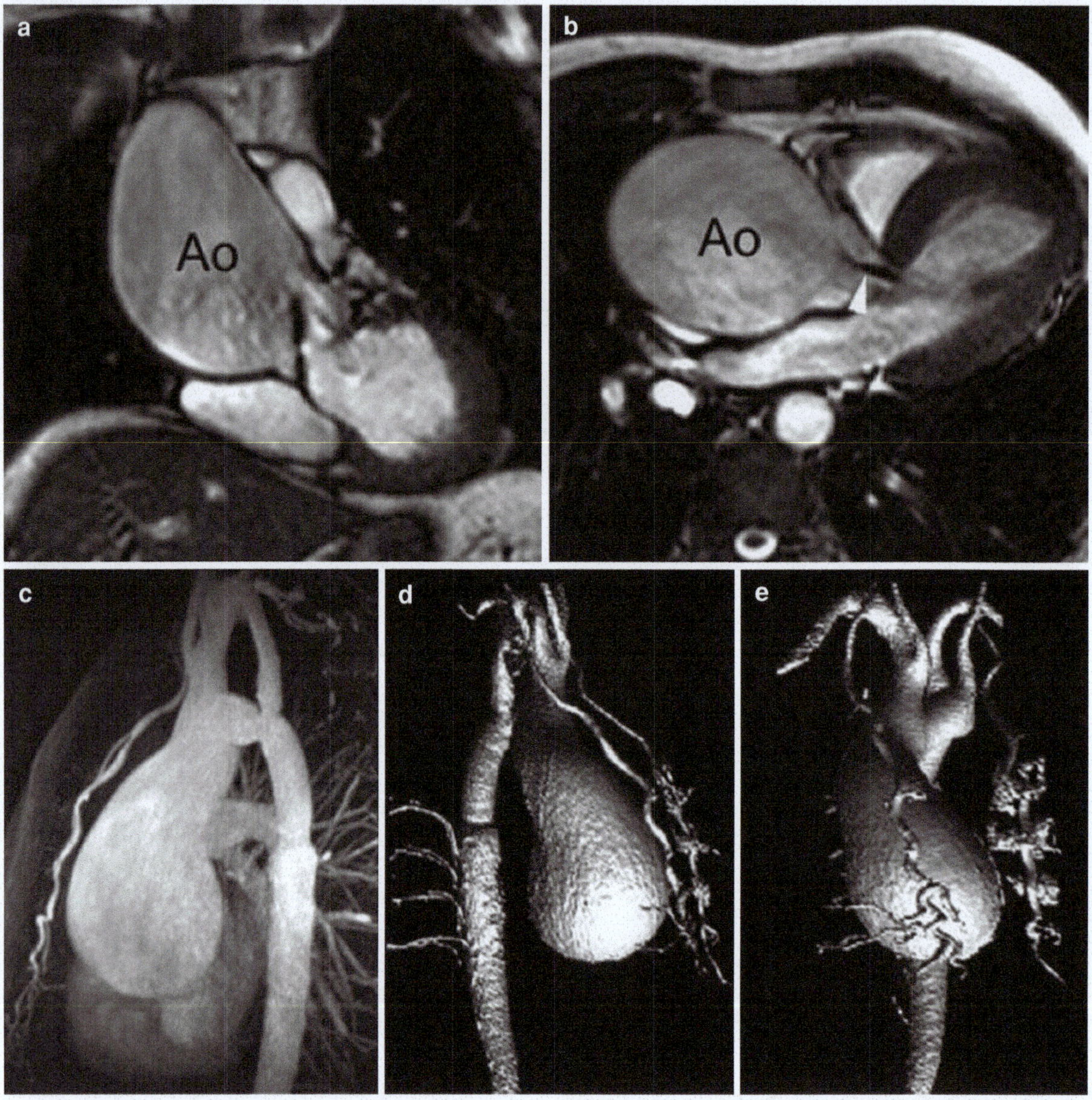

Fig. 21 Aneurysm of the ascending aorta in a 42-year-old man with history of previous surgical correction for aortic coarctation, and concomitant bicuspid aortic valve. **a** Bright-blood cine in the coronal view **b** and LV outflow tract view. **c** ceMRA maximum-intensity projection view **d, e** and volume-rendered view . A huge, fusiform aneurysm (85 mm) of the ascending aorta is clearly visible. The 3D-geometry can be best appreciated on the 3D volume-rendered views. On cine MRI **a**, **b** an important aortic regurgitation is shown (*arrowhead*). Note also the contour abnormalities of the aortic isthmus and proximal descending aorta from the previous surgical repair of the aortic coarctation

medical treatment for descending aortic involvement (Nienaber et al. 2004), and others adopting a more conservative approach with watchful waiting. MRI is extremely useful for follow-up of this group of patients. Features indicating surgery should be performed include: (Lansman et al. 2010)

- Persistent pain;
- New associated ulceration;
- Progression to aortic dissection;
- Maximum aortic diameter greater than or equal to 50 mm;
- Progressive aortic dilatation on follow-up;
- Increasing aortic wall thickness greater than or equal to 10 mm;

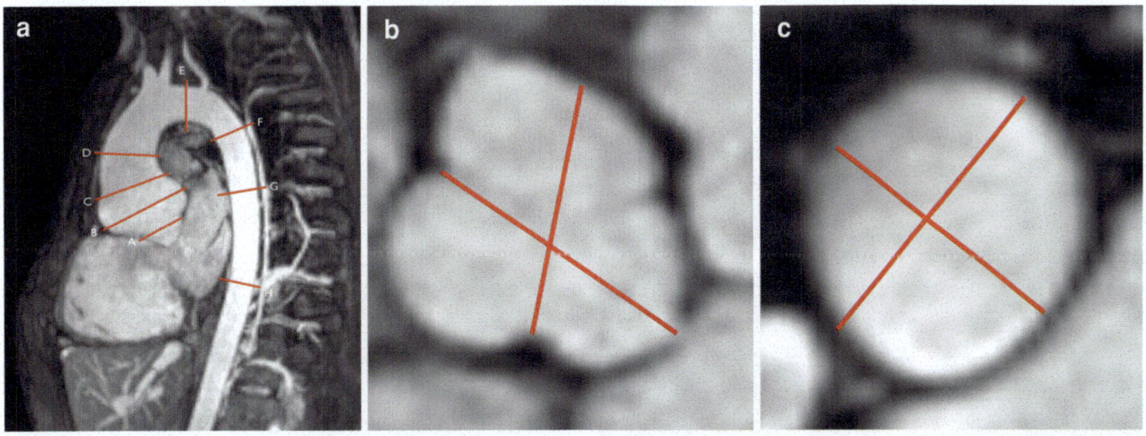

Fig. 22 Selected multiplanar reformat images from a 3D whole-heart volume in a patient with connective tissue disease, and a dilated aortic root. **a** Sagittal oblique view showing the positions to perform aortic measurements. A—aortic annulus, B—aortic sinuses, C—sinotubular junction, D—mid-ascending aorta, E—transverse arch, F—proximal descending aorta, G—mid descending aorta, H—descending aorta at diaphragm. **b** True short axis of the aortic sinuses (B) at the widest point showing measurements made from aortic cusp to opposite commissural junction. **c** True short axis of the mid-ascending aorta (D) showing maximum and minimum dimensions

Table 4 Revised ghent criteria for diagnosis of Marfan syndrome

In the absence of family history the following are diagnostic of Marfan syndome:
1. Aortic root dilatation (Z score 2 or more) or dissection *AND* ectopia lentis
2. Aortic root dilatation (Z score 2 or more) or dissection *AND* fibrillin mutation
3. Aortic root dilatation (Z score 2 or more) or dissection *AND* systemic features (7 or more points on the systemic features scoring scale)
4. Ectopia lentis *AND* fibrillin mutation with known aortic root dilatation or dissection

- Increasing pleural or pericardial effusion;
- Proximal aortic root involvement including aortic regurgitation; and
- Failure to regress

3.1.5.1 Inflammation

MRI is an important tool for investigating inflammatory aortitis syndromes (Table 7), as it can assess changes to both the arterial lumen and wall (Fig. 30). Takayasu disease is a chronic vasculitis affecting the aorta and its major branches and the pulmonary arteries. It produces a variety of ischemic symptoms due to stenosis and thrombosis of major arteries. Acute progression of the disease can lead to destruction of the arterial media, formation of aneurysms, or arterial rupture. It can be divided into two stages, with an acute period of large vessel inflammation, followed by a chronic period of fibrosis and scarring (Fig. 31). In the acute inflammatory stage the wall becomes thickened. This is well demonstrated with both 3D whole-heart imaging and black-blood imaging. A decrease in wall thickening has been observed following treatment (Tanigawa et al. 1992).

3D ceMRA is excellent for demonstration of multiple arterial stenosis, and also for regions of aneurysmal dilatation, although it needs to be remembered that signal dropout from flow acceleration can overestimate stenosis. It is important to image from the head and neck vessels down to the iliac vessels. Careful interrogation of all branches including the abdominal vessels, and branch pulmonary arteries is needed.

Following gadolinium, patterns of aortic mural enhancement are variable (Choe et al. 2000). In the acute phase, the aortic wall and surrounding adventitia enhance more than the myocardium, suggesting active disease (Fig. 32). Late gadolinium enhancement can also be shown within the wall, although the presence or absence of enhancement of the arterial wall is not necessarily a reliable tool for assessing disease activity (Andrews et al. 2004).

Cine imaging is useful for demonstrating regions of flow acceleration, and can be used to assess regional

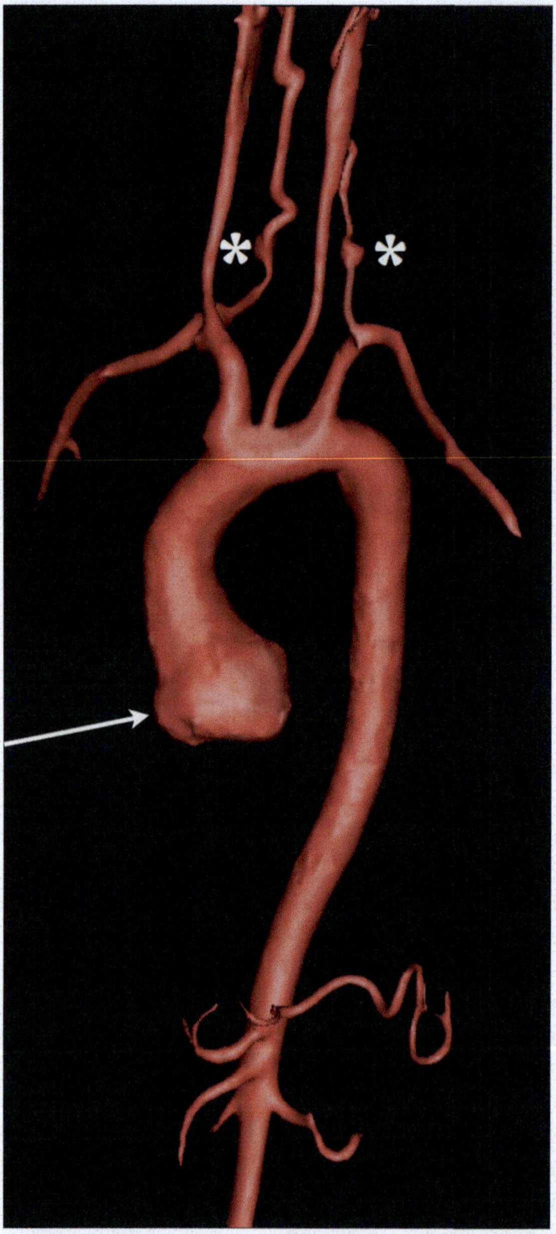

Fig. 23 Volume-rendered 3D reconstruction from a ceMRA of the aorta in a Marfan subject—oblique sagittal view. In Marfan syndrome, dilatation usually starts at the sinuses of Valsalva (*arrow*), so this measurement is critical for follow-up. Effacement of the sinotubular ridge occurs in Marfan syndrome, annuloaortic ectasia and syphilis, but not in post-stenotic dilatation secondary to aortic stenosis. Note also in this patient, there are bilateral saccular aneurysms of the vertebral arteries (*asterisks*)

Table 5 Causes of aortic dissection

Hypertension
Coarctation
Iatrogenic injury
Valvular disease
Marfan syndrome

Table 6 Classification of aortic dissection

Debakey et al. (1965)
Type I
Intimal tear in ascending aorta; terminates distal to brachiocephalic artery.
Type II
Intimal tear in ascending aorta; terminates proximal to brachiocephalic artery
Type III
Intimal tear at or distal to left subclavian artery
Stanford
Type A
Involves ascending aorta + descending aorta; needs immediate surgery
Type B
Involves descending aorta only.
Svensson et al. (1999)
Class 1
Classical aortic dissection with an intimal flap between true and false lumen
Class 2
Medial disruption with formation of intramural hematoma/ hemorrhage
Class 3
Discrete subtle dissection without hematoma eccentric bulge at tear site
Class 4
Plaque rupture leading to aortic ulceration, penetrating aortic atherosclerotic ulcer with surrounding hematoma, usually subadventitial
Class 5
Iatrogenic and traumatic dissection

Note
Types I and II and A require urgent surgery
Types III and B can be treated medically if uncomplicated

wall stiffness. In addition, it is important to assess the aortic valve for regurgitation, and ventricular function and mass to assess the effect of ventricular arterial interaction. PC-MRI can be used to measure maximum velocity across regions of narrowing to evaluate the need for intervention.

MRI is of particular importance in follow-up. New regions of stenosis can be demonstrated even in

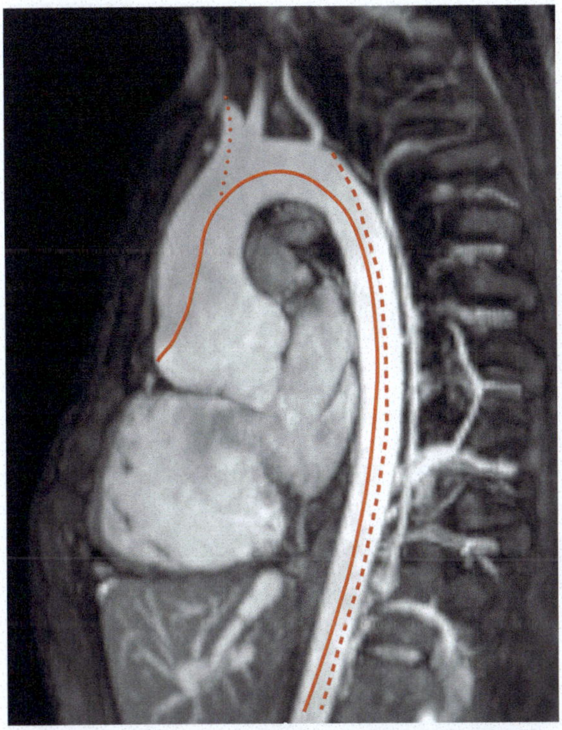

Fig. 24 Multiplanar reformat image from a 3D whole-heart volume in a patient with connective tissue disease, and a dilated aortic root same patient as Fig. 21 in "Congenital Heart Disease". Schema for origin and type of aortic dissection; left anterior oblique orientation. Type A (*red line*)—(60%) originate a few centimeters above the aortic valve, along the right anterolateral aspect of the aorta, where hydrodynamic and torsional forces are greatest. The dissection may extend into the head and neck vessels (*dotted red line*) or extend into the descending aorta (*solid red line*). Type B (*striped red line*)—(40%) originate in the descending thoracic aorta just beyond the insertion of the ligamentum arteriosum (anchorage of the relative mobile arch to the thoracic cage)

patients with clinical remission (Tann et al. 2008). Therapeutic effectiveness of medical and surgical intervention can be assessed, including treatment with steroids, the patency of bypass grafts, and any restenosis after percutaneous intervention.

3.1.6 Aortic Trauma

Acute aortic injury occurs following major trauma such as road traffic accidents and is associated with a significant mortality. Any delay in diagnosis and treatment can lead to death. The most common site of aortic injury is the region just beyond the isthmus where the relatively mobile thoracic aorta is joined by the ductal ligament and is the site of greatest strain. In one study, MRI demonstrated 100% accuracy for detecting traumatic lesions, compared with 84% for X-ray angiography and 69% for standard CT (Fattori et al. 1996). MRI can detect the hemorrhagic component of the lesion by the high signal intensity of acute blood, with black-blood imaging of the aorta in sagittal plane helping to prognosticate by differentiating between partial and complete lesions (Fattori and Nienaber 1999). In all forms of imaging, care should be made not to interpret a prominent ampulla (site of previous ligamentum arteriosus insertion) as a site of aortic injury. However, despite the high accuracy of MRI in assessing acute patients, its use is usually limited. Patients who have acute aortic injury are usually critically unwell, and often have multiple concomitant injuries, including fractures, which need to be imaged quickly, and hence multi-detector CT is the modality of choice in this setting.

Some of these aortic lesions; however, may not manifest themselves immediately after the trauma. Often, these patients may present many years later with symptoms that are caused by complications of a previous often forgotten chest trauma. The most frequent delayed complication of the thoracic aorta is a chronic saccular pseudoaneurysm originating from the distal aortic arch. The size of the pseudoaneurysm is consistent and about 3–5 cm. The most common site of disease is the isthmus just distal to the left subclavian artery at the attachment of the ductal ligament medial and anterior to the aortic isthmus. This is related to different shear forces during rapid deceleration between the somewhat fixed descending aorta and relatively mobile heart and aortic arch (Sevitt 1977). A distinction has to be made between the immediately fatal rupture of the postero-lateral wall of the isthmus and the disruption at the anteromedial wall. It is possible that the expanding hematoma from a medial tear could be contained by the pulmonary artery and the left main stem bronchus inferiorly (Gundry et al. 1984). The adherence of the mediastinal parietal pleura to these structures may limit expansion of the hematoma laterally. Because of the medial tear, the pseudoaneurysm typically forms in a saccular configuration adjacent to the descending aorta and the rest of a normal arch.

Compression of the pseudoaneurysm on the airways or recurrent laryngeal nerve will cause symptoms of dyspnea or hoarseness, but pseudoaneurysms are often an incidental finding on routine chest X-ray

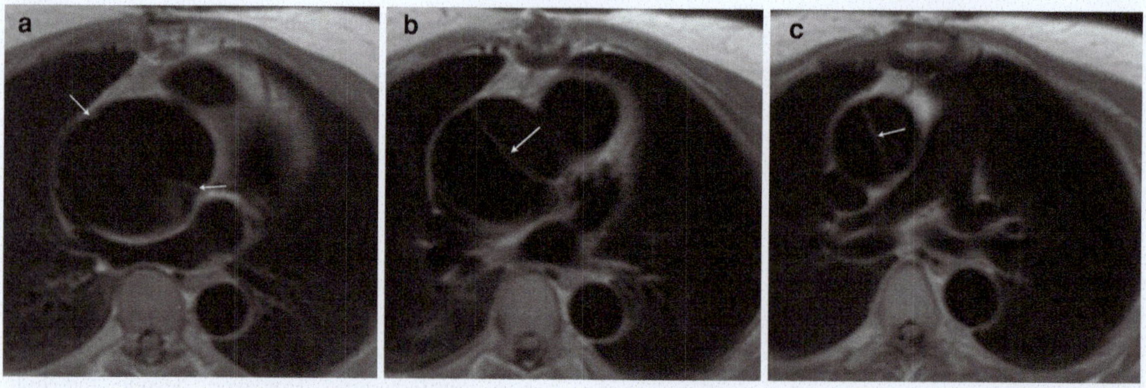

Fig. 25 Type II De Bakey aortic dissection in a patient with an aneurysm of the ascending aorta. Black-blood axial images from **a** foot to **c** head . The aortic dissection flap is restricted to the ascending aorta (*arrow*). Careful analysis of aneurysms of the ascending aorta not infrequently shows underlying dissections limited to the aneurysm (Svensson et al. 1999)

Fig. 26 Type B Stanford aortic dissection. Axial images in the same plane with; **a** Black-blood sequence, **b** bright-blood sequence, and PC-MRI, **c** magnitude image, **d** velocity map. The false lumen (*star*) is the large lumen, and has less flow within it on the velocity map

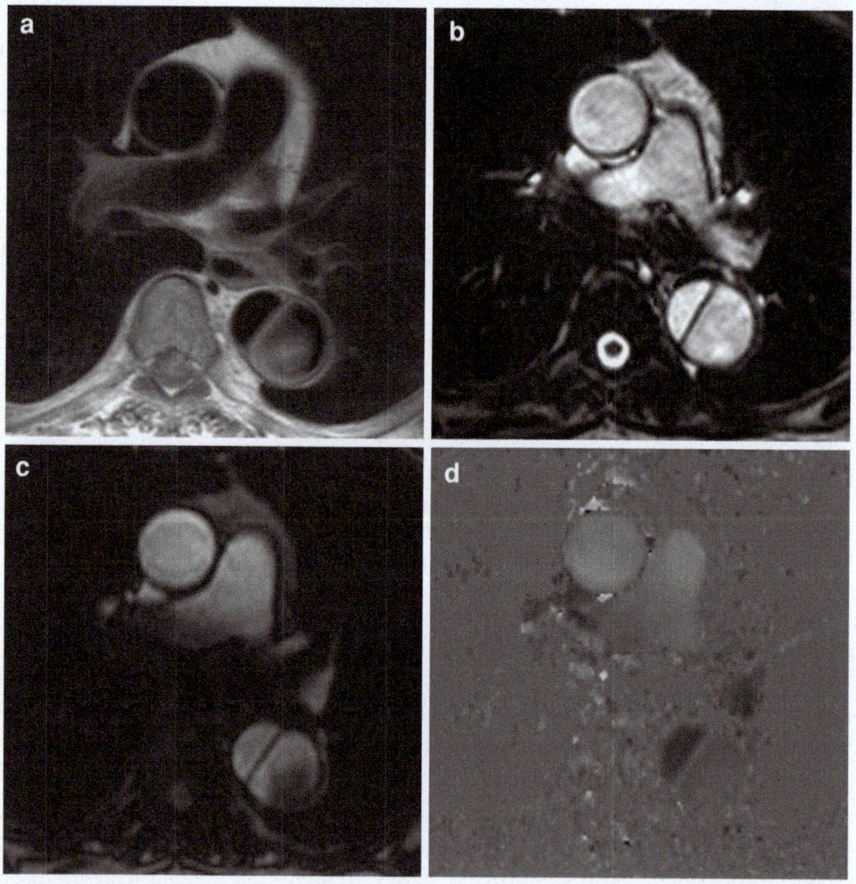

films. Because the exact time required for the acute lesion to convert into a pseudoaneurysm is not known, a chronic traumatic pseudoaneurysm is defined as existing 3 months or more after the injury. MRI should be considered one of the preferred imaging techniques to confirm the presence of, and to evaluate the precise location and extent of a pseudoaneurysm. Also the presence of a mural thrombus partially, or rarely completely, obliterating the aneurismal lumen can be depicted. Imaging with MRI may be helpful

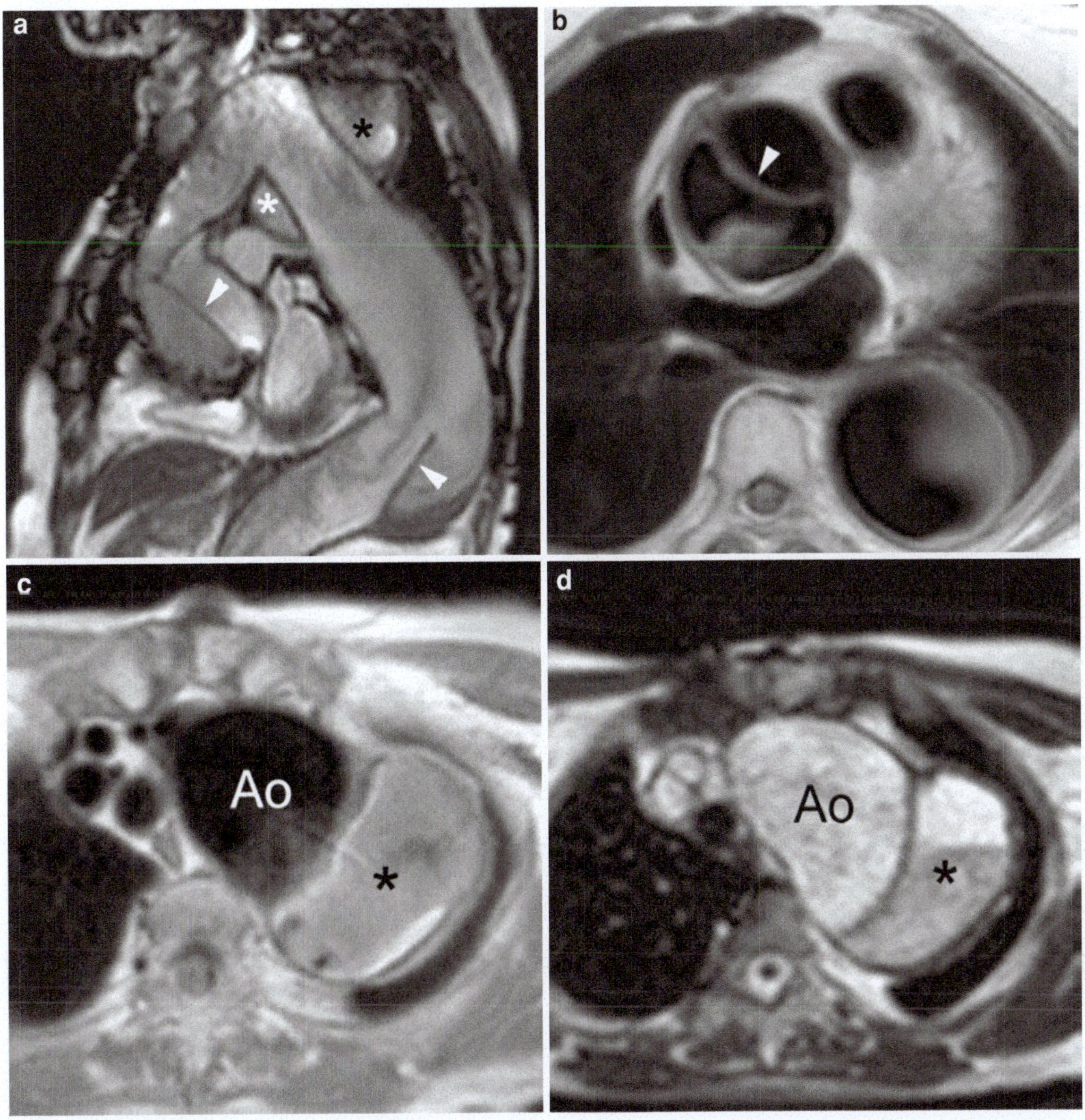

Fig. 27 Residual aortic dissection with multiple large pseudoaneurysms in a patient's post-Bentall operation. **a** Oblique sagittal bright-blood image through the aorta, showing ascending and descending aorta dissection flaps (*white arrowheads*), and several pseudoaneurysms (*star*). **b** Black-blood axial image through the ascending aorta showing a dissection flap (*white arrowhead*). **c** Axial Black-blood and bright-blood **d** images in the same plane at the level of the aortic arch showing a large psuedoaneurysm (*black star*)

for demonstrating the relationship of the saccular pseudoaneurysm to the aorta and to the origin of the left subclavian artery. This is of great importance for the operative procedure, as clamping of the left subclavian artery should be avoided during the repair of the pseudoaneurysm, or prior to an aortic stent placement. A combination of 3D whole-heart imaging and 3D contrast-enhanced MR angiography is the best strategy to study chronic post-traumatic aneurysms.

3.1.7 Aortic and Pulmonary Stent, and Percutanous Valve Imaging

Endovascular stent placement is increasingly used to treat aortic and pulmonary artery stenoses and

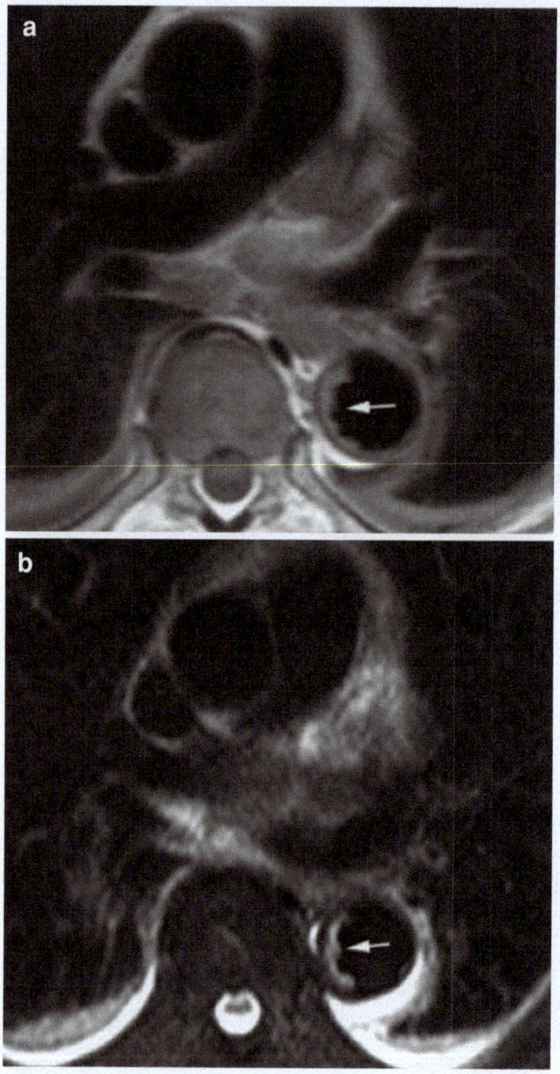

Fig. 28 Extensive atherosclerotic disease of the descending aorta. **a** Axial T1w image and **b** T2w fat-saturation image shows irregular centrally ulcerated plaque (thickness 5 mm) along the medial border of the descending aorta (*arrow*). Further ulceration may evolve toward a penetrating ulcer when the entire aortic wall is ulcerated

aneurysms (Dake et al. 1998; Hamdan et al. 2001; Baerlocher et al. 2008). Stent insertion is also an important part of percutaneous heart valve replacement (Lurz et al. 2008; Piazza et al. 2008). These metallic implants are safe to image under MRI, (Hilfiker et al. 1999; Engellau et al. 2000). A recognized complication of stent implantation is stenosis, which often requires re-intervention. Therefore, visualization of the stent lumen is a necessary part of follow-up. Conventional X-ray angiography can be used to image stents; however, conventional X-ray angiography is not suitable for routine surveillance because of the invasive nature of the procedure. CT is an accurate non-invasive alternative to catheterization, but there are concerns regarding the long-term health effects of ionizing radiation exposure, especially when multiple assessments need to be performed in long-term follow-up.

MRI is susceptible to artifacts related to the stent material, the stent orientation, and the type of MRI acquisition (Bartels et al. 2002; Hagspiel et al. 2005; Lenhart et al. 2000). In certain situations these artifacts prevent visualization of the stent lumen. In a recent in vitro study, high flip-angle through-plane spoiled GRE cine imaging, b-SSFP cine imaging, and high flip-angle ceMRA sequences were shown to be accurate methods of assessing stent stenosis (Fig. 33). Interestingly, black-blood sequences perform poorly in subjective identification of stent lesions, as it does not allow visualization of the vessel lumen (Nordmeyer et al. 2010a), not necessary because of metal artifact, but because the metallic stent acts as a Faraday cage.

In assessing stents, it is important to evaluate not only the presence of stenosis, and procedural complications, but also to look for the presence of leak, either endo-leak, or valvar and paravalvar leak in the case of valved stents. It is also necessary to look for the functional consequences of this in terms of increased ventricular preload, and afterload.

3.2 Pulmonary Arteries

Imaging of pulmonary artery anatomy is crucial for surgical planning and follow-up in patients with complex congenital heart disease (see "Congenital Heart Disease"). Imaging of the branch pulmonary arteries can be difficult on echocardiography, in particular in older patients and post-surgical patients, and MRI can provide a non-invasive alternative to X-ray cardiac catheterization for the assessment of the pulmonary arteries (Canter et al. 1989). MRI can define the size, patency, confluence, and character of the extraparenchymal pulmonary arteries, and has been shown to be 100% sensitive and specific for the diagnosis of main and branch pulmonary artery hypoplasia or stenosis as well as discontinuous or absent branch pulmonary arteries (Powell et al. 2000) (Fig. 34).

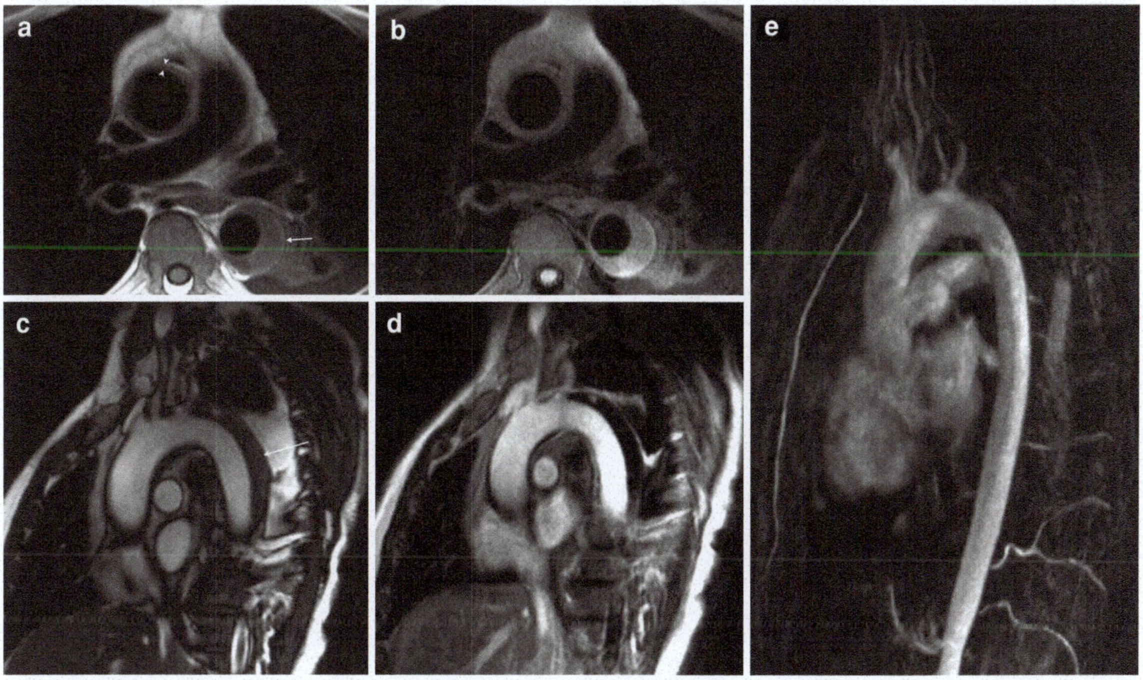

Fig. 29 Type A intramural hematoma. **a** Black-blood axial image showing circumferential thickening of the ascending aorta (*arrowhead*) with eccentric extension into the descending aorta (arrow), secondary to intramural hematoma. **b** T2-weighted fat-saturation image in the same imaging plane as (**a**). **c** Oblique sagittal bright-blood image clearly demonstrating the large eccentric thickening of the descending aorta (*arrow*). **d** late Gd MRI in the same imaging plane as (**d**). **e** maximum-intensity projection from a ceMRA appears relatively normal (except for sparsity of vertebral and intercostal arteries in proximal part of descending aorta), emphasizing the need for using other imaging sequences when investigating aortic pathology with MRI. However, in this case the 'normal' appearance of the ceMRA helps differentiate from a thrombosed false lumen in descending aorta, where there is usually some leakage of contrast into the 'false lumen' in proximal descending aorta on ceMRA

Three-dimensional ceMRA is essential to adequately evaluate the hilar and intrapulmonary segments of the central pulmonary arteries and aortopulmonary collaterals (Wang et al. 1996). In patients with respiratory distress, time-resolved MRA might be more suitable (Vogt et al. 2003). ceMRA is particularly good at demonstrating aortopulmonary collateral vessels. These may originate from the aorta or its main branches including the brachiocephalic arteries, subclavian and internal mammary arteries and intercostals, and also from the subdiaphragmatic aorta (Hernandez 2002). Three-dimensional whole-heart imaging is an alternative method for assessing the central pulmonary vasculature, although the distal vessels are usually not well seen because of a small field of view. In situations where 3D assessment is not feasible, 2D black-blood and cine imaging techniques may suffice for delineating central pulmonary arteries.

In cases of RVOT obstruction the central pulmonary arteries may be hypoplastic or if atretic, not identifiable. Focal branch stenosis proximal to the pulmonary hila may be identified directly. In cases of supravalvular pulmonary stenosis, the pulmonary

Table 7 Causes of aortic inflammation

Syphilitic aortitis
Rheumatic aortitis
Rheumatoid arthritis
Ankylosing spondylitis
Psoriatic arthritis
Reiter's syndrome
Behçet's syndrome
Relapsing polychondritis
Inflammatory bowel disease
Takayasu's arteritis
Giant cell arteritis
Atherosclerosis

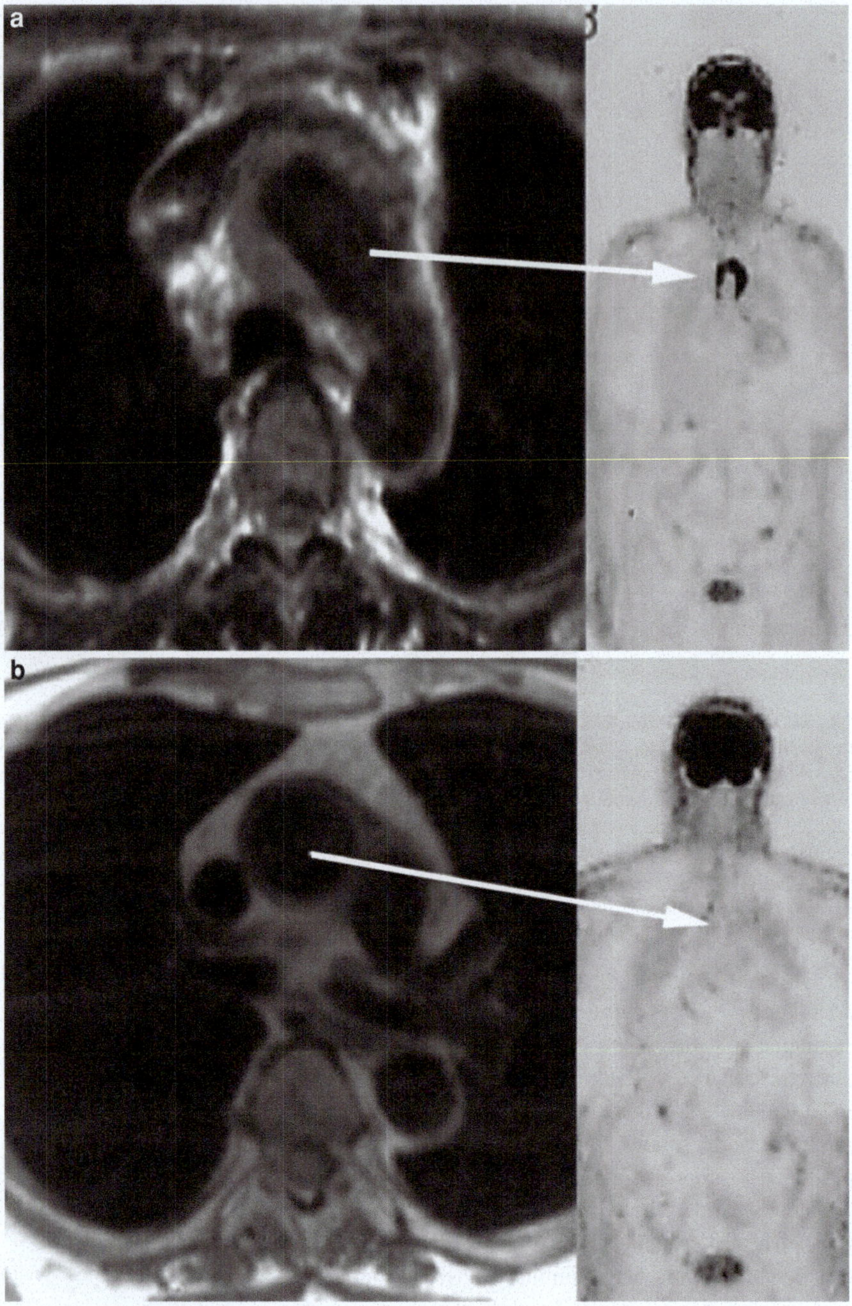

Fig. 30 Giant cell aortitis in a 62-year-old woman. Axial T1w image after administration of Gadolinium (*left*) and coronal FDG-PET (*right*) **a** at initial presentation and **b** after six weeks of corticosteroid treatment. Strong enhancement is found in the thickened wall of the ascending aorta. This inflammatory thickened aortic wall shows high glucose metabolism on FDG-PET (**a**). After corticosteroid treatment (**b**) wall thickness has nearly normalized, and no abnormal glucose metabolism is found on FDG-PET

trunk and central pulmonary arteries (as an isolated lesion or in association with Williams or Noonan's syndromes), may exhibit diffuse or focal wall thickening. Similarly, pulmonary arterial banding results in focal pulmonary artery narrowing. MRI can also be useful in the assessment of hypoplastic lung syndrome, demonstrating reduced lung volume, and identifying associated lesions including; hypoplastic supplying pulmonary artery; partial anomalous pulmonary venous drainage (Scimitar vein); and pulmonary sequestration.

Dilatation of the pulmonary trunk, with or without left or right pulmonary arterial enlargement may be seen in patients with pulmonary valve stenosis, and in patients with pulmonary regurgitation, either as a result of transannular patch pulmonary artery

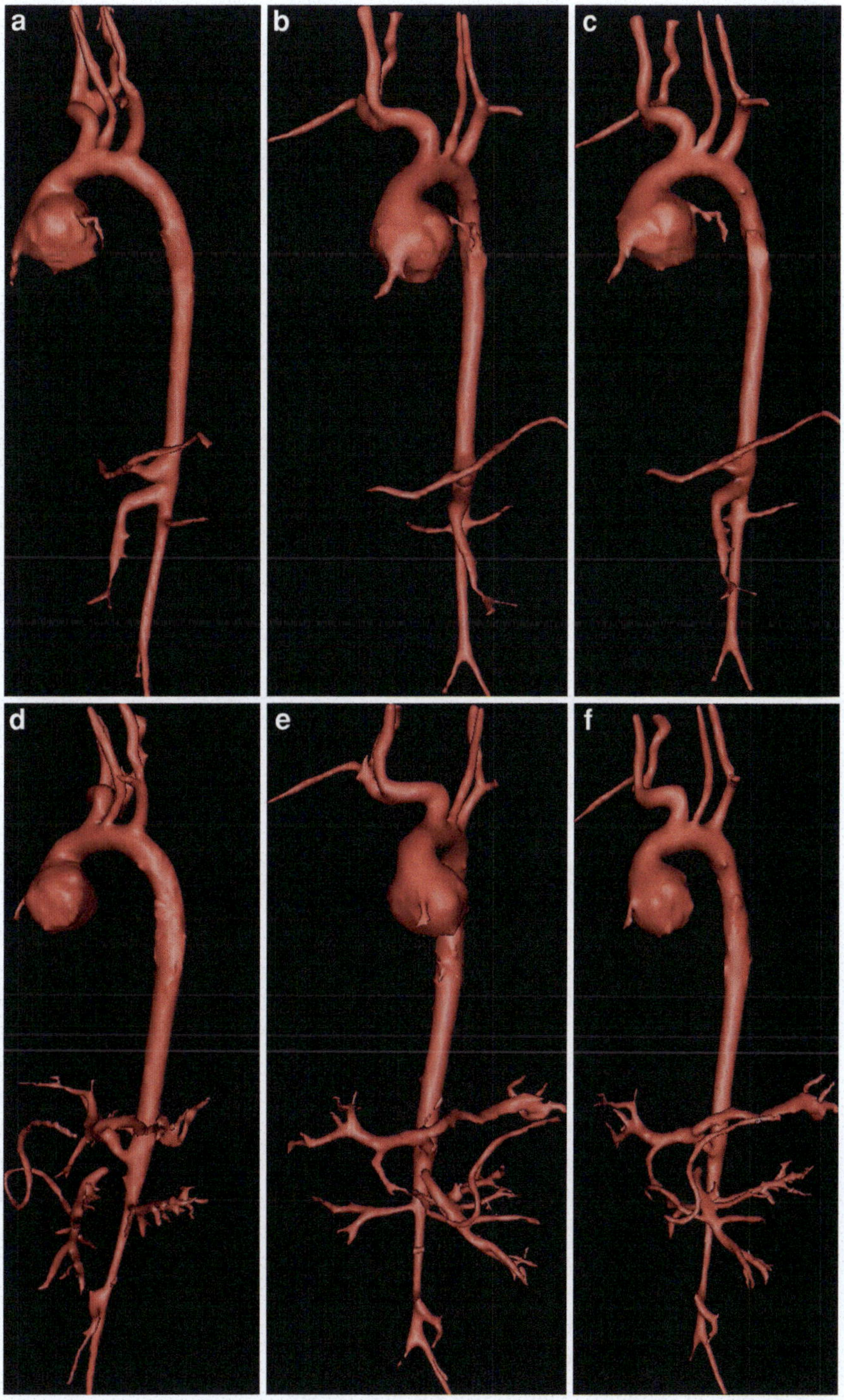

Fig. 31 Volume-rendered images from a ceMRA in a 2-year-old girl with Takayasu disease **a–c** (*top row*) taken at presentation, and **d–f** (*bottom row*) taken 4 months later while on medical therapy. **a**, **d** sagittal view, **b**, **e** anterior view, **c**, **f** sagittal oblique. At presentation, the aortic root is dilated, and there is mild narrowing of the origin of the left common carotid artery. Four months later, there has been progressive narrowing of the left common carotid origin. The origin of the celiac axis is now moderately narrowed, and the superior mesenteric artery origin is occluded. Multiple abdominal collaterals are now seen. The infra-renal aorta has progressively narrowed, and the right common iliac artery is severely narrowed

augmentation, or increased stroke volume. Aneurysmal dilatation of the pulmonary trunk and branch pulmonary arteries with absent or rudimentary pulmonary valve tissue and severe pulmonary regurgitation is characteristic of tetralogy of Fallot with absent pulmonary valve syndrome. The resulting tracheo-bronchial compression by the grossly dilated pulmonary arteries and occasionally aorto-pulmonary collaterals (Knauth et al. 2004) can be a cause of significant morbidity and mortality.

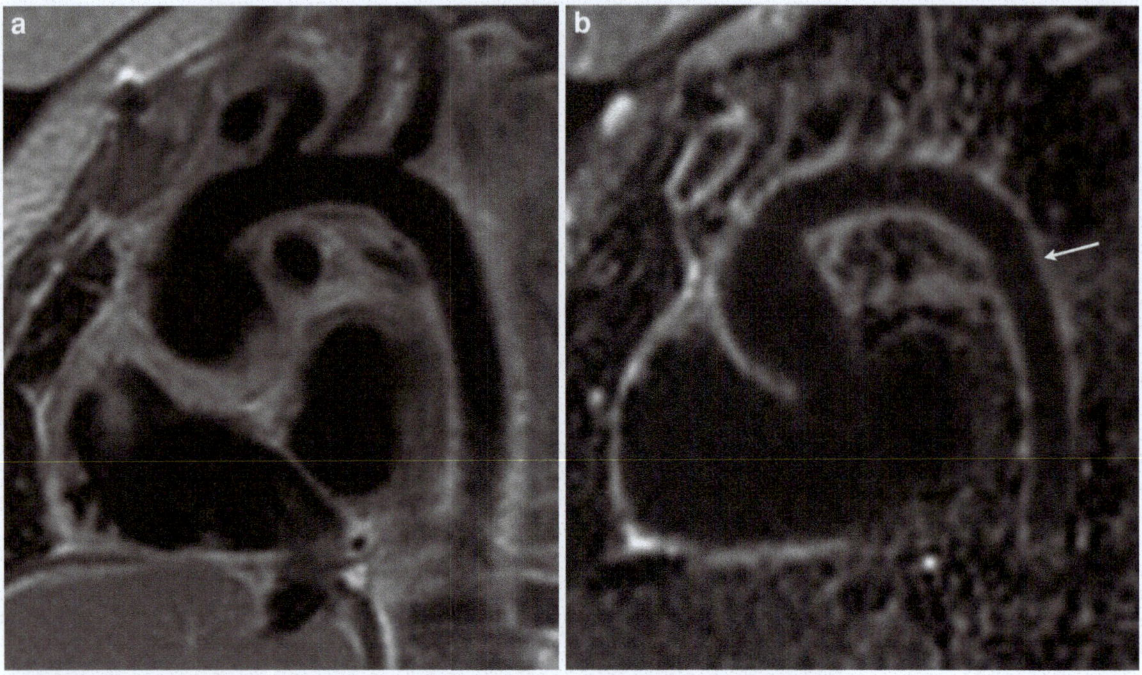

Fig. 32 **a** Black-blood sagittal oblique aortic image, and **b** late Gd sagittal oblique aortic image in the same patient as Fig. 31 in "Congenital Heart Disease", showing a dilated aortic root, and mild narrowing of the origin of the left common carotid, and left subclavian arteries, which is associated with increased wall thickening, and extensive late Gd enhancement of the whole aortic wall (*arrow*)

Pulmonary arterial anomalies, such as pulmonary artery sling can also be shown on MRI (Beekman et al. 1998) (Fig. 35). In pulmonary artery sling, the left pulmonary artery arises from the posterior aspect of the right pulmonary artery to the right of the trachea, before coursing to the left hilum between the esophagus and trachea. The ductal ligament is between the main pulmonary artery and descending aorta to the left of the trachea. The sling is almost always associated with airway abnormalities, through a combination of direct tracheal compression with resultant long-segment tracheobronchial stenosis, and also abnormal branching pattern of the tracheobronchial tree (Fiore et al. 2005). Although MRI is diagnostic, CT is generally preferred because of shorter scanning times, and better airway visualization in what is an extremely unwell group of patients.

Diagnosis of pulmonary embolism using breath-hold 3D ceMRA is now possible but it is crucial to acquire the data in a reasonably short breath-hold, as most patients with pulmonary embolism tend to be dyspneic. One study revealed 100% diagnostic accuracy (Grist et al. 1993; van Beek et al. 2003). Another major advantage is that MRA of the pulmonary vasculature can be complemented by MR venography of the pelvic and femoral veins (Carpenter et al. 1993). In patients with difficulty in breath holding, time-resolved MRA can be used. Pulmonary emboli are identified as filling defects in the pulmonary arteries, and can be seen to a segmental level. Furthermore, wedge-shaped perfusion defects can also be seen. Time-resolved MRA is particularly useful for the assessment of patients who are allergic to iodinated contrast, or with a mild degree of renal impairment as low volumes of gadolinium can be used (Ersoy et al. 2007). Despite these studies, the wide availability and ease of use of CT pulmonary angiography means that CT is currently the imaging modality of choice for direct visualization of the pulmonary vasculature in suspected pulmonary embolus (Kanne and Lalani 2004).

3.3 Pulmonary Veins

Abnormal pulmonary venous connections are accurately depicted by MRI either partial anomalous venous connection or total anomalous venous connection (Prasad et al. 2004) (Figs. 36, 37). Total

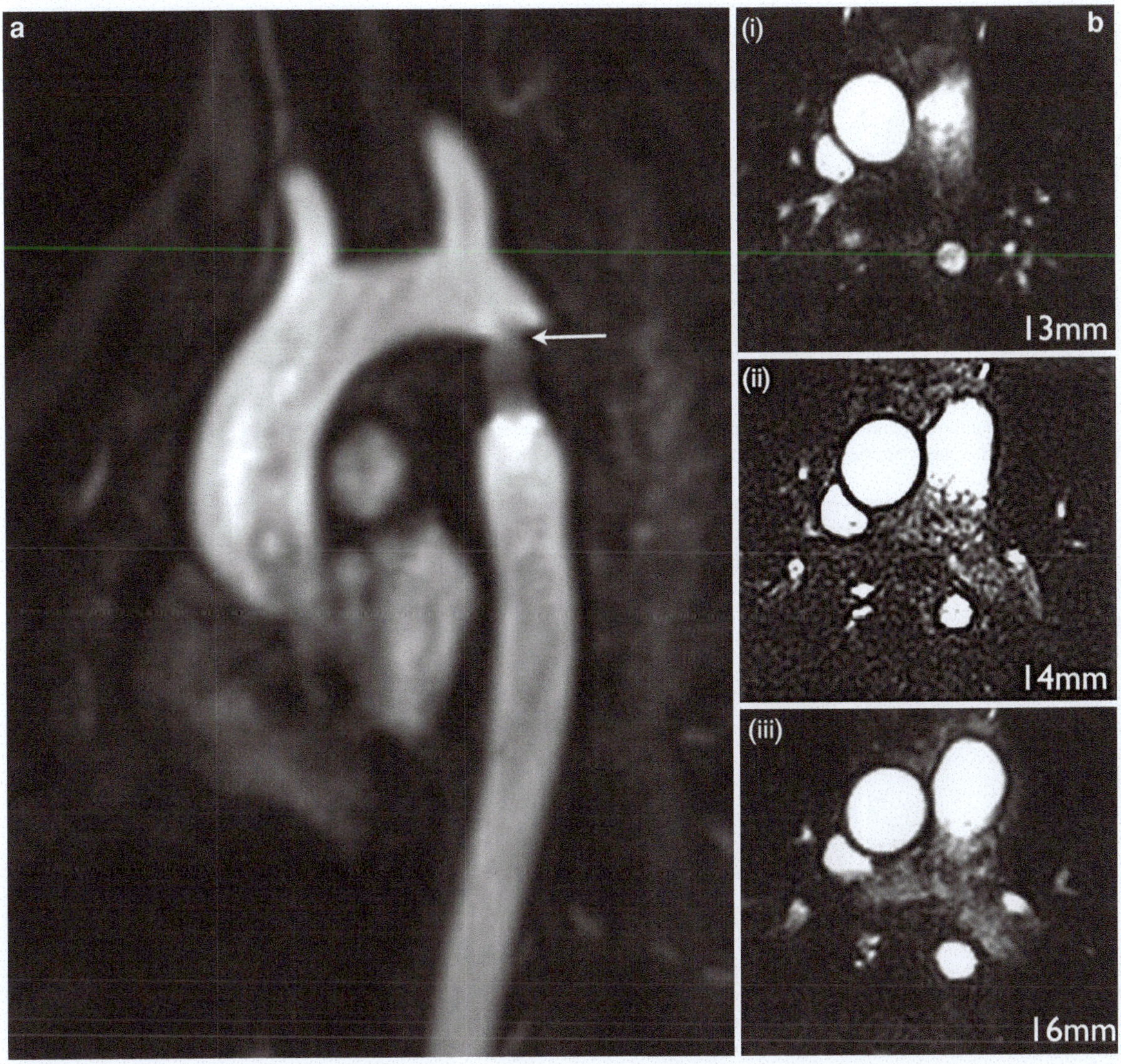

Fig. 33 Stent imaging in a 54-year-old patient with a stainless steel coarctation stent. **a** high flip-angle (75°) ceMRA sagital oblique MPR shows mild proximal stent narrowing (*arrow*). **b** selected through-plane high flip-angle (75°) cine images from a stack through the stent. The mild proximal narrowing is confirmed (13 mm internal luminal diameter image (i) 16 mm internal luminal diameter image (iii))

anomalous pulmonary connection can either be supracardiac, cardiac, or infracardiac (Figs. 38, 39). While 3D ceMRA and 3D whole-heart imaging (Pilleul and Merchant 2000, Greil et al. 2002) are most useful, axial black-blood, single-shot bright-blood acquisitions (Masui et al. 1991) and cine imaging (White et al. 1998) can also be used to evaluate anomalous pulmonary venous anatomy. Pulmonary venous connections with a tortuous course can be particularly difficult to follow by echocardiography. However, MRI with volume-rendered reconstruction shows these vessels readily, and should be considered the diagnostic tool of choice (Festa et al. 2006). Flow imaging of the aorta and pulmonary artery should be performed to calculate the shunt. It is important to note that partial anomalous venous drainage is often associated with a sinus venous atrial septal defect.

Other pulmonary abnormalities include pulmonary venous varix, which may appear as a dilated tubular structure confluent with the left atrium (Wildenhain and Bourekas 1991), and pulmonary arterio-venous malformations.

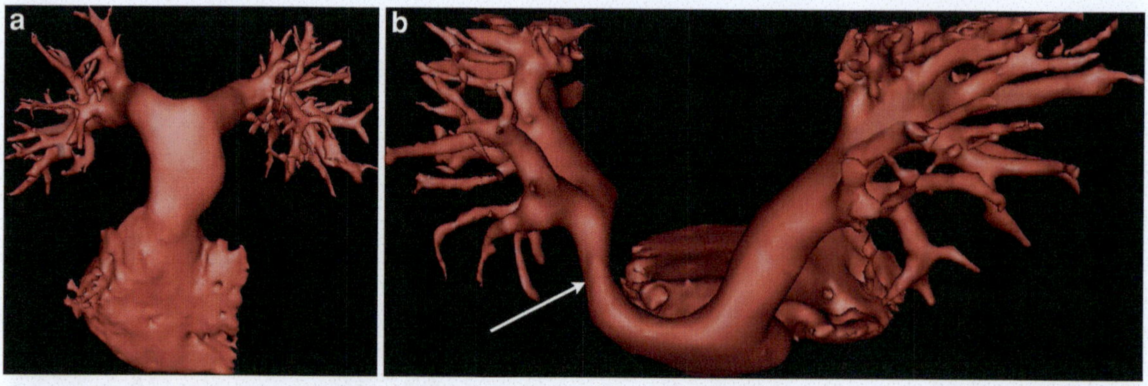

Fig. 34 Volume-rendered 3D reconstruction from a ceMRA of a complex pulmonary artery stenosis in a patient with transposition of the great arteries following the arterial switch operation. **a** Anterior view, and **b** superior oblique view, showing flattening of the distal main pulmonary artery, and narrowing of the right pulmonary artery (*arrow*)

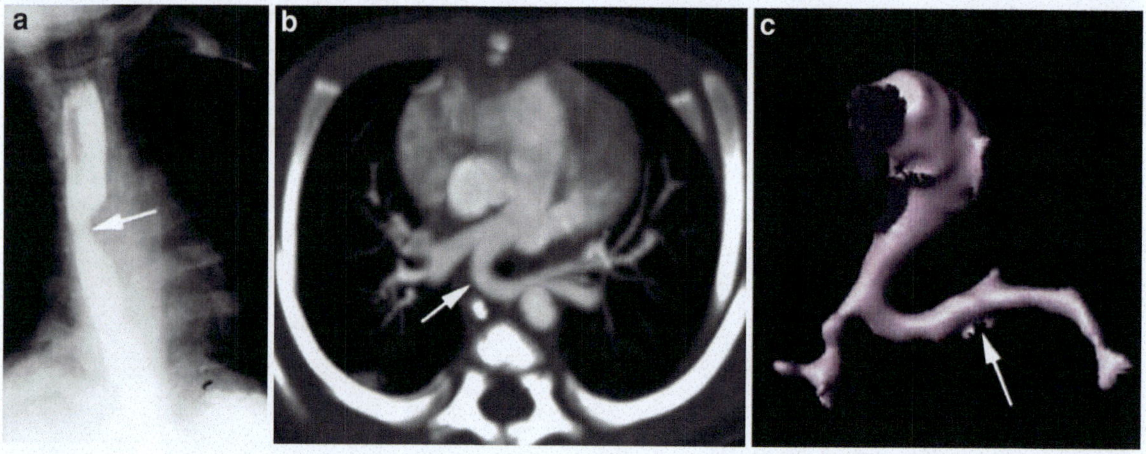

Fig. 35 Left pulmonary artery sling. **a** Right anterior oblique projection from a barium swallow showing anterior esophageal indentation (*arrow*). **b** Axial image from a post-contrast multi-slice CT scan showing the left pulmonary artery sling, originating from the mid-portion of the right pulmonary artery and passing behind the trachea (*arrow*). **c** Volume-rendered 3D reconstruction from ceMRA of left pulmonary artery sling (*arrow*) viewed from below. (Figure a, b courtesy of Dr. Cathy Owens, Department of Clinical Radiology, Great Ormond Street Hospital for Children, whom maintains copyright)

Pulmonary vein stenosis is a rare condition in children, and even rarer in adults, although with the advent of radiofrequency ablation therapy for atrial fibrillation more cases are being seen. Other causes include mediastinal abnormalities such as malignancy and fibrosing mediastinitis. In children more than half of patients have associated congenital heart disease. External compression is well-described secondary to dilatation of the left atrium, dilatation of the descending aorta (O'Donnell et al. 2003), and more specifically dilatation of the right atrium in Fontan patients (McElhinney et al. 1996; Hegde et al. 2004). It may also occur following surgical reimplantation of an anomalous pulmonary vein (Latson and Prieto 2007). Pulmonary veins can become focally stenosed at the atrial junction, or exhibit long-segment hypoplasia (Fig. 40).

Three-dimensional ceMRA is a good first-line technique for evaluation of pulmonary vein stenosis, although stenosis tends to be overestimated because of signal dropout from flow acceleration. Three-dimensional whole-heart imaging performed following gadolinium gives a higher blood-pool signal because of the T1 shortening effect of gadolinium, and is often extremely useful, both for the pulmonary venous stenosis, and for assessing for external compression. Cine imaging can be used to look for flow acceleration. Both 3D whole-heart and cine imaging

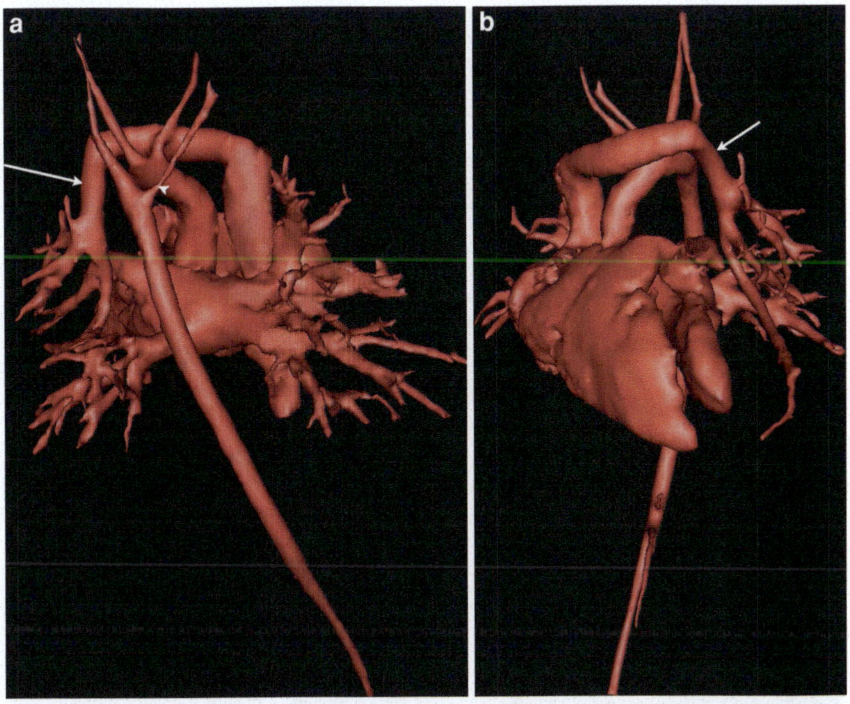

Fig. 36 Volume-rendered 3D reconstructed ceMRA of a patient with anomalous pulmonary venous drainage of the left upper pulmonary vein to the brachiocephalic vein (*arrow*). **a** Posterior view, and **b** anterior view. Note also the aberrant right subclavian artery (*arrowhead*)

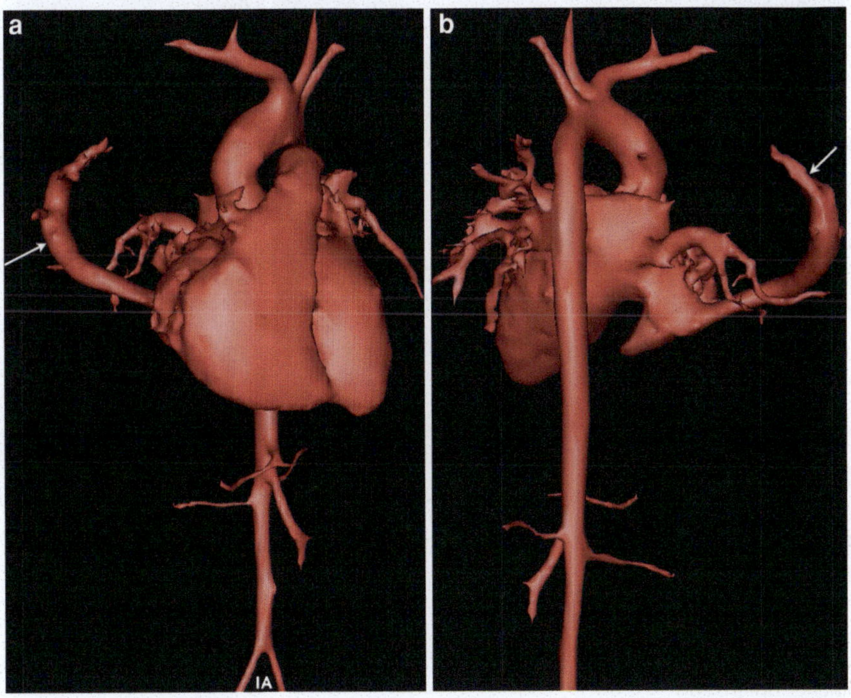

Fig. 37 Volume-rendered 3D reconstructed ceMRA of a patient with Scimitar syndrome. The pulmonary arteries have been removed to visualize the anomalous pulmonary venous drainage more clearly. The right-sided Scimitar vein (*arrow*) drains to the right atrial/IVC junction. **a** Anterior view, and **b** posterior view with the RV removed

can suffer from signal dropout in the pulmonary veins due to a combination of off-resonance, and pulmonary venous flow. Acquiring the 3D whole-heart in late diastole, when there is minimal pulmonary venous inflow (Hu et al. 2010), and keeping the TR to a minimum will improve the pulmonary venous signal. PC-MRI is also helpful in delineating the site and hemodynamic severity of pulmonary venous

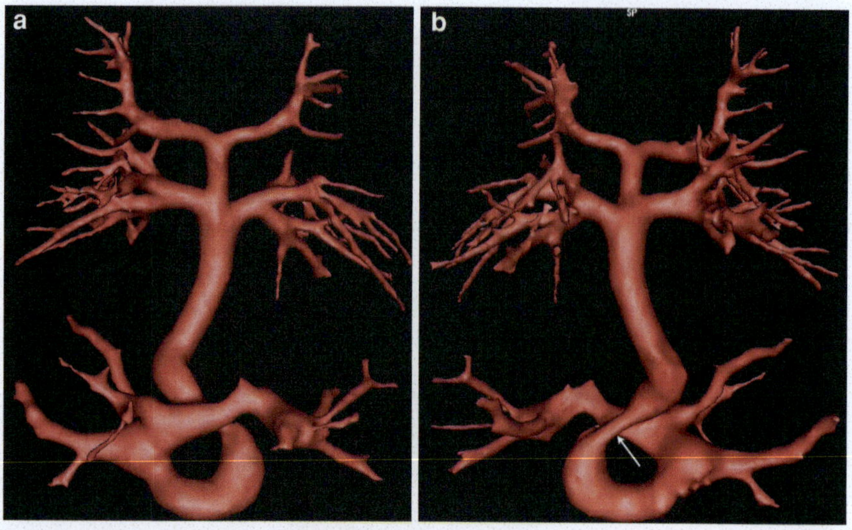

Fig. 38 Volume-rendered 3D reconstructed ceMRA of a patient with infra-cardiac total anomalous pulmonary venous connection to the portal vein. **a** Anterior view, and **b** posterior view. Note the narrowing of the pulmonary vein as it has passed through the diaphragm (*arrow*)

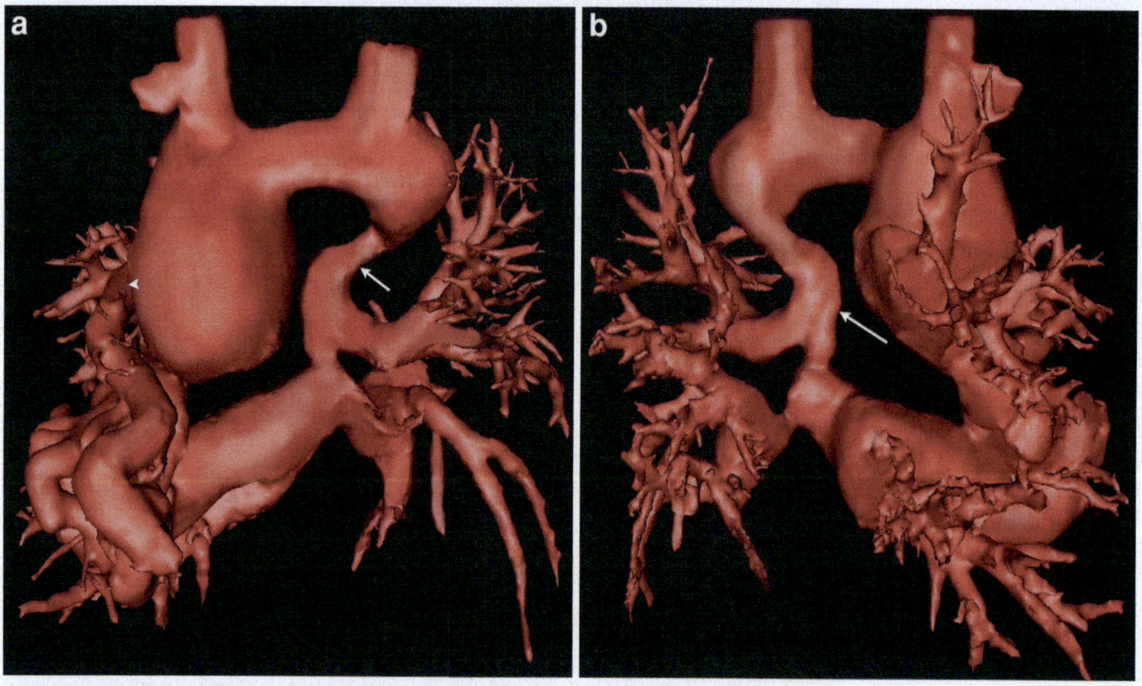

Fig. 39 Volume-rendered 3D reconstructed ceMRA of a patient with supra-cardiac total anomalous pulmonary venous connection. **a** Anterior view, and **b** posterior view. There are connections both to the brachiocephalic vein on the left (*arrow*), and the right-sided SVC (*arrowhead*). The right- and left-sided pulmonary veins join across the midline

obstruction (Videlefsky et al. 2001; Roman et al. 2005). Time-resolved MRA offers a potential additional tool for the evaluation of pulmonary vein stenosis. The dynamic nature of this imaging technique means that it is possible to detect slow transit of contrast through the region of lung with restrictive venous drainage. CT is a good technique for pulmonary vein assessment, and is particularly good at assessing mediastinal causes of compression. However, there is concern regarding ionizing radiation, particularly in young children, if repeated studies are needed.

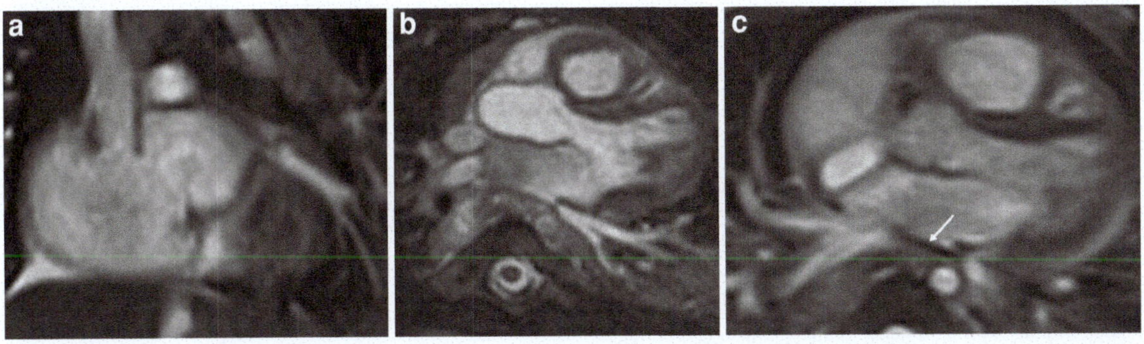

Fig. 40 Selected images from a patient with isolated left pulmonary venous stenosis. **a** Coronal oblique 3D whole-heart image **b** axial oblique 3D whole-heart image, and **c** cine image showing flow acceleration (*arrow*)

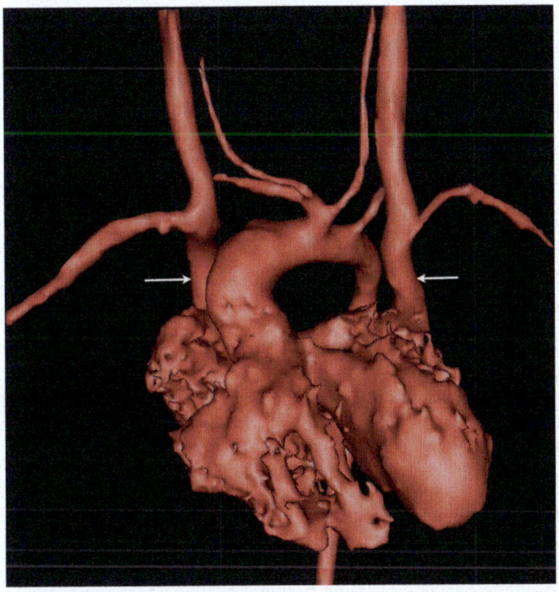

Fig. 41 Volume-rendered image of a patient with bilateral SVCs (*arrows*), and no bridging vein

Table 8 Cardiovascular MR imaging protocol for the aorta

1. Scout imaging
2. Single-shot black-blood stack
3. 4-chamber cine
4. Short Axis cine imaging quantification of LV function and mass
5. 3D ceMRA
6. 3D whole-heart volume
7. Cines of LVOT, aorta-in-plane, and aortic valve
8. Black-blood images of the aorta-in-plane (oblique sagittal view)
9. High flip-angle through-plane spoiled gradient echo bright-blood imaging if stents are present
10. PC-MRI both through-plane and in-plane at the site of any narrowings, and in the aortic root to assess for aortic valvular disease, and compare with ventricular stroke volumes.

3.4 Systemic Veins

MRI is superior to echocardiography in its ability to delineate systemic venous structures and therefore is very useful in the anatomic and hemodynamic evaluation of cardiac heterotaxia in infants and children (White 2000).

Systemic venous abnormalities that can be diagnosed and should be looked for on MRI include anomalous left brachiocephalic vein, left inferior vena cava, duplication of the inferior vena cava, persistence of left superior vena cava and thrombosis of the superior caval vein (Hernandez 2002). The innominate vein coursing posterior to the aorta can sometimes be mistaken for the right pulmonary artery (Didier et al. 1999). Three-dimensional whole-heart (Razavi et al. 2003) and 3D ceMRA will help in comprehensive evaluation of systemic venous abnormalities. The demonstration of a left SVC as well as azygos continuation is of importance in surgical planning, particularly in cases of functional single ventricle in which cavopulmonary shunts (Fontan operation) may be required (see "Congenital Heart Disease") (Fig. 41).

MRI is an excellent technique for examining the systemic venous system for stenoses and occlusions, and is particularly useful in the examination of patients who may have superior vena cava syndrome and in planning access for central venous catheters

Table 9 Cardiovascular MR-imaging protocol for the pulmonary arteries

1. Scout imaging
2. Single-shot black-blood stack
3. 4-chamber cine
4. Short Axis cine imaging quantification of RV function
5. 3D ceMRA
6. 3D whole-heart volume
7. Cines of RVOT, pulmonary trunk, and branch PAs
8. High flip-angle through-plane spoiled gradient echo bright-blood imaging if stents are present
9. PC-MRI through any narrowings (in-plane, through-plane), across the proximal pulmonary trunk to assess pulmonary valvular function, and across the branch pulmonary arteries to assess differential pulmonary blood flow

Table 10 Cardiovascular MR imaging protocol for the systemic and pulmonary veins

1. Scout imaging
2. Single-shot black-blood stack
3. 3D ceMRA
4. 3D whole-heart volume
5. In-plane cines of systemic and pulmonary veins
6. PC-MRI to look for flow acceleration, and alteration of normal pulmonary venous waveform

(Kim et al. 2008). Three-dimensional ceMRA (Hartnell et al. 1995; Lebowitz et al. 1997), and high-resolution bright-blood imaging (Spuentrup et al. 2001) have all been shown to be very useful for venography. Time-resolved MRA can also be used, and has the advantage of demonstrating the dynamic opacification of collateral vessels (Kim et al. 2008).

4 Conclusion

MRI is now well recognized as the optimal imaging modality for assessing and monitoring a wide variety of diseases of the great vessels and surrounding structures. However, the imaging modality of choice, may vary between centers, and is influenced by local availability and expertise. A variety of new techniques and faster pulse sequences have made cardiovascular MRI appealing to both Cardiologists and Radiologists especially for the assessment of great vessels of the chest.

4.1 The Future

MRI is increasingly being used to evaluate atherosclerosis plaques. In vivo characterization of atherosclerosis plaque components in human aorta is now possible (Toussaint 2002). Good correlation has also been found between multi-contrast MRI and TEE for aortic plaque quantification and characterization (Fayad 2003). There is growing interest in developing contrast agents that specifically target and identify components of vulnerable plaque (Flacke et al. 2001). The progression of atherosclerosis especially by positive arterial remodeling has been demonstrated in transgenic mouse models (Choudhury et al. 2002).

Angiogenesis is thought to be a critical feature of plaque development in atherosclerosis (Winter et al. 2003). In a recent study, targeted paramagnetic nanoparticles were developed for non-invasive molecular imaging of angiogenesis in an animal model at 3-Tesla field strength. It is hoped that MR molecular imaging of angiogenesis with targeted nanoparticles could provide a sensitive, high-resolution signal for monitoring progression and treatment of cardiovascular disease (Cai et al. 2010).

The high spatial resolution of MRI and improved contrast agents is giving MRI the edge over positron emission tomography (PET), other nuclear techniques and CT in the field of molecular imaging. MRI, therefore, holds the promise of becoming a valuable tool to image the presence or activity of specific molecules in vivo (Weissleder and Mahmood 2001).

Another area of interest is the response of the cardiovascular system to stress. Routinely, only heart rate and blood pressure are measured during exercise. However using MRI, by measuring aortic flow and blood pressure simultaneously, one can assess systemic vascular resistance, and total arterial compliance. This has been recently demonstrated during exercise (Steedon et al. 2010), and during mental stress (Jones et al. 2011). Stress may be used to unmask early signs of vascular disease in at-risk groups. The ability to noninvasively measure vascular resistance and compliance further improves the sensitivity of exercise testing. Thus, this technique may allow the identification of at-risk individuals.

5 Keypoints

- When available, MRI is the non-invasive method of choice for assessing the great vessels of the thorax.
- Three-dimensional sequences such as 3D ceMRA and 3D whole-heart imaging are extremely important for anatomical delineation. The ability to perform post-processing techniques on these data sets is a powerful tool for clinical decision-making.
- A combination of techniques should be used in all patients to avoid missing important pathology.
- Assessment of ventricular function and mass is useful to understand the functional significance of vascular abnormalities.
- Congenital vascular malformations are frequently associated with both valvular and intra-cardiac anomalies.
- Abnormal branching patterns of the great vessels may cause significant obstruction to swallowing and breathing, and a high index of suspicion is needed to rule out vascular rings.
- Careful scrutiny is needed to exclude dissection in patients with aortic dilatation, and in the follow-up of those with penetrating ulceration and intramural hematoma.
- Imaging stents is possible with MRI, and it is worth trying before resorting to CT, as it provides additional functional information.
- Imaging protocols for the great vessels are outlined in Tables 8, 9, 10

References

Andrews J, Al-Nahhas A, Pennell DJ et al (2004) Non-invasive imaging in the diagnosis and management of Takayasu's arteritis. Annals Rheumatic Dis 63:995–1000

Araoz PA, Reddy GP, Tarnoff H, Roge CL, Higgins CB (2003) MR findings of collateral circulation are more accurate measures of hemodynamic significance than arm-leg blood pressure gradient after repair of coarctation of the aorta. JMRI 17:177–183

Bartels LW, Bakker CJ, Viergever MA (2002) Improved lumen visualization in metallic vascular implants by reducing RF artifacts. Magn Reson Med 47:171–180

Becker AE, Becker MJ, Edwards JE (1970) Anomalies associated with coarctation of aorta: particular reference to infancy. Circulation 41:1067–1075

Bernard Y, Zimmermann H, Chocron S et al (2001) False lumen patency as a predictor of late outcome in Aortic Dissection. Am J Cardiol 15;87(12):1378–1382

Baerlocher L, Kretschmar O, Harpes P et al (2008) Stent implantation and balloon angioplasty for treatment of branch pulmonary artery stenosis in children. Clin Res Cardiol 97:310–317

Beekman RP, Hazekamp MG, Sobotka MA et al (1998) A new diagnostic approach to vascular rings and pulmonary slings: the role of MRI. Magn Reson Imaging 16:137–145

Bogaert J, Gewillig M, Rademakers F et al (1995) Transverse arch hypoplasia predisposes to aneurysm formation at the repair site after patch angioplasty for coarctation of the aorta. J Am Coll Cardiol 26:521–527

Bogaert J, Meyns B, Rademakers F et al (1997) Aortic dissection: contribution of MR angiography for evaluation of the abdominal aorta and its branches. Eur Radiol 7:695–702

Bogaert J, Kuzo R, Dymarkowski S et al (2000) Follow-up of patients with previous treatment for coarctation of the thoracic aorta: comparison between contrast-enhanced MR angiography and fast spin-echo MR imaging. Eur Radiol 10:1847–1854

Bogaert J, Dymarkowski S, Budts W, Daenen W, Gewillig M (2001) Graft dilatation after redo surgery for aneurysm formation following patch angioplasty for coarctation of the aorta. Europ J Thorac Cardiovasc Surg 19 :274–278

Buonocore MH, Bogren H (1991) Optimized pulse sequence for magnetic resonance measurment of aortic cross-sectional areas. Magn Reson Imaging 9(3):435–447

Cai K, Caruthers SD, Huang W et al (2010) MR molecular imaging of aortic angiogenesis. JACC Cardiovasc Imag 3(8): 824–832

Canter CE, Gutierrez FR, Mirowitz SA, Martin TC, Hartmann A F Jr (1989) Evaluation of pulmonary arterial morphology in cyanotic congenital heart disease by magnetic resonance imaging. Am Heart J 118:347–354

Carpenter JP, Holland GA, Baum RA, Owen RS, Carpenter JT, Cope C (1993) Magnetic resonance venography for the detection of deep venous thrombosis: comparison with contrast venography and duplex Doppler ultrasonography. J Vasc Surg 18:734–741

Carr J, Simonetti O, Bundy J et al (2001) Cine MR angiography of the heart with segmented true fast imaging with steady-state precession. Radiology 219:828–834

Carr JC, Finn JP (2003) MR imaging of the thoracic aorta. Magn Reson Imaging Clin N Am 11:135–148

Chien D, Saloner D, Laub Anderson C M (1994) High resolution cine MRI of vessel distension. J Comput Assisst Tomogr. 18(4):576–580

Choe YH, Han BK, Koh EM et al (2000) Takayasu's arteritis: assessment of disease activity with contrast- enhanced MR imaging. AJR 175:505–511

Choudhury RP, Fuster V, Badimon JJ, Fisher EA, Fayad ZA (2002) MRI and characterization of atherosclerotic plaque: emerging applications and molecular imaging. Arterioscler Thromb Vasc Biol 22:1065–1074

Clough RE, Schaeffter T, Taylor PR (2010) Magnetic Resonance imaging for aortic dissection. Eur J Vasc Endovasc Surg 39:514–517

Dake MD, Miller DC, Mitchell RS, Semba CP, Moore KA, Sakai T (1998) The "first generation" of endovascular stent-grafts for patients with aneurysms of the descending thoracic aorta. J Thorac Cardiovasc Surg 116:689–704

Daniels SR, James FW, Loggie JM et al (1987) Correlates of resting and maximal exercise systolic blood pressure after repair of coarctation of the aorta: a multivariable analysis. Am Heart J 113:349–353

DeBakey ME, Henly WS, Cooley DA et al (1965) Surgical management of dissecting aneurysms of the aorta. J Thorac Cardiovasc Surg 49:130–148

De Leval MR, Elliott MJ (2006) Vascular rings. In: Stark JF, de Leval MR, Tsang VT (eds) Surgery for Congenital Heart Defects. Wiley-Blackwell, London, pp 307–318

Didier D, Ratib O, Beghetti M, Oberhaensli I, Friedli B (1999) Morphologic and functional evaluation of congenital heart disease by magnetic resonance imaging. JMRI 10:639–655

Dietl CA, Torres AR, Favaloro RG, Fessler CL, Grunkemeier GL (1992) Risk of recoarctation in neonates and infants after repair with patch aortoplasty, subclavian flap, and the combined resection-flap procedure. J Thorac Cardiovasc Surg 103:724–732

Dymarkowski S, Bosmans H, Marchal G, Bogaert J (1999) 3D MR angiography of thoracic outlet. Am J Roentgenol 173: 1005–1008

Earls JP, Rofsky NM, DeCorato DR, Krinsky GA, Weinreb JC (1996) Breath-hold single-dose gadolinium-enhanced three-dimensional MR aortography: usefulness of a timing examination and MR power injector. Radiology 201: 705–710

Edwards JE (1948) Anomalies of the derivatives of the aortic arch system. Med Clin North Am 33:925–949

Elefteriades JA, Farkas EA (2010) Thoracic aortic aneurysm. clinically pertinent controversies and uncertainties. JACC 55:841–857

Engellau L, Olsrud J, Brockstedt S et al (2000) MR evaluation ex vivo and in vivo of a covered stent-graft for abdominal aortic aneurysms: ferromagnetism, heating, artifacts, and velocity mapping. JMRI 12:112–121

Erbel R, Alfonso F, Boileau C et al (2001) Diagnosis and management of aortic dissection. Recommendations of the Task Force on Aortic Dissection, European Society of Cardiology. Eur Heart J 22:1642-1681

Ersoy H, Goldhaber SZ, Cai T et al (2007) Time-resolved MR angiography: a primary screening examination of patients with suspected pulmonary embolism and contraindications to administration of iodinated contrast material. AJR Am J Roentgenol 188(5):1246–1254

Fatouraee N, Amini AA (2003) Regularization of flow streamlines in multislice phase-contrast MR imaging. IEEE Trans Med Imag 22:699–709

Fattori R, Celletti F, Bertaccini P et al (1996) Delayed surgery of traumatic aortic rupture. Role of magnetic resonance imaging. Circulation 94:2865–2870

Fattori R, Nienaber CA (1999) MRI of acute and chronic aortic pathology: pre-operative and post-operative evaluation. JMRI 10:741–750

Fattori R, Bacchi Reggiani L, Pepe G et al (2000) Magnetic resonance imaging evaluation of aortic elastic properties as early expression of Marfan syndrome. JCMR 2:251–256

Faust RA, Remley KB, Rimell FL (2001) Real-time, cine magnetic resonance imaging for evaluation of the pediatric airway. Laryngoscope 111:2187–2190

Fayad ZA (2003) MR imaging for the noninvasive assessment of atherothrombotic plaques. Magn Reson Imaging Clin N Am 11:101–113

Festa P, Ait-Ali L, Cerillo AG et al (2006) Magnetic resonance imaging is the diagnostic tool of choice in the preoperative evaluation of patients with partial anomalous pulmonary venous return. Int J Cardiovasc Imaging 22:685–693

Finn JP, Baskaran V, Carr JC et al (2002) Thorax: low-dose contrast-enhanced three-dimensional MR angiography with subsecond temporal resolution–initial results. Radiology 224:896–904

Fiore AC, Brown JW, Weber TR, Turrentine MW (2005) Surgical treatment of pulmonary artery sling and tracheal stenosis. Ann Thorac Surg Jan 79(1):38–46 Discussion

Flacke S, Fischer S, Scott MJ et al (2001) Novel MRI contrast agent for molecular imaging of fibrin: implications for detecting vulnerable plaques. Circulation 104:1280–1285

Forbat SM, Mohiaddin RH, Yang GZ et al (1995) Measurement of regional aortic compliance by MR Imaging: a study of reproducibility. J Magn Reson Imaging 5(6):635–639

Francois CJ, Shors SM, Bonow RO, Finn JP (2003) Analysis of cardiopulmonary transit times at contrast material-enhanced MR imaging in patients with heart disease. Radiology 227: 447–452

Ganaha F, Miller DC, Sugimoto K et al (2002) Prognosis of aortic intramural hematoma with and without penetrating atherosclerotic ulcer: a clinical and radiological analysis. Circulation 106:342–348

Gaubert JY, Moulin G, Mesana T et al (1995) Type A dissection of the thoracic aorta: use of MR imaging for long-term follow-up. Radiology 196:363–369

Giordano U, Giannico S, Turchetta A et al (2005) The influence of different surgical procedures on hypertension after repair of coarctation. Cardiol Young 15:477–480

Gomes AS, Lois JF, George B, Alpan G, Williams RG (1987) Congenital abnormalities of the aortic arch: MR imaging. Radiology 165:691–695

Gotzsche CO, Krag-Olson B, Nielsen J et al (1994) Prevalence of cardiovascular malformations and association with karyotypes in Turner's syndrome. Arch Dis Child 71:433–436

Greil GF, Powell AJ, Gildein HP, Geva T (2002) Gadolinium-enhanced three-dimensional magnetic resonance angiography of pulmonary and systemic venous anomalies. J Am Coll Cardiol 39:335–341

Greil GF, Kramer U, Dammann F et al (2005) Diagnosis of vascular rings and slings using an interleaved 3D double-slab FISP MR angiography technique. Pediatr Radiol 35: 396–401

Grist TM, Sostman HD, MacFall JR et al (1993) Pulmonary angiography with MR imaging: preliminary clinical experience. Radiology 189:523–530

Groenink M, de Roos A, Mulder BJ et al (2001) Biophysical properties of the normal-sized aorta in patients with Marfan syndrome: evaluation with MR flow mapping. Radiology 219:535–540

Gundry SR, Burney RE, Mackenzie JR, Jafri SZ, Shirazi K, Cho KJ (1984) Traumatic pseudoaneurysms of the thoracic aorta. Anatomic and radiologic correlations. Arch Surg 119:1055–1060

Hagan PG, Nienaber CA, Isselbacher EM et al (2000) The International Registry of Acute Aortic Dissection (IRAD): new insights into an old disease. JAMA 283:897–903

Hagspiel KD, Leung DA, Nandalur KR et al (2005) Contrast-enhanced MR angiography at 1.5 T after implantation of platinum stents: in vitro and in vivo comparison with conventional stent designs. Am J Roentgenol 184:288–294

Hamdan MA, Maheshwari S, Fahey JT, Hellenbrand WE (2001) Endovascular stents for coarctation of the aorta: initial results and intermediate-term follow-up. J Am Coll Cardiol 38:1518–1523

Hartnell GG, Hughes LA, Finn JP, Longmaid H E 3rd (1995) Magnetic resonance angiography of the central chest veins. A new gold standard? Chest 107:1053–1057

Hegde SR, Taylor AM, Muthurangu VM, Miquel ME, Razavi R (2004) The use of MRI in detecting pulmonary vein compression in patients with Fontan circulation. In: ECR conference proceedings 14(suppl 2): B-531

Hernandez RJ (2002) Magnetic resonance imaging of mediastinal vessels. Magn Reson Imaging Clin N Am 10:237–251

Hilfiker PR, Quick HH, Pfammatter T, Schmidt M, Debatin JF (1999) Three-dimensional MR angiography of a nitinol-based abdominal aortic stent graft: assessment of heating and imaging characteristics. Eur Radiol 9:1775–1780

Higgins CB, Sakuma H (1996) Heart disease: functional evaluation with MR imaging. Radiology 199:307–315

Ho VB, Foo TK (1998) Optimization of gadolinium-enhanced magnetic resonance angiography using an automated bolus-detection algorithm (MR SmartPrep). Original investigation. Invest Radiol 33:515–523

Ho VB, Choyke PL, Foo TK et al (1999) Automated bolus chase peripheral MR angiography: initial practical experiences and future directions of this work-in-progress. JMRI 10:376–388

Holmqvist C, Stahlberg F, Hanseus K et al (2002) Collateral flow in coarctation of the aorta with magnetic resonance velocity mapping: correlation to morphological imaging of collateral vessels. JMRI 15:39–46

Hope TA, Markl M, Wigstrom L et al (2007) Comparison of flow patterns in ascending aortic aneurysms and volunteers using four-dimensional magnetic resonance velocity mapping. J Magn Reson Imaging 26:1471–1479

Hope MD, Meadows AK, Hope TA et al (2010) Clinical evaluation of aortic coarctation with 4D flow MR imaging. J Magn Reson Imaging 31:711–718

Hoschtitzky JA, Anderson RH, Elliot MJ (2009) Paediatric Cardiology, 3rd edn. Churchill-Livingstone, Edinburgh, pp 945–966 Chap. 46

Hu P, Stoeck CT, Smink J et al (2010) Noncontrast SSFP Pulmonary vein magnetic resonance angiography: Impact of off-resonance and flow. J Magn Reson Imaging 32:1255–1261

Jones A, Steeden JA, Pruessner JC et al (2011) Detailed assessment of the haemodynamic response to psychosocial stress using real-time MRI. J Magn Reson Imaging 33(2): 448–454

Kaemmerer H, Theissen P, Konig U, Sechtem U, de Vivie ER (1993) Follow-up using magnetic resonance imaging in adult patients after surgery for aortic coarctation. Thorac Cardiovasc Surg 41:107–111

Kanne JP, Lalani TA (2004) Role of computed tomography and magnetic resonance imaging for deep venous thrombosis and pulmonary embolism. Circulation 109(12 Suppl 1): I15–21

Kersting-Sommerhoff BA, Sechtem UP, Schiller NB, Lipton MJ, Higgins CB (1987) MR imaging of the thoracic aorta in Marfan patients. J Comput Assist Tomogr 11:633–639

Kim CY, Mirza RA, Bryant JA et al (2008) Central veins of the chest: Evaluation with time resolved MR angiography. Radiology. 247(2):558–566

Knauth AL, Marshall AC, Geva T, Jonas RA, Marx GR (2004) Respiratory symptoms secondary to aortopulmonary collateral vessels in tetralogy of Fallot absent pulmonary valve syndrome. Am J Cardiol 93:503–505

Korosec FR, Grist TM, Mistretta CA (1996) Time-resolved contrast-enhanced 3D MR angiography. Magn Reson Med 36:345–351

Knyshov GV, Sitar LL, Glagola MD et al (1996) Aortic aneurysms at the site of the repair of coarctation of the aorta: a review of 48 patients. Ann Thorac Surg 61:935–939

Krishnam MS, Tomasian A, Lohan DG et al (2008) Low-dose, time resolved, contrast-enhanced 3D MR angiography in cardiac and vascular diseases: correlation to high spatial resolution 3D contrast-enhanced MRA. Clin Rad 63: 744–755

Lansman SL, Saunders PC, Malekan R et al (2010) Acute aortic syndrome J Thorac Cardiovasc Surg. 2010 140(6 Suppl): S92–97

Latson LA, Prieto LR (2007) Congenital and acquired pulmonary vein stenosis. Circulation 115(1):103–108

Lebowitz JA, Rofsky NM, Krinsky GA, Weinreb JC (1997) Gadolinium-enhanced body MR venography with subtraction technique. Am J Roentgenol 169:755–758

Lee VS, Resnick D, Bundy JM et al (2002) Cardiac function: MR evaluation in one breath hold with real-time true fast imaging with steady state precession. Radiology 222: 835–842

Leeson CP, Robinson M, Francis JM et al (2006) Cardiovascular magnetic resonance imaging for non-invasive assessment of vascular function: validation against ultrasound. J Cardiovasc Magn Reson 8(2):381–387

Lenhart M, Volk M, Manke C et al (2000) Stent appearance at contrast-enhanced MR angiography: invitro examination with 14 stents. Radiology 217:173–178

Leung DA, Debatin JF (1997) Three-dimensional contrast-enhanced magnetic resonance angiography of the thoracic vasculature. Eur Radiol 7:981–989

Loeys BL, Dietz HC, Braverman AC et al (2010) The revised Ghent nosology for the Marfan Syndrome. J Med Genet 47:476–485

Lohan DG, Krishnam M, Saleh R et al (2008) MR imaging if the thoracic aorta. Magn Reson Imaging Clin N Am 16(2): 213–234

Lurz P, Coats L, Khambadkone S et al (2008) Percutaneous pulmonary valve implantation: impact of evolving technology and learning curve on clinical outcome. Circulation 117:1964–1972

Markl M, Alley MT, Pelc NJ (2003a) Balanced phase-contrast steady-state free precession (PC-SSFP): a novel technique for velocity encoding by gradient inversion. Magn Reson Med 49:945–952

Markl M, Chan FP, Alley MT et al (2003b) Time-resolved three-dimensional phase-contrast MRI. JMRI 17:499–506

Martinez JE, Mohiaddin RH, Kilner PJ et al (1992) Obstruction in extracardiac ventriculopulmonary conduits: value of nuclear magnetic resonance imaging with velocity mapping and Doppler echocardiography. J Am Coll Cardiol 20: 338–344

Masui T, Seelos KC, Kersting-Sommerhoff BA, Higgins CB (1991) Abnormalities of the pulmonary veins: evaluation with MR imaging and comparison with cardiac angiography and echocardiography. Radiology 181:645–649

Masui T, Katayama M, Kobayashi S et al (2000) Gadolinium-enhanced MR angiography in the evaluation of congenital cardiovascular disease pre- and postoperative states in infants and children. JMRI 12:1034–1042

McElhinney DB, Reddy VM, Moore P, Hanley FL (1996) Revision of previous Fontan connections to extracardiac or intraatrial conduit cavopulmonary anastomosis. Ann Thorac Surg 62:1276–1283

Mohiaddin RH, Schoser K, Amanuma M, Burman ED, Longmore DB (1990) MR imaging of age-related dimensional changes of thoracic aorta. J Comput Assist Tomogr 14:748–752

Mohiaddin RH, Kilner PJ, Rees S et al (1993) Magnetic resonance volume flow and jet velocity mapping in aortic coarctation. J Am Coll Cardiol 22:1515–1521

Mohiaddin RH, McCrohon J, Francis JM et al (2001) Contrast-enhanced magnetic resonance angiogram of penetrating aortic ulcer. Circulation 103:18–19

Muthurangu V, Lurz P, Critchley JD et al (2008) Real-time assessment of right and left ventricular volumes and function in patients with congenital heart disease by using high spatiotemporal resolution radial k-t-SENSE. Radiology 248(3):782–791

Nayler GL, Firmin DN, Longmore DB (1986) Blood flow imaging by cine magnetic resonance. J Comput Assist Tomogr 10:715–722

Nienaber CA, Con Kodolitsch Y, Nicolas V et al (1993) The diagnosis of aortic dissection by non-invasive imaging procedures. N Engl J Med 328:1–9

Nienaber CA, Richartz BM, Rehders T, Ince H, Petzsch M (2004) Aortic intramural haematoma: natural history and predictive factors for complications. Heart 90:372–374

Nielsen JC, Powell AJ, Gauvreau K et al (2005) Magnetic resonance imaging predictors of coarctation severity. Circulation 111:622–628

Nordmeyer J, Gaudin R, Tann OR et al (2010a) MRI may be sufficient for noninvasive assessment of great vessel stens: an in vitro comparison of MRI, CT, and conventional angiography. Am J Roentgenol 195(4):865–871

Nordmeyer S, Riesenkampff E, Crelier G et al (2010b) Flow-sensitive four-dimensional cine magnetic resonance imaging for offline blood flow quantification in multiple vessels: a validation study. Am J Roentgenol 32:677–683

O'Donnell CP, Lock JE, Powell AJ, Perry SB (2003) Compression of pulmonary veins between the left atrium and the descending aorta. Am J Cardiol 91:248–251

Oppelt A, Graumann R, Barfuss H (1986) FISP–a new fast MRI sequence. Electromedica 54:15–18

Ou P, Celermajer DS, Jolivet O et al (2008) Increased central aortic stiffness and left ventricular mass in normotensive young subjects after successful. Coartation repair 155(1): 187–193

Pereles FS, Kapoor V, Carr JC et al (2001) Usefulness of segmented trueFISP cardiac pulse sequence in evaluation of congenital and acquired adult cardiac abnormalities. AJR 177:1155–1160

Piazza N, Grube E, Gerckens U et al (2008) Procedural and 30-day outcomes following transcatheter aortic valve implantation using the third generation (18 Fr) corevalve revalving system: results from the multicentre, expanded evaluation registry 1-year following CE mark approval. EuroIntervention 4:242–249

Pilleul F, Merchant N (2000) MRI of the pulmonary veins: comparison between 3D MR angiography and T1-weighted spin echo. J Comput Assist Tomogr 24:683–687

Pitt MP, Bonser RS (1997) The natural history of thoracic aortic aneurysm disease: an overview. J Card Surg 12(2 Suppl): 270–278

Powell AJ, Chung T, Landzberg MJ, Geva T (2000) Accuracy of MRI evaluation of pulmonary blood supply in patients with complex pulmonary stenosis or atresia. Int J Card Imaging 16:169–174

Prasad SK, Soukias N, Hornung T et al (2004) Role of magnetic resonance angiography in the diagnosis of major aortopulmonary collateral arteries and partial anomalous pulmonary venous drainage. Circulation 109:207–214

Prince MR (1994) Gadolinium-enhanced MR aortography. Radiology 191:155–164

Prince MR, Narasimham DL, Jacoby WT et al (1996) Three-dimensional gadolinium-enhanced MR angiography of the thoracic aorta. AJR 166:1387–1397

Razavi R, Baker E (1999) Magnetic resonance imaging comes of age. Cardiol Young 9:529–538

Razavi RS, Hill DL, Muthurangu V et al (2003) Three-dimensional magnetic resonance imaging of congenital cardiac anomalies. Cardiol Young 13:461–465

Riederer SJ, Bernstein MA, Breen JF et al (2000) Three-dimensional contrast-enhanced MR angiography with real-time fluoroscopic triggering: design specifications and technical reliability in 330 patient studies. Radiology 215:584–593

Roche KJ, Krinsky G, Lee VS, Rofsky N, Genieser NB (1999) Interrupted aortic arch: diagnosis with gadolinium-enhanced 3D MRA. J Comput Assist Tomogr 23:197–202

Roman KS, Kellenberger CJ, Macgowan CK et al (2005) How is pulmonary arterial blood flow affected by pulmonary venous obstruction in children? A phase-contrast magnetic resonance study. Pediatr Radio. 35:580–586

Roman MJ, Devereux RB, Niles NW et al (1987) Aortic root dilatation as a cause of isolated, severe aortic regurgitation. Prevalence, clinical and echocardiographic patterns, and relation to left ventricular hypertrophy and function. Ann Intern Med 106:800–807

Roos-Hesselink JW, Scholzel BE, Heijdra RJ et al (2003) Aortic valve and aortic arch pathology after coarctation repair. Heart 89:1074–1077

Samanak M, Slavik Z, Zborilova B et al (1989) Prevalence, treatment and outcome of heart disease in live-born children: A prospective analysis of 91823 live-born children. Pediatr Cardiol 10:205–211

Scheffler K, Lehnhardt S (2003) Principles and applications of balanced SSFP techniques. Eur Radiol 13:2409–2418
Schlesinger AE, Krishnamurthy R, Sena LM et al (2005) Incomplete double aortic arch with atresia of the distal left arch: distinctive imaging appearance. AJR Am J Roentgenol 184(5):1634–1639
Schmidta M, Theissen P, Klempt G et al (2000) Long-term follow-up of 82 patients with chronic disease of the thoracic aorta using spin-echo and cine gradient magnetic resonance imaging. Magn Reson Imaging 18:795–806
Senzaki H, Iwamoto Y, Ishido H et al (2008) Arterial haemodynamics in patients after repair of tetralogy of Fallot: influence on left ventricular after load and aortic dilation. Heart 94:70–74
Sevitt S (1977) The mechanisms of traumatic rupture of the thoracic aorta. Br J Surg 64:166–173
Simonetti OP, Finn JP, White RD et al (1996) "Black-blood" T2-weighted inversion-recovery MR imaging of the heart. Radiology 199:49–57
Smith DE, Matthews MB (1955) Aortic valvular stenosis with coarctation of the aorta, with special reference to the development of aortic stenosis upon congenital bicuspid valves. Br Heart J 17:198–206
Sonnabend SB, Colletti PM, Pentecost MJ (1990) Demonstration of aortic lesions via cine magnetic resonance imaging. Magn Reson Imaging 8(5):613–618
Sorensen TS, Korperich H, Greil GF et al (2004) Operator-independent isotropic three-dimensional magnetic resonance imaging for morphology in congenital heart disease: a validation study. Circulation 110(2):163–169
Spuentrup E, Buecker A, Stuber M, Gunther RW (2001) MR-venography using high resolution True-FISP.
Rofo Fortschr Geb Rontgenstr Neuen Bildgeb Verfahr 173: 686–690
Steeden JA, Atkinson D, Taylor AM et al (2010) Assessing vascular response to exercise using a combination of real-time spiral phase contrast MR and noninvasive blood pressure measurements. J Magn Reson Imaging 31(4):997–1003
Stehling MK, Holzknecht NG, Laub G et al (1996) Single-shot T1 and T2 weighted magnetic resonance imaging of the heart with black blood: preliminary experience. MAGMA 4:231–240
Stemerman DH, Krinsky GA, Lee VS, Johnson G, Yang BM, Rofsky NM (1999) Thoracic aorta: rapid black-blood MR imaging with half-Fourier rapid acquisition with relaxation enhancement with or without electrocardiographic triggering. Radiology 213:185–191
Summers RM, Sostman HD, Spritzer CE, Fidler JL (1996) Fast spoiled gradient-recalled MR imaging of thoracic aortic dissection: preliminary clinical experience at 1.5 T. Magn Reson Imaging 14:1–9
Svensson LG, Labib SB, Eisenhauer AC, Butterly JR (1999) Intimal tear without hematoma. An importantvariant of aortic dissection that can elude current imaging techniques. Circulation 99:1331–1336
Szolar DH, Sakuma H, Higgins CB (1996) Cardiovascular applications of magnetic resonance flow and velocity measurements. JMRI 6:78–89
Tangcharoen T, Bell A, Hegde S et al (2011) Detection of coronary artery anomalies in infants and young children with congenital heart disease by using MR imaging. Radiology 259(1):240–247
Tanigawa K, Eguchi K, Kitamura Y et al (1992) Magnetic resonance imaging detection of aortic and pulmonary artery wall thickening in the acute stage of Takayasu arteritis. Improvement of clinical and radiologic findings after steroid therapy. Arthritis Rheum 35:476–480
Tann OR, Tulloh RMR, Hamilton MCK (2008) Takayasu's disease: a review. Cardiol Young 18(3):250–259
Toussaint JF (2202) MRI characterization of atherosclerotic arteries: diagnosis of plaque rupture. J Neuroradiol 29: 223–230
van Beek EJ, Wild JM, Fink C, Moody AR, Kauczor HU, Oudkerk M (2003) MRI for the diagnosis of pulmonary embolism. JMRI 18:627–640
Van Grimberge F, Dymarkowski S, Budts W, Bogaert J (2000) Role of magnetic resonance in the diagnosis of subclavian steal syndrome. J Magn Reson Imaging 12:339–342
Van Mierop LH, Kutsche LM (1986) Cardiovascular anomalies in DiGeorge syndrome and importance of neural crest as a possible pathogenetic factor. Am J Cardiol 58:133–137
Van Praagh R, Bernhard WF, Rosenthal A, Parisi LF, Fyler DC (1971) Interrupted aortic arch: surgical treatment. Am J Cardiol 27(2):200–211
Van Son JA, Julsrud PR, Hagler DJ et al (1993) Surgical treatment of vascular rings: the Mayo Clinic experience. Mayo Clin Proc 68(11):1056–1063
Videlefsky N, Parks WJ, Oshinski J et al (2001) Magnetic resonance phase-shift velocity mapping in pediatric patients with pulmonary venous obstruction. J Am Coll Cardiol 38:262–267
Vilacosta I, Aragoncillo P, Canadas V et al (2009) Acute aortic syndrome: a new look at an old conundrum. Heart 95: 1130–1139
Voges I, Jerosch-Herold M, Hedderich J, et al (2010) maladaptive aortic properties in children after palliation of hypoplastic left heart syndrome assessed by cardiovascular magnetic resonance imaging. Circulation 122: 1068–1076
Vogt FM, Goyen M, Debatin JF (2003) MR angiography of the chest. Radiol Clin North Am 41:29–41
Von Kodolitsch Y, Csosz SK, Koschyk DH et al (2003) Intramural hematoma of the aorta: predictors of progression to dissection and rupture. Circulation 107:1158–1163
von Schulthess GK, Higashino SM, Higgins SS, Didier D, Fisher MR, Higgins CB (1986) Coarctation of the aorta: MR imaging. Radiology 158:469–474
Wang Y, Rossman PJ, Grimm RC, Wilman AH, Riederer SJ, Ehman RL (1996) 3D MR angiography of pulmonary arteries using real-time navigator gating and magnetization preparation. Magn Reson Med 36:579–587
Warnes CA, Williams RG, Bashore TM et al (2008) ACC/AHA 2008 Guidelines for the Management of Adults With Congenital Heart Disease: Executive Summary: a report of the American College of Cardiology/American Heart Association Task Force on Practice Guidelines (Writing committee to develop guidelines for the management of adults with congenital heart disease): Developed in Collaboration with the American Society of Echocardiography, Heart Rhythm Society, International Society for Adult Congenital Heart Disease, Society for Cardiovascular Angiography and Interventions, and Society of Thoracic Surgeons Circ 118:2395–2451

Weinberg PM, Whitehead KK (2010) Aortic arch anomalies. In: Fogel MA (ed). Principles and practice of cardiac magnetic resonance in congenital heart disease form function and flow, Wiley-Blackwell (Chapter 11)

Weissleder R, Mahmood U (2001) Molecular imaging. Radiology 219:316–333

White CS, Baffa JM, Haney PJ, Campbell AB, NessAiver M (1998) Anomalies of pulmonary veins: usefulness of spin-echo and gradient-echo MR images. Am J Roentgenol 170:1365–1368

White CS (2000) MR imaging of thoracic veins. Magn Reson Imaging Clin N Am 8:17–32

Wildenhain PM, Bourekas EC (1991) Pulmonary varix: magnetic resonance findings. Cathet Cardiovasc Diagn 24: 268–270

Winter PM, Morawski AM, Caruthers SD et al (2003) Molecular imaging of angiogenesis in early-stage atherosclerosis with alpha(v)beta3-integrin-targeted nanoparticles. Circulation 108:2270–2274

Zanotti G, Vricella L, Cameron D (2008) Thoracic aortic aneurysm syndrome in children. Semin Thorac Cardiovasc Surg Pediatr Card Surg Annu 11(1):11–21

MR Guided Cardiac Catheterization

Vivek Muthurangu and Andrew M. Taylor

Contents

1 **Introduction** 657

2 **Rationale for MR Guided Cardiac Catheterization** 658

2.1 Increased Anatomical Information 658

2.2 Increased Functional Information 658

2.3 Reduced X-ray Exposure 658

3 **Requirements for MR Guided Cardiac Catheterization** 659

3.1 Interventional MR Suite 659

3.2 Devices and Delivery Systems 660

3.3 Real-Time Imaging 660

3.4 Catheter Visualization 662

3.5 X-Ray/MR Fusion Technology 663

3.6 Safety Procedures for Interventional MR 663

4 **Applications of MR Guided Cardiac Catheterization** 664

4.1 Experimental Animal Studies 664

4.2 Human Diagnostic MR Guided Cardiac Catheterization 664

4.3 Human Interventional MR Guided Cardiac Catheterization 666

5 **Conclusion** 666

6 **Key Points** 666

References 666

V. Muthurangu (✉) · A. M. Taylor
UCL Centre for Cardiovascular Imaging and Great Ormond Street Hospital for Children, London, WC1N 3JH, UK
e-mail: v.muthurangu@ucl.ac.uk

Abstract

This chapter will address recent developments in MR guided cardiac catheterization and give the reader a better understanding of this novel technique. The rationale behind the development of MR guided cardiac catheterization will be explained with respect to improved anatomical information, increased physiological information and reduced x-ray exposure. In addition, the technical requirements and MR guided cardiac catheterisation will be discussed. Finally, animal and human studies using MR guided cardiac catheterisation will be discussed.

1 Introduction

For the past half century, cardiac catheterization has been the 'gold standard' diagnostic method in cardiology.Furthermore, interventional cardiac catheterization is a growth area particularly in structural heart disease. However, cardiac (MRI) is increasingly replacing diagnostic cardiac catheterization as a method of assessing cardiac anatomy, measuring blood flow and quantifying ventricular function. In fact, cardiac MRI is now often regarded as a 'gold standard' for functional assessment of the heart (Muthurangu et al. 2005b). Nevertheless, diagnostic cardiac catheterization is still necessary when intracardiac or intra-vascular pressure measurements are necessary or if selective angiography is required. Currently, X-ray fluoroscopy is the imaging modality of choice for guiding cardiac catheterization with some interventions also utilizing echocardiography.

J. Bogaert et al. (eds.), *Clinical Cardiac MRI*, Medical Radiology. Diagnostic Imaging,
DOI: 10.1007/174_2011_423,

However, there are problems with this approach, which could be solved by using MRI during catheterization. In this chapter the role of MRI in the catheterization laboratory will be reviewed. By the end of this chapter, the reader should have a greater understanding of the current state and future possibilities of MR guided cardiac catheterization.

2 Rationale for MR Guided Cardiac Catheterization

A fundamental question prior to developing any new medical technology is—Why do we need a new technology? The next section will develop the three main arguments for MR guided cardiac catheterization.

2.1 Increased Anatomical Information

Fluoroscopy provides excellent visualization of catheters, guidewires, devices and bony structures. However, it is less suited to delineating the soft tissue structures of the heart and vessels. Furthermore, it only provides 2D projection images, making it more difficult to perceive the position of catheters in the third dimension. Of course, invasive angiography can provide lumenographic views of the anatomy, which when combined with the operator's knowledge of the anatomy can provide sufficient information for many interventions. However, there are several problems with this traditional approach to catheterization. First, it is highly dependant on the operators 'mental image' of the anatomy. This is sufficient in patients with relatively normal anatomy and in whom simple catheter procedures are being performed. However, in patients with complex anatomy (congenital heart disease, complex electrophysiology) the lack of true anatomical information makes the intervention more difficult. This not only prolongs the procedure, but also increases the small risk of perforating the heart or great vessels. Furthermore, as interventions become more ambitious the need for accurate delineation of cardiac anatomy becomes more pressing. In fact, some novel interventions may not be clinically possible without better imaging. In many centers, MRI has become the optimum way to assess cardiac anatomy. This is due to excellent visualization of soft tissue structures, unrestricted 2D imaging and true 3D imaging capabilities. These properties of MRI make it particularly attractive as a possible additional or replacement imaging modality for cardiac catheterization.

2.2 Increased Functional Information

Cardiac catheterization is important in the assessment of ventricular and vascular hemodynamics. For instance, invasive pressures and blood flow measurements are used to calculate pulmonary vascular resistance (PVR), which is a vital part of the diagnostic work-up in patients with pulmonary hypertension. Unfortunately, the currently used invasive methods of flow quantification (i.e. the Fick method, and thermodilution) are associated with significant inaccuracies (Dhingra et al. 2002). Velocity encoded phase contrast MR is a very accurate method of measuring flow and has the benefit of being reliable in the presence of regurgitation and shunts (Hundley et al. 1995). Thus, MRI used in combination with invasive pressures could be used to more accurately calculate PVR (Schalla et al. 2003). MR guided cardiac catheterization also allows other physiological parameters to be assessed. One good example is pressure volume (P–V) loops, which require the simultaneous measurement of ventricular volumes and pressures. It has been shown that cardiac MRI is the most accurate and reproducible method of quantifying ventricular volumes. Thus, P–V loops constructed using this technique should be able to accurately gauge abnormal ventricular hemodynamics in disease.

2.3 Reduced X-ray Exposure

Medical exposure to ionizing radiation is recognized as a significant health risk for both patients and health care professionals. In adults, the UK National Radiation Protection Board have calculated the mean risk of developing a solid tumor after single cardiac catheterization procedure is ~1 in 2,500 (NRPB 1999). The risk of radiation is amplified in patients with severe structural heart disease for the following reasons. First, interventions in structural heart disease often take longer than in adult ischemic disease. This is due to both the greater complexity of the interventions and the more difficult anatomy of the

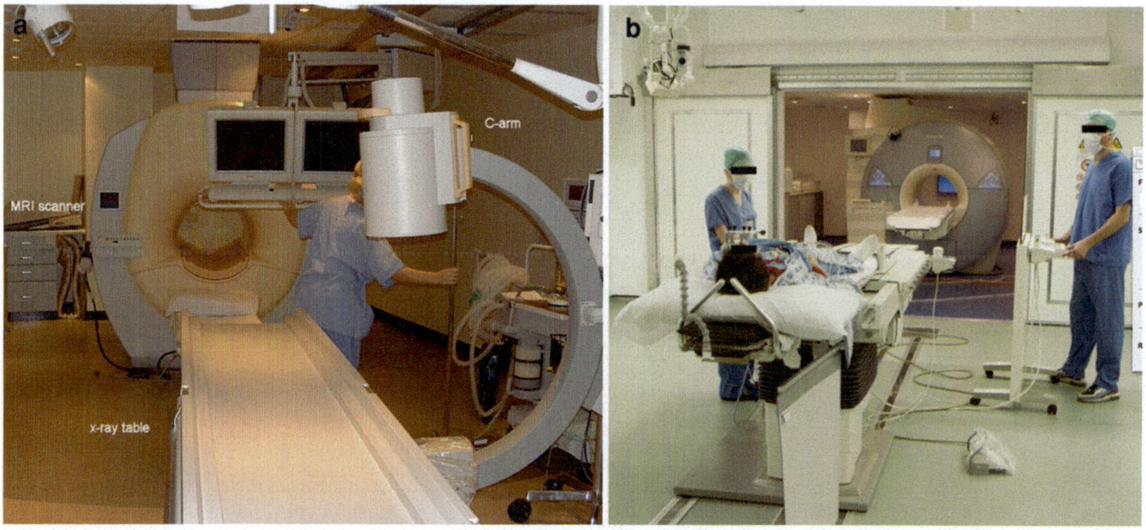

Fig. 1 **a** Photograph of an XMR suite in a single room RF shielded room. (Courtesy of Reza Razavi, Kings' College London). **b** Photograph of an XMR suite consisting of a separate catheterization laboratory and MRI scanner. The two rooms are separated by RF shielded doors

patients. Unfortunately, this problem is likely to be exacerbated by the increasing intricacy of new interventions. Second, many patients with congenital heart disease are children or young adults and thus they have a greater risk of malignancy after radiation exposure. For instance if exposure occurs at five years of age, the risk of malignancy is increased to $\sim$1 in 1,000. Finally, patients with structural heart disease are likely to have several catheterizations throughout their lives multiplying the risk of developing radiation exposure related health problems. Thus, there is a need to reduce exposure to ionizing radiation during cardiac catheterization. The development of real-time MRI offers the possibility of catheter guidance without exposure to X-ray radiation. Reduction and eventual elimination of the ionizing radiation exposure during cardiac catheterization is one of the main driving forces in the development of MR guided cardiac catheterization.

3 Requirements for MR Guided Cardiac Catheterization

3.1 Interventional MR Suite

There are many specialist pieces of equipment required for MR guided cardiac catheterization. However, it can be argued that the most important is the interventional MR suite. Currently, interventional MRI is in its infancy and therefore cannot be carried out without the possibility of reverting to traditional X-ray fluoroscopy. Thus, most interventional MRI suites incorporate X-ray imaging facilities and are often referred to as XMR suites. There are two common designs for XMR suites. The simplest solution is to include the X-ray equipment in the RF shielded MR scanner room (Fig. 1a), with the patient being transferred between the two imaging modalities by some form of moveable tabletop (Razavi et al. 2003). This requires the scanner room to be enlarged so that the X-ray equipment can be placed safely outside the five Gauss line. The enlarged room also enables ferromagnetic materials to be used in the 'X-ray side' of the room without risk of attraction by the static magnetic field. For this solution to work, the X-ray intensifier must be shielded to prevent magnetic distortion, while all X-ray equipment must be shut down during MR scanning to prevent RF interference. The main problems with this solution are: (1) bringing ferromagnetic equipment into the scanner room increases the risk of accidental transfer to the 'MR side' of the room, and (2) the enlarged RF shielded room is significantly more expensive than a normal MR scanner suite. The second solution is to have separate MR scanner and cardiac catheterization suites separated by RF shielded doors (Fig. 1b) (Lurz et al. 2009). In this solution, both facilities can be

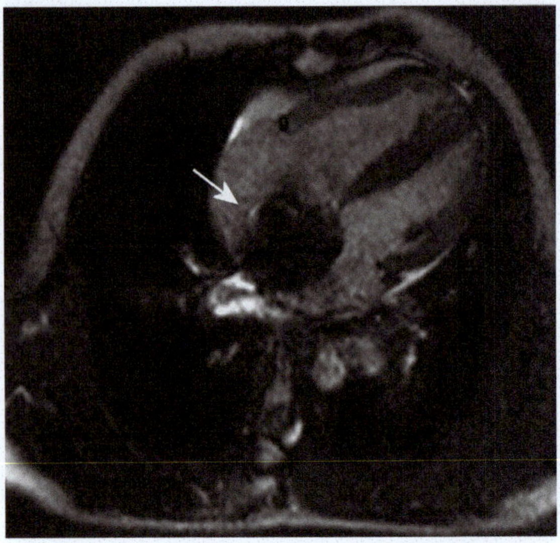

Fig. 2 Cine image of an ASD device immediately post placement. Note the large area of signal loss associated with the metallic device

operated independently and the only specialization required is RF shielded doors. However, there are disadvantages including: further transfer distance for patients, requirement for two anesthetic machines, and the larger total floor space required. Both solutions have been installed in various centers and the choice is mainly dependant on the requirements of the Institution. Irrespective of the solution chosen, it is important that a suitable MR scanner is used. Most importantly, the configuration of the scanner must allow sufficient access to the patient in order to perform catheter manipulation. Several vertical bore 'open' scanners are currently marketed for the interventional MR. However, in most there is still considerable distance between the operator and the patient, making patient access difficult. Wide, short, horizontal bore scanners may be a better solution as the operator has better access to the patient. Of course it is also important that the MR scanner produces high-quality cardiac images. Unfortunately, the earliest examples of short-bore scanners did not have good enough gradients or magnetic field homogeneity to be useful interventional MR scanners. However, newer models can produce excellent images, while maintaining relatively short bore lengths (120 cm) and large diameters (70 cm). Another vital consideration is the need for in-room control. Most MR scanners are controlled from a control room outside the RF cage. However, in interventional MR the operator must be able to view real-time MR images and easily instruct changes in scanning to follow the catheter. Thus, interventional MR scanners must have some form of in-room control and display that allows complete control of the MR scanner.

3.2 Devices and Delivery Systems

Almost all interventional devices (i.e. stents and ASD devices) are MR compatible after insertion. In fact, several groups have performed cardiac MRI immediately after device implantation with no adverse affect of device function (Razavi et al. 2003) (Fig. 2). However, most device delivery systems are not MR compatible, due to the presence of metallic guide wires. Guide wires enable proper positioning and delivery of devices and are traditionally metallic as this provides the right combination of stiffness, flexibility and strength. Unfortunately, long metallic guide wires are known to heat up during MR scanning. Currently, this is the biggest impediment to the development of MR guided cardiac catheterization. Thankfully several solutions are on the horizon, including active detuning and decoupling during scanning, integration of serial transformers into guide wires (Weiss et al. 2010), and the use of novel non-conductive material such as fiberglass (Tzifa et al. 2010). These MR compatible guide wires are currently in various stages of regulatory approval and may well revolutionize MR guided cardiac catheterization.

3.3 Real-Time Imaging

Real-time imaging is a prerequisite for MR guided interventions. The majority of studies into MR guided cardiac catheterization use real-time b-SSFP sequences for catheter and anatomical visualization (Schalla et al. 2003). In the normal cardiac imaging, cine MRI is performed using cardiac gating. However, for real-time imaging data must be acquired continuously with each k-space frame being filled in a sequential manner. The temporal resolution is therefore dependent on the time taken to fill a single k-space frame. This in turn is dependant on TR and the number of phase encoding steps. In b-SSFP imaging, TR is already short and therefore increased temporal resolution

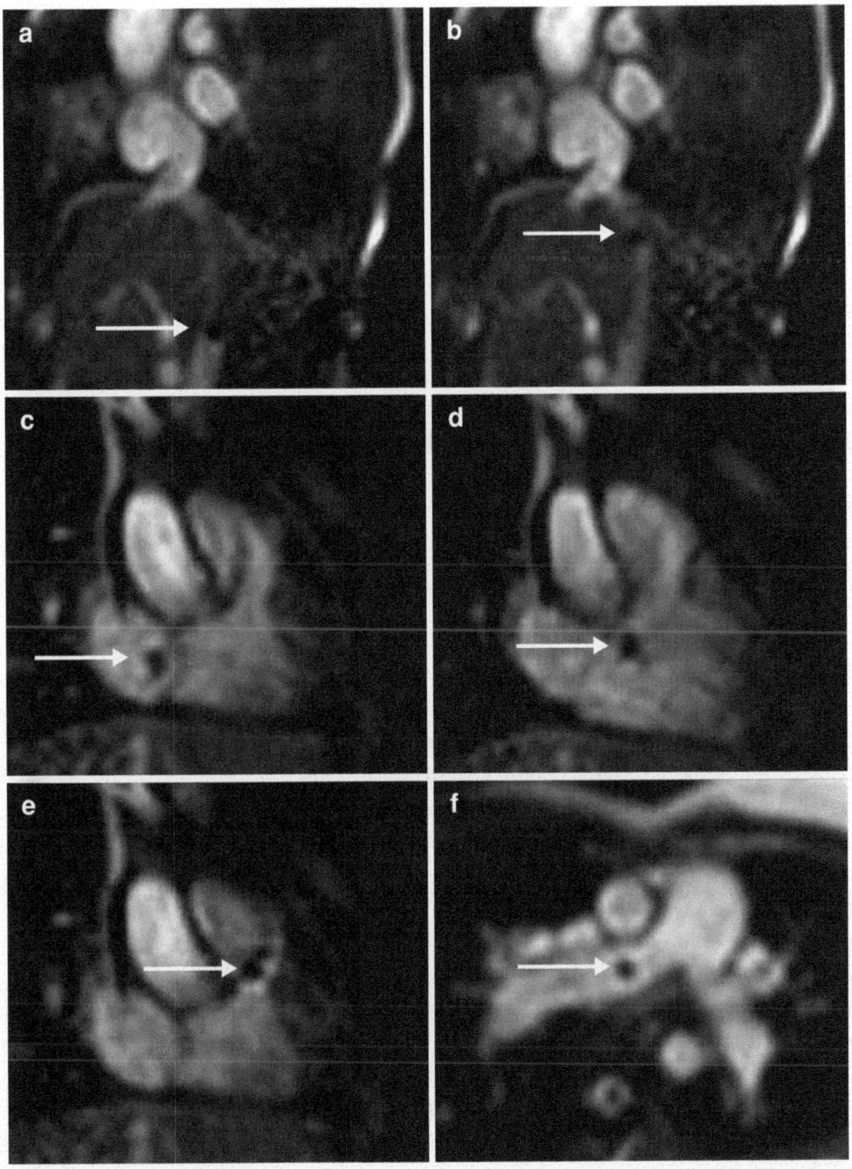

Fig. 3 Frames of MR guided cardiac catheterisation. Imaging sequence: real time b-SSFP. *White arrows* point to the signal void produced by the CO_2 filled balloon tip. **a** Catheter in inferior vena cava. **b** Catheter at inferior vena cava right atrial junction. **c** Catheter in right atrium. **d** Catheter in right ventricle. **e** Catheter in right ventricular outflow tract. **f** Catheter in right pulmonary artery

requires a reduction in the number of phase encode steps. This can be accomplished without changing spatial resolution by utilizing a rectangular FOV (i.e. 60% of FOV) in conjunction with the partial Fourier technique. However, it is usually also necessary to choose a lower imaging matrix (i.e. 128 × 128), which will reduce spatial resolution. Utilizing the techniques described above a temporal resolution of 100 ms can be achieved, translating into a frame rate of 10fps (Miquel et al. 2004). This temporal resolution is sufficient for simple interventions (Fig. 3), but is probably not sufficient for more complex interventions. Another method of increasing temporal resolution is to undersample k-space and use information from multiple coils or temporal correlations to remove aliasing (i.e. SENSE or *k-t* BLAST) (Hansen et al. 2006). However, in MR guided cardiac catheterization, real-time acquisition must be coupled with real-time reconstruction. Unfortunately, for techniques like SENSE and *k-t* SENSE, reconstruction is computationally intensive and real-time image display is difficult. Thankfully, the advent of parallel computing, particularly on graphical processing units, is making real-time reconstruction of heavily undersampled data possible (Sorensen et al. 2009). Thus it is probable that in the future, real-time techniques with a similar spatial and temporal resolution to traditional gated cardiac MR could be used for interventions. A further requirement of interventional MR is the ability to interactively change the imaging plane to follow the catheter. This can be accomplished either automatically or manually depending on the mechanism of catheter tracking. Several groups are actively developing methodologies to improve the ability to visualize and track catheters within the heart. These include tracking multiple points on the catheter on an overlaid 3D MR angiogram and real-time acquisition of multiple perpendicular planes through the thorax (McVeigh et al. 2005). It is the development of these real-time acquisition and visualization techniques that have made MR guided cardiac catheterization a possibility.

3.4 Catheter Visualization

Catheters can be visualized using either active or passive methods. Passive catheter visualization relies on inherent properties of the catheter to provide either local signal enhancement or loss. In b-SSFP sequences the blood is bright and therefore techniques that rely on signal loss/voids are commonly used. The main method used clinically is to create a signal void using standard balloon catheter filled with CO_2. The signal void produced by CO_2 is due to inherent lack of signal rather than magnetic susceptibility and thus signal void produced is approximately the same size as the balloon itself (Fig. 3). The benefit of this approach is that it uses standard catheter laboratory equipment and thus, poses no greater safety risk to the patient (Miquel et al. 2004). An alternative method of producing negative contrast is by visualizing magnetic susceptibility artefacts. The benefit of this approach is that the signal void will be larger than the marker. For instance, paramagnetic dysprosium chelates have placed along the length of the catheter enabling visualization of the resultant susceptibility artefact (Bakker et al. 1997). In theory, any agent that provides a susceptibility artefact [e.g. iron oxide (Mekle et al. 2006)] could be used in this way, producing negative contrast against the 'bright blood' signal. The problem with negative contrast techniques is that non–ambiguous catheter localization is difficult in the presence of flow related signal void artefacts. Positive contrast techniques based on off-resonance imaging or susceptibility dependant rephasing have been developed (Dharmakumar et al. 2006; Seppenwoolde et al. 2003). Such methods allow more non-ambiguous catheter discrimination. However, sequences that enable positive contrast imaging of susceptibility artefacts are complex and difficult to perform in the real-time environment (Dharmakumar et al. 2006; Seppenwoolde et al. 2003).

A more fruitful approach may be imaging of nuclei such as ^{19}F or hyperpolarized ^{13}C (Kozerke et al. 2004; Olsson et al. 2006). These isotopes have no or low abundance in the human body and therefore inherently produce positive contrast with very little or no background signal, when introduced into the body. This allows non-ambiguous discrimination of the catheter and more importantly automatic catheter tracking. It has been recently shown that tracking of a perflurocrabon filled balloon tip was possible using three 1D ^{19}F projections (Kozerke et al. 2004). Interleaving ^{19}F projection imaging with conventional proton real-time SSFP imaging allowed superimposition of tracking data and 2D anatomy (Kozerke et al. 2004). This method could be extended to visualize the whole catheter in real-time within a dynamic 3D roadmap.

The other approach is to use active catheter visualization and tracking techniques (Fig. 4). Active devices are connected to the scanner and comprise of micro-coils or loopless antennae, which can be used for signal reception. Automatic tracking of micro-coil tips is possible using three 1D projections. Projection imaging can be interleaved with bSSFP imaging for superimposition of tracking data onto real-time anatomy. As loopless antennae receive signal from the surrounding protons during conventional 2D imaging they can be visualized along their length and superimposed onto the image from the surface coil (Lederman 2005). Thus, these active techniques have significant advantages over passive catheter visualization. Unfortunately, the fundamental problem with active devices is its susceptibility to heating within the MR environment. Several techniques are under development to solve this problem, but currently they are not suitable for human work.

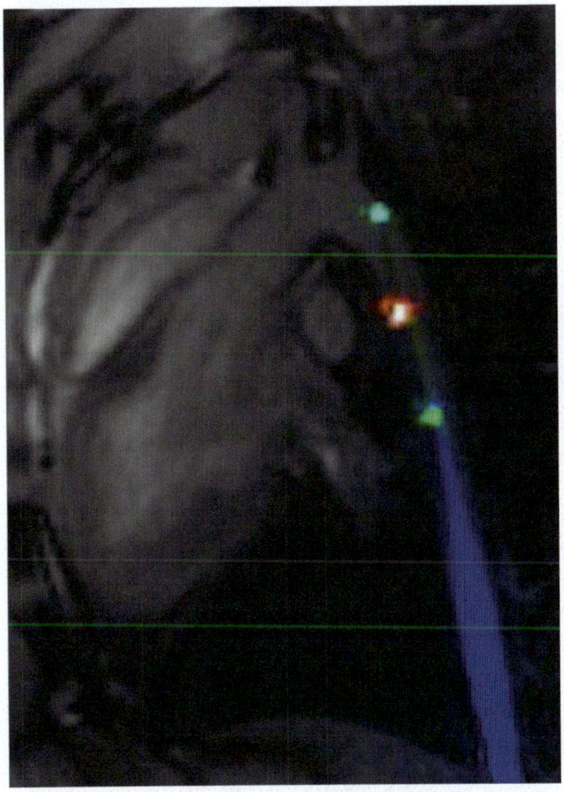

Fig. 4 b-SSFP images of an active catheter inserted percutaneously from the femoral artery, through the aorta, and towards the left subclavian artery. Device-related signal is evident with independent catheter receiver channels allowing colorized reconstruction of the catheter (first and third coil, *green*; middle coil, *red*; catheter shaft, *blue*). (Courtesy Ozgur Kocaturk, NHLBI, NIH)

3.5 X-Ray/MR Fusion Technology

As previously stated, the lack MRI compatible delivery systems make true interventional cardiac MRI difficult in humans. Thus, there is a need for an interim solution that uses the power of MRI to improve cardiac catheterization procedures. This can be achieved by X-ray/MR fusion, which uses MR data to provide anatomical roadmap during fluoroscopy-guided procedures (Rhode et al. 2003) (Fig. 5). The benefit of this fusion approach is that 3D MR information can be used to improve visualization during 2D projection fluoroscopic imaging. A necessity for this approach is accurate registration of MR and X-ray space to prevent misalignment of MR overlays during catheterization. It is also important that these overlays automatically respond to positioning of the X-ray suite c-arms. This can be achieved by using MR and X-ray visible fiducial markers and real-time display of various 3D MRI data depending on the position of the patient and the c-arms. Several centers have demonstrated the use of fusion technology to aid congenital interventions (Ratnayaka et al. 2009) as well as electrophysiological studies (Rhode et al. 2003).

3.6 Safety Procedures for Interventional MR

There is a great deal of literature on MRI hazards and safety issues and a comprehensive review and discussion of the subject is outside the scope of this Chapter. However, this area is probably one of the most important in MR guided cardiac catheterization. Traditional catheterization utilizes many ferromagnetic objects, from scissors to introducer needles. In the MRI environment these would be attracted to the magnet leading to possible projectile injuries. Of course, it is not feasible to replace all the ferromagnetic objects used during cardiac catheterization. Thus, in units with XMR suites the initial part of the procedure (i.e. intravascular sheath insertion) is performed in the 'X-ray side' of the room before transfer to the MR side of the room. Prior to transfer mechanisms must be in place to ensure that no ferromagnetic equipment is transferred over with the patient. Other safety features include: (1) Compulsory MR safety training for all staff involved in interventional MR procedures; (2) Clear demarcation of the ferromagnetic safe and unsafe areas by different color floor covering; (3) Restricted entrance to the facility during an interventional MR procedure - this may include prior agreement on which staff members should cross into the MR side of the room; (4) Tethering of all Ferromagnetic equipment to the walls - all ferromagnetic equipment should be outside the five Gauss line, tethering prevents accidental placement within the magnetic field; (5) A safety officer present in the interventional suite throughout the procedure to ensure the safety protocols are adhered to, especially at the time of patient transfer. The interventional MR environment is an intrinsically dangerous environment. However, when the correct safety procedures are instigated catheterization can be performed in a safe and reliable manner.

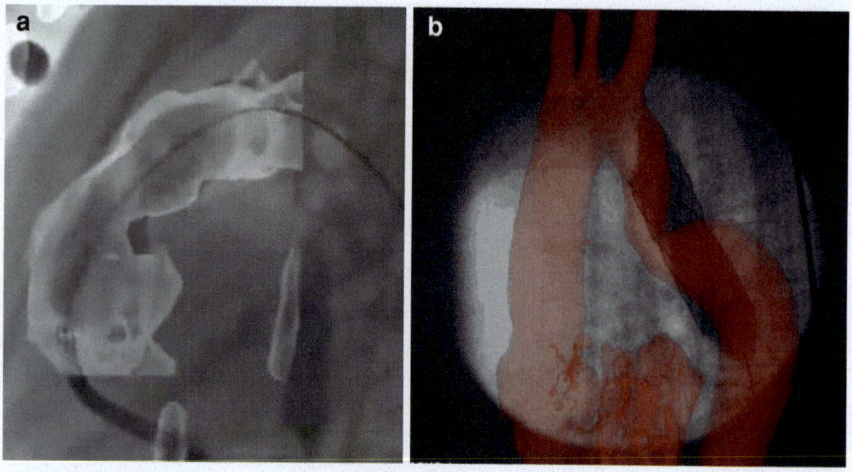

Fig. 5 **a** Roadmap of the right ventricular outflow tract derived from an MR angiogram and used during percutaneous pulmonary valve implantation. Registration of the MR and X-ray data was performed using fiducial markers. **b** Roadmap of the aorta derived from an MR angiogram and used during percutaneous stent implantation

4 Applications of MR Guided Cardiac Catheterization

4.1 Experimental Animal Studies

There have been a number of studies performed demonstrating the possibility of MR guided cardiac catheterization in animal models. Simultaneous measurement of invasive pressure and MR flow has been demonstrated in a porcine model of atrial septal defect (ASD) (Schalla et al. 2003). In this study, active catheter techniques were used to manipulate the catheter into the right heart from the inferior vena cava. Post mortem analysis revealed no cardiac damage associated with catheterization. The majority of other studies have centered on MR guided cardiac interventions. These include placement of ASD/VSD occluders (Schalla et al. 2005), valve stents in the aortic and pulmonary position (Kuehne et al. 2004a) and intra-myocardial injection of stem cells (Dick et al. 2003). These studies have demonstrated that interventional device placement under passive and active MR guidance is feasible in animal models and bring the benefits of greater anatomical information. In addition, they demonstrate the benefit of physiological monitoring with MR prior to and after the intervention (i.e. the measurement of valvar regurgitation in valve stent placement). Unfortunately, as previously noted, most of the delivery systems used in these studies are not currently suitable for human use due to safety issues with heating. Until MR compatible guide wires and delivery systems are available, solely MR guided placement of devices in humans is difficult. However, the availability of the real-time techniques described above coupled with passive catheter visualization and PCMR do make MR guided diagnostic catheterization in humans a possibility.

4.2 Human Diagnostic MR Guided Cardiac Catheterization

There have been a number of studies demonstrating the feasibility of diagnostic MR guided cardiac catheterization. Most have revolved around pulmonary vascular resistance (PVR) studies in patients with pulmonary hypertension (Muthurangu et al. 2004). Traditionally, PVR is calculated using invasive pressure and flow measurements. However, as previously pointed out invasive flow techniques like thermodilution and the Fick method are prone to inaccuracy. During MR guided cardiac catheterization flow it is possible to measure pulmonary artery flow using phase contrast MRI. This technique is known to be accurate and may represent the in vivo reference standard for assessment of flow. Thus, combining phase contrast MRI data with invasive pressure measurements may be a better way to assess PVR (Fig. 6). In the first demonstration of this technology, standard balloon wedge catheters were used during MR guided cardiac catheterization. The benefit of these catheters is that they contain no metal so there is no risk of RF heating. Furthermore, the balloon tip can be filled with CO_2 enabling visualization of the catheter tip as previously described. The catheter was navigated into the pulmonary artery to measure

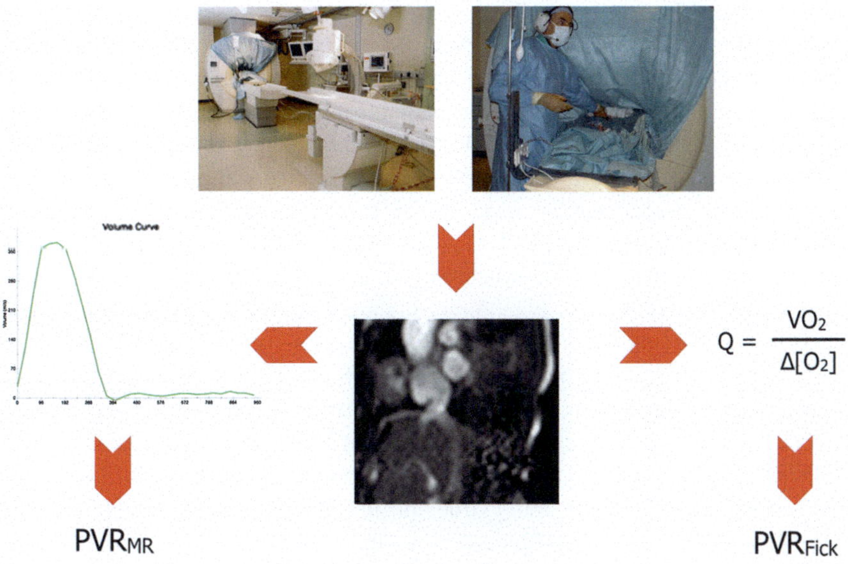

Fig. 6 Assessing pulmonary vascular resistance during MR guided cardiac catheterization. In this experiment PVR was calculated using MR derived flows and Fick derived flows—the data suggests the MR is more reliable particularly in the presence of oxygen

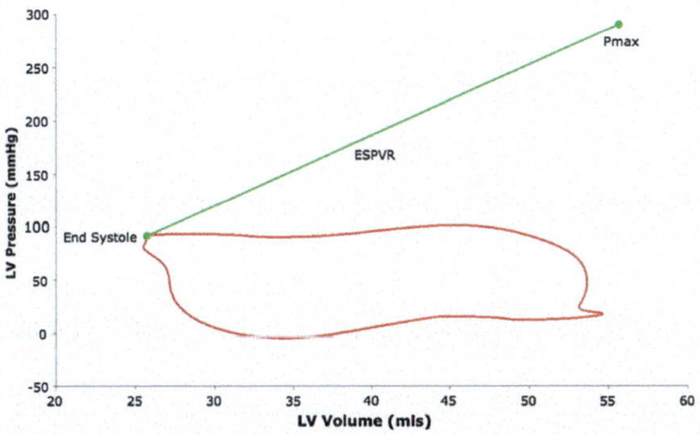

Fig. 7 Example of pressure volume constructed using simultaneously acquired pressure and MR volumetric data. Maximum pressure is calculated using the single beat method, which allows calculation load independent contractility

invasive pulmonary artery pressure. Once the catheter was in place, pulmonary artery flow was measured and combined with invasive pressure measurement to calculate PVR. This study showed a significant discrepancy between PVR, calculated using Fick derived flow and MR derived flow, particularly in the presence of oxygen. This appeared secondary to inaccuracies in the Fick method and suggests that MR may be superior to the traditional Fick method. Further work has demonstrated the utility of this MR technique in a more homogeneous population of patients with moderate/severe pulmonary hypertension (Kuehne et al. 2005). In this study, the investigators also demonstrated the improved precision of phase contrast MR over thermodilution methods. Several groups are now routinely performing all clinical PVR studies using a combination of MR and invasive pressure measurements. Another benefit of using MR to assess physiological parameters during diagnostic catheterization is that it allows other more sophisticated measurements to be made. A good example is pulmonary arterial compliance, which has been measured during MR guided cardiac catheterization, and may provide added information over PVR in patients with pulmonary hypertension (Muthurangu et al. 2005a). Another example is construction of pressure volume (P–V) loops through simultaneous measurement of ventricular volumes and pressures (Kuehne et al. 2004b) (Fig. 7). It has been shown that cardiac MR is an accurate and reproducible method of quantifying ventricular volumes. Thus, P–V loops constructed using cardiac MR data should also be accurate and reproducible. The feasibility of constructing MR derived P–V loops has been demonstrated in patients with pulmonary hypertension. However, measuring these more sophisticated parameters using MR does raise some problems. Firstly, only fluid filled catheters can be used in the MR environment. Unfortunately, fluid filled catheters have well known problems with dampening and resonance, which can affect the shape of the pressure curve. This does not have a major affect on mean pressure, but may be problematic when constructing P–V loops (Fig. 7). Thus, to really make MR guided cardiac catheterization clinically usable, MR compatible micromanometers must be developed. Several groups are developing such devices based on fiber-optic transmission and these should be available in the near future. A second problem is how to combine real-time pressure data with gated flow and cine data acquired over several cardiac cycles. For accurate production of P–V loops and similar metrics, it is vital that pressure and MR data are synchronized and this is an area where more work is required. It should be noted that MR guidance is not necessary to harness the power of MR for physiological assessment. Some groups with XMR suites would catheterize under X-ray guidance (which is currently quicker than MR guidance) and then transfer to MR for flow or volume assessment. This is particularly true in unstable patients with PH whose procedure time must be limited. Nevertheless, both MR guided and MR augmented diagnostic cardiac catheterization have the potential to significantly change practice.

4.3 Human Interventional MR Guided Cardiac Catheterization

A recent development in MR guided cardiac catheterization is the availability of plastic/fiber glass-based guide wires. These are intrinsically MR compatible and can be covered in iron oxide for passive visualization. Using such a guide wire the first fully MR guided intervention in humans has now been performed (Tzifa et al. 2010). The intervention performed was balloon angioplasty of stenotic pulmonary valves, and the guide wire was utilized to aid manipulation of the balloon catheter. Visualization was accomplished using real-time b-SSFP. This is an extremely exciting development that finally opens up the possibility of MR guided cardiac interventions. Further work is now being done on improving guide wire properties and incorporating it into more delivery systems and defining wire safety.

5 Conclusion

The feasibility of using MR guided cardiac catheterization in humans has been demonstrated. However, a number of issues still need to be addressed before MR guided cardiac interventions enter widespread clinical use. Further developments by catheter manufacturing companies are needed in order to provide specific products for MR interventions. Currently, catheters are designed for use in the X-ray environment and, consequently, many contain ferromagnetic components (e.g. braiding in catheters) or long conducting materials (e.g. guidewires) that are potentially hazardous in the MR environment. Non-braided balloon catheters can be used in the MR environment; however, they often lack the desired torque and steerability. In addition, catheter visualization and tracking must be improved so that the whole length of the catheter can be automatically tracked. Once these issues have been resolved MR guided cardiac catheterization will be possible in all patients. This should bring the benefits of elimination of exposure to X-ray radiation, better anatomical visualization and increased physiological information.

6 Key Points

MR guided cardiac catheterization has the benefits of: 1) reduced X-ray exposure; 2) better functional information; and 3) better soft tissue delineation.

Currently this technology is impeded by the lack of MR compatible delivery devices and poor catheter visualization.

However, it already has an important part to play in diagnostic cardiac catheterization such as assessment of pulmonary vascular resistance.

References

Bakker CJ, Hoogeveen RM, Hurtak WF, Van Vaals JJ, Viergever MA, Mali WP (1997) MR-guided endovascular interventions: susceptibility-based catheter and near-real-time imaging technique. Radiology 202:273–276

Dharmakumar R, Koktzoglou I, Li D (2006) Generating positive contrast from off-resonant spins with steady-state free precession magnetic resonance imaging: theory and proof-of-principle experiments. Phys Med Biol 51:4201–4215

Dhingra VK, Fenwick JC, Walley KR, Chittock DR, Ronco JJ (2002) Lack of agreement between thermodilution and fick cardiac output in critically ill patients. Chest 122:990–997

Dick AJ, Guttman MA, Raman VK, Peters DC, Pessanha BS, Hill JM, Smith S, Scott G, Mcveigh ER, Lederman RJ (2003) Magnetic resonance fluoroscopy allows targeted delivery of mesenchymal stem cells to infarct borders in Swine. Circulation 108:2899–2904

Hansen MS, Baltes C, Tsao J, Kozerke S, Pruessmann KP, Eggers H (2006) k-t BLAST reconstruction from non-Cartesian k-t space sampling. Magn reson medicine : official j Soc Magn Reson Medicine/Soc Magn Reson Medicine 55:85–91

Hundley WG, Li HF, Hillis LD, Meshack BM, Lange RA, Willard JE, Landau C, Peshock RM (1995) Quantitation of cardiac output with velocity-encoded, phase-difference magnetic resonance imaging. Am J Cardiol 75:1250–1255

Kozerke S, Hegde S, Schaeffter T, Lamerichs R, Razavi R, Hill DL (2004) Catheter tracking and visualization using 19F nuclear magnetic resonance. Magn Reson Med 52:693–697

Kuehne T, Yilmaz S, Meinus C, Moore P, Saeed M, Weber O, Higgins CB, Blank T, Elsaesser E, Schnackenburg B, Ewert P, Lange PE, Nagel E (2004a) Magnetic resonance imaging-guided transcatheter implantation of a prosthetic valve in aortic valve position: Feasibility study in swine. J Am Coll Cardiol 44:2247–2249

Kuehne T, Yilmaz S, Steendijk P, Moore P, Groenink M, Saaed M, Weber O, Higgins CB, Ewert P, Fleck E, Nagel E, Schulze-Neick I, Lange P (2004b) Magnetic resonance imaging analysis of right ventricular pressure-volume loops: In vivo validation and clinical application in patients with pulmonary hypertension. Circulation 110:2010–2016

Kuehne T, Yilmaz S, Schulze-Neick I, Wellnhofer E, Ewert P, Nagel E, Lange P (2005) Magnetic resonance imaging guided catheterisation for assessment of pulmonary vascular resistance: in vivo validation and clinical application in patients with pulmonary hypertension. Heart 91:1064–1069

Lederman RJ (2005) Cardiovascular interventional magnetic resonance imaging. Circulation 112:3009–3017

Lurz P, Nordmeyer J, Muthurangu V, Khambadkone S, Derrick G, Yates R, Sury M, Bonhoeffer P, Taylor AM (2009) Comparison of bare metal stenting and percutaneous pulmonary valve implantation for treatment of right ventricular outflow tract obstruction: use of an X-ray/magnetic resonance hybrid laboratory for acute physiological assessment. Circulation 119:2995–3001

Mcveigh ER, Guttman MA, Kellman P, Raval AN, Lederman RJ (2005) Real-time, Interactive MRI for cardiovascular interventions. Acad Radiol 12:1121–1127

Mekle R, Hofmann E, Scheffler K, Bilecen D (2006) A polymer-based MR-compatible guidewire: a study to explore new prospects for interventional peripheral magnetic resonance angiography (ipMRA). J Magn Reson Imaging 23:145–155

Miquel ME, Hegde S, Muthurangu V, Corcoran BJ, Keevil SF, Hill DL, Razavi RS (2004) Visualization and tracking of an inflatable balloon catheter using SSFP in a flow phantom and in the heart and great vessels of patients. Magn Reson Med 51:988–995

Muthurangu V, Taylor A, Andriantsimiavona R, Hegde S, Miquel ME, Tulloh R, Baker E, Hill DL, Razavi RS (2004) Novel method of quantifying pulmonary vascular resistance by use of simultaneous invasive pressure monitoring and phase-contrast magnetic resonance flow. Circulation 110:826–834

Muthurangu V, Atkinson D, Sermesant M, Miquel ME, Hegde S, Johnson R, Andriantsimiavona R, Taylor AM, Baker E, Tulloh R, Hill DL, Razavi RS (2005a) Measurement of total pulmonary arterial compliance using invasive pressure monitoring and MR flow quantification during MR guided cardiac catheterization. Am J Physiol Hear Circ Physiol 289(3):1301–1306

Muthurangu V, Semesant M, Atkinson D, Hill D, Razavi R (2005b) A non-invasive method of calculating pulmonary vascular resistance using MR flow data. J Cardiovasc Magn Reson 7:104

NRPB (1999) Guidelines on patient dose to promote the optimisation of protection for diagnostic medical exposures. National Radiation Protection Board.

Olsson LE, Chai CM, Axelsson O, Karlsson M, Golman K, Petersson JS (2006) MR coronary angiography in pigs with intraarterial injections of a hyperpolarized 13C substance. Magn Reson Med 55:731–737

Ratnayaka K, Raman VK, Faranesh AZ, Sonmez M, Kim JH, Gutierrez LF, Ozturk C, Mcveigh ER, Slack MC, Lederman RJ (2009) Antegrade percutaneous closure of membranous ventricular septal defect using X-ray fused with magnetic resonance imaging. JACC Cardiovasc interv 2:224–230

Razavi R, Hill DL, Keevil SF, Miquel ME, Muthurangu V, Hegde S, Rhode K, Barnett M, Van Vaals J, Hawkes DJ, Baker E (2003) Cardiac catheterisation guided by MRI in children and adults with congenital heart disease. Lancet 362:1877–1882

Rhode KS, Hill DL, Edwards PJ, Hipwell J, Rueckert D, Sanchez-Ortiz G, Hegde S, Rahunathan V, Razavi R (2003) Registration and tracking to integrate X-ray and MR images in an XMR facility. IEEE Trans Med Imaging 22:1369–1378

Schalla S, Saeed M, Higgins CB, Martin A, Weber O, Moore P (2003) Magnetic resonance–guided cardiac catheterization in a swine model of atrial septal defect. Circulation 108:1865–1870

Schalla S, Saeed M, Higgins CB, Weber O, Martin A, Moore P (2005) Balloon sizing and transcatheter closure of acute atrial septal defects guided by magnetic resonance fluoroscopy: assessment and validation in a large animal model. J Magn Reson Imaging 21:204–211

Seppenwoolde JH, Viergever MA, Bakker CJ (2003) Passive tracking exploiting local signal conservation: the white marker phenomenon. Magn Reson Med 50:784–790

Sorensen TS, Atkinson D, Schaeffter T, Hansen MS (2009) Real-time reconstruction of sensitivity encoded radial magnetic resonance imaging using a graphics processing unit. IEEE Trans Med Imaging 28:1974–1985

Tzifa A, Krombach GA, Kramer N, Kruger S, Schutte A, Von Walter M, Schaeffter T, Qureshi S, Krasemann T, Rosenthal E, Schwartz CA, Varma G, Buhl A, Kohlmeier A, Bucker A, Gunther RW, Razavi R (2010) Magnetic resonance-guided cardiac interventions using magnetic resonance-compatible devices: a preclinical study and first-in-man congenital interventions. Circ Cardiovasc Interv 3(6):585–592

Weiss S, Wirtz D, David B, Krueger S, Lips O, Caulfield D, Pedersen SF, Bostock J, Razavi R, Schaeffter T (2010) In vivo evaluation and proof of radiofrequency safety of a novel diagnostic MR-electrophysiology catheter. Magn Reson Med 65:770–777

Cardiovascular Modeling

Giovanni Biglino, Silvia Schievano, Vivek Muthurangu, and Andrew Taylor

Contents

1 **Introduction** 669

2 **Engineering Modeling Techniques** 670
2.1 In vitro Modeling 670
2.2 In silico Modeling 672
2.3 Virtual Surgery 675

3 **The Usefulness of MR in This Context** 675

4 **MR and Cardiac Modeling** 676
4.1 Valve Stenting 676
4.2 Valve Modeling and Assessment 679
4.3 Congenital Heart Disease 681
4.4 Cardiac Resynchronization Therapy 684
4.5 Virtual Physiological Human 687

5 **Discussion** 687

6 **Conclusion** 689

7 **Key Points** 689

References 689

Abstract

Modeling of the cardiovascular system is increasingly used to provide information that is not easily measured in humans or that can be used to predict treatment outcomes. Importantly, cardiac MRI can not only provide much of the data necessary to build such models, but can also be used to provide much of the data necessary to validate these processes. This will be a relatively novel area of work for most in the field of imaging, and this chapter will outline the basic principles and types of models that are currently available, and demonstrate their use with in specific examples.

1 Introduction

Over the last decade modeling of the cardiovascular system has received a huge amount of attention from the engineering, computer scientist and medical communities (Virtual Physiological Human, Health-e-Child–http://www.health-e-child.org, Sim-e-Child–http://www.sim-e-child.org and EuHeart–http://www.euheart.eu to name but a few). The aim of modeling is to improve our understanding of the cardiovascular system by providing new information that cannot be measured easily in humans and by using models to predict what may happen over time or following treatments. One important area may be the use of human anatomy to enable optimization of new devices or surgical treatments. The advantage of MR imaging in these processes is that it can provide much of the information required to build computational and in vitro models (3D and 4D anatomy, flow data

G. Biglino · S. Schievano · V. Muthurangu · A. Taylor (✉)
Centre for Cardiovascular Imaging, UCL Institute of Cardiovascular Science and Great Ormond Street Hospital for Children, Great Ormond Street, WC1N 3JH, London, UK
e-mail: a.taylor76@ucl.ac.uk

J. Bogaert et al. (eds.), *Clinical Cardiac MRI*, Medical Radiology. Diagnostic Imaging,
DOI: 10.1007/174_2011_424, © Springer-Verlag Berlin Heidelberg 2012

and ventricular function), while at the same time providing the follow-up data necessary to validate predictive modeling. The interaction between clinicians, imagers, engineers and computer scientists is crucial for this field, with each group of specialists needing to learn the advantages and limitations of the data and the modeling methodologies.

In 1996, MR was used to construct a model of myocardial perfusion (Larsson et al. 1996). In this study, which presents a more refined model based on previous work by the same group (Larsson et al. 1994), MR was used to estimate perfusion using gadolinium as an intravenous bolus injection. Another example of the utility of MR data for modeling, rather than diagnostic purpose, is its use for visualization and analysis of blood flow patterns. In 1999, a study showed features such as helical paths in the ascending aorta in systole or vortices within an ascending aorta graft (Buonocore and Bogren 1999). Even earlier, in 1992, a model was already setup to show flow trajectories for internal carotid and cerebral aneurysm application (Napel et al. 1992). Such patterns that were modeled on 2D flow data can now be seen using new 4D MR flow techniques, bringing cardiovascular MR modeling and validation full circle.

Nowadays, the technical advances in terms of both software and hardware render MR data even more appealing and easily handled for modeling applications. The aim of this chapter is to provide an introduction and overview of modeling terminology and technologies and to describe those aspects of MR imaging that are valuable for cardiovascular modeling.

2 Engineering Modeling Techniques

The definition of a *model* is neither simple nor concise. In 1985, a Committee on Models for Biomedical Research (National Research Council 1985) quoted R. Ransom's classification of different models (Ransom 1981), including:

- *Paper and pencil*, or *static*, models
- *Mathematical* models
- *Computer* models normally animated as *simulations*
- *Substitute systems*, or *surrogate*, models.

Models and experiments can also be classified as:

- In vivo: the experiment is carried out in the living organism;
- In vitro: the system is reproduced, with a varying degree of approximation, on the bench; or
- In silico: the experiment is performed by means of a computer simulation.

Without further discussing the concept of a biomedical model, advantages and limitations of the in vitro and in silico will be described, together with a more recent technique here defined as *virtual surgery* and followed by the potential of employing MR data in this context.

2.1 In vitro Modeling

In vitro cardiac modeling consists of creating a physical representation of part of the circulation. The main advantages of such an approach are that:

- Tests can be performed multiple times with high reproducibility,
- Variables can be studied in isolation if necessary,
- They are relatively low cost,
- There is the possibility of testing a component or a device under extreme conditions ("worst case scenario") or under a gradually varied range of conditions ("parametric study"), and
- They represent an ethical alternative to animal studies (Hanson et al. 2007; Morrison et al. 2010). The main disadvantages are the lack of homeostasic and autoregulatary mechanisms and the lack of histological information.

Experimental cardiac modeling can be broadly split into 3 area:

- *Mock circulatory systems* (also referred to as mock circuits, or loops), usually for hydrodynamics testing and device testing,
- *Visualization experiments*, for particle tracking or flow patterns analysis,
- *Rapid prototyping*, for experimental reconstruction of an anatomical model or manufacturing of test sections.

Mock circulatory systems are widely used in the cardiovascular field. They consist of any system which contains arterial, capillary and venous networks connected in their usual and natural sequence (Skalak 1972). It is important to note that the design and the level of detail of such bench experiments depends on the purpose of the study (Skalak 1972). For this reason, mock loops of varying complexity are described in the literature: from loops containing all the main components of the circulation including the

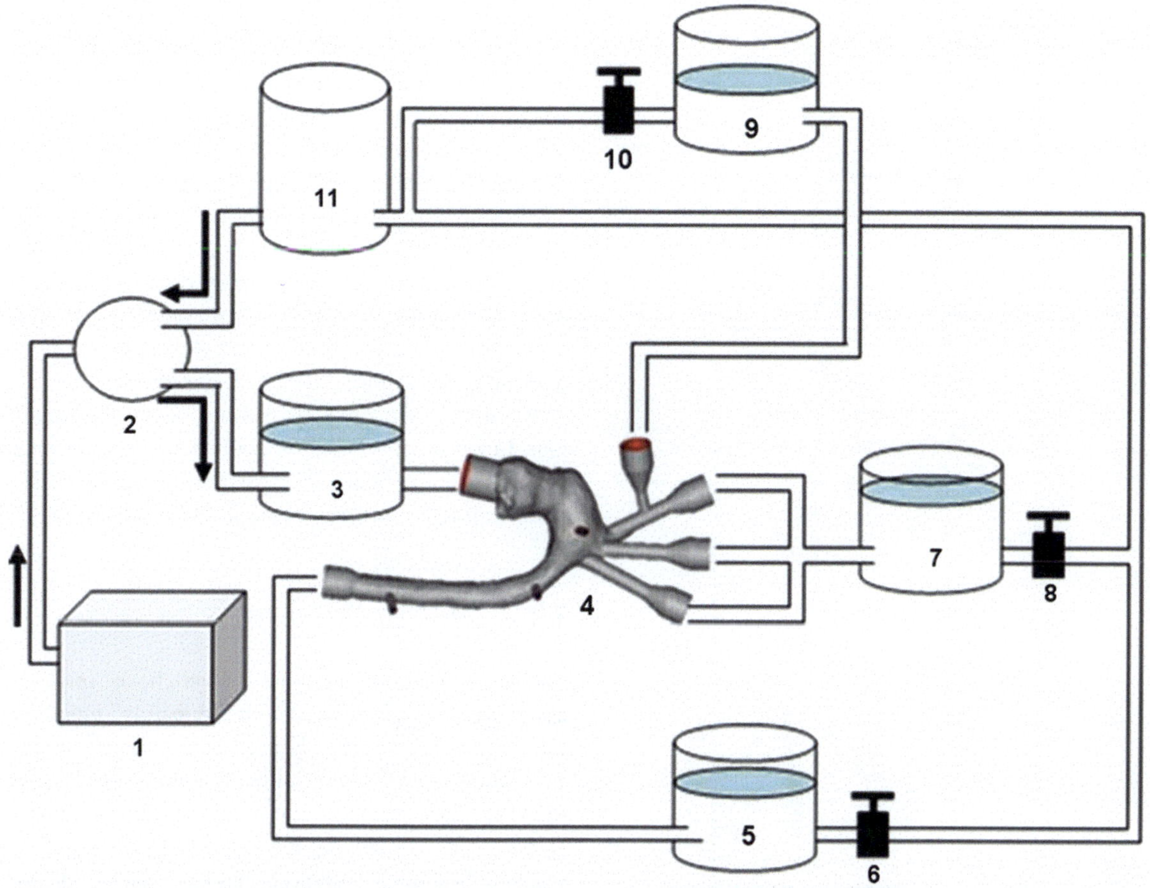

Fig. 1 Schematic representation of a pediatric mock loop simulating first stage palliation of hypoplastic left heart syndrome. Components: PC-controlled piston (*1*) driving a Berlin Heart Excor device (*2*) simulating the single ventricle, proximal compliance chamber (*3*), patient-specific rapid prototyped model (*4*), lower body compliance (*5*), lower body resistance (*6*), upper body compliance (*7*), upper body resistance (*8*), pulmonary compliance (*9*), pulmonary resistance (*10*), atrial chamber (*11*). Image from Biglino et al. (2011a, b)

four heart chambers, valves and atrial/ventricular septal defects (Timms et al. 2011) to loops focusing only on one side of the heart, such as the left heart circulation loop presented in Fig. 1 (De Paulis et al. 2005; Fries et al. 2006), and experiments including the effect of respiration (Camp et al. 2007). All these circuits, example in Fig. 2, include resistive and compliant elements, which are commonly based on variations of the Windkessel theory. The Windkessel model is analogous to an electrical circuit, with pressure representing electrical potential and flow representing current (Hales 1733; Frank 1899). One major use of mock loops is to study cardiac assist devices, such as axial flow pumps (Camus et al. 2007; Nakatani et al. 1994), centrifugal pumps (Jahanmir et al. 2009; Takami 2006) and counterpulsators (Bowles et al. 1991; Kolyva et al. 2010; Papaioannou et al. 2004). They are also useful to study heart valves (Scharfscherdt et al. 2009) in the aortic (Kuehnel et al. 2005), mitral (Jimenez et al. 2005) and pulmonary (Gohean et al. 2006) positions, as well as being used as "bioreactors" for bioengineering tissue valves (Bowles et al. 2010; Dumont et al. 2002). Finally, mock loops are an extremely effective teaching tool (Pantalos et al. 2010; Zannoli et al. 2009).

Visualization experiments are carried out in similar setups to mock loops, usually with some adaption to accommodate a method to visualize flow. Particle image velocimetry (PIV) is an optical measurement technique used to obtain high temporal resolution velocity information from particles suspended in flowing blood (Raffel et al. 2007). It has been successfully used to

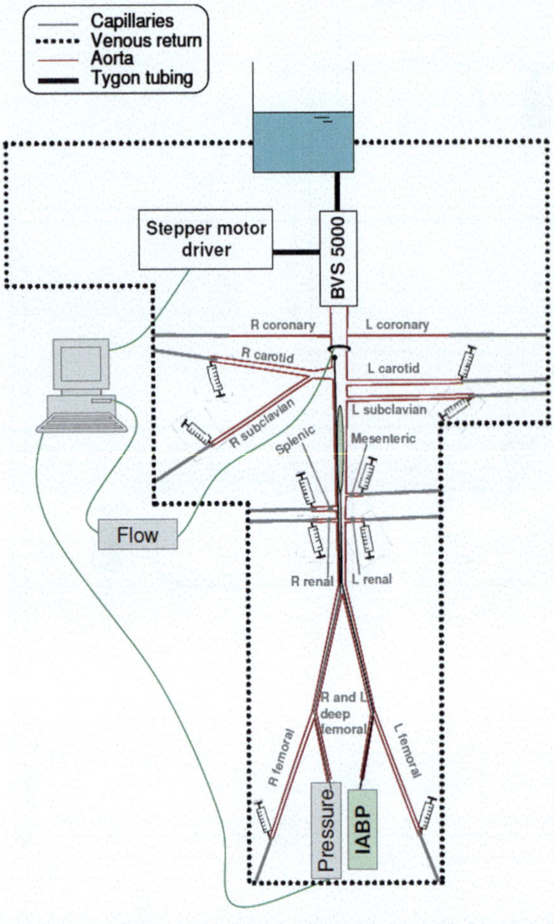

Fig. 2 Schematic overview of a compact and complete mock circulatory system for intra-aortic balloon pump (IABP) testing. A 14-branch polyurethane aorta is attached to a ventricular assist device (BVS 5000, Abiomed) which simulated the left atrium and left ventricle. Physiological distribution of compliance and peripheral resistance is implemented by means of air chambers (syringes) of varying air volume and capillary tubes of varying length, respectively. Image from Kolyva et al. (2010)

investigate flow through prosthetic valves (Kaminsky et al. 2007; Vermeulen et al. 2009). An example of PIV measurement applied to studying the flow distribution in the pulmonary arteries after the Fontan procedure is shown in Fig. 3. Ink studies, albeit less refined than PIV, can also provide valuable qualitative information, such as in the case of stenotic and regurgitant jets (Krabill et al. 1989). High-speed cameras alone can also be useful to gain detailed time information on the mechanical behavior of a device (Biglino et al. 2010).

Rapid prototyping describes the layer-by-layer fabrication of a three-dimensional (3D) model from a computer-aided design (Laoui and Shaik 2003). Its relevance in the context of in vitro modeling is linked to its ability to create detailed model, down to patient-specific level. A rapid prototyped model is thus useful as a test section within a mock circulatory loop. Test sections in fact can be either simplified morphologies (Bowles et al. 1991; Vismara et al. 2009) or patient-specific phantoms (Biglino et al. 2011a; de Zélicourt et al. 2005; Kitajima et al. 2008). They can also be either rigid (de Zélicourt et al. 2005; Ensley et al. 1999) or compliant (Biglino et al. 2011b; Kolyva et al. 2010; Segers et al. 1998) depending on the purpose of the experiment.

Finally, in vitro models can also serve the important function of validation tools for computational studies (Matthys et al. 2007; Medvitz et al. 2009). The latter is briefly outlined in the following paragraph.

2.2 In silico Modeling

Advances in computational power have rendered computational simulations an appealing modeling tool, which is increasingly used in the cardiovascular field. It has the advantage of being more cost-effective than in vitro testing and has greater flexibility. However, computational modeling lacks the ability to evaluate biological responses and adaptations, and the evaluation of complex loading and boundary conditions can be computationally expensive (Morrison et al. 2010).

In silico models can be divided into 4 main areas:

- *Finite element analysis* (FEA), or *finite element method* (FEM)
- *Computational fluid dynamics* (CFD)
- *Fluid structure interaction* (FSI)
- *Multiscale modeling*.

FEA is a computational method used to determine the spatial distribution of one or more mechanical variables in a tissue structure. The structure being modeled is divided into finite elements that are arranged in a *mesh* (Cook et al. 2002). FEA has been applied to different areas of cardiovascular modeling, and recent examples include: stress analysis of carotid atherosclerotic plaques (Teng et al. 2011); studying pulmonary autograft dilatation following the Ross procedure (Matthews et al. 2011); simulation of cardiac torsion (Bagnoli et al. 2011); study of the forces exerted by angioplasty balloons (Capelli et al. 2010a); FEA of various percutaneous aortic valve stent

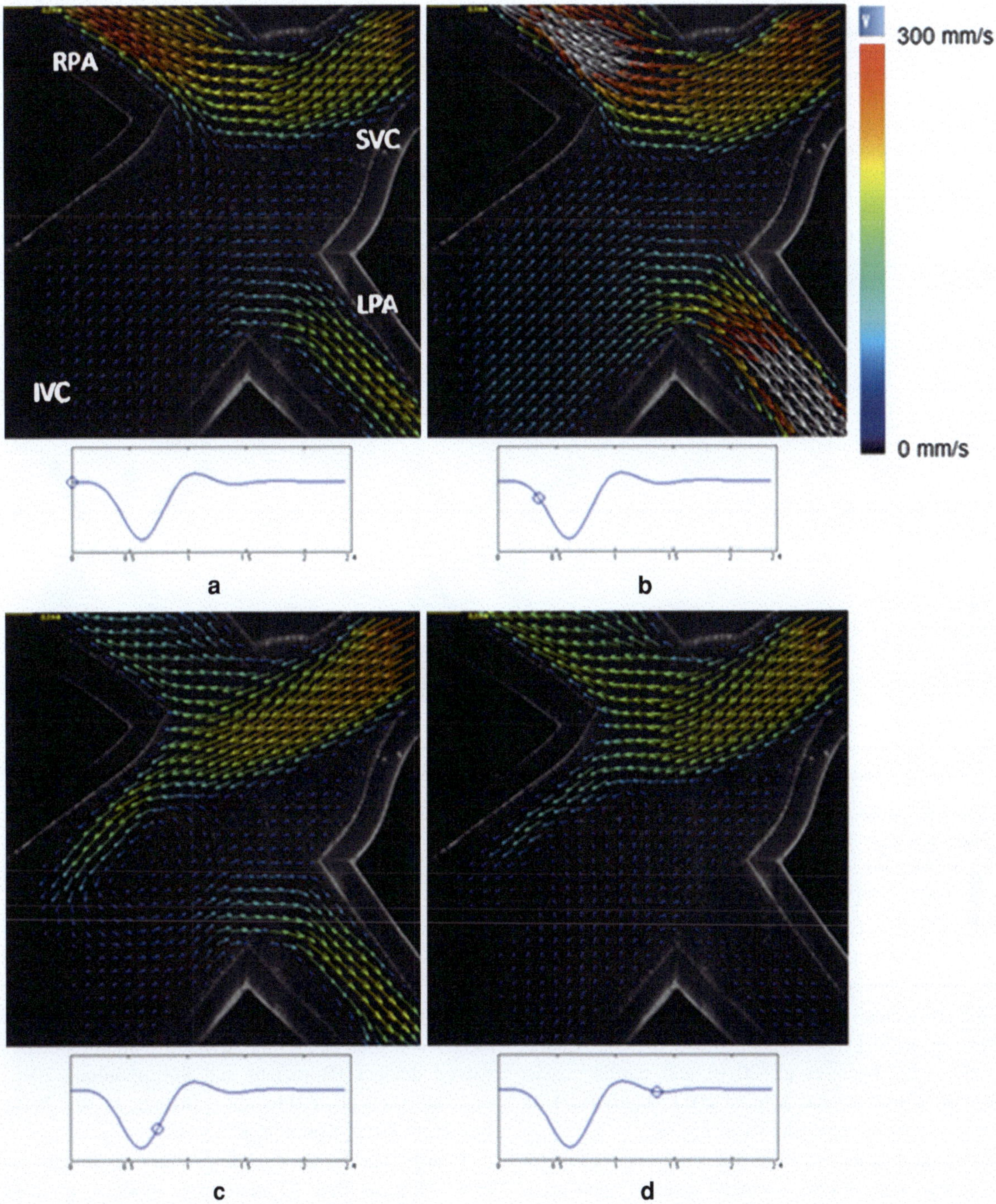

Fig. 3 Particle Image Velocimetry (PIV) assessing the flow passing through a total cavopulmonary connection (TCPC) in an artificial heart flow simulator, showing the distribution of flow into right pulmonary artery (*RPA*) and left pulmonary artery (*LPA*) from the inferior and superior venae cavae (*IVC* and *SVC*). Image from Chiulli et al. (2012)

designs using different biomaterials and varying loads (Kumar and Mathew 2011) and FEA of the tricuspid valve (Stevanella et al. 2010).

CFD aims to model problems that involve viscous fluid flows. Computational studies have looked at flow phenomena in different areas of the circulation,

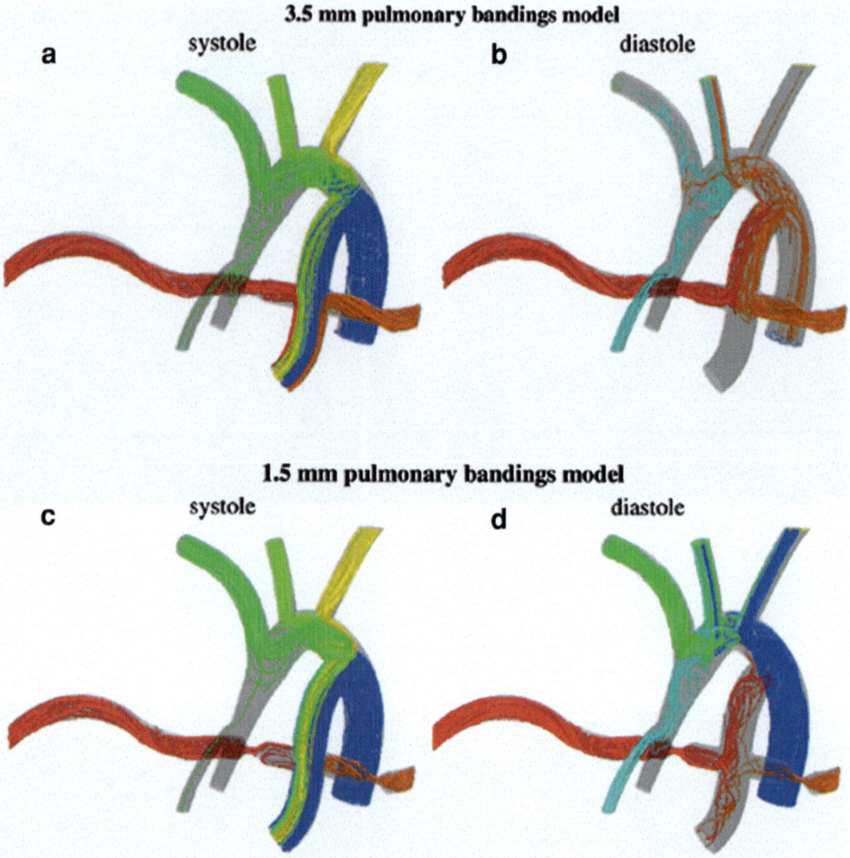

Fig. 4 In silico simulation of hybrid Norwood procedure, using CFD to compare the effects of different pulmonary bandings. **a** and **b**: 3.5 mm pulmonary bandings and 7.0 mm ductus arteriosus during systole and diastole. **c** and **d**: 1.5 mm pulmonary bandings and 7.0 mm ductus arteriosus during systole and diastole. Image modified from Corsini et al. (2011)

such as pulsatile flow in the carotid artery bifurcation (Perktold et al. 1991) and the way in which endothelial cells are stimulated by fluid forces (Satcher et al. 1992). CFD models have become more refined with increasing computational power and recent work covers different areas, including cerebral and abdominal aneurysms (Cebral et al. 2011; O'Rourke and McCullough 2010), coronary circulation (Chaichana et al. 2011), congenital heart disease (Ladisa et al. 2010; Qian et al. 2010) and cardiac assist devices (Filipovic and Schima 2011; Medvitz et al. 2007). An example is shown in Fig. 4.

The application of FEM for solids and CFD for fluids has achieved an advanced level of sophistication, but the interaction of fluids and solids poses a more complex problem. These so-called fluid structure interactions essentially consists of coupling the solid domain and the fluid domain, aiming to provide a more realistic simulation. In fact, several phenomena in the cardiovascular system present a FSI problem, including opening and closure of heart valves, ventricular ejection and vessel/myocardial interaction in the coronary circulation (Chen et al. 2010). Different methods can be applied for this purpose (Chen et al. 2010; van de Vosse et al. 2003). Recent FSI studies have investigated problems such as stress analysis of atherosclerotic plaque in the carotid artery (Gao et al. 2009) and stent re-stenosis in the coronary circulation (Selvarasu et al. 2011), but the majority have focused on heart valve dynamics and prosthetic-valved devices (Borazjani and Sotiropoulous 2010; de Tullio et al. 2011a, b; Einstein et al. 2010; Lau et al. 2010; Simon et al. 2010).

Finally, *multiscale* modeling refers to simulations in which a detailed 3D anatomical model is coupled with a Windkessel-like model for the concurrent simulation of local and global dynamics (Formaggia et al. 1999; Quarteroni and Veneziani 2003). A multiscale model links detailed fine scale information, to macroscale effects (i.e. function, pathology) of tissues and entire organs (Chapman 2009). In the case of the heart, for instance, the scale hierarchy could be: body,

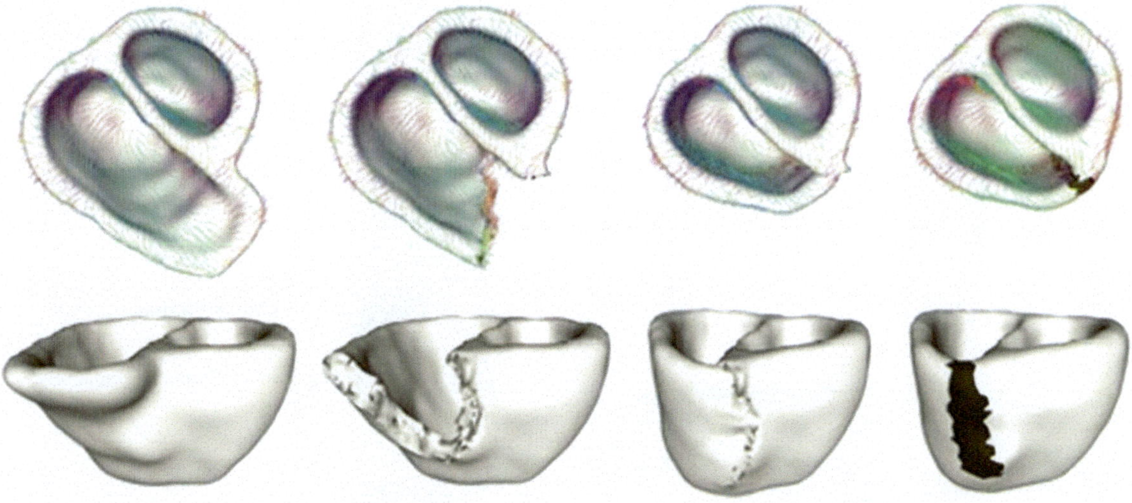

Fig. 5 Example of virtual right ventricle volume reduction surgery, showing (*from left to right*) the original mesh, resection, attachment, and the final mesh. *Colour* lines indicate fibre orientation. The *black* area (*right*) indicates postoperative scar. Image from Mansi et al. (2009)

organ, tissue, cell and ion channel (Chapman 2009). Different areas of cardiovascular research are nowadays tackled with a multiscale approach, including dynamics of healthy and diseased valves (Weinberg et al. 2010), the effect of aortic valvular and arterial stenoses on global hemodynamics (Liang et al. 2009), ventricular arrhythmias (Arevalo et al. 2007) and congenital single ventricle physiology (Bove et al. 2008; Hsia et al. 2009; Laganá et al. 2005).

2.3 Virtual Surgery

When referring to *virtual surgery* it is here intended to indicate a fast computational model combined with image processing algorithms and an interactive surgical simulation platform to simulate the direct post-operative effects of different therapies (Mansi et al. 2009; Taylor et al. 1999). One interesting, recent example is the evaluation of two techniques for pulmonary valve replacement, virtually comparing the minimally invasive approach to open-heart surgery with direct right ventricle volume reduction (Mansi et al. 2009). In this application, the myocardial geometry is reconstructed, defining the orientation of fibers and applying models of myocardial electrophysiology and of cardiac motion to the recreated volume. Once the model is complete, the different interventions can be simulated in real time using appropriate software platform (see example of virtual suture of the right ventricle in Fig. 5). The model also maps fiber orientation to the post-operative scenario.

The ability to simulate the surgical outcomes of different procedures can be extremely important, especially in the case of complex surgeries. An example could be the simulation of surgical palliation of hypoplastic left heart syndrome. Following the Norwood operation, or stage 1 palliation (Norwood 1991), the surgeon can opt for either a bidirectional Glenn anastomosis (Hopkins et al. 1985) or a hemi-Fontan procedure (Douglas et al. 1999). These are different surgeries, whose outcome can be compared in silico (Bove et al. 2003). The result of simulations carried out in idealized Glenn and hemi-Fontan geometries is shown in Fig. 6. In essence: the clinician provides the engineer with preoperative information, the engineer returns different virtual postoperative scenarios and, based on the latter, the clinician evaluates potetial surgical alternatives.

3 The Usefulness of MR in This Context

MR imaging can be an integral and useful component of in vitro, in silico and virtual surgery modeling techniques for cardiac applications. MR can in fact provide two types of information for this purpose:

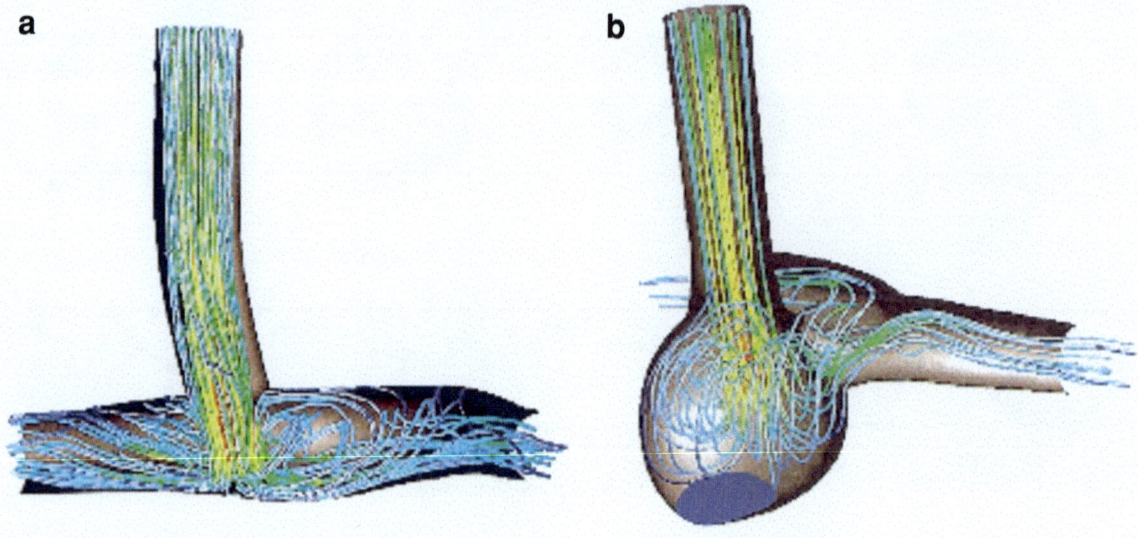

Fig. 6 Computational comparison of surgical outcomes for stage 2 palliation of hypoplastic left heart syndrome. **a**: bidirectional Glenn operation. **b**: hemi-Fontan procedure. Path lines correspond to superior vena cava injection for both models. Lines are colour-coded with reference to velocity magnitude (*red* = high velocity, *blue* = low velocity). Image from Bove et al. (2003)

- Anatomical, and
- Functional

In the case of anatomical information, MR images can be analyzed with commercially available software in order to recreate the 3D anatomical models of the anatomy of interest. This process has been clearly outlined by Schievano et al. with regard to the reconstruction of a right ventricular outflow tract (RVOT) anatomy (Schievano et al. 2007b). The outcome of such a procedure for cardiovascular applications is a 3D volume of blood in the region of interest, or the lumen of a vessel. Depending on the application (e.g. rapid prototyping a physical model, 3D geometry for multiscale modeling) the vessel wall can be extruded to a desired wall thickness.

In the case of functional information, PC-MRI can be used to derive quantitative flow data (Saleh et al. 2007). This technique was first described almost thirty years ago (Moran 1982) and since then it has been further developed and refined, and validated both in vitro (Lotz et al. 2005) and in vivo (Firmin et al. 1987). Interestingly, less than ten years ago, PC-MRI was still indicated as "a well-known, but undervalued method of obtaining quantitative information on blood flow" (Lotz et al. 2002). A crucial point of the technique concerns the definition of the contours of the vessel where velocity and flow are going to be estimated (Burkart et al. 1994; Kozerke et al. 1999; Odille et al. 2011).

So, while MR anatomical data can be essential in *constructing* a model, MR functional data can be vital for *validating* the outcome of an experiment.

4 MR and Cardiac Modeling

The following sections will describe recent advances in the use of MR for experimental, computational and virtual cardiac modeling.

4.1 Valve Stenting

4.1.1 Patient Selection

The anatomical information derived from MR can be extremely useful in assessing a patient population and determining suitability to a certain treatment. A good example of this application is found in the context of percutaneous pulmonary valve implantation (PPVI). In 2000, Bonhoeffer et al. performed the first PPVI in a patient (Bonhoeffer et al. 2000) and this procedure was quickly established as a successful alternative to surgical valve replacement (Coats et al. 2006; Khambadkone et al. 2005; Lurz et al. 2008).

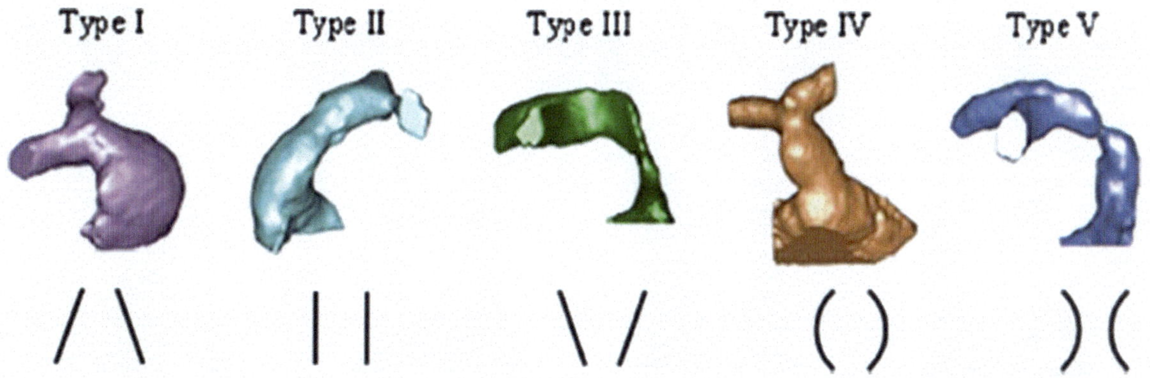

Fig. 7 Classification of right ventricular outflow tract morphologies as proposed by Schievano et al. based on anatomy reconstruction from MR data. Type I ("pyramidal") was most prevalent (49% of study population) but percutaneous pulmonary valve implantation was not performed in this group

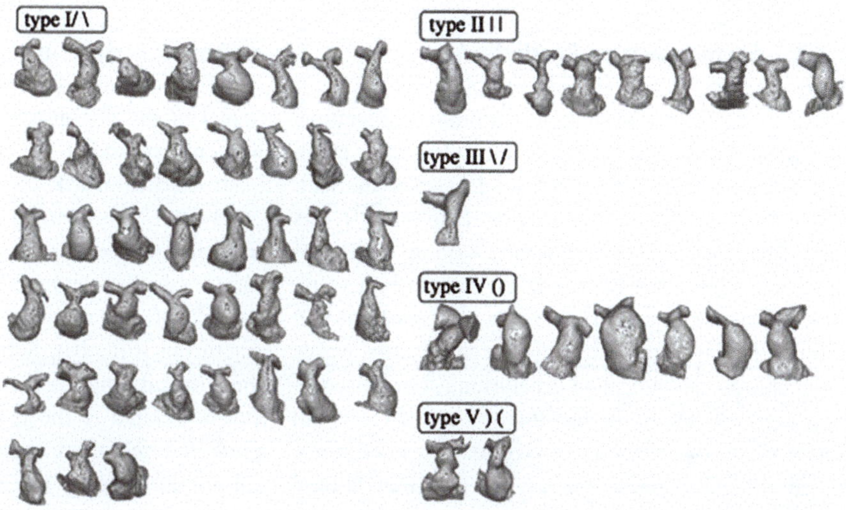

Fig. 8 Patient-specific reconstruction of RVOT anatomies from MR data and classification of RVOT morphology for assessment of second-generation percutaneous pulmonary valve implantation

However, it emerged that the success of the procedure was highly influenced by the dimensions, the morphology and the dynamics of the RVOT. This was demonstrated by Schievano et al. (2007b), who proposed a classification of RVOT morphologies, based on MR information (Schievano et al. 2007a).

This classification is shown in Fig. 7. In conclusion, patient selection was shown to be profoundly affected by morphological factors and according to this work only 15% patients were recommended PPVI instead of invasive surgery.

Recently, a second-generation device was introduced (Bonhoeffer et al. 2008). with the aim of deployment in patients with larger pulmonary arteries. To verify whether the new device was indeed suitable for a wider range of morphologies, Capelli et al. carried out patient-specific FEA mimicking virtual PPVI (Capelli et al. 2010b). To do this, MR images of 62 patients who had undergone surgical pulmonary valve replacement were used to reconstruct a range of 3D RVOT anatomies. The 62 resulting anatomies were classified according to the same classification proposed by Schievano et al. (Fig. 8) and were used as the as the substrate for virtual implantation of the second-generation PPVI stent-graft (Fig. 9). The advantage of this in silico technique was multiple stent designs could be tested in multiple anatomies. In this way, the study assessed the patients' suitability for the procedure while also exploring potential optimization of the device itself. Results showed that between 37 and 63% patients could benefit from the percutaneous procedure depending on the design of the stent-graft.

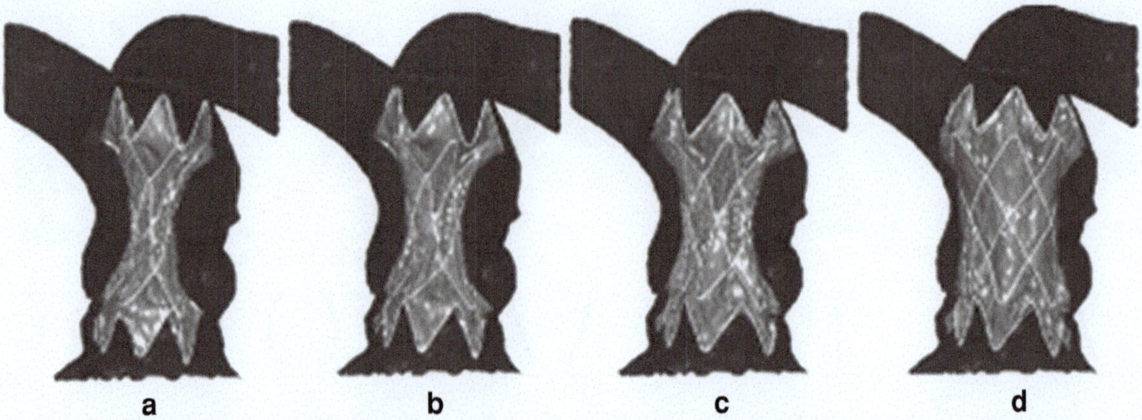

Fig. 9 Finite element simulation of stent-graft release in a patient-specific anatomy, showing progressive phases of deployment, namely (**a**) crimped position, (**b**) stent release, (**c**) contact with the arterial wall and (**d**) final configuration

4.1.2 Stent Fracture Prediction

Stent fracture is a common complication of stent implantation for different cardiovascular applications (Breinholt et al. 2008; Lim et al. 2008; Rits et al. 2008). In the context of PPVI—described in Sect. 4.1.1—the first-generation device (Melody^{TM}) has been shown to be prone to fracture, with up to 20% of stent being fractured in follow up (Nordmeyer et al. 2007). This is despite the fact that experimental and animal testing suggested a potential for valve degeneration but not stent fracturing., This discrepancy could be due to the fact that the in vitro tests did not correctly replicate the in vivo loading conditions, or on the other hand due to the fact that animal experiments were not representative of the human pathological anatomy. Hence, the problem was tackled from a FEM perspective (Schievano et al. 2007c, 2010a, b).

A computational study was performed using MR data from a patient with significant pulmonary homograft stenosis and mild pulmonary regurgitation. This patient was successfully treated with first-generation PPVI; however, stent fractures were detected three months after the procedure. Preoperative MR data, which included ce-MRA of the RVOT, were used to reconstruct the RVOT morphology in 3D. Biplane fluoroscopy images were used to reconstruct the 3D shape and deformation of the stent in situ. Three scenarios were simulated:

- Stent expanded up to 20 mm internal diameter, corresponding to the balloon diameter used clinically during deployment;
- Stent expanded up to 22 mm internal diameter, corresponding to the maximum deployment diameter of the first-generation PPVI device;
- Stent expanded in the RVOT anatomy reconstructed from MR.

Overall, the simulations showed that deployment in a patient-specific anatomy influences the configuration of the device, predicting a more realistic "map" of the regions with a higher likelihood of fracturing (Fig. 10). Schievano et al. underlined that the clinical implication of identifying such regions can be related to the fact that patients with a higher predicted risk of fracturing may require more frequent follow up to verify the integrity of the device.

4.1.3 First-in-man: Implantation of a Novel Device

When a new device for PPVI was first introduced in order to suit larger diameter RVOT morphologies (Sect. 4.1.1), modeling was not only useful for the process of patient selection, but it was also crucial in practicing the procedure and identifying the best access route for implantation. This was achieved by means of a rapid prototyped patient-specific model.

In the first-in-man procedure, the patient-specific anatomy of RVOT, pulmonary trunk and proximal pulmonary arteries was reconstructed from imaging data (in this specific case, 4D CT data was available, but the reconstruction process was identical). This data was then used to create a hollow resin-based 3D phantom, which was extremely useful in studying access routes and device placement. In fact, the

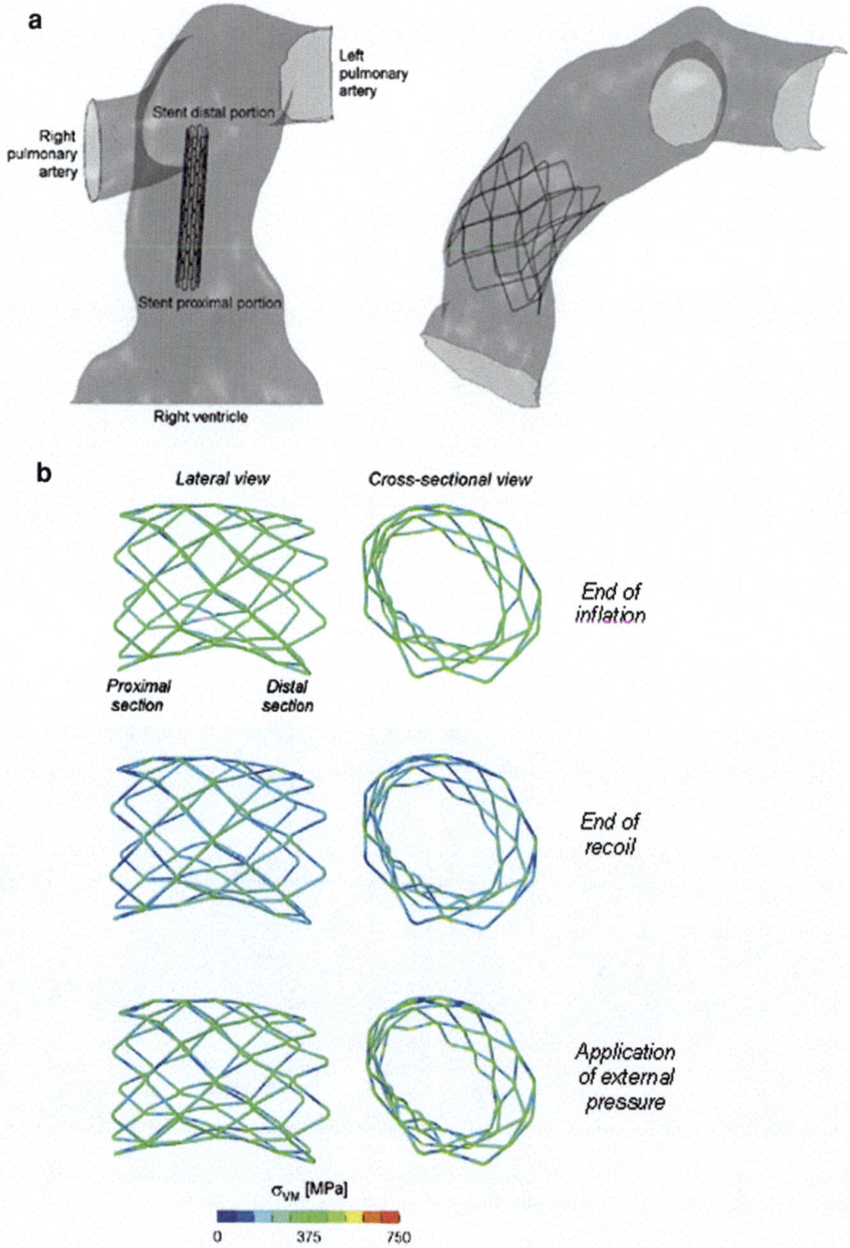

Fig. 10 Virtual stent deployment in a reconstructed patient-specific RVOT anatomy (**a**) and computation of von Mises stresses (**b**)

implanters were able to identify both an optimal approach and approaches that would in all likelihood be unsuccessful (shown in Fig. 11).

While a surgeon has direct visual access to the area of interest, the interventional cardiologist traditionally does not have such visual information, but in this case a rapid prototyped model provided a visualization tool to test correct positioning of the guide wire and practice the implantation in vitro prior first-in-man procedure.

4.2 Valve Modeling and Assessment

4.2.1 Aortic Flow with Mechanical Heart Valve

Flow in the ascending aorta is characterized by complex patterns. Some parameters useful in the analysis of flow pattern and general hemodynamics (e.g. wall shear stress) cannot be directly measured in vivo. Their evaluation is facilitated by a combined approach involving MR imaging and CFD modeling.

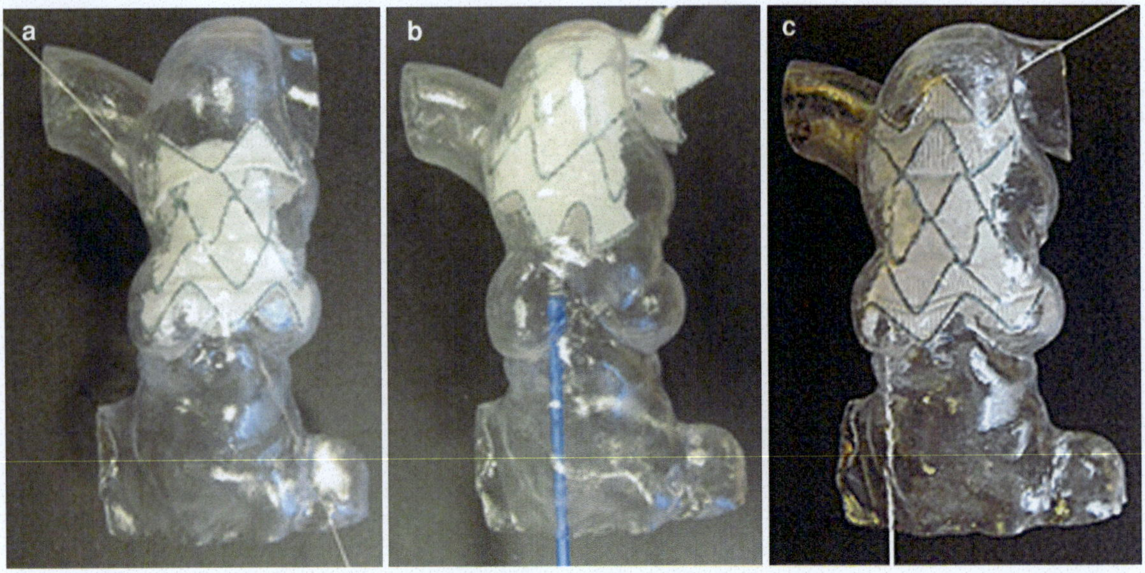

Fig. 11 First-in-man implantation of a novel device for PPVI. A rapid prototyped, transparent experimental model aided the interventional cardiologist both visually and practically in planning the best access route, in this case via the left pulmonary artery (**b**, **c**) instead of the right pulmonary artery (**a**)

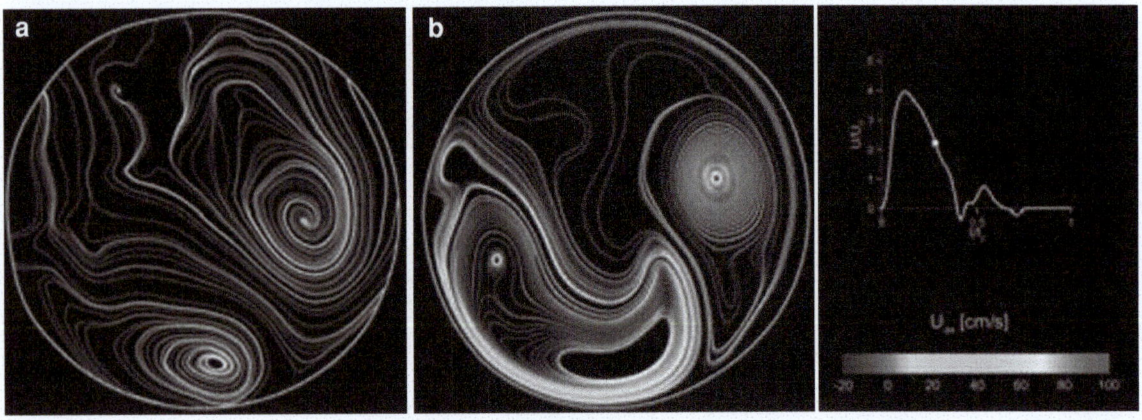

Fig. 12 Healthy aortic valve scenario, streamlines at the outlet of the aortic model during systolic deceleration, comparing MR measurements (**a**) and CFD result (**b**). Image from Leuprecht et al. (2003)

For instance, a study by Leuprecht et al. employing this method investigated axial and secondary flows in the ascending aorta, focusing on the effect of the presence of cardiovascular implants (Leuprecht et al. 2003). Their work compared blood flow downstream an artificial aortic valve implanted in a patient-specific model with blood-flow characteristics in the ascending aorta of a healthy volunteer. They highlighted that this comparison is especially relevant considering the late complications associated with mechanical valve prostheses and their different hemodynamics compared to native valves, as shown both in vitro (Woo and Yoganathan 1985) and in vivo (Hasenkam et al. 1988). In addition, they noted that mechanical valves still present an advantage over biological valves in terms of their durability, especially for young patients.

In this study, velocity observations from the computational model were validated against MR data, with additional MR measurements of the three-directional velocity field at the outlet of the model. The velocity contours showed good qualitative agreement, especially for high systolic velocities. Figure 12 shows velocity streamlines at the outlet of the model comparing CFD and MR. With respect to the MR data, CFD modeling can also provide additional important information of wall shear stress distribution. However, MR data is fundamental for validating the CFD model.

The major difference in the computational models of the healthy subjects and the patient with an artificial valve was substantially higher values of aortic shear stress. This would have been extremely difficult to assess with MR alone and is important as wall shear stress is linked with endothelial gene expression and the pathogenesis of atherosclerosis (Cunningham and Gotlieb 2005).

This study exemplifies how realistic anatomic models can be obtained from MR data and used for CFD simulation of flow with or without a prosthetic valve. Comparison of flow patterns between MR and CFD results can help validating the model. Once the model is validated, stress analysis can yield additional information in silico.

4.2.2 Mitral Valve Modeling

Early FEM models of the mitral valve (Kunzelman et al. 1993) have evolved into more sophisticated simulations, e.g. including more realistic mitral leaflets (Prot et al. 2009). Recent studies also aim to include the valve into a ventricular model. To do this CFD models based on MR imaging data and including the valves (Schenkel et al. 2009) must be created. The geometry in the model is patient-specific, as is derived from MR images. However, the valve geometry, as well as spatially and timing-dependent changes of the leaflets' shape, cannot be derived from the MR data. Valves are therefore usually represented as a 2D model. The orifice area can be derived from 3D echo scans of healthy valves (aortic and mitral) and then adapted to the size measured in the MR examination. Such CFD results show an asymmetric jet through the mitral valve during diastole, the jet leading to the formation of the initial vortex ring. This is in conformity with in vivo observations.

A more refined model of the mitral apparatus is proposed by Wenk et al. who created a computational model of the left ventricle, mitral valve and chordae tendineae (Wenk et al. 2010). Data for the creation of the model was obtained from MR images of a sheep that developed moderate mitral regurgitation after postero-basal myocardial infarction. Following a previously described protocol (Guccione et al. 2006), ventricular pressure was measured with a non-ferromagnetic transducer-tipped pressure catheter. Ventricular surfaces were contoured on the MR images and the annulus and leaflets of the mitral valve were identified using custom software, while the chordae tendineae could not be identified and consequently could not be contoured. Nonetheless, the chordae were computationally reconstructed from anatomic images of a mitral valve from an excised heart. Surface meshes of the valve leaflets were based on the information gained from the MR images. The posterior and anterior mitral valve leaflets were assigned different thickness and material properties, since the anterior leaflet has higher relative stiffness. The basal and marginal chordae were also assigned different material properties, and were connected directly between the papillary muscles and the leaflets, without branching. The model is shown in Fig. 13. Simulations were able to show the presence of mitral regurgitation as a gap between the leaflets and to show the effect of displacement of the papillary muscle on ischemic regurgitation. The authors stated that, with further improvements such as refining the anatomical detail and implementing FSI, the model may be used to plan clinical trials and to potentially optimize surgery for ischemic mitral regurgitation.

4.3 Congenital Heart Disease

4.3.1 Single Ventricle Physiology: The Y-graft

The single ventricle physiology, caused by congenital heart defects such as hypoplastic left heart syndrome and tricuspid atresia, is characterized by one functioning pumping chamber and saturated pulmonary venous blood mixed with desaturated systemic venous blood. This otherwise fatal physiology is often palliated with a staged surgical approach. In hypoplastic left heart syndrome, the first stage involves reconstruction of the hypoplastic aortic arch and sourcing pulmonary blood flow according to different options (Norwood 1991; Sano et al. 2003; Galantowicz and Cheatham 2005). The second stage, or bidirectional Glenn (Hopkins et al. 1985), involves anastomosis of the superior vena cava (SVC) into the pulmonary arteries (PAs). Finally, the third stage, or Fontan procedure (Fontan and Baudet 1971), involves connecting the inferior vena cava (IVC) to the PAs either

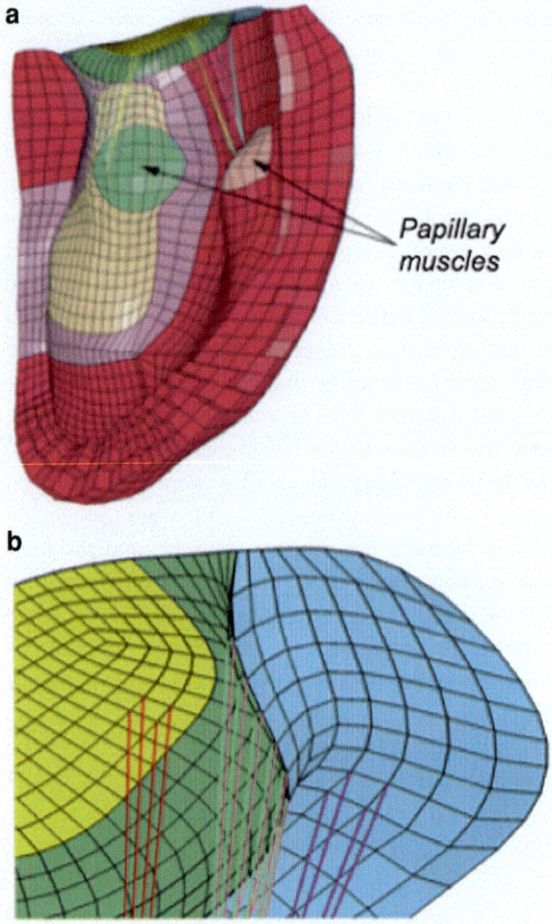

Fig. 13 Finite element mitral valve model derived from MR data. Interior view of the left ventricle showing the chordae attached to the papillary muscles (**a**) and more detailed view of the valve (**b**), showing chordae attachments at the mid-section of the anterior (*green* and *yellow*) and posterior (*blue*) leaflets. Images modified from Wenk et al. (2010)

with an extracardiac conduit or with an intracardiac baffle (the lateral tunnel), resulting in the total cavopulmonary connection (TCPC). At the end of the three-staged palliation, oxygenated and deoxygenated blood are separated. The complex Fontan surgery has evolved over the years, as the surgeons were gaining experience. Recently, an extracardiac Fontan was performed using a Y-shaped graft (Okano et al. 2002). Following this, Marsden et al. investigated the performance of the Y-graft design and variations of the design by making use of a patient-specific approach based on reconstructions from MR data (Marsden et al. 2009).

In such studies, acquisition of MR angiography data is the first step toward the creation of a virtual surgery paradigm. Anatomical information can be acquired using 3D ce-MRA or b-SSFP whole-heart techniques. Flows in the caval veins can be assessed using PC-MRI. This MR data can then be processed to extract geometric information and create an anatomical patient-specific model as described below:

- Creation of centerline paths in the vessels of interest
- Creation of perpendicular segmentations of the vessel lumen
- The 2D segmentations are lofted together, thus generating a solid model
- The solid model is discretized into a tetrahedral mesh for FEM use.

These steps are shown in Fig. 14. In the specific study by Marsden et al. a patient-specific anatomy was constructed, using data from a child who had a traditional extracardiac Fontan with anastomosis of IVC and SVC to the PAs (''T-junction'' configuration). Three geometric models were derived from it: (1) left PA offset, (2) small Y-graft and (3) large Y-graft. The four models are shown in Fig. 15 and represent the four options for virtual surgery. Flow inlet boundary conditions were imposed according to patient-specific flows derived from MR data, while resistance values were set so to match pressure values from the catheterization data. This highlights that the input in the simulation can be strictly patient-specific when setting the model, then parameters can be varied for evaluation purposes, as in this case in fact flow was increased incrementally simulating different levels of exercise.

Results showed that the large Y-graft design improved pressure levels, energy efficiency and flow distribution, compared to the offset and T-junction designs. This was observed both at rest and during exercise. Although, clinical trials are mandatory before the actual benefit of a novel technique can be proven, these results are compelling and create the foundations for further clinical studies and in vivo validation.

Further work on the Y-graft from the same group also involved performing an optimization study on a model Y-graft design problem, by using formal design optimization methods (Yang et al. 2010). This was carried out on an idealized anatomy. A modeling-directed trial of the Y-graft surgery is now underway.

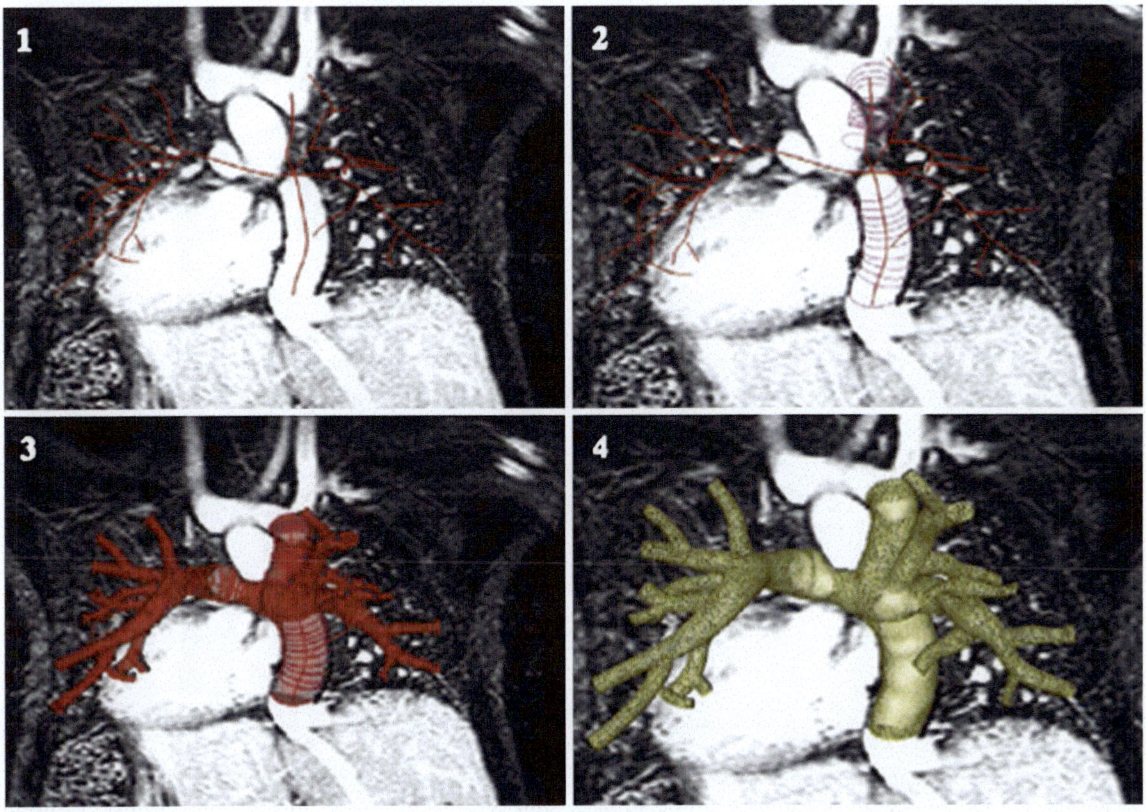

Fig. 14 Y-graft model construction from MR data: (**1**) Creation of centerlines, (**2**) perpendicular segmentations of the vessel's lumen, (**3**) lofting of the segmentations resulting in a solid model, (**4**) discretization of the solid model in a tetrahedral mesh. Image from Marsden et al. (2009) (provided with author's permission)

4.3.2 Single Ventricle Physiology: Hepatic Baffle Design

Following the superior cavopulmonary palliation of single ventricle diseases, complications such as pulmonary arteriovenous malformations (PAVMs) may arise. This is particularly true in patients with interrupted IVC and azygous continuation, with a likelihood of about 1 in 5 after the Kawashima procedure (de Zélicourt et al. 2011). Arteriovenous malformations can be prevented if hepatic blood is directed into the pulmonary arteries. Shah et al. proposed completion of the TCPC as potential way to solve PAVMs, increasing hepatic blood flow to the lungs (Shah et al. 1997). Taking full advantage of the predictive power of virtual surgery, a comparative study in planning the Fontan surgery in single ventricle patients with interrupted IVC was performed, in order to investigate the options to prevent or revert PAVMs (de Zélicourt et al. 2011).

In this study, the anatomies of the study population were reconstructed in 3D from MR data. These 3D morphological models were then used for testing virtual surgery options. The efficiency of different surgeries was quantified in silico. The surgical options that were finally simulated are all realistic and took into consideration the anatomical space available for potentially performing each operation, namely:

- Intra-/extra-cardiac grafts
- Bifurcated Y-grafts
- Hepatic vein-to-azygous shunts
- Azygous-to-hepatic vein shunts.

Inflow boundary conditions were imposed using phase contrast MR data. Each option was tested over a wide range of PAs flow ratios in order to evaluate hepatic flow distribution, ultimately reflecting PAVMs evolution. Hepatic flow distribution was assessed quantifying the flux of hepatic particles exiting through the left and right PA.

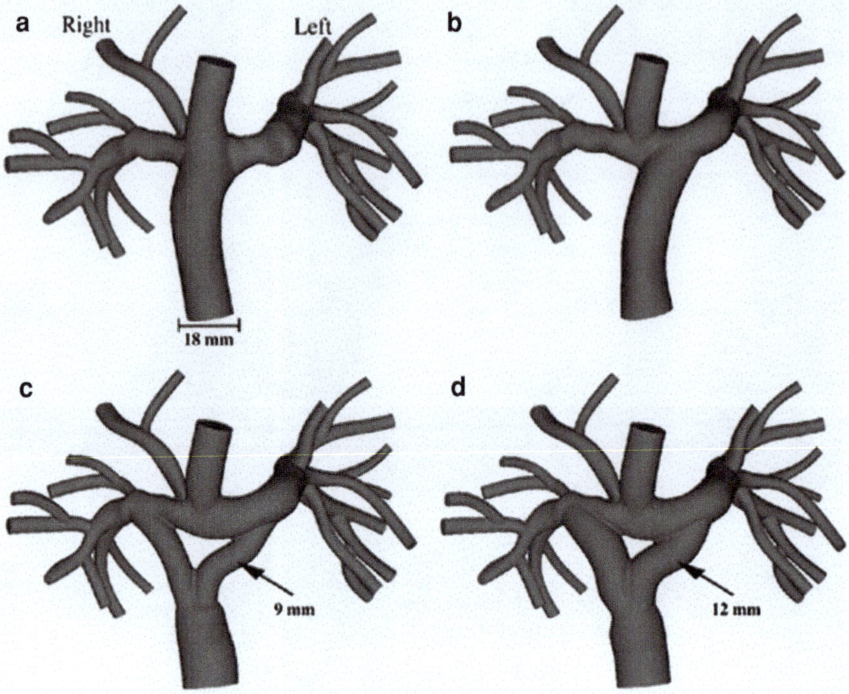

Fig. 15 Model comparison for virtual surgery: patient-specific Fontan model with T-junction (**a**), left PA offset (**b**), small Y-graft (**c**) and large Y-graft (**d**). Image from Marsden et al. (2009) (provided with author's permission)

An example of virtual surgery outcomes for one of the patient-specific anatomies examined in this study is shown in Fig. 16. The authors remarked that virtual determination of the best surgery thus involves both detailed anatomical analysis and flow distribution analysis, and observed that the measured flow rates may evolve as the patient ages.

4.3.3 Tetralogy of Fallot: Ventricle Modeling

"How to construct patient-specific ventricle models based on limited information and make reliable assessment of ventricle function is a great challenge to the cardiovascular research community" (Tang et al. 2010). Ventricle modeling and related patient-specific virtual surgery can be a resourceful tool in studying Tetralogy of Fallot, for both surgical planning and optimization. Recent advances in the field involve mechanical ventricle modeling and constructing patient-specific computational ventricle models based on in vivo cardiac MR images.

It has been hypothesized that right ventricle volume reduction and scar tissue trimming in pulmonary valve replacement can improve recovery of the ventricular function. Virtual surgery has been very useful in exploring this hypothesis (Tang et al. 2010). MR data can be used to construct preoperative patient-specific ventricle models. Such models can include both ventricles, scar, patch, anisotropic material properties and fiber orientation. Flow and stress distribution can then be simulated using FSI. Virtual surgery involves adjusting the preoperative morphology (i.e. scar tissue trimming) and the outcome is assessed in terms of ventricle stroke volume and ejection fraction. MR data can then be used to validate the post-operative outcome (Fig. 17).

An example of virtual surgery is shown in Fig. 18. Virtual patch modeling showed that employing a smaller patch resulted in 50% lower stress levels and 40% lower strain levels in comparison to a larger patch. This is a desirable outcome in terms of ventricular function and recovery (Tang et al. 2010).

4.4 Cardiac Resynchronization Therapy

Cardiac resynchronization therapy (CRT) "aims to treat the electrical substrate in symptomatic heart failure patients with reduced LV ejection fraction and wide QRS complex" (Strik et al. 2011). Pooled data from six studies has shown that CRT reduces all-cause mortality by 28% and new hospitalizations for worsening heart failure by 37% (Rossi et al. 2008). Additional insight into the

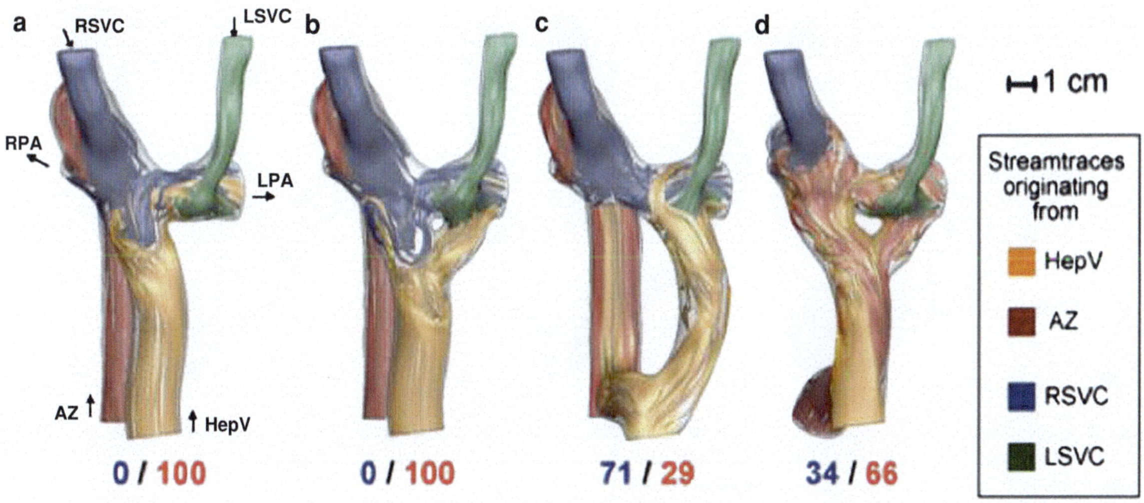

Fig. 16 Flow patterns and hepatic flow distribution for different virtual surgery options in a patient-specific anatomy reconstructed from MR images. The simulated surgical options are an intra-atrial connected opposite to the RSVC (**a**), a Y-graft (**b**), an H-connection using an extracardiac to the LSVC and an hepatic vein-to-azygous shunt (**c**), and an azygous-to-hepatic vein shunt in combination with a Y-graft (**d**). AZ = azygous; HepV = hepatic veins; LPA = left pulmonary artery; RPA = right pulmonary artery; RSVC = right superior vena cava; LSVC = left superior vena cava. The ratios indicate the proportion of hepatic flow traveling to the left and right pulmonary artery. Image from de Zélicourt et al. (2011)

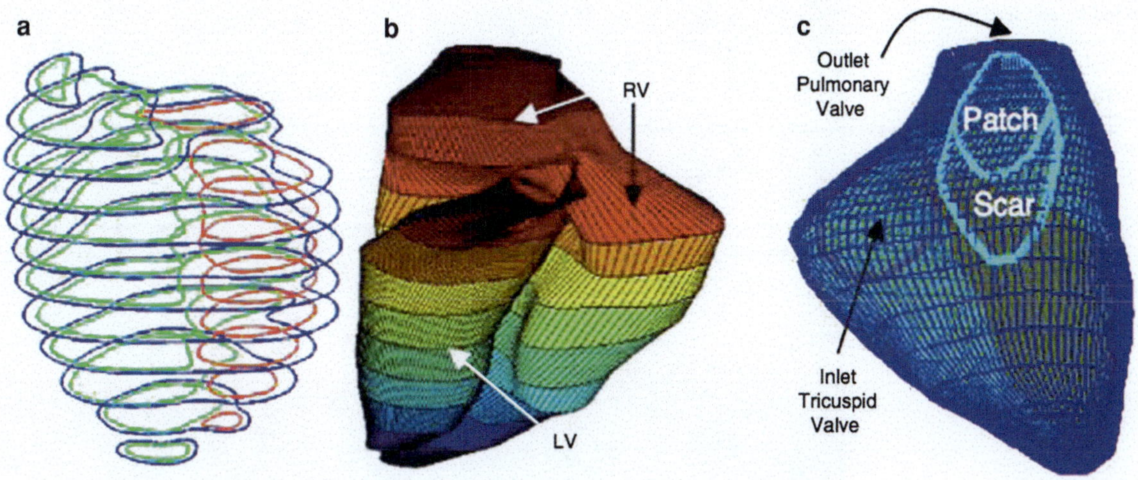

Fig. 17 Example of reconstructed 3D anatomy of right and left ventricle, showing segmented ventricular contours from MR (**a**), ventricular inner surfaces (**b**) and the location of the valves and of the patch (**c**), in the context of ventricle modeling for Tetralogy of Fallot. Image from Tang et al. (2010)

response to CRT can be provided by MR imaging and nuclear imaging, and variables with potential prognostic and therapeutic values include: evaluation of cardiac dyssynchrony, scar, cardiac sympathetic function, myocardial blood flow, myocardial glucose and oxidative metabolism (Aggarwal et al. 2009).

In addition to providing insight into CRT response, cardiac MR images registered with fluoroscopic images during the procedure can also guide CRT device implantation (Duckett et al. 2010). This process allows the operator to place the left ventricular lead while avoiding scar regions, which represents an

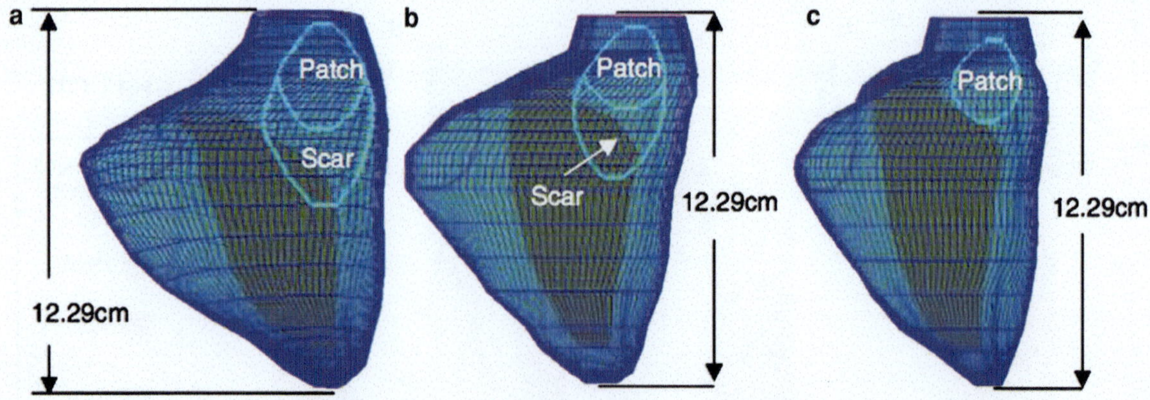

Fig. 18 Example of virtual surgery for Tetralogy of Fallot: pre-operative ventricle model (**a**); patch model with conventional patch and minimum scar tissue trimming (**b**); patch model with smaller patch and more substantial scar tissue trimming (**c**). Image from Tang et al. (2010)

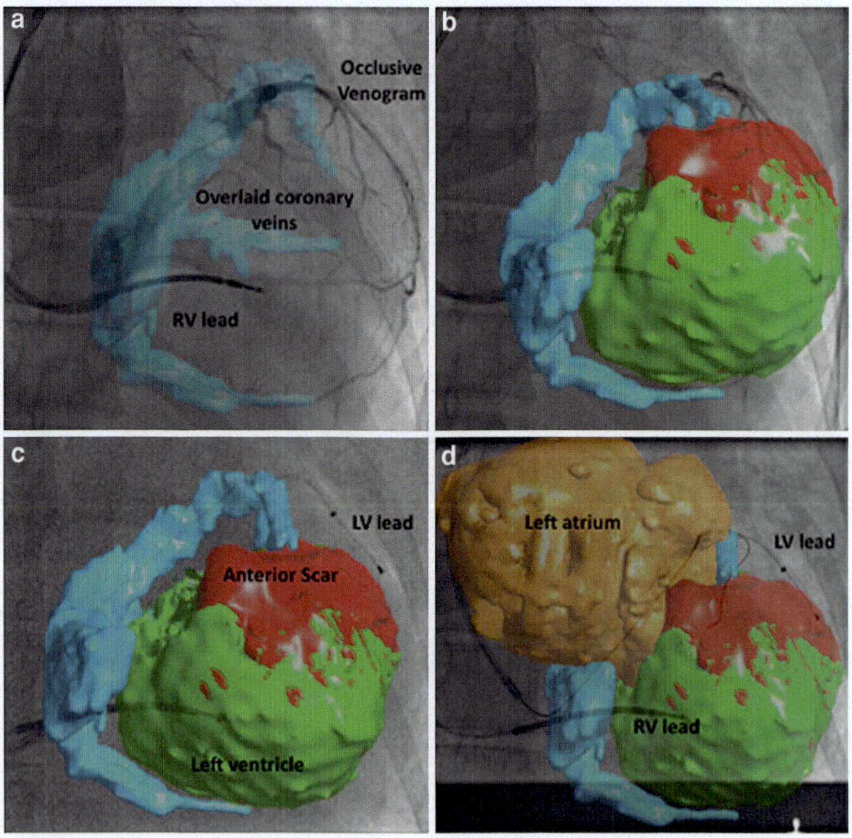

Fig. 19 Superimposition of MR images of whole heart, coronary veins and scar and fluoroscopy image to guide lead implantation in CRT, showing coronary venous anatomy and scar overlaying on the occlusive venogram (**a** and **b**) and lead position with respect to ventricle and scar (**c** and **d**). LV = left ventricle, RV = right ventricle. Image from Duckett et al. (2010)

important advance since the position of the lead affects response to CRT (Fig. 19).

The usefulness of anatomical MR data in this context is also reported in a similar study, in which a detailed cardiac model was generated and registered to the X-ray fluoroscopy for seven patients, resulting in successful left lead implantation in all patients (Ma et al. 2010). In this case:

- Whole heart MR images provided detailed anatomical models, down to the coronary veins;
- Cine MR images provided information on ventricular motion and regions of late activation;

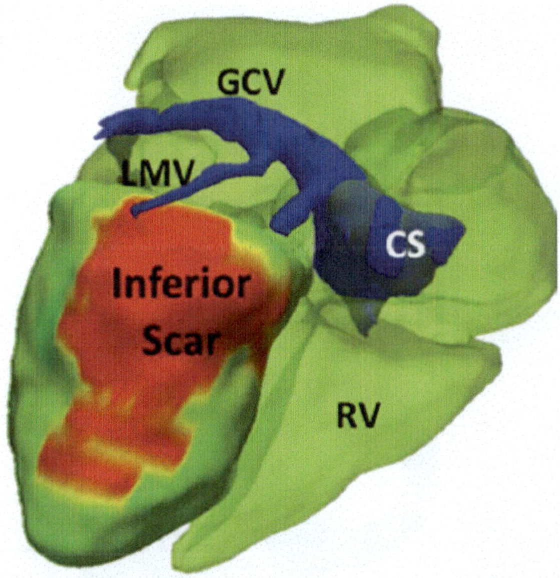

Fig. 20 Segmented whole heart providing clear visualization of coronary venous anatomy and scar identification in CRT. CS = coronary sinus; LMV, left marginal vein; GCV, great cardiac vein; RV, right ventricle. Image from Duckett et al. (2011)

- Late Gadolinium enhancement images highlighted scar regions.

A more recent study from the same group (Duckett et al. 2011) proposed a slow infusion protocol of gadolinium to assess coronary venous anatomy and myocardial scar with MR imaging. Excellent visualization of the coronary venous anatomy was achieved in fourteen CRT patients (an example is shown in Fig. 20). MR veins visualization strongly correlated with venography.

4.5 Virtual Physiological Human

The Virtual Physiological Human (VPH) is a European research network concerned with multidisciplinary research and the integration of models and data across the various relevant levels of physiological structure (www.vph-noe.eu, last accessed June 2011). As part of the cardiac modeling section of VPH, the "Virtual pathological heart of the virtual physiological human" (VPH2) project aims to "develop a patient-specific computational model and simulation of the human heart to assist the cardiologist and the cardiac surgeon in defining the severity and extent of disease in patients with post-ischemic left ventricular dysfunction, with or without ischemic mitral regurgitation" (www.vph-noe.eu/vph-projects, last accessed June 2011). Modeling within this project relies on MR data. The "mitral valve tool", for instance, can both *assess* the biomechanics of a mitral valve based on the geometry recreated from MR images and also *predict* the effect of annuloplasty on the mitral valve (www.vph2.eu, last accessed June 2011).

Another part of VPH, namely "Multi-level patient-specific artery and atherogenesis model for outcome prediction, decision support treatment, and virtual hand-on training" (ARTreat), aims to create a patient-specific computational model of the vascular system in order to improve the prediction of atherosclerosis progression (www.vph-noe.eu/vph-projects, last accessed June 2011). In this case, MR data is used to construct patient-specific representations of the patients' carotid arterial trees (www.artreat.org, last accessed June 2011). High-resolution MR imaging can be employed not only for morphological assessment of atherosclerotic plaques, but also as a source of geometrical data for biomechanical stress analysis. In a recent study on 70 patients, MR-based stress analysis was shown to potentially identify high-risk patients with vulnerable plaques (Sadat et al. 2011). An example of plaque stress analysis is shown in Fig. 21.

5 Discussion

Several examples of the use of MR imaging in cardiac modeling have been proposed, ranging from optimizing surgeries for congenital heart diseases to assessment of a device's mechanical performance. MR can in fact provide both anatomical and functional data, the first essential for recreating a 3D model down to patient-specific accuracy, the second equally important for either imposing boundary conditions or validating results obtained through a simulation or an experiment.

Engineering modeling in the cardiac field can be performed on the bench or virtually. In vitro experiments, computational simulations and virtual surgery are not self-exclusive. On the contrary, it has been underlined that a synergy of in vitro and in silico experiments can be conducive to more thorough and substantial modeling (Morrison et al. 2010), taking advantage of the respective benefits of each modeling

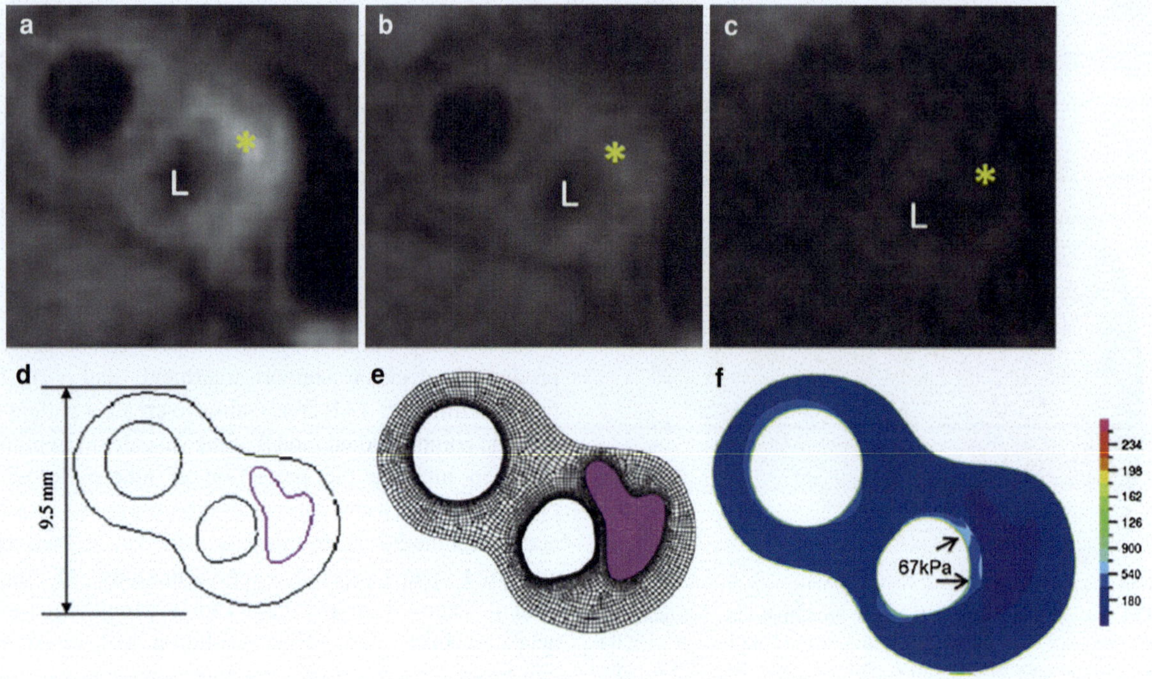

Fig. 21 Example of the use of MR images for stress analysis of atherosclerotic plaques in the carotid artery. Symptomatic plaque at T_1 (**a**), proton density (**b**) and STIR (**c**) weightings. L indicates lumen and the yellow star indicates lipid content. Contours as exported into appropriate software (ADINA 8.6) for biomechanical simulation (**d**). A mesh is generated, identifying the plaque (**e**). Stress distribution in the plaque with maximum critical stress at the vulnerable site (**f**). Image from Sadat et al. (2011)

mode, or using one of the steps as a validation tool (e.g. validating a computational model against data gathered in a mock circulatory system).

With regard to in silico studies, the fundamental importance of setting boundary conditions has been repeated abundantly in the literature. MR data is useful in this regard, as it can provide boundary conditions for a computational model (e.g. setting patient-specific flow values).

Both experimentally and computationally the engineer is bound to simplify the physiological model. As it can also be appreciated from the examples reported in this chapter, there are different levels of assumptions: a model can be patient-specific but there are studies employing simplified geometries; the effect of respiration on blood flow has been simulated in mock loops (Camp et al. 2007) or computationally (Marsden et al. 2009), but is not included in several models; fiber orientation is not included in some ventricular models. The refinement of modeling techniques is leading to a place where, while inevitably some assumptions have to be imposed, more sophisticated simulations are performed and the results are more clinically meaningful. From the experimental point of view, for example, while rigid phantoms have been undeniably valuable as in the case of aiding the interventional cardiologist in identifying the optimal access for a new device implantation (Sect. 4.1.3), rapid prototyping and manufacturing techniques also allow the construction of more realistic compliant models that, albeit still not representing biological properties of blood vessels, can replicate the arterial Windkessel (Biglino et al. 2011a). From the computational point of view, virtual surgery is carried out more and more to patient-specific level, aiming to identify "tailored" solutions, as an optimal universal solution appears to be unlikely, especially for complex surgeries (e.g. Fontan).

With respect to the models themselves, the completeness of a mock circulatory system or the exquisite details of a computational simulation remain a *medium* and do not represent a *goal* in themselves. As appreciated from the examples reported in this chapter, and from several others in the literature, cardiovascular modeling is not an engineering exercise, but a multidisciplinary field of crosstalk between imaging, physiology, surgery, mathematics and mechanics.

6 Conclusion

Magnetic resonance imaging has become an integral part of engineering modeling for cardiac solutions. It provides both the anatomical information necessary to construct a model and the functional data to validate it. At present, MR-based models are used for understanding the fluid mechanics of vessels and valves, investigating complex fluid–solid interactions, testing cardiovascular devices and optimizing surgical practice, with exciting developments especially in the field of virtual surgery. From an engineering point of view, it remains true that "the ideal model will be as simple as possible and as complex as necessary for the particular question raised" (Garny et al. 2005).

7 Key Points

- Cardiovascular modeling is in its infancy, but shows much promise for providing data that is difficult or impossible to measure, or allowing for virtual treatments to be performed and outcomes predicted in a patient-specific way.
- MR imaging is central for data acquisition to build cardiovascular models and for the validation of these models in the long-term.
- Cardiovascular modeling requires a close collaboration between engineers, computer scientists, imagers and clinicians.

Acknowledgments We would like to gratefully acknowledge Fondation Leducq, British Heart Foundation, Royal Academy of Engineering/EPSRC and National Institute for Health Research UK for their support.

References

Aggarwal NR, Martinez MW, Gersh BJ, Chareonthaitawee P (2009) Role of cardiac MRI and nuclear imaging in cardiac resynchronization therapy. Nat Rev Cardiol 6(12):759–770

Arevalo H, Rodriguez B, Trayanova N (2007) Arrhythmogenesis in the heart: multiscale modeling of the effects of defibrillation shocks and the role of electrophysiological heterogeneity. Chaos 17(1):015103

Bagnoli P, Malagutti N, Gastaldi D, Marcelli E, Lui E, Cercenelli L, Costantino ML, Plicchi G, Fumero R (2011) Computational finite element model of cardiac torsion. Int J Artif Organs 34(1):44–53

Biglino G, Kolyva C, Whitehorne M, Pepper JR, Khir AW (2010) Variations in aortic pressure affect the mechanics of the intra-aortic balloon: an in vitro investigation. Artif Organs 34(7):546–553

Biglino G, Schievano S, Baker C, Giardini A, Figliola R, Taylor AM, Hsia TY (2011a) A patient-specific paediatric mock circulatory system: investigating the circulation following the Norwood procedure. ASAIO J–Abstracts of the 57th annual conference 57(2):69–105

Biglino G, Verschueren P, Zegels R, Taylor AM, Schievano S (2011b) Quantification of TangoPlus FullCure 930® compliance for printing patient-specific vascular models. ASAIO J–Abstracts of the 57th annual conference 57(2): 69–105

Bonhoeffer P, Boudjemline Y, Saliba Z, Merckx J, Aggoun Y, Bonnet D, Acar P, Le Bidois J, Sidi D, Kachaner J (2000) Percutaneous replacement of pulmonary valve in a right-ventricle to pulmonary-artery prosthetic conduit with valve dysfunction. Lancet 356(9239):1403–1405

Bonhoeffer P, Huynh R, House M, Douk N, Kopcak M, Hill A, Rafiee N (2008) Transcatheter pulmonic valve replacement in sheep using a grafted self-expanding stent with tissue valve. Circulation 118:S_812

Borazjani I, Sotiropoulos F (2010) The effect of implantation orientation of a bileaflet mechanical heart valve on kinematics and hemodynamics in an anatomic aorta. J Biomech Eng 132(11):111005

Bove EL, de Leval MR, Migliavacca F, Guadagni G, Dubini G (2003) Computational fluid dynamics in the evaluation of hemodynamic performance of cavopulmonary connections after the Norwood procedure for hypoplastic left heart syndrom. J Thorac Cardiovasc Surg 126(4):1040–1047

Bove EL, Migliavacca F, de Leval MR, Balossino R, Pennati G, Lloyd TR, Khambadkone S, Hsia TY, Dubini G (2008) Use of mathematic modeling to compare and predict hemodynamic effects of the modified Blalock-Taussig and right ventricle-pulmonary artery shunts for hypoplastic left heart syndrome. J Thorac Cardiovasc Surg 136(2):312–320

Bowles CT, New SEP, Van Loon R, Dreger SA, Biglino G, Chan C, Parker KH, Chester AH, Yacoub MH, Taylor PM (2010) Hydrodynamic evaluation of a bioreactor for tissue engineering heart valves. Cardiovascular Eng Technol 1(1):10–17

Bowles CT, Shah SS, Nishimura K, Clark C, Cumming DV, Pattison CW, Pepper JR, Yacoub MH (1991) Development of mock circulation models for the assessment of counter-pulsation systems. Cardiovasc Res 25(11):901–908

Breinholt JP, Nugent AW, Law MA, Justino H, Mullins CE, Ing FF (2008) Stent fractures in congenital heart disease. Catheter Cardiovasc Interv 72(7):977–982

Buonocore MH, Bogren HG (1999) Analysis of flow patterns using MRI. Int J Card Imaging 15(2):99–103

Burkart DJ, Felmlee JP, Johnson CD, Wolf RL, Weaver AL, Ehman RL (1994) Cine phase-contrast MR flow measurements: improved precision using an automated method of vessel detection. J Comput Assist Tomogr 18(3):469–475

Camp TA, Stewart KC, Figliola RS, McQuinn T (2007) In vitro study of flow regulation for pulmonary insufficiency. J Biomech Eng 129(2):284–288

Camus JM, Campomar G, D'Attellis C, Silvestrini M, Varela L, De Forteza E (2007) In vitro evaluation of an axial flow pump: mock-pump interaction and an approach to control. Int J Artif Organs 30(1):34–43

Capelli C, Nordmeyer J, Schievano S, Lurz P, Khambadkone S, Lattanzio S, Taylor AM, Petrini L, Migliavacca F, Bonhoeffer P (2010a) How do angioplasty balloons work: a computational study on balloon expansion forces. EuroIntervention 6(5):638–642

Capelli C, Taylor AM, Migliavacca F, Bonhoeffer P, Schievano S (2010b) Patient-specific reconstructed anatomies and computer simulations are fundamental for selecting medical device treatment: application to a new percutaneous pulmonary valve. Philos Transact A Math Phys Eng Sci 368(1921): 3027–3038

Cebral JR, Mut F, Weir J, Putman C (2011) Quantitative characterisation of the hemodynamic environment in ruptured and unruptured brain aneurysms. AJNR Am J Neuroradiol 32(1):145–151

Chaichana T, Sun Z, Jewkes J (2011) Computation of hemodynamics in the left coronary artery with variable angulations. J Biomech [Epub ahead of print]

Chapman SJ (2009) Multiscale mathematical modelling in medicine and biology. Proceedings of the 18th world IMACS/MODSIM congress, Cairns, Australia, 13–17th July, pp 13–22

Chen HY, Zhu L, Huo Y, Liu Y, Kassab GS (2010) Fluid-structure interaction (FSI) modeling in the cardiovascular system. In: Computational cardiovascular mechanics – Modeling and application in heart failure. Eds. Guccione JM, Kassab GS, Ratcliffe MB. Springer, New York, USA

Chiulli JA, Conover T, Xue Z, Zhao Y, Hsia TY, Figliola RS (2012) An in vitro multi-scale model of the Fontan circulation with respiration effects. J Biomech Eng (in press)

Coats L, Khambadkone S, Derrick G, Sridharan S, Schievano S, Mist B, Jones R, Deanfield JE, Pellerin D, Bonhoeffer P, Taylor AM (2006) Physiological and clinical consequences of relief of right ventricular outflow tract obstruction late after repair of congenital heart defects. Circulation 113(17): 2037–2044

Cook RD, Malkus DS, Plesha Witt RJ (2002) Concepts and applications of finite element analysis. 4th edition. Wiley, New York

Corsini C, Cosentino D, Pennati G, Dubini G, Hsia T-Y, Migliavacca F (2011) Multiscale models of the hybdrid palliation for hypoplastic left heart syndrome. J Biomech 44(4):767–770

Cunningham KS, Gotlieb AI (2005) The role of shear stress in the pathogenesis of atherosclerosis. Lab Invest 85(1): 9–23

De Paulis R, Schmitz C, Scaffa R, Nardi P, Chiariello L, Reul H (2005) In vitro evaluation of aortic valve prosthesis in a novel valved conduit with pseudosinuses of Valsalva. J Thorac Cardiovasc Surg 130(4):1016–1021

de Tullio MD, Afferrante L, Demelio G, Pascazio G, Verzicco R (2011a) Fluid-structure interaction of deformable aortic prostheses with a bileaflet mecanical valve. J Biomech 44(9): 1684–1690

de Tullio MD, Pascazio G, Weltert L, De Paulis R, Verzicco R (2011b) Evaluation of prosthetic-valved devices by means of numerical simulations. Philos Transact A Math Phys Eng Sci 369(1945):2502–2509

de Zélicourt DA, Haggerty CM, Sundareswaran KS, Whited BS, Rossignac JR, Kanter KR, Gaynor JW, Spray TL, Sotiropoulos F, Fogel MA, Yoganathan AP (2011) Individualized computer-based surgical planning to address pulmonary arteriovenous malformations in patients with a single ventricle with an interrupted inferior vena cava and azygous continuation. J Thorac Cardiovasc Surg 141(5):1170–1177

de Zélicourt DA, Pekkan K, Wills L, Kanter K, Forbess J, Sharma S, Fogel M, Yoganathan AP (2005) In vitro flow analysis of a patient-specific intraatrial total cavopulmonary connection. Ann Thorac Surg 79(6):2094–2102

Douglas WI, Goldberg CS, Mosca RS, Law IH, Bove EL (1999) Hemi-Fontan procedure for hypoplastic left heart syndrome: outcome and suitability for Fontan. Ann Thorac Surg 68(4):1361–1367

Duckett SG, Chiribiri A, Ginks MR, Sinclair S, Knowles BR, Botnar R, Carr-White GS, Rinaldi CA, Nagel E, Razavi R, Schaeffter T (2011) Cardiac MRI to investigate myocardial scar and coronary venous anatomy using a slow infusion of dimeglumine gadobenate in patients undergoing assessment for cardiac resynchronization therapy. J Magn Reson Imaging 33(1):87–95

Duckett SG, Ginks M, Knowles BR, Chiribiri A, Ma YL, Razavi R, Schaeffter T, Carr-White G, Rinaldi CA, Rhode K (2010) A novel cardiac MRI protocol to guide successful cardiac resynchronization therapy implantation. Circ Heart Fail 3(4):e18–e21

Dumont K, Yperman J, Verbeken E, Segers P, Meuris B, Vandenberghe S, Flameng W, Verdonck PR (2002) Design of a new pulsatile bioreactor for tissue engineered aortic heart valve formation. Artif Organs 26(8):710–714

Einstein DR, Del Pin F, Jiao X, Kuprat AP, Carson JP, Kunzelman KS, Cochran RP, Guccione JM, Ratcliffe MB (2010) Fluid-structure interactions of the mitral valve and left heart: comprehensive strategies, past, present and future. Int J Numer Methods Eng 26(3–4):348–380

Ensley AE, Lynch P, Chatzimavroudis GP, Lucas C, Sharma S, Yoganathan AP (1999) Toward designing the optimal total cavopulmonary connection: an in vitro study. Ann Thorac Surg 68(4):1384–1390

Filipovic N, Schima H (2011) Numerical simulation of the flow field within the aortic arch during cardiac assist. Artif Organs 35(4):E73–E83

Firmin DN, Nayler GL, Klipstein RH, Underwood SR, Rees RS, Longmore DB (1987) In vivo validation of MR velocity imaging. J Comput Assist Tomogr 11(5):751–756

Fontan F, Baudet E (1971) Surgical repair of tricuspid atresia. Thorax 26(3):240–248

Formaggia L, Nobile F, Quarteroni A, Veneziani A (1999) Multiscale modelling of the vascular system: a preliminary analysis. Comp Visc Sci 2:75–83

Frank O (1899) Die Grundform des arteriellen Pulses. Zeitschrift fur Biologie 27:483–526

Fries R, Graeter T, Aicher D, Reul H, Schmitz C, Böhm M, Schäfers HJ (2006) In vitro comparison of aortic valve movement after valve-preserving aortic replacement. J Thorac Cardiovasc Surg 132(1):32–37

Galantowicz M, Cheatham JP (2005) Lessons learned from the development of a new hybrid strategy for the management of hypoplastic left heart syndrome. Pediatr Cardiol 26(3): 190–199

Gao H, Long Q, Graves M, Gillard JH, Li ZY (2009) Carotid arterial plaque stress analysis using fluid-structure interactive simulation based on in vivo magnetic resonance images of four patients. J Biomech 42(10):1416–1423

Garny A, Noble D, Kohl P (2005) Dimensionality in cardiac modeling. Prog Biophys Mol Biol 87(1):47–66

Gohean J, Figliola R, Camp T, McQuinn T (2006) Comparative in vitro study of bileaflet and tilting disk valve behaviour in the pulmonanry position. J Biomech Eng 128(4):631–635

Guccione JM, Walker JC, Beitler JR, Moonly SM, Zhang P, Guttman MA, Ozturk C, McVeigh ER, Wallace AW, Saloner DA, Ratcliffe MB (2006) The effect of anteroapical aneurysm plication on end-systolic three-dimensional strain in the sheep: a magnetic resonance imaging tagging study. J Thorac Cardiovasc Surg 131(3):579–586

Hales S (1733) Statistical Essays: Containing Haemostatics, vol II. Innys and Manby, London, UK

Hanson BM, Levesley MC, Watterson K, Walker PG (2007) Hardware-in-the-loop simulation of the cardiovascular system, with assist device testing application. Med Eng Phys 29(3):367–374

Hasenkam JM, Pedersen EM, Ostergaard JH, Nygaard H, Paulsen PK, Johannsen G, Schurizek BA (1988) Velocity fields and turbulent stresses downstream of biological and mechanical aortic valve prostheses implanted in pigs. Cardiovasc Res 22(7):472–483

Hopkins RA, Armstrong BE, Serwer GA, Peterson RJ, Oldham HN Jr (1985) Physiological rationale for a bidirectional cavopulmonary shunt A versatile complement to the Fontan principle. J Thorac Cardiovasc Surg 90(3):391–398

Hsia TY, Migliavacca F, Pennati G, Balossino R, Dubini G, de Leval MR, Bradley SM, Bove EL (2009) Management of a stenotic right ventricle-pulmonary shunt early after the Norwood procedure. Ann Thorac Surg 88(3):830–837

http://kheradvar.eng.uci.edu/research.php, last accessed May 2011

Jahanmir S, Hunsberger AZ, Ren Z, Heshmat H, Heshmat C, Tomaszewski MJ, Walton JF (2009) Design of a small centrifugal blood pump with magnetic bearings. Artif Organs 33(9):714–726

Jimenez JH, Soerensen DD, He Z, Ritchie J, Yoganathan AP (2005) Mitral valve function and chordal force distribution using a flexible annulus model: an in vitro study. Ann Biomed Eng 33(5):557–566

Kaminsky R, Kallweit S, Weber HJ, Claessens T, Jozwik K, Verdonck P (2007) Flow visualization through two types of aortic prosthetic heart valves using stereoscopic high-speed particle image velocimetry. Artif Organs 31(12):869–879

Khambadkone S, Coats L, Taylor A, Boudjemline Y, Derrick G, Tsang V, Cooper J, Muthurangu V, Hedge SR, Razavi RS, Pellerin D, Deanfield J, Bonhoeffer P (2005) Percutaneous pulmonary valve implantation in humans: results in 59 consecutive patients. Circulation 112(8):1189–1197

Kitajima HD, Sundareswaran KS, Teissevre TZ, Astary GW, Parks WJ, Skrinjar O, Oshinski JN, Yoganathan AP (2008) Comparison of particle image velocimetry and phase contrast MRI in patient-specific extracardiac total cavopulmonary connection. J Biomech Eng 130(4):041004

Kolyva C, Biglino G, Pepper JR, Khir AW (2010) A mock circulatory system with physiological distribution of terminal resistance and compliance: application for testing the intra-aortic balloon pump. Artif Organs doi: 10.1111/j.1525-1594.2010.01071.x. [Epub ahead of print]

Kozerke S, Botnar R, Oyre S, Scheidegger MB, Pedersen EM, Boesiger P (1999) Automatic vessel segmentation using active contours in cine phase contrast flow measurements. J Magn Reson Imaging 10(1):41–51

Krabill KA, Sung HW, Tamura T, Chung KJ, Yoganathan Ap, Sahn DJ (1989) Factors influencing the structure and shape of stenotic and regurgitant jets: an in vitro investigation using Doppler color flow mappaing and optical flow visualization. J Am Coll Cardiol 13(7):1672–1681

Kuehnel RU, Puchner R, Pohl A, Wendt MO, Hartrumpf M, Pohl M, Albes JM (2005) Characteristic resistance curves of aortic valve substitutes facilitate individualized decision for a particular type. Eur J Cardiothorac Surg 27(3):450–455

Kumar GP, Mathew L (2011) Stent biomaterial and design selection using finite element analysis for percutaneous aortic valve replacement. Artif Organs 35(2):166–175

Kunzelman KS, Cochran RP, Chuong C, Ring WS, Verrier ED, Eberhart RD (1993) Finite element analysis of the mitral valve. J Heart Valve Dis 2(3):326–340

Ladisa JF, Taylor CA, Feinstein JA (2010) Aortic coarctation: recent developments in experimental and computational methods to assess treatments for this simple condition. Prog Pediatr Cardiol 30(1):45–49

Laganà K, Balossino R, Migliavacca F, Pennati G, Bove EL, de Leval MR, Dubini G (2005) Multiscale modeling of the cardiovascular system: application to the study of pulmonary and coronary perfusions in the univentricular circulation. J Biomech 38(5):1129–1141

Laoui T, Shaik SK (2003) Rapid prototyping techniques used to produce medical models/implants. In: Proceedings of teh 4th international conference on rapid prototyping and virtual prototyping and applications. Centre for rapid design and manufacture, Buckinghamshire Chilterns University College, UK, pp 23–32 June 20

Larsson HB, Stubgaard M, Søndergaard L, Henriksen O (1994) In vivo quantification of the unidirectional influx constant for Gd-DTPA diffusion across the myocardial capillaries with MR imaging. J Magn Reson Imaging 4(3):433–440

Larsson HB, Fritz-Hansen T, Rostrup E, Søndergaard L, Ring P, Henriksen O (1996) Myocardial perfusion modeling using MRI. Magn Reson Med 35(5):716–726

Lau KD, Diaz V, Scambler P, Burriesci G (2010) Mitral valve dynamics in structural and fluid-structure interaction models. Med Eng Phys 32(9):1057–1064

Leuprecht A, Kozerke S, Boesiger P, Perktold K (2003) Blood flow in the human ascending aorta: a combined MRI and CFD study. J Eng Math 47:387–404

Liang F, Takagi S, Himeno R, Liu H (2009) Multi-scale modeling of the human cardiovascular system with applications to aortic valvular and arterial stenoses. Med Biol Eng Comput 47(7):743–755

Lim HB, Hur G, Kim SY, Kim YH, Kwon SU, Lee WR, Cha SJ (2008) Coronary stent fracture: detection with 64-section

multidetector CT angiography in patients and in vitro. Radiology 249(3):810–819
Lotz J, Döker R, Noeske R, Schüttert M, Felix R, Galanski M, Gutberlet M, Meyer GP (2005) In vitro validation of phase-contrast flow measurements at 3 T in comparison to 1.5 T: precision, accuracy, and signal-to-noise ratios. J Magn Reson Imaging 21(5):604–610
Lotz J, Meier C, Leppert A, Galanski M (2002) Cardiovascular flow measurement with phase-contrast MR imaging: basic facts and implementation. Radiographics 22(3):651–671
Lurz P, Coats L, Khambadkone S, Nordmeyer J, Boudjemline Y, Schievano S, Muthurangu V, Lee TY, Parenzan G, Derrick G, Cullen S, Walker F, Tsang V, Deanfield JE, Taylor AM, Bonhoeffer P (2008) Percutaneous pulmonary valve implantation: impact of evolving technology and learning curve on clinical outcome. Circulation 117(15):1964–1972
Ma YL, Duckett S, Chinchapatnam P, Shetty A, Rinaldi CA, Schaeffter T, Rhode KS (2010) Image and physiological data fusion for guidance and modelling of cardiac resynchronization therapy procedure. In: STACOM'10/CESC'10 Proceedings of the first international conference on statistical atlases and computational models of the heart, and international conference on cardiac electrophysiological simulation challenge, Camara O, Pop M, Rhode K, Sermesant M, Smith N (eds), Springer Berlin, Heidelberg
Mansi T, André B, Lynch M, Sermesant M, Delingettes H, Boudjemline Y, Ayache N (2009) Virtual pulmonary valve replacement interventions with a personalised cardiac electromechanical model. In: Recent advances in the 3D physiological human, Eds. Magnenat-Thalmann N, Zhang JJ, Feng DD. Springer, London, UK
Marsden AL, Bernstein AJ, Reddy VM, Shadden SC, Spilker RL, Chan FP, Taylor CA, Feinstein JA (2009) Evaluation of a novel Y-shaped extracardiac Fontan baffle using computational fluid dynamics. J Thorac Cardiovasc Surg 137(2): 394–403
Matthews PB, Jhun CS, Yaung S, Azadani AN, Guccione JM, Ge L, Tseng EE (2011) Finite element modelling of the pulmonary autograft at systemic pressure before remodelling. J Heart Valve Dis 20(1):45–52
Matthys KS, Alastruey J, Peiró J, Khir AW, Segers P, Verdonck PR, Parker KH, Sherwin SJ (2007) Pulse wave propagation in a model human arterial network: assessment of 1-D numerical simulations against in vitro measurements. J Biomech 40(15):3476–3486
Medvitz RB, Kreider JW, Manning KB, Fontaine AA, Deutsch S, Paterson EG (2007) Development and validation of a computational fluid dynamics methodology for simulation of pulsatile left ventricular assist devices. ASAIO J 53(2):122–131
Medvitz RB, Reddy V, Deutsch S, Manning KB, Paterson EG (2009) Validation of a CFD methodology for positive displacement LVAD analysis using PIV data. J Biomech Eng 131(11):111009
Moran PR (1982) A flow velocity zeugmatographic interlace for NMR imaging in humans. Magn Reson Imaging 1(4):197–203
Morrison T, Dreher M, Ibrahim N, Nagaraja S, Takai E, Wu C (2010) Computational modelling in device submissions: where we are and where we want to go. Workshop on computer methods for cardiovascular devices, Washington D.C., USA, June 10–11
Nakatani T, Anai H, Araki K, Wakisaka Y, Taenaka Y, Tatsumi E, Akagi H, Masuzawa T, Baba Y, Eya K, Toda K, Takano H (1994) In vitro and in vivo assessment of an intravenous axial flow pump for right heart assist. ASAIO J 40(3):M723–M727
Napel S, Lee DH, Frayne R, Rutt BK (1992) Visualizing three-dimensional flow with simulated streamlines and three-dimensional phase-contrast MR imaging. J Magn Reson Imaging 2(2):143–153
National Research Council (1985) A new perspective. Committee on models for biomedical research. Board on basic biology. Commission on life sciences. National Academy Press, Washington
Nordmeyer J, Khambadkone S, Coats L, Schievano S, Lurz P, Parenzan G, Taylor AM, Lock JE, Bonhoeffer P (2007) Risk stratification, systematic classification, and anticipatory management strategies for stent fracture after percutaneous pulmonary valve implantation. Circulation 115(11):1392–1397
Norwood WI Jr (1991) Hypoplastic left heart syndrome. Ann Thorac Surg 52(3):688–695
O'Rourke MJ, McCullough JP (2010) An investigation of the flow field withing patient-specific models of an abdominal aortic aneurysm under steady inflow conditions. Proc Inst Mech Eng H 224(8):971–988
Odille F, Steeden JA, Muthurangu V, Atkinson D (2011) Automatic segmentation propagation of the aorta in real-time phase contrast MRI using nonrigid registration. J Magn Reson Imaging 33(1):232–238
Okano T, Yamagishi M, Shuntoh K, Yamada Y, Hayashida K, Shinkawa T, Kitamura N (2002) Extracardiac total cavopulmonary connection using a Y-shaped graft. Ann Thorac Surg 74(6):2195–2197
Pantalos GM, Ionan C, Koenig SC, Gillars KJ, Horrell T, Sahetya S, Colyer J, Gray LA Jr (2010) Expanded pediatric cardiovascular simulator for research and training. ASAIO J 56(1):67–72
Papaioannou TG, Mathioulakis DS, Stamatelopoulos KS, Gialafos EJ, Lekakis JP, Nanas J, Stamatelopoulos SF, Tsangaris SG (2004) New aspects of the role of blood pressure and arterial stiffness in mechanical assistance by intra-aortic balloon pump: in vitro data and their application in clinical practice. Artif Organs 28(8):717–727
Perktold K, Resch M, Peter RO (1991) Three-dimensional numerical analysis of pulsatile flow and wall shear stress in the carotid artery bifurcation. J Biomech 24(6):409–420
Prot V, Haaverstad R, Skallerud B (2009) Finite element analysis of the mitral apparatus: annulus shape effect and chordal force distribution. Biomech Model Mechanobiol 8(1):43–55
Qian Y, Liu JL, Itatani K, Miyaji K, Umezu M (2010) Computational hemodynamic analysis in congenital heart disease: simulation of the Norwood procedure. Ann Biomed Eng 38(7):2302–2313
Quarteroni A, Veneziani A (2003) Analysis of a geometrical multiscale model based on the coupling of PDE's and ODE's for blood flow simulations. Multiscale Model Simul: a SIAM Interdiscip J 1(2):173–195
Raffel M, Willert CE, Wereley ST, Kompenhans J (2007) Particle image velocimetry: a practical guide. 2nd edition. Springer, New York, USA
Ransom R (1981) Computers and embryos: models in developmental biology. John Wiley and sons, New York

Rits J, van Herwaarden JA, Jahrome AK, Krievins D, Moll FL (2008) The incidence of arterial stent fractures with exclusion of coronary, aortic, and non-arterial settings. Eur J Vasc Endovasc Surg 36(3):339–345
Rossi A, Rossi G, Piacenti M, Startari U, Panchetti L, Morales MA (2008) The current role of cardiac resynchronization therapy in reducing mortality and hospitalization in heart failure patients: a meta-analysis from clinical trials. Heart Vessels 23(4):217–223
Sadat U, Teng Z, Young VE, Graves MJ, Gaunt ME, Gillard JH (2011) High-resolution magnetic resonance imaging-based biomechanical stress analysis of carotid atheroma: a comparison of single transient ischaemic attack, recurrent transient ischaemic attacks, non-disabling stroke and asymptomatic patient groups. Eur J Vasc Endovasc Surg 41(1):83–90
Saleh RS, Lohan DG, Nael K, Grover-McKay M, Finn P (2007) Cardiovascular MRI at 3T. Appl Radiol 36(11):10–26
Sano S, Ishino K, Kawada M, Arai S, Kasahara S, Asai T, Masuda Z, Takeuchi M, Ohtsuki S (2003) Right ventricle-pulmonary artery shunt in first-stage palliation of hypoplastic left heart syndrome. J Thorac Cardiovasc Surg 126(2): 504–509
Satcher RL Jr, Bussolari SR, Gimbrone MA Jr, Dewey CF Jr (1992) The distribution of fluid forces on model arterial endothelium using computational fluid dynamics. J Biomech Eng 114(3):309–316
Scharfschwerdt M, Thomschke M, Sievers HH (2009) In vitro localization of initial flow-induced thrombus formation in bileaflet mechanical heart valves. ASAIO J 55(1):19–23
Schenkel T, Malve M, Reik M, Markl M, Jung B, Oertel H (2009) MRI-based CFD analysis of flow in a human left ventricle: methodology and application to a healthy heart. Ann Biomed Eng 37(3):503–515
Schievano S, Migliavacca F, Coats L, Khambadkone S, Carminati M, Wilson N, Deanfield JE, Bonhoeffer P, Taylor AM (2007a) Percutaneous pulmonary valve implantation based on rapid prototyping of right ventricular outflow tract and pulmonary trunk from MR data. Radiology 242(2): 490–497
Schievano S, Coats L, Migliavacca F, Norman W, Frigiola A, Deanfield J, Bonhoeffer P, Taylor AM (2007b) Variations in right ventricular outflow tract morphology following repair of congenital heart disease: implications for percutaneous pulmonary valve implantation. J Cardiovasc Magn Reson 9(4):687–695
Schievano S, Petrini L, Migliavacca F, Coats L, Nordmeyer J, Lurz P, Khambadkone S, Taylor AM, Dubini G, Bonhoeffer P (2007c) Finite element analysis of stent deployment: understanding stent fracture in percutaneous pulmonary valve implantation. J Interv Cardiol 20(6):546–554
Schievano S, Taylor AM, Capelli C, Coats L, Walker F, Lurz P, Nordmeyer J, Wright S, Khambadkone S, Tsang V, Carminati M, Bonhoeffer P (2010a) First-in-man implantation of a novel percutaneous valve: a new approach to medical device development. EuroIntervention 5(6): 745–750
Schievano S, Taylor AM, Capelli C, Lurz P, Nordmeyer J, Migliavacca F, Bonhoeffer P (2010b) Patient specific finite element analysis results in more accurate prediction of stent fractures: application to percutaneous pulmonary valve implantation. J Biomech 43(4):687–693
Segers P, Dubois F, De Wachter D, Verdonck P (1998) Role and relevancy of a cardiovascular simulator. Cardiovasc Eng 3(1):48–56
Selvarasu NK, Tafti DK, Vlachos PP (2011) Hydrodynamic effects of compliance mismatch in stented arteries. J Biomech Eng 133(2):021008
Shah MJ, Rychik J, Fogel MA, Murphy JD, Jacobs ML (1997) Pulmonary AV malformations after superior cavopulmonary connection: resolution after inclusion of hepatic veins in the pulmonary circulation. Ann Thorac Surg 63(4): 960–963
Simon HA, Ge L, Sotiropoulos F, Yoganathan AP (2010) Numerical investigation of the performance of three hinge designs of bileaflet mechanical heart valves. Ann Biomed Eng 38(11):3295–3310
Skalak R (1972) Synthesis of a complete circulation. In: Bergel D.H. Cardiovascular fluid dynamics, Vol 2. Academic Press, USA, pp 341–376
Stevanella M, Votta E, Lemma M, Antona C, Redaelli A (2010) Finite element modelling of the tricuspid valve: a preliminary study. Med Eng Phys 32(10):1213–1223
Strik M, Ploux S, Vernooy K, Prinzen FW (2011) Cardiac resynchronization therapy. Circ J 75(6):1297–1304
Takami Y (2006) In vitro study to estimate particle release from a centrifugal blood pump. Artif Organs 30(5):371–376
Tang D, Yang C, Geva T, Del Nido PJ (2010) Image-based patient-specific ventricle models with fluid-structure interaction for cardiac function assessment and surgical design optimization. Prog Pediatr Cardiol 30(1–2):51–62
Taylor CA, Draney MT, Ku JP, Parker D, Steele BN, Wang K, Zarins CK (1999) Predictive medicine: computational techniques in therapeutic decision-making. Comput Aided Surg 4(5):231–247
Teng Z, Sadat U, Ji G, Zhu C, Young VE, Graves MJ, Gillard JH (2011) Lumen irregularity dominates the relationship between mechanical stress condition, fibrou-cap thickness, and lumen curvature in carotid atherosclerotic plaque. J Biomech Eng 133(3):034501
Timms DL, Gregory SD, Greatrex NA, Pearcy MJ, Fraser JF, Steinseifer U (2011) A compact mock circulation loop for the in vitro testing of cardiovascular devices. Artif Organs 35(4):384–391
van de Vosse FN, de Hart J, van Oijen CHGA, Bessems D, Gunther TWM, Segal A, Wolters BJBM, Stijnen JMA, Baaijens FPT (2003) Finite-element-based computational methods for cardiovascular fluid-structure interaction. J Eng Math 47(3–4):335–368
Vermeulen M, Kaminsky R, Van Der Smissen B, Claessens T, Segers P, Verdonck P, Van Ransbeeck P (2009) In vitro flow modelling for mitral valve leakage quantification. 8th international symposium on particle image velocimetry. Merbourne, Victoria, Australia, August 25–28
Vismara R, Laganà K, Migliavacca F, Schievano S, Coats L, Taylor A, Bonhoeffer P (2009) Experimental setup to evaluate the performance of percutaneous pulmonary valved stent in different outflow tract morphologies. Artif Organs 33(1):46–53
Weinberg EJ, Shahmirzadi D, Mofrad MR (2010) On the multiscale modeling of heart valve biomechanics in health and disease. Biomech Model Mechanobiol 9(4): 373–387

Wenk JF, Zhang Z, Cheng G, Malhotra D, Acevedo-Bolton G, Burger M, Suzuki T, Saloner DA, Wallace AW, Guccione JM, Ratcliffe MB (2010) First finite element model of the left ventricle with mitral valve: insights into ischemic mitral regurgitation. Ann Thorac Surg 89(5):1546–1553

Westerhof N, Lankhaar JW, Westerhof BE (2009) The arterial Windkessel. Med Biol Eng Comput 47(2):131–141

Westwood JD (ed) (2007) Medicine meets virtual reality 15 – in vivo, in vitro, in silico: designing the next medicine. IOS press, Amsterdam, Netherlands

Woo YR, Yoganathan AP (1985) In vitro pulsatile flow velocity and turbulent shear stress measurements in the vicinity of mechanical aortic heart valve prostheses. Life Support Syst 3(4):283–312

Yang W, Feinstein JA, Marsden AL (2010) Constrained optimization of an idealized Y-shaped baffle for the Fontan surgery at rest and exercise. Comput Methods Appl Mech Eng 199(33–36):2135–2149

Zannoli R, Corazza I, Branzi A (2009) Mechanical simulator of the cardiovascular system. Phys Med 25(2):94–100

General Conclusions

J. Bogaert, S. Dymarkowski, A. M. Taylor, and V. Muthurangu

Contents

1 Standardized Protocols for Cardiovascular MRI Including Structured Reporting 695

2 Recommendations for Training and Accreditation in Cardiovascular MRI 696

3 Appropriateness Criteria for Cardiovascular Magnetic Resonance 697

4 General Key Points 699

References 700

J. Bogaert (✉) · S. Dymarkowski
Department of Radiology and Medical Imaging Research Center (MIRC), University Hospitals Gasthuisberg, Catholic University of Leuven, Herestraat 49, 3000 Leuven, Belgium
e-mail: jan.bogaert@uzleuven.be

A. M. Taylor · V. Muthurangu
Centre for Cardiovascular Imaging, UCL Institute of Cardiovascular Science and Great Ormond Street Hospital for Children, London, UK

Abstract

Since 2004 when the first edition of this textbook was published, there have been no 'major' leaps in the field on cardiovascular MRI. This is in contrast to the previous decade with for example the advent of the contrast-enhanced delayed/late enhancement imaging technique, which provided a paradigm shift in the assessment of cardiac diseases. However, over the last decade, cardiovascular MRI has matured and become an established rather than an emerging technique in many areas of cardiovascular imaging. To some extent this has shifted the focus from exploring the potential of MRI to unravel and understand cardiac diseases towards determining standardized protocols for cardiovascular MRI including structured reporting, defining appropriateness criteria, as well as recommendations for training and accreditation in the field. In this concluding chapter, these issues will be emphasized.

1 Standardized Protocols for Cardiovascular MRI Including Structured Reporting

Standardized protocols with structured reporting in cardiovascular MRI are crucial to achieve the highest possible output of a cardiac MRI study, to harmonize studies between centres as well as between imaging modalities. In several chapters of this textbook, we provided practical study protocols with standard and optional MRI sequences as well as a list of key points that cardiac imagers can use as guides in daily clinical

J. Bogaert et al. (eds.), *Clinical Cardiac MRI*, Medical Radiology. Diagnostic Imaging,
DOI: 10.1007/174_2011_397,

routine. In addition, we would like to refer to two review papers recommended by the society for cardiovascular magnetic resonance (SCMR) providing standardized protocols for cardiovascular magnetic resonance imaging (Kramer et al. 2008) and a practical framework for reporting the results of these kinds of examinations (Hundley et al. 2009). Both papers provide a brief, but well-structured overview of the requirements for cardiovascular MRI, including stress and safety equipment, general and disease-specific protocols, as well as the essential components that should be mentioned in the final report, which are based on previously published guidelines from professional societies (ACC/AHA/ACR and others) (Douglas et al. 2009; Hendel et al. 2009). Besides these 'official' papers, several optimized, comprehensive approaches for studying different cardiac diseases have been presented and are discussed elsewhere in this textbook (e.g., see, "Ischemic Heart Disease").

2 Recommendations for Training and Accreditation in Cardiovascular MRI

Besides the need for defining standards for data acquisition and reporting, there is a drive to set standards for training and accreditation in cardiovascular MRI. Because cardio-(vascular) MRI has become a part of daily routine, there is a growing interest amongst cardiologists/radiologists in training as well as board-certified cardiologists/radiologists to get trained in cardio-(vascular) MRI and complementary techniques, such as cardiac CT. Initiatives endorsed by the SCMR (Pohost et al. 2008), the European society of cardiology (ESC) (http://www.escardio.org/education/coresyllabus/Documents/esc-core-curriculum.pdf), by the working group on cardiovascular magnetic resonance of the European society of cardiology (Plein et al. 2011), and the ACCF 2008 Training statement on multimodality noninvasive cardiovascular imaging by the American college of cardiology foundation (ACCF)/American heart association (AHA)/American college of physician (ACP) Task force on clinical competence and training (Thomas et al. 2008) nowadays provide recommendations for training of individuals wishing to perform and report cardiovascular MRI studies ('Individual Certification') as well as for the accredition of centres performing these studies and wishing to offer training in cardiovascular MRI ('Institutional Certification'). Individual certification of competency in cardiovascular MRI can be obtained at 3 levels (Table 1):

Level 1 competency is the most basic level and reflects core cardiovascular MRI training that should be obtained and by all cardiology/radiology trainees. This level provides basic background knowledge in cardiovascular MRI, sufficient to select the appropriate cardiovascular MRI indications for patients with known or suspected cardiovascular diseases and to interpret these exams in the clinical context.

Level 2 competency is the level required for an individual wishing to report cardiovascular MRI studies with local or remote support from a Level 3 certified individual. It is recommended that Level 2 certification should only be issued after completion of specialty training.

Level 3 competency is required for individuals wishing to perform, interpret, and report cardiovascular MRI studies fully independently, to lead a cardiovascular MRI laboratory and to supervise cardiovascular MRI training programmes in an accredited cardiovascular MRI training centre.

To achieve Level 2 and Level 3 for the working group on cardiovascular magnetic resonance of the European society of cardiology, the candidates should prepare a log book consisting of 150 (Level 2) or 300 (Level 3) clinical MRI cases accrued over a 12-month period, should have primarily reported at least 50 (Level 2) or 100 (Level 3) exams, candidates must pass a written exam ('European CMR exam'), and should be trained in basic cardio-pulmonary life support (BCLS) and advanced cardio-pulmonary life support (ACLS) (for a detailed description see Plein et al. 2011). Re-certification every 3 years is recommended. Regarding MRI in patients with congenital heart disease and adult/grown-up congenital heart disease, however, it is emphasized that because of the complexity of cardiovascular MRI findings and the need for appropriate pathophysiological understanding, specific training in this domain is needed (Kilner et al. 2010). These studies should be included in Level 2 (25 cases) or Level 3 (50 cases), and allow trained individuals to recognize these conditions and to refer to a specialist if required.

To ensure the quality of training in cardiovascular MRI training, and to harmonize standards of training throughout countries, *institutional accreditation* is

Table 1 Summary of recommendations for individual certification in cardiovascular MRI

Level	Duration of training	Cases	CMR	CME	Other
1	1 month	50+	No	20	
2	3 months (can be split)	150+ (log book)	Yes	50	BCLS, ACLS
3	12 months	300+ (log book)	Yes	50	BCLS, ACLS

Abbreviations *BCLS* basic cardiac life support, *ACLS* advanced cardiac life support
(Adapted from Plein et al. 2011)

required. Recently, the Working Group on Cardiovascular Magnetic Resonance of the European Society of Cardiology (Plein et al. 2011), has proposed requirements for institutional accredition, including, besides the annual number/diversity of cardiovascular MRI studies, level of training, etc., also issues such as safety and quality control. Initiatives, such as the EuroCMR registry, represent first steps toward quality control assessment by centralized expert reading (Bruder et al. 2009; Wagner et al. 2010).

Similar initiatives taken by the European society of cardiac radiology (ESCR) and endorsed by the European society of radiology (ESR) have recently (2011) led to standardize training and expertise in cardiac radiology across Europe with the possibility to obtain a European board cardiac radiology (EBCR) (for details see www.escr.org). Besides an oral and written centralized exam at the time of the annual ESCR meeting, the candidates must present an RIS documentation or logbook with the total record of their experience in cardiac imaging. Minimum qualifications required as entry criterium are experience in at least 100/300 (life-cases/data-base cases) cardiac CT and 100/300 cardiac MRI studies. At least 50 of the CT life-cases should be contrast-enhanced scans. Up to 50 life-cases and 150 database cases of other cardiac imaging modalities can be submitted towards the experience required. Moreover, because of the rapid evolution in both cardiac CT and MRI the EBCR diploma needs to be renewed every 5 years.

A last issue is to streamline and harmonize training in noninvasive cardiac imaging (i.e. echocardiography, nuclear medicine, cardiac CT, and cardiac MRI). The continuous developments in medical technology and clinical research constantly expand the range of diagnostic tests and diagnostic measurements urging for evidenced-based choice of diagnostic imaging modalities (see Sect. 3), collaboration between imaging subspecialities, and joint educational programmes (Fraser et al. 2006; Thomas et al. 2008).

3 Appropriateness Criteria for Cardiovascular Magnetic Resonance

Regularly updated appropriateness criteria defined by an expert panel blending scientific evidence and practical experience aim to guarantee quality of cardiovascular care and to ensure effective use of diagnostic imaging tools. In 2006, the ACCF/ACR/SCCT/SCMR/ASNC/NASCI/SCAI/SIR appropriateness criteria for cardiac CT and cardiac MRI were published (Hendel et al. 2006). An appropriate imaging study is defined as one in which the expected incremental information, combined with clinical judgment, exceeds the expected negative consequences by a sufficiently wide margin for a specific indication that the procedure is generally considered acceptable care and a reasonable approach for the indication. Negative consequences include the risks of the procedure and the downstream impact of the poor test performance such as delay in diagnosis (false negatives) or inappropriate diagnosis (false positives). For each indication a 1–9 score was used, whereby a score 7–9 was appropriate for that specific indication, whereas a score 4–6 or a score 1–3 was considered uncertain and inappropriate, respectively (Hendel et al. 2006). Similar initiatives to define the clinical indications for cardiovascular MRI were presented in 2004 by a consensus panel report by the working group on CMR of the European society of cardiology and the SCMR (Pennell et al. 2004), using four classes for recommendation (i.e., 3 clinical classes and one investigational class). In 2010, an expert consensus paper on cardiovascular MRI was published reviewing the use of cardiac MRI for assessing patients with cardiovascular diseases, highlighting the capabilities and advantages of this technique relative to other imaging techniques, and to propose new recommendations

Table 2 Current clinical position of MR among the cardiac imaging modalities

	MRI	Echocardiography		MDCT	Nuclear	X-ray
		TTE	TEE		cardiology	angiography
Cardiac anatomy						
Pericardium						
Thickness	+++	+	++	++	0	–
Effusion	+++	++	+++	+++	0	∓
Calcifications	+	+	+	+++	0	-/+
Inflammation	+++	+	+	++	+	0
Myocardium						
Thickness	+++	++	++	+++	+	+
Mass	+++	+	+	+++	0	0
Tissue characterization	++(+)	+	+	+	+	–
Cardiac cavities						
Endoluminal masses	+++	++	+++	++(+)	0	++
Volume quantification	+++	++	++	++(+)	++	++
Cardiac valves						
Number of leaflets	+++	++	+++	+++	0	++
Valve integrity	+(+)	++	+++	++	0	+
Perivalvular space (e.g. abscess)	++	++	+++	++	0	+
Intra-and extracardiac communications						
Patent foramen ovale	+	+	+++	+	0	0
Patent ductus arteriosus	++	++	++	++	0	++
Atrial septal defect	++	++	+++	++	0	++
Ventricular septal defect	++	++	+++	++	0	+++
Extracardiac spaces	+++	+(+)	+(+)	+++	0	0
Cardiac function						
Systolic function						
Global	+++	++	++	++	++(+)	++
Regional	+++	++	++	+	++	+(+)
Stress imaging	+++	+++	+++	+	++	++
Diastolic function	++(+)	+++	+++	0	+	+
Strain analysis	++	++[b]	0	0	0	
Valvular function						
Valve stenosis	++	++(+)	++(+)	0	0	++(+)
Valve regurgitation	++(+)	++	++(+)	0	+	++
Myocardial perfusion	++(+)	+(+)	+(+)	+	++(+)	–
Ischemic myocardial damage						
Myocardial edema	+++	–	–	–	–	–
Myocardial ischemia	++(+)	++	++	0	++(+)	+
Myocardial stunning	++	++	++	0	++	+

(continued)

Table 2 (continued)

	MRI	Echocardiography		MDCT	Nuclear	X-ray
		TTE	TEE		cardiology	angiography
Myocardial hibernation	++(+)	++	++	0	++(+)	+
Myocardial infarction	+++	+	+	+	++	+
Myocardial metabolism	++[c]	0	0	0	++	0
Coronary arteries						
Anatomy	++	+	–	++	0	++(+)
Patency	+	–	–	+(+)	0	+++
Calcifications	–	–	–	+++	0	+
Wall imaging and characterization	+	-	-(+++)[a]	+(+)	0	0
Flow and flow reserve	+	–	-(+++)[a]	–	+	+
Great vessels						
Anatomy	+++	+(+)	++(+)	+++	0	+++
Vessel wall						
Thickness	+++	+	++	+++	0	+
Integrity	++(+)	+	++	++	+	–
Vessel lumen	+++	+	++(+)	+++	0	+++
Flow pattern	+++	+	++(+)	+	0	++
Compliance	++	+	+	0	0	0

+++ Excellent; ++ good; + average; – poor; *0* not possible
[a] Intracoronary echo-Doppler, [b] tissue Doppler imaging, [c] MR spectroscopy
Abbreviations *MDCT* multi-detector CT, *MRI* magnetic resonance imaging

for the use of cardiovascular magnetic resonance for those situations where guidelines were unavailable (Hundley et al. 2010). In Table 2, we summarized and compared the clinical value of MRI amongst the other cardiac imaging techniques using a five-point score. This table has been updated since the 2004 edition with up- or down-scaling of the value of MRI with regard to its competitors depending on the evolution of techniques over the last years. It largely reflects the recommendations and appropriateness criteria, is based on the most recent literature, but also on personal experience, and serves as a guideline for the clinician in choosing the most appropriate diagnostic imaging modality for a particular cardiovascular problem.

4 General Key Points

- The key to a successful cardiac MRI exam is a thorough knowledge of the technique of cardiovascular MRI, and cardiovascular anatomy and physiology in normal and pathological conditions.
- Correct patient positioning, and adequate ECG triggering are crucial to obtain the optimal image quality.
- Use the strengths of MRI to compete with other cardiac imaging techniques.
- Use a combination of black-blood and bright-blood imaging in different imaging planes to study cardiac anatomy/morphology.
- Always consider the heart as a dynamic structure, exhibiting a repetitive process of ejection and filling. To fully appreciate the cardiac function, both processes should be evaluated.
- Cine MRI is currently the reference technique for assessment of global and regional cardiac function.
- Phase-contrast MRI allows to accurately quantify flow velocities and volumes in vessels and through cardiac valves.
- Hemodynamically significant coronary artery stenoses can be accurately assessed by first-pass myocardial perfusion imaging, and incremental dobutamine/atropine stress MRI.

- Myocardial edema can be detected by T2w-imaging techniques.
- Late Gd imaging is the best approach to image tissue necrosis, inflammation and fibrosis in patients with ischemic/non-ischemic myocardial diseases, and other cardiac pathology as pericardial inflammation.
- Coronary MR angiography is indicated to explore the origin and proximal course of the epicardial coronary arteries, but is not yet clinically useful to detect and quantify coronary artery stenoses.
- MRI is a highly valuable technique to image and to determine the etiology of cardiac masses.
- In valvar heart disease patients, MRI is of great interest to assess valvar morphology and to evaluate the functional implications on valvular flow patterns and the remainder of the heart.
- The role of MRI in congenital heart disease is primarily in the postoperative assessment and follow-up of patients.
- MRI and CT are currently the preferential techniques to assess the thoracic great vessels.
- Interventional MR (XMR) is emerging tool that provides valuable information in selected cases.

References

Bruder O, Schneider S, Nothnagel D et al (2009) EuroCMR (European cardiovascular magnetic resonance) registry. Results of the German pilot phase. J Am Coll Cardiol 54:1457–1466

Douglas PS, Hendel RC, Cummings JE et al (2009) ACCF/ACR/AHA/ASE/ASNC/HRS/NASCI/RSNA/SAIP/SCAI/SCCT/SCMR 2008 Health policy statement on structured reporting in cardiovascular imaging. Circulation 119:187–200

Fraser AG, Buser PT, Bax JJ et al (2006) The future of cardiovascular imaging and non-invasive diagnosis. A joint statement from the European association of echocardiography, the working groups on cardiovascular magnetic resonance, computers in cardiology, and nuclear cardiology, of the European society of cardiology, the European association of nuclear medicine, and the association for European paediatric cardiology. Eur Heart J 27:1750–1753

Hendel RC, Patel MR, Kramer CM et al (2006) ACCF/ACR/SCCT/SCMR/ASNC/NASCI/SCAI/SIR 2006 Appropriateness criteria for cardiac computed tomography and cardiac magnetic resonance imaging. J Am Coll Cardiol 48:1475–1797

Hendel RC, Budoff MJ, Cardella JF et al (2009) ACC/AHA/ACR/ASE/ASNC/HRS/NASCI/RSNA/SAIP/SCAI/SCCT/SCMR/SIR 2008 Key data elements and definitions for cardiac imaging: a report of the American college of cardiology/American heart association task force and clinical data standards (writing committee to develop clinical data standards for cardiac imaging). Circulation 119:154–186

Hundley WG, Bluemke D, Bogaert JG et al (2009) Society for cardiovascular magnetic resonance guidelines for reporting cardiovascular magnetic resonance examinations. J Cardiovasc Magn Reson 11:5

Hundley WG, Bluemke DA, Finn JP et al (2010) ACCF/ACR/AHA/NASCI/SCMR 2010 Expert consensus document on cardiovascular magnetic resonance. A report of the American college of cardiology foundation task force on expert consensus documents. Circulation 121:2462–2508

Kilner PJ, Geva T, Kaemmerer H, Trindade PT, Schwitter J, Webb GD (2010) Recommendations for cardiovascular magnetic resonance in adults with congenital heart disease from the respective working groups of the European society of cardiology. Eur Heart J 31:794–805

Kramer CM, Barkhausen J, Flamm SD, Kim RJ, Nagel E (2008) Standardized cardiovascular magnetic resonance imaging (CMR) protocols, society for cardiovascular magnetic resonance: board of trustees task force on standardized protocols. J Cardiovasc Magn Reson 10:35

Pennell DJ, Sechtem UP, Higgins CB et al (2004) Clinical indications for cardiovascular magnetic resonance (CMR): consensus panel report. Eur Heart J 25:1940–1965

Plein S, Schulz-Menger J, Almeida A et al (2011) Training and accreditation in cardiovascular magnetic resonance in Europe: a position statement of the working group on cardiovascular magnetic resonance of the European society of cardiology. Eur Heart J 32:793–798

Pohost GM, Kim RJ, Manning WJ (2008) Task force 12: training in advanced cardiovascular imaging (cardiovascular magnetic resonance (CMR)) Endorsed by the society for cardiovascular magnetic resonance. J Am Coll Cardiol 51:408

Thomas JD, Zoghbi WA, Beller GA et al (2008) ACCF 2008 Training statement on multimodality noninvasive cardiovascular imaging. J Am Coll Cardiol 53:125–146

Wagner A, Bruder O, Schneider S, et al (2010) Current variables, definitions and endpoints of the European cardiovascular magnetic resonance registry. J Cardiovasc Magn Reson 11:43

Index

A
Acceleration time, 360–361
Accreditation in cardiovascular MRI, 696–697
Acquisition
  multi-phase, 17–18
  real-time, 20
  single-phase, 17
  single-shot, 20
  window, 17, 120
Acute coronary syndrome, 204, 228, 249–250, 317
Acyanotic heart disease, 571, 578
Adenosine, 33, 183, 527
Afterload (ventricular), 282
AICD, 58–60
Airway compression, 625–626
ALCAPA, 537, 599–600
Alcohol cardiotoxicity, 330–331
Aliasing, 10, 292
Allograft rejection, 376–380
Amphetamines, 331
Ampulla cardiomyopathy, 320–321
Amyloid heart disease, 323–325
Anatomy *see* cardiac anatomy
Anderson-fabry disease, 327
Aneurysm
  aortic, 627–629
  atrial septum, 447–448
  HCM, 290
  sinus of valsalva, 444, 448–449
Angiosarcoma, 430–431
Annulo-aortic ectasia of aortic root, 628
Anomalous origin of the left coronary artery (ALCAPA), 537, 599–600
Antracycline cardiotoxicity, 331–332
Aorta (aortic), 619–640
  aneurysm, 627–629
  arch, 624–627
  coarctation, 620–624
  dissection, 630–632, 636
  image planes, 99
  inflammation, 635–637, 641
  intramural hematoma, 632–635
  marfan syndrome, 629–630, 635
  MR imaging protocol, 649
  stent, 639–640
  ulcers/ulceration, 632–635
  supravalvular stenosis, 577–578
  trauma, 637–639
  valve (*see also* valve(s)/valvular), 79, 476–484
  valve implantation, 481–484, 679–680
Aortitis (inflammatory), 635–637, 641
(LV) apical ballooning, 320–321
Appendages *see* atrium
Appropriateness criteria, 697–699
ARVC/D *see* arrhythmogenic right ventricular cardiomyopathy/dysplasia
Arrhythmia(s), 282, 284, 293
Arrhythmia rejection window, 18
Arrhythmogenic right ventricular cardiomyopathy/dysplasia, 76, 125, 304–309, 314
Arterial spin-labelling also arterial tagging, 171
Arterial switch operation, 584–587
ASD *see* atrium
Athlete's heart, 279, 282
ATP (adenosine triphosphate), 33, 380, 500–502
Atrium (atrial)
  appendage (left-right), 71–73, 389, 570
  enlargement, 291
  function, 145–147
  morphological left atrium, 73, 454–455
  morphological right atrium, 71–73, 451
  septal aneurysm, 447–448
  septal defect (asd), 573–574, 664
  septum, 73–75
  situs, 71–74, 570
  stent (placement), 639–640
  switch operation, 587–588
  volume(s), 145–147
Atrioventricular groove, 80
Atrioventricular septal defect (ASVD), 574–575
Autoimmune disease, 336–337

B
Baffle, 587–588
Balanced FFE *see* b-SSFP
Balanced steady-state free precession technique *see* b-SSFP

J. Bogaert et al. (eds.), *Clinical Cardiac MRI*, Medical Radiology. Diagnostic Imaging,
DOI: 10.1007/978-3-642-23035-6, © Springer-Verlag Berlin Heidelberg 2012

B (*cont.*)
Bicuspid aortic valve diseasem, 481–482, 628
Bidirectional cavo-pulmonary connection (BCPC), 593–596
Bio-effects, 55
Biomarkers, 369–373
Black-blood (*see* also dark-blood), 6, 21, 70, 277, 370, 385, 522, 558–561, 616–617, 622
Blalock-Taussig (BT) shunt, 591
Blood flow, 359–360
Blood oxygen level-dependent (BOLD), 35, 225
Body axes, 95
Bolus-track technique, 612–614
Breath-hold cardiac MRI, 61
Bright-blood, 27, 70, 116–117, 277, 522
Bronchogenic cyst, 438
b-SSFP, 25–28, 70, 117, 174, 277, 357, 563
Bull's-eye plot, 104–105

C
^{13}C, 32, 662
CABG *see* coronary artery bypass graft
Cancer treatment-induced cardiac toxicity, 331–333
Carcinoid tumor/carcinoid heart syndrome, 498
Cardiac anatomy, 69–89
  atrium (atria), 71–75
  coronary arteries, 80–81
  great vessels, 82–89
  gross cardiac anatomy, 70–71
  imaging planes, 93–102
  MRI techniques, 70
  pericardium, 81–82
  ventricle(s), 75–79
  valve(s), 79–80
  Variant(s), 452–456
Cardiac axes, 95–98
Cardiac failure *see* heart failure
Cardiac function
  accuracy of measurements, 125–127
  atria, 145–147
  basic principles, 110–114
  cardiac image plane, 122–123
  comparison with other techniques, 127–128
  delineation techniques, 123–125
  diastolic, 141–147, 394
  global function, 114–129
  heart failure, 369–370
  MRI sequence design, 116–120
  normal values, 151–155
  phase-contrast MRI, 128–129, 142–145
  post-processing techniques, 149–150
  regional function, 129–140
  right ventricle, 125, 357–359
  stress imaging, 225–228
  systolic, 114–140
  tagging, 130–134
Cardiac hypertrophy, 279–284
Cardiac image plane, 94–103
Cardiac mass(es)
  clinical presentation, 412
  computed tomography, 415
  echocardiography, 415
  MRI techniques, 415–418
  non-tumoral causes, 439–452
  normal cardiac anatomy and variants, 452–456
Cardiac gating, 16–17
Cardiac metastasis, 433–437
Cardiac morphology *see also* cardiac anatomy
Cardiac output, 380
Cardiac pacemaker, 58–60
Cardiac resynchronization therapy, 255, 369–370, 373–376, 684–687
Cardiac tamponade, 390–391
Cardiac thrombus (*see also* thrombus formation), 439–443
Cardiac tumors
  benign, 418–430
  classification, 418
  extracardiac, 437–438
  malignant, 430–433
  paracardiac, 437–438
  primary, 418–433
  secondary, 433–439
Cardiomyopathy
  etiology, 275–276, 284
  ampulla, 320–321
  diabetic, 337–338
  dilated, 297–302
  hypertrophic, 284–297
  inflammatory, 312–320
  iron-overload, 325–327
  ischemic, 250–256
  non-compaction, 310
  peripartum, 321–323
  primary, 284–323
  restrictive, 302–304, 385, 394–395, 402–405
  secondary, 323–338
  stress, 320–321
  tachycardia-induced, 321–323
  tako-tsubo, 320–321
  uremic, 338
Cardiovascular modeling, 669–689
Cartesian (filling), 12, 23
Caseous calcification of the mitral annulus, 449–450
Catheter tracking/visualization, 662
Caval vein *see also* vena(e) cava(e) and systemic veins, 86–87, 649–650
Cemra (contrast-enhanced MR angiography), 23–24, 361, 515–516, 567, 581, 612–616, 621–623
Chagas' (heart) disease, 319
Chiari network, 453
Chronic fibrosing pericarditis *see* constrictive pericarditis
Chronic ischemic cardiomyopathy, 250–255
Chronic obstructive airways disease (COPD), 363
Chronic stable plaque, 204
Churg-strauss syndrome, 335–336, 539
Cine MRI, 27, 120, 207, 277, 357, 385, 470–472, 475, 616
Circumferential shortening, 111
Claustrophobia, 66
Coarctation *see* aortic coarctation
Cocaine, 331
Coil
  placement, 60–61

sensitivity, 15
Collagen, 279, 298
Collateral circulation/flow, 623, 643
Common arterial trunk, 590–591
Compliance
myocardial, 112
pericardial, 405
Computational fluid dynamics, 672–675
Computed tomography (CT), 363, 399, 415, 446, 467, 545, 567, 587, 630–631
Congenital heart disease
acyanotic, 571–578
clinical indications for MRI, 554–558
coronary arteries, 599–600
cyanotic, 578–591
future directions, 602–603
modeling, 681–684
MRI protocols, 556–562
(role of) cardiovascular CT, 600–602
sequence optimization, 569
sequential segmental analysis, 569–571
Congenitally corrected transposition of the great arteries (CCTGA), 588–589
Congenital diverticulum, 339–340
Constrictive pericarditis, 303, 332, 393–406
Continuity equation, 476, 480
Contractility (myocardial), 357
Contractility reserve, 252
Contraction (myocardial), 111–112
Contraindications to MRI, 66
Contrast agent(s) (or media)
blood-pool (or intravascular), 37, 178
(for) coronary artery imaging, 523–525
dose ranging, 35, 219–220
endogenous, 180
extracellular, 35, 178
intracellular, 39
magnetic susceptibility, 180
molecular imaging, 45
multipurpose, 39
necrosis-avid, 39
negative, 34, 662
plaque, 44
positive, 34, 662
precautions, 62–63
T1-enhancing, 180
thrombus-specific, 44
Contrast-enhanced inversion recovery MRI, 5–6
Contrast-enhanced mr angiography *see* ceMRA
Cor pulmonale *see* pulmonary hypertension
Coronary artery
anatomy, 80
blood flow (reserve), 168, 527–528
bypass graft (CABG), 528, 543–545
congenital anomaliesm, 534–537
cookbook or practical approach, 528–532
CT angiography, 545
disease (CAD), 223–228
distribution pattern, 106
imaging planes, 102–103, 523, 529
imaging in congenital heart diseases, 537–538, 587
motion, 516–520
MR imaging strategies, 513–527
plaque imaging, 44–45, 546
post-processing techniques, 532–533
stenosis (detection), 540–542
stent imaging, 542–543
vasculitis, 538–539
vasodilator reserve, 169
wall imaging, 521–522
X-ray (or catheter-based) angiography, 512–513
Coronary sinus, 71, 527–528
Coronary vein(s), 375, 686
Coupling *see* ventricular coupling
Crista supraventricularis *see also* supraventricular crest, 75
Crista terminalis *see also* terminal crest, 71, 453
CRT *see* cardiac resynchronization therapy
Cross-fiber, 112, 138
(coronary) CT angiography, 545, 587
CT *see* computed tomography
Cyanotic heart disease, 578–591
Cyclophosphamide, 332–333
Cyst
bronchogenic, 438
hydatid, 450–451
pericardial, 386, 451
thymic, 438, 455

D

Dark blood *see* black blood
Dark-rim artifact, 185
DeBakey classification for aortic dissection, 630
Delayed enhancement *see* late Gd MRI
DENSE (displacement encoding with stimulated echoes), 135, 293
Deoxyhemoglobin, 35
Dephasing, 4, 370
Dermatomyositis, 337
Devices and delivery systems, 660
Diastole (diastolic)
(dys)function, 142–148, 282, 292, 303, 394–395
heart failure, 141, 303, 370
principles, 112–114
Dipyridamole, 183, 527
DIR (double inversion recovery), 6
Dissection *see* aortic dissection
Dobutamine, 225–228, 252
Double aortic arch, 626–627
Double inversion recovery (DIR), 6
Double outlet right ventricle, 589–590
Dressler's syndrome, 244, 393
Dual-bolus, 174, 180–181
Duchenne muscular dystrophy, 338
Ductus arteriosus, 86
Dysprosium (Dy^{3+}), 33
Dyssynchrony (ventricular), 114, 373–374

E

Early Gd imaging, 216
Ebstein's anomaly, 496–498

E (*cont.*)
ECG
monitoring, 61
myocardial infarction, 240–241
triggering, 516
Echinococcosis, 450–451
Echocardiography, 415
Echo-planar imaging (EPI), 13–14
Echo-sharing *see also* view sharing
Edema imaging, 211–213, 229, 316–317, 376
Edward's hypothetical double aortic arch, 626
Effusive-constrictive pericarditis, 399–400
Ejection fraction
global, 110, 115, 377
regional, 139
EMB *see* endomyocardial biopsy
End-diastolic volume, 115
End-systolic volume, 115
Endocardial border, 123–125
Endocarditis, 443–444, 469
Endocrine disorders, 337–338
Endomyocardial biopsy (EMB), 278, 306, 315, 333, 376
Endomyocardial disease, 328–330
Endomyocardial fibrosis, 328–330
Engineering modeling techniques, 670–675
EPI (echo-planar imaging), 13–14, 174–175
Epicardial border, 123–125
Ethanol, 330–331
Eustachian valve, 71, 453
Extracellular (fluid space) contrast agent(s), 35, 525

F
^{19}F, 32, 662
False tendon(s), 456
Faraday cage, 561, 640
Fast spin echo (FSE), 21
Fat suppression, 308, 446, 522–523
Fatty infiltration/replacement
atrial septum, 446
ARVC/D, 308
myocardium, 277
Ferromagnetic object, 54–55, 663
FFE *see* spoiled-GE
Fiber (myocardial), 111–112, 138
Fibro(fatty) replacement, 305, 308
(papillary) fibroelastoma, 421
Fibroma, 425
Fibrosis *see* myocardial fibrosis
Fick principle/method, 664
Field of view, 10–12
Field inhomogeneity, 4, 561
FIESTA *see* b-SSFP
Finite element analysis, 672–674
First-pass imaging, 170–171
FLASH *see* spoiled—GE
Flow
measurement, 25
quantification, 25
velocity, 360
4D flow, 502
Fluid structure interaction, 672–675
Fontan, 597–599
Foramen ovale, 73
Foreign body granuloma, 407, 451–452
Foreign device(s), 456–457
Fossa ovalis, 73
Four-chamber view (4Ch), 95
Fourier transformation, 10
Free-breathing scans, 61
Friedreich's ataxia, 338
FSE (fast spin echo), 21
Function *see also* cardiac function

G
Gadolinium (Gd)(Gd^{3+}), 23, 33, 213
Gating
cardiac, 16–17
navigator, 19–20
retrospective, 18
Gauss line, 55–57
Geometric assumption, 115
Glenn, 593–596, 676
Glycogen storage disease, 327–328
Gossypiboma, 407, 451–452
Gradient echo (GRE), 22–25, 174, 562–563
Granulomatosis with polyangiitis, 335
GRAPPA, 15–16
Great vessels, 82, 86–89, 98–102, 611–651

H
^{1}H, 32
H(a)emochromatosis (myocardial), 325
HASTE (half (Fourier) acquisition single shot turbo spin echo), 21
Heart failure, 250–255, 291, 367–381, 412
Heart transplantation, 376–381
Heavy metals, 330–331
Hemangioma (cardiac), 427–428
Hematoma, 407, 632–635
Hemi-Fontan, 593–596
Hemorrhagic infarction, 236–238
Hibernating myocardium, 206
High field strength imaging, *see* magnetic field
Horizontal long-axis (HLA), 95
Hydatid cyst, 450–451
Hypertrabeculation, 309
Hypertrophic cardiomyopathy *see* cardiomyopathy
Hypertrophy (cardiac/ventricular/myocardial), 279–284, 298, 377
Hypoplastic left heart syndrome (HLHS), 591–593

I
IHD *see* ischemic heart disease
Image (imaging)
breath hold, 19
dynamic, 16
foldover, 10–11
parallel, 15, 23

plane(s), 94–103, 122–123
radial, 14
reconstruction, 8–16
self-gated, 121
signal, 32
3D, 14–15
Infarct(ion) *see* myocardial infarction
Infiltrative (myocardial) disease, 323–328
Inflammatory pericarditis *see also* pericardial inflammation
Inflow enhancement, 117–119
Infundibulum, 75
Interactive imaging, 103–104
Interatrial septum *see* atrium (atrial septum)
Interventional MR suite, 659–660, 663
Interventricular septum *see* ventricular septum
Intramural hematoma, 632–635
Inversion pulse, 4
Inversion-recovery (IR), 4–7, 176
contrast-enhanced, 5–6
short tau (STIR), 5
spectral inversion (SPIR), 5
Inversion time or delay (TI), 220
IR *see* inversion recovery
Iron (Fe^{3+}), 33
Iron overload cardiomyopathy, 325–327
Ischemic cascade, 204
Ischemic cardiomyopathy, 250–255
Ischemic heart disease (IHD)
imaging strategies, 207–223
pathophysiology, 204–207
practical MRI recipes, 256–258
prognosis assessment, 255–256

J
Jeopardized myocardium, 204, 229–231

K
Kawasaki disease, 538–539, 599
Keyhole imaging, 176
Kommerell's diverticulum, 627
K-space, 9–16, 17, 176, 516
κ-space fillings strategies, 12–15
K-t blast, 16, 103, 121, 176, 661
K-t sense, 16, 121, 176, 236, 357, 563–564, 661

L
Larmor frequency, 2
Lake louise criteria, 316
Late Gd imaging, 216, 278, 298, 308, 312, 362, 375, 393, 417, 441, 481, 567–568
Left anterior descending coronary artery (LAD), 80, 102–103
Left atrium *see* atrium
Left circumflex coronary artery (LCx), 80, 102–103
Left common carotid artery, 81
Left coronary artery (LCA), 80, 102–103
Left heart, 96–98
Left main stem coronary artery (LM), 80, 102–103
Left subclavian artery, 81
Left ventricular segmentation, 104–105
Left ventricular inflow/outflow tract view, 96
Left ventricular outflow tract view, 96
Ligamentum arteriosus, 86
Lipoma, 420–421
Lipomatous hypertrophy of the interatrial septum, 446
Lipomatous metaplasia, 277
Liquefaction necrosis of the mitral annulus calcification, 449–450
Löffler endocarditis, 328–330
Longitudinal shortening, 111
Look-locker, 220
Lung fibrosis, 363
LV non-compaction cardiomyopathy, 309–312
Lyme disease, 319
Lymphoma (cardiac), 432–433

M
Magnetic
gradient, 55
field (strength), 2, 54–55, 181–183, 221, 498–500, 526
Magnetic resonance spectroscopy, 500, 502
Magnetic susceptibility, 180
Magnetization
preparation (pulses), 4–8, 522–523
transfer contrast (MTC) pulses, 523
Magnetohyodrodynamic effect, 61
Major aortopulmonary collaterals (MAPCAs), 583, 601
Malignant fibrous histiocytoma, 431
Malignant pericardial mesothelioma, 433
Manganese (Mn^{2+}), 33, 213
MAPCAs (major aortopulmonary collaterals), 583, 601
Marfan syndrome, 629–630, 635
Medical device(s), 58–60
Mesothelioma (malignant pericardial), 433
Metabolic storage disease(s), 327–328
Metastasis *see* cardiac metastasis
Microvascular obstruction *see* MVO
(tumor) mimics, 439–452
Mirror-image branching, 627
Mitral (or LV) valve (*see also* valve(s)/valvular), 79, 96, 291, 484–487, 681
Mitral-aortic intervalvular fibrosa, 77, 444
Model, 670
Moderator band, 75, 453
Molecular imaging with MRI, 45
Motion
artifact, 516
compensation, 16, 516–518
MPI *see* myocardial perfusion
MR angiography *see* MRA
MRCA *see* coronary MR angiography
MR coronary angiography *see* coronary MR angiography
MR-guided cardiac catheterization, 657–666
MR signal, 2, 3
MRA (MR angiography), 27–28, 34
MRCA (MR coronary angiography), 27–28
Muscular cleft(s), 289
Multipurpose contrast agents, 39
Multiscale modeling, 674–675

M (*cont.*)
Mustard procedure, 587–588
MVO (*see* also no-reflow), 220, 232–236
Myocardial blood flow, 168
Myocardial bridging, 537
Myocardial contractility (intrinsic), 140
Myocardial contrast echocardiography, 170
Myocardial edema, 316–317, 376
Myocardial fat (imaging), 223, 308
Myocardial fibrosis, 278, 293, 301, 312, 481
Myocardial hypertrophy *see* hypertrophy
Myocardial inflammation, 308
Myocardial infarction, 312–316
  aborted, 231
  acute, 214–216
  complications, 243–247
  enhancement patterns, 241–243
  expansion, 206
  healed, 216–217
  healing, 247
  hemorrhage, 236–238
  imaging, 229–230
  papillary muscle, 247
  peri-procedural, 248
  practical MRI recipes, 256–258
  remodeling, 206, 247
  right ventricular, 238–240
  silent, 240
  size, 232
  tissue heterogeneity, 238
  transmural extent, 232
  unrecognized, 240
Myocardial ischemia, 293
Myocardial mass, 358
Myocardial perfusion
  analysis, 185–192
  applications, 192–195, 378
  in ischemic heart disease, 210–211, 224–225
  MR techniques, 171–174
  pathophysiology, 168–169
  reserve (MPR), 225, 378
  (semi-)quantification, 188–192
Myocardial relaxation, 112
Myocardial reperfusion, 205
Myocardial reperfusion injury, 205–206, 233
Myocardial salvage, 230–231
Myocardial scar, 374–376
Myocardial siderosis, 325
Myocardial signal nulling, 176–177
Myocardial stiffness, 302–303
Myocardial strain *see* strain
Myocardial tethering, 112
Myocardial tagging *see* tagging
Myocardial trabeculations, 298, 309
Myocardial viability, 251–255
Myocardial wall *see* wall
Myocardium at risk, 204, 229–231
Myocarditis, 302, 312–320
Myofibrillar disarray, 284
Myopathies, 338
Myxoma, 418–420

N
^{23}Na, 32
NACA *see* necrosis—avid contrast agents
Navigator-echo acquisition(s), 514–515
NE *see* navigator-echo
Necrosis-avid contrast agent(s) (NACAs), 39–44, 213
Neonatal cardiac MRI, 62
Nephrogenic systemic fibrosis (NSF), 62–63, 338–339
Neurological/neuromuscular disorders, 338
(LV) non-compaction cardiomyopathy, 309–312
No-reflow, 185, 232–236
Normal values, cardiac function, 115, 151–156, 569
Norwood procedure, 591, 674
NSF *see* nephrogenic systemic fibrosis
Nuclear medicine, 169–170

O
Oblique sinus, 82, 386
One-stop shop cardiac MRI, 32, 42
Osteosynthesis material, 60
Oval fossa, 73
Overload, 282

P
^{31}P, 32, 379
Pacemaker (cardiac), 58–60
Pacemaker wires, 60
Pacing, 374–375
Papillary fibroelastoma, 421
Papillary muscle(s), 95, 247, 456
Paraganglioma, 425
Parallel imaging, 15–16, 23
Parietal band, 75
Partial anomalous pulmonary venous return, 573
Partial fourier, 13
Particle image velocimetry, 673
Patent ductus arteriosus (PDA), 591
Patient positioning, 60–61
Patient preparation, 60–66, 558
PC-MRI *see* phase contrast MRI
PCr (phosphocreatine), 33, 380, 500
Pectinate muscles/ridges, 454
Pediatric cardiac MRI, 62
Penetrating aortic ulceration, 632–635
Percutaneous valve implantation, 491–495, 639–640, 676–677
Perfusion *see* myocardial perfusion
Pericardiocentesis, 390
Pericarditis *see* also pericardial inflammation
  constrictive, 393–406
  effusive-constrictive, 399–400
  focal constrictive, 400–401
  inflammatory, 386
  inflammatory-constrictive, 400
  minimally thickened constrictive, 401
  occult constrictive, 401
  post-infarction, 244, 393
Pericardium (pericardial)
  anatomy, 81–82, 384, 456

calcification(s), 399
compliance, 405
congenital anomalies, 386–390
cyst, 386
defect, 387–388
diverticulum, 390
effusion/effusive pericardial disease, 380, 390–393
inflammation, 393
layer(s), 82, 384
masses, 406–407
motion/mobility, 406
MRI techniques, 384, 386
normal, 81–82, 386
paraganglioma, 425–427
physiology, 384, 394
recess(es), 82, 386
sac, 81–82, 386
sinus(es), 82, 386
stretch, 390–391
tamponade, 390–391
thickness/width, 82, 386, 390, 399
Peripartum cardiomyopathy *see* cardiomyopathy
Peri-procedural necrosis, 248
Perivalvular extension of infection, 444–446
Perfusion *see* myocardial perfusion
Perivalvular extension of infection, 444, 446, 449
PET (positron emission tomography), 170
Phase contrast MRI (PC-MRI), 24–25, 128–129, 278, 292, 385, 402–403, 418, 472–473, 475–476, 486–487, 527–528, 564–566, 580, 598, 619, 622–623
congenital heart disease, 564–566, 580, 598, 622–623
coronary blood flow, 527–528
diastolic function, 141–142
great vessels, 619
myocardium, 144–145
technique, 24–25
valve disease, 472–473, 475–476
ventricular inflow pattern(s), 142–144
ventricular stroke volume assessment, 128–129
venous flow patterns, 143–144
Phase sensitive inversion-recovery (PSIR), 221
Phase-shift MRI *see* phase contrast MRI
Pheochromocytoma, 425–427
Phenotype (phenotypic), 276
Phosphocreatine *see* PCr
Polymyositis, 337
Postprocessing techniques, 149–150, 580
Pregnancy and MRI, 63–66
Preload, 282
Preparation pulse(s), 520, 522, 524
Pressure-volume (PV) loop, 665
Prosthetic valve(s), 60, 444, 456, 498–500
Proton density, 33
Pseudo-aneurysm, 627–628, 637–639
Pulmonary artery, 86, 99–102, 359, 640–644
distensibility, 359
mrimaging protocols, 650
pressure, 356
sling, 644, 646
stenosis, 577–578
Pulmonary atresia, 582–584
Pulmonary hypertension, 125, 355–364, 665
Pulmonary trunk, 86, 492
Pulmonary valve *see* also valve(s)/valvular, 487, 495
Pulmonary vascular resistance, 356, 664
Pulmonary vein(s), 87–88, 644–648, 650
Pulmonary veno-occlusive disease, 363
Pulse sequence, 12–13

Q
Q-tip sign, 455
Qp:Qs, 564, 572, 619

R
Radial imaging, 14
Radial tagging, *see* tagging
Radial thickening, 111
Radiofrequency (RF), 55
Radiotherapy (radiation therapy), 332–333, 393
Real-time MRI, 20, 70, 103–104, 121, 277–278, 357, 370, 385, 402–406, 563–564, 660–662
Recommendations for training, 696–697
Recreational drugs, 330–331
Rectangular field of view, 13
Regurgitation *see* valve regurgitation
Rejection *see* allograft rejection
Relaxation
longitudinal, 33
transverse, 3, 33
myocardial, 112
ventricular, 292–293
Remodeling, 247, 358
Repetition time (TR)
Reproducibility (of measurements), 109, 125
Resolution, 10–12, 120
Resonance, 2
Respiratory gating, 19
Respiratory motion, 177–178, 401
Restrictive cardiomyopathy *see* cardiomyopathy
Restrictive filling pattern, 92, 361, 380, 401–403
Rhabdomyoma, 421–425
Rhabdomyosarcoma, 431
Right aortic arch, 626–627
Right atrium *see* atrium
Right coronary artery (RCA), 80, 102–103
Right heart, 98
Right ventricle
volume, function, mass, 125, 357, 358, 489, 579, 675
Right ventricular outflow tract tachycardia, 308–309
Right ventricular outflow tract, 98, 492, 493, 641, 677, 679
Risk stratification, 300

S
Safety issue(s), 54–60, 663
Sano-type repair, 592
Sarcoidosis (cardiac), 333–335
Sarcoma(s) (cardiac), 430–432
Saturation recovery (sr), 7–8, 177
SCD *see* sudden cardiac death

S (*cont.*)
Scimitar syndrome, 647
Segment or segmented acquisition, 17, 117
Segmentation (left ventricle), 104–105, 129–130, 207, 228
SENC (strain-encoded MRI), 134–135, 373
Senning procedure, 587–588
SENSE (sensitivity encoding), 15, 103, 661
Septal bounce, 404
Septal (ventricular) configuration, 358, 359, 403, 406
Septal excursion, 403, 406
Septomarginal band, 75
Septomarginal trabeculation, 75
Septoparietal trabeculation(s), 75
Sequence (cardiac), 20–28
Serum markers, 241
Shear motion, 111
Shim coils, 4
Shimming, 4
Short-axis (SA) plane, 95
Short tau inversion recovery (STIR), 5
Shunt quantification, 571–572
Siderosis (myocardial), 325
Simpson's rule, 115
Single bolus, 180–181
Single-phase imaging, 13
Single shot acquisition, 20
(functionally) single ventricle, 591–599, 681–684
Sinus(es) of valsalva, 448–449
Slice
  selection, 12
  track(ing), 403
(C)SPAMM, 132–134, 374
Spatial encoding, 8–16
Spatial resolution, 525–526
Specific absorption rate (SAR), 55
SPECT (single photon-emission computed tomography), 169–170
Spectral inversion recovery (SPIR), 5
Spectroscopy, 379–380
Spin, 1–2
Spin-lattice relaxation, 3
Spin-spin interactions, 3
Spin echo (SE), 20–22, 70
SPIR (spectral inversion recovery), 5
Spiral (filling/trajectory), 14
Spoiled gradient echo (GRE), 22–25
SR (saturation recovery), 7
Standardized protocols for cardiovascular MRI, 695–696
Stanford classification for aortic dissection, 630
Steady-state free precession *see* balanced steady-state free Precession (b-SSFP)
Steal-phenomenon, 183
Stent
  fracture prediction, 678
  placement, 639–640
  virtual stent deployment, 679
Stiffness, 292, 302–303
Stir (short tau inversion recovery), 5
(myocardial) storage disease, 323–328
Strain (myocardial)
  analysis, 137–139
  imaging, 130–137
  principles, 110–111
  strain rate, 130
Stress imaging
  adverse effects, 183–185
  (in) congenital heart disease, 569
  contraindications, 183–185
  dobutamine, 225–228, 252–253, 569
  for detection of myocardial ischemia, 183–185
  for assessment of myocardial viability, 252–255
  function, 149
  monitoring, 61–62, 227
  patient preparation, 183–185, 225–228
  perfusion imaging, 183–185, 210–221, 224–225, 569
  termination criteria, 227
Stress-strain relation, 148–149
Stroke volume, 115, 128–129, 358
Stunned myocardium, 206
Substance abuse, 330–331
Sudden cardiac death (SCD), 280, 284, 291, 314
(congenital) supravalv(ul)ar aortic stenosis, 577–578
Supraventricular crest *see also* crista supraventricularis, 75
Surgical clip(s), 60
Susceptibility effect *see also* T2* shortening effect, 34
Svensson classification for aortic dissection, 630
Systemic lupus erythematosus, 336
Systemic sclerosis, 336
Systemic veins *see also* caval veins, 86–87, 649–650
Systolic (dys)function, 111–112, 292

T
T1, 3
T1-enhancing contrast media, 180
T1 map, 279, 301
T1 relaxation time *see also* longitudinal relaxation time, 277
T1-weighting (T1w MRI), 21–22, 70, 277, 416
T2, 3
T2*, 4, 174, 298, 326, 370–373
T2 map, 298
T2 preparation (T2 prep), 8, 523
T2 relaxation time *see also* transverse relaxation time, 277, 326, 370
T2* shortening *see* also susceptibility effect, 34
T2-weighted short-tau inversion-recovery (STIR) technique, 211–212
T2-weighting (T2w MRI), 22, 277, 298, 385, 419
Tagging (myocardial), 130–134, 141, 293, 373–374
Takayasu's arteritis, 540, 635
Tako-tsubo cardiomyopathy, 320–321
Tamponade *see* cardiac tamponade
TE *see* also echo time
Temporal resolution, 120
Tendinous chords, 456
Teratoma (pericardial), 428–430
Terminal crest *see also* crista terminalis, 71, 453
Tetralogy of fallot, (ToF), 125, 578–582, 684
Textiloma, 451–452
TGA *see* transposition of the great arteries
Thebesian valve, 71, 453

Thermal injury, 55
Thromboembolism, 361, 412
Thrombus (formation), 243–244, 417, 439–443, 468–469
Through-plane motion, 121
TI *see* inversion time
Time-resolved ceMRA, 615–616
Tissue heating, 55
Torsion (ventricular, myocardial), 111, 113, 282, 293
Total anomalous pulmonary venous return, 573
Total cavo-pulmonary connection (TCPC), 591, 597–599, 682
Toxicity, 330–331
TR *see* also repetition time
Trabeculations (endocardial), 123–125, 309
Tracheo-bronchial malacia, 626
Trachea-esophageal compression, 626, 643
Transcatheter aortic valve implantation, 481–484
Transient LV dysfunction, 320–321
Transplant vasculopathy, 380
Transposition of the great arteries (TGA), 584, 589
Transverse (T2) relaxation time *see* T2 relaxation time
Transverse sinus, 82, 386
Triangle of dysplasia, 305
Tricuspid (or RV) valve, 360, 495–498
Triggering *see* gating
Triple inversion recovery (TIR), 7, 212, 385
Thromboembolism, 256
Thrombus formation, 380
TrueFISP *see* b-SSFP
TSE (turbo spin echo), 21
Turbo FLASH, 22–25
Turbo spin echo, 21
Twisting (ventricular, myocardial), 113–114

U
Uhl' anomaly, 309

V
Valve(s)/valvular
- anatomy (morphology), 468–469
- aortic, 79, 476–484, 679–681
- area, 480, 487
- (atrio)ventricular valve(s), 79
- computed tomography, 467
- echocardiography, 466–467
- implantation, 481–484, 491–495, 639–640, 664, 676–677
- leaflet(s), 79, 468
- mitral, 79, 484–487, 681
- mixed valvular disease, 498
- prosthetic, 60, 456–457, 498–500
- pulmonary, 79, 360, 487–495, 677–679
- regurgitation, 244, 360–361, 457, 469–475, 476–480, 484–486, 487–491
- semilunar valves, 79
- stenosis, 475–476, 480–481, 486–487
- stenting, 676
- tricuspid, 79, 360, 495–498
- tumors, 421
- vegetations, 443–444
- velocity mapping, 472–473, 486–487
- X-ray angiography, 467

Vascular distension, 359
Vascular ring, 625–627
Vasculitis, 335–336, 635
VCATS (volume coronary arteriography using targeted Scans), 515
Vectorcardiogram or vectrocardiography (VCG), 61
Vein(s) *see* pulmonary/systemic/coronary vein(s)
Velocity-encoding, 25
Velocity mapping *see* PC-MRI
Velocity time integral (VTI), 476
Vena(e) cava(e) *see also* caval or systemic veins, 86–87, 649–650
Ventricle (ventricular)
- borderline left or right ventricle, 591
- compliance, 142–144
- coupling, 147–148, 278, 384, 403–405
- filling, 112–113, 303
- hypertrophy *see* hypertrophy
- (interventricular) dependence, 147–148, 384, 403–405
- inflow pattern(s), 142–144, 402
- mass/volume, 115–116, 142
- morphological left ventricle, 77–78, 456, 570
- morphological right ventricle, 75–77, 453–454, 570
- relaxation, 147
- remodeling, 247
- right ventricle volume, function, mass, 125, 489, 579
- septal defect (VSD), 575–577, 578, 582–584, 589–591, 664
- septum, 78–79, 358–359, 584
- single, 591–599, 681–684

Ventriculoarterial connection, 570–571
Ventriculoarterial discordance, 584
Venturi effect, 292
Vertical long-axis plane (VLA), 95
View-sharing *see* also echo-sharing
Virtual surgery, 675
Virtual physiological human, 687
Volumetric quantification, 115, 472, 489, 579
VSD *see* ventricular

W
Wall motion, 129
Wall stress, 148–149, 282, 298
Wall thickening
- systolic, 112, 129

Wall thickness, 281–282, 289–290
Wegener's granulomatosis, 335
Whole heart MR angiography, 566–567, 616, 622
Williams syndrome, 577–578
Wrap, 10–11

X
XMR, 659–660
X-ray angiography/fluoroscopy, 659
X-ray exposure, 658–659

Y
Y-graft model, 681–684

The manufacturer's authorised representative in the EU is Springer Nature Customer Service Centre GmbH, Europaplatz 3, 69115 Heidelberg, Germany. If you have any concerns regarding our products, please contact ProductSafety@springernature.com

Printed and bound by CPI Group (UK) Ltd, Croydon, CR0 4YY

25/09/2026

02222883-0001